Handbook of Behavior, F

Victor R. Preedy • Ronald Ross Watson
Colin R. Martin
Editors

Handbook of Behavior, Food and Nutrition

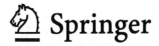 Springer

Editors
Prof. Victor R. Preedy
King's College London
Department Nutrition & Dietetics
150 Stamford St.
London SE1 9NH
UK

Prof. Ronald Ross Watson
University of Arizona
Health Sciences Center
Department of Health Promotion Sciences
1295 N. Martin Ave.
Tucson, AZ 85724-5155
USA

Prof. Colin R. Martin
University of the West of Scotland
Ayr Campus
KA8 0SR Ayr
UK

ISBN 978-1-4939-3982-4   ISBN 978-0-387-92271-3 (eBook)
DOI 10.1007/978-0-387-92271-3
Springer New York Dordrecht Heidelberg London

Springer is part of Springer Science+Business Media (www.springer.com)

This book is dedicated to Miss Caragh Brien, my wonderful daughter.

Colin R. Martin

Foreword

The Editors are to be commended for bringing together what is arguably the best and most comprehensive text book on the complex interrelationships between the brain, behaviour, food selection and choice. There are more than 200 chapters describing not only how behaviour affects our food selection but also how what we eat affects how we behave. Content covers genetics, sensory factors, endocrine and neuro-endocrine processes, neurology, behaviour, psychology, physiology, the act of eating, food choice, selection, preferences, appetite, pregnancy, human development, children and adolescents, ageing, anorexia nervosa, bulimia nervosa, obesity, nutrient excess and toxicity, alcoholism, quality of life, body image and much more. The authors have helpfully included chapters on changing eating behaviour and attitudes. The International Handbook of Behavior, Food and Nutrition can truly be said to be research based, theoretical, factual, scientific, academic and practical.

The International Handbook of Behavior, Food and Nutrition is without doubt a quality text attractive to the wide range of practitioners and intelligent readers with an interest in these areas. These contributions are a testament not only to the skills of the authors, but the Editorial attributes of Professor Preedy, Watson and Martin. They have marshalled together a truly international team of experts. I especially like the structuring of the chapters. Each contribution has a mini-dictionary, "key facts" and "summary points" to facilitation the navigation across fields of interest.

This is a cross-disciplinary book of tremendous importance to the health of individuals and society at large and deserves wide dissemination.

The Editors and all the authors are to be congratulated.

Prof Betty Kershaw DBE FRCN
Emeritus Dean
The School of Nursing and Midwifery
The University of Sheffield
United Kingdom

Preface

In this book the Editors aims to disseminate important data pertaining to the modulatory effects of foods and nutritional substances on behavior and neurological pathways and visa versa. This ranges from the neuroendocrine control of feeding to the effects of disease on the brain. The importance of this book pertains to the fact that food is an essential component of cultural heritage but the effects of perturbations in the food-cognitive axis can be quite profound. The complex inter-relationship between neuropsychological processing, diet and behavioural outcome is explored within the context of the most contemporary psychobiological research in the area. This comprehensive psychobiologically and pathology-themed text examines the broad spectrum of diet, behavioural and neuropsychological interactions from normative function to occurrences of severe and enduring psychopathology. The Editors have taken a scientific and objective stand and included chapters that scrutinize the relationships between the brain, behaviour, food and nutrition in a scientific and rational way.

In very simple terms this books addresses limitations in other works that may individually look at the one-way-traffic of either food and behavior. This book examines via two-way-traffic at multiple levels. For example, it examines at both preclinical and clinical levels, genes and populations, and how (a) components in food will affect our sensory responses and (b) how our behavior and sensory responses affect what foods we eat, their pattern of consumption and so on. This book consists of over 200 chapters, and is conveniently divided into 5 main sections to represent the various specialty areas, namely:

General, normative aspects and overviews
Pathological and abnormal aspects
Specific conditions and diseases
Changing eating behaviour and attitudes
Selective methods

The Editors recognize the difficulty in assigning chapters to specific sections. For example in order to describe normative features, abnormal aspects of diet and behavior may also be described. Chapters on food choice may have coverage on the developing brain, behavior and neuroendocrinology. Thus, some chapters can potentially be assigned to several sections. However, this is resolved with the excellent indexing systems that Springer is renowned for. The chapters are well illustrated with numerous tables and figures.

This book represents a multidisciplinary "one-stop-shop" of information with suitable indexing of the various pathways and processes. The chapters are written by national or international experts or specialists in their field. The Editors recognize that very often experts in one field may be novices in another. To bridge this knowledge-divide the authors have incorporated sections on "Applications to other areas health and disease", "Key Facts or Features" and "Summary Points" This reference book is for nutritionists, dietitians, food scientists, behavioral scientists, psychologists, doctors, nurses, physiologists, health workers and practitioners, college and university teachers and lecturers, undergraduates and graduates.

Contents

Volume 1

Volume 2

Volume 3

Volume 4

Part XXIV: Starvation and Nutrient Deficiency

Volume 5

Contributors

Gian Franco Adami, M.D.
Department of Surgery, University of Genova, Largo Rosanna Benzi 8,
Genova 16132, Italy

W. Stewart Agras, M.D.
Department of Psychiatry and Behavioral Sciences, Stanford University,
School of Medicine, Stanford, CA, USA

Rexford S. Ahima, M.D., Ph.D.
Institute for Diabetes, Obesity and Metabolism, School of Medicine, University
of Pennsylvania School of Medicine, 712A Clinical Research Building, 415 Curie
Boulevard, Philadelphia, PA 19104

Jennie C. Ahrén
Center for Health Equity Studies, CHESS, Karolinska Institutet/Stockholm
University, Sveavagen 160, 106 91, Stockholm, Sweden

Akira Akabayashi
Graduate School of Medicine, Department of Stress Sciences and Psychosomatic
Medicine, The University of Tokyo, Tokyo, Japan

Takashi Akamizu
Translational Research Center, Kyoto University Hospital, Kyoto University
School of Medicine, 54 Shogoin-Kawaharacho, Sakyo-ku, Kyoto 606-8507, Japan

Samir Al-Adawi, M.Sc., Ph.D.
Department of Behavioral Medicine, College of Medicine and Health Sciences,
Sultan Qaboos University, Al-Khoudh 123, Muscat, Sultanate of Oman

Abdulmajid Ali
General Surgery Department, Ayr Hospital, Ayr, UK

J. Alaghband-Zadeh
Department of Clinical Biochemistry, King's College Hospital, London, UK

Thomas R. Alley
Department of Psychology, 418 Brackett Hall, Clemson University, Clemson,
SC 29634-1355, USA

Kelly C. Allison, Ph.D.
Department of Psychiatry, Center for Weight and Eating Disorders,
University of Pennsylvania School of Medicine, Philadelphia, PA, USA

Ibrahim Al-Zakwani, Ph.D.
Department of Pharmacy College of Medicine and Health Sciences, Sultan Qaboos
University, Muscat, Sultanate of Oman

Oliver Amft, Ph.D.
ACTLab, Signal Processing Systems, Faculty of Electrical Engineering,
Eindhoven University of Technology, NL-5600 MB Eindhoven, The Netherlands

Joel G. Anderson
Department of Nutrition, University of North Carolina at Greensboro, Greensboro,
NC, USA

Helma Antony
School of Medical Science, Griffith University, Gold Coast Campus, Southport,
Queensland, Australia

Gastón Ares
Sección Evaluación Sensorial, Departamento de Ciencia y Tecnología de Alimentos,
Facultad de Química. Universidad de la República (UdelaR),
Gral. Flores 2124. C.P. 11800, Montevideo, Uruguay

Akihiro Asakawa
Department of Psychosomatic Internal Medicine, Kagoshima University Graduate
School of Medical and Dental Sciences, Kagoshima, Japan

Rheanna N. Ata, B.A.
Department of Psychology, University of South Florida, 4202 E. Fowler Avenue,
PCD 4118G, Tampa, FL 33620-8200

John Atkinson
West of Scotland University, Paisley, UK

Nicole M. Avena, Ph.D.
Department of Psychiatry, University of Florida, Gainesville, FL 32608, USA
and
Department of Psychology and Program in Neuroscience, Princeton University,
Princeton, NJ 08540, USA

Mary Ballard, Ph.D.
Department of Psychology, Appalachian State University, Boone, NC 28608, USA

Pauline Banks
School of Health, Nursing and Midwifery, University of the West of Scotland,
Beech Grove, Ayr, UK

Tom Baranowski, Ph.D.
Children's Nutrition Research Center, Department of Pediatrics,
Baylor College of Medicine, 1100 Bates Street, Houston TX 77030, USA

Stephanie Bauer
Center for Psychotherapy Research, University Hospital Heidelberg, Heidelberg,
Germany

Louise A. Baur, B.Sc.(Med), M.B.B.S. (Hons), Ph.D., FRACP
Discipline of Paediatrics and Child Health, University of Sydney, Sydney,
NSW 2006, Australia
and
Weight Management Services, The Children's Hospital at Westmead, Westmead,
NSW 2145, Australia

Christian Beaulieu
Department of Biomedical Engineering, 1098 Research Transition Facility,
University of Alberta, Edmonton, Alberta T6G 2V2, Canada

Stephen C. Benoitm, Ph.D.
Department of Psychiatry, University of Cincinnati, Cincinnati, OH, USA

David Benton
Department of Psychology, University of Wales Swansea, Swansea SA2 8PP,
Wales, UK

Pere Berbel
Instituto de Neurociencias, Universidad Miguel Hernández and Consejo Superior
de Investigaciones Científicas, Campus de Sant Joan, Apartado de Correos 18,
Sant Joan d'Alacant, 03550 Alicante, Spain

Lynda Bergsma, Ph.D.
Mel & Enid Zuckerman College of Public Health, University of Arizona,
P.O. Box 245209, Tucson, Arizona 85724

Daniel M. Bernstein
Department of Psychology, Kwantlen Polytechnic University,
12666 – 72nd Avenue, Surrey, BC, Canada

Monelle Bertrand
Unité de Nutrition, CHU Larrey, Toulouse cedex

Carole A. Bisogni
Division of Nutritional Sciences, 183 MVR Hall, Cornell University, Ithaca,
NY 14853, USA

Christine E. Blake
Department of Health Promotion, Education, and Behavior, Arnold School
of Public Health, University of South Carolina, Columbia, SC, USA

Eva Blomstrand
The Åstrand Labaratory, The Swedish School of Sport and Health Sciences,
Box 5626 114 86 Stockholm, Sweden

Miriam E. Bocarsly
Department of Psychology, Princeton University, Princeton, NJ, USA

Sandra D.M. Bot, Ph.D.
Department of General Practice and the EMGO Institute for Health and Care
Research, VU University Medical Center, Amsterdam, the Netherlands

Wayne A. Bowers, Ph.D.
Department of Psychiatry, University of Iowa, 2916 John Pappajohn Pavilion,
Iowa City, IA 52242

L. Mallory Boylan, Ph.D., RD, LD
Department of Nutrition, Hospitality & Retailing, Texas Tech University, Lubbock, TX, USA

Emma J. Boyland
Kissileff Laboratory for the Study of Human Ingestive Behaviour, School of Psychology, Eleanor Rathbone Building, Bedford Street South, University of Liverpool, Liverpool, L69 7ZA, UK

Christophe Breton
Neurostress (EA4347), Equipe Dénutritions Maternelles Périnatales, Bâtiment SN4, Université des Sciences et Technologies de Lille, France

Marie-Claude Brindisi, M.D.
Endocrinology and Nutrition Department, CHU le Bocage (Dijon University Hospital), BP 77908, 21079 Dijon Cedex

Russell Brown
Department of Obstetrics & Gynaecology, IWK Health Centre, Dalhousie University, Halifax, NS, Canada

Thomas A. Brunner
ETH Zurich, Institute for Environmental Decisions, Consumer Behavior, Universitaetsstrasse, Zurich, Switzerland

Eleanor J. Bryant
Centre for Psychology Studies, Social Sciences and Humanities, Richmond House, University of Bradford, West Yorkshire, BD7 1DP, UK

S. Alexandra Burt, Ph.D.
Department of Psychology, Michigan State University, East Lansing, MI, USA

Pietro Caliandro
Institute of Neurology, Largo F. Vito 1, 00168, Roma, Italy
and
Fondazione Pro Iuventute Don Carlo Gnocchi, Roma, Italy

Maria Valeria Camboni, Bpsych
Department of Psychology, University of Cagliari, Cagliari, Italy

Jameason D. Cameron
Behavioral and Metabolic Research Unit, School of Human Kinetics, University of Ottawa, Ottawa, Ontario, Canada

L. Arthur Campfield, Ph.D.
Department of Food Science and Human Nutrition, College of Applied Human Sciences, Colorado State University, Fort Collins, CO 80523-1571, USA

Lucia Camporese, PsyD
AIDAP Verona, Via Sansovino, Verona, Italy

Mehmet Cansev
Uludag University Medical School, Department of Pharmacology, Gorukle, 16059 Bursa, Turkey

Antonio Capurso, M.D.
Department of Geriatrics, Center for Aging Brain, Memory Unit, University of Bari, Bari, Italy

Cristiano Capurso
Department of Geriatrics, University of Foggia, Foggia, Italy

Céline Caquineau
Centre for Integrative Physiology, University of Edinburgh, Edinburgh, UK

Daniel P. Cardinali, M.D., Ph.D.
Departamento de Docencia e Investigación, Pontificia Universidad Católica Argentina, Buenos, Aires, Argentina

Amanda Carson
School of Health, Nursing and Midwifery, University of the West of Scotland, Beech Grove, Ayr, UK

Natalie A. Ceballos
Department of Psychology, Texas State University, San Marcos, TX, USA

Kim M. Cecil, Ph.D.
Cincinnati Children's Environmental Health Center at the Cincinnati Children's Hospital Medical Center, Departments of Radiology, Pediatrics, Neuroscience and Environmental Health, University of Cincinnati College of Medicine, Cincinnati, OH, USA
and
Cincinnati Children's Hospital Medical Center, Department of Radiology/Imaging Research Center MLC 5033, 3333 Burnet Avenue, Cincinnati, OH 45229, USA

Hellas Cena, M.D.
Department of Health Sciences, Section of Human Nutrition, University of Pavia, Pavia, Italy

Elena Centis, Ph.D.
Clinical Dietetics, University of Bologna, Bologna, Italy

Antonio Cepeda-Benito
Department of Psychology, Henderson Hall, Texas A&M University, College Station, TX, USA

Seung Hun Cha
School of Medicine, Department of Biological Chemistry, The Johns Hopkins University, Baltimore, MD, USA

Evonne J. Charboneau, M.D.
School of Medicine, Vanderbilt University, Nashville, TN, USA

Christine Charrueau, PharmD, Ph.D.
Laboratoire de Pharmacie Galénique EA 2498, Faculté des Sciences Pharmaceutiques et Biologiques, Université Paris Descartes, Paris Cedex, France

Catherine Chaumontet
INRA, CNRH-IdF, UMR914 Nutrition Physiology and Ingestive Behavior, Paris,
France
and
AgroParisTech, CNRH-IdF, UMR914 Nutrition Physiology and Ingestive Behavior,
Paris, France

Anastasia Chellino, B.S.
Health Psychology, Ingestive Behavior Laboratory, Pennington Biomedical
Research Center, Baton Rouge, LA, USA
and
Department of Natural Sciences, University of Education Heidelberg, Heidelberg,
Germany

Hui Chen
Faculty of Science, Department of Medical and Molecular Bioscience, University
of Technology, Sydney, Australia
and
School of Medical Sciences, Department of Pharmacology, University of New
South Wales, Sydney, Australia

Kai-Chun Cheng
Department of Psychosomatic Internal Medicine, Kagoshima University Graduate
School of Medical and Dental Sciences, Kagoshima, Japan

Sergio Chieffi
Department of Experimental Medicine, Section of Human Physiology, and Clinical
Dietetic Service, Second University of Naples, Naples, Italy

W.I. Cho
Department of Food and Animal Biotechnology, College of Agriculture and Life
Sciences, Seoul National University, San 56-1 Sillim-dong, Gwanak-gu,
Seoul 151-921, Korea

Derrick L. Choi, B.S.
Department of Psychiatry, University of Cincinnati, Cincinnati, OH, USA

Chin Moi Chow
Delta Sleep Research Unit, Discipline of Exercise and Sport Science,
The University of Sydney, Lidcombe NSW 1825, Australia

Yvonne Christley
School of Health, Nursing and Midwifery, University of the West of Scotland,
Beech Grove, Ayr, UK

J.K. Chun
Department of Food and Animal Biotechnology, College of Agriculture and Life
sciences, Seoul National University, Seoul, Korea

Cicero G. Coimbra
Laboratory of Clinical and Experimental Pathophysiology, Department of
Neurology and Neurosurgery, Federal University of São Paulo (UNIFESP),
São Paulo SP BRAZIL

Anna M. Colacicco, Ph.D.
Department of Geriatrics, Center for Aging Brain, Memory Unit, University of
Bari, Bari, Italy

Nelson Barros Colauto
Laboratório de Biologia Molecular, Universidade Paranaense, Praça Mascarenhas
de Moraes, Umuarama-PR, Brazil

Cian E. Collins, FRCSI (Ophth), MRCOphth
Princess Alexandra Eye Pavilion, Chalmers Street, Edinburgh EH3 9HA

Mark Conner
Institute of Psychological Sciences, University of Leeds, Leeds, UK

James R. Connor, Ph.D.
Milton S. Hershey Medical Center, Pennsylvania State University, Hershey, PA, USA

Richard W.I. Cooke
School of Reproductive and Developmental Medicine, University of Liverpool,
First Floor, University Department, Liverpool Women's Hospital,
Crown Street, Liverpool, L8 7SS, UK

John Correa, B.S.
Health Psychology, Ingestive Behavior Laboratory, Pennington Biomedical
Research Center, Baton Rouge, LA, USA

Vassiliki Costarelli, BSc, MSc, Ph.D, R.Nutr.
Human Ecology Laboratory, Department of Home Economics and Ecology,
Harokopio University, 70 El. Venizelou Ave, 17671 Kallithea, Athens, Greece

Mihai Covasa
INRA, Écologie et Physiologie du Système Digestif, 78350 Jouy-en-Josas, France

Ronald L. Cowan M.D., Ph.D.
School of Medicine, Vanderbilt University, Nashville, TN, USA

Sabrina Crepin
Service de Toxicologie et Pharmacologie - Pharmacovigilance, Centre Hospitalier
Universitaire, F-87042 Limoges, France

Kristen M. Culbert, M.A.
Department of Psychology, Michigan State University, East Lansing, MI, USA

Maria Czyzewska
Department of Psychology, Texas State University, 601 University Drive,
San Marcos, TX, USA

Alessia D'Introno, Ph.D.
Department of Geriatrics, Center for Aging Brain, Memory Unit,
University of Bari, Bari, Italy

Ippeita Dan
Sensory & Cognitive Food Science Laboratory, National Food Research Institute,
Kannondai, Tsukuba, Ibaraki, Japan

Daniel Rigaud, M.D.
Department of Endocrinology and Nutrition, CHU Le Bocage (Dijon University Hospital), BP 77908, 21079 Dijon Cedex, France

Nicolas Darcel
INRA, CNRH-IdF, UMR914 Nutrition Physiology and Ingestive Behavior, Paris, France
and
AgroParisTech, CNRH-IdF, UMR914 Nutrition Physiology and Ingestive Behavior, Paris, France

Undurti N. Das, M.D., FAMS
UND Life Sciences 13800 Fairhill Road, #321, Shaker Heights, OH, 44120, USA
Jawaharlal Nehru Technological University, Kakinada- 533 003, Andhra Pradesh, India

Christopher Davids
Department of Psychology, Cornell College, Mt. Vernon, IA, USA

Fiona Davies, B.A. (Hons), M.Psych. (Applied)
Weight Management Services, The Children's Hospital at Westmead, Westmead, Australia
and
Gymea Lily Psychotherapy Centre, Sutherland, Australia

Caroline Davis
Department of Psychiatry, University Health Network, Toronto, Ontario, Canada

Jon F. Davis, Ph.D.
Department of Psychiatry, University of Cincinnati, Genome Research Institute Building E, Lab 334, 2170 East Galbraith Road, 45237 Cincinnati, OH, USA

Gwenaelle Diene
Centre de référence du syndrome de Prader-Willi, Hôpital des Enfants, Toulouse Cedex, France

Bruno De Luca
Department of Experimental Medicine, Section of Human Physiology, and Clinical Dietetic Service, Second University of Naples, Naples, Italy

Mary Jane De Souza, Ph.D., FACSM
Women's Health and Exercise Laboratory, Noll Laboratory, Department of Kinesiology, Penn State University, University Park, PA 16802, USA

Fabien Delahaye
Neurostress (EA4347), Equipe Dénutritions Maternelles Périnatales, Bâtiment SN4, Université des Sciences et Technologies de Lille, France

Sylvie Deloof
Neurostress (EA4347), Equipe Dénutritions Maternelles Périnatales, Bâtiment SN4, Université des Sciences et Technologies de Lille, France

Jean-Claude Desport
Université de Limoges, Institut de Neuroépidémiologie et de Neurologie Tropicale,
EA 3174 NeuroEpidémiologie Tropicale et Comparée, Limoges, France
and
Service de Gastro-Hépato-Entérologie, Unité de Nutrition, Centre Hospitalier
Universitaire, Limoges, France

Silvia Di Domizio, R.D.
Clinical Dietetics, University of Bologna, Bologna, Italy

D.A.J. Dijck-Brouwe
University Medical Center Groningen, Groningen, the Netherlands

Atsu S.S. Dorvlo, Ph.D.
Department of Mathematics and Statistics, Sultan Qaboos University, Muscat,
Sultanate of Oman

Éric Doucet
Behavioral and Metabolic Research Unit, School of Human Kinetics,
University of Ottawa, Ontario, Ottawa, Canada, K1N 6N5

Alison J. Douglas
Centre for Integrative Physiology, University of Edinburgh, Hugh Robson Building,
George Square, Edinburgh, EH8 9XD, UK

Ronald G. Downey, Ph.D.
Kansas State University, Manhattan, KS, USA

Vicky Drapeau
Department of physical education, Laval University, Quebec City, Canada

Robert Drewett
Science Laboratories, Durham University, South Road, Durham, DH1 3LE, UK

Tim Duffy
School of Health, Nursing and Midwifery, University of the West of Scotland,
Beech Grove, Ayr, UK

Audrey DunnGalvin, Ph.D., Reg.Psychol.Ps.S.I.
Clinical Investigations Unit, Department of Paediatrics and Child Health,
Cork University Hospital, University College Cork (UCC), Wilton, Cork, Ireland

Holiday Durham, Ph.D., RD
Pennington Biomedical Research Center, Louisiana State University, Baton Rouge,
LA, USA

Isabelle Dutriez-Casteloot
Neurostress (EA4347), Equipe Dénutritions Maternelles Périnatales, Bâtiment SN4,
Université des Sciences et Technologies de Lille, France

Louise Dye
Human Appetite Research Unit, Institute of Psychological Sciences,
University of Leeds, LS2 9JT, UK

Nina Eikelis, Ph.D.
Human Neurotransmitters Laboratory, Vascular and Hypertension Division, Baker
IDI Heart and Diabetes Institute, Melbourne, Victoria 8008, Australia

Mark Ellrichmann, M.D.
Department of Medicine I, University Hospital Schleswig Holstein, Campus Kiel,
Schittenhelmstr 12, 24105 Kiel, Germany

Enzo Emanuele, M.D.
Department of Health Sciences, Section of Psychiatry, University of Pavia, Pavia, Italy

Keith M. Erikson
Department of Nutrition, University of North Carolina at Greensboro, Greensboro,
NC 27402-6170, USA

Charlotte Erlanson-Albertsson, M.D., Ph.D.
Appetite Control Unit, Division of Diabetes, Endocrinology and Metabolism,
Department of Experimental Medical Science, Lund University, BMC B11,
SE-221 84, Lund, Sweden

Gabriella Morreale de Escobar
Instituto de Investigaciones Biomédicas Alberto Sols, CSIC and Universidad
Autónoma de Madrid, and Center for Biomedical Research on Rare Diseases
(CIBERER), Madrid, Spain

Ana I. Esquifino, Ph.D.
Departamento de Bioquímica y Biología Molecular III, Universidad Complutense,
28040 Madrid, Spain

Christine Feinle-Bisset
Discipline of Medicine, Royal Adelaide Hospital, Adelaide, South Australia, Australia

Dorianne Feldman, M.D., MSPT
Department of Physical Medicine and Rehabilitation, School of Medicine, Johns
Hopkins University, Baltimore, MD

Marlís González Fernández, M.D., Ph.D.
Department of Physical Medicine and Rehabilitation, School of Medicine,
Johns Hopkins University, Baltimore, MD

M. Carmen Fernández
Departamento de Personalidad, Evaluación y Tratamiento Psicológico, Facultad de
Psicología, Universidad de Granada, Granada, Spain

Elizabeth Ferris
University of Arizona, Mel & Enid Zuckerman College of Public Health, Tucson,
AZ, USA
and
Department of Psychiatry, Center for Weight and Eating Disorders,
University of Pennsylvania School of Medicine, Philadelphia, PA, USA

Mick P. Fleming
School of Health, Nursing and Midwifery, University of the West of Scotland,
Beech Grove, Ayr, UK

Eduardo Fonseca-Pedrero
Department of Psychology, University of Oviedo, Centro de Investigación
Biomédica en Red de Salud Mental, CIBERSAM, Plaza Feijoo, s/n, Oviedo, 33003,
Spain

Georg Förster
Department of Psychology, University of Würzburg, Würzburg, Germany

Joanna S. Fowler, Ph.D.
Medical Department, Brookhaven National Laboratory, Upton, New York, USA

Vincenza Frisardi, M.D.
Department of Geriatrics, Center for Aging Brain, Memory Unit, University of
Bari, Bristol, UK

Gilles Fromentin
INRA, CNRH-IdF, UMR914 Nutrition Physiology
and Ingestive Behavior, F-75005 Paris, France
and
AgroParisTech, CNRH-IdF, UMR914 Nutrition Physiology
and Ingestive Behavior, F-75005 Paris, France
and
UMR 914 INRA/AgroParisTech, 16 rue Claude Bernard,
75231 Paris Cedex 05, France

Toshikatsu Fujii
Department of Behavioural Neurology and Cognitive Neuroscience, Tohoku
University Graduate School of Medicine, Sendai, Japan

Tahany M. Gadalla, Ph.D., M.Sc., MMath
Factor-Inwentash Faculty of Social Work, University of Toronto, 246 Bloor Street
West, Toronto, Ontario, Canada, M5S 1V4

Salah Gariballa, M.D., FRCP
Department of Internal Medicine, Faculty of Medicine and Health Sciences, UAE
University, Al-Ain, United Arab Emirates

Michael K. Georgieff, M.D.
Department of Pediatrics, Neonatology Division & Center for Neurobehavioral
Development, School of Medicine, University of Minnesota, 420 Delaware St. SE,
MMC 39 (for mail), D-136 Mayo Building (for courier), Minneapolis,
MN 55455, USA

E.L. Gibson
Clinical and Health Psychology Research Centre, Department of Psychology,
Whitelands College, Roehampton University, Holybourne Avenue,
London SW15 4JD, UK

Giuseppe Derosa, M.D., Ph.D.
Department of Internal Medicine and Therapeutics, University of Pavia, Pavia, Italy

Cheryl Glover
School of Health, Nursing and Midwifery, University of the West of Scotland,
Ayr Campus, Beech Grove, Ayr, UK

Bertrand Godet
Service de Neurologie, Centre Hospitalier Universitaire, Limoges, France

Dina Gohar
Department of Psychology, University of Pennsylvania, Philadelphia, PA, USA

Iratxe Gonzalez

Oscar Gonzalez-Perez, M.D., Ph.D
Laboratory of Neuroscience, School of Psychology, University of Colima,
Av. Universidad 333, Colima, Col 28040, México
and
Neuroscience Department, Centro Universitario de Ciencias de la Salud,
University of Guadalajara, Guadalajara, Jal 44340, México

E. González-Reimers
Servicio de Medicina Interna, Hospital Universitario de Canarias, Ofra s/n 38320,
La Laguna, Tenerife, Canary Islands, Spain

S.A. van Goor
University Medical Center Groningen, Nijlandspark 26, 9301 Bz Roden,
The Netherlands

Amy A. Gorin, Ph.D.
Department of Psychology, Center for Health, Intervention, and Prevention,
University of Connecticut, 2006 Hillside Road, Storrs, CT 06269-1248, USA

Alja Gössler
Department of Pediatric and Adolescent Surgery, General Hospital Klagenfurt,
St.Veiter Str. 47, 9020 Klagenfurt, Austria

Reiko Graham
Department of Psychology, Texas State University, San Marcos, TX, USA

Riccardo Dalle Grave, M.D.
Department of Eating and Weight Disorder, Villa Garda Hospital,
Via Montebaldo 89, I-37016 Garda (VR), Italy

Michael W. Green
Nutrition and Behaviour Laboratory, Psychology Department, School of Life and
Health Sciences, Aston University, Birmingham, UK, B4 7ET

Melinda A. Green
Department of Psychology, Cornell College, 106E Law Hall,
600 First Street West, Mt. Vernon, IA 52314

G. Grugni
Department of Auxology, IRCCS 'S. Giuseppe Hospital'-Verbania, Roma, Italy

Rubem Carlos Araújo Guedes, M.D., Ph.D.
Departamento de Nutrição, Universidade Federal de Pernambuco,
BR-50670901, Recife, PE, Brazil

Matthieu J. Guitton, Ph.D.
Centre de Recherche Université Laval Robert-Giffard (CRULRG), 2601
Chemin de la Canardière F-6517, Québec, QC, G1J 2G3, Canada
and
Faculty of Pharmacy, Laval University, Quebec City, QC, Canada

Alissa A. Haedt, M.A.
Department of Psychiatry, University of Iowa, Iowa City, IA, USA

Jason C.G. Halford
Kissileff Laboratory for the Study of Human Ingestive Behaviour,
School of Psychology, University of Liverpool, Liverpool, UK

John Hall, Ph.D.
Deakin Business School, Deakin University, Melbourne, Victoria, Australia

Hélène Hanaire
Unité de Nutrition, CHU Larrey, Toulouse cedex

Rhona M. Hanning, Ph.D., RD
Department of Health Studies and Gerontology, University of Waterloo, Waterloo,
Ontario, Canada

Joanne A. Harrold
Kissileff Laboratory for the Study of Human Ingestive Behavior, School
of Psychology, University of Liverpool, Liverpool, UK

Sybil L. Hart, Ph.D.
Texas Tech University, Department of Human Development and Family Studies,
Lubbock, TX 79409-1230

Jenni Harvey
Division of Medical Sciences, Centre for Neuroscience, Ninewells Hospital
and Medical School, University of Dundee, Dundee DD1 9SY, UK

Kenji Hashimoto
Division of Clinical Neuroscience, Chiba University Center for Forensic
Mental Health, 1-8-1 Inohana, Chiba 260-8670, Japan

Michio Hashimoto
Department of Environmental Physiology, Shimane University Faculty of Medicine,
Izumo, Shimane 693–8501, Japan

Remco C. Havermans
Department of Clinical Psychological Science, Maastricht University, Maastricht,
6200 MD, The Netherlands

Narasimha Hegde, Ph.D.
Department of Nutritional Sciences, Pennsylvania State University, University Park,
PA, USA

Christopher Herrera
Delta Sleep Research Unit, Discipline of Exercise and Sport Science,
The University of Sydney, Lidcombe, Australia

Marion Hetherington
Institute of Psychological Sciences, University of Leeds, Leeds,
West Yorkshire, UK

Takashi Higuchi
Department of Integrative Physiology, University of Fukui, Eiheij-cho, Matsuoka,
Fukui, 910-1193, Japan

Anke Hinney
Klinik für Psychiatrie und Psychotherapie des Kindes- und Jugendalters, LVR-
Klinikum Essen, Kliniken und Institut der Unisitat Duisburg-Essen, Essen, Germany

Angelica Lindén Hirschberg, M.D., Ph.D.
Department of Obstetrics and Gynaecology, Karolinska University Hospital,
Stockholm, Sweden

Claude Marcel Hladik
UMR CNRS/MNHN 7206, Eco-Anthropologie et Ethnobiologie, Brunoy, France

Bartley G. Hoebel
Department of Psychology, Princeton University, Princeton, NJ, USA

Wilhelm Hofmann
University of Chicago, Booth School of Business,
5807 South Woodlawn Avenue, Chicago, IL 60615

Pleunie Hogenkamp
Division of Human Nutrition, TI Food and Nutrition, Wageningen University
and Research Centre, Wageningen, the Netherlands

Eef Hogervorst, Ph.D.
School of Sport, Exercise and Health Sciences, Loughborough University,
Ashby Road, Loughborough, Leicestershire, United Kingdom

R.H. Holloway, B.Sc. (Med), M.B.B.S., M.D., FRACP
Discipline of Medicine, University of Adelaide, Adelaide, Australia

Chang Hyung Hong
Department of Psychiatry and Ajou Institute of Aging, Ajou University School
of Medicine, San 5, Wonchun-dong, Youngtong-gu, Suwon-si, 443-749, Korea

Mary Hostler
Program Secretary, Cancer Research Center Hawaii, Prevention and
Control Program, University of Hawaii at Manoa, Honolulu, HI, USA

Jonathan O'B. Hourihane, M.B., D.M., MRCPI, FRCPCH
Clinical Investigations Unit, Department of Paediatrics and Child Health, Cork
University Hospital, University College Cork (UCC), Wilton, Cork, Ireland

Alexa Hoyland
Human Appetite Research Unit, Institute of Psychological Sciences, University
of Leeds, Leeds, UK

Wallace Huffman, Ph.D.
Department of Economics, Iowa State University, Ames, IA 50011, USA

Ethan E. Hull, Ph.D.
Children's Hospital of Pittsburgh, Pittsburgh, PA

Michael Huncharek, MD, MPH
Meta-Analysis Research Group, 10 Sasanqua Circle, Columbia, SC 29209, USA

Teresa Iannaccone
Department of Experimental Medicine, Section of Human Physiology, and Clinical
Dietetic Service, Second University of Naples, Naples, Italy

Melinda J. Ickes, Ph.D.
Health Promotion & Education, University of Cincinnati, Cincinnati, OH, USA

Bruno P. Imbimbo, Ph.D.
Research and Development Department, Chiesi Farmaceutici, Parma, Italy
and
Department of Geriatrics, University of Foggia, Foggia, Italy

Syed A. Imran
Department of Physiology & Biophysics, Dalhousie University, Halifax, NS,
Canada

Sheila M. Innis
Department of Paediatrics, Child and Family Research Institute, University
of British Columbia, 950 West 28th Avenue, Vancouver, BC V5Z 4H4, Canada

Akio Inui
Department of Psychosomatic Internal Medicine, Kagoshima University Graduate
School of Medical and Dental Sciences 8-35-1 Sakuragaoka, Kagoshima 890-8520,
Japan

Shera C. Jackson, M.S., CLC
Department of Human Development and Family Studies, Texas Tech University,
Lubbock, TX, USA

Sanjay Jaju, M.D. M.Phil.
Directorate of Research & Studies, DG Planning, Ministry of Health (HQ), Muscat,
Sultanate of Oman

Anita Jansen
Department of Clinical Psychological Science, Maastricht University, P.O. Box 616,
6200 MD Maastricht, The Netherlands

Margaret Jastran
Division of Nutritional Sciences, Cornell University, Ithaca, NY, USA

Aminah Jatoi, M.D.
Department of Oncology, Mayo Clinic, 200 First Street SW, Rochester,
Minnesota, USA

Vickii B. Jenvey
School of Psychology, Psychiatry, Monash University, Building 17, Clayton,
Victoria 3800, Australia

Amanda Jepson
Department of Psychology, Cornell College, Mt. Vernon, IA, USA
and
Neuroscience Department, Centro Universitario de Ciencias de la Salud, University
of Guadalajara, Guadalajara, Jal, México

Amy R. Johnson
Department of Nutrition, University of North Carolina at Chapel Hill, Chapel Hill,
NC, USA

Fiona Jones
Department of Psychology, University of Bedfordshire, Luton, LU1 3JU, UK

Michelle P. Judge, Ph.D., RD
School of Nursing, University of Connecticut, 231 Glenbrook Rd, Unit 2026,
Mansfield, CT, USA

Alexei B. Kampov-Polevoy, M.D., Ph.D.
Department of Psychiatry, University of North Carolina at Chapel Hill, 237 Medical
School Wing B, Campus Box 7160, Chapel Hill, NC 27599-7160

Natalie Kanakam
Institute of Psychiatry, King's College London, London, UK
and
Department of Academic Psychiatry, Eating, Disorder Research Unit,
Guy's Hospital, London, UK

Masanori Katakura
Department of Environmental Physiology, Shimane University Faculty
of Medicine, Izumo, Shimane, Japan
and
Meta-Analysis Research Group, Columbia, SC, USA

Patrick G. Kehoe, Ph.D.
Dementia Research Group, Institute of Clinical Neurosciences, The John James
Building, Frenchay Hospital, University of Bristol, Bristol, UK

A.R. Kelles, Ph.D.
Department of Nutrition, New York Chiropractic College, Seneca Falls,
New York, USA

Eva Kemps
School of Psychology, Flinders University, GPO, Adelaide, SA 5001, Australia

Alexandra P.F. Key, Ph.D.
Vanderbilt Kennedy Center for Research on Human Development, 230 Appleton
Place, Peabody Box 74, Vanderbilt University, Nashville, TN 37203

Joan Khoo
Discipline of Medicine, Royal Adelaide Hospital, Adelaide, South Australia,
Australia

Hiroe Kikuchi
Educational Physiology Laboratory, Graduate School of Education, The University
of Tokyo, Tokyo, Japan

Atsushi Kimura
Sensory & Cognitive Food Science Laboratory, National Food Research Institute,
Kannondai, Tsukuba, Ibaraki, Japan

Neil King
Human Movement Studies & Institute of Health and Biomedical Innovation,
Queensland University of Technology, Brisbane, Queensland, Australia

Kelly L. Klump, Ph.D.
Department of Psychology, Michigan State University, East Lansing, MI, USA

Y. Kodra
National Centre for Rare Diseases, Istituto Superiore di Sanità, Roma, Italy

Anna Kokavec, Ph.D.
School of Psychological Science, La Trobe University, Bendigo, Australia, 3552

Hitoshi Komuro
Department of Neurosciences/NC30, Lerner Research Institute, The Cleveland
Clinic Foundation, 9500 Euclid Avenue, Cleveland, OH 44195, USA

Yutaro Komuro
Department of Neurosciences/NC30, Lerner Research Institute, The Cleveland
Clinic Foundation, Cleveland, OH, USA

Takashi Kondoh, Ph.D.
Institute of Life Sciences, Ajinomoto Co., Inc., Kawasaki, Japan
and
AJINOMOTO Integrative Research for Advanced Dieting, Graduate School
of Agriculture, Kyoto University, Kyoto, Japan
and
Institute of Psychiatry, King's College London, London, UK
and
Department of Academic Psychiatry, Eating Disorders Research Unit,
Guy's Hospital, London, UK

Karel Krafka
Department of Pediatric and Adolescent Surgery, General Hospital Klagenfurt,
Klagenfurt, Austria

David Kugler
Department of Psychology, Cornell College, Mt. Vernon, IA, USA

Jyrki T. Kuikka
Imaging Center, Kuopio University Hospital, FIN-70211 Kuopio, Finland

Tatsuro Kumada
Department of Neurosciences/NC30, Lerner Research Institute, The Cleveland
Clinic Foundation, Cleveland, OH, USA

Angela B. Kydd
School of Health Nursing and Midwifery, University of the West of Scotland,
Hamilton Campus, Almada Street, Hamilton, Lanarkshire, ML3 0JB, UK

Christine Laborie
Neurostress (EA4347), Equipe Dénutritions Maternelles Périnatales,
Bâtiment SN4, Université des Sciences et Technologies de Lille, France

Virginie F. Labrousse
Psynugen, Université Bordeaux 2, INRA, UMR1286, CNRS, UMR5226, Bâtiment
UFR Pharmacie – 2ème Tranche – 2ème Etage, Case courrier 34, 33076
BORDEAUX Cedex

Jeroen Lakerveld
Department of General Practice and the EMGO Institute for Health and Care
Research, VU University Medical Center, van der Boechorststraat 7, 1081 BT,
Amsterdam, The Netherlands

Sylvia M.S. Chung Chun Lam
Riddet Institute, Massey University, Private Bag 11-222, Palmerston North,
New Zealand

Gavin Lambert, Ph.D.
Human Neurotransmitters Laboratory, Vascular and Hypertension Division,
Baker IDI Heart and Diabetes Institute, Melbourne, Australia

Carol J. Lammi-Keefe, Ph.D., RD
Human Nutrition and Food, School of Human Ecology, Louisiana State University,
Baton Rouge, LA, USA

Daniel Lamport
Human Appetite Research Unit, Institute of Psychological Sciences,
University of Leeds, Leeds, UK

M. Daniel Lane
Department of Biological Chemistry, School of Medicine, The Johns Hopkins
University, Baltimore, Maryland 21205

Brenda Larson, M.D.
Department of Oncology, Mayo Clinic, 200 First street SW, Rochester, Minnesota,
USA

Antonio Laverde
Laboratório de Química de Produtos Naturais, Universidade Paranaense, Praça
Mascarenhas de Moraes, Umuarama-PR, Brazil

Clare Lawton
Human Appetite Research Unit, Institute of Psychological Sciences, University of
Leeds, Leeds, UK

Sophie Laye, Ph.D.
Psychoneuroimmunology, nutrition and genetics (Psynugen), Université Bordeaux 2,
INRA, UMR1286, CNRS, UMR5226, Bâtiment UFR Pharmacie – 2ème Tranche –
2ème Etage, Case courrier 34, 146 rue Léo Saignat, 33076 BORDEAUX, Cedex

Catherine Lebel
Department of Biomedical Engineering, 1098 Research Transition Facility,
University of Alberta, Edmonton, Alberta

Edward B. Lee, M.D., Ph.D.
Institute for Diabetes, Obesity and Metabolism, School of Medicine, University of
Pennsylvania, Philadelphia, PA, USA

Kang Soo Lee
Department of Psychiatry, Bundang Cha hospital, CHA University, Bundang-gu,
Seongnam-si, Kyounggi-do, Korea

Louis Lefebvre
Department of Biology, McGill University, Montreal, Quebec, Canada

David S. Leland, Ph.D.
Department of Psychology, University of Wisconsin - Eau Claire, 105 Garfield Ave,
Eau Claire, WI 54702, USA

Serafín Lemos-Giráldez
Department of Psychology, Centro de Investigación Biomédica en Red de Salud
Mental (CIBERSAM), University of Oviedo, Oviedo, Spain

Gareth Leng
Centre for Integrative Physiology, University of Edinburgh, George Square,
Hugh Robson Building, EH8 9XD Edinburgh, UK

William R. Leonard
Department of Anthropology, Northwestern University, 1810 Hinman Avenue,
Evanston, IL 60208, USA

Jean Lesage
Neurostress (EA4347), Equipe Dénutritions Maternelles Périnatales, Bâtiment SN4,
Université des Sciences et Technologies de Lille, France

Moira S. Lewitt
Faculty of Science & Technology, University of the West of Scotland,
Paisley Campus, PA1 2BE, Paisley, Scotland, UK

Ying Li
Department of Neurosciences/NC30, Lerner Research Institute, The Cleveland
Clinic Foundation, Cleveland, OH, USA

Ying-Xiao Li
Department of Psychosomatic Internal Medicine, Kagoshima University Graduate
School of Medical and Dental Sciences, Kagoshima, Japan

S.W. Lim
Department of Biological System Engineering, University of Wisconsin-Madison,
Madison, WI, USA

Giani Andrea Linde
Laboratório de Biologia Molecular, Universidade Paranaense, Praça Mascarenhas
de Moraes, 4282, CEP 87.502-210, Umuarama-PR, Brazil

Katajun Lindenberg
Center for Psychotherapy Research, University Hospital Heidelberg, Bergheimer
Straße 54, 69115 Heidelberg, Germany

Diana M. Lindquist, Ph.D.
Department of Radiology/Imaging Research, Cincinnati Children's Hospital
Medical Center, Cincinnati, OH, USA

Yoav Littner
Department of Neonatology, Cleveland Clinic Children's Hospital, The Cleveland
Clinic Foundation, Cleveland, OH, USA

Elizabeth F. Loftus
Department of Psychology, University of California at Irvine, Irvine, CA, USA

Antonio Carlos Lopes
Department of Medicine, Federal University of São Paulo (UNIFESP), São Paulo, Brazil

Alison Bryant Ludden, Ph.D.
Psychology Department, College of the Holy Cross, Worcester, MA, USA

D. A. de Luis
Institute of Endocrinology and Nutrition, Medicine School and
Unit of Investigation, Hospital Rio Hortega. Hospital Clinico,
University of Valladolid, Valladolid, Spain

Marie-Amélie Lukaszewsk
Neurostress (EA4347), Equipe Dénutritions Maternelles Périnatales, Bâtiment SN4,
Université des Sciences et Technologies de Lille, France

Colleen Taylor Lukens, Ph.D.
Pediatric Feeding and Swallowing Center, The Children's Hospital of Philadelphia,
34th Street & Civic Center Boulevard, Philadelphia, PA 19104, USA

Jennifer D. Lundgren, Ph.D.
Department of Psychology, University of Missouri-Kansas City, 4825 Troost
Avenue, Ste. 124, Kansas City, Missouri, 64110, USA

Christine-Johanna Macare
Institute of Psychiatry, King's College London, London, UK
and
Department of Academic Psychiatry, Eating, Disorder Research Unit,
Guy's Hospital, London, UK

Ian G. Macreadie
Bio21 Institute, University of Melbourne, 30 Flemington Road,
Melbourne, VIC 3010, Australia

Sandra Maestro
Division of Child Neuropsichiatry, Stella Maris Scientific Institute, University of
Pisa, Italy

Mario Maj
Department of Psychiatry, University of Naples SUN, Naples, Italy

Alexandros Makriyannis
Center for Drug Discovery, Northeastern University, Boston, MA, USA

Izaskun Marañon
Navarra Health Service (Osasunbidea), Itsasargi 11-3, 20280 Hondarribia, Spain

Glenn R. Marland
School of Health, Nursing and Midwifery, University of the West of Scotland, Dumfries Campus, Dudgeon House, Bankend Road, Dumfries, DG1 4ZN, UK

Monica Mars
Division of Human Nutrition, TI Food and Nutrition/Wageningen University and Research Centre, Wageningen, the Netherlands

Corby K. Martin, Ph.D.
Ingestive Behavior Laboratory, Pennington Biomedical Research Center, 6400 Perkins Rd., Baton Rouge, LA, USA

Colin R. Martin
School of Health, Nursing and Midwifery, University of the West of Scotland, Ayr Campus, Beech Grove, Ayr, KA8 0SR, UK

Catia Martins
Department of Cancer Research and Molecular Medicine, Faculty of Medicine, Norwegian University of Science and Technology, Trondheim, Norway

Giulio Marchesini, M.D.
Unit of Metabolic Diseases & Clinical Dietetics, "Alma Mater Studiorum" University, University of Bologna, Policlinico S. Orsola, Via Massarenti 9, I-40138, Bologna, Italy

Rebecca Marzocchi, M.D.
Clinical Dietetics, University of Bologna, Bologna, Italy

Alessandra Mauri
Nutrition, Metabolism and Diabetes Unit, Ospedale Ca' Foncello,Treviso, Italy

Sylvain Mayeur
Neurostress (EA4347), Equipe Dénutritions Maternelles Périnatales, Bâtiment SN4, Université des Sciences et Technologies de Lille, France

F. Joseph McClernon, Ph.D.
Health Behavior Neuroscience Research Program, Investigator, Center for Nicotine and Smoking Cessation Research, Duke University Medical Center, Durham, NC, USA

Patrick O. McGowan
Department of Psychiatry, McGill University, Montreal, QC, Canada

Peter J. McLaughlin
Department of Psychology, University of Connecticut, Storrs, CT, USA
and
Department of Psychology, Edinboro University of Pennsylvania, Edinboro, PA, USA

James S. McTaggart
Department of Physiology, Anatomy and Genetics, University of Oxford, Oxford, UK

Michael J. Meaney
Sackler Program for Epigenetics and Psychobiology, Douglas Institute – Research, Montreal, QC, Canada

Giovanni Messina
Department of Experimental Medicine, Section of Human Physiology, and Clinical Dietetic Service, Second University of Naples, Naples, Italy

Jessie L. Miller
Department of Psychiatry and Behavioural Neurosciences, Offord Centre for Child Studies, McMaster University, Chedoke Site, Central Building, 3rd Floor, 1200 Main Street West, Hamilton, Ontario, Canada, L8N 3Z5

Robert R. Miller, Jr.
Biology Department, Hillsdale College, 278 N. West St., Dow Science 213, Hillsdale, MI 49242-1205, USA

Emmanuelle Mimoun
Centre de référence du syndrome de Prader-Willi/Hôpital des Enfants/ 330 av de Grande Bretagne/TSA 70034/31059 Toulouse Cedex 9/France

Paola Miotto, M.D.
Eating Disorders Unit, Department of Psychiatry, Conegliano, TV, Italy

Katsumi Mizuno, M.D., Ph.D.
Department of Pediatrics, Showa University of Medicine, 1-5-8 Hatanodai, Shinagawa-ku, Tokyo, 142-8666, Japan

Markus Moessner
Center for Psychotherapy Research, University Hospital Heidelberg, Heidelberg, Germany

Christophe Moinard, Ph.D.
Laboratoire de Biologie de la Nutrition EA 4466, Faculté des Sciences Pharmaceutiques et Biologiques, Université Paris Descartes, 4 avenue de l'Observatoire 75270 Paris Cedex 06, France

Marcellino Monda, M.D.
Department of Experimental Medicine, Section of Human Physiology, and Clinical Dietetic Service, Second University of Naples, Via Costantinopoli 16, 80138 Naples, Italy

Naresh Mondraty
Wesley Eating Disorders Centre, Wesley Hospital, 85 Milton Street, Ashfield, Sydney NSW, 2131 Australia

Marie-Odile Monneuse
Centre National de la Recherche Scientifique, UMR CNRS/MNHN 7206: Eco-Anthropologie et Ethnobiologie, Musée National d'Histoire Naturelle Département HNS - CP135, 57 rue Cuvier, 75231 Paris Cedex 05, France

Chiara Montalto
Division of Child Neuropsichiatry, Stella Maris Scientific Institute, University of Pisa, Italy

Palmiero Monteleone
Department of Psychiatry, University of Naples SUN, Largo Madonna delle Grazie, 80138 Naples, Italy

Carmen C. Moran
School of Psychology & National Wine and Grape Industry Centre, Charles Sturt University, Wagga Wagga, NSW, Australia

Silvia Moreno
Departamento de Psicología, Facultad de Humanidades y Ciencias de la Educación, Universidad de Jaén, Jaén, Spain

Linda Morgan
Division of Nutritional Sciences, Faculty of Health and Medical Sciences, University of Surrey, Guildford, UK

Etsuro Mori
Department of Behavioural Neurology and Cognitive Neuroscience, Tohoku University Graduate School of Medicine, Sendai, Japan

Béatrice Morio, Ph.D.
UMR1019 Nutrition Humaine, INRA, 63120 Saint Genès Champanelle, France
and
Université Clermont 1, UFR Médecine, 63000 Clermont-Ferrand, France

Margaret J. Morris
Department of Pharmacology, School of Medical Sciences, University of New South Wales, Sydney, NSW 2052, Australia

Paul J. Moughan
Riddet Institute, Massey University, Palmerston North, New Zealand

Leonardo Munari
Dipartimento di Farmacologia Preclinica e Clinica, Universita' di Firenze, Florence, Italy

Filippo Muratori
Division of Child Neuropsichiatry, Stella Maris Scientific Institute, University of Pisa, IRCCS Stella Maris, Via dei Giacinti, 2-56018 Calambrone, Pisa, Italy

F.A.J. Muskiet
University Medical Center Groningen, Groningen, the Netherlands

Sabine Naessén, M.D., Ph.D.
Department of Obstetrics and Gynaecology, Karolinska University Hospital, SE-171 76 Stockholm, Sweden

Naoko Narita, M.D., Ph.D.
Institute of Education, Bunkyo University, 3337 Minamiogishima, Koshigaya-City, Saitama, 343-8511, Japan

Masaaki Narita, M.D., Ph.D.
Developmental and Regenerative Medicine, Mie University, Tsu, Mie, Japan

Chantal Nederkoorn
Department of Clinical Psychological Science, Maastricht University, Maastricht, the Netherlands

N.Q. Nguyen, M.B.B.S., FRACP, Ph.D.
Department of Gastroenterology and Hepatology, Royal Adelaide Hospital, North Terrace, Adelaide, SA, 5000, Australia

Heather M. Niemeier, Ph.D.
Department of Psychology, University of Wisconsin Whitewater, Whitewater, WI, USA

Giel Nijpels, M.D., Ph.D.
Department of General Practice and the EMGO Institute for Health and Care Research, VU University Medical Center, Amsterdam, the Netherlands

Chiara Nuccitelli, Ph.D.
Clinical Dietetics, University of Bologna, Bologna, Italy

Daryl B. O'Connor
Institute of Psychological Sciences, University of Leeds, LS2 9JT, UK

Teresia O'Connor, M.D., MPH
Children's Nutrition Research Center, Department of Pediatrics, Baylor College of Medicine, Houston, TX, USA

Barry O'Mahony, Ph.D.
School of Hospitality, Tourism and Marketing, Victoria University, Melbourne City, Vic 8001, Australia

Kaeko Ogura
Department of Pediatrics, National Rehabilitation Center for Persons with Disabilities, 1, Namiki 4-chome, Tokorozawa, Saitama 359-8555, Japan
and
Department of Behavioural Neurology and Cognitive Neuroscience, Tohoku University Graduate School of Medicine, Sendai, Japan

Ken Ohashi
Graduate School of Medicine, Department of Metabolic Diseases, The University of Tokyo, Tokyo, Japan

Chuma O. Okere
Department of Biological Sciences, Clark Atlanta University, Atlanta, GA, USA

Leonardo A. Ortega
Department of Psychology, Texas Christian University, Fort Worth, TX, USA

Sarah E. Overington, Ph.D.
Department of Biology, McGill University, 1205 Avenue Docteur Penfield, Montreal, Quebec, Canada H3A 1B1

Agostino Paccagnella
Nutrition, Metabolism and Diabetes Unit, Ospedale Ca' Foncello, 31100 Treviso, Italy

L. Padua
Institute of Neurology, Università Cattolica, Roma, Italy
and
Fondazione Pro Iuventute Don Carlo Gnocchi- Roma, Italy

Mercedes Paíno
Department of Psychology, Centro de Investigación Biomédica en Red de Salud
Mental (CIBERSAM), University of Oviedo, Oviedo, Spain

Francesco Panza, M.D., Ph.D.
Department of Geriatrics, Center for Aging Brain, Memory Unit,
University of Bari, Policlinico, Piazza Giulio Cesare, 11, 70124 Bari, Italy

Mauricio R. Papini
Department of Psychology, Texas Christian University, Fort Worth, TX 76129

Timo Partonen, M.D., Ph.D.
Mood, Depression and Suicidal Behaviour Unit, Department of Mental Health and
Substance Abuse Services, National Institute for Health and Welfare, Helsinki, Finland

Elettra Pasqualoni, R.D.
Department of Eating and Weight Disorder, Villa Garda Hospital, Garda, Italy

Elettra Pasqualoni, R.D.
AIDAP Verona, Via Sansovino, Verona, Italy

Patrick Pasquet
UMR CNRS/MNHN 7206: Eco-Anthropologie et Ethnobiologie, Brunoy, France

Maria Beatrice Passani
Dipartimento di Farmacologia Preclinica e Clinica, Universita' di Firenze, Viale
Pieraccini 6, Florence, Italy

Kendra Patrick
Michigan State University, East Lansing, MI, USA

Karen Patte
Faculty of Health, York University, Toronto, Ontario, Canada

Nicole L.M. Pernat
Department of Psychology, Kwantlen Polytechnic University, Surrey, BC, Canada

Jennifer E. Phillips, Jaime A. Pineda, Ph.D.
Department of Cognitive Science and Group in Neuroscience, University of
California, San Diego, CA, USA

J. Pinkney, M.D., FRCP
Department of Diabetes and Endocrinology, Royal Cornwall Hospital, Peninsula
College of Medicine and Dentistry, Truro, Cornwall, UK

Pierluigi Politi
Department of Health Sciences, Section of human nutrition and dietetics,
University of Pavia, Via Bassi 21, I-27100 Pavia, Italy

Kathleen A. Potter
Department of Biochemistry and Molecular Biology, Medical University of South Carolina, Charleston, SC, USA

Michael L. Power, Ph.D.
Research Department, American College of Obstetricians and Gynecologists, Washington, DC 20090–6920
and
Nutrition Laboratory, Conservation Ecology Center, Smithsonian National Zoological Park, MRC 5503 Washington, DC 20013-7012

Antonio Preti, M.D.
Department of Psychology, University of Cagliari, via is Mirrionis 1, 09123 Cagliari, Italy
and
Centro Medico Genneruxi, Via Costantinopoli 42, 09129 Cagliari, Italy

Pierre-Marie Preux
Université de Limoges, Institut de Neuroépidémiologie et de Neurologie Tropicale, EA 3174 NeuroEpidémiologie Tropicale et Comparée, Limoges, France

Kathryn Proulx, Ph.D., PMHCNS-BC
Mental Health Services, University of Massachusetts, Hills North, Amherst, MA 01103

Sarah E. Racine, M.A.
Department of Psychology, Michigan State University, East Lansing, MI, USA

Tri Budi W. Rahardjo, Ph.D.
Center for Health Research, University of Indonesia, Jakarta, Indonesia

Sayali C. Ranade
National Brain Research Centre, National Highway-8, Near NSG Campus, Nainwal Mode, Manesar, Haryana 122050, India

Patrick A. Randall
Department of Psychology, University of Connecticut, Storrs, CT, USA

Christoph Randler
Biology, Department of Natural Sciences, University of Education Heidelberg, Im Neuenheimer Feld 561–2, D-69120 Heidelberg, Germany

L.R. Ranganath, FRCPE, FRCPath, Ph.D.
Department of Clinical Chemistry, Royal Liverpool University Hospital, Prescot Street, Liverpool, L7 8XP, UK

Mohammad Tariqur Rahman
Department of Biomedical Science, Kulliyyah of Science, International Islamic University Malaysia (IIUM), Jalan Istana, Bandar Indera Mahkota, 25200 Kuantan, Malaysia

Carmen Rasmussen
Department of Pediatrics, Glenrose Rehabilitation Hospital, Edmonton, Alberta

Christopher K. Rayner
Discipline of Medicine, Royal Adelaide Hospital, Adelaide, South Australia,
Australia

Katherine Read
Department of Psychology, Cornell College, Mt. Vernon, IA, USA

Caroline Reid
Centre for Addiction and Mental Health, University of Toronto, Toronto, Ontario,
Canada

Thomas Reinehr
Department of Paediatric Nutrition Medicine, Vestische Hospital for Children
and Adolescents, University of Witten/Herdecke, Dr. F. Steiner Str. 5, 45711
Datteln, Germany

Britta Renner
Department of Psychology, University of Konstanz, Konstanz, Germany

Jared Edward Reser
University of Southern California, Psychology Department, SGM 501, 3620 South
McClintock Ave., Los Angeles, CA 90089-1061, USA

Caroline Reverdy
AUXIME - ODOROSMÊ, Les Grandes Roches, 69490, Saint Romain de Popey,
France
and
PANCOSMA, R&D Department, 6 Voie des Traz, 1218 Le Grand Saconnex,
Switzerland

Paul Richardson
Brain, Behaviour & Cognition Research Group, Psychology, Sheffield Hallam
University, Collegiate Campus, Sheffield, UK S10 2BP

A. Rinehart
New York Chiropractic College, Seneca Falls, New York, USA

Reeta Rintamäki, M.D., Ph.D.
National Institute for Health and Welfare, Department of Mental Health and
Substance Abuse Services, Mood, Depression and Suicidal Behaviour Unit, 30
(Mannerheimintie 166), FI-00271 Helsinki, Finland

Patrick Ritz, M.D., Ph.D.
Unité de Nutrition, CHU Larrey, TSA 30030, F-31059 Toulouse cedex 9, France

Rachel E. Roberts
Discipline of Medicine, School of Medicine, King's College London, 2nd Floor,
Henriette Raphael House, Guy's Campus, London Bridge, London, SE1 1UL, UK

Marcia L. Robertson
Department of Anthropology, Northwestern University, Evanston, IL, USA

Denise Robertson
Division of Nutritional Sciences, Faculty of Health and Medical Sciences,
University of Surrey, Guildford, UK

Athena Robinson, Ph.D.
Department of Psychiatry and Behavioral Sciences, Stanford University, School of
Medicine, 401 Quarry Road, Stanford, CA 94305-5722

Sonia Rodríguez-Ruiz
Departamento de Personalidad, Evaluación y Tratamiento Psicológico, Facultad de
Psicología, Universidad de Granada, Campus de la Cartuja s/n, 18071, Granada, Spain

Dana L. Rofey, Ph.D.
Children's Hospital of Pittsburgh, 3414 Fifth Avenue, Room 128, Pgh, PA 15213, USA

Ariz Rojas, M.A.
Department of Psychology, University of South Florida, Tampa, FL, USA

Susanne de Rooij, Ph.D.
Department of Clinical Epidemiology and Biostatistics, Room J1b 210.1,
Academic Medical Centre, University of Amsterdam, Meibergdreef 9,
1100 DD, Amsterdam, The Netherlands

Matthew Rousu, Ph.D.
Department of Economics, Susquehanna University, Selinsgrove, PA, USA

C.W. le Roux
Department of Metabolic Medicine, Imperial College Faculty of Medicine, London, UK

Paul Rozin
Department of Psychology, University of Pennsylvania, 3720 Walnut St,
Philadelphia, PA 19104-6241, USA

J.A. Rycroft
Unilever Research and Development, Colworth House, Sharnbrook, Bedford, UK
and
Department of Experimental Medicine, Section of Human Physiology, and Clinical
Dietetic Service, Second University of Naples, Naples, Italy

Perminder Sachdev
University of New South Wales, Neuropsychiatric Institute, The Prince of Wales
Hospital, Randwick, NSW, Australia

John D. Salamone
Department of Psychology, University of Connecticut, 406 Babbidge Road,
Storrs, CT 06269-1020, USA

Anthony J. Saliba
National Wine and Grape Industry Centre, Charles Sturt University,
Locked Bag 588, Wagga Wagga, NSW, 2678, Australia

F. Santolaria-Fernández
Servicio de Medicina Interna, Hospital Universitario de Canarias, Tenerife, Canary
Islands, Spain

Fumiyo Sato
Corporate Research & Development Group, SHARP Corporation

Nūn Sava-Siva Amen-Ra, M.A., Ph.D.
Amenta Academy of Theoretical Sciences (AATS), 25101Chimney-House Court,
Damascus, MD, USA

Donna Scarborough, Ph.D., CCC-SLP
Department of Speech Pathology and Audiology, Miami University, 26 Bachelor Hall,
Oxford, OH 45056, USA

Sigfrido Scarpa
Dip. di Chirurgia "P. Valdoni", Centro di Ricerca in Neurobiologia "Daniel Bovet"
CriN, Sapienza Università di Roma, via Antonio Scarpa, 14, 00161 Roma, Italy

Jennifer L. Scheide
Women's Health and Exercise Laboratory, Noll Laboratory, Department of
Kinesiology, Penn State University, University Park, PA, USA

Susan M. Schembre, Ph.D., RD
Cancer Research Center Hawaii, Prevention and Control Program, University
of Hawaii, Manoa, 677 Ala Moana Blvd. Suite 200, Honolulu, Hawaii 96813

Anna Schierberl Scherr, B.A.
Center for Health, Intervention, and Prevention, Department of Psychology,
University of Connecticut, Storrs, CT, USA

Gessica Schiavo
Nutrition, Metabolism and Diabetes Unit, Ospedale Ca' Foncello, Treviso, Italy

Jay Schulkin
Nutrition Laboratory, Conservation Ecology Center, Smithsonian National
Zoological Park, Washington DC

Harald T. Schupp
Department of Psychology, University of Konstanz, 78457 Konstanz, Germany

C.M. Schweitzer, M.D., Ph.D.
Department of Internal Medicine, TweeSteden Ziekenhuis, Tilburg

Christina L. Scott, Ph.D.
Whittier College, 13406 E. Philadelphia St. Whittier, CA 90608, USA

Kristen N. Segovia
Department of Psychology, University of Connecticut, Storrs, CT, USA

Claudio A. Serfaty
Laboratory of Neural Plasticity, Fluminense Federal University, 100180,
Niterói, RJ, 24001-970, Brazil

Justine Joan Sheppard, Ph.D.
Department of Biobehavioral Sciences, Teachers College, Columbia University,
525 W. 120th Street, New York, NY 10027

Hossain Md Shahdat
Department of Environmental Physiology, Shimane University Faculty of Medicine,
Izumo, Shimane, Japan
and
Department of Biochemistry and Molecular Biology, Jahangirnagar University,
Savar, Dhaka, Bangladesh

Manoj Sharma, M.B.B.S, Ph.D.
Health Promotion & Education, University of Cincinnati, Cincinnati,
OH 45221-0068, USA

Jason Shogren, Ph.D.
Department of Economics and Finance, University of Wyoming, Laramie, WY, USA

Lauren B. Shomaker, Ph.D.
Department of Medical and Clinical Psychology, Uniformed Services University of
the Health Sciences, Bethesda, MD, USA
and
Unit on Growth and Obesity, Program in Developmental Endocrinology and
Genetics, Eunice Kennedy Shriver National Institute of Child Health and Human
Development, National Institutes of Health Department of Health and Human
Services, Bethesda, MD, USA

M. Shroff, Ph.D.
Department of Health Promotion, Education, and Behavior, University of South
Carolina, Columbia, SC, USA

Susana Sierra-Baigrie
Department of Psychology, University of Oviedo, Plaza Feijoo, s/n, Oviedo
33003 Spain

Kelly Siglin
Department of Psychology, Cornell College, Mt. Vernon, IA, USA

Bruno Simmen
UMR CNRS/MNHN 7206, Eco-Anthropologie et Ethnobiologie, Brunoy, France
and
Department of Biochemistry and Molecular Biology, Jahangirnagar University,
Savar, Dhaka, Bangladesh

Julia Simner
School of Philosophy, Psychology and Language Sciences, University
of Edinburgh, 7 George Square, Edinburgh, EH8 9JZ, UK

Rita Sinigaglia-Coimbra
Electron Microscopy Center, Federal University of São Paulo (UNIFESP),
São Paulo, Brazil
and
Laboratory of Clinical and Experimental Pathophysiology,
Department of Neurology and Neurosurgery, Federal University of São Paulo
(UNIFESP), São Paulo, Brazil

Kelly Sink
Department of Psychology, University of Connecticut, Storrs, CT, USA

Gudrun V. Skuladottir
Department of Physiology, Faculty of Medicine, School of Health Sciences,
University of Iceland, Vatnsmyrarvegi 16, IS-101 Reykjavik, Iceland

Alexandra C. Smith
Department of Food Science and Human Nutrition, College of Applied Human
Sciences, Colorado State University, Fort Collins, CO, USA

Veronique de Smedt-Peyrusse
Psynugen, Université Bordeaux 2, INRA, UMR1286, CNRS, UMR5226, Bâtiment
UFR Pharmacie – 2ème Tranche – 2ème Etage, Case courrier 34, 33076
BORDEAUX Cedex

Françoise J. Smith
Department of Food Science and Human Nutrition, College of Applied Human
Sciences, Colorado State University, Fort Collins, CO, USA

Marek Smulczyk
The Maria Grzegorzewska Academy of Special Education, Institute of Applied
Psychology, 40 Szczesliwicka Street, 02-353 Warsaw, Poland

J. Josh Snodgrass
Department of Anthropology, University of Oregon, Eugene, OR, USA

Harriëtte M. Snoek
Behavioural Science Institute, Radboud University Nijmegen,
The Netherlands
and
Agricultural Economics Research Institute, Wageningen University and Research
Center, P.O. Box 8130, 6700 EW Wageningen, The Netherlands

Vincenzo Solfrizzi, M.D., Ph.D.
Department of Geriatrics, Center for Aging Brain, Memory Unit, University
of Bari, Policlinico, Piazza Giulio Cesare, 11, 70124 Bari, Italy

Annette Stafleu
TI Food and Nutrition/TNO Quality of Life, 3700 AJ Zeist, The Netherlands

J.E.R. Staddon
Department of Psychology and Neuroscience, Duke University, Durham, NC, USA
and
Department of Psychology, University of York, York, UK

Malgorzata Starzomska
The Maria Grzegorzewska Academy of Special Education, Institute of Applied
Psychology, 40 Szczesliwicka Street, 02-353 Warsaw, Poland

Andreas Stengel, M.D.
CURE: Digestive Diseases Research Center, David Geffen School of Medicine,
University of California, Los Angeles, Building 115, Room 117, Los Angeles,
CA, USA

Ashley Stillman
Department of Psychology, Cornell College, Mt. Vernon, IA, USA

Wolfgang Stroebe
Department of Social and Organizational Psychology, Utrecht University, Utrecht, the Netherlands

James Stubbs
Slimming World, Alfreton, Derbyshire, UK

Albert J. Stunkard, M.D.
Center for Weight and Eating Disorders, Department of Psychiatry, School of Medicine, University of Pennsylvania, 3535 Market Street, Philadelphia, PA, 19104-3309, USA

Shiro Suda, M.D., Ph.D.
Research Center for Child Mental Development, Hamamatsu University School of Medicine, Hamamatsu, Shizuoka, Japan

Alessandro Suppini, Ph.D.
Clinical Dietetics, University of Bologna, Bologna, Italy

Nan M. Sussman, Ph.D.
Department of Psychology, College of Staten Island, City University of New York, Staten Island, New York

Timothy Swartz
INRA, Écologie et Physiologie du Système Digestif, 78350 Jouy-en-Josas, France

Moshe Szyf
Sackler Program for Epigenetics and Psychobiology,
and
Department of Pharmacology and Therapeutics, McGill University, 3655 Sir William Osler Promenade, room 1309, Montreal, QC, Canada H3G 1Y6

Yvette Taché, Ph.D.
CURE: Digestive Diseases Research Center and Center for Neurovisceral Sciences & Women's Health, Digestive Diseases Division, David Geffen School of Medicine at UCLA and VA Greater Los Angeles Healthcare System, Los Angeles, CA, USA

Domenico Tafuri
Department Studies of Institutions and Territorial Systems, Faculty of Movement Science, University of Naples "Parthenope", Naples, Italy
and
Faculty of Movement Science, University of Naples "Parthenope", Naples, Italy

Nori Takei, M.D., M.Sc., Ph.D.
Research Center for Child Mental Development and United Graduate School of Child Development, Hamamatsu University School of Medicine, 1-20-1 Handayama, Higashi-ku Hamamatsu Shizuoka, 431-3192 Japan
and
Division of Psychological Medicine, Institute of Psychiatry, London, SE5 8AF, UK

Masato Takii
Department of Psychosomatic Medicine, Graduate School of Medical Sciences,
Kyushu University, 3-1-1 Maidashi, Higashi-ku, Fukuoka, 812-8582, Japan

Yoshiyuki Takimoto
Graduate School of Medicine, Department of Stress Sciences and Psychosomatic
Medicine, The University of Tokyo, Tokyo, Japan

Marian Tanofsky-Kraff, Ph.D.
Department of Medical and Clinical Psychology, Uniformed Services University of
the Health Sciences, Bethesda, MD, USA
and
Unit on Growth and Obesity, Program in Developmental Endocrinology and
Genetics, Eunice Kennedy Shriver National Institute of Child Health and Human
Development, National Institutes of Health, Department of Health and Human
Services, Bethesda, MD, USA

D. Taruscio
National Centre for Rare Diseases, Istituto Superiore di Sanità, Roma, Italy
and
Fondazione Pro Iuventute Don Carlo Gnocchi, Roma, Italy

Maithe Tauber
Centre de référence du syndrome de Prader-Willi, Hôpital des Enfants, 330 av de
Grande Bretagne, TSA 70034, 31059 Toulouse Cedex 9, France

Raed Tayyem
General surgery department, Ayr Hospital, Ayr, UK

Mami Tazoe, M.S.
The Department of Clinical Psychology, Japan Lutheran College, Mitaka, Tokyo,
Japan

Ababyue Tegene
US Department of Agriculture, Economic Research Service, Washington DC

Frank Telang, M.D.
Neuroimaging Laboratory, National Institute on Alcohol Abuse and Alcoholism,
Upton, New York, USA

Salvadeo Sibilla Anna Teresa, M.D.
Department of Internal Medicine and Therapeutics, University of Pavia, Pavia, Italy

Panayotis K. Thanos, Ph.D.
Behavioral Neuropharmacology & Neuroimaging Laboratory, National Institute on
Alcohol Abuse and Alcoholism, Upton, New York, USA
and
Medical Department, Brookhaven National Laboratory, Upton, New York, USA

David R. Thompson
Department of Health Sciences and Department of Cardiovascular Sciences,
University of Leicester, Leicester, UK

J. Kevin Thompson, Ph.D.
Department of Psychology, University of South Florida, Tampa, FL, USA

Marika Tiggemann
School of Psychology, Flinders University, Adelaide, Australia

Daniel Tomé
INRA, CNRH-IdF, UMR914 Nutrition Physiology and Ingestive Behavior, Paris, France
and
AgroParisTech, CNRH-IdF, UMR914 Nutrition Physiology and Ingestive Behavior, Paris, France

Kunio Torii
Institute of Life Sciences, Ajinomoto Co., Inc., Suzuki-cho 1-1, Kawasaki-ku, Kawasaki 210-8681, Japan

Phu V. Tran, Ph.D.
Center for Neurobehavioral Development, Neonatology Division & Center for Neurobehavioral Development, School of Medicine, Department of Pediatrics, University of Minnesota, MN, USA

Janet Treasure
Institute of Psychiatry, King's College London, London, United Kingdom
and
Department of Academic Psychiatry, Eating Disorder Research Unit, Guy's Hospital, Bermondsey Wing, SE1 9RT, London, United Kingdom

Angelo Tremblay
Division of Kinesiology, Laval University, Quebec City, QC, Canada

Nhan Truong, Ph.D.
Ismail H. Ulus
Department of Pharmacology, Acibadem University Medical School, Gulsuyu Mahallesi, Maltepe, Istanbul, Turkey

Erica L. Unger, Ph.D.
Department of Nutritional Sciences, Pennsylvania State University, University Park, PA 16802

Tracy Vaillancourt
Faculty of Education and School of Psychology, University of Ottawa, Ottawa, Ontario, Canada
and
Department of Psychology, Neuroscience, & Behaviour, McMaster University, Hamilton, Ontario, Canada

Olga van den Akker
Department of Psychology, Middlesex University, The Town Hall, The Burroughs, Hendon, London, NW4 4BT, UK

Koert van Ittersum, Ph.D.
Georgia Institute of Technology, Atlanta, GA, USA

V. Kiran Vemuri
Center for Drug Discovery, Northeastern University, Boston, MA, USA

Gianluigi Vendemiale
Department of Geriatrics, University of Foggia, Foggia, Italy
and
Internal Medicine Unit, IRCSS Casa Sollievo dalla Sofferenza, San Giovanni
Rotondo, Puglia, Italy.

R.H. Verheesen, M.D.
Regionaal Reuma Centrum Z.O. Brabant, Máxima Medisch Centrum,
Ds. Th. Fliednerstraat 1, 5631 BM Eindhoven, The Netherlands

Claudia Vicidomini
Department of Experimental Medicine, Section of Human Physiology,
and Clinical Dietetic Service, Second University of Naples, Naples, Italy

Didier Vieau
Environment Périnatal et Croissance (EA4489), Equipe Dénutritions Maternelles
Périnatales, Bâtiment SN4, 2ème étage, Université des Sciences et Technologies de
Lille, 59655 Villeneuve d'Ascq, France

Andrea Viggiano
Department Studies of Institutions and Territorial Systems, Faculty of Movement
Science, University of Naples "Parthenope", Naples, Italy
and
Faculty of Movement Science, University of Naples "Parthenope", via Medina,
Naples, Italy

Valentina Viglione
Division of Child Neuropsichiatry, Stella Maris Scientific Institute,
University of Pisa, Italy

Jaime Vila
Departamento de Personalidad, Evaluación y Tratamiento Psicológico,
Facultad de Psicología, Universidad de Granada, Granada, Spain

Piergiuseppe Vinai, M.D.
"GNOSIS" No Profit Research Group, V Langhe 64, 12060, Magliano Alpi,
CN, Italy

Vivianne H.M. Visschers
ETH Zurich, Institute for Environmental Decisions, Consumer Behavior,
Universitaetstrasse 22 CHN J75.2, 8092 Zurich, Switzerland

Nora D. Volkow, M.D.
Office of Director, National Institute on Drug Abuse, Rockville, MD, USA

Yuji Wada
Sensory & Cognitive Food Science Laboratory, National Food Research Institute,
2-1-12, Kannondai, Tsukuba, Ibaraki 305-8642, Japan

Bai-Ren Wang
Institute of Neuroscience, Fourth Military Medical University, Xi'an, China

Gene-Jack Wang, M.D.
Medical Department, Building 490, Brookhaven National Laboratory, Upton,
New York, 11973 USA

Brian Wansink, Ph.D.
Cornell University, 110 Warren Hall, Ithaca, NY 14853-7801, USA

Carolina Werle, Ph.D.
Grenoble Ecole de Management CERAG, Grenoble, France

Stephen Whybrow
Faculty of Health and Medical Sciences, University of Surrey, Guildford,
GU2 7XH, UK

Reinout W. Wiers
Department of Psychology, University of Amsterdam, Amsterdam, the Netherlands

Karen Wight
Faculty of Health, York University, 223 Bethune College, 4700 Keele Street,
Toronto, Canada
and
Centre for Addiction and Mental Health, University of Toronto, Toronto, Canada

Michael Wilkinson
Department of Obstetrics & Gynaecology, IWK Health Centre, Dalhousie
University,
University Avenue, Halifax, NS, Canada, B3K 6R8
and
Department of Physiology & Biophysics, Dalhousie University, Halifax, NS,
Canada, B3H 1X5
and
Division of Endocrinology and Metabolism, Victoria General Hospital,
Department of Medicine, Dalhousie University, Halifax, NS, Canada, B3H 2Y9

Gary Wittert
Discipline of Medicine, Royal Adelaide Hospital, Adelaide, South Australia,
Australia

Sarah J. Woodruff, Ph.D., CEP
Department of Kinesiology, University of Windsor, 401 Sunset Avenue, Windsor,
Ontario N9B 3P4, Canada

Li-Ze Xiong
Department of Anesthesiology, Xijing Hospital, Fourth Military Medical University,
15 West Changle Rd, Xi'an, 710032, P.R. China

Yajun Xu
Department of Nutrition and Food Hygiene, School of Public Health, Peking
University Health Science Center, No. 38 Xue Yuan Road, Hai Dian District,
Beijing 100191, China

Yoshiharu Yamamoto
Educational Physiology Laboratory, Graduate School of Education,
The University of Tokyo

Jack A. Yanovski, M.D., Ph.D.
Section on Growth and Obesity, Program in Developmental Endocrinology
and Genetics,
Eunice Kennedy Shriver National Institute of Child Health and Human
Development,
National Institutes of Health, Department of Health and Human Services,
9000 Rockvile Pike, MSC 1103, Hatfield CRC, room IE-3330, Bethesda,
Maryland 20892-1103, USA

Amina Yesufu-Udechuku, Ph.D.
CORE, Clinical Health Psychology, University College London, London, UK

Kazuhiro Yoshiuchi
Graduate School of Medicine, Department of Stress Sciences and Psychosomatic
Medicine, The University of Tokyo, Tokyo, Japan

B.S. Zanutto
IIBM-Universidad de Buenos Aires, and IBYME-CONICET, Argentina

Steven H. Zeisel, M.D., Ph.D.
University of North Carolina at Chapel Hill, Nutrition Research Institute,
500 Laureate Way, Kannapolis, North Carolina 28081

Jie Zhao
Department of Nutrition and Food Hygiene, School of Public Health, Peking
University Health Science Center, Beijing, China

Zheng-Hua Zhu
Department of Anesthesiology, Xijing Hospital, Fourth Military Medical University,
Xi'an, China
and
Centro Medico Genneruxi, Cagliari, Italy

Nicolien Zijlstra
Division of Human Nutrition, TI Food and Nutrition/Wageningen University
and Research Centre, Wageningen, the Netherlands

Part XXIV
Starvation and Nutrient Deficiency

Chapter 141
Diet-Related Behavioral Mechanisms in Times of Economic Constraint

A.R. Kelles, M. Shroff, and A. Rinehart

Abbreviations

SES	Socioeconomic status
CVD	Cardiovascular disease
DM	Diabetes mellitus
CHD	Coronary heart disease
BMR	Basal metabolic rate
WHO	World Health Organization
DHHS	Department of Health and Human Services
USDA	Unites States Department of Agriculture
CDC	Centers for Disease Control
FSP	Food Stamp Program
WIC	Special Supplemental Nutrition Program for Women, Infants, and Children
SNAP	Supplemental Nutrition Assistance Program
FAO	Food and Agriculture Organization
HIV	Human immunodeficiency virus
AIDS	Acquired immunodeficiency syndrome
GHI	Global hunger index
IFPRI	International Food Policy Research Institute

141.1 Introduction

Obesity is a global epidemic with a rapidly increasing predominance among low-income populations. Unfortunately, low-income populations are also the least capable of dealing with the health and economic consequences directly associated with obesity and indirectly with obesity-related chronic diseases (Russell 2004; Leive and Xu 2008). Increases in chronic disease prevalence among low-income populations could ultimately lead to overall reduced quality of life as well as a substantial increase in days of work lost in the global work force (Goudge et al. 2009). Similar to the impact of obesity,

A.R. Kelles (✉)
Department of Nutrition, New York Chiropractic College, Seneca Falls, New York, USA
e-mail: akelles@nycc.edu

V.R. Preedy et al. (eds.), *Handbook of Behavior, Food and Nutrition*,
DOI 10.1007/978-0-387-92271-3_141, © Springer Science+Business Media, LLC 2011

chronic undernutrition, still prevalent in many developing countries, leads to increased infectious disease risk and is associated with substantial days of work lost (McIntyre et al. 2006).

To curtail the global trend towards decreased health among low-income populations it is important to understand the mechanism by which economic constraint leads to adverse disease outcomes. Research has identified several possible pathways, such as the impact of economic constraint on accessibility/usage of healthcare services, physical activity, and dietary behaviors (Gordon-Larsen et al. 2006; Nelson et al. 2006; Goudge et al. 2009; Larson et al. 2009; Pollack and Armstrong 2009). A goal of this chapter is to explore specifically the mechanism by which economic constraint influences dietary behaviors among low-income populations. This information can be incorporated into the development of efficient and effective interventions and policies aimed at improving health status among the poor. Creating policy measures to support low-income populations, however, is complicated because dietary behavior responses to economic constraint differ substantially depending on the local, national, and international environmental contexts. For example, economic constraint in a developed country setting often leads to the consumption of high-energy but low-nutrient dense diets (Drewnowski and Darmon 2005). The impact of economic constraint in some developing country settings may resemble a developed country yet for others it may lead to an overall insufficient intake of both micronutrients and total calories (Hakeem 2001; Popkin 2001; Shafique et al. 2007; Vorster et al. 2007; Ntandou et al. 2009). Due to the diversity in dietary behavior response to economic constraint, we will explore this relationship in both a developed and developing country setting.

The accessibility of resources such as foodstuffs/food markets, transportation, safe environment, and healthcare is not solely influenced by the economic ability of an individual or family. In fact, the relationship between dietary choices and economic constraint differ substantially by the economic, social, and political state of an individual's or family's environment. More specifically the relationship differs for those in a developing versus a developed country setting and within countries by the level of urbanicity (Vorster 2002; Popkin 1998). There is a global nutrition phenomenon, referred to as the nutrition transition, documenting a shift from undernutrition to overnutrition as the economic wealth of a developing country increases (Popkin 1998). This transition is accompanied by an increase in food availability particularly in urban areas. The increase in food availability results in an increase in overconsumption, particularly of highly processed carbohydrates, animal fats, and a concurrent decrease in fresh fruits and vegetables (see Fig. 141.1). Compounding the emergence of this unhealthy lifestyle is a population shift from active to sedentary transportation as well as agriculture to service-oriented occupations leading to an overall sedentary population. These changes in both dietary and physical activity patterns lead to a shift in disease prevalence from infectious diseases to the emergence of obesity and related chronic diseases such as cardiovascular disease (CVD), hypertension, diabetes mellitus (DM Type 2), and many types of cancers (Ntandou et al. 2009; Misra and Khurana 2008). This phenomenon is often referred to as the epidemiologic transition (see Fig. 141.2) (Manton 1988; Mathers and Loncar 2006; Stuckler 2008). Occurring with the increased economic growth on a national level is the decrease in both fertility and mortality leading to a shift towards an aging population structure. This change is known as the demographic transition and is in part a result of increased active family planning, increased number of women in the work force, and overall improvements in sanitation and healthcare (Manton 1988; Mathers and Loncar 2006). An aging population, concurrent with the increase in obesogenic lifestyles, leads to the increase in obesity and chronic diseases versus infectious diseases found in middle- and high-income developed countries.

Within a country, both accessibility to and affordability of food resources affect the dietary behaviors of economically constrained populations. Food accessibility and affordability are in turn dependent on contextual wealth and development of a given geographic area. In a developed country, accessibility to resources, although an issue, may not be as much a limiting factor to healthy dietary

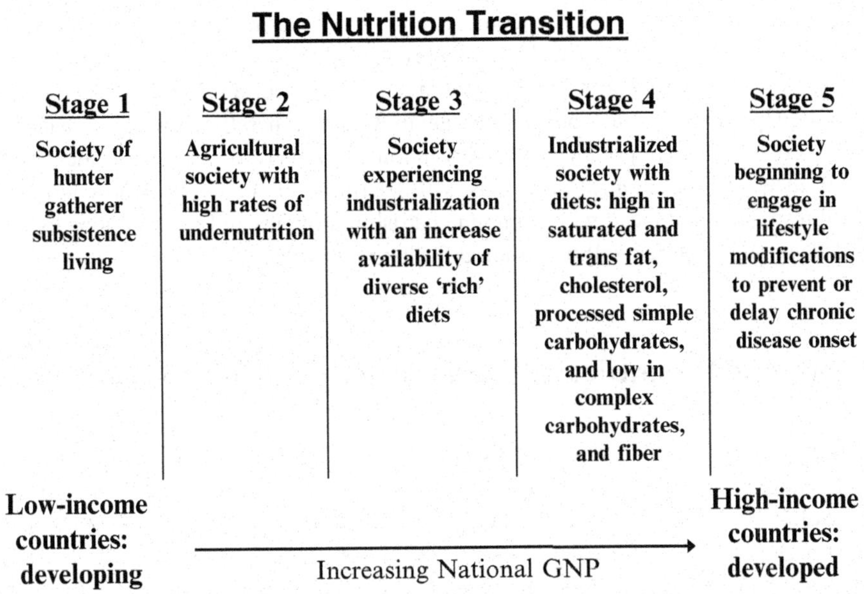

The Nutrition Transition
Stage 1
Society of hunter gatherer subsistence living
Stage 2
Agricultural society with high rates of undernutrition
Stage 3
Society experiencing industrialization with an increase availability of diverse 'rich' diets
Stage 4
Industrialized society with diets: high in saturated and trans fat, cholesterol, processed simple carbohydrates, and low in complex carbohydrates, and fiber
Stage 5
Society beginning to engage in lifestyle modifications to prevent or delay chronic disease onset
Low-income countries: developing
Increasing National GNP
High-income countries: developed

Fig. 141.1 Key features of the nutrition transition. This figure represents the general dietary trends observed depending on the wealth and development of a country. The trend can be used to compare the expected dietary patterns between countries but can also be used to represent the changes that occur as a country experiences increases in wealth and development and transitions from a preindustrial to a highly industrial economy

Stages of Demographic, Epidemiologic, and Nutrition Change
Nutrition Transition
High prevalence of undernutrition
Receding famine, Introduction of processed foods and away from home food consumption
High prevalence of overnutrition
Epidemiologic Transition
High prevalence of infectious disease
Receding pestilence occurring with improved environmental conditions
High prevalence of chronic diseases
Demographic Transition
High fertility and mortality
Reduced mortality, reduced fertility due to active family Planning, and changing age structure
Low fertility and mortality
Low-income countries: developing
Increasing National GNP
High-income countries: developed

Fig. 141.2 The dietary and disease patterns as well as the population structure for countries at varying stages of wealth and development. These trends are inextricably intertwined and occur simultaneously as a country undergoes transition from a preindustrial to a highly industrialized country

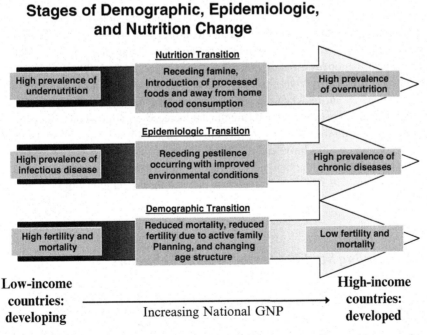

behaviors as affordability among low-income groups (Darmon and Drewnowski 2008). Within a developing country context, however, there is substantial diversity in the availability of resources often, depending on the urbanicity of the environment (Dixon et al. 2007). In low- and middle-income developing countries, in a more urban environment, generally there is a greater access to resources. To create effective policies and interventions, it is therefore crucial to identify the local and national environmental context since this will determine to some extent how individuals and families will respond when faced with economic hardship. Policies and interventions in both developed and developing countries will be explored further in this chapter.

141.2 Developed Countries: Trends in Obesity and Related Diseases

In the past century, the prevalence of chronic disease has increased steadily in developed countries where people have ready access to energy-dense diets. In 1960, the estimated obesity prevalence in the US was 13.4%, but by 2000 this number had risen to 30.9% (Flegal et al. 2002). It is now estimated that roughly 2/3rds of Americans are overweight or obese (Ogden et al. 2006). As a result, researchers recently projected a decrease in the life expectancy for the twenty-first century (Olshansky et al. 2005). Similar trends exist throughout Britain and Europe (Seidell 2000). It is well documented that obesity is significantly correlated with an increased risk of many chronic diseases such as CVD, endocrine disorders, many forms of cancer, pulmonary disorders, musculoskeletal disorders, gastrointestinal, hepatic and reproductive disorders (Brown et al. 2009). In the last decade new research has identified substantial metabolic activity in adipose tissue indicating a neuroendocrine link between obesity and chronic diseases such as CVD and diabetes (Ohman et al. 2009; Korner et al. 2009). We now know that adipose tissue releases chronic disease-related inflammatory mediators known as adipokines such as adiponectin and aromatase. For example, research indicates that Adiponectin may be the causal link between abdominal fat and atherosclerosis (Hansen et al. 2009). Aromatase, which promotes the conversion of estrogen to a carcinogenic metabolite, is now targeted using drug inhibitors as a post-menopausal breast cancer treatment (Maccio et al. 2009). Screening for overweight status can help identify high-risk individuals; however, the estimated accuracy of this tool is continually modified as our understanding of the neuroendocrine nature of adipose tissue expands. For example, a recent study in Japan found significant increases in visceral fat associated with a high risk of coronary heart disease (CHD) even among subjects with a low to normal estimated BMI (Popkin 1994). These findings have lead to a proposed lowering of the BMI cutoffs for overweight status in Asian populations (International Diabetes Institute 2000). New findings such as these also remind us that we are still in the early stages of uncovering the relationship between obesity and chronic disease.

141.2.1 Identifying Modifiable Obesogenic Behaviors

Given the strong correlation between obesity and chronic disease risk it is crucial that researchers identify modifiable behaviors leading to obesity that can be targeted by policies and interventions. Studies indicate that the rising rates of obesity are largely a result of the energy-dense diets associated with technological innovations, urbanization and improved socioeconomic status (SES) (Bleich et al. 2008). Specifically, technological advances in agriculture, food-preparation, cooking appliances, and food storage have led to significant decreases in the price of food. Greater reductions in

Table 141.1 Key features of diet quality (Kant 1996; Arvaniti and Panagiotakos 2008)

1. Diet quality, independent of diet quantity, is critical in the prevention of chronic diseases such as obesity. There are innumerable studies that have identified an association between chronic disease risk and specific dietary attributes such as the distribution of energy among the different macronutrients or the dietary adequacy of specific micronutrients
2. Diet quality is an overall balance of macronutrients with an intake of micronutrients to meet recommended levels relative to total energy intake
3. Several scoring systems exist to measure diet quality. Each system is aimed at measuring diet quality or the adherence to national dietary recommendations or guidelines constructed with the specific aim of chronic disease risk reduction (e.g. cardiovascular disease (CVD), hypertension, and cancer), including:
   (a) *Healthy Eating Index (HEI)* – was developed by the US Department of Agriculture and based on the Dietary Guidelines for America and the Food guide pyramid. The HEI has 10 component scores each with a maximum diet quality adherence score of 10, including:
       (i) Five components measure adherence to the recommended servings of each of the following major food groups: grains, vegetables, fruits, milk, and meat
       (ii) Dietary fat intake as a percent of total energy
       (iii) Saturated fat intake as a percent of total energy
       (iv) Cholesterol intake
       (v) Sodium intake
       (vi) Measure of dietary diversity
       Although the HEI provides a measure of overall dietary quality, several large scale studies found a lack of association with diet quality measured by the HEI and chronic disease risk. This lack of association may be due in part to the exclusion of food components that play a protective role such as fiber and essential fatty acids.
   (b) *Diet Quality Index (DQI)* – was specifically designed to measure diet quality as a reflection of chronic disease risk based on scientific guidelines provided by the scholars in the diet and health area. The components include:
       (i) Three components based on recommendations of dietary lipid intake (total fat, saturated fat, and cholesterol)
       (ii) Two components based on recommendations for simple and complex carbohydrate intake
       (iii) Although weighted less heavily in the total score, several components were included based on dietary protein, calcium, sodium, fluoride and supplement use
   This Index was revised (DQI-R) to include the most current US dietary guidelines and modified (DQI-I) to take into consideration diet characteristics such as: adequacy, variety, moderation, and overall balance

Several scoring systems have been created to quantify dietary quality for research and public policy purposes. This table outlines several of these indices

food prices have occurred for sweets, fats, and sugar-sweetened caloric beverages than for fresh fruits and vegetables (Drewnowski and Darmon 2005). This price disparity in turn has promoted the consumption of calorie-rich and nutrient-poor diets among low-income populations. To improve diet quality (see Table 141.1), researchers have estimated 35–40% additional food costs for low-income families (Jetter and Cassady 2005).

141.2.2 Defining the Environmental Context Associated with Obesogenic Behaviors

Various national policies and interventions exist to reduce the consumption of energy-dense foods, yet obesity continues to rise in developed countries like the United States, Canada, France, Germany, Great Britain, and several Scandinavian countries (Popkin 1994). Rising obesity trends may be due in part to a lack of consideration for the environmental context where obesity predominates.

Interventions directly targeting obesogenic behaviors often do not take into consideration underlying household factors such as SES that may influence an individual or family's ability for behavior change. In developed countries, higher rates of obesity are observed in low- versus high-income populations leading to an increased risk of many chronic diseases among the poor (Popkin 2004). This may be a direct result of the poor quality diets observed in many low-income populations. Compared to high-income families, economically constrained families are less likely to consume whole grains, lean meats, fish, low-fat dairy products, and fresh fruits and vegetables. Additionally, these low-income families tend to consume higher quantities of fatty meats, refined grains, and added fats (Darmon and Drewnowski 2008). Diets high in these energy-dense foods are associated with increased obesity risk as well as CVD and type II diabetes (Mendoza et al. 2007).

In general, as the economic status of an individual or family decreases there is an increased reliance on cheaper high-calorie diets rather than the more expensive nutrient-dense diets. Fruits and vegetables, which tend to be the most expensive foods per calorie, provide high quantities of micronutrients and fiber and thus improve the overall quality of a diet. However, fruits and vegetables are often prohibitively expensive for low income families, particularly given their relatively short shelf-life. Affordable high-calorie diets tend to consist of highly processed foods with longer shelf-lives that are high in simple sugars, saturated and trans- fats. Additionally, high-calorie foods are generally better tasting and convenient to prepare (Mendoza et al. 2007). Unfortunately, these highly processed foods are typically less satiating and therefore lead to overconsumption of total calories (Drewnowski and Darmon 2005). As a result, low-income families often meet or exceed calorie needs, but are deficient in micronutrients which come primarily from the more expensive fruits and vegetables (Andrieu et al. 2006).

141.3 Developed Countries: Why Low SES Leads to Poor Health Outcomes

There are multiple factors thought to link the effect of SES to health outcomes. Low SES groups receive less nutrition education and have poor access to healthcare services (Heck and Parker 2002; Devoe et al. 2007). Low-income families also commonly seek care for health problems later than middle or high-income families due to rapidly rising healthcare costs (Bodenheimer 2005). This leads to later diagnoses and ultimately more expensive healthcare interventions. Despite an increasing need of medical care for chronic diseases related to poor diet and sedentary lifestyles, there is a shortage of physicians interested in meeting this demand. Physicians report a lack of time, poor patient compliance, insufficient training, and lack of adequate insurance reimbursement as barriers to appropriately addressing care needs for the obese (Tsai et al. 2006). Additionally, technological innovation leading to the development of labor-saving household devices and passive forms of transportation has been estimated to contribute up to 40% of current weight gain in the United States (Lakdawalla and Philipson 2002).

141.3.1 Impact of SES on Dietary Behaviors

One of the most significant factors leading to poor health in developed countries is the impact of SES on diet behaviors. Individual and household SES is more dynamic than previously thought as families fall in and out of poverty due to unforeseen economic events and household expenses (Cornia 1994; Lokshin and Popkin 1999). Economic events can lead to periods of food insecurity characterized by a general decrease in food availability and a concurrent reduction in diet quality due to decreased purchasing power. Generally, low-income families experience food insecurity at higher rates than middle and high-income families because they are more susceptible to falling either temporarily or permanently in to poverty during periods of economic crisis (Cornia 1994; Lokshin and Popkin 1999). Further, psychosocial problems associated with food insecurity can contribute to disease-promoting diet behavior. Specifically, individuals from poorer families experience higher levels of loneliness, boredom, and depression which can lead to behaviors such as excessive snacking, skipped meals, and sedentarianism (Darmon and Drewnowski 2008). Economic constraints can present a conflict between competing priorities such as food preferences and affordability of these foods (Dore et al. 2003) adding to the psychological stress. Wealth disparity, increased household size, unexpected family expenses, loss of food stamp benefits, and unemployment can also lead to food insecurity among families (Rose 1999). Additionally low-income families report a lack of cooking skills, lack of motivation (Dibsall et al. 2003; Henry et al. 2006) and disinterest in cooking (Henry et al. 2006) as barriers to healthy eating.

141.3.2 Who Is the Most Severely Impacted?

During periods of economic duress, the nutritional status of adults typically declines first as a result of prioritizing their children's nutritional needs over their own (Messer and Ross 2002). Despite efforts of parents to ensure adequate nutrition for their children, lower rates of breastfeeding among low-income families as compared to middle- and high-income families often results in poor childhood nutritional status. Given that dietary habits are established in childhood, children of low-income families are at particular risk of establishing lifelong poor quality dietary habits particularly during economic crises (Wang et al. 2002; Nicklas 1995). Poor dietary quality in childhood decreases overall immune function, increases the rate of dental caries, and can lead to cognitive deficiencies (Nelson 2000) and can permanently downregulate basal metabolic rate (BMR) increasing the risk of adult onset obesity.

141.4 Developed Countries: Pathways by Which Socioeconomic Status Affects Diet Quality

There are multiple proposed pathways linking the effect of SES to decreased diet quality and poor health outcomes (see Fig. 141.3). Low-income groups receive less nutrition education (Variyam et al. 1996) and have poor access to healthcare services (Devoe et al. 2007). Physical access to healthy foods is recognized as a significant factor in diet-related disease for low-income groups (Gittelsohn and Sharma 2009). Proximity to supermarkets that offer a variety of fruits, vegetables, and low-fat dairy products exist in lower concentrations in economically impoverished areas and can limit accessibility to healthy food choices for low-income families (Larson et al. 2009). Additionally, concentration of fast food restaurants is higher in low-income neighborhoods (Smoyer-Tomic et al. 2008). The low walkability and perceived safety of low-income neighborhoods limits access to facilities offering fresh produce, low-fat dairy products, and unprocessed lean meats and poultry (Maziak et al. 2008; Mujahid et al. 2008a, b). Low-income individuals from urban environments are subject to long commute times and have low vehicle ownership which dramatically decreases accessibility of large food markets (Larson et al. 2009). Further, reduced wages force many low-income individuals to work extended hours decreasing both the time available to travel to distant grocery stores and

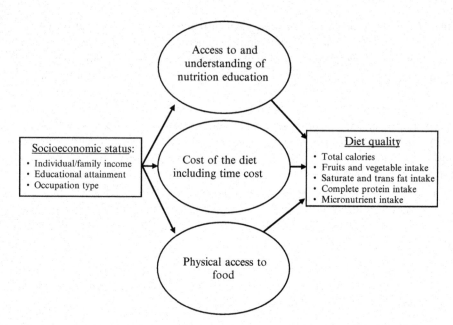

Fig. 141.3 Etiologic mechanism by which socioeconomic status (SES) impacts dietary quality. This figure illustrates the impact of SES on diet quality in developed countries. Nutrition education as well as accessibility and affordability of food are all intermediary factors linking low SES to poor diet. These factors are therefore key potential areas for interventions designed to successfully promote dietary change

prepare fresh home-prepared meals (Jabs and Devine 2006). Physical access to food stores can be complicated in districts that span large rural areas (Sharkey 2009). Quality of roads, tight district budgets, and work and commuting schedules can also complicate access for low-income families. Overall limited physical access to healthy food choices promotes the consumption of unhealthy prepackaged shelf-stable processed foods exacerbating the excess intake of total calories and insufficient micronutrient observed in low-income populations. As with food insecurity, individuals in urban versus rural areas experience more stress, which feeds psychosocial elements of disease-promoting dietary behaviors (Quine et al. 2003).

Food choices are made primarily on the basis of cost, taste, and convenience, rather than health and variety (Glanz et al. 1998). The high cost of nutrient-dense foods is likely the most significant determinant of inadequate consumption of fruits and vegetables, high quality lean meats and dairy products (Drewnowski and Specter 2004). The percentage of total family income accounting for food purchases inside and outside of the home is lowest for US families. Despite food expenditures accounting for the lowest percentage of the family budget, US families consume one of the most energy-dense diets in the world (Meade and Rosen 1996). Food costs take up a greater percentage of low- versus high-income family budgets creating an incentive for low-income families to purchase prepackaged and prepared calorie-rich foods to satisfy dietary needs. In contrast, unless consumed relatively quickly, the more expensive fresh foods such as fruits and vegetables are more likely to spoil than processed foods posing a highly inefficient use of money for overworked low-income families (Dowler 1997). Furthermore, low-income families tend to purchase highly processed fatty meats (Guenther et al. 2005) and high-fat dairy products (Prattala et al. 2003) such as hot dogs, prepackaged hamburgers, and processed cheese products due to cost and time limitations. Compared to dietary guidelines from the US Department of Health and Human Services (DHHS) and Department of Agriculture (USDA), a significant proportion of low-income families consume an excess of unhealthy fats and added sugars (DHHS and USDA 2005; Darmon and Drewnowski 2008). Overall, low-income families in developed countries often meet or exceed calorie needs, but fall far short of dietary guidelines of 400 g of fruits and vegetables set by the World Health Organization (WHO 2010). Consequently, this insufficient intake of fruits and vegetables leads to inadequate micronutrient intakes among many low-income individuals and families (Andrieu et al. 2006). The consumption of low quality diets in response to the high cost of nutrient-dense diets has been observed in other developed countries such as the UK, France, and Denmark (Darmon et al. 2004).

141.5   Developed Countries: Public Policies and Interventions to Promote Health

A combination of environment reconfiguration, public policy initiatives, and multilevel economic strategies may be required to reduce the prevalence of obesogenic dietary and physical activity behaviors (see Table 141.2) (Sallis and Glanz 2009). Historically, policy recommendations in developed countries have focused on reducing calorie consumption (Bleich et al. 2008), increasing fruit and vegetable consumption (WHO 2010), and increasing physical activity (CDC 2009). Decreasing total calories by limiting dietary fat has had limited success. Instead of decreasing total calories, individuals commonly substitute fatty foods with high-glycemic foods that make weight loss difficult and that contributes to diet-related disease (Pawlak et al. 2002). On the other hand, limiting carbohydrates in the diet is difficult to sustain and may be associated with high intake of saturated fats (Strychar 2006). Consumption of fruits and vegetables is a major determinant of dietary energy-density due to their high water and micronutrient content. Increasing intake of fruits and vegetables along with whole-grains and fish has been consistently associated with improved health outcomes (Kant 2004). Altering the food environment to improve accessibility to health food choices and subsidizing specific fruits and vegetables may help increase diet quality for low-income populations (Powell et al. 2009). Point-of-purchase techniques (e. g. health information and detailed menu labeling where purchasing decisions are made) in addition to subsidies for fresh produce may be important components to policies that support individual food preference yet promote healthy dietary habits. Such campaigns could be utilized in worksites, universities, grocery stores, and restaurants, but few adequate research trials have been conducted to evaluate the effectiveness of such efforts (Seymore et al. 2004). As a mechanism to prevent weight gain, stimulate weight loss and maintain weight loss, a recent Center for Disease Control (CDC) and Prevention task force proposed recommendations to improve physical activity in communities (CDC 2009). Such an evidence-based campaign would combine billboards, radio, television, newspapers, mailings, self-management education, worksite programs, tenant-based rental assistance programs, center-based programs for low-income children, enhanced school-based physical education, and behavioral and social support interventions. Many of these tools have been tested and have successfully increased physical activity levels individually but they have not been evaluated as a comprehensive intervention.

141.5.1   Public Policies and Interventions Aimed at Dietary Behavior Change

Awareness of health assistance programs and services in the digital age can be problematic for low-income individuals. In rural areas, low-income individuals are much less likely to use internet resources to acquire health information (Miller 2009). Low-income groups will benefit from government-sponsored programs that equalize access and provide incentives for purchasing healthy, nutrient-dense foods.

Table 141.2 Examples of developed country government-sponsored food interventions targeting low-income individuals and families

National program	Type of intervention	Governing body	Target audience	Program goal	Potential limitation
Expanded Food, Nutrition and Food Stamp Education Program	Nutrition-related education program only	USDA Cooperative State Research, Education, and Extension Service	Low-income families with a particular focus on youth	Educate families on healthy food choices	Can fail to take into account individual preferences, behavior patterns, and high cost/accessibility of healthy food
Food Stamp Program (FSP)/Supplemental Nutrition Assistance Program (SNAP)	Direct assistance to supplement food purchasing power only	USDA Food and Nutrition Service	Employed low-income individuals and families	Reduce food insecurity among low-income families	Subject to social restraints such as complex application forms, lengthy time required for participation, cultural and language barriers, as well as social stigma
Special Supplemental Nutrition Program for Women, Infants, and Children (WIC)	Nutrition-related education and direct assistance to supplement food purchasing power	USDA Food and Nutrition Service	Low-income pregnant, breastfeeding and nonbreastfeeding postpartum women, and their infants and children of ages up to 5 years old	Reduce incidence of low birth weight and iron deficiency anemia among infants	May not reach adequate number of at risk population due to age and gender restrictions. Limited sources of fruits and vegetables covered by subsidies
Housing Assistance Program	Indirect nonfood subsidy	Department of Housing and Urban Development	State housing credit agencies provide affordable housing to 35,000 low-income households	Increase food budgets and improve overall diet quality	Limited impact on food purchasing practices towards healthier food choices

This table summarizes the existing US government programs aimed at improving dietary quality of low-income individuals and families. There are a wide range of program methods used to address poor dietary practices in developed country settings. However programs that include subsidizing targeted healthy food choices as well as providing general nutrition education may result in the most successful sustainable improvements in dietary quality in low-income populations

Programs focusing on diet education alone have been largely ineffective with respect to improving diet quality. Often, dietary advice does not take into account individual preferences and long-standing behavior patterns or the prohibitive costs of healthy food choices. Governmental programs such as the Expanded Food and Nutrition Education Program, and the Food Stamp Education Program rely exclusively on educational tools to low-income families as a means of improving food choices. Their recommendations often focus on strategies and foods with low palatability and convenience for families (Lino 2001). In place of dietary advice, studies from the UK and US have shown that providing vouchers for purchasing fruit and vegetables was a simple and effective way of increasing fruit and vegetables intakes for groups of low-income women (Burr et al. 2007; Herman et al. 2006). Unfortunately, the effectiveness of assistance programs can be limited significantly by social restraints. For example, form requirements, time required for participation, cultural and language barriers, and social stigmas can deter qualifying individuals from taking part in food assistance programs. The magnitude of the perceived assistances from the program also plays a role in sign-on rates. These barriers to utilization are difficult to quantify and measure. However, experts suggest that linking related aid/benefits into the same program may increase utilization and ultimately improve overall effectiveness (Remler and Glied 2003).

The US Food Stamp Program (FSP), now known as the Supplemental Nutrition Assistance Program (SNAP), helps low-income individuals and families purchase healthy foods and provides education on healthy eating practices and methods to incorporate physical activities into daily routines (USDA 2009). Low-income households that are enrolled in an FSP have a significantly lower incidence of food insecurity (Rose 1999). However, high dietary energy-density has also been found in diets of FSP recipients (Mendoza et al. 2006). To satisfy family dietary needs, recipients often ensure calorie-sufficiency foremost (Wilde et al. 2000) and ultimately fail to shift purchase behavior toward healthier foods (Drewnowski 2003). Additionally, food stamp recipients tend to consume more added sugars, meats, and fats and failed to improve intake of fruits, vegetables, grains, and dairy products after receiving assistance (Wilde et al. 2000). Subsidizing lean deli meats as well as specific fruits and vegetables might also improve diet quality in these low-income populations (Dore et al. 2003).

The Special Supplemental Nutrition Program for Women, Infants, and Children (WIC) program is another federally sponsored program managed at the state level that acts to provide nutritious foods, information on healthy eating, and appropriate health referrals for low-income women, infants, and children up to age 5 (FNS USDA 2009). WIC has lead to higher birth weight and lower incidence of iron deficiency anemia in infants born to participants of this program (Owen and Owen 1997). WIC provides assistance for the purchasing of milk, cheese, eggs, iron-fortified cereal, fruit juice, and adds canned tuna and fresh carrots for breastfeeding women. WIC does not provide subsidies for other fruit and vegetables. A pilot initiative which added an additional $10 weekly-voucher to the WIC program was highly utilized among program recipients and increased fruit and vegetable consumption by 0.8–1.4 servings per day depending on the purchasing environment (Herman et al. 2006) (see Table 149.1).

141.5.2 Public Policies and Interventions Created to Impact Purchasing Power

Indirect attempts, such as housing subsidies have been used to increase the percentage of family budgets available for the purchase of healthy food. However, despite improvements in housing subsidies, available income for food spending remained inadequate to promote the consumption of a nutritious diet (Kirkpatrick and Tarasuk 2007). In general, government-sponsored programs and subsidies aimed at increasing overall purchasing power have had limited impact on the improvement of diet quality in low-income populations. An increase in economic resources tends to increase the quantity of less-expensive, energy-dense foods that are purchased rather than stimulating the purchase of healthy food choices. To be successful, future policy initiatives should be multilevel strategies to enhance accessibility to healthy food choices, provide subsidies for foods such as fresh fruits and vegetables, provide nutrition education, and promote the participation in existing government assistance program.

141.5.3 Individual/Family-Initiated Dietary Behavior Change

A recent study in Russia shows that there are some behavior modifications that are undertaken by individuals and families outside the context of government assistance to retain dietary habits during times of economic constraint. During a recent economic crisis, total energy intake of low income children remained robust, but diet composition shifted suggesting that low-income families purchased significantly less-expensive foods and prepared more meals at home. Both low and high-income families conserved diet structure by purchasing foods which provided more calories per unit cost (Dore et al. 2003). Specifically, low-income families demonstrated economic resilience by increasing consumption of less-expensive eggs and dairy products in order to provide stable sources of protein (Dore et al. 2003). This information can be used to subsidize targeted foods to ensure that families are able to purchase sufficient high quality calories.

141.6 Developing Countries: The Current Health Situation

Developing countries are characterized by low-scoring human indices such as life expectancy, per capita income, and level of literacy. Within a developing country context, the proportion of the population facing intermittent and/or chronic economic constraint far outnumbers the proportions observed in developed countries. A substantial percent of economically constrained individuals and families fall below the World Bank defined cut point for poverty, $2.00 per person per day and even the extreme poverty cut point of $1.25 in many low and middle-income countries (WB 2007). A disproportionate number of this impoverished population resides in rural areas. In contrast, many urban centers in developing countries are experiencing economic growth with a steadily growing middle-class superimposed over the urban poor. Typically, rural areas have poor transportation systems, health care infrastructure, sanitation conditions, and educational programs, which inhibit rural area growth and development. In contrast, urban centers are rapidly developing transportation infrastructure, organized healthcare systems, and educational programs including access to a diverse array of higher education institutions. Overall, economic opportunities for growth are limited in rural areas due to accessibility to resources. Similar to the dynamics observed in developed countries, populations in many developing country urban areas are limited primarily by the affordability of resources and existing services.

141.6.1 Environmental Context Underlying Obesity and Chronic Disease Trends

This widespread disparity in economic development, resource availability, and affordability of goods in developing countries also impacts dietary behaviors and ultimately health (see Fig. 141.4). Unlike developed nations, these countries are experiencing a rapid shift in health outcomes with increasing

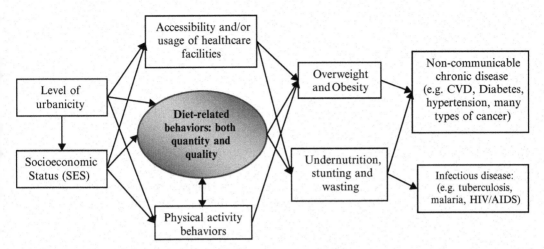

Fig. 141.4 The etiologic pathway from the socio-economic status of low-income populations leading to health status in developing countries. This figure emphasizes that, given the tremendous range of accessibility and affordability of resources (which is highly dependent on regional urbanization), there are multiple disparate pathways leading to the contrasting health outcomes of either chronic or infectious disease in developing countries. As a result blanket national policies to address malnutrition have the potential of addressing one form of malnutrition and ignoring or even exacerbating the other. Therefore, it is recommended that policy makers identify the specific etiologic framework underlying the disease status of an area and customize interventions to specific target populations

rates of obesity and chronic diseases (Popkin 2007). In economically middle-income countries of Latin America and parts of Asia, more than one third of the population is overweight (Popkin 2007). Although low-income countries in sub-Saharan Africa and south Asia are still struggling with a high prevalence of undernourished people there is a rapid rise of obesity in the urban areas (Popkin 2007). The shift from undernutrition to overnutrition is commonly referred to as the nutrition transition and the trend from infectious to chronic disease is referred to as the epidemiologic transition (Popkin 2006a). These shifts, however, occur superimposed over persistent undernutrition and infectious disease among certain low-income subpopulations. Two major factors influencing this disparity is the level of national wealth (determined by per capita income) and regional urbanization within the country both of which affect food availability as well as income potential and purchasing power. Substantial growth and development has occurred in many middle-income countries, particularly in urban centers, which has accelerated the nutrition and epidemiologic transitions towards overconsumption and increasing chronic disease prevalence. Although not as progressed, even in low-income countries where severe undernutrition persists, increases in obesity and chronic disease are occurring in response to the globalization of market systems (Gillespie and Haddad 2003). One stark difference between the urban populations in developing versus developed nations is that many adults in low and middle-income countries were chronically undernourished during the crucial developmental stages from childhood to early adulthood. Severe undernutrition during physiologic development can cause a permanent lowering of an individual's BMR. Therefore with an increased accessibility to western highly processed diets accompanying national development, these adults are even more prone to obesity than their low-income developed country counterparts.

The food accessibility and affordability in low and middle-income countries differs substantially depending on the level of urbanization of a particular region. In urban areas of developing countries food accessibility is less of a challenged than affordability. Like the developed country poor, low-income urban populations are rapidly shifting towards consumption of highly processed foods that are cheap, convenient, energy-dense, and micronutrient-poor with the exception of sodium which typically exists in excesses of recommendations (Popkin 1998, 2001). Income limitations restrict low-income individuals and families from purchasing expensive fruits, vegetables, and high quality lean animal products. In contrast, rural populations struggle with the accessibility as well as the affordability of nutrient-rich quality foods.

141.6.2 Rising Global Food Prices Cause a Further Decline in Diet Quality

The recent global trend of rising food prices is negatively impacting access to food in developing nations at an alarming rate. Specifically, rising food prices impact both dietary convergence and dietary adaptation – terms used by researchers to explain the change in dietary pattern among population in developing countries (FAO 2004; Hawkes 2006). Dietary convergence refers to a reduction in the diet diversity found in a majority of traditional diets to a narrow range of globally accessible staple grains, meats and poultry, edible oils, salt, and sugar (FAO 2004). For example, a dramatic increase in the consumption of meat and poultry products as well as edible oils and processed high-glycemic index foods has replaced the more traditional rice and vegetable-based diet in many Asian countries (Ding and Malik 2008). A similar shift has occurred in Colombia in the last decade due to the increased production of poultry in response to a national policy which increased the import of cheap animal feed. In India, dietary convergence is characterized by increases in the consumption of quality protein sources such as eggs and milk. However, significant increases in the consumption of salty snacks, edible oils, and processed sugary foods such as baked goods and candy has also occurred in India (FAO 2004).

Dietary convergence is a function of rising food prices coupled with changes in individual or family income. Essentially, the price of a commodity influences availability and in turn consumer demand, thus creating a cyclical pattern to the availability, affordability, and consumption of specific food products. This pattern is heavily influenced by the national political environment and the government strategies towards food trade. Ultimately, products which are produced in high quantity on a global scale such as edible oils and processed sugary foods are relatively cheaper than traditional foods that are produced in much smaller quantities, thus tipping the scales towards less healthy dietary choices.

Dietary adaptation occurs in the population due to the changes in lifestyle such as increase use of transportation, eating out for convenience, and relying on cheaper foods to achieve calorie needs (FAO 2004). Adaptation is an individualized lifestyle change in response to environment changes such as: increasing food marketing and advertisements, increasing accessibility to convenient street food or fast food outlets and an increasing prevalence of supermarkets. Although dietary adaptation is less common among the severely/chronically poor in developing countries it is becoming rapidly more prevalent in intermittently poor and middle income groups. For example, recent increases in advertisements of calorie-rich low-nutrient foods in Brazil have lead to significant increases in energy-dense diets in middle-class communities. In the Philippines and other Asian countries, the change from traditional meal patterns to habits based on convenience is leading to increased consumption of processed foods high in fat, sugar, and low in micronutrients (FAO 2004; Rayner et al. 2007).

141.7 Developing Countries: Implications for Policy Makers

Given the substantial income disparity within developing countries and the complex web of environmental factors influencing dietary behavior patterns, policy makers should consider a multi-pronged strategy to address malnutrition. Low-income populations are not equipped to handle the increased chronic disease risk associated with the emerging obesity occurring as a result of increased food accessibility and affordability (Popkin 2009). As described previously, however, the level of food accessibility and affordability is highly influenced by the level of national wealth and regional urbanization. Therefore, each developing country should customize policies and programs for the disparate economic and geographic populations facing the nutrition and epidemiological transition.

National policies created to improve the health and dietary patterns of economically-constrained groups that target only a segment of the population can often create more problems than they address (Ng et al. 2008). In particular, this is true for middle-income countries where the dual-burden of undernutrition and overnutrition occur in the same communities and in many cases in the same households. For example, in Chile, a government program designed to reduce undernutrition, exacerbated the problem of obesity for specific subgroups in urban areas of the country. In contrast, a government program in Mauritius aimed at the prevention of CVD in areas of high-risk individuals, successfully decreased obesity rates in this population (FAO 2004). As the nutrition transition continues throughout the developing world, governments must design targeted programs to address persistent undernutrition while simultaneously developing programs to address the growing prevalence of obesity and chronic diseases (see Table 141.3).

Table 141.3 Examples of developing country government-sponsored food programs and policies targeting low-income populations

Country	Type of program/ policy	Target audience	Program goal	Observed outcomes
Bangladesh	Challenging the Frontiers of Poverty Reduction	Ultra poor communities in rural Bangladesh	Reduction of poverty to create a foundation for sustainable economic developments to support long term diet and health improvements	Increase intake of grains and vegetables but no reduction in mortality
Mauritius	Health Promotion program through Ministry of Health supported by health policy change	National level program to improve health status in both urban and rural environments	Reduction of cardiovascular diseases (CVD)	Increase in obesity rates due to switching of oils but reduction in cholesterol levels
Republic of Korea	Mass media campaigns to promote traditional foods and diets	Rural communities	Retain traditional diets and increase intake of vegetables and grains	Increase fresh fruit and vegetable consumption and reduce fat intake particularly animal fats
Brazil	Trade liberalization	Agrarian regions	To allow foreign investment, reduce farm tax, and lower import taxes on fertilizers and pesticides	Increase production of soybean oil to become second largest soybean exports but contribute to high consumption of soybean oil around the world

This table summarizes existing policies and programs aimed at improving health and dietary quality of low-income individuals and families in developing countries. With the given diversity of health challenges faced by urban versus many rural populations, government and nongovernmental programs will need to customize policies and interventions, e.g. programs to increase accessibility of fruits and vegetable in rural areas and a distinct program to decrease consumption of edible oils in the urban settings

141.7.1 Public Policies and Interventions Aimed at Dietary Behavior Change

An integral component of a multifaceted developing-country intervention strategy should include nutrition education programs to elucidate the negative health consequences of diets excessive in processed fats, and sugar, and deficient in micronutrient-rich fruits and vegetables. Given that traditional diets in many developing countries were inherently high in unprocessed grains, vegetable oils and fruits and vegetables, a strategy could be to preserve and reinforce the consumption of these already culturally-accepted dietary practices. For example, the Republic of Korea's Ministry of Rural Development has successfully preserved traditional dietary practices in rural communities through nutrition education on the importance of fruits and vegetables reinforced by the use of traditional Korean food recipes (Popkin et al. 2001). This has lead to decreased rates of obesity in this country in spite of the improved economic condition in the country.

The impact of economic independence on food industry dynamics and its consequent effect on the health of a population must be considered in the process of creating developing country health policy. The food industry in a country not only depends on agricultural productivity but on national and international food trade policies as well. Before making drastic changes, policy makers must carefully examine the possible consequences of modifying trade restriction and regulations in the food industry. Often it is assumed that removal of trade restrictions will automatically benefit a low-income population. For example, in Brazil, the government recently altered policies around the production of soybean oil in the country. Multiple changes were made including: opening the market to foreign investors, removing the export tax on soybean oil, restructuring the taxation for soybean farmers, and levying taxes on the imports of fertilizers and pesticides. This resulted in the reduction of prices of the edible oil not only within Brazil but also globally. This price reduction lead to significant increases in oil consumption in Brazil and is now believed to be one of the causes of increased obesity within the country. This policy also increased soybean oil consumption globally and is believed to have caused the destruction of local oilseed production in India and China, thus negatively impacting the national economies of these countries (Popkin et al. 2001; Hawkes 2006; Rayner et al. 2007).

141.7.2 Public Policies and Interventions Aimed at Overall Poverty Reduction

Given that poverty is a primary cause of poor diet quality in developing countries, programs aimed at alleviating poverty may significantly reduce malnutrition. Specifically, policy makers should consider programs to improve population quality of life by encouraging local farming, increasing accessibility to micro-finance schemes, improving the health care infrastructure, and establishing sustained educational systems (Russell 2004; Popkin 2009). Policies geared towards local community culture and practices may have an advantage over national programs with respect to improving the quality of dietary behaviors and lifestyles. Currently, in many sub-Saharan African and Asian countries, local farmers who do not produce sufficient quantities to support their communities, are becoming more dependent on foods imported via global trade. This has lead to a significant increased consumption of processed foods high in fats and sugar. To prevent this trend, governments should invest in local farming by subsidizing specific crops for poor farmers in a manner that supports local habits as well as fertilizers that will allow them to grow these crops. Often, they may not be in line with the globalization of food trade markets but it will allow the local farmer to sustain their local diets and enable a correspondingly healthy lifestyle (Rayner et al. 2007). Micro-finance schemes, such as the programs designed by Nobel Peace prize winner Mohammed Yunus, have dramatically improved the quality of life of the ultra-poor in rural Bangladesh (Haseen 2007). This financial support has allowed rural populations to become financially viable and revive local industry of agriculture and goods. To combat poverty and malnutrition in developing countries it is also to improve the health care infrastructure promoting a healthier population free from debilitating infectious conditions such as HIV/Acquired Immunodeficiency Syndrome (AIDS), tuberculosis, and malaria. The cost of these diseases can be substantial and government and nongovernmental organizations should consider expanding the preventive services to rural populations where low-income groups predominate (Russell 2004).

Possibly the most important public policy strategy is the need for education in developing country communities – both in terms of overall education and nutritional education. The basic primary and secondary programs serve a dual purpose of building an intellectually stronger future generation as well as increasing awareness of basic nutritional needs and the hazards of inappropriately consumed foods. Institutions should have both nutritional education and hands on food-related programs as part of both the primary and secondary curriculum.

141.8 Conclusion

In recent decades rapid increases in obesity and associated chronic diseases have occurred with a disproportionately high rate of increase among low-income populations. For developed countries where affordability is a significant barrier to good nutrition, nutrient dense foods such as fruits and vegetables are prohibitively expensive for economically-constrained population. As a result low-income individuals and families rely heavily on cheap highly processed energy-dense foods. Although policies and programs exist to help alleviate food insecurity, these policies and programs have had limited success in improving the nutrient density of diets among the poor. To curb overconsumption and improve diet quality, developed country policies and interventions must address the price barrier as well as provide nutrition-based education typical of traditional interventions. In developing countries, barriers to quality nutrition include both the affordability of as well as accessibility to nutrient-rich food commodities. In urban centers where economic growth has lead to food environments similar to those found in developed countries a majority of low-income families rely on highly processed convenience foods high in fats and sugars and low in nutrients to meet energy needs. This has lead to tremendous increases in obesity and chronic disease prevalence. Low-income populations in rural developing country settings face an added barrier of food accessibility. In times of economic crisis, low-income individuals and families are more likely to experience intermittent or chronic periods of food insecurity. As a result, infectious diseases associated with chronic undernutrition are still common in rural areas of developing countries. Given the dramatic variance in dietary behavior response to economic constraint in developing countries, policies and interventions must be customized by region and take into consideration the specific barrier to quality nutrition.

Summary Points

- Obesity is a global epidemic with a rapidly increasing predominance among low-income populations. Unfortunately, low-income populations are also the least capable to deal with the health and economic consequences directly associated with obesity and indirectly with obesity-related chronic diseases.

- One of the most recognized etiologic pathways influencing obesity risk is the impact of income status on dietary behaviors and subsequent nutritional status which in turn impacts obesity risk.
- An individual or family's dietary behavior response to economic constraint is dependent on the local, national, and international environmental context.
- In developed countries, economic constraint tends to result in selective purchasing of relatively cheap processed foods high in refined carbohydrates, saturated fats, and trans fats with a concurrent decrease in expensive fruits and vegetables, lean meats, and low-fat dairy products. Consequently many low-income individuals are malnourished consuming excess calories and insufficient micronutrients.
- In many urban settings of middle-income developing countries the relationship between economic constraint and dietary behavior modification closely resembles the pattern observed in developed countries. In rural settings dietary behavior change in response to economic constraints tends to resemble patterns observed more commonly in low-income developing countries.
- In low-income developing countries, researchers have observed substantial food insecurity resulting in diets insufficient in both total calories and micronutrients among poor populations facing periods of economic constraint. This is particularly evident in rural areas where a lack of purchasing power is compounded by a lack of food availability.
- The prohibitively high cost of fruit and vegetable as well as quality meat and dairy products is at the root of insufficient intake among economically constrained populations. For this reason policies and interventions aimed at providing nutrition education as a means of improving diet quality have had negligible success.
- To be effective, policies and interventions to improve nutritional status in economically constrained populations must take in to consideration the environmental context driving the dietary behavior changes.
- In a developed country context: policies and interventions that increase economic resources for food purchasing successfully reduce incidence of food insecurity, but fail to increase consumption of nutrient-dense foods such as lean meats and fish, whole grains, and fruits and vegetables.
- Given the availability of resources, incorporating subsidies for targeted foods such as fruits and vegetables into existing or new polices and interventions may substantially increase the potential for success in developed countries.
- In developing countries there is a wide range of accessibility to and affordability of healthy food choices and is highly dependent on the urbanization of a region
- In developing countries policy makers must identify whether the cause of malnutrition is an accessibility or affordability issue to create successful sustainable interventions, e.g. if the barrier to diet quality is affordability using a food-specific subsidy might be appropriate whereas an accessibility barrier might require agricultural-based support

---

Key Terms

Nutrition transition: A phenomenon in low and middle-income countries where decreases in undernutrion concurrent with emerging overnutrition occur with increases in national gross domestic product.

Epidemiologic transition: A phase of development in a country context where a recession in the prevalence of infectious disease occurs simultaneously with an increase in the incidence of chronic noncommunicable diseases. Typically this transition is accompanied by improved national healthcare, sanitation, family participation in active family planning, and an increase in women working outside the home.

Demographic transition: The transformation in a country where steady decreases in initially high birth and death rates are observed resulting in a shift towards an older population structure. This shift occurs most commonly as a country transitions from a preindustrial agrarian-focused economy to one that is highly industrialized.

Food insecurity: A state where an individual or family lives in with intermittent or chronic hunger due to sporadic access to food and is in fear of starvation.

Poverty: Defined by the world bank as $2.00 per person per day and for extreme poverty $1.25 per person per day.

References

Andrieu E, Darmon N, Drewnowski A. Eur J Clin Nutr. 2006;60:434–6.
Arvaniti F, Panagiotakos D. Crit Rev Food Sci Nutr. 2008;48:317–27.
Bleich S, Cutler D, Murray C, Adams A. Ann Rev Public Health. 2008;29:273–95.
Bodenheimer T. Ann Intern Med. 2005;142:847–54.
Brown WV, Fujioka K, Wilson PWF, Woodworth KA. Am J Med. 2009;122:S4–11.
Burr ML, Trembeth J, Jones KB, Geen J, Lynch LA, Roberts ZE. Public Health Nutr. 2007;10:559–65.
Centers for Disease Control and Prevention (CDC). 2009. http://www.thecommunityguide.org/pa/
Cornia GA. Am Econ Rev. 1994;84:297–302.
Darmon N, Drewnowski A. Am J Clin Nutr. 2008;87:1107–17.
Darmon N, Briend A, Drewnowski A. Public Health Nutr. 2004;7:21–7.
Devoe JE, Baez A, Angier H, Krois L, Edlund C, Carney PA. Ann Fam Med. 2007;5:511–8.
Dibsall LA, Lambert N, Bobbin RF, Frewer LJ. Public Health Nutr. 2003;6:159–68.
Ding EL, Malik VS. Global Health. 2008;4(4):8.
Dixon J, Omwega AM, Friel S, Burns C, Donati K, Carlisle R. J Urban Health.2007; 84:i118–29.
Dore AR, Adair LS, Popkin BM. J Nutr. 2003;133:3469–75.
Dowler E. Food Policy. 1997;22:405–17.
Drewnowski A. J Nutr. 2003;133:838S–40S.
Drewnowski A, Specter SE. Am J Clin Nutr. 2004;79:6–16.
Drewnowski A, Darmon N. Am J Clin Nutr. 2005;82:265S–73S.
Flegal KM, Carroll MD, Ogden CL, Johnson CL. JAMA 2002;288:1723–7.
Food and Agricultural Organization of Unites States (FAO). Globalization of food systems in developing countries: impact on food security and nutrition. 2004.
Gillespie S, Haddad L. The double burden of malnutrition in Asia. New Delhi: Sage; 2003.
Gittelsohn J, Sharma S. Am J Prev Med. 2009;36:S161–5.
Glanz K, Basil M, Maibach E, Goldberg J, Snyder D. J Am Diet Assoc. 1998;98:1118–26.
Gordon-Larsen P, Nelson MC, Page P, Popkin BM. Pediatrics 2006;117:417–24.
Goudge J, Gilson L, Russell S, Gumede T, Mills A. BMC Health Serv Res. 2009;9:75.
Guenther PM, Jensen HH, Batres-Marquez SP, Chen C-F. J Am Diet Assoc. 2005;105:1266–74.
Hakeem R. Eur J Clin Nutr. 2001;55:400–6.
Hansen T, Ahlstrom H, Soderberg S, Hulthe J, Wikstrom J, Lind L, Johansson L. Atherosclerosis 2009;205:163–7.
Haseen F. Asia Pac J Clin Nutr. 2007;16(Suppl 1):58–64.
Hawkes C. Global Health. 2006;2(4):8.
Heck KE, Parker JD. Health Serv Res. 2002;37:171–84.
Henry H, Reimer K, Smith C, Reick M. J Am Diet Assoc. 2006;106:841–9.
Herman DR, Harrison GG, Jenks E. J Am Diet Assoc. 2006;106:740–4.
International Diabetes Institute. The Asia-Pacific perspective: redefining obesity and its treatment. Australia: health communications. Australia Pty; 2000.
Jabs J, Devine CM. Appetite 2006. [Epub ahead of print]. http://www.ncbi.nlm.nih.gov/pubmed/16698116
Jetter KM, Cassidy DL. AIC issues brief. 2005. http://aic.ucdavis.edu/pub/briefs/brief29.pdf
Kant AK. J Am Diet Assoc. 1996;96:785–91.
Kant AK. J Am Diet Assoc. 2004;104:615–35.

Kirkpatrick SI, Tarasuk V. Public Health Nutr. 2007;10:1464–73.

Korner J, Woods SC, Woodsworth KA. Am J Med. 2009;122:S12–18.

Lakdawalla D, Philipson T. NER Working Paper 8946. 2002. http://www.nber.org/papers/w8946

Larson NI, Story MT, Nelson MC. Am J Prev Med. 2009;36:74–81.

Leive A, Xu K. Bull World Health Organ. 2008;86:849–56.

Lino M. Fam Econ Nutr Rev. 2001;13:50–63.

Lokshin M, Popkin BM. Econ Dev Cult Change. 1999;47:803–29.

Maccio A, Mededdu C, Mantovani G. Obes Rev. 2009. [Epub ahead of print].

Manton KG. World Health Stat Q. 1988;41:255–66.

Mathers CD, Loncar D. PLoS Med. 2006;3:e442.

Maziak W, Ward KD, Stockton MB. Obes Rev. 2008;9:35–42.

McIntyre D, Thiede M, Dahlgren G, Whitehead M. Soc Sci Med. 2006;62:858–65.

Meade M, Rosen EM. Food Rev. 1996;19:39–43.

Mendoza JA, Drewnowski A, Cheadle A, Christakis DA. J Nutr. 2006;136:1318–22.

Mendoza JA, Drewnowski A, Christakis DA. Diabetes Care. 2007;30:974–9.

Messer E, Ross EM. Nutr Clin Care. 2002;5:168–81.

Miller EA. J Health Polit Policy Law. 2009;34:261–84.

Misra A, Khurana L. J Clin Endocrinol Metab. 2008;93:S9–30.

Mujahid MS, Diez Roux AV, Shen M, Gowda D, Sánchez B, Shea S, Jacobs DR Jr, Jackson SA. Am J Epidemiol. 2008a;167:1349–57.

Mujahid MS, Diez Roux AV, Morenoff JD, Raghunathan TE, Cooper RS, Ni H, Shea S. Epidemiology 2008b;19:590–8.

Nelson M. Proc Nutr Soc. 2000;59:307–15.

Nelson MC, Gordon-Larsen P, Song Y, Popkin BM. Am J Prev Med. 2006;31:109–17.

Ng SW, Zhai F, Popkin BM. Soc Sci Med. 2008;66(2):414–26.

Nicklas TA. Am J Med Sci. 1995;310:S101–8.

Ntandou G, Delisle H, Agueh V, Fayomi B. Nutr Res. 2009;29:180–9.

Ogden CL, Carroll MD, Curtin LR, McDowell MA, Tabak CJ, Flegal KM. JAMA 2006;295:1549–55.

Ohman MK, Wright AP, Wickenheiser KJ, Luo W, Eitzman DT. Curr Vasc Pharmacol. 2009;7:169–79.

Olshansky SJ, Passaro DJ, Hershow RC, Layden J, Carnes BA, Brody J, Hayflick L, Butler RN, Allison DB, Ludwig DS. N Engl J Med. 2005;352:1138–45.

Owen AL, Owen GM. J Am Diet Assoc. 1997;97:777–82.

Pawlak DB, Ebbeling CB, Ludwig DS. Obes Rev. 2002;3:235–43.

Pollack CE, Armstrong K. Arch Intern Med. 2009;169:945–9.

Popkin BM. Nutr Rev. 1994;52:285–98.

Popkin BM. Public Health Nutr. 1998;1:5–21.

Popkin BM. J Nutr. 2001;131:871S–3S.

Popkin BM. Nutr Rev. 2004;62:S140–3.

Popkin BM. Public Health Nutr. 2006a;5(1A):205–14.

Popkin BM. Sci Am. 2007;297(3):88–95.

Popkin BM. Nutr Rev. 2009;67(Suppl 1):S79–82.

Popkin BM, Horton S, Soowan K. Food Nutr Bull. 2001;22(S4):47–51.

Powell LM, Zhao Z, Wang Y. Health Place. 2009. [Epub ahead of print].

Prattala RS, Groth MV, Oltersdorf US, Roos GM, Sekula W, Tuomainen HM. Eur J Pub Health. 2003;13:124–32.

Quine S, Bernard D, Booth M, Kang M, Usherwood T, Alperstein G, Bennett D. Rural Remote Health. 2003;3:245.

Rayner G, Hawkes C, Lang T, Bello W. Health Promot Int. 2007;21(S1):67–74.

Remler DK, Glied SA. Am J Public Health. 2003;93:67–74.

Rose D. J Nutr. 1999;129:517S–20S.

Russell S. Am J Trop Med Hyg. 2004;71:147–55.

Sallis JF, Glanz K. Milbank Q. 2009;87:123–54.

Seidell JC. Br J Nutr. 2000;83:S5–8.

Seymore JD, Yaroch AL, Serdula M, Blank HM, Khan LK. Prev Med. 2004;39:S108–36.

Shafique S, Akhter N, Stallkamp G, de Pee S, Panagides D, Bloem MW. Int J Epidemiol. 2007;36:449–57.

Sharkey JE. Am J Prev Med. 2009;36:S151–5.

Smoyer-Tomic KE, Spence JC, Raine KD, Amrhein C, Cameron N, Yasenovskiy V, Cutumisu N, Hemphill E, Healy J. Health Place. 2008;14:740–54.

Strychar I. CMAJ. 2006;174:56–63.

Stuckler D. Milbank Q. 2008;86:273–326.

Tsai AG, Asch DA, Wadden TA. J Am Diet Assoc. 2006;106:1651–5.

US Department of Agriculture (USDA). FNS Supplemental Nutrition Assistance Program (SNAP). 2009. http://www.fns.usda.gov/FSP/

US Department of Health and Human Services and US Department of Agriculture. Dietary guidelines for Americans, 2005. 6th ed. Washington, DC: US Government Printing Office; 2005.

Variyam JN, Blaylock J, Smallwood DM. Stat Med. 1996;15:23–35.

Vorster HH, Kruger A, Venter CS, Margetts BM, MacIntyre UE. Cardiovasc J Afr. 2007;18:282–9.

Vorster HH. Public Health Nutr. 2002;5:239–43.

Wang Y, Bently ME, Zhai F, Popkin BM. J Nutr. 2002;132:430–8.

Wilde PE, McNamara PE, Ranney CK. USDA/ERS FANR Report No. 9. 2000.

World Bank. Understanding poverty. 2007. http://web.worldbank.org/WBSITE/EXTERNAL/TOPICS/EXTPOVERTY/0,,contentMDK:20153855~menuPK:373757~pagePK:148956~piPK:216618~theSitePK:336992,00.html

World Health Organization (WHO). Promoting fruit and vegetable consumption around the world. 2010. http://www.who.int/dietphysicalactivity/fruit/en/index.html

Chapter 142
Food Deprivation: A Neuroscientific Perspective

Harald T. Schupp and Britta Renner

Abbreviations

AgRP	Agouti-related protein
BOLD	Blood oxygenation level dependent
EEG	Electroencephalography
ERP	Event related potential
fMRI	Functional magnetic resonance imaging
LiCL	Lithium chloride
LPP	Late positive potential
MNE	Minimum norm estimate
Nc	Nucleus
NPY	Neuropeptide Y
PET	Positron emission tomography
POMC	Proopiomelanocortin
rCBF	Regional cerebral blood flow
ROI	Region of interest

142.1 Introduction

The Russian physiologist Pavlov considered eating as the most powerful relationship an organism has to its surrounding world (Pavlov 1953). This "food connection" is heavily regulated by internal state variables such as hunger. Prolonged periods of starving are one of the most tragic experiences of humanity and even mild conditions of food deprivation clearly affect consummatory behavior as reflected in the saying "hunger is the best spice".

Everybody knows about the effects of deprivation. The effects appear intuitively so obvious that the phenomenon receives paradoxically rather too little than too much attention. Consider for instance the work of Pavlov and Skinner, in which food stimuli play a central role. The empirical finding that the contingent pairing of a tone and food establishes new behaviors is nowadays taught in high school. After training, the dog salivates to a previously neutral stimulus. Similarly, knowledge

H.T. Schupp (✉)
Department of Psychology, University of Konstanz, 78457 Konstanz, Germany
e-mail: harald.schupp@uni-konstanz.de

V.R. Preedy et al. (eds.), *Handbook of Behavior, Food and Nutrition*,
DOI 10.1007/978-0-387-92271-3_142, © Springer Science+Business Media, LLC 2011

about the Skinner box, in which rats may learn to vigorously press a button to obtain food, is well perceived in the public. Imagine what would happen, if the animals were tested while satiated? The simple answer is they would probably not learn to press the button or to salivate. The role of deprivation in these learning principles is easily overlooked. However, Pavlov was very clear in his writing by stating that even the most avaricious dog will not learn the salivary response when satiated (Pavlov 1953). Accordingly, internal state variables have profound effects on responding to and learning about food cues.

In humans, the effects of prolonged periods of reduced food consumption were investigated in the Minnesota semi-starvation experiment, which was conducted during Second World War by Keys and colleagues (Keys et al. 1950). Food intake was greatly limited for several months resulting in pronounced loss of body weight (~25 kg). The experiment revealed massive physiological and psychological effects of semi-starvation. One notable finding is that food became the most important thing in life (Keys et al. 1950). Preoccupation with food and episodes of binge eating may be also induced by voluntary restricting food intake as in dieting and restrained eating (Polivy 1996). However, deprivation need not be sustained over long periods to affect the human feeding system. Acute food deprivation is associated with increased food consumption compared to nondeprived control groups (Spiegel et al. 1989; Drobes et al. 2001; Mauler et al. 2006) and increases the reinforce value of food in behavioral choice paradigms (Raynor and Epstein 2003).

142.2 Deprivation and the Feeding System: Conceptual Considerations

Deprivation affects almost every aspect related to food intake. Animal research over the past decade allows sketching a basic scheme of the feeding system providing a conceptual framework for the understanding of the effects of food deprivation on ingestive behaviors. As illustrated in Fig. 142.1, the organization of goal-directed ingestive behaviors rests on the integration of information about internal state (e.g., food deprivation), cues from the environment (e.g., availability of palatable food), and behavioral state (e.g., circadian rhythm). Furthermore, ingestive behavior is temporally organized in distinct appetitive and consummatory phases (cf., Timberlake 2001). To obtain food, one has first to look for potential food sources. A general search mode occurs when the subject does not know where to look for food. Exploratory behaviors bring the organism close to food and a focal search mode is engaged readying the organism for consummatory behaviors of chewing and swallowing. Ethological observations reveal reflexive-stereotypic behaviors during food consumption, while appetitive behaviors are more variable and non-stereotypic. These motivational stages differ in many respects such as temporal and spatial proximity to food consumption, engagement of distinct perception-action units, and specific cues sensitizing the engagement of stages. Recent research also suggests that the weighting of external and internal information differs among motivational stages. When food was readily available, consumption was controlled by the palatability of the food independent whether the animal underwent food restriction (~85% of normal weight) or not. Conversely, measurement of anticipatory locomotor behaviors revealed significant deprivation effects, which were independent from food palatability (Barbano and Cador 2005).

Great progress has been made to delineate mechanisms how information about internal state is represented in the brain and controls ingestive behaviors. The brain perceives an array of interosensory signals conveying information about the availability of food and nutrients generated by the gastrointestinal tract, postabsorptive sites (pancreas, liver, muscle), and stored nutrients in adipose tissue (Woods et al. 2000; Berthoud and Morrison 2008). While it is recognized that multiple brain regions are important for perceiving internal state, specific nuclei in the hypothalamus are consid-

Basic Scheme of the Feeding System

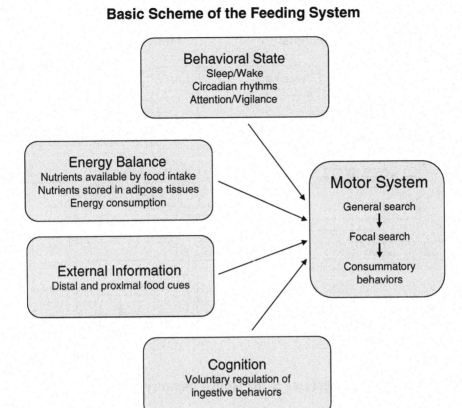

Fig. 142.1 Conceptual framework of the organization of the feeding system (Based on Swanson 2000; Timberlake 2001)

ered as key sites for the integration of metabolic-related information. The nucleus (Nc) arcuatus is assumed to integrate metabolic information via two populations of neurons (Neuropeptide Y (NPY)/ Agouti-related Protein (AgRP), Proopiomelanocortin (POMC)). These neurons are sensitive to a number of metabolic-related information (e.g., leptin, insulin, ghrelin) and exert opposite actions on feeding behavior. Efferents from these neurons to the paraventricular, lateral, and ventromedial hypothalamus provide a gateway for the translation of metabolic information to adaptive feeding responses as these neurons project widely through the entire brain (Swanson 2000; Watts and Swanson 2002; Berthoud and Morrison 2008). Based on anatomical, developmental, genetic, and functional data, Swanson introduced the concept of the behavioral control column in the rostral hypothalamus, which is considered as key motor control structure for motivated behaviors of feeding, reproduction, and defense (Swanson 2000). Consistent with its presumed role for ingestive behaviors, the paraventricular Nc affects many brain regions implicated in the selection, planning, and execution of specific somatic motor behaviors (cortical, striatal, and pallidal motor structures, brain stem motor nuclei), endocrine and autonomic responses and behavioral state regulation (see Fig. 142.2a). Overall, distinct nuclei in the rostral hypothalamus appear critical for the representation of internal state and provide mechanisms how food deprivation exerts motivational control on ingestive behaviors.

The incentive value of food is dynamically adjusted according to variations in internal state of energy balance. Even the tastiest food item is not consumed when satiated. This finding requires that

Neural Mechanisms of the Feeding System

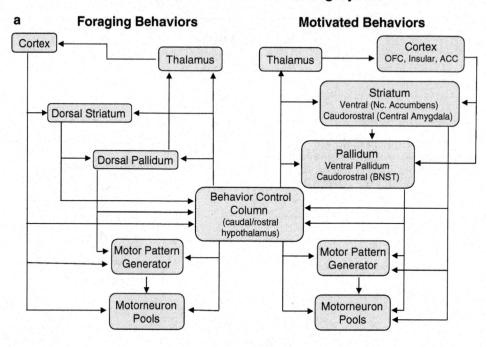

a   **Foraging Behaviors**   **Motivated Behaviors**

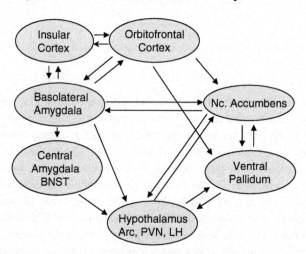

b   **Key Structures of the Motive Circuitry**

Fig. 142.2 (**a**) Illustration of the concept of the behavioral control column in the medial zone of the hypothalamus. The rostral segment is thought to regulate basic classes of motivated behaviors (ingestive, reproductive, defensive). Exploratory or foraging behaviors are assumed to involve the caudal segment (The graph is based on Swanson (2000) and Watts & Swanson (2002) and the reader is directed to these sources for details) (**b**) Schematic diagram of key structures of the motive circuitry implicated in the perception of reward and the activation of adaptive behavioral responses

reward perception is at least in some neural structures profoundly dependent on internal state of energy balance. Many neural structures sensitive to food reward have been revealed in the past decade. In the rat, a motive circuitry has been delineated responding to appetitive food stimuli including regions in the orbitofrontal cortex, insular cortex, amygdala, Nc. Accumbens, ventral pallidum, ventral tegmental area, and dorsal thalamus (see Fig. 142.2b; Kalivas and Nakamura 1999; Holland and Gallagher 2004; Berridge and Kringelbach 2008; Smith et al. 2009). While the specific contributions of these structures to the organization of motivated behaviors remains to be determined, unique contributions among selected structures in controlling ingestive behaviors have been demonstrated. For instance, recent research has revealed "hedonic hot spots" in the Nc. accumbens and ventral pallidum of the rat brain with different functions in instrumental responding to and consumption of food and hedonic liking responses measured by facial expression (Smith et al. 2009). Furthermore, core structures of the motive circuitry are differentially implicated in the phenomenon of classically conditioned eating. In the learning phase, a cue is repeatedly presented when hungry rats are allowed to eat. During testing, presentation of this cue can stimulate eating even when the rat is satiated. A recent study suggests that this phenomenon relies on direct pathways from orbitofrontal cortex and basolateral nuclei of the amygdala but not from Nc. accumbens (Petrovich et al. 2005). Furthermore, new learning induced by devaluation of the food with LiCL (lithium chloride) is abolished when the orbitofrontal cortex but not the amygdala is lesioned before the devaluation procedure (Pickens et al. 2003). Thus, the orbitofrontal cortex seems to be critical for learning about changes in the stimulus-reinforcement contingencies. Further differentiation among the contribution of neural structures of the motive circuitry is suggested when considering the inhibition of the feeding response by fear. Specifically, inhibition of feeding by presenting a classically conditioned fear stimulus is abolished when leasoning the central (but not the basolateral) nuclei of the amygdala (Petrovich et al. 2009). Overall, an interconnected network of neural structures has been revealed which mediates reward perception and provides gateways to the engagement of feeding motivation and the organization of appropriate motor responses. In humans, a growing number of studies investigated the hypothesis that core structures of reward perception are sensitive to incentive value using functional neuroimaging (e.g., Arana et al. 2003; Killgore et al. 2003; Kringelbach et al. 2003; Beaver et al. 2006; Porubská et al. 2006; Schienle et al. 2009). Despite notable differences, the findings support the notion that incentive value modulates neural activity in core structures of reward processing.

142.3 Food Deprivation and Incentive Value

The understanding of the neural organization of reward perception provides a roadmap for the neuroscientific examination of deprivation effects in humans. Early studies investigating fasting and satiation effects on brain activity revealed that neural activity decreased among other regions in several structures of the motive circuitry including orbitofrontal cortex, insular cortex, basal ganglia, and hypothalamus in satiated as compared to hungry state (Tataranni et al. 1999; Delparigi et al. 2002, 2005). These findings imply that hunger may have profound effects on resting state activity of the motive circuitry in the absence of external stimulation.

More recent studies investigated the effects of food deprivation on food-related stimulus processing. Incentive motivation theory posits that incentive value of food items is modulated by physiological drive states (Toates 1981). According to this hypothesis, core structures of the motive circuitry are expected to show increased activity to food-related stimuli in deprived as compared to satiated state. To identify relevant studies, a literature research on public databases (PubMed, Web of Science) was conducted using a variety of key words (e.g., hunger, deprivation, eating, food). Nine studies were identified, which directly contrasted deprived and satiated state and measured brain activity in the motive circuitry to the presentation of food-related stimuli (Tables 142.1 and 142.2).

Hemodynamic measures were used in all studies with functional magnetic resonance imaging (fMRI) being more common than positron emission tomography (PET), in particular in most recent

Table 142.1 Schematic overview of fMRI- and PET-studies investigating deprivation effects on food stimulus processing

	N	Hours of deprivation (h)	Day time of session	Manipulation check	Assessment of eating	Method	Task	Stimuli
LaBar et al. (2001)	9 (8 women)	~8	5:00–8:00pm	Self-report		1.5 T fMRI Event-related Design	Control task	Pictures of foods and objects
Uher et al. (2006)	18 (10 women)	~24	12:30–1:30pm	Self-report Biochemical measures	Three Factor Eating Questionnaire	1.5 T fMRI Event-related & Block-Design	Evaluative rating task	Pictures of Foods and Objects; Taste of chicken broth, chocolate milk, saliva
Goldstone et al. (2009)	20 (10 women)	~16	11:00–12:00 am	Self-report	Dutch Eating Behavior Questionnaire SCOFF	3 T fMRI Block-Design	Evaluative rating task	Pictures of low- and high-caloric foods and objects
Hinton et al. (2004)	12 (0 women)	~18	12:30–1:30pm	Self-report Biochemical measures		PET Block-Design	Evaluative rating task	Low and high incentive menus
Piech et al. (2009)	8 (3 women)	~6	6:00–7:00pm	Self-report	History of eating disorder	1.5 T fMRI Event-related Design	Evaluative rating task	Low and high incentive menus
Morris and Dolan (2001)	10 (1 woman)	~16	4:00–5:00pm	Self-report Biochemical measures	History of eating disorder	PET Block-Design	Picture recognition task	Pictures of foods and objects
Mohanty et al. (2008)	7	~8	?	Self-report	Restrained Eating	3 T fMRI Mixed Event-related Design	Spatial attention task	Food and object pictures
Siep et al. (2009)	12 (12 women)	~18	1:00–3:00pm	Self-report	History of eating disorder; Restrained Eating	3 T fMRI Block-Design	Attention task: Attend taste, Attend objects, Attend bars	Pictures of low- and high caloric foods and objects
Haase et al. (2009)	18 (9 women)	~12	11:00–12:00am	Self-report	Three Factor Eating Questionnaire	3 T fMRI Event-related	No task	Taste stimuli: caffeine, saccharin, sucrose, sodium chloride, guanosin 5' monophosphate

Summary of selected methodological aspects of fMRI- and PET-studies examining food deprivation

Table 142.2 Key findings of deprivation effects

Study	Effect	Orbitofrontal cortex	Insular cortex	Amygdala	Striatum	Hypothalamus	Other regions
LaBar et al. (2001)	DEP			L			Fusiform R, Parahipp R
Uher et al. (2006)	Vision: DEP						Fusiform LR
Goldstone et al. (2009)	DEP x CAL	LR	LR	LR	LR, ventral		Hipp, ACC, DLPFC
	DEP: High vs. low CAL	LR	LR	LR	LR, ventral		
	SAT: High vs. low CAL						
Hinton et al. (2004)	DEP		L	R	LR	L	Thal L, Brainstem, ACC R
	Incentive	L		L			
	DEP x Incentive	L					
Piech et al. (2009)	Incentive	L, medial		L			
	DEP x Incentive	L, lateral					Cerebellum R
Morris and Dolan (2001)	Hunger		R, anterior	R, anterior	R, NAcc	R	Parahipp R, PCC LR, Brainstem PC R, Peristriate cortex L
Mohanty et al. (2008)	DEP x Picture			R			Fusiform, PCC
Siep et al. (2009)	DEP x Picture	LR, medial L, lateral	R		L		DLPFC R, MPFC R, Postcen L
Uher et al. (2006)	Taste: DEP		L, anterior				
Haase et al. (2009)	DEP: Sucrose	R	R	R	R		Parahipp LR, Thal R, Hipp LR
	DEP: Saccharin						Parahipp R, Thal R, Hipp R
	DEP: Caffeine				L	LR	Parahipp LR, Thal LR, Hipp R
	DEP: Citric acid	R	LR	LR	LR	R	Parahipp LR, Thal L, Hipp LR

This table summarizes the main findings of deprivation effects in structures of the motive circuitry and other brain regions

DEP deprivation, *CAL* calorie, *SAT* satiated, *L* left, *R* right, *ACC* anterior cingulate cortex, *DLPFC* dorsolateral prefrontal cortex, *Fusiform* fusiform gyrus, *Hipp* hippocampus, *MPFC* medial prefrontal cortex, *NAcc* nucleus accumbens, *PC* parietal cortex, *PCC* posterior cingulate cortex, *Parahipp* parahippocampal cortex, *Postcen* postcentral gyrus, *Thal* thalamus

studies. Accordingly, before considering empirical findings, basic principles of fMRI are briefly summarized. The technique is not measuring neural activity directly but associated epiphenomena, the local vascular response. Neuronal activation is associated with an increase in blood flow (cf., Logothetis 2008). For poorly understood reasons, the delivery of oxygenated hemoglobin is larger than local oxygen consumption. Oxygenated and deoxygenated hemoglobin have different magnetic properties and changes in their relative concentration can be revealed by magnetic resonance signals. Like other brain imaging methods assessing blood flow, temporal resolution is on the order of seconds as the changes in blood flow are relatively slow. However, spatial resolution is high as the brain is divided in small cubes (e.g., $1 \times 1 \times 1$ mm). The subtraction method is used to disclose deprivation effects on food cue processing in which the Blood Oxygenation Level Dependent (BOLD) signal to food cues under deprived versus satiated state is contrasted.

Three studies examined the processing of food and control pictures in deprived and satiated state. The first of these studies observed increased BOLD activity in the amygdala when viewing food pictures in a deprived state (LaBar et al. 2001). In contrast, Uher and colleagues (2006) observed no differential activity in the motive circuitry elicited by food pictures as a function of deprivation. A recent study revealed that deprivation effects in the motive circuitry may appear specifically to high-incentive food pictures (Goldstone et al. 2009). Pronounced increases in activation of orbitofrontal and insular cortex, amygdala, and striatum were observed when contrasting high- and low incentive stimuli during deprived but not satiated state. Presenting symbolic visual representations of food items, in particular of high incentive value, is accordingly sufficient to elicit motivational responding in humans. Two further studies relied to an even greater extent on the presentation of symbolic stimuli and mental imagery. Specifically, a restaurant-like situation was realized, in which participants' brain activity was measured while they read and chose between menus items consisting of entrée, dinner, and dessert which were tailored individually to be of low and high incentive value (Hinton et al. 2004; Piech et al. 2009). A PET-study revealed that food deprivation was associated with increased BOLD activity in several structures of the motive circuitry (see Table 142.2). Furthermore, regions in the orbitofrontal cortex were particularly activated when reading high incentive menu items in a deprived state (Hinton et al. 2004). Using an event-related fMRI design, a follow-up study revealed two regions in orbitofrontal cortex, which were similarly showing an interaction of incentive value and motivational state. In addition, irrespective of food deprivation, amygdala activation was increased for menu items of high compared to low incentive value (Piech et al. 2009). Overall, food deprivation increases the incentive value of visual representations of food-related stimuli in the motive circuitry, possibly specifically for high-incentive stimuli.

Deprivation effects on the processing of taste stimuli were investigated in two studies. The study by Uher and colleagues (2006) included a taste condition in which processing of chicken broth and chocolate milk was compared to a control condition (artificial saliva). Deprivation did not alter the activity in structures of the motive circuitry when processing these complex gustatory stimuli. Studying pure taste stimuli, a recent study revealed deprivation effects in the motive circuitry (Haase et al. 2009; see Table 142.2), which, however, were most pronounced for the highly pleasant sucrose and mildly unpleasant citric acid stimuli. Overall, these studies reveal a pattern of findings similar to studies examining visual processing.

From a theoretical perspective, these studies revealed deprivation effects on food stimulus processing either in passive viewing or in active attention conditions, which were low in processing demand. Recent research suggests that task focus may have pronounced effects on food processing even when comparing passive viewing with evaluative rating tasks (Bender et al. 2009). It is therefore interesting to consider studies in which deprivation effects were investigated while participants performed explicit tasks. The first of these studies (Morris and Dolan 2001) used PET to explore whether food deprivation specifically enhances the recognition of food pictures. Blocks of either food or non-food pictures were presented and participants' task was to indicate whether the seen pictures was included in a memory set presented immediate before the scanning took part. Furthermore, participants were initially tested in a deprived state and fed to satiety in the course of the experiment. Hunger ratings were positively correlated with BOLD activity in the insular cortex, Nc. Accumbens, and hypothalamus, irrespective whether participants viewed food or object pictures. Specificity for food picture processing was seen in the right posterior orbitofrontal cortex, which showed a positive relationship to hunger ratings. Several regions in the brain showed a relationship to memory performance, category-independent (e.g., orbitofrontal cortex) and category-dependent (e.g., left amygdala, insula), which, however, was not modulated by the motivational state. A second study examined the effects of spatial attention and food deprivation (Mohanty et al. 2008). The attention task consisted of valid, invalid, and neutrally cued responses to laterally presented target stimuli (donuts or tools) and foils (danishes and screws). In a mixed event-related paradigm, food and nonfood pictures were shown in separate blocks. Deprivation increased BOLD activity in the amygdala to blocks containing food pictures in a deprived as compared to a satiated state (see Table 142.2 for other regions). This finding was specific to food picture processing and not observed in blocks presenting tool items. A further aim of this study was to examine the relationship of anticipatory activity in neural structures of the spatial attention network and speed of responding. Deprivation specifically modulated anticipatory activity in parietal and posterior cingulate cortex during blocks of food targets. Furthermore, medial sectors of the orbitofrontal cortex were related to the performance in the attention task when hungry and lateral orbitofrontal cortex during satiety. A third study examined deprivation effects on the processing of high and low caloric food and object pictures in the context of an explicit object-based attention task (Siep et al. 2009). In separate blocks, attentional focus was directed either toward food items, towards the color of the picture, or to bars positioned at lateral sites of the pictures. A strict analysis revealed no significant three-way interaction of picture type, attention focus and deprivation. Less stringent analysis revealed that regions in the insular cortex, medial and inferior orbitofrontal cortex, and striatum showed an interaction between picture type (low calorie, high calorie food, objects) and deprivation. In these structures, low compared to high calorie stimuli seemed to elicit increased activity in the satiated state, while high compared to low calorie stimuli elicit increased activity in the deprived state. Furthermore, these effects were independent from the attention task. With regard to the effects of paying attention to food, activity in amygdala and orbitofrontal cortex was increased when food pictures where task relevant, however, the effect was similarly pronounced for low- and high calorie stimuli. Overall, deprivation effects were investigated in active task contexts by several studies adapting established paradigms from cognitive neuroscience. Albeit preliminary, evidence for modulations of incentive value by food deprivation seems ambiguous. Embedding food items in the structure of cognitive tasks may diminish their salience. The use of a passive viewing condition is recommended in order to determine the activation of structures of the motive circuitry independent from explicit task demands. Furthermore, although food stimuli are task-relevant in these studies, there are striking differences to natural situations in which goal-relevance of food stimuli serves to support adaptive behaviors.

One reading of the information depicted in Table 142.2 is that core structures of the motive circuitry are sensitive to both incentive value of food stimuli and internal state. However, there is considerable variety in experimental findings across studies. No single structure received unanimous support and positive findings showed considerable variability with regard to hemispheric lateralization. Consideration of methodological variables might be particularly informative to identify issues, which need to be addressed in future research (see Table 142.1).

The number of participants pronouncedly varied across studies raising the concern that differences in findings may simply arise because of differences in statistical power. While hours of deprivation greatly varied across studies (6–24 h), there seems no simple relationship to the observation of deprivation effects. However, considering also the great variance with regard to time of testing, circadian rhythm might moderate the effects of food deprivation on food-related stimulus processing. Overall, a paradigmatic approach seems valuable to empirically delineate appropriate sample sizes and hours of deprivation and to reveal circadian rhythm effects.

The majority of studies presented visual stimuli. Food pictures were presented in six studies with most recent studies varying caloric content of the stimulus materials. Written descriptions of menus (starter, entrée, dessert) were used in two studies, which individually varied preference for the menus. Obviously, the quality of stimulus materials is of great importance in revealing deprivation effects. The development of freely shared stimulus materials, calibrated according to major dimensions of eating and ingestion might facilitate progress in the field, similar to the development of the International Affective Picture Series (IAPS, Lang et al. 2008) in the domain of emotion research.

In summary, insights about the neural organization of the feeding system derived from animal research can serve as theoretical foundation to investigate the neural organization of the human feeding system in general, and regarding the effects of deprivation in particular. The rather small number of studies provides promising evidence for the hypothesis that core structures of the motive circuitry, associated with reward perception and adaptive behavior organization, are sensitive to variations in internal state. However, given the importance of deprivation, the widespread practice of voluntary restricting food intake by dieting and restrained eating, a much larger database is needed to realize the potential of the neuroscientific perspective on the understanding of both basic mechanism of food intake regulation and eating-related disorders.

142.4 Overfeeding, Satiation and Incentive Value

A complementary perspective on the effects of deprivation is provided by studies investigating sensory-specific satiety and overfeeding (see Tables 142.3 and 142.4). Several studies examined the phenomenon of sensory-specific satiety, which denotes that the incentive value and rated pleasantness decreases to food, which is eaten to satiety to a greater extent than for other foods. In an fMRI-study (O'Doherty et al. 2000), processing of vanilla and banana odors was investigated in two sessions (pre- and post-meal), which were identical with the exception that the second session took part after eating bananas to satiety. The orbitofrontal cortex was related to olfactory sensory-specific satiety showing a specific decrease in BOLD signal to banana odors in the post- as compared to the pre-meal condition. These findings are consistent with single cell recording in the orbitofrontal cortex of macaques, which revealed that olfactory neurons decreased responding to food odors eaten to satiety (Critchley and Rolls 1996). A further PET- study investigated changes in brain activity related to eating chocolate. Specifically, brain activity was measured while participants were given a single piece of chocolate immediately before the scanning period, tracking the hedonic experience of chocolate from being highly pleasurable to being highly aversive (Small et al. 2001). Among other regions (see Table 142.4), medial orbitofrontal cortex, insular cortex, and striatal regions showed a decrease in activity with increasing satiety. Of particular interest, lateral orbitofrontal cortex showed opposite effects, i.e., enlarged activity when chocolate was perceived as highly aversive. Accordingly, adding further evidence for the role of orbitofrontal cortex and sensory-specific satiety, medial and lateral orbitofrontal cortex appear to be selectively responsive during states in which approach and avoidance dispositions were dominant. Effects of sensory-specific satiety were furthermore investigated in the context of associative conditioning paradigm, in which odors were paired with task-relevant visual stimuli (Gottfried et al. 2003). Devaluation affected several structures of the motive circuitry

Table 142.3 Schematic overview of fMRI- and PET-studies investigating effects of satiation, and overfeeding

Study	N	Effect	Manipulation check	Method	Task	Stimuli
O'Doherty, et al. (2000)	5	Sensory-specific satiety	Self-report	3 T fMRI Block-Design	No task	Vanilla and banana odors
Small et al. (2001)	9 (5 women)	Sensory-specific satiety	Self-report	PET Block-Design	Evaluative rating task	Pieces of chocolate
Gottfried et al. (2003)	13	Sensory-specific satiety	Self-report	1,5 T fMRI Event-related Design	Reaction time task (CS) and Implicit associative conditioning	CS: Visual images US: Odors
Holsen et al. (2005)	9 children (5 women)	Pre- vs. Post meal		3 T fMRI Block-Design	Memory task	Pictures of foods, animals and objects
Cornier et al. (2007)	25 (13 women)	2 days of overfeeding	Control of food intake	3 T fMRI Block-Design	No task	Pictures of high- and low incentive foods and objects
Cornier et al. (2009)	22, thin (10 women) 19, reduced obese (10 women)	2 days of overfeeding	Control of food intake	3 T fMRI Block-Design	No task	Pictures of high- and low incentive foods and objects

Summary of selected methodological aspects of fMRI- and PET-studies examining satiation and overfeeding

Table 142.4 Key findings of effects due to satiation and overfeeding

Study	Effect	Orbitofrontal cortex	Insular Cortex	Amygdala	Striatum	Hypothalamus	Other regions
O'Doherty et al. (2000)	Pre-> post-meal	R					
Small et al. (2001)	rCBF decreases with decreasing reward value	LR, medial	LR		LR		ITG LR, MTG LR, OTG/Cereb LR, Hipp L, Thal L
	rCBF increases with decreasing reward value	R, lateral					Precen LR, IFG L, Cing, Parahipp R, SMA R, MFG, middle FC L
Gottfried et al. (2003)	Pre-> post-meal	L, rostral / R, caudal	R, anterior	L	L, ventral		ACC R
Holsen et al. (2005)	Motivational State x Picture Type	R, medial / LR lateral	L	R	R		MFG L, Oper LR, Parahipp R, Cing, Fusiform L, IFG R, SFG LR, ITG R, Postcen LR, Precen LR, Supra LR, Cereb/Fusiform R
Cornier et al. (2007)	EU>OF: (High Val> Low Val)					L	IVC R
Cornier et al. (2009)	Thin Subjects: EU>OF: (High Val > Obj)		X			X	
	(Thin > Reduced Obese): (EU>OF): (High Val > Obj)		LR			R	IVC R

This table summarizes effects of satiation and overfeeding on the activation of structures of the motive circuitry and other brain regions

EU eucaloric state, *OF* overfeeding, *High Val* high incentive food picture, *Low Val* low incentive food picture, *Obj* object picture, *L* left, *R* right, *ACC* anterior cingulate cortex, *Cereb* cerebellum, *Cing* cingulate cortex, *Fusiform* fusiform gyrus, *IFG* inferior frontal gyrus, *ITG* inferior temporal gyrus, *IVC* inferior visual cortex, *MFG* medial frontal gyrus, *middle FC* middle frontal cortex, *MTG* medial temporal gyrus, *OTG* occipitotemporal gyrus, *Oper* basal operculum, *Parahipp* parahippocampal gyrus, *PCG* posterior cingulate gyrus, *Postcen* postcentral gyrus, *Precen* precentral gyrus, *SFG* superior frontal gyrus, *SMA* supplementary motor area, *Supra* supramarginal gyrus, *Thal* thalamus, *rCBF* regional cerebral blood flow

(amygdala, ventral striatum, orbitofrontal cortex, insular cortex, see Table 142.4). Furthermore, regions in the amygdala and orbitofrontal cortex showed decreased BOLD signals specifically to the visual stimuli associated with the devalued odor while other brain regions (ventral striatum, insular cortex) showed both decreases and increases to visual stimuli paired with devalued and nondevalued odors, respectively. Investigating children, Holsen and colleagues (2005) presented food and object pictures in two sessions (pre- and post-meal) with participants eating a meal (500 kcal) in between the sessions. Amygdala, orbitofrontal cortex, and insular cortex showed a selective decrease to food pictures when comparing pre- and post-meal sessions. Two further studies investigated the effects of overfeeding on the processing of food (low and high incentive) and control pictures (Cornier et al. 2007; Cornier et al. 2009). Towards this end, participants were tested even after 2 days of either eucaloric or overfed (30% above eucaloric) energy intake. Overfeeding attenuated responding to high as compared to low incentive food pictures in the hypothalamus and inferior visual cortex (Cornier et al. 2007). These results were extended in a recent study investigating thin and obese participants, which reduced weight by 8% (Cornier et al. 2009). Regarding thin participants, food compared to object pictures elicited increased BOLD signals among other structures in orbitofrontal cortex, insular cortex, and ventral striatum in the eucaloric state. Overfeeding for 2 days resulted in reduced activity in these structures reaching significance in the insular cortex and hypothalamus. These effects of overfeeding were attenuated in obese participants. Overall, core structures of the reward matrix, in particular regions of the orbitofrontal cortex, showed a decrease in activity when fed to satiety.

142.5 The Motivational Regulation of Attention

The feeding system controls the organization of ingestive behaviors. Internal state and the perception of food-related cues from the immediate environment prime unique sets of perceptual-motor units that increase sensitivity to relevant stimuli at the appetitive and consummatory behavioral stage. According to this perspective, food deprivation effects operate at multiple levels, by increasing incentive value of food stimuli, and by regulating attention processes.

However, attention is not a unitary phenomenon but refers to a collection of disparate functional processes. For instance, recent research has begun to detail food deprivation effects on spatial attention mechanisms and object-based attention, which imply distinct neural mechanisms (Mohanty et al. 2008; Siep et al. 2009). Furthermore, attention is not only regulated according to explicit instructions by varying the task relevance of food stimuli, but is also passively captured by stimuli according to their motivational and emotional significance (Öhman 1986). When related to current motivational needs, stimuli may reflexively capture attentional resources to facilitate efficient responding.

Support for the obligatory nature of the motivational regulation of attention processes has been obtained in a study, in which food pictures were passively viewed, and participants performed an easy control task (detecting an occasional flicker of the images). Food deprivation enhanced the activity in higher order visual-associative regions (fusiform gyrus) when processing food pictures (LaBar et al. 2001). Conceptually similar results were observed when pictures were evaluated according to their likeability after viewing the pictures (Uher et al. 2006), but not when ratings of appealingness were made during picture viewing (Goldstone et al. 2009). Accordingly, although not explicitly designed to address the issue, there is some evidence that deprivation enhances attention processes to need-related food stimuli.

Two recent studies explicitly assessed the hypothesis that deprivation (24 h) sensitizes the processing of food cues (Stockburger et al. 2008, 2009a). Event-related brain potentials (ERPs) were measured in these studies, which provide a voltage measurement of neural activity that can be recorded non-invasively from multiple scalp regions. More specific, ERPs are considered to reflect summed post-synaptic potentials generated in the process of neural transmission and passively conducted through the brain and skull to the skin surface where they contribute to the electroencephalogram (EEG). Since ERPs are usually hidden in the larger background EEG activity, it is necessary to use multiple stimulus presentations and stimulus-locked signal averaging to extract the ERP signal from the background EEG activity. Biophysical considerations suggest that large-amplitude ERP components reflect widespread, synchronous sources in cortical regions. Brain activity locked to the processing of a stimulus becomes apparent as positive and negative deflections in the ERP waveform. The amplitude and latency of specific ERP components provide information regarding the strength and time course of underlying neural processes. Furthermore, given appropriate spatial sampling, the topography of ERP components can be used to estimate the neural generator sites by advanced analytic tools such as L2-Minimum-Norm-Estimate (L2-MNE; Junghöfer et al. 2006).

The first study was specifically designed to determine whether motivational state modulates early visual attention processes (Stockburger et al. 2008). A rapid serial presentation technique was used in which stimuli were presented for 330 ms without any perceivable interstimulus gap. Thus, this paradigm induces perceptually demanding conditions, which are deemed as necessary to reveal attention effects. Food stimuli were interspersed in a stream of pleasant, neutral, and unpleasant control stimuli drawn from various categories of human experience, which served as control stimuli to determine the specificity of deprivation effects on food picture processing. Results showed that deprivation specifically modulated the relatively early processing of food pictures. Between 170 and 320 ms, the ERP waveform revealed enhanced posterior positive deflections for food pictures in hungry compared to satiated state (Fig. 142.3a). MNE source calculations revealed that these deprivation effects on food processing were associated with primary activations in posterior perceptual representation networks. In addition, secondary activations were suggested over anterior brain regions (Fig. 142.3b). However, spatial resolution was insufficient to determine whether this finding

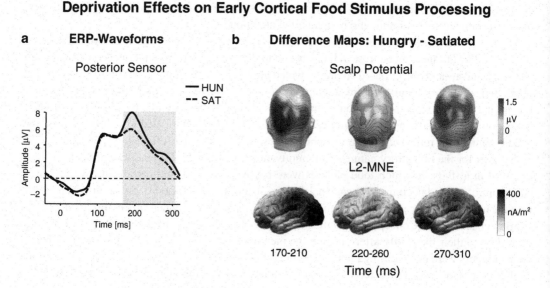

Fig. 142.3 (a) Representative ERP-waveforms for food pictures in the hungry (*red lines*) and satiated (*black lines*) states. (b) Scalp potential (*back view*) and L2-Minimum Norm estimates maps (right lateral view) show differences in processing food pictures in deprived and satiated state (Based on Stockburger et al. 2008)

relates to orbitofrontal activations, which were observed when comparing food cue processing in hungry and satiated state and food stimuli varying in their incentive value (O'Doherty et al. 2000; Morris and Dolan 2001; Arana et al. 2003). These findings suggest that perceptual stimulus processing is gated in specific ways according to motivational state. According to a functional perspective, ERP modulations in this time window have been considered to reflect a call for processing resources in later capacity-limited processing stages implicated in conscious stimulus recognition (cf. Öhman 1986; Schupp et al. 2006).

These later processing stages related to working memory and stimulus recognition were the focus of another study in which food and flower pictures were presented as rapid serial stream for 660 ms (Fig. 142.4a and b; Stockburger et al. 2009a). A consistent body of evidence revealed that emotionally relevant pictures elicit increased late positive potentials (LPP) between 350 and 700 ms post-stimulus (Schupp et al. 2006). Similarly, food deprivation specifically enhanced the LPP component to food pictures (Fig. 142.4c). The assumption that increased positive potentials to food pictures in a hungry state reflects enhanced processing is supported by L2-MNE analyses, which revealed increased dipole strength over extended posterior visual processing regions (Fig. 142.4d). Thus, consistent with its presumed relation to conscious stimulus recognition, the LPP is linked to widespread activation broadcasting stimulus information to many associative cortical regions rather than reflecting local processing (Del Cul et al. 2007). Overall, in a state of food deprivation, food pictures seem to elicit a state of heightened selective attention in a capacity-limited processing stage, which is a critical gateway for the stimulus representation in working memory and conscious stimulus recognition. Furthermore, these findings were observed while participants passively viewed the stimulus materials and the food images were not task relevant. Consequently, the motivational regulation of visual processing appears to be a spontaneous and involuntary phenomenon, important characteristics of automatic processes.

Overall, electrophysiological measures of brain activity allow delineating the regulation of attention processes at the level of distinct processing stages. Internal motivational state sensitizes responding to need-related stimuli in processing stages mandatory for stimulus recognition. This mechanism seems highly adaptive from a functional perspective. The selective responding and evaluation of need-relevant stimuli is critical for the efficient organization of food-related behaviors.

142.6 Food Deprivation and the Startle Reflex

To obtain reliable measures of brain activity related to stimulus processing, neuroimaging methods require repeated stimulus presentations. Accordingly, in the case of food deprivation, stimuli are presented while participants are denied access to food. Unfortunately, the motivational orientation elicited in these protocols is potentially ambiguous. On the one hand, viewing food-related stimuli in deprived state may prompt associated appetitive responses. Alternatively, a state of frustrative non-reward may be induced, if participants are denied the immediate consumption of food.

Studies utilizing the startle probe methodology (see Table 142.5) may help to resolve this issue (Drobes et al. 2001; Mauler et al.2006). This research builds upon the notion that responding to emotionally and motivationally significant stimuli is organized by two basic brain circuits, one prompting appetitive responding and pleasant affects, and the other determining withdrawal and defense behaviors and unpleasant affect. The measurement of the defensive startle reflex allows inferring the engagement of basic motive systems, which is potentiated when elicited during an aversive state and inhibited during pleasant states. In their study, Drobes and colleagues (2001) presented a series of food pictures as well as emotional and neutral control pictures varying level

Deprivation Effects on Later Cortical Food Stimulus Processing

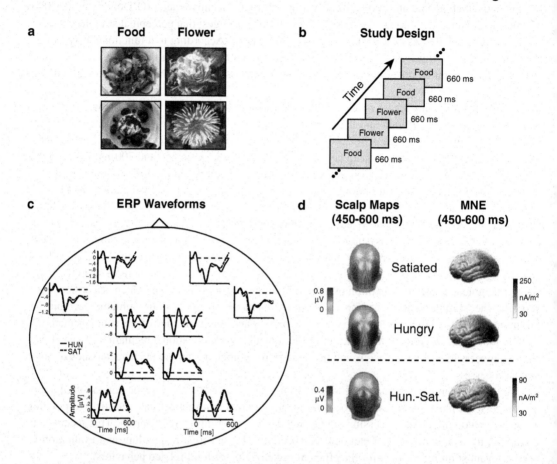

Fig. 142.4 (**a**) Representative examples of the food and flower stimuli. (**b**) Illustration of the rapid serial visual presentation paradigm. Food and flower pictures were presented for 660 ms without perceivable interstimulus gap. (**c**) Representative ERP-waveforms for food pictures in the hungry (*red lines*) and satiated (*black lines*) states. (**d**) Scalp potential (*back view*) and L2-Minimum Norm estimates maps (right lateral view) show the topography of the LPP component for food and the difference between the hungry and satiated states (Based on Stockburger et al. 2009a)

Table 142.5 Key features of the startle reflex

1. The startle reflex is a defense response that prevents organ injury and interrupts ongoing mental and behavioral activity
2. The startle reflex is a whole body response that consists of rapid flexor movements cascading throughout the body
3. The reflex is elicited by sudden, unexpected, and intense stimuli. In the laboratory, acoustic stimuli (e.g., 50 ms duration, 90–110 dB loudness, and instantaneous rise time) are often used to elicit the reflex
4. Rapid eye closure is among the most reliable components of the startle response in humans and measured by recording the electrical activity of the orbicularis oculi muscle
5. The acoustic blink reflex shows an onset latency of ~20–40 ms and usually peaks between 50 and 100 ms
6. While the startle reflex is an obligatory response, its magnitude varies as a function of emotional, motivational, and attentional processes

This table lists the key features of the startle reflex

of food deprivation across subjects (0, 6, 24h). In a nondeprived state, food pictures revealed inhibited startle responses as compared to the other picture materials suggesting that these cues prompt an appetitive approach disposition. In contrast, startle reflexes elicited during food picture viewing were potentiated for both deprivation levels as compared to the nondeprived group. These findings were considered to reflect an aversive motivational reaction, which is attributed to a state of frustrative non reward, i.e., participants were not allowed immediate consumption (Drobes et al. 2001). However, another line of studies revealed that the active imagination of pleasant scenes triggered enhanced startle reflexes compared to neutral imagery contents (Miller et al. 2002). An alternative interpretation of the Drobes et al. (2001) and Mauler et al. (2006) findings is accordingly, that viewing food pictures elicited vivid imagination in the participants. Resolving the issue is of great theoretical importance and the startle probe methodology may serve as promising tool to disambiguate motivational orientation elicited by internal deprivation state and external food cue reactivity.

142.7 Applications to Other Areas of Health and Disease

Revealing the effects of food deprivation with regard to incentive value and attention processes provides highly relevant information for the obesity pandemic. The voluntary restriction of food intake for regulating body weight is an increasing phenomenon in many Western cultures. Such attempts in dieting and restrained eating are often accentuated towards foods considered as fattening (e.g., sweets, high-fat food). Specific food restrictions may be also due to moral and health concerns as is the case for instance in vegetarianism. It seems highly informative to determine the specificity of food restrictions on the processing of food stimuli with particular emphasis of affective attitudes and short- and long-term effects. For instance, a recent event-related brain potential study revealed the increased attention capture of meat pictures in vegetarians refraining from eating meat for several years (Stockburger et al. 2009b). Understanding food deprivation effects may be furthermore relevant in understanding eating disorders such as anorexia nervosa and bulimia.

Summary Points

- At the core of the feeding system are neural circuits that were laid down early during evolutionary history, in primitive cortex, sub-cortex, and midbrain.
- These motivational circuits are engaged by unconditioned food-related stimuli, determine general mobilization and approach behaviors of the organism, and mediate the shaping of the feeding system by learning and experience.
- Internal state variables exert a profound effect on the feeding system and neuroimaging methods appear promising to provide novel insights into the operation of food deprivation.
- Hemodynamic studies were reviewed providing some support for the notion that food deprivation increases the incentive value of food-related stimuli in core structures of the motive circuitry. There is evidence that these effects appear most robust for high-incentive stimuli.
- Furthermore, attention to need-related stimuli is regulated by motivational state. Event-related potential studies delineate motivated attention processes with high temporal resolution suggesting that deprivation effects facilitate perceptual processing in stages related to stimulus recognition and working memory representation.

- Guided by animal research about the neural organization of the feeding system, electrophysiological, hemodynamic, and reflex measures of brain activity provide a window to probe deprivation effects on food stimulus processing.
- Given the sparse number of relevant studies, a considerable research effort is needed to reveal consistent and reliable findings related to deprivation.
- Understanding these effects seems important when considering that attempts to regulate body weight and eating-related disorders often include the voluntary restriction of food intake.

Key Terms

Ingestive behavior: Ingestive behaviors are comprised by appetitive and consummatory phases which depend on the integration of information about internal state, cues from the environment, behavioral state, and cognition.

Incentive motivation: Incentives arouse motivated behaviors and form the target for goal-direct behaviors. Incentive motivation is determined by external stimuli and internal states.

Motive circuitry: Cortical, subcortical, and brainstem neural structures implicated in reward perception and activation of adaptive behaviors.

Functional magnetic resonance imaging: Neural activity is coupled with blood oxygenation level dependent (BOLD) signal changes that can be measured with MRI. Assessment of short-term changes can be used to infer functional neural activity associated with food stimulus processing in core structures of the motive circuitry.

Motivated attention: In natural environments, attention is dictated by motivational significance of salient stimuli and internal states.

Event-related brain potentials: Electrophysiological recordings of brain activity associated with food stimulus processing. Providing a high temporal resolution, event-related potential recordings allow measuring the motivational regulation of attention by food deprivation.

Acknowledgments We thank Tobias Flaisch and Christoph Becker for their feedback on an earlier version of this manuscript. This work was supported by the German Research Foundation (grant Schu 1074/11-2, Schu 1074/10-3), by the European Community FP7 (grant 'TEMPEST', 223488), and the German Federal Ministry of Education and Research (grant 'EATMOTIVE', 0315671).

References

Arana FS, Parkinson JA, Hinton E, Holland AJ, Owen AM, Roberts AC. J Neurosci. 2003;23:9632–8.
Barbano MF, Cador M. Behav Neurosci. 2005;119:1244–53.
Beaver JD, Lawrence AD, van Ditzhuijzen J, Davis MH, Woods A, Calder AJ. J Neurosci. 2006;26:5160–6.
Bender G, Veldhuizen MG, Meltzer JA, Gitelman DR, Small DM. Eur J Neurosci. 2009;30:327–38.
Berridge KC, Kringelbach, ML. Psychopharmacology 2008;199:457–80.
Berthoud HR, Morrison C. Annu Rev Psychol. 2008;59:55–92.
Cornier MA, Von Kaenel SS, Bessesen DH, Tregellas JR. Am J Clin Nutr. 2007;86:965–71.
Cornier MA, Salzberg AK, Endly DC, Bessesen DH, Rojas DC, Tregellas JR. PLoS One. 2009;4:e6310.
Critchley HD, Rolls ET. J Neurophysiol. 1996;75:1673–86.
Del Cul A, Baillet S, Dehaene S. PLoS Biol. 2007;5:2408–23.
Delparigi A, Gautier JF, Chen K, Salbe AD, Ravussin E, Reiman E, Tataranni, PA. Ann N Y Acad Sci. 2002;967:389–97.
Delparigi A, Chen K, Salbe AD, Reiman EM, Tataranni PA. NeuroImage. 2005;24:436–43.
Drobes DJ, Miller EJ, Hillman CH, Bradley MM, Cuthbert BN, Lang PJ. Biol Psychol. 2001;57:153–77.

Goldstone AP, de Hernandez CG, Beaver JD, Muhammed K, Croese C, Bell G, Durighel G, Hughes E, Waldman AD, Frost G, Bell JD. Eur J Neurosci. 2009;30:1625–35.

Gottfried JA, O'Doherty J, Dolan RJ. Science 2003;301:1104–7.

Haase L, Cerf-Ducastel B, Murphy C. NeuroImage 2009;44:1008–21.

Hinton EC, Parkinson JA, Holland AJ, Arana FS, Roberts AC, Owen AM. Eur J Neurosci. 2004;20:1411–8.

Holland PC, Gallagher M. Curr Opin Neurobiol. 2004;14:148–55.

Holsen LM, Zarcone JR, Thompson TI, Brooks WM, Anderson MF, Ahluwalia JS, Nollen NL, Savage CR. NeuroImage 2005;27:669–76.

Junghöfer M, Peyk P, Flaisch T, Schupp HT. Prog Brain Res. 2006;156:123–43.

Kalivas PW, Nakamura M. Curr Opin Neurobiol. 1999;9:223–7.

Keys A, Brozek J, Henschel A, Mickelson O, Taylor HL. The biology of human starvation. 2 vols. Minneapolis: University of Minnesota Press; 1950.

Killgore WD, Young AD, Femia LA, Bogorodzki P, Rogowska J, Yurgelun-Todd DA. NeuroImage 2003;19:1381–94.

Kringelbach ML, O'Doherty J, Rolls ET, Andrews C. Cereb Cortex. 2003;13:1064–71.

Lang PJ, Bradley, MM, Cuthbert BN (2008). International affective picture system (IAPS): Affective ratings of pictures and instruction manual. Technical Report A-8. University of Florida, Gainesville, FL.

LaBar KS, Gitelman DR, Parrish TB, Kim YH, Nobre AC, Mesulam MM. Behav Neurosci. 2001;115:493–500.

Logothetis NK. Nature 2008;12:869–78.

Mauler BI, Hamm AO, Weike AI, Tuschen-Caffier B. J Abnorm Psychol. 2006;115:567–79.

Miller MW, Patrick CJ, Levenston GK. Psychophysiology 2002;39:519–29.

Mohanty A, Gitelman DR, Small DM, Mesulam MM. Cereb Cortex. 2008;18:2604–13.

Morris JS, Dolan RJ. J Neurosci. 2001;21:5304–10.

O'Doherty J, Rolls ET, Francis S, Bowtell R, McGlone F, Kobal G, Renner B, Ahne G. Neuroreport 2000;11:893–7.

Öhman A. Psychophysiology 1986;23:123–45.

Pavlov IP. Zwanzigjährige Erfahrungen mit dem objektiven Studium der höheren Nerventätigkeit (des Verhaltens) der Tiere. Berlin: Akademischer; 1953.

Petrovich GD, Holland PC, Gallagher M. J Neurosci. 2005;25:8295–302.

Petrovich GD, Ross CA, Mody P, Holland PC, Gallagher M. J Neurosci. 2009;29:15205–12.

Pickens CL, Saddoris MP, Setlow B, Gallagher M, Holland PC, Schoenbaum G. J Neurosci. 2003;23:11078–84.

Piech RM, Lewis J, Parkinson CH, Owen AM, Roberts AC, Downing PE, Parkinson JA. PLoS One. 2009;4:e6581.

Polivy J. J Am Diet Assoc. 1996;96:589–92.

Porubská K, Veit R, Preissl H, Fritsche A, Birbaumer N. NeuroImage 2006;32:1273–80.

Raynor HA, Epstein LH. Appetite 2003;40:15–24.

Schienle A, Schäfer A, Hermann A, Vaitl D. Biol Psychiatry. 2009;65:654–61.

Schupp HT, Flaisch T, Stockburger J, Junghofer M. Prog Brain Res. 2006;156:31–51.

Schupp HT, Stockburger J, Codispoti M, Junghöfer M, Weike AI, Hamm AO. J Neurosci. 2007;27:1082–9.

Siep N, Roefs A, Roebroeck A, Havermans R, Bonte ML, Jansen A. Behav Brain Res. 2009;198:149–58.

Small DM, Zatorre RJ, Dagher A, Evans AC, Jones-Gotman M. Brain 2001;124:1720–33.

Smith KS, Tindell AJ, Aldridge JW, Berridge KC. Behav Brain Res. 2009;196:155–67.

Spiegel TA, Shrager EE, Stellar E. Appetite 1989;13:45–69.

Stockburger J, Weike AI, Hamm AO, Schupp HT. Behav Neurosci. 2008;122:936–42.

Stockburger J, Schmalzle R, Flaisch T, Bublatzky F, Schupp HT. NeuroImage 2009a;47:1819–29.

Stockburger J, Renner B, Weike A, Hamm AO, Schupp HT. Appetite 2009b;52:513–6.

Swanson LW. Brain Res. 2000;886:113–64.

Tataranni PA, Gautier JF, Chen K, Uecker A, Bandy D, Salbe AD, Pratley RE, Lawson M, Reiman EM, Ravussin E. Proc Natl Acad Sci USA. 1999;96:4569–74.

Timberlake W. In: Mowrer RR, Klein SB, editors. Handbook of contemporary learning theories. Mahwah: Erlbaum; 2001. p. 155–209.

Timberlake W, Allison J. Psychol Rev. 1974;81:146–64.

Toates FM. Appetite 1981;2:35–50.

Uher R, Treasure J, Heining M, Brammer MJ, Campbell IC. Behav Brain Res. 2006;169:111–9.

Watts AG, Swanson LW. In: Gallistel CR, Pashler H, editors. Stevens' handbook of experimental psychology, volume 3, learning, motivation, and emotion. New York: Wiley; 2002. p. 563–631.

Woods SC, Schwartz MW, Baskin DG, Seeley RJ. Annu Rev Psychol. 2000;51:255–77.

Chapter 143
Symptoms of Starvation in Eating Disorder Patients

Riccardo Dalle Grave, Elettra Pasqualoni, and Giulio Marchesini

Abbreviations

DSM   Diagnostic and Statistical Manual of Mental Disorders
NOS   Not otherwise specified

143.1 Introduction

The DSM-IV classification of eating disorders includes three main diagnostic categories: anorexia nervosa, bulimia nervosa, and eating disorders not otherwise specified (NOS) (American Psychiatric Association 1994). Underweight is a key diagnostic criterion for anorexia nervosa, but could be present in a subgroup of patients with eating disorder NOS (e.g., underweight patients that meet all DSM-IV criteria for AN except amenorrhea (Dalle Grave et al. 2008b) or the overevaluation of shape and weight (Dalle Grave et al. 2008c)). Severe weight loss and dietary restriction (i.e., a persistent caloric intake lower than energy expenditure) could also be present in a subgroup of not underweight eating disorder patients with bulimia nervosa or eating disorder NOS with an history of obesity.

Keys and his colleagues in their classic two-volume, 1,385-page text *The Biology of Human Starvation* (Keys et al. 1950) gave a detailed description of the symptoms of dietary restriction and underweight, traditionally called "starvation symptoms," reported by young male volunteers. The observation that many symptoms reported by the volunteers were similar to those found in patients with anorexia nervosa improved the understanding and the treatment of eating disorders (Garner 1997). Today, it is widely accepted that many symptoms, once attributed to the psychopathology of anorexia nervosa, are the mere consequences of severe weight loss and caloric restriction.

R. Dalle Grave (✉)
Department of Eating and Weight Disorder, Villa Garda Hospital,
Via Montebaldo 89, I-37016 Garda (VR), Italy
e-mail: rdalleg@tin.it

V.R. Preedy et al. (eds.), *Handbook of Behavior, Food and Nutrition*,
DOI 10.1007/978-0-387-92271-3_143, © Springer Science+Business Media, LLC 2011

The chapter has three main aims: (1) to review the symptoms associated with underweight and dietary restriction; (2) to describe the role of underweight and dietary restriction in the maintenance of eating disorder psychopathology; (3) to analyze the clinical implications of these symptoms in the treatment of eating disorders.

143.2 Symptoms Associated with Underweight and Dietary Restriction (Starvation Symptoms)

The Minnesota study is considered the key reference on the effect of dietary restriction and weight loss in normal weight individuals. The study was carried out at the University of Minnesota between November 19, 1944 and December 20, 1945 (Keys et al. 1950). The study was designed to evaluate the physiological and psychological effects of severe and prolonged dietary restriction and the effectiveness of nutritional rehabilitation strategies. The principal aim of the study was to guide the assistance to famine victims in Europe and Asia during and after the World War II by using the data derived by a laboratory simulation of severe famine.

More than 100 men were ready to volunteer in the study as an alternative to military service. Of this initial sample, 36 men with the best physical and psychological health and with a high motivation to participate were selected (Keys et al. 1950). The participants were all white males in the age range from 22 to 33 years. Of the 36 volunteer individuals, 25 were members of the Historic Peace Churches (Mennonites, Church of the Brethren, and Quakers).

The study was divided in three phases: a control period of 12 weeks, 24 weeks of semistarvation, and 12 weeks of rehabilitation. During the control period the mean daily caloric intake of the participants was 3,492 calories, during the period of semistarvation the calories were decreased to a mean of 1,570, and during the period of rehabilitation they were re-increased to normal levels. In the semistarvation period, participants were fed foods most likely consumed in European famine areas and lost approximately 25% of their body weight.

Complete data are available only for 32 participants because 4 participants interrupted the study during or at the end of the second phase of semistarvation. The individual reactions to semistarvation and to the weight loss were heterogeneous, but in most cases the participants experienced dramatic effects (see Table 143.1).

143.2.1 Behavioral Effects

Toward the end of the starvation phase the participants spent almost 2 h to eat a meal that they previously consumed in few minutes. Many participants read cookbooks and collected recipes. Some increased coffee and tea consumption, drank large amount of water or soups to increase their fullness, and developed specific eating rituals (e.g., eating very slowly, cutting the food in small pieces, mixing the food in a bizarre way, ingesting hot food). The use of salt, spices, and gums increased, and also nail-biting and smoking. Many of these behaviors persisted also during the 12-week weight restoration phase.

During the semistarvation period, all participants reported a significant increase hunger. However, some were able to tolerate it, while others had bulimic episodes followed by self-criticism. In the weight restoration phase, when participants had access to a large amount of foods, some lost control eating, ingesting more or less than necessary. After 5 months of rehabilitation, most of the participants normalized their eating habits, but a subgroup continued to eat large amount of foods.

Table 143.1 Starvation effects reported by the Minnesota Study (Keys et al. 1950)

Behavioral effects
- Eating rituals (eating very slowly, cutting the food in small pieces, mixing the food in a bizarre way, ingesting hot food).
- Reading cookbooks and collecting recipes
- Increasing coffee and tea consumption
- Increasing the use of salt, spices, gums, hot soup, and water
- Nail-biting
- Increased smoking
- Bulimic episodes
- Increasing exercise to avoid the reduction of the caloric content of the diet
- Self-mutilation

Psychological effects
- Impairment of concentration capacity
- Poor insight and critical judgment
- Preoccupation about thought on food and eating
- Depression
- Mood lability
- Irritation
- Hunger
- Anxiety
- Apathy
- Psychotic episodes
- Personality changes

Social effects
- Social withdrawal
- Loss of sexual appetite

Physical effects
- Abdominal pain
- Gastrointestinal discomfort
- Sleep disturbances, vertigo
- Headache
- Strength reduction
- Hypersensitivity to light and noises
- Edema
- Cold intolerance
- Paresthesia
- Reduction of basal metabolism
- Reduce of heart and respiratory frequency.

Many participants reduced their habitual level of physical activity and complained that they had less energy. However, some individuals used intense exercise to be allowed a larger amount of food or to avoid a reduction in the caloric content of the diet.

143.2.2 Psychological Effects

Most of the participants showed marked cognitive and emotional changes. They reported a decreased concentration capacity, insight, and critical judgment, while no changes in intellectual ability were observed. The impairment in concentration capacity was probably due to the presence of recurrent thoughts on food and eating that were reported by most of the participants.

Some suffered periods of depression, while others had frequent periods of mood changes. A subgroup became irritated and developed episodes of hunger explosion. Anxiety and apathy were common, and in a subgroup of participants the emotional disturbances became so severe that the authors coined the term "starvation neurosis" to describe them. The emotional changes were confirmed by the Minnesota Multiphasic Personality Inventory that showed a significant increase in depression, hysteria, and hypochondria. Two participants developed psychotic symptoms and one self-mutilated three fingers of his hand to modulate his mood. In general, the emotional changes did not disappear immediately after rehabilitation, but persisted for many weeks. However, some participants did not show any psychological deterioration during the entire study period.

143.2.3 Social Effects

Starvation had also a large effect on social functioning. Participants become inward-looking and self-focused, which led to social isolation. In general, they also reported a loss of sexual appetite, another effect that could have contributed to social withdrawal.

143.2.4 Physical Effects

The most frequent symptoms reported by participants during the dietary restriction phase were abdominal pain, difficult digestion, sleep disturbances, vertigo, headache, strength reduction, hypersensitivity to light and noises, edema, cold intolerance, sight and hearing alterations, and paraesthesias. Participants showed a marked reduction in their basal metabolism (almost a 40% decrease), as well as in heart and respiratory frequency. During the weight restoration phase their basal metabolic rate increased proportionally to the increased caloric intake and they regained their baseline body weight after a weight loss of 25% or more of initial body weight.

143.2.5 Comments by Participants to the Minnesota Starvation Experiment

In 2003–2004, 18 of the 36 participants were still alive and were interviewed by researchers of The Johns Hopkins School of Medicine, Baltimore, MD (Kalm and Semba 2005). Participants were in their 80s when interviewed and each spoke passionately when discussing why they chose to be a conscientious objector and to participate in the experiment. Although the data of the study have been reported with scientific details in *The Biology of Human Starvation* book, participants painted a more vivid picture of their daily lives during the experiment (Kalm and Semba 2005). They reported that, after an initial enthusiasm, they suffered great changes in their personalities during semistarvation. They became increasingly irritable and impatient with one another and began to suffer the physical effect of caloric restriction. They also reported an increase of introversion, less energy, dizziness, extreme tiredness, cold intolerance, muscle soreness, hair loss, reduced coordination, ringing in their ears, and poor concentration. Food became an obsession for all the participants, and several men confirmed that interest in women and dating was lost soon after study began. Despite the difficulties of starvation, they reported a strong determination to continue the study, and suggested different reasons for their dedication, including religious reasons, discipline, and will power (Kalm and Semba 2005).

For some men, the rehabilitation period was considered the most difficult part of the experiment. They reported that symptoms of dizziness, apathy, and lethargy were the first to decrease, while feelings of tiredness, loss of sex drive, and weakness were much slower to improve. They reported not being back to normal by the end of the 3-month recovery period. Many overate after they left Minnesota and became obese. They estimated that the time to achieve a full recovery ranged from 2 months to 2 years (Kalm and Semba 2005). However, none of the participants believed they experienced any negative long-term health effects as a result of the experiment (Kalm and Semba 2005).

143.3 Starvation Symptoms in Eating Disorders

The starvation study had a fundamental role in improving our understanding of eating disorders because many symptoms observed in the volunteers are similar to those reported by underweight eating disorder patients. However, to date no study has evaluated the prevalence of starvation symptoms in eating disorder individuals. Table 143.2 reports the prevalence of starvation symptoms in the

Table 143.2 Prevalence of starvation symptoms in the last 28 days reported by 50 consecutive patients with anorexia nervosa (mean BM 15.3 kg/m² – range 11.7–17.4 kg/m²)

Symptoms	Percent (%)
Preoccupation with thoughts about eating and eating	90
Irritability	82
Anxiety	78
Depression	76
Mood changes	66
Sleep disturbance	66
Social withdrawal	56
Weakness	56
Gastrointestinal discomfort	56
Cold intolerance	56
Impaired concentration	54
Apathy	50
Heightened satiety	50
Low body temperature	38
Eating very slowly	38
Reduction in sexual interest	38
Heightened sensation of fullness	36
Heightened sensation of hunger	32
Cutting the food in small pieces	30
Collecting cookbooks and recipe books	28
Increasing the consumption of coffee or tea or spice	28
Personality changes	28
Hoarding food	24
Eating hot food	24
Noise intolerance	22
Tingling	20
Edema at the legs	18
Binge eating	16
Light intolerance	16
Hearing voices in the head	4
Hallucinations	0

last 28 days reported by 50 outpatients with anorexia nervosa consecutively assessed before starting treatment at the Department of Eating and Weight Disorder, Villa Garda Hospital. Starvation symptoms were assessed with the Starvation Symptoms Check List (see Appendix). About 90% of the patients reported preoccupation with thoughts about food and eating, and 82% irritability. Other symptoms reported by at least 50% of patients were anxiety, depression, mood changes, sleep disturbances, social withdrawal, weakness, gastrointestinal discomfort, cold intolerance, impaired concentration, apathy, and heightened satiety.

143.4 Interaction of Starvation Symptoms with Eating Disorder Psychopathology

The effects of starvation symptoms in individuals with eating disorders are different from those observed in subjects without these disorders. In the absence of eating disorder psychopathology, starvation symptoms lead individuals to focus their attention primarily towards food searching, and when food becomes available, they eat without being concerned about losing their control of body shape and weight. On the contrary, the presence of the eating disorder psychopathology (i.e., the overvaluation of shape, weight, and their control) (Fairburn et al. 2003) interacts with starvation symptoms maintaining the eating disorder (see Table 143.3 for the proposed general mechanisms).

In particular, it has been suggested that some symptoms of starvation stimulate further dietary restriction by undermining the person's sense of being in control over their eating, shape, weight, or themselves in general (Fairburn et al. 1999), while other symptoms exaggerate the tendency to use control over eating as an index of self-control in general (Shafran et al. 2003). It has also been proposed that some eating disorder individuals interpret the symptoms of starvation as a positive sign of being in control and as evidence that they are working hard to achieve their goal of controlling eating, shape, and weight (Shafran et al. 2003). Support for these hypotheses is provided by two studies. The first study found that patients with eating disorders were significantly more likely to interpret four symptoms of starvation (hunger, poor concentration, heightened satiety, and reduction in rate of weight loss) as a proof of control (Shafran et al. 2003). The second study found that a significantly higher proportion of inpatient eating disorder patients interpret the symptoms of hunger, heightened satiety, and dizziness in terms of control when compared to nonclinical participants (Dalle Grave et al. 2007) (see Table 143.4 for clinical examples).

Table 143.3 Proposed mechanisms through which starvation symptoms maintain the eating disorder psychopathology (Dalle Grave et al. 2007; Shafran et al. 2003; Fairburn 2008)

1. Underweight and dietary restriction symptoms increase the need to get control over their eating, shape, weight, or themselves in general.
2. Preoccupation with food and eating keeps the eating disorder mindset permanently "in place"
3. Social withdrawal and loss of previous interests prevent the development of other domains of self-evaluation
4. The maintenance of underweight requires the adoption of a hypocaloric diet that maintains the preoccupation with food and eating
5. Indecisiveness makes it difficult for patients to decide whether to change (procrastination)
6. Heightened need for routine and predictability interferes with change
7. Heightened feeling of fullness makes it difficult to increase the amount of food.

Table 143.4 Examples of how eating disorder patients may interpret some starvation symptoms

Symptoms	Dysfunctional interpretation of eating disorder patients
Hunger	I am controlling my diet
	I have to increase my attention to avoid losing control over eating
Sense of fullness	I eat too much, I have to reduce the calories of my diet
Binge eating	I am weak, I have to increase my control over eating
Reduction in the rate of weight loss	I am losing control over my weight. I have to reduce the amount of food I eat
Mood instability	I am not in control. I have to increase my control over eating, weight, and shape
Dizziness	It is a positive sign that I am losing weight
Poor concentration	I am losing control. I have to increase my control over eating

143.5 Clinical Implications

The knowledge of starvation symptoms and how they interact with eating disorder psychopathology have important implications both for the understanding and the treatment of eating disorders.

Clinicians should be informed that many psychosocial symptoms reported by underweight eating disorder patients are the consequences of dietary restriction and underweight and not the expression of their eating disorder psychopathology. These symptoms are not related only to food and eating, but extend to the whole range of psychosocial functions. Since many symptoms reported by eating disorder patients, often suggested to be the cause of their disorder, are indeed the consequences of underweight and dietary restriction, clinicians should be aware that the weight must be completely restored before a final assessment of the psychological functions and personality of their patients is accurately performed (Garner 1998).

Patients should be educated on the starvation symptoms and on the Minnesota study (Garner 1997; Garner et al. 1997). This recommendation is based on the assumptions that patients with eating disorders often have misconceptions about the cause of their symptoms and may be less likely to continue their efforts to maintain underweight if they informed about the scientific data on the maintenance of their disorder (Garner 1998). They also should be helped to change their dysfunctional interpretation of starvation symptoms, since a subgroup of patients tend to view some of these symptoms as a positive sign of being in control (Shafran et al. 2003; Fairburn et al. 1999). Finally, they should be helped to achieve a healthy body weight since the maintenance of caloric restriction and underweight is a mechanism maintaining their eating disorder psychopathology (Fairburn 2008). Educational material on starvation symptoms for underweight eating disorders patients (Garner 1997) and manuals for clinicians describing the procedures and the strategies to address underweight and caloric restriction in eating disorder patients are available (Dalle Grave et al. 2008a; Fairburn 2008).

143.6 Applications to Other Areas of Health and Disease

The dissemination of the knowledge about symptoms associated with underweight and caloric restriction could help to improve the assessment and the treatment of the following conditions associated with underweight and low calorie intake (the list is not complete):

- AIDS
- Alcoholism
- Alzheimer's disease

- Anxiety
- Cancer
- Celiac disease
- Chronic heart disease
- Chronic lung disease
- Chronic renal disease
- Clinical depression
- Cystic fibrosis
- Dementia
- Denture difficulties
- Dysphagia
- Infections
- Inflammatory bowel disease
- Lactose intolerance
- Malabsorption
- Poverty and lack of food
- Stomach ulcer
- Stomatitis
- Systemic lupus erythematous
- Schizophrenia
- Tuberculosis
- Uncontrolled diabetes mellitus

Summary Points

- Underweight is a key diagnostic criterion for anorexia nervosa, but could be present in a subgroup of patients with eating disorder NOS (e.g., underweight patients who meet all DSM-IV criteria for anorexia nervosa except amenorrhea or the overvaluation of shape and weight).
- Severe weight loss and dietary restrictions are also present in a subgroup of nonunderweight eating disorder patients with bulimia nervosa or eating disorder NOS with previous obesity.
- Underweight and dietary restrictions are associated with several physical and psychosocial symptoms ("starvation symptoms").
- Many psychosocial symptoms observed in underweight eating disorder individuals are the consequences of underweight and dietary restriction and not the expression of their psychopathology or personality.
- The most frequent starvation symptoms reported by eating disorder patients are preoccupation with thoughts about food and eating and irritability.
- Starvation symptoms interact with eating disorder psychopathology stimulating further dietary restrictions by undermining the individuals' sense of being in control over their eating, shape, weight, or themselves in general
- Some eating disorder individuals interpret the symptoms of starvation as a positive sign of being in control and as evidence that they are working hard to achieve their goal of controlling eating, shape, and weight.
- The treatment of eating disorder patients with underweight and/or caloric restrictions should include education on starvation symptoms, strategies to change their dysfunctional interpretation of starvation symptoms, and to favor weight regain

Definitions and Explanations

Dietary restriction: Persistent caloric intake lower than energy expenditure
Eating disorders: Persistent disorder of eating behavior and/or of behaviors aimed to modify or control the shape and weight, associated with an overvaluation of shape and weight and with significant physical and psychosocial impairment not secondary to any medical or psychiatric condition known.
Overvaluation of shape and weight and their control: Judging themselves predominantly or even exclusively in term of weight, shape, and their control (it is considered the core psychopathology of eating disorders).
Starvation symptoms: Symptoms associated with dietary restriction and underweight.
Starvation neurosis: Emotional disturbances associated with dietary restriction and underweight.

Key Points

1. The presence of starvation symptoms should always be evaluated in eating disorder patients.
2. The weight must be completely restored before carrying out an accurate assessment of the psychological functions and personality of eating disorder patients
3. Eating disorder patients should be educated that the maintenance of dietary restriction and underweight is associated with severe physical and psychosocial impairment.
4. Since starvation symptoms are potent mechanisms maintaining eating disorder psychopathology, the treatment of underweight eating disorders should <u>always</u> address underweight and dietary restriction.

Appendix: Starvation Symptoms Check List

Riccardo Dalle Grave

Instructions: The following questions are concerned with the past 28 days only. Please read each questions with attention. Please answer all the questions circling the appropriate number on the right. Thank you

On how many of the past 28 days ...	No. days	1–5 days	6–12 days	13–15 days	16–22 days	23–27 days	Every day
1. Have you spent much time thinking about eating and food?	1	2	3	4	5	6	7
2. Have you collected cookbooks and recipes?	1	2	3	4	5	6	7
3. Have you cut food into small pieces?	1	2	3	4	5	6	7
4. Have you hoarded food?	1	2	3	4	5	6	7
5. Have you eaten very slowly?	1	2	3	4	5	6	7
6. Have you eaten hot food?	1	2	3	4	5	6	7
7. Have you increased the consumption of coffee or tea or spice?	1	2	3	4	5	6	7

(continued)

Appendix (continued)

On how many of the past 28 days …	No. days	1–5 days	6–12 days	13–15 days	16–22 days	23–27 days	Every day
8. Have you eaten a large amount of food with the sensation of losing control over eating?	1	2	3	4	5	6	7
9. Have you been depressed?	1	2	3	4	5	6	7
10. Have you been anxious?	1	2	3	4	5	6	7
11. Have you been irritable?	1	2	3	4	5	6	7
12. Have you had mood changes?	1	2	3	4	5	6	7
13. Have you heard voices in your head?	1	2	3	4	5	6	7
14. Have you had hallucinations?	1	2	3	4	5	6	7
15. Have you noticed some change in your personality?	1	2	3	4	5	6	7
16. Have you been withdrawn socially?	1	2	3	4	5	6	7
17. Have you found it difficult to concentrate?	1	2	3	4	5	6	7
18. Have you been apathetic?	1	2	3	4	5	6	7
19. Have you had sleep disturbances?	1	2	3	4	5	6	7
20. Have you felt weak?	1	2	3	4	5	6	7
21. Have you had gastrointestinal discomfort?	1	2	3	4	5	6	7
22. Have you been intolerant to noise?	1	2	3	4	5	6	7
23. Have you been intolerant to light?	1	2	3	4	5	6	7
24. Have you felt your legs or other part of your body swollen?	1	2	3	4	5	6	7
25. Have you had a low body temperature?	1	2	3	4	5	6	7
26. Have you felt some tingling?	1	2	3	4	5	6	7
27. Have you felt a reduction of sexual interest?	1	2	3	4	5	6	7
28. Have you felt cold?	1	2	3	4	5	6	7
29. Have you felt an increase in hunger?	1	2	3	4	5	6	7

(continued)

Appendix (continued)

On how many of the past 28 days …	No. days	1–5 days	6–12 days	13–15 days	16–22 days	23–27 days	Every day
30. Have you felt an increase in your sense of satiety?	1	2	3	4	5	6	7
31. Have you felt full after eating?	1	2	3	4	5	6	7

In females:
How many periods have you had in the last 3 months?...................
Have you been taking the "pill" ?...................

References

American Psychiatric Association. Diagnostic and statistical manual of mental disorders 4th ed. Washington, D.C: American Psychiatric Association; 1994.

Dalle Grave R, Bohn K, Hawker D, Fairburn CG. In Fairburn CG, editors. Cognitive behavior therapy and eating disorders. New York: Guilford Press 2008a: p. 231–44.

Dalle Grave R, Calugi S, Marchesini G. Behav Res Ther. 2008b;46:1290–94.

Dalle Grave R, Calugi S, Marchesini G. Int J Eat Disord. 2008c; 41:705–12.

Dalle Grave R, Di Pauli D, Sartirana M, Calugi S, Shafran R. Eat Weight Disord. 2007;12:108–13.

Fairburn CG. Cognitive Behavior Therapy and Eating Disorders. New York: Guilford Press; 2008.

Fairburn CG, Cooper Z, Shafran R. Behav Res Ther. 2003;41:509–28.

Fairburn CG, Shafran R, Cooper Z. Behav Res Ther. 1999;37:1–13.

Garner DM. In: Garner DM, Garfinkel PE, editors. Handbook of treatment for eating disorders. New York: Guilford Press; 1997. p. 145–177.

Garner DM, Vitousek K, Pike K. In: Garner DM, Garfinkel PE, editors. Handbook of treatment for eating disorders. New York: Guilford Press; 1997. p. 94–144.

Garner DM. Health Weight J. 1998;12:68–72.

Kalm LM, Semba RD. J Nutr. 2005;135:1347–52.

Keys A, Brozek J, Henschel A, Mickelsen O, Taylor HL. The biology of human starvation. Minneapolis: University of Minnesota Press; 1950.

Shafran R, Fairburn CG, Nelson L, Robinson PH. Behav Res Ther. 2003;41:887–94.

Chapter 144
Epigenetics and Nutrition: B-Vitamin Deprivation and its Impact on Brain Amyloid

Sigfrido Scarpa

Abbreviations

AD	Alzheimer Disease
C	Cytosine
CpG	Cytosine-Guanine Dinucleotides
SAM	S-Adenosylmethionine
SAH	S-Adenosylhomocysteine
HCY	Homocysteine
GSH	Glutathione
DNMT	DNA-Methyltransferase
ATP	Adenosyntriphosphate
CBS	Cystathionine-Beta-Synthase
B6	B6 Vitamin
B12	B12 Vitamin
B9	B9 Vitamin, Tetrahydrofolate
MP	Methylation Potential
APP	Amyloid-Precursor-Protein
Abeta	Beta Amyloid
PS1	Presenilin 1, Gamma-Secretase
BACE	Beta-Secretase
PD	Parkinson's Disease
ADMA	Asymmetric Dimethylarginine
NO	Nitric Oxide
DDAH	Dimethylarginine-Dimethylaminohydrolase
NOS	Nitric Oxide Synthase
PP2A	Phosphatase-2A
Tau	Tau Protein
TgCRND8	Transgenic Mice Carrying a Human Transgene with a Double Mutation Swedish/Indiana

S. Scarpa (✉)
Dip. di Chirurgia "P. Valdoni", Centro di Ricerca in Neurobiologia
"Daniel Bovet" CriN, Sapienza Università di Roma,
via Antonio Scarpa, 14, 00161 Roma, Italy
e-mail: sigfrido.scarpa@uniroma1.it

V.R. Preedy et al. (eds.), *Handbook of Behavior, Food and Nutrition,*
DOI 10.1007/978-0-387-92271-3_144, © Springer Science+Business Media, LLC 2011

144.1 Introduction

B vitamin deficiency, namely B12, B9 (folate), and B6, is linked to hyperhomocysteinemia, to brain amyloid overproduction and to aging in one of the most devastating disease in the elderly: Alzheimer's Disease (AD).

Aging is a progressive decrease of the physiological capacity to react to stress arising from the environment, leading to increased susceptibility and vulnerability to disease. Although the activity of the brain and the individual psychology plays a major role for such phenomena through unknown mechanisms, the physiology of aging it appears must be controlled by epigenetic mechanisms that made it possible for evolution to increase our lifespan. When approaching the maximum potential lifespan humans have to face physiological modifications and diseases most likely due to alteration of those epigenetic mechanisms that enhance early survival but could be disadvantageous later in life (Egger et al. 2004; Troen 2003). One of these is evidently AD, which increases proportional to lifespan. The study of non-DNA sequence-related heredity, as epigenesis can be defined, is becoming the epicenter of modern medicine because it is beginning to clarify the relationship between genetic background, environment, aging, and disease. Although DNA sequence remains essentially the same, the epigenetic state may vary among tissues and during the lifetime; in other words, it may be responsible for phenotypic plasticity in age-related modifications. Vitamin deficiency, either due to defective nutrition or to pathology, is among the elements capable of modifying the epigenetic mechanisms in the direction of disease. The new fact is that alteration of these mechanisms is not measurable by genetic defect or pathogenic elements, but could result in the modification of gene expression regulation. Over-production of brain amyloid due to hypomethylation of at least one specific gene promoter has been shown in recent years in several publications (Fuso et al. 2007, 2009; Scarpa et al. 2003, 2006). In these papers, the authors demonstrated that B vitamin deficiency (B6, B12, and folate) may be responsible for amyloid overproduction, whether in brains of transgenic mice or in human cell culture. Widespread loss of DNA methylation was observed in colorectal cancers in 1983 and thereafter a large number of reports of either hypomethylation of oncogenes or hypermethylation of oncosuppressor genes, which may result in a variety of cancers. The most fascinating aspect of epigenesis is the possibility of reversing its changes, unlike sequence mutations in disease, which could lead to a host of new therapeutic tools.

In this review the impact of those nutritional elements – B vitamins and catabolites like homocysteine – that may influence epigenetic mechanisms by altering the metabolism of methyl donor, will be discussed.

144.2 DNA Methylation

The study of DNA methylation in aging is extremely topical because of its implication in tumorigenesis, since cancer onset increases with aging. The general decrease in total genomic methylcytosine during aging in various organisms and the apparently finite number of cell divisions, characteristic of most somatic cells, reinforces the view of overall methylcytosine loss as a cellular timing mechanism that triggers senescence. Nevertheless, it is important to underline the fact that the methylation status of the majority of examined genes seems to be intact during aging. The alterations in CpG island methylation are crucial to modulate binding of transcription factors and methyl-DNA binding proteins. Aberrant methylation of CpG islands in the promoter region may contribute to the progressive inactivation of growth-inhibitory genes during aging, resulting in the clonal selection of cells with a growth advantage towards cancer development. Alterations in DNA methylation during aging can depend on alterations in dietary status. The great influence of nutritional components on health and lifespan is largely accepted. Among the various mechanisms by which nutritional elements could affect the progress of senescence, two pathways involve DNA methylation: the first concerns the supply of metabolites of the S-adenosylmethionine cycle (SAM, folic acid, and B vitamins), whereas the second refers to elements able to directly modify the DNA-methyltransferase (DNMT) activity (selenium, cadmium, and nickel). Clear indications of methylation alterations come from studies on aging, on various noncommunicable diseases (Prader-Willi, Angelman's, and Beckwith-Wiedemann syndromes) and on various diseases related to aging (Down's syndrome, Alzheimer's, Parkinson's, and Huntington's diseases). Changes in chromatin structure are related to epigenetic modifications that consist of DNA methylation, histone post-transcriptional modifications (methylation, acetylation, and phosphorylation) and ATP-mediated chromatin modifications. In proliferating cells, DNA is principally found as euchromatin in actively transcribed loci like the growth regulatory genes. Conversely, it has been proposed that reassembly of repressive chromatin domains (heterochromatin) may contribute to cellular senescence. The main tool of epigenetic control on gene expression seems to lie in the CpG sequence, irrespective of whether this sequence contains a methyl group bound on C (Razin and Riggs 1980). We should bear in mind that although most studies have been dedicated to DNA, methylation processes have to do also with RNA, proteins, and lipids (Chiang et al. 1996). Regulation of gene expression through DNA methylation consists of the methylation or demethylation of cytosines in CpG sequences that eventually present in the gene promoters of those genes whose regulation is controlled by methyl groups. There is a basic difference between sequences that are normally unmethylated (Bergman and Mostoslavsky 1998), like CpG islands (Cross et al. 1997), and the CpG moieties belonging to genes expressed during development that are silenced later by methylation for physiological reasons. The former may become methylated for a pathogenetic mechanism, for example in the inactivation of oncosuppressor genes in cancer, and the latter may gradually lose their methylation and therefore overexpress genes that should be downregulated.

144.3 Epigenetic Mechanisms

At the molecular level, the biochemical modifications of DNA and histone proteins are the major epigenetic mechanisms. Additional mechanisms, involving RNA interference and prion proteins contribute as well to epigenetic regulation (Levenson and Sweatt 2006), but will not be included here. Essentially, chromatin modifications comprise DNA methylation at cytosine–guanine dinucleotides and post-translational modifications of histone proteins. Post-translational histone modifications, because of their chemical properties, influence the condensation of chromatin and therefore modulate the accessibility of DNA to the transcriptional machinery. DNA methylation is functionally most relevant when present in sequences rich in CpG dinucleotides: the CpG islands. These regions with more than 500 base pairs in size and with a C+G density higher than 55% (Takai and Jones 2002) have been conserved during evolution because they are normally unmethylated. The completion of human genome sequencing revealed that about 50% of all genes contain CpG islands within their regulatory elements (Venter et al. 2001) and they are stably methylated in transcriptionally silenced genes. Epigenetic control of gene expression by cytosine methylation is made possible by the activity of DNA methyltransferases (DNMTs) (Hitchler and Domann 2007). These enzymes catalyze transmethylation of cytosines by transferring methyl groups from S-adenosylmethionine (SAM) to position 5 of the pyrimidine ring with production of 5-MeC in DNA. Cytosine methylation in mammalian genomes is mainly carried out by three DNMTs: DNMT1, DNMT3a, and DNMT3b. Maintenance

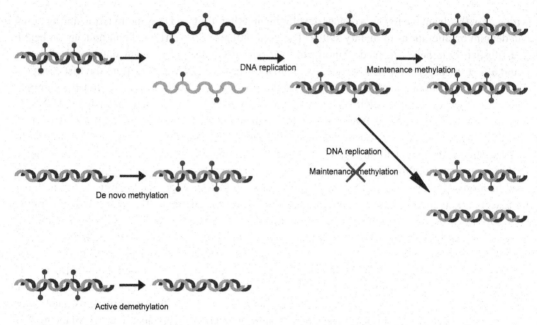

Fig. 144.1 Schematic representation of DNA methylation. DNA methylation and demethylation mechanisms: maintenance methylation, passive demethylation, de novo methylation, and active demethylation

methylation is catalyzed by DNMT1 and occurs rapidly following DNA replication. DNMT1 has the primary role of passing on epigenetic control of gene expression to daughter cells (Kautiainen and Jones 1985). De novo DNA methylation is catalyzed by DNMT3a and DNMT3b, which are primarily responsible for initiating new epigenetic events regulating gene expression. De novo methylation can occur anytime following DNA replication (Fig. 144.1). This epigenetic event can be passed on during future cell divisions. These enzymes were identified and cloned in 1998 (Okano et al. 1998, 1999; Xie et al. 1999).

144.4 DNA Demethylation

Soon after Holliday and Pugh proposed that DNA methylation could control gene expression (Holliday and Pugh 1975) it became clear that, besides the possibility of inhibiting DNA methylases (maintenance and de novo), to obtain demethylation, global demethylation known to occur during early embryogenesis has to rely on an active mechanism (Kapoor et al. 2005). The author of this chapter participated in the first study showing active demethylating activity in cell culture (Razin et al. 1986). Since then three active demethylation mechanisms have been proposed, none of which has been widely accepted (Kress et al. 2001). The first is direct replacement of the methyl moiety by a hydrogen atom. The other two both involve DNA repair processes: the second mechanism proposes the removal of methyl-C by nucleotide excision followed by replacement with an unmethylated one (Weiss et al. 1996; Weiss and Cedar 1997), the third one postulated the participation of RNA molecules and appears to have gained support by key experimental observations, although the demethylase involved has not yet been cloned. Having ascertained that DNA undergoes the establishment of an inherited methylation pattern in adult organisms (Fig. 144.2), with the formation of stably activated

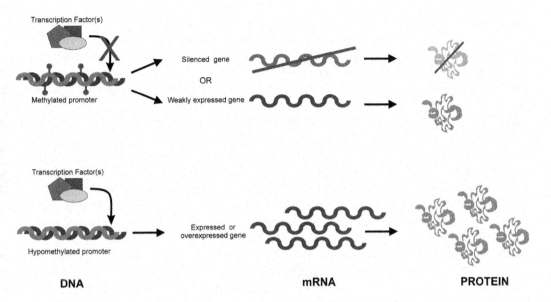

Fig. 144.2 Schematic model of methylation-dependent gene expression

genes (mostly demethylated), stably silenced genes (mostly fully methylated), and genes with specific methylation patterns able to be induced by reassessment of methyl moieties, it should be explained what mechanisms control the donation of methyl groups.

144.5 Central Role of SAM

In the last fifty years SAM has been shown to be perhaps the most frequently used substrate, after ATP, and therefore occupies a central position in human health, disease, and aging. SAM is known to be the primary methyl-donor present in eukaryotes and it is involved in methylation of target molecules as DNA, RNA, proteins, lipids, and polyamines synthesis (Fontecave et al. 2004; Lu 2000). SAM is probably second only to ATP in the variety of reactions in which it is involved; the most important ones are transmethylation, transsulfuration, and aminopropylation, which occur due to the presence of the high-energy sulfonium ion, which activates each of the attached carbons toward nucleophilic attack. SAM was discovered in 1951 by Giulio Cantoni as an important molecule in methylation reactions (Cantoni 1951, 1953; Kresge et al. 2005). It is a conjugate of methionine at the sulfur atom with adenosine, a reaction catalyzed by methionine–adenosyltransferase. SAM appears to be altered in some neurological disorders, including AD (Bottiglieri and Hyland 1994). About 95% of SAM is engaged in methylation reactions. It is then transformed in S-adenosylhomocysteine (SAH) and further hydrolyzed into homocysteine (HCY) and adenosine. The reaction is strongly reversible and HCY, if not rapidly transformed in methionine or cystathionine, forms SAH, which is a potent inhibitor of methyl-transferases. These metabolic alterations may be responsible for the generalized reduction of DNA methylations observed in aging. HCY exerts a pathogenic effect, at very high concentrations, through the alteration of oxidative metabolism, but it can even generate a pathological situation at concentrations just above normal by modifying the methylation pattern. Remethylation of homocysteine to form methionine, along with the transsulfuration pathway prevents HCY accumulation. Accumulation of homocysteine has been a great concern for human health since hyperhomocysteinemia is present both in cardiovascular diseases and dementia. Many clinical studies have been undertaken to verify whether supplementation of human nutrition with B vitamins to lower homocysteine would be beneficial for health (Mason et al. 2008; Refsum and Smith 2008; Smith et al. 2008; Smith 2008). There seems to be a growing consensus that lowering homocysteine with vitamin supplementation does not solve the problem. Probably not enough attention has been paid to SAM production and SAH accumulation. The SAM metabolism is strictly controlled by B12 and B9 (tetrahydrofolate), except when remethylation of homocysteine to methionine occurs through betaine reaction, in its transmethylation pathway. Betaine reaction though seems to be absent in the brain. The second pathway, derived from SAM catalytic reactions to form homocysteine, is trans-sulfuration where B6 vitamin plays a fundamental role in the transformation of homocysteine to L-cystathionine to finally produce glutathione (Fig. 144.3). To mention another SAM activity, it has been shown (Lichtenthaler et al. 1999) that it functions as an allosteric activator of cystathionine beta-synthase (CBS), by increasing the enzyme activity about threefold. Low SAM concentrations generate low CBS activity, with the result that HCY is directed toward the transmethylation pathway. The result is lesser glutathione production. This alteration is exerted by poor uptake of B6 vitamin.

The most common alteration of this metabolism is the decreased uptake of vitamin B (folate, B12, and B6) with consequent HCY accumulation and SAM/SAH alteration. Diminished uptake of B12 and folate can be determined by a number of nutritional events as well as by pathological ones. *Helicobacter pylori*, which is very common in the population and very hard to eradicate, is known to

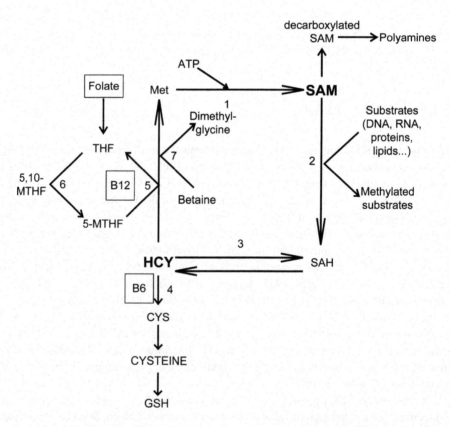

Fig. 144.3 SAM metabolism. *Met* Methionine, *SAM* S-adenosylmethionine, *SAH* S-adenosylhomocysteine, *HCY* Homocysteine, *CYS* Cystathionine, *GSH* Glutathione, *THF* Tetrahydrofolate, *MTHF* methyltetrahydrofolate, *B12* Vitamin B12, *B6* Vitamin B6, (1) Methionine adenosyltransferase (MAT); (2) Methyltransferase(s); (3) SAH hydrolase; (4) Cystathionine-β-synthase (CBS); (5) Methionine synthase; (6) Methylenetetrahydrofolate reductase (MTHFR); (7) Betaine homocysteine methyltransferase (BHMT)

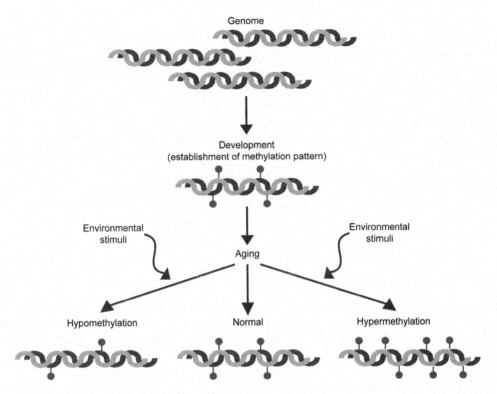

Fig. 144.4 Modifications of DNA methylation pattern with aging. DNA methylation pattern is established during embryonal development and tissue differentiation. Environmental stimuli occurring during the lifespan could generate abnormal modifications of the DNA methylation pattern in specific genes

have this effect. The result will again be the alteration of the SAM metabolism. Accumulation of amyloid protein in the brain is a clear example of this alteration. SAH increase affects SAM/SAH ratio; this is an important indicator of cellular methylation status and is usually indicated as Methylation Potential (MP) (Chiang et al. 1996; Fuso et al. 2008; Lee and Wang 1999). Although there is some disagreement about this parameter, biochemically, SAH concentration is an undiscussed indicator for appropriate methylation.

Aside of the physiological function, these epigenetic phenomena may be influenced by alterations of metabolites and of the enzymes part of the methyl-donor (SAM) metabolic cycle which may be responsible for reduced brain concentrations in elderly (Morrison et al. 1996). The consequent demethylation and overexpression of genes would not be regulated, but rather induced by reduced synthesis of the methyl-donor or by inhibition of methylases. Recent experiments on TgCRND8 mice seem to show the second hypothesis to be the most common. With the aging of an organism, the general decrease of DNA methylation can lead to overactivation of methylation-controlled genes (Fig. 144.4).

144.6 SAM and Brain Amyloid

Alzheimer's Disease (AD) is becoming one of the most common pathologies in the aging population, leading also to increased social cost and impact, because of the increase in life expectation. Besides a familial (genetic) form of the disease, which has an early onset, the higher percentage of cases is represented by the sporadic occurrence of AD with onset at an advanced age.. Whereas it is becoming increasingly evident which is the pool of molecules involved in the pathogenesis, the causes of this form of AD are not yet well understood. Alzheimer's disease is neuropathologically characterized by the presence of amyloid plaques and neurofibrillary tangles in the brain. Amyloid plaques are extracellular deposits primarily composed of amyloid beta-peptide, which is derived from amyloid beta-precursor protein (APP) by sequential cleavages at beta-secretase and gamma-secretase sites. Neurofibrillary tangles represent intracellular bundles of self-assembled hyperphosphorylated tau protein. In recent years, hyperhomocysteinemia has began to be widely considered a risk factor in AD and this may be ascribed to alteration of the S-adenosylmethionine/homocysteine (SAM/HCY) metabolism (Seshadri et al. 2002). In fact, a frequently observed condition in AD-affected people is the increase of haematic HCY along with the decrease of B12, B6, and folate uptake (Bottiglieri 1996; Joosten 2001; Quadri et al. 2004; Selhub et al. 2000). In AD, the loss of precise control through gene methylation may alter a delicate equilibrium among the three enzymes (alpha-, beta-, and gamma-secretases) known to be involved in the production of either amyloid-beta or other nondangerous catabolites (De Strooper 2000). It is well established that alpha-secretase cleavage of APP does not produce the amyloidogenic peptides and that, on the contrary, they are produced by the activity of beta-secretases that generate an N-terminal soluble fragment and a C-terminal fragment that is sequentially cleaved by gamma-secretase to produce A-beta peptides (Tabaton and Tamagno 2007; Vassar et al. 1999; Vassar 2005). The alteration of SAM/SAH ratio is tightly related to the altered expression of two genes involved in APP metabolism, finally producing the accumulation of A-beta peptide in the senile plaque. Previous papers in cell culture showed that two of the genes responsible for amyloid-beta production (PS1 and BACE, i.e., gamma and beta secretases) are upregulated by vitamin B deficiency; exogenous SAM administration can restore the normal gene expression, thus reducing amyloid levels (Fig. 144.5) (Cavallaro et al. 2006; Fuso et al. 2005; Scarpa et al. 2003, 2006). Moreover, a study on mice carrying the transgenic beta-amyloid-protein precursor (APP) showed that vitamin B deprivation was able to induce PS1 and BACE upregulation and increased Abeta deposition (Fuso et al. 2008). Accumulation of HCY and DNA hypomethylation are metabolically related since the lack of transformation of HCY to methionine reverts the metabolism to SAH, which is a strong inhibitor of DNA methyltransferases, therefore inducing DNA hypomethylation (Chiang et al. 1996). Therefore, hypomethylation may be a mechanism through which HCY exerts its toxicity in AD and promotes amyloidogenesis.

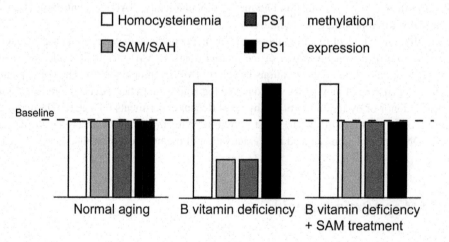

Fig. 144.5 Effect of B vitamin deficiency and SAM supplementation in TgCRND8 Alzheimer mice. Vitamin B deficiency causes hyperhomocysteinemia, decrease of SAM/SAH ratio and PS1 methylation, and upregulation of PS1 mRNA expression. SAM treatment, although it cannot completely revert high HCY can normalize the other parameters

144.7 SAM and Oxidative Stress

Increasing evidence demonstrates that oxidative stress is implicated in a number of age-related disorders among which are AD, Parkinson's disease (PD), and atherosclerosis. Hyperhomocysteinemia is a risk factor for atherosclerotic vascular disease and AD as well, and it is associated with increased oxidative stress. The central nervous system is particularly vulnerable to free radical damage owing to high brain oxygen consumption, its abundant polyunsaturated fatty acid content, and its relative paucity of anti-oxidant enzymes compared with other tissues (Guidi et al. 2006; Migliore et al. 2005; Vitvitsky et al. 2006; Zafrilla et al. 2006). Increased concentrations of HCY in the plasma of AD patients are associated with an increase of asymmetric dimethylarginine (ADMA) and a decrease in nitric oxide (NO) plasma concentrations, through inhibition of DDAH (dimethylarginine dimethylaminohydrolase, the enzyme that converts ADMA into citrulline and dimethylamine). ADMA is an endogenous inhibitor of nitric oxide synthase (NOS), and it is synthesized during the process of protein arginine methylation by SAM and subsequent hydrolysis. ADMA accumulation impairs cerebral blood flow. Brain infarcts and atherosclerosis increase the incidence and the severity of symptoms of AD patients; therefore, accumulation of ADMA may contribute to the development of AD by increasing the incidence of atherosclerosis and stroke (Selley 2003; Siroen et al. 2006; Stuhlinger et al. 2001). Moreover, the toxic effect of HCY in atherosclerosis is mainly due to the stimulation of inflammatory response through oxidative reactions, since HCY is involved in the synthesis of GSH, the major cellular antioxidant.

144.8 SAM and Tau Protein

Microtubule-associated tau protein is a phosphoprotein whose phosphorylation is regulated. The main physiological function of tau is the promotion of the assembly and stabilization of the microtubular network, which is essential for normal axonal transport of vesicles within the neuron. In humans, tau protein undergoes several post-translational modifications, such as abnormal phosphorylation, which plays a significant role in the formation of neurofibrillary pathology. Phosphorylated tau has a reduced capability of binding to microtubules and hyperphosphorylation contributes to the formation of pathological tau filaments. This leads to destabilization of the microtubular network and subsequent impairment of microtubule-associated axonal transport. The modification of tau by phosphorylation is regulated by the equilibrium between kinase and phosphatase enzymes. Previous works suggest that a decrease in Phosphatase 2A (PP2A) activity, rather than an increase in kinase activity, is crucial for the elevated levels of aberrant protein phosphorylation in AD. PP2A is abundantly expressed in the brain and its abnormal function has been demonstrated to be associated with AD. Expression of a mutant form of PP2A in mouse brain causes a marked decrease in PP2A activity and induces AD-like hyperphosphorylation of tau at specific serine/threonine residues (Kins et al. 2001). In vivo, PP2A enzymes predominantly exist as heterotrimers containing a catalytic subunit (C), a scaffolding subunit (A), and a regulatory subunit (B). The highly conserved carboxyl-terminal sequence of the C subunit can undergo post-translational modifications like methylation on the Leu-309 residue by a specific methyltransferase (PPMT). This modification critically modulates the binding of regulatory B subunits to the (AC) core enzyme, thereby affecting PP2A substrate specificity, targeting, and cellular function (Evans and Hemmings 2000; Wei et al. 2001; Yu et al. 2001). It has been observed that PPMT expression and PP2A methylation become downregulated in AD (Sontag et al. 2004). Nicola et al. 2010 showed that alteration in the SAM/HCY cycle results in decreased PP2A methylation. Reduced PP2A methylation is associated with B subunit down regulation and accumulation of phosphorylated tau (Sontag et al. 2007;

Zhang et al. 2008). Moreover, other papers showed that PP2A mRNA expression levels were increased in AD fibroblast (Zhao et al. 2003). These data suggest a double regulation both at gene and protein level.

144.9 Conclusions

Amyloid-beta has erroneously been considered toxic, but although several functions have been recently postulated, it is not yet clear which is the main one. Abeta becomes dangerous only when abundant and in oligomeric or polymeric forms. Dimers and trimers of beta-amyloid are now considered the first cause of AD onset and memory loss. These observations have quite changed the diffused idea that assigned the onset of AD to senile plaques. Recently it was demonstrated (Fuso et al. 2008) that the two genes responsible for Amyloid-beta production, beta (BACE) and gamma (PS1) secretases, are regulated by vitamin B deficiency and by SAM supplementation. Moreover, we showed that feeding either neuroblastoma cells with culture medium deficient of B12, B6, and folate, or TgCRND8 transgenic mice with food deficient in the same vitamins increased Abeta production (Fuso et al. 2005, 2008). The administration of methyl-donor has the opposite effect: it reduced significantly Abeta levels by remethylating the genes (Fuso et al. 2010). It is evident that whereas genetic factors are clearly associated with early-onset form of AD, epigenetic factors could be more easily linked to late-onset AD, since the epigenome is prone to changes during development and also aging (Bird 2007; Dolinoy 2007). The gene control mechanism here described is being studied in vivo for therapeutic applications (Table 144.1).

Table 144.1 Key epigenetic mechanisms possibly involved in Alzheimer's disease

Gene	Epigenetic modification	Treatment suggested	References
APP	APP cleavage product (AICD) recruits HAT TIP60 suggesting potential hyperacetylation.	None	Cao and Sudhof (2001)
	APP-induced death of cortical neurons causes H3 and H4 hypoacetylation.	None	Rouaux et al. (2003)
PS1	PS1 mutations prevent CBP degradation resulting in abnormal gene expression, potentially through hyperacetylation.	Substitution of PS1-mediated enzymatic activity	Marambaud et al. (2003)
	PS1 conditional knockout mice have decreased CBP level and CBP-mediated gene expression.	None	Saura et al. (2004)
	Hypomethylation of PS1 promoter increases Abeta production.	SAM administration reverses hypomethylation silencing gene and reduces Abeta production.	Fuso et al. (2009); Scarpa et al. (2003)
BACE	Vitamin B deficiency increases BACE expression and induces Abeta production.	Treatment with methyl-donor reduces BACE expression by unknown mechanism, thus reducing Abeta production	Fuso et al. (2008)

This table lists three genes implicated in Abeta production. APP is the large protein (695 amino acids) originating the 39–42 polypeptide fragment (Abeta). PS1 is presenilin 1 enzyme involved in gamma-secretase cut of APP. PS1 is also involved with Notch1 control, a factor necessary for stem cells maturation; which is the reason why knock-out of this gene cannot be applied as therapy. Beta-secretase (BACE) operates the second cut to form Abeta fragment

Although it is not clear if specific vitamins could be used as preventive therapy in the pathologies treated in this chapter, since depending on the dosage they could become responsible of the development of subclinical tumors, it will be very interesting to test clinically the use of SAM for the prevention and arrest of AD. This is only one of the cases in which gene silencing could be induced to repair or prevent pathologic outcomes due to an epigenetic disorder.

144.10 Applications to Other Areas of Health and Disease

The epigenetic mechanism outlined in this chapter will have a large number of applications. Considering the number of genes that may be controlled by methylation and the possibility to silence them by supplying the methyl-donor, it is evident that several other diseases may be studied in this respect to identify a possible target. The most delicate field seems to be cancer, since DNA methylation involvement has been shown in a large body of publications, but with contrasting results.

Summary Points

- Homocysteine accumulation is one of the key features in two major pathologies: neurodegenerative diseases and cardiovascular diseases.
- Diminished uptake of vitamins, both for nutritional or pathological reasons (helicobacter pylori), may be the main cause of AD.
- Several recent trials have shown that administration of vitamins to patients is not a sufficient remedy to control AD.
- If the hypothesis of a general loss of methyl groups in the elderly is correct, few epigenetic mechanisms are involved in these pathologies.
- The main remedy for hypomethylation of genes responsible for beta-amyloid production could be the reestablishment of correct concentrations of the main methyl-donor (SAM).
- The best indicator of altered SAM metabolism in the brain is SAH and homocysteine accumulation.
- Since the main source of SAM in humans is the liver, prevention of AD should point to liver diseases.

Key Terms

Epigenetic: DNA methylation at cytosine–guanine dinucleotides, post-translational modifications of histone proteins, RNA interference, and methylation; lipid methylation and prion proteins contribute as well to epigenetic regulation.

Transmethylation: remethylation of homocysteine to methionine where the methyl-donor is methyl-tetra-hydrofolate.

Transsulfuration: transformation of homocysteine to cystathionine; final product will be GSH, the main antioxidant agent in the body.

Gene silencing in epigenetics: the remethylation of cytosines in CpG sites or CCGG belonging to a gene promoter inactivates gene expression. It may be reversed.

Abeta: beta amyloid protein. It may be composed of 39 to 43 amino-acids. The latter is most dangerous since it aggregates more easily to form senile plaques.

Tau protein: is a phosphoprotein whose phosphorylation is regulated. The physiological function of tau is the promotion of assembly and the stabilization of a microtubular network, which is essential for normal axonal transport of vesicles within the neuron.

Vitamin B12 and folate (B9): are cofactors in the transformation of homocysteine to methionine where methyltetrahydrofolate is the methyl donor.

Vitamin B6: is cofactor of cystathionine beta-synthase transforming homocysteine in cystathionine. The end product is GSH (glutathione).

References

Bergman Y, Mostoslavsky R. Biol Chem. 1998;379:401–7.
Bird A. Nature. 2007;447:396–8.
Bottiglieri T. Nutr Rev. 1996;54:382–90.
Bottiglieri T, Hyland K. Review Acta Neurol Scand Suppl. 1994;154:19–26.
Cantoni GL. J Biol Chem. 1951;189:745–54.
Cantoni GL. J Biol Chem. 1953;204:403–16.
Cao X, Sudhof TC. Science. 2001;293:115–20.
Cavallaro RA, Fuso A, D'Anselmi F, Seminara L, Scarpa S. J Alzheimers Dis. 2006;9:415–9.
Chiang PK, Gordon RK, Tal J, Zeng GC, Doctor BP, Pardhasaradhi K, McCann PP. FASEB J. 1996;10:471–80.
Cross SH, Meehan RR, Nan X, Bird A. Nat Genet. 1997;16:256–9.
De Strooper B. Alzheimer's disease. Nature. 2000;405:627:9.
Dolinoy DC. Pharmacogenomics. 2007;8:5–10.
Egger G, Liang G, Aparicio A, Jones PA. Nature. 2004;429:457–63.
Evans DR, Hemmings BA. Mol Gen Genet. 2000;264:425–32.
Fontecave M, Atta M, Mulliez E. Trends Biochem Sci. 2004;29:243–9.
Fuso A, Seminara L, Cavallaro RA, D'Anselmi F, Scarpa S. Mol Cell Neurosci. 2005;28:195–204.
Fuso A, Cavallaro RA, Zampelli A, D'Anselmi F, Piscopo P, Confaloni A, Scarpa S. J Alzheimers Dis. 2007;11:275–90.
Fuso A, Nicolia V, Cavallaro RA, Ricceri L, D'Anselmi F, Coluccia P, Calamandrei G, Scarpa S. Mol Cell Neurosci. 2008;37:731–46.
Fuso A, Nicolia V, Pasqualato A, Fiorenza MT, Cavallaro RA, Scarpa S. Changes in Presenilin 1 gene methylation pattern in diet-induced B vitamin deficiency. Neurobiol Aging. 2010 Epub ahead of print.
Guidi I, Galimberti D, Lonati S, Novembrino C, Bamonti F, Tiriticco M, Fenoglio C, Venturelli E, Baron P, Bresolin N, Scarpini E. Neurobiol Aging. 2006;27:262–9.
Hitchler MJ, Domann FE. Free Radic Biol Med. 2007;43:1023–36.
Holliday R, Pugh JE. Science. 1975;187:226–32.
Joosten E. Clin Chem Lab Med. 2001;39:717–20.
Kapoor A, Agius F, Zhu JK. FEBS Lett. 2005;579:5889–98.
Kautiainen TL, Jones PA. Biochemistry. 1985;24:5575–81.
Kins S, Crameri A, Evans DR, Hemmings BA, Nitsch RM, Gotz J. J Biol Chem. 2001;276:38193–200.
Kresge N, Tabor H, Simoni RD, Hill RL. J Biol Chem. 2005;280:e35.
Kress C, Thomassin H, Grange T. FEBS Lett. 2001;494:135–40.
Lee ME, Wang H. Trends Cardiovasc Med. 1999;9:49–54.
Levenson JM, Sweatt JD. Cell Mol Life Sci. 2006;63:1009–16.
Lichtenthaler SF, Multhaup G, Masters CL, Beyreuther K. FEBS Lett. 1999;453:288–92.
Lu SC. Int J Biochem Cell Biol. 2000;32:391–5.
Marambaud P, Wen PH, Dutt A, Shioi J, Takashima A, Siman R, Robakis NK. Cell. 2003;114:635–45.
Mason JB, Cole BF, Baron JA, Kim YI, Smith AD. Lancet. 2008;371:1335–6.
Migliore L, Fontana I, Colognato R, Coppede F, Siciliano G, Murri L. Neurobiol Aging. 2005;26:587–95.
Morrison LD, Smith DD, Kish SJ. J Neurochem. 1996;67:1328–31.
Nicolia V, Fuso A, Cavallaro RA, Di Luzio A, Scarpa SJ. Alzheimers Dis. 2010;19:895–907.
Okano M, Xie S, Li E. Nat Genet. 1998;19:219–20.
Okano M, Bell DW, Haber DA, Li E. Cell. 1999;99:247–57.
Quadri P, Fragiacomo C, Pezzati R, Zanda E, Forloni G, Tettamanti M, Lucca U. Am J Clin Nutr. 2004;80:114–22.
Razin A, Riggs AD. DNA methylation and gene function. Science. 1980;210:604–10.
Razin A, Szyf M, Kafri T, Roll M, Giloh H, Scarpa S, Carotti D, Cantoni GL. Proc Natl Acad Sci U.S.A. 1986;83:2827–31.
Refsum H, Smith AD. Am J Clin Nutr. 2008;88:253–4.

Rouaux C, Jokic N, Mbebi C, Boutillier S, Loeffler JP, Boutillier AL. EMBO J. 2003;22:6537–49.

Saura CA, Choi SY, Beglopoulos V, Malkani S, Zhang D, Shankaranarayana Rao BS, Chattarji S, Kelleher RJ, III, Kandel ER, Duff K, Kirkwood A, Shen J. Neuron. 2004;42:23–36.

Scarpa S, Fuso A, D'Anselmi F, Cavallaro RA. FEBS Lett. 2003;541:145–8.

Scarpa S, Cavallaro RA, D'Anselmi F, Fuso A. Review J Alzheimers Dis. 2006;9:407–14.

Selhub J, Bagley LC, Miller J, Rosenberg IH. Am J Clin Nutr. 2000;71:614S–20S.

Selley ML. Neurobiol Aging. 2003;24:903–7.

Seshadri S, Beiser A, Selhub J, Jacques PF, Rosenberg IH, D'Agostino RB, Wilson PW, Wolf PA. N Engl J Med. 2002;346:476–83.

Siroen MP, Teerlink T, Nijveldt RJ, Prins HA, Richir MC, van Leeuwen PA. Annu Rev Nutr. 2006;26:203–28.

Smith AD. Food Nutr Bull. 2008;29:S143–72.

Smith AD, Kim YI, Refsum H. Am J Clin Nutr. 2008;87:517–33.

Sontag E, Hladik C, Montgomery L, Luangpirom A, Mudrak I, Ogris E, White CL, III. J Neuropathol Exp Neurol. 2004;63:1080–91.

Sontag E, Nunbhakdi-Craig V, Sontag JM, Diaz-Arrastia R, Ogris E, Dayal S, Lentz SR, Arning E, Bottiglieri T. J Neurosci. 2007;27:2751–9.

Stuhlinger MC, Tsao PS, Her JH, Kimoto M, Balint RF, Cooke JP. Circulation. 2001;104:2569–75.

Tabaton M, Tamagno E. Cell Mol Life Sci. 2007;64:2211–8.

Takai D, Jones PA. PNAS. 2002;99:3740–5.

Troen BR. Mt Sinai J Med. 2003;70:3–22.

Vassar R. Subcell Biochem. 2005;38:79–103.

Vassar R, Bennett BD, Babu-Khan S, Kahn S, Mendiaz EA, Denis P, Teplow DB, Ross S, Amarante P, Loeloff R, Luo Y, Fisher S, Fuller J, Edenson S, Lile J, Jarosinski MA, Biere AL, Curran E, Burgess T, Louis JC, Collins F, Treanor J, Rogers G, Citron M. Science. 1999;286:735–41.

Venter JC, Adams MD, Myers EW, Li PW, Mural RJ, Sutton GG, Smith HO, Yandell M, Evans CA, Holt RA, Gocayne JD, Amanatides P, Ballew RM, Huson DH, Wortman JR, Zhang Q, Kodira CD, Zheng XH, Chen L, Skupski M, Subramanian G, Thomas PD, Zhang J, Gabor Miklos GL, Nelson C, Broder S, Clark AG, Nadeau J, McKusick VA, Zinder N, Levine AJ, Roberts RJ, Simon M, Slayman C, Hunkapiller M, Bolanos R, Delcher A, Dew I, Fasulo D, Flanigan M, Florea L, Halpern A, Hannenhalli S, Kravitz S, Levy S, Mobarry C, Reinert K, Remington K, Abu-Threideh J, Beasley E, Biddick K, Bonazzi V, Brandon R, Cargill M, Chandramouliswaran I, Charlab R, Chaturvedi K, Deng Z, Di F, V, Dunn P, Eilbeck K, Evangelista C, Gabrielian AE, Gan W, Ge W, Gong F, Gu Z, Guan P, Heiman TJ, Higgins ME, Ji RR, Ke Z, Ketchum KA, Lai Z, Lei Y, Li Z, Li J, Liang Y, Lin X, Lu F, Merkulov GV, Milshina N, Moore HM, Naik AK, Narayan VA, Neelam B, Nusskern D, Rusch DB, Salzberg S, Shao W, Shue B, Sun J, Wang Z, Wang A, Wang X, Wang J, Wei M, Wides R, Xiao C, Yan C, Yao A, Ye J, Zhan M, Zhang W, Zhang H, Zhao Q, Zheng L, Zhong F, Zhong W, Zhu S, Zhao S, Gilbert D, Baumhueter S, Spier G, Carter C, Cravchik A, Woodage T, Ali F, An H, Awe A, Baldwin D, Baden H, Barnstead M, Barrow I, Beeson K, Busam D, Carver A, Center A, Cheng ML, Curry L, Danaher S, Davenport L, Desilets R, Dietz S, Dodson K, Doup L, Ferriera S, Garg N, Gluecksmann A, Hart B, Haynes J, Haynes C, Heiner C, Hladun S, Hostin D, Houck J, Howland T, Ibegwam C, Johnson J, Kalush F, Kline L, Koduru S, Love A, Mann F, May D, McCawley S, McIntosh T, McMullen I, Moy M, Moy L, Murphy B, Nelson K, Pfannkoch C, Pratts E, Puri V, Qureshi H, Reardon M, Rodriguez R, Rogers YH, Romblad D, Ruhfel B, Scott R, Sitter C, Smallwood M, Stewart E, Strong R, Suh E, Thomas R, Tint NN, Tse S, Vech C, Wang G, Wetter J, Williams S, Williams M, Windsor S, Winn-Deen E, Wolfe K, Zaveri J, Zaveri K, Abril JF, Guigo R, Campbell MJ, Sjolander KV, Karlak B, Kejariwal A, Mi H, Lazareva B, Hatton T, Narechania A, Diemer K, Muruganujan A, Guo N, Sato S, Bafna V, Istrail S, Lippert R, Schwartz R, Walenz B, Yooseph S, Allen D, Basu A, Baxendale J, Blick L, Caminha M, Carnes-Stine J, Caulk P, Chiang YH, Coyne M, Dahlke C, Mays A, Dombroski M, Donnelly M, Ely D, Esparham S, Fosler C, Gire H, Glanowski S, Glasser K, Glodek A, Gorokhov M, Graham K, Gropman B, Harris M, Heil J, Henderson S, Hoover J, Jennings D, Jordan C, Jordan J, Kasha J, Kagan L, Kraft C, Levitsky A, Lewis M, Liu X, Lopez J, Ma D, Majoros W, McDaniel J, Murphy S, Newman M, Nguyen T, Nguyen N, Nodell M. Science. 2001;291:1304–51.

Vitvitsky V, Thomas M, Ghorpade A, Gendelman HE, Banerjee R. J Biol Chem. 2006;281:35785–93.

Wei H, Ashby DG, Moreno CS, Ogris E, Yeong FM, Corbett AH, Pallas DC. J Biol Chem. 2001;276:1570–7.

Weiss A, Cedar H. Genes Cells. 1997;2:481–6.

Weiss A, Keshet I, Razin A, Cedar H. Cell. 1996;86:709–18.

Xie S, Wang Z, Okano M, Nogami M, Li Y, He WW, Okumura K, Li E. Gene. 1999;236:87–95.

Yu XX, Du X, Moreno CS, Green RE, Ogris E, Feng Q, Chou L, McQuoid MJ, Pallas DC. Mol Biol Cell. 2001;12:185–99.

Zafrilla P, Mulero J, Xandri JM, Santo E, Caravaca G, Morillas JM. Curr Med Chem. 2006;13:1075–83.

Zhang CE, Tian Q, Wei W, Peng JH, Liu GP, Zhou XW, Wang Q, Wang DW, Wang JZ. Neurobiol Aging. 2008;29:1654–65.

Zhao WQ, Feng C, Alkon DL. Neurobiol Dis. 2003;14:458–69.

Chapter 145
Reinforcement and Food Hedonics: A Look at How Energy Deprivation Impacts Food Reward

Jameason D. Cameron and Éric Doucet

145.1 Introduction

Why is it that amidst the plethora of seemingly conscious choices we make throughout our days that we often find it irresistible to reach for that next chip? After all, aren't *we* in control here? When asked such seemingly simple questions it appears as though problems such as helpless overeating – or just as germane, the command involved in dietary restriction – seems to be plainly a matter of psychological weakness and purposeful cognitive control. But, as will be discussed throughout this chapter, there is much more to feeding behavior and stable body energy reserves than self-control. In order to comprehend the physiological and psychological components involved in the uncomplicated act of eating (or not eating!) a bag of potato chips it is necessary to focus on the myriad of mechanisms that are in motion when anticipating, approaching, ingesting, and reflecting about food.

Upon closer investigation it will be argued in the following pages that a significant amount of the variation in the individual response to a similar food environment can begin to be explained not only at the gene level, but also by examining psychobiological differences in the evaluation of food *reward*. Specifically, by highlighting the potential differences in responding between lean and obese animals – spanning studies from rodents to primates (including humans) – both to the hedonic evaluation of food and to the reinforcing value of food, this chapter will attempt to describe some of the intricacies behind one the most integrated of all behaviors, feeding. Furthermore, another underlying theme will be the discussion of how energy deprivation, defined as either acute or chronic, can impact the two abovementioned components of food reward.

Beginning with the advent of agricultural practices and modernized with industrial production of food, modern-day humans are now unique to the animal kingdom in that feeding, for much of the affluent world, occurs for reasons other than sustained periods of energy deprivation. The pursuit of pleasure – or the hedonics (from the Greek word *delight*) of food – is what often guides feeding behavior. But what belies the physiology and psychobiology of what amounts to abhorrent feeding patterns still remains elusive. What is clear, however, is that when energy deprivation is prolonged there is a degree of disinhibition with respect to appetite: not only does palatable food become more salient but items that would normally not be selected can also become attractive. A plethora of research has since emerged on how homeostatic-like elements – states of nutritional need – can alter the pleasure of a sensation of food. This concept was coined as *alliesthesia* and has since received much attention.

É. Doucet (✉)
Behavioral and Metabolic Research Unit, School of Human Kinetics,
University of Ottawa, Ontario, Ottawa, Canada, K1N 6N5
e-mail: eric.doucet@uottawa.ca

V.R. Preedy et al. (eds.), *Handbook of Behavior, Food and Nutrition*,
DOI 10.1007/978-0-387-92271-3_145, © Springer Science+Business Media, LLC 2011

Often a combination of sight, smell, touch, and previous exposure to the food stimulus, the rewarding quality of food is therefore represented by an active process of the brain that is defined by a composite reaction to the food, and as a result is not simply a physical property of the taste stimulus itself (Berridge 1996). Furthermore, the actual reward corresponds to, and is divided by, what are believed to be three separate psychological concepts ("*wanting*," "*liking*," and learning) which are underpinned by distinct neurobiological mechanisms. Each of these dissociable components describes independent qualities that define a rewarding stimulus, and each will be elaborated on in the following sections.

As a final introductory note, it must be clarified that contrary to the view that obesity is only about behavioral control (or lack thereof), that feeding behavior is not entirely a conscious process. The *Milieu Intérieur* is constantly responding to the ebb and flow of blood-borne (chemical) and mechanical (distension) signals and their sensory afferents; incentive stimuli in the external environment along with learned associations both external and internal add salience to edible objects; genotypic variations amongst several hundred genes predispose behavioral outcomes in particular environments; and the whole of the hierarchy from blood to brain necessitates access to the basal motor system to coordinate the action of hand-to-mouth. In the end this chapter is guided by the unresolved questions regarding how each level of the aforementioned hierarchy impacts the rewarding characteristics of feeding. This chapter will also serve as an analysis of the degree to which reinforcement/"wanting" and palatability/"liking" may reflect underlying nutritional needs (e.g., chronic energy deprivation) or to what extent these components of food reward can be reflected independently of need state (e.g., weight-stable and energy replete).

145.2 Reinforcement

145.2.1 *Episodic Nature of Feeding: Beyond Homeostasis*

Prior to beginning a discussion about the intricacies of defining and describing the rewarding attributes of a food stimulus there is a need to introduce the physiology of feeding in relatively general terms. At the behavioral level food intake is episodic (i.e., not continuous). This indicates that there must be physiologically distinct messengers that bring an animal to begin and to end a meal. In fact, nearly half a century of research has shown that there are hormonal signals released by the gastrointestinal tract – peripheral short-term feeding signals – resulting from, or prior to, a single bout of eating. These short-term signals are divided into orexigenic signals (e.g., the peptide hormone ghrelin) that convey the overall message to eat, and this in contrast with anorexigenic signals (e.g., the peptide hormones cholecystokinin and peptide YY) that convey the message of fullness (see Table 145.1). These peripheral feeding signals released from the physical act of consuming foodstuffs are first processed within the nuclei of the hindbrain (primarily, the nucleus of the solitary track, NTS). In a reciprocal manner, these stimuli are transmitted and converge to the real-time processing stations of the hypothalamus and associated cortico-limbic structures eventually leading to goal-directed motor programs that either facilitate or impede the further ingestion of food. Furthermore, there is extensive evidence that these peripheral meal-to-meal signals act directly on the arcuate nucleus of the hypothalamus by crossing the highly selective blood brain barrier, or indirectly at the arcuate through second messenger signaling. It must also be noted that there are metabolic signals such as excursions in blood glucose that can act to promote feeding. Classic work on glycemia first demonstrated in rats was extended to humans and showed that arteriovenous differences (rate of utilization) of glucose correlated with hunger and energy intake (Van Itallie et al. 1953). Although there is continued controversy on the action and mechanism of glucose's role in feeding, it appears that this metabolic signal also has downstream effects at the hypothalamus. The hypothalamus

Table 145.1 A brief list of the peripheral feeding signals implicated in the short- and long-term modulation of energy intake (Modified from Cameron and Doucet (2007). With permission)

Feeding signal	Primary site of secretion	Effect on food intake
Long term		
Insulin	Pancreatic β cells	Decreased energy intake
Leptin	Adipocytes	Decreased energy intake
Short term		
CCK	Endocrine I cells of the proximal Small Intestine	Decreased energy intake
PYY_{3-36}	Enteroendocrine L cells of the ileum & colon	Decreased energy intake
GLP-1	Enteroendocrine L cells of the proximal Small Intestine	Decreased energy intake
Ghrelin	Oxyntic X/A cells of the stomach	Increased energy intake

Of all the feeding signals, ghrelin is the only peptide hormone that is an orexigenic feeding signal
CCK cholecystokinin, PYY_{3-36} peptide YY, *GLP-1* glucagon-like peptide 1

acts as a primary relay station that influences three major systems: the autonomic nervous system, the endocrine system, and the nested brain areas involved in motivational systems. As previously noted, when considering feeding behavior – on a very primitive level – this response can be deconstructed and thought of as motivational states (or drives) that are based upon bodily needs. More than this, whether it is to quench one's thirst or to eat in response to severe hunger pangs, these drives often force the body into action.

Overall, there are two main points to consider regarding the short-term regulation of energy intake: meal size and frequency. What is noticed in free-feeding laboratory conditions is that meal size predicts the interval until the following eating episode. This so-called "postprandial relationship" suggests that meal size is determined via adjustments to the interval to the next meal – not dependent on mere convenience or learned time cues. Conversely, and in most cases in the Western world, meals are scheduled at specific times of the day, resulting in no significant relationship between meal size and intermeal interval (de Castro 2000). In this so-called "preprandial relationship" there is however a relationship between the intermeal interval and meal size; what can be extrapolated is that under daily circumstances, the episodic quality of feeding is lead by associative learning. However, as the period of deprivation (intermeal) increases there may be a shift to respond in a drive-induced manner. What this indicates is that there need not be a deprivation or homeostatic signal in order to initiate a drive state or to continue consummatory behavior; once an animal learns simple stimulus–response relationships, stimuli that were once meaningless become powerful cues with the potential to initiate goal-directed motor programs. Simply put, humans *learn* how and when to initiate feeding: we discover very early that the general feeling of malaise created by the rumbling of a hunger pang or light-headedness of hypoglycemia are often associated with a lack of food. And humans, like snakes and snails, learn by reinforcement.

145.2.2 Reinforcement: Psychological Theory

Although there is no single definition of reinforcement, the concept at its most basic level – in a purely behaviorist sense – can be defined by an environment–behavior relation resulting in the strengthening of an association. As an example, a foraging animal may be experiencing some form of vitamin deficiency and randomly come across a *novel* food containing the deprived vitamin. Prior to having experienced the positive postingestive consequences of that food stimulus – without the paired experience of assuaging the metabolic requirement for the vitamin – there existed no incentive value to the object. Without previous exposure there is no goal, or direction to behavior. This definition becomes inadequate (or incomplete), however, given the evidence that the taste of sweet or salty food can be innately rewarding (Berridge 1996), and therefore considered a "primary reward/primary reinforcer." As an example, newborn babies (and chimps and rats) demonstrate stereotypical responses of "liking" of sweet foods. In the above examples, then, sweet/salty foods are innate incentive stimuli, which are analogous to unconditioned stimuli, and the initially neutral food containing the vitamin (the conditioned stimuli) becomes a predictor of reward (Berridge and Robinson 1998).

In the field of psychology some of the most used descriptors for a *reinforcer* label it as a goal and an incentive, or a stimulus that is approached or attained (Salamone and Correa 2002). Furthermore, implicit in any definition of a reinforcer is the ability for a stimulus to motivate behavior once the stimulus reward association is imprinted. The motivation to obtain the goal object (e.g., food) is not merely an immeasurable psychological concept but can be categorized (e.g., anticipatory, appetitive, etc.) and the neurotransmitters mapped. In fact, the role of midbrain dopamine projections will be argued as being one avenue for explaining the neurophychology of motivation – and specifically the incentive contribution to food reward – in the etiology of what today me be considered maladaptive behavior.

145.2.3 Food as a Reward

The concept that food can serve as a natural *reward* is not hard to grasp in the subjective sense that many foods have the quality of inducing a sense of gratified pleasure. This is most easily measured in humans because an experimenter can simply ask a subject to rate this pleasure/palatability on an analogue scale, for example. But the first neurophysiological evidence for the role of food as a *reward* emerged from brain stimulation studies during the late 1960s and throughout the 1970s. These studies demonstrated that humans would work to obtain electrical stimulation of some sites of the brain (including the lateral hypothalamus (Olds 1977; Rolls 1975), which was by definition rewarding. What is more, the rewarding quality of the brain stimulation appeared to mimic the rewarding quality of food; interestingly, it was found that animals would work harder to obtain brain stimulation when hungry (Hoebel 1969), but when an animal was fed to satiety, it was later found that the group of lateral hypothalamic neurons under observation ceased to respond to food (Rolls et al. 1986). It must be noted that evidence offered with human brain *reward* stimulation suggested that while the experience was certainly rewarding – patients could be found compulsively self-stimulating over thousands of repeated presses – there was no evidence of self-described pleasure in either case (Heath 1972; Portenoy et al. 1986). Observations such as these helped to lay the framework that disentangled the concept that rewards must be pleasurable; it is part of the *incentive salience* hypothesis (described below) that attempts to verify that under various circumstances (e.g., addiction) a *reward* need not be both pleasurable and desired at the same time.

The work on brain stimulation was extended to psychomotor stimulants and eventually it was discovered that the rewarding effects of both of these sources of unnatural reward could be blocked by dopamine antagonists. Eventually it was later confirmed that food *reward* – a natural *reward* – could be similarly attenuated (Wise et al. 1978), and thus began the explosion of studies examining how dopamine modulates feeding and food reward. The following subsections will describe some of the theoretical views of dopamine's role in feeding and reinforcement. The focus will then shift to an examination of the potential role that reinforcement (and dopamine) plays in obesity and how peripheral signals of energy deprivation (e.g., the "hunger hormone" ghrelin and the adiposity-marker hormone leptin) may modulate reinforcement through altered dopamine function.

145.2.3.1 The Dopamine Hypothesis of Feeding: From Anhedonia to Incentive Salience

The accepted hypothesis that is now entrenched in fields spanning from neuroscience to clinical psychology is what has been termed the dopamine hypothesis, or applied to food intake, the dopamine hypothesis of feeding. In brief, via dopamine signaling arising from the ventral tegmental area of the midbrain there is downstream communication with limbic and prefrontal cortex brain areas that act to focus attention on salient environmental stimuli and to promote learning associations, thereby facilitating specific behavioral output such as feeding. The thesis is that dopamine neurons form the backbone of the network of the brain's natural reinforcement system. Indeed, food consumption, in likeness with drug consumption, increases brain dopamine levels in not only in animals, but also in humans (Wang et al. 2002). A more detailed account of the effects of altered levels of dopamine in the brain is presented in Fig. 145.1. The *exact* role that dopamine plays in reward is, however, still open to debate.

Dopamine is both a hormone and neurotransmitter that occurs in a wide variety of animals, including humans. It is one of the primary neurotransmitters in the mammalian brain, where it controls cognition, emotion, locomotor activity, food intake and endocrine regulation (Missale et al. 1998). In the brain there are three major dopaminergic pathways but the most relevant to this discussion is the reward related circuit – the mesolimbic pathway – originating in the midbrain ventral tegmentum and extending to several limbic structures, including the nucleus accumbens, the amygdala, and the hippocampus (Berthoud 2007). Part of the dopamine hypothesis of food intake is based on the initial

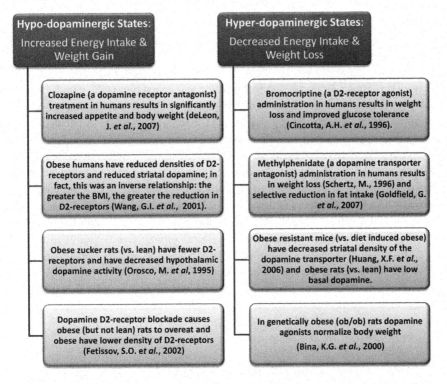

Fig. 145.1 Key points describing dopamine's role in feeding behavior. A look at how altered levels of the neurotransmitter dopamine, by pharmacological or genetic manipulation, can impact normal feeding behavior and body weight regulation in humans and in rodents. Note that a dopamine receptor antagonist *blocks* dopamine signaling by postsynaptic inhibition; oppositely, a dopamine transporter antagonist *promotes* signaling by flooding the synapse with dopamine (References are, from left side (de Leon et al. 2007; Fetissov et al. 2002; Orosco et al. 1995; Wang et al. 2001) and from the right side (Bina and Cincotta 2000; Cincotta and Meier 1996; Goldfield et al. 2007; Hauge et al. 1991))

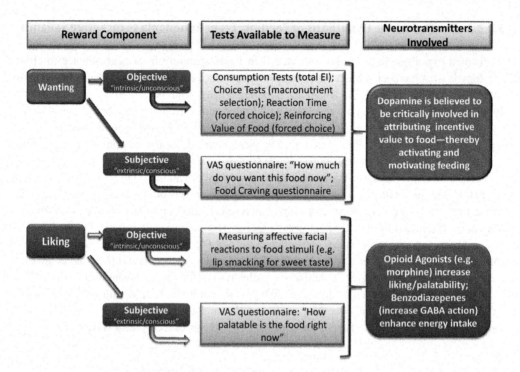

Fig. 145.2 A representation of the dissociable qualities of food reward according to the "incentive salience hypothesis" and the means by which each process can be quantitatively assessed in the laboratory. Note that EI is an abbreviation for energy intake.

work performed on animals subjected to the dopamine antagonist pimozide, which eventually led to the "Anhedonia (Greek for *without pleasure*) Hypothesis." This hypothesis stated, amongst other findings, that neuroleptics (specifically dopamine D2-receptor blockers) appeared to selectively blunt the rewarding impact of food stimuli by decreasing the pleasure of the reinforcer (Wise 1982). While other groups have arrived at many of the same conclusions – in that dopamine is required for *normal* motivation and reward – there appears to be some disagreement regarding the precise role of dopamine in reinforcement or reward. All of the intricacies of the various theories cannot be covered here; however, the view that appears most persuasive has been painstakingly developed (for review see (Berridge and Robinson 1998)) and asserts that dopamine is *not* necessary for 1) hedonic activation (i.e., normal affective reactions described as subjective/objective "liking") and, 2) for reward learning (i.e., relation between the conditioned stimulus and the unconditioned stimulus), but it *is* important for the attribution of the incentive salience of rewards. In fact, these three psychological processes are the foundation of the "incentive salience hypothesis," which offers a further description suggesting that these three processes are all dissociable qualities of reward that can be separated into components of "wanting" and "liking" (see Fig. 145.2)

145.2.3.2 "Wanting" and "Liking": Measuring Perceptual and Motivational Qualities of Food Reward

According to the "incentive salience hypothesis," there is a change at the neurological level that describes *perceptual* (e.g., cognitive) and motivational (e.g., unconscious) components that accompany the shift from a stimulus being neutral to something that is attractive and can energize and motivate behavior (Berridge et al. 2009). The relevance for the study of feeding is that tools can be devised that measure the level of attraction to a stimulus/reinforcer and how much behavior it will support. One method that has been designed to examine *explicit* "liking"/ "wanting" and *implicit* "wanting" of food is the recent development of a forced choice computer-based procedure (Finlayson et al. 2007). This task presents photographic food stimuli of 20 different items varying along two dimensions – fat (high or low) and taste (savoury or sweet). From this computer task implicit "wanting" is measured by the speed with which one stimulus is chosen in preference to an alternative and is additionally measured by relative preference (e.g., fat vs. sweet).

In an attempt to determine whether acute energy deprivation influences food reward this forced choice paradigm was utilized at times pre- and post a standard lunch meal. The objective was to look for a state (hungry vs. satiated) dependent dissociation between "wanting" and "liking." The main findings noted that in a hungry state (3–4 h acute energy deprivation) subjects "wanted" fat (particularly high fat) and savoury food more so than fat and sweet food, but this trend was reversed and subjects "wanted" low fat sweet after the completion of an ad libitum pizza lunch. A separate study from the same group looked at the impact of meal-induced satiation on the dissociable qualities of food reward and discovered that once again implicit "wanting" for low fat sweet foods increased following a lunch meal and that "liking" for sweet foods did not decrease as much as that for fat foods (Finlayson et al. 2008). The general trend of decreased "liking" as one progresses from a hungry to satiated state is consistent with the notion of alliesthesia, a concept that will be discussed in greater detail in Sect. 145.3.

Under study designs similar to those just discussed (state-dependent), recent results from neuroimaging studies offer promising descriptions of what might be occurring in areas of the brain implicated in reward. With fMRI analysis, it was discovered that satiated normal weight women show a stronger BOLD response in the striatum and OFC – reward centers that can be viewed in Figs. 145.4 and 145.6 in Sect. 145.3 – when presented with images of low calorie foods. When hungry, however, these brain areas showed a stronger bold response to high calorie foods (Siep et al. 2009). In a separate fMRI study subjects were tested 3 h after the ingestion of a standardized meal by either infusing the "hunger hormone" ghrelin or a saline control prior to looking at food pictures (Malik et al. 2008). Ghrelin (and not saline) increased the response to food cues in the amygdala, the OFC, and the striatum. Consequently, as demonstrated by these fMRI data, the state-dependent results reported with the forced choice paradigm reported in the previous paragraph may be in part explained by a homeostatic-like influence on reward processing. To be sure, a study combining the "wanting/liking" computer task with fMRI neuroimaging and peripheral injections of ghrelin/leptin or neuropharmacological manipulation of dopamine would be of the highest impact. Unfortunately no such work has yet been performed.

145.2.3.3 The Relative-Reinforcing Value of Food & Energy Deprivation: Do Dopamine-Related Polymorphisms Impact Feeding?

In yet another definition of a reinforcing stimulus, one can describe a reinforcer as a stimulus that increases the rate of a behavior that it follows. The reinforcing value of a stimulus refers to how much behavior the stimulus will support (Epstein et al. 2007a). This can be objectively observed as the increased willingness – a quantitative measure – to work at a progressive ratio computer task to obtain a desirable food stimulus (vs. some alternative). As an example, a computer can be set up with a screen that alternates between two different choices (typically a healthy food and palatable snack food) that can be navigated with a mouse pad. It is called the relative-reinforcing value of food because the probability of earning food points varies across schedules and is contingent on performing simple button presses on a computer joystick. The reinforcement schedule typically remains at a variable ratio (VR2) for all five trials for the healthy food, but increases progressively for the palatable snack food at VR2, VR4, VR8, VR16, and VR32 across the five trials. Thus, on average the reinforcement schedule for the healthy food is set to reinforce every second button push (VR2), and this remains the same across all trials; the reinforcement schedule for the snack food doubles across each trial, such that in the final trial (VR32) snacks were reinforced on every 32nd button press. Essentially, if subject 1 stops responding for the snack food at 16 button presses per point and subject 2 continues to respond for snack points at 32 button pushes per point, then the snack food is said to be twice as reinforcing for subject 2, as they must work twice as hard to obtain the reinforcer.

What is interesting is that comparing obese and lean individuals with this relative-reinforcing value of food paradigm, it was noted that not only did obese subjects work harder for palatable food items (vs. sedentary activities or healthy foods), but they also demonstrated an increased willingness to work for the reinforcer. In fact, this increase in the reinforcing value of food predicted ad libitum intake in the obese independently of rated pleasantness (Saelens and Epstein 1996; Temple et al. 2008). What this suggests is that the measure of motivation to work to obtain, i.e., implicit "wanting" as measured by button-presses, can in some instances be a better predictor of energy intake than explicit subjective accounts of "liking." It appears as though at the behavioral level the combination of consummatory and appetitive motivation can trump orosensory reward. Indeed a troubling finding is the observance that not only do the obese find food more reinforcing (they work more for food than for sedentary activity compared to lean) (Saelens and Epstein 1996), but obese persons also find high-fat foods more reinforcing than low-fat foods when compared to normal weight controls (Epstein et al. 1991). The reinforcing value of food, in turn, can influence how much food is eaten at an ad libitum buffet. What is more, individuals who are categorized as high in food reinforcement (i.e., spend more time at a variable ratio task working for palatable food vs. bland or nonfood items) eat more in an all-you-want-to-eat environment compared to individuals low in food reinforcement (Epstein et al. 2004a). It is unclear, however, whether these findings represent a cause or consequence of excess energy reserves.

One almost inescapable consequence of obesity is sustained periods of energy depletion or dieting. It is well known from psychological studies of reinforcement that food deprivation (and even drug deprivation) increases the reinforcing value of food. Obese and lean individuals alike pass through perturbations in body weight as a result of the prolonged interplay between energy intake, energy expenditure, and the overall involvement of gene and environment interactions. Indeed, results from an energy deprivation in lean individuals ranging in the time of ~13–20 h indicated that in this relatively short period of deprivation the reinforcing value of a palatable snack food significantly increased from the baseline measure in the fed state (Raynor and Epstein 2003). As an ecologically relevant example, if a lean person begins to regularly skip meals, then food is likely to become more reinforcing when it is finally approached. It is unknown if this phenomenon would persist with chronic periods of energy deprivation, but one could postulate that such behavior would lead to body weight gain according to the connection between the reinforcing value of food and energy intake (Raynor and Epstein 2003). Obese individuals experiencing the same feeding patterns theoretically would be even more vulnerable to weight gain, as food is already more reinforcing to begin with. What is fascinating is evidence suggests that polymorphisms of genes involved in the normal regulation of the neurotransmitter dopamine may be involved in a "high-food reinforcement" phenotype, or even related to excess energy reserves.

As a member of the catecholamine family, dopamine is synthesized from the amino acid tyrosine (produced in the liver from phenylalanine), mainly by nervous tissue and the medulla of the adrenal glands. Following the synthesis of dopamine (see Fig. 145.3) there is vesicle packaging in the nerve terminal that prepares this monoamine neurotransmitter for synaptic release. When a dopaminergic

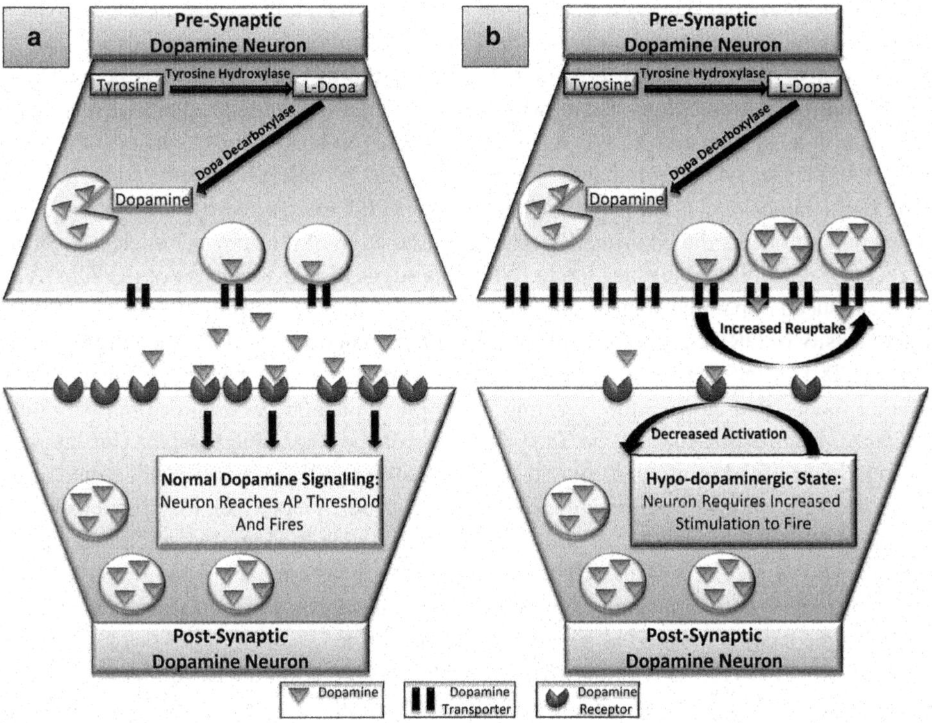

Fig. 145.3 A stylized representation of midbrain dopamine neurons representing (**a**) a typical neuron with a normal propagation of action potential (AP) and (**b**) a neuron with impeded postsynaptic signaling (a "hypodopaminergic state") due to polymorphisms of the dopamine receptor and transporter. The dopamine transporter is responsible for the reuptake of dopamine and the 10/10 allele is hypothesized to result in decreased synaptic dopamine due to *increased* transporter density (i.e., increased reuptake). Also believed to be involved in impaired dopamine signaling, the Taq1A allele of DRD2 results in *decreased* density of dopamine D2-receptors (see **b**)

neuron is sufficiently excited, dopamine is released into the synaptic cleft where it interacts with the postsynaptic receptors causing the depolarization of the postsynaptic cell and initiating a new action potential. Dopamine availability is dependent on its metabolism, release, transport, and receptor binding. Consequently, by looking at the genes involved at any one of these stages there is an opportunity to indirectly investigate brain dopamine levels – in effect looking at markers of neurotransmitter activity (Epstein et al. 2007b) – and how behavior may be resultantly impacted.

The dopamine transporter gene (SLC6A3) codes for a membrane spanning dopamine transporter protein (DAT) that mediates reuptake of dopamine from the synapse into surrounding neurons. There are multiple alleles for this DAT protein and it appears that the 10-repeat homozygous polymorphism is associated with increased dopamine transporter density and transport (Fuke et al. 2001) when compared with the 9-repeat/10- repeat allele. The hypothesis posits that due to simple mendellian genetics, people who received the same 10-repeat allele (i.e., 10/10 genotype) from both parents have lower levels of postsynaptic dopamine. This is further evidenced from in vivo PET studies in humans showing that individuals with the 9-repeat/10-repeat genotype displayed a mean 22% reduction of DAT protein availability compared with 10-repeat homozygous individuals (Heinz et al. 2000). Individuals with the 10/10 genotype can also be at increased risk to obesity. It was found that African Americans with the 10/10 genotype had an odds of having BMI values ≥ 30 kg/m^2 that were 5.2 times greater than African Americans with the 9/9 or 9/10 genotype (Epstein et al. 2002).

Another polymorphism believed to result in decreased dopamine signalling occurs due to an alteration in the ANKK1 gene, known as the Taq1A restriction fragment length polymorphism. To remain consistent with existing literature–and due to the fact that ANKK1 is believed to be in linkage disequilibrum with DRD2–Taq1A will be acknowleged as being linked to DRD2. Specifically, there are three *Taq1* A variants (A1/A1, A1/A2, and A2/A2) and compared to carriers of the *Taq1* A2 allele, in vivo imaging had shown that people with the *Taq1* A1 allele have reduced brain dopamine signaling (Pohjalainen et al. 1998). With further in vivo (PET imaging) evidence, the mechanism of action is thought to be mediated primarily with the association of the *Taq1* A1 allele with decreased DRD2 receptor density (Noble et al. 1991). What this suggests is that carriers of the *Taq1* A1 allele experience reduced dopamine signaling in the brain; indeed, it has recently been demonstrated that decreased density of DRD2 is strongly associated with human obesity, in inverse proportion to BMI (Wang et al. 2001). Linking physiology with behavior, current research has revealed that the reinforcing value of food – analogous to the "wanting" component of food reward – can not only influence energy intake, but the presence of the *Taq1* A1 allele of the dopamine receptor can interact with obesity to influence food reinforcement (Epstein et al. 2004b, 2007b). Subjects identified as high in food reinforcement who were carriers of the A1 allele consumed more food than participants high in food reinforcement without the A1 allele and participants low in food reinforcement with or without the A1 allele (Epstein et al. 2007b). Although these data are preliminary, what this suggests is that using a behavioral genetic approach to understand the interaction between genotype, obesity, and food reinforcement can be viewed as a viable research venture.

Taken together, individuals with the *Taq1* A1 or the 10/10-repeat alleles are hypothesized to be less sensitive to stimulation of dopamine-regulated reward circuits – analogous to a reward-deficiency syndrome (Noble et al. 1994) – and by enduring a hypodopaminergic state are more likely to seek reinforcers, whether it be food or drug (Blum et al. 1996). In fact, this represents one view of dopamine's involvement in food reward and it fits well with much of the literature presented thus far. Although it is a very hedonistic view of feeding behavior, it is a tenable hypothesis that overeating has emerged as a compensatory mechanism to ameliorate a deficiency in the reward circuitry (Wang et al. 2002). Others contend a somewhat opposing view that focuses on an individual's sensitivity to reward, as measured by a psychobiological questionnaire. It is argued that individuals with high levels (hyperdopaminergia) of synaptic dopamine are more sensitive and have a greater capacity for reward, thereby making them more likely to engage in pleasurable behaviors (Davis and Fox 2008). In the end, it is not clear whether the dopamine hypothesis of feeding is best explained by hypodopaminergic states as described by a reward deficiency syndrome, or by hyperdopaminergic states as described by heightened reward sensitivity, or by both.

145.2.4 Peripheral Feeding Signals Impact Brain Dopamine: Evidence That Energy Deprivation Can Impact the Motivational Component of Food Reward

A promising path has been paved with respect to adiposity signals and their possible role in mediating food reward. When leptin is administered intraventricularly in rodents, it attenuates the rewarding impact of food-restriction-sensitive stimulation (Fulton et al. 2000), where animals significantly decrease rates of brain stimulation reward. What is interesting is that this rewarding effect is potentiated by chronic food deprivation and that the ability of this deprivation to enhance brain stimulation reward is proportional to the degree of weight loss (Carr and Wolinsky 1993). In effect, with greater weight loss animals will continue pressing the lever for ever smaller amounts of stimulation, which is translated into a leftward shift in the rate–frequency curve. Further, intracerebroventricular leptin administration causes a rightward shift in this curve, restoring the reward value to predeprivation levels (Fulton et al. 2000), but to initially respond to the deprivation, an absolute weight loss of approximately 10% was required. It may be that long-term adiposity signals like leptin actively signal reward pathways of current body reserves, thereby intrinsically making food more attractive – more rewarding – when a significant loss of body energy reserves or a similar signal (decreased leptin) is detected.

New developments into the study of leptin and ghrelin – signals of energy surfeit and deficit, respectively – have indicated that these feeding signals may play complimentary roles in the dopamine hypothesis of feeding. Mesolimbic brain circuits have recently been shown to express the long form of the leptin receptor (the main leptin receptor, OB-Rb); more than this, it has been demonstrated that OB-Rb mediated signaling modified dopamine signaling and food intake. When leptin was administered directly to the ventral tegmental area (VTA) – the central hub of dopaminergic neurons – rats decreased food intake; oppositely, when the OB-Rb was knocked out in this area, feeding was increased, especially of highly palatable chow (Hommel et al. 2006). In contrast, but consistent with its role in feeding, when ghrelin is injected into the VTA rats show a robust dose dependent feeding response (Naleid et al. 2005). Taken together, what emerges is the neurological foundation that connects dopaminergic pathways of reward with short- and long-terms feeding signals. Leptin inhibits the firing of VTA dopamine neurons and ghrelin triggers tonic dopamine release, resulting in decreased and increased feeding, respectively. Food reward appears to be impacted by homeostasis and dopamine plays an integral role in the appetitive motivation to feed. Another possible role for dopamine that cannot be discounted is that it has indirect downstream action on another neurotransmitter. Indeed, there is evidence that ghrelin can impact the opioid system in the rat (Sibilia et al. 2006). The point here is that dopamine is only one piece of the grand puzzle that describes the intricate network underlying food reward.

145.3 Food Hedonics

145.3.1 Palatability: The Multimodal Representation of Taste

Taste perception is transmitted by cranial nerves, which propagate information about the touch, temperature and pain sensation on the tongue (Kringelbach 2004). The afferent taste signal progresses from cranial nerves to the NTS, continuing to the thalamus and then to the primary taste cortex; higher order taste assimilation is believed to be accomplished by the connections of the primary taste cortex with the secondary taste cortex (i.e., the orbitofrontal cortex) (Baylis et al. 1995). With respect to the pleasantness of the taste of foods, the responsiveness of the taste neurons in the NTS and in the primary taste cortex (see Fig. 145.4) do not seem to be affected by states of deprivation and repletion (Rolls et al. 1988; Yaxley et al. 1988). What this implies is that these areas do not reflect the hedonics of feeding, but instead represent sensory qualities of food independent of motivational state. Therefore the identity and intensity of food taste is made explicit in the primary taste cortex, but it is with the rich interconnectivities of the orbitofrontal cortex (OFC) that the hedonic component of the rewarding value of food finally is coded. In short, evidence from primates indicates that the identity of a taste and its intensity are represented separately from its pleasantness (Rolls 2007).

The OFC can be subdivided into two regions: the posterior region, restricted to the limbic functions and considered part of the limbic system, and an anterior region, restricted to inhibitory control over the amygdala (Borod 2000). In order for peripheral feeding related signals to influence food pleasantness – and by convention, food reward – this must occur from the processing of the stimuli

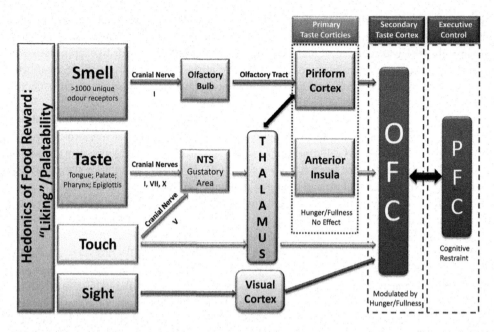

Fig. 145.4 A schematic diagram of pathways demonstrating the multimodal representation of taste and olfaction in the brain. Note that cranial nerve I is the olfactory nerve; cranial nerve VII is the facial nerve; cranial nerve X is the vagus nerve; and cranial nerve V is the trigeminal nerve (which transmits the mouthfeel of fats and oils); OFC is the orbitofrontal cortex; and PFC is the prefrontal cortex

at the level at or beyond the secondary taste cortex (Rolls et al. 1990). Efferent connections from the OFC include the amygdala, the hippocampus, the lateral hypothalamus, the striatum, and the ventral tegmental area (Kandel et al. 2000). What is interesting is that each of these brain areas is influenced by ghrelin, leptin, and dopamine. Interconnected within this network of neuromodulators and feeding-related signals lies what is believed to be a path toward describing reward signaling, or in the context of energy deprivation, *alliesthesia* (discussed below).

Pioneering work performed on primates indicated that responses from a group of OFC neurons to glucose taste decreased to zero when the monkey ate glucose to satiety; concurrently, over the course of administration of glucose the animal's behavior changed from positive to negative affective reactions (Rolls et al. 1989). Furthermore, it was demonstrated that this decrease in neural activity was specific to the ingesta, i.e., the authors discovered a piece of the neural foundation of *sensory specific satiety* (Rolls et al. 1989). What remains unclear is the role that information from the primary taste cortex and from adjacent limbic areas impacts the change in pleasantness of a food stimulus that occurs with continuous exposure over a meal or from refeeding after chronic energy deprivation.

Another area that requires clarification is to what degree the decisions regarding when, what, and with whom to eat are conscious. Indeed, much of the expression of appetite and eating is not explicit, and therefore outside of introspection. Studies from rats, to chimps, to human infants have demonstrated that "liking" of sweet foods can be implicit – and this was accomplished by measuring stereotypical facial reactions to the sweet stimuli (Steiner et al. 2001). Sweet tastes elicit a positive hedonic pattern of evaluation primarily described by tongue protrusions (licking/smacking of lips) and paw licking (Grill and Berridge 1985). Since "liking" is considered a basic evaluative reaction of the brain with objective behavioral indicators it can be implicitly measured by affective measures to the food *reward*; alternatively, the hedonic impact of "liking" can be explicitly measured in humans by describing their reaction to the food stimulus (e.g., analogue scales). A pleasant stimulus is a rewarding stimulus and for the most part feeding is a rewarding action. The "liking" component of food reward has its biological underpinnings in at least two major neurotransmitter families defined by opioid, and endocannabinoid systems. The best studied in humans is the opioid modulation of palatability. Specifically, opioid receptor antagonists (e.g., naltrexone and naloxone) reduce the pleasantness of foods (Bertino et al. 1991; Drewnowski et al. 1992) and agonists (e.g., DAMGO and morphine) increase the pleasantness (Atkinson 1987; Levine and Atkinson 1987). This hedonic pleasure/palatability component of reward is represented in the brain mainly by pallidal circuits (Yeomans and Gray 2002) and by circuits within the shell of the nucleus accumbens (Pecina and Berridge 2005) (see *striatum* in Fig. 145.6).

145.3.2 Peripheral Feeding Signals and Taste Processing

There is limited data regarding the potential role of gut peptides (peripheral feeding signals) in taste processing. Studies on rats have indicated that PYY_{3-36}, a hormone released by L-cells of the distal colon, produced a dose-dependent conditioned taste aversion to a sweet solution (Chelikani et al. 2006; Halatchev and Cone 2005). Similarly, another peptide released by intestinal L-cells, GLP-1, also has the potential to produce a robust conditioned taste aversion to saccharine (Thiele et al. 1997). What is intriguing is that CCK, a "satiety hormone" like PYY and GLP-1, can actually produce a conditioned flavour *preference* at low doses in rats (Perez and Sclafani 1991). The authors interpreted this preference to the positive postingestive consequences of satiety. It is possible that the taste aversion with PYY and GLP-1 could be an artifact of nausea that has been reported in human subjects; nonetheless, there is evidence that these gut-peptide messengers are involved in taste-processing.

The hormone produced by the OB gene, leptin, has also been demonstrated to have a role in the hedonic evaluation of food. Specifically, leptin receptors were identified in taste cells and exogenous administration of leptin inhibited sweet taste responses in lean mice but not in db/db mice (lacking a functional leptin receptor) (Ninomiya et al. 2002). Evidence of a separate role for leptin in *olfactory processing* has also emerged from data on rats showing how nutritional status impacts olfactory perception. Specifically, intracerebroventricular leptin administration (mimicking satiety) dose dependently increases consumption of an aversive odorized drink, suggesting that leptin decreases odor sensitivity (Julliard et al. 2007). Taken together, leptin appears to play a role in *taste* and *olfactory* processing that is dependent on nutritional status. What this suggests is that when rodents are energy-replete and leptin levels are high there is a corresponding decrease in sensitivity to taste and to olfactory stimuli. Although there are limited data, human studies have also indicated that leptin is expressed and may play a functional role in the salivary glands and the oral cavity; the expression of the long form of the leptin receptor has also been discovered in the membranes of glandular cells and in the salivary ducts (Bohlender et al. 2003).

The role that *serum* leptin may play in food hedonics in humans has only been superficially investigated. In a group of six men and 20 women offered a standardized high carbohydrate breakfast, palatability was positively correlated to fasting serum leptin independently of BMI and body fat mass (Raynaud et al. 1999). One interpretation of these results is that palatability would be independent of need state, as those who had the highest leptin levels (indicating caloric surfeit) rated food as tasting most pleasant. Contrarily, these results could be demonstrative of the large variation in body composition in this study. With nearly half of the subjects being obese there could be a resistance to leptin that could not be easily detected.

In a study examining the impact of fasting leptin concentration on energy intake and macronutrient preference it was found that high fasting serum leptin was associated with lower preference for chocolate as well as lower energy intakes and specifically fat intake (Karhunen et al. 1998). These findings remained significant after adjusting leptin concentrations for body fat mass and dietary underreporting. In a more recent study consisting of a chronic energy deprivation (8 week weight loss trial) and a repeated measure looking at food hedonics pre- and post weight loss, there was no significant relationship between serum leptin and rated pleasantness (Cameron et al. 2008). What this study did demonstrate, however, was that after the 8 weeks of caloric deprivation (−700 kcal/day) subjects rated the same foods as more pleasant to taste. Of note, both types of food presented to the subjects – vegetables and fruits vs. desserts – increased in hedonic valance. After weight loss both healthy food and "junk" food tasted better.

145.3.3 Energy Deprivation and Palatability: Evidence from Alliesthesia

A question that remains to be answered is the extent to which homeostatic components (a need-state) can impact the quality of orosensory reward, thereby enhancing food hedonics. Much of the research on this topic uses a preload paradigm that assesses the impact of a pretest snack on the subsequent ad libitum energy intake and rated palatability. The rationale behind this test supposes that if palatability is dependent on a need-state, then a preload of high energy density (vs. low) would have a greater impact on palatability of the ad libitum meal (i.e., meal becomes less pleasant following energy dense preload). There are conflicting data, but it appears that the short term manipulation of satiety does not reliably impact palatability. For example, subjects not only rated food as being less pleasant following a high energy preload (vs. low), but they consumed less total weight and calories in ad libitum feeding following the preload (Johnson and Vickers 1993) and similar findings were noted in a separate study (Booth et al. 1982).

On the other hand, several studies employing similar preload paradigms have demonstrated a lack of change in palatability with need state (Birch and Deysher 1986; Yeomans et al. 1998). Specifically, when a soup preload was covertly manipulated with maltodextrin and administered 30 min prior to ad libitum feeding, subjects did not rate the palatability lower than the trial where plain soup was consumed (Yeomans et al. 1998). However, with the added maltodextrin it was noted that subjects had lower hunger and higher fullness ratings prior to beginning ad libitum feeding. Similarly, a study of children aged 3–5 and adults 25–35 years old showed no change in pleasantness with respect to preload energy density, but both groups displayed sensory specific satiety during the lunch feeding (Birch and Deysher 1986). While the preload paradigm may be examining possible short-term signaling of need (free)-state, a far better manipulation that is unfortunately studied even less is increasing the deprivation state (e.g., chronic energy deprivation). As alluded to in much of this chapter, feeding repeatedly takes place without any measurable changes in body energy reserves, and most often according to learned cues (see Fig. 145.5). In order to truly examine how the "*internal milieu*" impacts food reward there most likely needs to be a prolonged perturbation in energy balance over days and weeks.

Some of the pioneering efforts examining energy deprivation and palatability were conducted by Michel Cabanac, the coiner of the term alliesthesia. In his seminal paper on hedonics (1971) he tested changes in gustative and olfactive perception at the subjects' normal weight, at 10% below this weight, and then again after the subject returned to normal weight. To reduce the body weight by 10% the energy intake was limited to 500–800 kcal per day until the weight was achieved, and this reduced weight was maintained for several weeks prior to the test day. In short, alliesthesia was measured by the change in subjective pleasantness ratings for multiple ingestions of sweet tasting sucrose solutions. When subjects were at their normal weight and after ingesting 200 ml of a 25% aqueous solution of glucose, these stimuli became unpleasant (negative alliesthesia). However, when subjects lost 10% of their body weight alliesthesia could no longer be demonstrated, and 50 g of glucose was insufficient to cause the negative affective ratings. Finally, the return to normal body weight restored the change in sensation from pleasant to unpleasant.

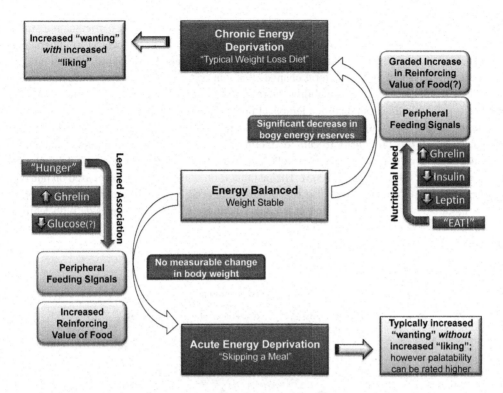

Fig. 145.5 Key Features representing the Ying and Yang of food reward as a function of energy deprivation. When there is no measurable change in body weight, it is believed that peripheral signals act as *cues* to feed, but chronic energy deprivation results in exaggerated responses from peripheral signals. It may be that significant changes in body energy reserves changes mere cues into powerful signals that motivate appetitive and consummatory feeding behavior

Corroborating these results are findings from deprivation periods of much shorter duration. By manipulating the period of energy deprivation with two separate test days, one day with a 3.5 h period of deprivation and another with an overnight fast of approximately 12–15 h, Spiegel et al. (1989) found that the deprivation period impacted palatability, consistent with alliesthesia. These results were consistent with obese and lean subjects. Germaine to this chapter are two major findings from this study: (1) the longer deprivation period resulted in increased palatability ratings and increased rate and quantity of food eaten ad libitum and (2) obese persons experienced a greater increase in palatability than lean persons, but lean individuals increased ad libitum feeding more than obese individuals.

145.4 Conclusions and Theoretical Integration

Food intake is the result of a multimodal representation of the sensory information about the food stimulus: in the brain there is a continuum consisting of the visual exteroreception of the sight of food, to the interoreception of primary and secondary taste corticies' evaluation of taste, temperature, texture, and viscosity. While energy deprivation can have an impact at several of these levels, humans also eat for reasons other than nutritional needs. For most of the developed countries meals are entrained to a schedule thereby eliminating what might be real signals of energy deprivation – this fact has raised to attention that such feeding may anticipate and prevent the development of significant metabolic changes (Woods 1991). The study of feeding behavior, and in particular the study of subjective hedonic experience and objective measures of motivation, are central to understanding how appetite regulation can be compromised in certain individuals. Furthermore, with an integrated picture of physiological and behavioral changes that can occur as a result of caloric deprivation – particularly with regard to food palatability and reinforcement – what emerges is a better understanding of how palatable food can disrupt attempts at body weight regulation.

Epidemiological data suggests that some people are more susceptible to weight gain (Ravussin and Kozak 2004); this propensity to gain, maintain, or lose weight under similar environments has been attributed to various susceptibility levels such as metabolic, behavioral, psychological, physiologic, and genetic (Blundell et al. 2005). The fact that food intake is not merely based on nutritional or homeostatic requirements but is also very much influenced by its reinforcing properties presupposes a modulating role for dopamine in everyday feeding (Carr 2007) alongside with leptin and ghrelin (Figlewicz 2003) (see Fig. 145.6).

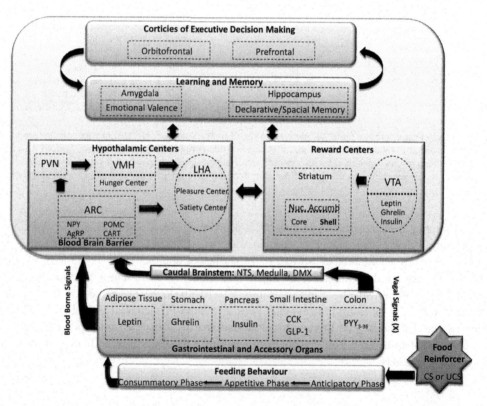

Fig. 145.6 An integrated summary of all the concepts discussed throughout this chapter: with the introduction of a food reinforcer begins the appetitive motivation to seek and finally to consume the food stimulus. When fasted for an extended period of time peripheral feeding-related signals from gastrointestinal and accessory organs are proposed to drive feeding behavior in a powerful manner via the ARC and the activation of neuropeptides that trigger hunger signals (e.g., NPY and AgRP). Conversely, when in the sated state, the nucleus accumbens and VTA may continue to promote consummatory behavior in the absence of hunger, i.e., as conditioned associations and learning interact with the reward pathways to increase implicit wanting. Equally as plausible, the palatability of food signaled by the Insular and Orbitofrontal corticies could also trigger eating in the absence of hunger. Abbreviations: *PVN* paraventricular nucleus, *LHA* lateral hypothalamic area, *ARC* arcuate nucleus, *NPY* neuropeptide Y, *AgRP* agouti-related peptide, *POMC* pro-opiomelanocortin, *CART* cocaine and amphetamine-related transcript, *Nuc. Accumb* Nucleus accumbens (Modified from Cameron and Doucet (2007). With permission)

If it can be shown with more fecundity that a biological basis exists for differences in the reward experienced in feeding, then as an example, individualized treatment and prevention programs for weight loss could differentially help those who are high in food reinforcement versus someone low in food reinforcement (Epstein et al. 2007a). Furthermore, there needs to be more data regarding the change in orosensory reward that may occur with chronic energy deprivation. One of the messages behind this chapter is that hedonic feeding results from discordance between appetitive motivation and inhibitory control. In order to help those trying to lose or maintain a specific level of body energy reserves, there needs to be a better understanding of the processes behind the rewarding qualities of food, both implicit and explicit. Behavioral strategies promoting dietary restraint – thereby shifting inhibitory control over appetitive motivation – may be what need to be promoted in a continual effort to inhibit weight gain in this modern obesogenic environment.

145.5 Applications to Other Areas of Health and Disease

Much of what has been described in this two part chapter was theoretical. Dissociating a psychological concept such as a reward into separable components of hedonic evaluation and motivation to obtain and consume does, however, have ecological validity. In particular, the tool described that measures the relative-reinforcing value of food can offer valuable information regarding the determinants of food choice. There are a lot of data showing that if access to a preferred food (such as cheesecake) is reduced, then people will choose a less preferred – although still enjoyable – alternative (such as yogurt). Applied in light of behavioral economics theory, if the price of a good that is typically purchased is increased, then as cost increases there will be a certain point where the consumer will *substitute* with something similar, though less expensive. A knee-jerk solution would be to tax foods with "empty calories" such as high fructose corn syrup, which in fact is occurring in some U.S. States. A better solution may be to promote the development of ready-to-eat healthy snacks such as the conveniently peeled and washed baby carrots, and to implement such foods across school cafeterias nationwide. At the very least, a goal should be to decrease the disparity in prices between fresh produce and the lower cost highly processed foods.

When considering the millions of people that start dieting each year, the fact that food reinforcement increases with energy deprivation has obvious concerns. The very thing that is supposed to help with weight loss (e.g., decreased energy intake) can act to increase the motivation to eat energy dense food. Although there are no definitive data to show that increased meal frequency (independent of energy intake) promotes weight loss, it may still be a good approach to prescribe such a diet in an attempt to control for overeating due to increased saliency of palatable food. To be sure, irregular meal patterns such as skipping meals can reinstate abhorrent binge-eating behavior in individuals recovering from bulimia nervosa. Nonetheless, a reduced calorie diet imposed with a greater frequency of meals may also leave individuals to choose a nonfood activity that is reinforcing (e.g., hiking) in the place of impulsively eating due to a perceived deprivation in energy and increased food reinforcement. The increased food reinforcement – and its predicting power of ad libitum feeding – experienced by the obese may also highlight the importance of limiting access to food in a strategic manner. Although there are no data about food reinforcement and success with weight loss, a valid hypothesis would be that for individuals high in food reinforcement (vs. low) a high meal frequency (e.g., six meals) diet of prepackaged meals would result in improved adherence to the diet and better appetite control vs. low meal frequency (e.g., three meals).

Regarding the forced-choice computer task that was developed in an attempt to measure *implicit* "wanting" and *explicit* "wanting" and "liking," there exists the potential to test the impact of various forms of energy deprivation on these reward-related variables. Useful information will no doubt emerge on how relative (macronutrient) preference or reaction time – two quantitative measures of implicit "wanting" – can be impacted by not only reduced energy intake but also by increased energy expenditure. A recent study examined the impact of energy deprivation by means of exercise on food reward and ad libitum energy intake with two counterbalanced sessions, one at 50 min of high intensity exercise and then other without exercise (Finlayson et al. 2009). Although there was no significant difference in the amount of food eaten by test day for this group of lean women, it was found that after the exercise session there was a subgroup of "compensators" who ate more after exercise and also displayed a significant increase in *implicit* "wanting." After exercise there was an unconscious *implicit* desire for the "compensators" to eat high-fat sweet foods. What is interesting is that a separate study with similar exercise intensity (but longer duration) also demonstrated that lean female subjects overcompensated for the exercise session (vs. an equicaloric lower intensity exercise) when given access to an ad libitum for the remainder of the day (Pomerleau et al. 2004). In both studies there was evidence that performing intense aerobic exercise results in increased energy intake, thereby acutely promoting *positive* energy balance. It may be that some individuals are more sensitive to substrate flux and the mobilization and utilization of glucose, making them more likely to select energy dense foods following intense aerobic work. Elucidating who would potentially be "compensators" from the onset of an exercise prescription, as measured by increased implicit "wanting," could not only help with recidivism but also with weight loss success. Extending these findings to obese individuals could potentially identify those who would benefit from performing a lower intensity exercise to attain/maintain weight loss.

Summary Points

- Variation in the individual response to a similar food environment can begin to be explained not only at the gene level, but also by examining psychobiological differences in the evaluation of food reward.
- When energy deprivation is prolonged there is a degree of disinhibition with respect to appetite: not only does palatable food become more salient but items that would normally not be selected can also become attractive.
- Short-term feeding-related signals are divided into orexigenic signals (e.g., the "hunger hormone" ghrelin) that convey the overall message to eat, and this in contrast with anorexigenic signals (e.g., CCK and PYY_{3-36}) that convey the message of fullness/satiety.
- Leptin appears to play a role in taste and olfactory processing that is dependent on nutritional status: when energy-replete and leptin levels are high there is a corresponding decrease in sensitivity to taste and to olfactory stimuli.
- There need not be a deprivation or homeostatic signal in order to initiate a drive state or to continue consummatory behavior; humans *learn* how and when to initiate feeding.
- The dopamine hypothesis states that dopamine neurons form the backbone of the network of the brain's natural reinforcement system acting to focus attention on salient environmental stimuli and to promote learning associations. Leptin and ghrelin may play complimentary roles in the dopamine hypothesis of feeding.
- *Incentive salience theory* suggests that dopamine is *not* necessary for subjective/objective "liking") *nor* for reward learning, but it *is* important for the attribution of the incentive salience of rewards.
- The measure of motivation to work to obtain, i.e., implicit "wanting," can in some instances be a better predictor of energy intake than explicit subjective accounts of "liking."
- In vivo imaging suggests that individuals with the *Taq1* A1 (dopamine transporter) or the 10/10-repeat (dopamine receptor) alleles can be less sensitive to stimulation of dopamine-regulated reward circuits – analogous to a reward-deficiency syndrome – by imposing a hypodopaminergic state.

- The "liking" component of food reward has its biological underpinnings in at least two major neurotransmitter families defined by opioid and endocannabinoid systems.
- A question that remains to be answered is the extent to which homeostatic components (nutritional need-states) can impact the quality of orosensory reward, thereby enhancing food hedonics.

Definitions

Acute vs. Chronic Energy Deprivation: Acute energy deprivation will be defined as a complete fasting period of several hours (but otherwise being relatively weight stable), whereas, chronic energy deprivation will be defined as a prolonged reduction in energy intake below that would maintain body weight stability.

Alliesthesia: From the words esthesia (*meaning sensation*) and allios (*meaning changed*). It is the modification of conscious sensations by changes in internal signals, reflected by afferent actions of peripheral receptors; plainly, a pleasant or unpleasant sensation depending on the subject's internal state.

Appetite: An internal state or a specific disposition to act. Appetite as it pertains to feeding can be conceptualized as the hunger-stimulated response to a particular food and implies knowledge of the item(s) to which the actions should be directed

Incentive Salience: A motivational process that does not involve a pleasure/hedonic component, but is limited to a drive process that defines the "wanting" component of a reward. It is primarily believed to be influenced by dopaminergic neurotransmission.

Reinforcer: In a Skinnerian sense reinforcement can be viewed as behavioral measures of learning: it is the strengthening of an observed behavioral response (stimulus–response associations) or the strengthening of a learned behavioral response (stimulus–stimulus associations). A reinforcer can be a goal or a commodity.

Relative-Reinforcing Value of Food: Describes how hard an individual is willing to work for food by measuring responses at a predetermined reinforcement schedule. It is *relative-reinforcing* due to the fact that there are alternatives, albeit in a forced choice methodology.

Reward: A psychological process that is contingent on a reinforcing stimulus. Reward can be dissociated into two qualities of a food stimulus: (1) a hedonic component of "liking"/palatability and (2) a reinforcing component that is sometimes described as "wanting"/incentive motivational component.

1. "Liking": Divided into *implicit liking*, which is measured objectively by affective facial reactions to various food stimuli, and *explicit liking*, which is measured by the subjective hedonic rating of orosensory pleasure (e.g., visual analogue scales).
2. "Wanting": Divided into *intrinsic wanting*, which can be measured by choice tests, reaction time, or reinforcement, and *extrinsic wanting*, which can be defined by the intent or desire to consume a specific food and measured subjectively on a visual analogue scale.

Satiation/Satiety: Satiation refers to the processes that lead to the termination of feeding, e.g., a within-meal interval, whereas, satiety refers to the state of inhibition of feeding, e.g., a between meal interval.

Sensory-Specific Satiety: With continued exposure to the same food item there is a discernable and rather abrupt change in the overall hedonic rating, i.e., the perceived sensory qualities of the item are not absolute though the change in liking is specific to the unchanging sensory characteristics of the item itself.

References

Atkinson RL. Fed Proc. 1987;46:178–82.
Baylis LL, Rolls ET, Baylis GC. Neuroscience. 1995;64:801–12.
Berridge KC. Neurosci Biobehav Rev. 1996;20:1–25.
Berridge KC, Robinson TE. Brain Res Brain Res Rev. 1998;28:309–69.
Berridge KC, Robinson TE, Aldridge JW. Curr Opin Pharmacol. 2009;9:65–73.
Berthoud HR. Physiol Behav. 2007;91:486–98.
Bertino M, Beauchamp GK, Engelman K. Am J Physiol. 1991;261:R59–63.
Bina KG, Cincotta AH. Neuroendocrinology. 2000;71:68–78.
Birch LL, Deysher M. Appetite. 1986;7:323–31.
Blum K, Braverman ER, Wood RC, Gill J, Li C, Chen TJ, Taub M, Montgomery AR, Sheridan PJ, Cull JG. Pharmacogenetics. 1996;6:297–305.
Blundell JE, Stubbs RJ, Golding C, Croden F, Alam R, Whybrow S, Le Noury J, Lawton CL. Physiol Behav. 2005;86:614–22.
Bohlender J, Rauh M, Zenk J, Groschl M. J Endocrinol. 2003;178:217–23.
Booth DA, Mather P, Fuller J. Appetite. 1982;3:163–84.
Borod J. The neuropsychology of emotion. Oxford: Oxford University Press; 2000.
Cabanac M. Science. 1971;173:1103–7.
Cameron J, Doucet E. Appl Physiol Nutr Metab. 2007;32:177–89.
Cameron JD, Goldfield GS, Cyr MJ, Doucet E. Physiol Behav. 2008;94:474–80.
Carr KD. Physiol Behav. 2007;91:459–72.
Carr KD, Wolinsky TD. Brain Res. 1993;607:141–8.
Chelikani PK, Haver AC, Reidelberger RD. Peptides. 2006;27:3193–201.
Cincotta AH, Meier AH. Diabetes Care. 1996;19:667–70.
Davis C, Fox J. Appetite. 2008;50:43–9.
de Castro JM. Nutrition. 2000;16:800–13.
de Leon J, Diaz FJ, Josiassen RC, Cooper TB, Simpson GM. J Clin Psychopharmacol. 2007;27:22–7.
Drewnowski A, Krahn DD, Demitrack MA, Nairn K, Gosnell BA. Physiol Behav. 1992;51:371–9.
Epstein LH, Bulik CM, Perkins KA, Caggiula AR, Rodefer J. Pharmacol Biochem Behav. 1991;38:715–21.
Epstein LH, Jaroni JL, Paluch RA, Leddy JJ, Vahue HE, Hawk L, Wileyto EP, Shields PG, Lerman C. Obes Res. 2002;10:1232–40.
Epstein LH, Wright SM, Paluch RA, Leddy J, Hawk LW, Jr, Jaroni JL, Saad FG, Crystal-Mansour S, Lerman C. Physiol Behav. 2004a;81:511–7.
Epstein LH, Wright SM, Paluch RA, Leddy JJ, Hawk LW, Jr, Jaroni JL, Saad FG, Crystal-Mansour S, Shields PG, Lerman C. Am J Clin Nutr. 2004b;80:82–8.
Epstein LH, Leddy JJ, Temple JL, Faith MS. Psychol Bull. 2007a;133:884–906.
Epstein LH, Temple JL, Neaderhiser BJ, Salis RJ, Erbe RW, Leddy JJ. Behav Neurosci. 2007b;121:877–86.
Fetissov SO, Meguid MM, Sato T, Zhang LH. Am J Physiol Regul Integr Comp Physiol. 2002;283:R905–10.
Figlewicz DP. Am J Physiol Regul Integr Comp Physiol. 2003;284:R882–92.
Finlayson G, King N, Blundell JE. Neurosci Biobehav Rev. 2007;31:987–1002.
Finlayson G, King N, Blundell J. Appetite. 2008;50:120–7.
Finlayson G, Bryant E, Blundell JE, King NA. Physiol Behav. 2009;97:62–7.
Fuke S, Suo S, Takahashi N, Koike H, Sasagawa N, Ishiura S. Pharmacogenomics J. 2001;1:152–6.
Fulton S, Woodside B, Shizgal P. Science. 2000;287:125–8.
Goldfield GS, Lorello C, Doucet E. Am J Clin Nutr. 2007;86:308–15.
Grill HJ, Berridge KC. Taste reactivity as a measure of the neural control of palatability. In: Sprague JM, Epstein LH, editors. Progress in psychobiology and physiological psychology. Orlando, FL: Academic Press; 1985. pp. 1–61.
Halatchev IG, Cone RD. Cell Metab. 2005;1:159–68.
Hauge XY, Grandy DK, Eubanks JH, Evans GA, Civelli O, Litt M. Genomics. 1991;10:527–30.
Heath RG. J Nerv Ment Dis. 1972;154:3–18.
Heinz A, Goldman D, Jones DW, Palmour R, Hommer D, Gorey JG, Lee KS, Linnoila M, Weinberger DR. Neuropsychopharmacology. 2000;22:133–9.
Hoebel BG. Ann N Y Acad Sci. 1969;157:758–78.
Hommel JD, Trinko R, Sears RM, Georgescu D, Liu ZW, Gao XB, Thurmon JJ, Marinelli M, DiLeone RJ. Neuron. 2006;51:801–10.
Johnson J, Vickers Z. Appetite. 1993;21:25–39.
Julliard AK, Chaput MA, Apelbaum A, Aime P, Mahfouz M, Duchamp-Viret P. Behav Brain Res. 2007;183:123–9.
Kandel E, Schwartz JH, Jessell M, Jessell TM. Principals of neural science. Appleton and Lange; East Norwalk, Connecticut, U.S.A. 2000.

Karhunen LJ, Lappalainen RI, Haffner SM, Valve RH, Tuorila H, Miettinen H, Uusitupa MI. Int J Obes Relat Metab Disord. 1998;22:819–21.

Kringelbach ML. Neuroscience. 2004;126:807–19.

Levine AS, Atkinson RL. Fed Proc. 1987;46:159–62.

Malik S, McGlone F, Bedrossian D, Dagher A. Cell Metab. 2008;7:400–9.

Missale C, Nash SR, Robinson SW, Jaber M, Caron MG. Physiol Rev. 1998;78:189–225.

Naleid AM, Grace MK, Cummings DE, Levine AS. Peptides. 2005;26:2274–9.

Ninomiya Y, Shigemura N, Yasumatsu K, Ohta R, Sugimoto K, Nakashima K, Lindemann B. Vitam Horm. 2002;64:221–48.

Noble EP, Blum K, Ritchie T, Montgomery A, Sheridan PJ. Arch Gen Psychiatry. 1991;48:648–54.

Noble EP, Noble RE, Ritchie T, Syndulko K, Bohlman MC, Noble LA, Zhang Y, Sparkes RS, Grandy DK. Int J Eat Disord. 1994;15:205–17.

Olds J. Drives and reinforcements: Behavioral studies of hypothalamic functions. New York: Raven Press; 1977.

Orosco M, Gerozissis K, Rouch C, Meile MJ, Nicolaidis S. Obes Res. 1995;3 Suppl 5:655S–65S.

Pecina S, Berridge KC. J Neurosci. 2005;25:11777–86.

Perez C, Sclafani A. Am J Physiol. 1991;260:R179–85.

Pohjalainen T, Rinne JO, Nagren K, Lehikoinen P, Anttila K, Syvalahti EK, Hietala J. Mol Psychiatry. 1998;3:256–60.

Pomerleau M, Imbeault P, Parker T, Doucet E. Am J Clin Nutr. 2004;80:1230–6.

Portenoy RK, Jarden JO, Sidtis JJ, Lipton RB, Foley KM, Rottenberg DA. Pain. 1986;27:277–90.

Ravussin E, Kozak L. Energy homeostasis. In: Hofbauer K, Keller U, Boss O, editors. Pharmacotherapy of obesity-options and alternatives.CRC Press: Boca Raton, FL; 2004. pp. 488.

Raynaud E, Brun JF, Perez-Martin A, Sagnes C, Boularan AM, Fedou C, Mercier J. Clin Sci (Lond). 1999;96:343–8.

Raynor HA, Epstein LH. Appetite. 2003;40:15–24.

Rolls ET. The brain and reward. Pergamon Press: Oxford; 1975.

Rolls ET. Proc Nutr Soc. 2007;66:96–112.

Rolls ET, Murzi E, Yaxley S, Thorpe SJ, Simpson SJ. Brain Res. 1986;368:79–86.

Rolls ET, Scott TR, Sienkiewicz ZJ, Yaxley S. J Physiol. 1988;397:1–12.

Rolls ET, Sienkiewicz ZJ, Yaxley S. Eur J Neurosci. 1989;1:53–60.

Rolls ET, Yaxley S, Sienkiewicz ZJ. J Neurophysiol. 1990;64:1055–66.

Saelens BE, Epstein LH. Appetite. 1996;27:41–50.

Salamone JD, Correa M. Behav Brain Res. 2002;137:3–25.

Sibilia V, Lattuada N, Rapetti D, Pagani F, Vincenza D, Bulgarelli I, Locatelli V, Guidobono F, Netti C. Neuropharmacology. 2006;51:497–505.

Siep N, Roefs A, Roebroeck A, Havermans R, Bonte ML, Jansen A. Behav Brain Res. 2009;198:149–58.

Spiegel TA, Shrager EE, Stellar E. Appetite. 1989;13:45–69.

Steiner JE, Glaser D, Hawilo ME, Berridge KC. Neurosci Biobehav Rev. 2001;25:53–74.

Temple JL, Legierski CM, Giacomelli AM, Salvy SJ, Epstein LH. Am J Clin Nutr. 2008;87:1121–7.

Thiele TE, Van Dijk G, Campfield LA, Smith FJ, Burn P, Woods SC, Bernstein IL, Seeley RJ. Am J Physiol. 1997;272:R726–30.

Van Itallie TB, Beaudoin R, Mayer J. J Clin Nutr. 1953;1:208–17.

Wang GJ, Volkow ND, Fowler JS. Expert Opin Ther Targets. 2002;6:601–9.

Wang GJ, Volkow ND, Logan J, Pappas NR, Wong CT, Zhu W, Netusil N, Fowler JS. Lancet. 2001;357:354–7.

Wise RA. Behav Brain Sci. 1982;5:39–87.

Wise RA, Spindler J, deWit H, Gerberg GJ. Science. 1978;201:262–4.

Woods SC. Psychol Rev. 1991;98:488–505.

Yaxley S, Rolls ET, Sienkiewicz ZJ. Physiol Behav. 1988;42:223–9.

Yeomans MR, Gray RW. Neurosci Biobehav Rev. 2002;26:713–28.

Yeomans MR, Gray RW, Conyers TH. Physiol Behav. 1998;64:501–6.

Chapter 146
Nutritional Deficiencies and Spatial Memory Function

Sayali C. Ranade

Abbreviations

CNS	Central Nervous System
PUFA	Poly Unsaturated Fatty Acids
DHA	Docosahexanoic Acid
AA	Arachidonic Acid
EFA	Essential Fatty Acid
DNA	Deoxyribonucleic Acid
RNA	Ribonucleic Acid
CED	Chronic Energy Deficiency
BMI	Body Mass Index
PEM	Protein Energy Malnutrition
ID	Iron Deficiency
RAM	Radial Arm Maze
PD	Protein Deficiency
CA	Cornu Ammonis
IUGR	Intra Uterine Growth Retardation
BDNF	Brain Derived Neurotrophic Factor
DMT-1	Dimetallic Transporter 1
MMSE	Mini Mental State Examination
WMS-R	Wechsler Memory Scale-Revised
WAIS-R	Wechsler Adult Intelligence Scale-Revised
ERPs	Event Related Potentials
RA	Retinoic Acid

S.C. Ranade (✉)
National Brain Research Centre, National Highway-8, Near NSG Campus, Nainwal Mode, Manesar,
Haryana 122050, India
e-mail: sayali@nbrc.res.in; ranade.sayali@gmail.com

V.R. Preedy et al. (eds.), *Handbook of Behavior, Food and Nutrition*,
DOI 10.1007/978-0-387-92271-3_146, © Springer Science+Business Media, LLC 2011

146.1 Overview

Food has classically been perceived as a means to provide energy and building material to the body. However, its role in development and maintenance of specific physiological systems has been suggested only recently. One such system which is sensitive to the effects of nutrition or lack of it is the nervous system. A healthy nervous system requires balanced intake of food. Nutrition is one of the major epigenetic factors that affects the development and functioning of the nervous system. It took long for the general acceptance of the concept that the food that you consume can have an effect on the structure and function of the brain.

The term "Nutrition" refers to the balanced intake of nutrients for proper functioning of all body systems. There could be either qualitative or quantitative deviation from this optimum food intake. The nervous system is extremely vulnerable to different types of nutritional insults. There is a wide range of defects induced by nutritional deficiencies on the nervous system. These include structural (brain size, hippocampal volume), cellular (cerebellar neurogenesis, oligodendrocyte maturation), biochemical (neurotransmitter synthesis and release), electrophysiological (excitation and inhibition levels of neurons), behavioral (antisocial/violent behavior), and cognitive (memory disturbances, learning impairment) defects. The deleterious consequences of malnutrition on the nervous system depend on various factors. The most important factors which affect the nature and severity of these defects are: type of deficiency, level of malnourishment, and timing of exposure. The interaction of these factors will decide the outcome of the nervous system's defects. There is an enormous amount of data available on the effects of nutritional deficiencies on CNS. These reports come primarily from case studies or experimentation done on children from several developing countries. In addition, animal models have also been used as they provide a great tool to study and understand the effects of malnutrition on the CNS and also the mechanisms involved therein.

146.2 Role of Different Nutrients in Normal Development and Function of the Nervous System

The role of optimum nutrition in the normal cognitive and psychological development of an individual was evidenced by studies carried out following the Dutch hunger winter of 1944–1945 and the Chinese famine of 1950. These natural experiments provide valuable information on the role of different nutritional factors in the normal psychological development of an individual. The strong evidence from these studies suggests a connecting link between neurodevelopmental disruption and increased risk of schizophrenia. Deficiency of several candidate nutrients has been implicated in the vulnerability of an offspring to different psychiatric disorders including schizophrenia. Although discussing the involvement of different nutrients in normal psychological development in detail is outside the scope of this chapter, these are perhaps initial evidences that confirm the role of optimum nutrition in the normal development of the nervous system.

The exact mechanism by which food and nutrients affect various aspects of brain development and functioning are not fully known. However, the voluminous literature available provides an insight on how specific nutrients could possibly affect various aspects of brain functioning.

The important nutrient groups that affect development and/or functioning of the nervous system are proteins, certain types of fatty acids, micronutrients like iron, zinc, certain vitamins, etc.

Several findings in humans support the hypothesis of links between n-3 polyunsaturated fatty acid (PUFA) status and psychiatric diseases. Essential fatty acids are an important component of nerve cell membranes and are also essential for neurotransmitter release (Arnold et al. 2000). The nutritionally essential PUFAs, docosahexanoic acid (DHA), and arachidonic acid (AA) are critical for the proper development of brain structure and function during early development (Neuringer et al. 1986). EFAs provide nutrients and healthy fats necessary for the formation of myelin sheaths that cover axons, allowing faster conduction of nerve impulse.

Protein deficiency causes a variety of effects on the nervous system. In general, proteins are required by the brain for synthesis of DNA, RNA, structural proteins, growth factors, and neurotransmitters. They also play a role in synapse formation and extension of neurites, besides increasing the efficacy of neurotransmitters. Protein deficiency causes defects in the development and maturation of the nervous system, motor function, and major cognitive functions. Reduced brain size and impaired spinal cord histology are a few effects of protein deficiency on CNS.

The essential micronutrients, vitamin E, vitamin C, and selenium, affect the nervous system by virtue of their antioxidant functions. They protect the brain from oxidative insults by scavenging free radicals. Vitamin B complex is also essential for general health of the nervous system. Vitamin B12 helps in the formation of neurons, B9 is involved in synthesis of neurotransmitters, and vitamin B1 is involved in glucose metabolism of the brain.

The minerals calcium, magnesium, as well as manganese, iodine, potassium, silicon, sodium, and sulfur are all important for nervous system health. Calcium and magnesium also have an important role to play in nerve impulse conduction. There is considerable evidence that iron is important for neurological functioning and development (Lozoff 1987; Beard et al. 1993).Iron is a co-factor for several enzymes involved in neurotransmitter synthesis (Larkin and Rao 1990). It is also required for proper myelination of the spinal cord and white matter of cerebellar folds (Larkin and Rao 1990). Zinc is also an important co-factor involved in neurotransmitter synthesis. It is known to be indirectly involved in dopamine metabolism (Arnold et al. 2000)

146.3 The Factors Affecting Nature and Severity of Nervous System Defects

146.3.1 Extent of Nutritional Deficiency

The importance of the various nutrients in the development and maintenance of a healthy nervous system is well established. It can therefore be intuitively anticipated that anything less than the optimum requirement would be detrimental and induce deficits in the normal structure and function of the nervous system. The lesser the availability of the nutrient, the more severe the defects.

In a study of the effect of early long-term undernutrition on rat spatial cognition, the group with the highest level of dietary restriction showed the poorest performance on a water maze behavioral task. This effect however was significant in older rats. These findings demonstrate that the severity of the defects seen in the nervous system is directly proportional to the level of undernutrition. These findings also suggest that deficiency takes a longer time to exert its effects (Yanai et al. 2004). Rats undernourished (8% protein diet against normal 20% protein diet) during their lactational period were hyperactive to shock as adults (Vendite et al. 1985).Severe protein malnourishment causes reduction in brain size which is proportional to the degree of malnourishment. Children who are exposed to mild to moderate undernutrition are known to show varying degree of emotional instability, depending on extent of undernutrition.

However, any severity of malnourishment below a certain level exerts effects which are more general and are not limited only to the nervous system. In our own experience, female mice kept on a diet of low protein (less than 8%) had difficulty in becoming pregnant (unpublished observation).

146.3.2 Types of Nutritional Deficiency

Nutritional deficiencies are of different types. Undernutrition refers to insufficient caloric intake (chronic energy deficiency-CED, with BMI <18.5), while malnutrition implies imbalance or complete absence of one or more essential food constituents. However the term "malnutrition" is used in a more general sense, covering both under nutrition and malnutrition. The effects of malnutrition and under-nutrition on nervous system development and functioning are often overlapping, but not always.

Undernutrition continues to be one of the major health hazards in developing countries and in certain sections of developed countries. Undernutrition affects several parameters of nervous system development and maintenance, including volumes of one or more brain regions (Ranade et al. 2008), their morphology, neurotransmitter metabolism, and even behavior.

Malnutritional deficiencies can be further divided into macronutrient and micronutrient deficiencies. Macronutrient deficiency is the complete absence or reduction in the amount of macronutrients in the diet.

Protein deficiency is one of the major macronutrient deficiency affecting millions of people worldwide. Protein energy malnutrition is a global problem. Nearly 20 million people worldwide suffer from various forms of PEM viz. marasmus, kwashiorkar. It is also known to induce several types of brain defects. Considerable evidence indicates that PUFAs like DHA and AA also cause some defects in visual and cognitive development (Uauy et al. 1990; Carlson et al. 1994). This can also be categorized under macronutrient deficiency.

Among the micronutrient deficiencies, iron deficiency has a significant effect on the nervous system. The brain is sensitive to dietary iron depletion and regulates iron flux homeostasis very tightly. Perinatal iron deficiency (ID) is known to produce learning and memory impairments as well as reduced psychomotor skills both in humans and animal models (Pollit 1989; Walter et al. 1989).Other micronutrient deficiencies include deficiencies of important vitamins (Vitamin A or vitamin E) and minerals (calcium, magnesium, zinc) which are essential for normal nervous system functioning.

Each of these deficiencies induces its own set of defects which could either be unique to that particular deficiency or may show common features with the defects induced by other malnutritional deficiencies.

146.3.3 Critical Period of Nutritional Deficiency

The effects of malnutrition and undernutrition are of great interest due to the widespread incidence of fetal and infantile nutritional deficiencies. There is a growing body of evidence which suggests that the effects of nutritional insult on the developing brain are long-lasting and lead to permanent deficits in learning and behavior (Van Gelder 1984; Strupp and Levitsky 1995; Galler 2001). These evidences mainly come from human studies as well as animal experimentation. The issue of timing of nutritional deficiency, therefore, is of great importance. It is generally seen that nutritional deficiencies early on in life tend to lead to permanent defects in the CNS as against nutritional inadequacies in the later part of life.

It has been observed that some nervous system defects remain irreversible even after complete restoration of optimum nutrition. This is a good indication of the presence of a "critical period" of nutritional deficiency. This "critical period" is a period during which nutritional deficiency causes maximum damage. Depending on the timing of exposure, any inadequacy during the critical period might interfere with basic developmental processes including cytogenesis, histogenesis, and functional maturation of the brain.

There is vast literature detailing the effect of perinatal malnutrition on the developing brain. "Perinatal" malnutrition refers to a large time window in terms of development. So it would be convenient to divide it further into smaller time frames in order to pinpoint specific brain defects occurring during particular developmental time points. Perinatal malnutrition can therefore be further divided into prenatal and postnatal malnutrition. Each of these can induce varying degree of defects in the developing nervous system, depending on the brain compartment involved during that particular time window. The brain compartment showing a high level of activity will be affected the most.

146.4 Spatial Memory: An Essence of Life

Yes! We all need it! We require it to go to our work place or movie theatre and get back home from there. We need it to locate objects around us and locate ourselves with respect to these objects. Grazing animals need it to locate food patches. Mice and frogs need it to save themselves from predators. What is it that is needed in all the above cases? It's spatial memory. Spatial memory is a highly specialized function of the brain that is vital for survival in all species, including humans.

Memory is the process of retention of acquired information. When this information is about the space surrounding you, it is considered as spatial memory. Literally, therefore, it means memory of the space around you. Spatial memory is an essential component of our daily life which helps us move around in our environment. It is remembrance of places visited and understanding your position with respect to your surrounding. The concept of spatial learning was first introduced by O'Keefe and Nadal. In their words "Spatial learning refers to the construction of a representation of the topographical layout of an environment, and enables goal-directed navigation on the basis of a cognitive map" (O'Keefe and Nadel 1978). In simpler words, it is the process of acquiring information related to the space around you and retaining it for future use. This process can be divided into three phases:

1. Acquisition: Wherein individuals gain information about their surroundings.
2. Retention: The acquired information is stored or retained in specialized compartments of the brain.
3. Retrieval: The stored information is retrieved or recalled for subsequent use.

Spatial memory has two components: one is "spatial" (the one related to space) while the other one is "mnemonic" (memory component). Both these components are equally important for proper spatial memory function. Impairment in any of these components significantly affects overall spatial memory function.

One of the most compelling problems in neuroscience today is to identify the mechanisms underlying memory function. The area of the brain which has been recognized to play a vital role in formation of spatial memory in particular is the hippocampus. The involvement of the hippocampus in spatial memory processes has been established in a variety of species such as birds and mammals, including humans.

The hippocampus is a cortical structure located deep in the temporal lobe. It is formed by two sheets of cortex interlocking each other and has a layered structure where rows of pyramidal cells are arranged along with these layers. The connections within the hippocampus generally follow this laminar format and are unidirectional. They form well characterized closed loops originating in the adjacent **entorhinal cortex**. The different cell layers and sections are defined by the series of connections made. The main pyramidal cell layers are the regions **CA1** and CA3 and the granule cell layer is the **dentate gyrus** (Figs. 146.1 and 146.2)

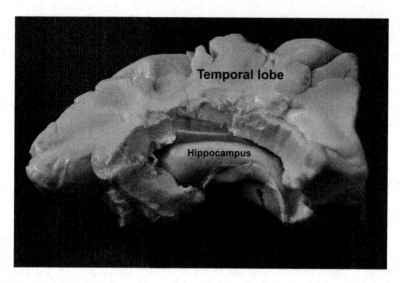

Fig. 146.1 A photograph showing human hippocampus, along with overlying temporal lobe. The hippocampus is one of the important structures involved in spatial memory function (Courtesy: Dr. Soumya Iyengar, National Brain Research Centre)

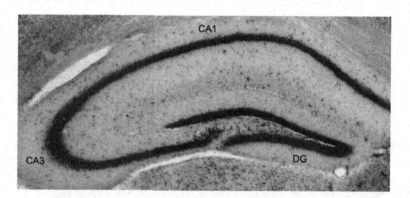

Fig. 146.2 A Nissl stained coronal section of rat hippocampus. Different subdivisions of hippocampus are seen viz. CA1, CA3 and Dentate gyrus (Courtesy: Dr. Shiv Kumar Sharma, National Brain Research Centre)

The hippocampus is a region of the brain which has both a prenatal and postnatal developmental window (Rice and Barone 2000). This course of development and the sequence of developmental processes are the same in both rodents and humans. There is a large increase in the size of the hippocampus during the first 4 postnatal weeks. The developmental processes occurring in the hippocampus during this period include neurogensis, myelination, proliferation of synapses, and dendritic remodeling (Altman and Bayer 1990). Normal progression of these processes is required for proper functioning of the hippocampus. Any deviation or disturbance in one or more of these processes can bring about defects in the normal functioning of the hippocampus, thereby affecting spatial memory function.

Although the initial knowledge about the involvement of the hippocampus in declarative memory came from patients with bilateral medial temporal lobe resection, further support and evidence indicating and confirming involvement of the hippocampus in spatial learning and memory (Witter and Amaral 1991) came from animal studies. Implication of the hippocampus in spatial memory function

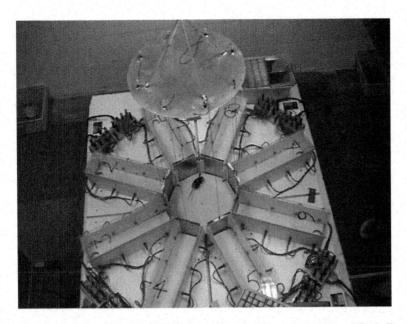

Fig. 146.3 Radial arm maze. A photograph of Radial Arm Maze apparatus at the National Brain Research Centre. Radial Arm Maze is an apparatus first designed by Samuel and Olton (1976). The apparatus is used to study spatial memory in laboratory animals or human subjects. The picture shows radial arm maze used for studying spatial memory in mice. It consists of a central platform with eight arms radiating from it. At the end of each arm is food cup in which a reward (in this case a chocoflake or a small food pellet) is kept. Each arm is separated from the central platform by a Guillotine door. All the Guillotine doors are attached to common pulley. Both central platform and arms are covered with transparent plexiglass covers. Different temporal domains of spatial memory viz. reference memory, working memory can be tested by employing different experimental paradigms (Courtesy: Professor V. Ravindranath, former Director, National Brain Research Centre)

is supported by lesion, reversible inactivation, early gene expression, and electrophysiological studies (Frankland and Bontempi 2005).

There are well developed protocols available for studying, establishing, and confirming the role of the hippocampus in spatial learning. A variety of paradigms are available for investigation of spatial learning, and perhaps the most commonly used are the Morris water maze(Morris et al. 1982) and the Radial Arm Maze (Olton and Samuelson 1976) (Figs. 146.3, 146.4, and 146.5).

Another important brain area involved in spatial memory function in primates, including humans, is the prefrontal cortex. This area is also vulnerable to malnutritional insults. The effect of malnutritional insults on prefrontal cortex has been studied with respect to delay in development and maturation of cognitive function. However, its specific role in spatial memory function following malnutritional deficiencies has not been studied so far.

146.5 Malnutrition and Spatial Memory

As described previously, the effect of malnutrition on spatial memory or for that matter on any other brain function can be divided broadly into two groups:

(a) Perinatal malnutrition
(b) Malnutrition in later stages of life

Fig. 146.4 A schematic representation of an 8-arm Radial Arm Maze. An 8-arm radial arm maze showing the central platform, arms radiating from it, and food cups located at the distal end of each arm

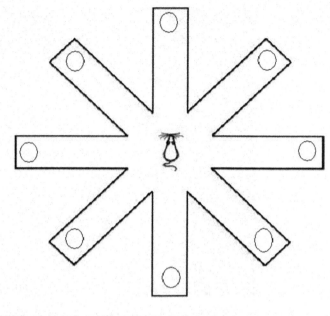

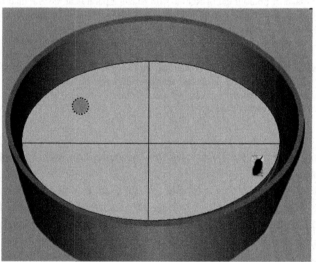

Fig. 146.5 A schematic representation of Morris Water maze designed to study spatial memory function in rodents. The Morris water navigation task is another behavioral procedure used to study spatial memory of laboratory rodents. The apparatus was devised by Professor Richard Morris. It consists of a small water pool, which contains a small escape platform submerged few millimeters below the water level. The pool is theoretically divided into four quadrants. Conspicuous visual cues are placed around the pool in plain sight of the animal. The animal is placed in the pool and it swims around the pool in search of an escape. Various parameters like total distance traveled, the time spent in each quadrant of the pool, the time taken to reach the platform are recorded. The improvement of performance on all these parameters will be measured over the period of time

There is a distinct difference between the types and severity of deficits induced by these two different time windows, and each window will result in an entirely different profile of the defects on CNS. The reasons for these differences are as follows: In the first group, where the developing brain is especially malleable, malnutrition has a more pronounced effect on brain structures and systems supporting cognitive function. These effects are more severe and long lasting. These effects are therefore more likely to be irreversible even after subsequent rehabilitation. In the latter group, because it is the developed brain that is exposed to malnutrition the effects are less severe and can be reversed at least to a certain extent with subsequent supplementation. It is thus logical and rational to consider both these groups separately.

146.5.1 Perinatal Malnutrition/Undernutrition and Spatial Memory

Malnutrition and/or undernutrition during infancy and childhood are problems prevalent in many parts of the world. Malnutrition neither produces gross anatomical abnormalities in the nervous system nor gross mental retardation or psychopathology. The effect of malnutrition shouldn't however be underrated for this reason. The malnutritional insults rather result in permanent suboptimal development leading to long-term learning and cognitive impairments. This is an equally serious problem. It is therefore important to study these effects. Animal studies provide a reasonable means of obtaining relevant information pertaining to the effects of malnutritional insults on the developing brain. These types of spatial memory defects have been studied at various levels of organization viz. structural, functional, biochemical, physiological, behavioral, and cognitive.

The defects underlying spatial memory function are best manifested at and therefore can be best studied at a behavioral level. Behavioral testing of rodents and primates are routinely done by using either the radial arm maze or the water maze paradigm. These behavioral protocols provide valuable insights into mechanisms underlying memory process. Behavioral defects are the manifestation of spatial memory dysfunction and the underlying cause could be a structural defect. Considering the involvement of the hippocampus in spatial memory function it is reasonable to study the hippocampus with respect to structural defects if any, followed by its functional implications.

Along with other areas of the brain which undergo rapid postnatal development, the hippocampus appears to be vulnerable to early undernutrition. This provides one more reason to study the hippocampus for possible defects. In spite of early undernutrition not producing brain lesions, deficits seen in the hippocampus by early undernutrition may show some related functional disability (Lynch et al. 1975). It is therefore important to study defects other than structural defects such as lesions, if any.

The type of deficiency one is subjected to, is one of the major deciding factors of the outcome of spatial memory deficits. Different types of deficiencies may or may not have similar effects on the system under consideration, in this case spatial memory function. Ranade et al. (2008) have shown that different types of malnourishment affect different domains of spatial memory function. Although these data have been shown with only three types of nutritional deficiencies; perinatal Chronic energy deficiency (CED), Protein deficiency (PD) and Iron deficiency (ID) and studied spatial memory function only at behavioral and gross anatomical levels, it is evident from this report that the type of deficiency has a significant role to play in deciding the specificity of defects seen. It is therefore important to study each type of deficiency specifically with respect to spatial memory function. Data from such studies will help in understanding the effects of specific types of malnutrition on spatial memory function.

146.5.1.1 Undernutrition and Spatial Memory Deficits

The effects of perinatal undernutrition on spatial memory or hippocampal function are inconsistent. Some studies, using radial arm maze or Morris water maze, report significant deficits in spatial memory function. However, others claim that spatial learning is completely unaffected by early undernutrition.

Jordan et al. (1981) have shown that perinatal undernutrition in rats affected their radial arm maze performance tested on an 8- and 16-arm apparatus, when tested at 90 days of age. Significant differences were seen on many parameters. Experimental animals showed less exploratory behavior and took more time to make choices when compared with control animals. Such deficits are similar to hippocampal dysfunction defects, which severely impair the performance of animals on similar spatial tasks.

Recent studies of the effects of developmental malnutrition in rats have suggested that hippocampal formation may be especially prone to irreversible neuroanatomical and neurophysiological alterations as well.

In another study, reduced cell numbers have been reported in the dentate gyrus and in the CA fields of the hippocampus proper (Lewis et al. 1979; Jordan et al. 1982) following perinatal undernutrition. In an altogether different paradigm of postnatal undernutrition it has been shown that lengthy periods of undernutrition affect the developmental growth curve of synapse formation and also alters the neuron: synapse ratio (Ahmed et al. 1987). Yanai et al. (2004) have reported the effect of different levels of dietary restriction on spatial cognition in rats. Animals were subjected to 80%, 60%, or 40% of free feeding and tested with Morris water maze place task throughout their lives. At a younger age, no significant difference was seen among the different experimental groups. However, at 9 months and thereafter, the 40% feeding group performed poorer than the other groups. This example also confirms the long-lasting nature of early undernutrition on spatial memory function.

On the other hand, Campbell and Bedi (1989) using Morris's test showed little evidence of any differences in the spatial learning abilities of rats previously undernourished from birth up to 60 days of age compared with well-fed age-matched controls. This is despite the fact that the same group had reported significant and persistent alterations in the morphology (viz. synapses per cell) of the dentate gyrus induced by undernutrition. The possible links between morphological and behavioral defects induced by perinatal undernutrition need to be established and confirmed.

146.5.1.2 Perinatal Protein Deficiency

It is well established that protein–calorie restriction, or protein malnutrition experienced during the early postnatal period leads to significant and often permanent changes in brain anatomy physiology, biochemistry, and behavior. The damages induced by protein deficiency include the damages to the maturation of the nervous system, motor function, and major cognitive functions. These effects have been observed in protein malnourished children all over the world. Exposure to protein deficiency even for a limited period may evoke permanent impairments of several brain functions. It has also been demonstrated (Ranade et al. 2008) that early protein malnourishment affects various aspects of hippocampal structure and function.

Protein deficiency can be induced in two ways.

(a) Protein malnourishment as a result of total undernutrition. Total reduced intake of food means reduced intake of proteins which culminates in protein deficiency.
(b) Protein malnourishment because of imbalanced diet i.e. diet doesn't contain the required amount of protein although there is optimum intake of food. That means there is no quantitative reduction in food intake.

The effects of both these conditions may sometimes have similar effects but sometimes may generate an entirely different profile of defects. Unless studied strictly under defined experimental conditions these two conditions are difficult to dissociate. So for this chapter these two conditions will not be explained separately. A series of studies have shown marked and lasting changes in the structure and function of the hippocampal formation in rats subjected to prenatal protein malnutrition.

The structural changes seen in the hippocampus include volume or area changes of the total hippocampus or certain subdivisions of it. Noback and Eisenman (1981) have reported a decreased width of the dentate gyrus as a result of protein–calorie restriction on the developing brain. Paula-Barbosa et al. (1988), in a study of long-term, postweaning undernutrition, reported a decrease in the width of the dentate gyrus and decreased granule cell packing density at 6, 12, and 18 months (Diaz-Cintra et al. 1991). Perinatal protein deficiency showed the highest reduction in hippocampal volume of F1-pups.This was in comparison with control as well as other deficiencies including CED and ID. This decrement was contributed maximally by the dentate gyrus and CA1 subdivisions of the hippocampus (Ranade et al. 2008).

These gross changes in the dimensions are a result of finer changes that occur at the cellular level. These changes include reduction in total cell number or decrease in certain population of cells. It could also be due to reduction in cell size of a certain population of cells. These changes at the cellular level either in isolation or in combination can bring about changes in the volume of the hippocampus.

Diaz-Cintra et al. (1991) have shown the effect of prenatal protein deprivation on the development of granule cells in rat at different ages. They showed significant reduction in the size of granule cells, a decreased number of synaptic spines, and reduced complexity of dendritic branching in the outer two thirds of the molecular layer. The effects persisted throughout the study period of 220 days.

The functional changes in hippocampus following early protein malnourishment include a reduction in the mean threshold to produce after discharge activity within the dentate gyrus. An even greater number of stimulations is required to elicit full convulsive motor seizures in response to perforant path kindling stimuli (Bronzino et al. 1991). Prenatal protein deprivation affected certain components of long-term potentiation (Austin et al.1986) in the dentate gyrus of adult rats.

Taken together, these results suggest the vulnerability of the hippocampus to prenatal protein insults. An important question however is whether these structural and functional defects together lead to any behavioral impairment or not. Reports suggesting the effect of protein malnourishment on behavioral parameters are inconsistent.

Barnes et al. (1966) studied learning behavior in rats that were subjected to different forms of nutritional deprivation in early life. The performance of these rats was tested on visual discrimination performance in a Y-maze at 6–9 months of age. The rats that were deprived both before and after weaning made significantly more errors in their choices than the normal controls. Rats born to females fed on 8% case in throughout pregnancy showed lower visuo-spatial memory performance. The rats were deprived either preweaning or postweaning or both. On the Y-maze task, double-deprived rats performed the worst. When these rats were tested for position reversal performance in the water maze shortly after weaning the maximum number of errors were made by the double-deprived rats. The results also showed gender biases. Valadares and Almeida (2005) tested rats fed with 16% (well-nourished) or 6% (malnourished) protein diets during the lactation phase on the Morris water-maze in procedures of spaced trials (1 trial/day), intermediate density (4, 8, 12 trials/day), and condensed trials (24 trials/day).The results showed that protein malnutrition caused deficits in spatial learning and memory in spaced but not in intermediate and condensed trials procedure. When tested again 7 and 28 days after training, malnourished animals showed significantly higher latency compared with well-nourished controls. In another study, mice which were maintained on a protein-deficient diet during both gestation and lactation were tested on the radial arm maze. The results showed a specific and significant negative effect on working memory compared to other malnourished groups (viz. CED and ID) and controls (Ranade et al. 2008). These findings are inconsistent with previous reports by Tonkiss and Galler (1990), who reported no effect on working memory of rats which were prenatally protein deprived. This working memory was tested on two different behavioral protocols of learning and memory. The differences in experimental paradigms as well as in malnutrition protocols may account for the differences in results in this case.

Taken together these results very clearly suggest vulnerability of the developing hippocampus to gestational and/or lactation protein deficiency at various organizational levels. The discrepancies seen in the effect of PD on spatial memory function at the behavioral level could arise partially from the differences in the malnutritional paradigm used and partially due to differences in the design of the spatial memory task. There is also a possibility of the existence of species-specific differences.

146.5.1.3 Iron Deficiency and Spatial Memory

Iron deficiency is the largest single-nutrient deficiency affecting millions of new born babies worldwide. The several reasons for intrauterine iron deficiency include IUGR, anemia, alcoholism, maternal diabetes mellitus, and maternal nutritional iron deficiency either prior to or during pregnancy.

Several human studies report that anemic children show lower scores on various cognitive tests. Recognition memory at birth and at follow-up seemed to be affected in children who were at risk for brain iron deficiency (ID) during the late fetal/early neonatal period of the development (Siddappa et al. 2004). Although ID is associated with long-term cognitive abnormalities (de-Regnier et al. 2000; Nelson et al. 2000) its direct role in spatial memory is supported by only a few studies. Animal models have shown irreversible behavioral abnormalities resulting from diet-induced iron deficiency during early development. B.T. Felt and B. Lozoff (1996). View Record in Scopus Cited By in Scopus (107) ID is also known to delay myelination, thus leading to behavioral deficits. Therefore, behavioral defects seen as a result of iron deficiency cannot be attributed solely to hippocampal dysfunction.

Iron deficiency is known to affect some of the developmental processes related to the hippocampus, including myelination (Lozoff 2000), proliferation, and maturation of synapses (Jorgenson et al. 2005), and dendritic remodeling. It can therefore be speculated that some functions of the hippocampus may be compromised as a result of these underlying structural changes. Spatial memory could be one of them. The link between ID and spatial memory function is indirect and speculative at this point of time. Another possibility is that iron deficiency could potentiate these effects on the hippocampus through other adverse effects like oxidative stress.

The wide range of effects of iron deficiency on the hippocampus includes decrease in hippocampal energy metabolism (deUngria et al. 2000), altered hippocampal iron concentration (Felt and Lozoff 1996), altered neurotransmission by altering glutamate and GABA concentration (Rao et al. 2003), disrupted dendritic morphogenesis in CA1 pyramidal neurons (Jorgenson et al. 2003), and maturation of synaptic function and efficacy (Jorgenson et al. 2005). In addition there is an alteration in the pattern of neurochemical profiling (Rao et al. 2003), which also suggests changes in energy status, neurotransmission, and even myelination. Fetal or neonatal iron deficiency is also known to lower BDNF function, thereby impairing neuronal differentiation in the hippocampus (Tran et al. 2008). All or some of these changes may underlie spatial memory deficits seen in ID.

There are a few studies which report direct involvement of iron deficiency in spatial memory function.In their study of the effect of different types of malnutrition on spatial memory function checked by the radial arm maze test, Ranade et al. (2008) have reported that reference memory is selectively affected in the ID model. F1-pups born to mothers who were kept on an iron-deficient diet for 6 weeks prior to conception and also during gestation and lactation were checked for their spatial memory performance at 8 weeks of age. These animals showed selective impairment of reference memory function leaving other functions like working memory intact. In a recent report by Carlson et al. (2009), the importance of iron in neuronal development and memory function has been shown in the mouse hippocampus. Double mutants of mouse DMT-1(Slc11a2) were not able to perform

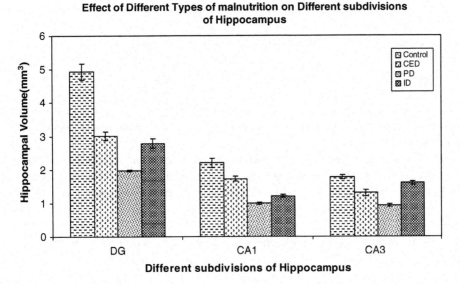

Fig. 146.6 Effect of different types perinatal malnutritional deficiencies on volumes of different hippocampal subdivisions. The *x*-axis shows different subdivisions of the hippocampus and *y*-axis shows a reduction in the volume of different hippocampal subdivisions with respect to control. This volume reduction was seen following perinatal malnutrition of different types viz. *CED* chronic energy deficiency, *PD* protein deficiency, *ID* iron deficiency. Results are expressed as mean ± SEM, *n* = 5 for each group (Reprinted from Ranade et al. 2007)

well on the difficult version of the spatial navigation task but were able to learn the easier version of it checked by the Morris water maze. No difference was found between the wild type and double mutant on learning of visual cued task.

From the above discussion it is clear that iron deficiency can cause a wide range of abnormalities in hippocampal structure and function. In addition, a strong correlation has been shown between iron deficiency and spatial memory dysfunction. However, a causal relationship between the two needs to be established. This can be achieved by suggesting a biologically plausible mechanism and studying it by using animal models. This will confirm the causal role of ID in spatial memory function (Fig. 146.6).

146.5.1.4 Other Perinatal Nutritional Deficiencies and Spatial Memory Function

Zinc deficiency occurs widely within the human population. In animal models, gestational or lactational zinc deficiency is found to produce various behavioral defects which include increased aggression (Halas et al. 1975.), increased food motivation (Halas et al. 1980), and impaired avoidance conditioning (Halas and Sandstead 1975). In their study carried out on rats Halas et al. (1985) showed the effect of perinatal zinc deficiency on learning and memory of young adult rats. Rats born to zinc-deficient mothers showed learning and memory deficits tested on the 17-arm radial arm maze. Pups which were born to zinc-deficient mothers showed significantly inferior working memory compared to the control group. No differences were seen in the reference memory of any of the experimental groups.

Choline is another important constituent which when deprived during fetal or neonatal development causes spatial memory deficits in addition to other nervous system defects. Choline is derived not only from diet but is also synthesized in the body. It influences cell proliferation and apoptosis, thereby altering brain structure and function. Choline supplementation in rats during pre- and postnatal development is known to enhance their spatial memory performance checked on the radial-arm maze (Meck et al.

1988) and water maze tasks (Schenk and Brandner 1995). Prenatally choline-supplemented and choline-deprived rats showed no difference in radial arm maze performance when the trials were spaced. Choline-deficient rats exhibited high levels of proactive interference as a function of mass trials suggesting that choline deprivation causes modification of discriminative abilities that distinguish between end of one trial and beginning of another and the capacity to remember location during a trial.

Transient vitamin D deficiency in rats is associated with subtle and discrete alterations in learning and memory. However, animals prenatally depleted of vitamin D showed impairment neither on spatial learning task in the radial arm maze nor on two-way avoidance learning in the shuttle box (Becker et al. 2005)

The initial evidence suggesting the importance of folate came from studies that established a link between increased risk of neurodevelopmental disorders and folate-deficient pregnant women (Smithells et al. 1976). Although cognitive defects following folate deficiency are well known, these defects do not pertain to spatial memory function. The mechanisms involved are also poorly understood.

Since the developing brain is an extremely transient system with its requirements very tightly regulated, any small modification or perturbation brings about a huge change in the outcome of this system at various levels. Nutritional factors which are major regulatory elements of this system have to be properly balanced in order to get the best out of it. It is therefore absolutely essential to strike the right balance of these nutrients to get the desired results of a normal functioning brain.

146.5.2 Late Age Nutritional Deficiencies and Effect on the Nervous System

In contrast to the developing brain the mature brain has long been thought to be resistant to malnutritional insults. Therefore, not much attention has been paid to the effect of nutritional deficiencies on the developed brain. But since it is evident from the literature that nutritional deficiencies not only affect development but also maintenance of the central nervous system, more efforts are being made to study the effect of nutritional deficiencies on the adult brain. A healthy diet is extremely important for the proper functioning of the developed nervous system as well. Exposure to nutritional deficiencies in adult life may not produce effects which are as severe as fetal or neonatal nutritional deficiencies. However, the adult nervous system is equally at risk to the hazardous effects of nutritional deficiencies.

A significant population of developing countries or certain socioeconomic groups of developed countries could very well serve as a model for adult malnutritional deficiency studies. However, there is a possibility that this is the same population which has also experienced fetal as well as neonatal malnutritional deficiency. So the results that one sees would be the cumulative effects of both perinatal as well as adult malnutritional insults. Population studies therefore don't offer much in terms of understanding the effects of malnutritional insults on adult brain. Once again, animal studies come as a great help. Most of our knowledge about these effects also comes from animal experimentation.

Two important deficiencies which are well studied with respect to their effects on the adult brain are protein deficiency and iron deficiency. However undernutrition is also known to have a significant effect on hippocampus-dependant cognitive function. A study carried out on 16 anorexia nervosa patients with same number of age-matched controls showed reduced hippocampal volume in anorexia nervosa patients (Connan 2006). This study did not report the link between the cause and consequence of hippocampal size and function. However, incorporation of endocrine, neuropsychological, and neuroimaging aspects in such studies would help in doing so.

In their study using a long-term low-protein diet model started in adult life, Paula-Barbosa et.al have shown that a low protein diet for an extended period of time in adult rats leads to a decrease in the numerical density of the dentate granule and CA3 pyramidal cells (Paula-Barbosa et al. 1988, 1989).The same group has further shown that the numerical density of synapses established by mossy fibers and the thorny excrescences of CA3 pyramidal cells was also decreased (Andrade et al. 1991). Paula-Barbosa further demonstrated that besides granule and CA3 pyramidal cells, the remaining neuronal populations of the hippocampal formation of the adult rat also show reduction in number as a result of long-term protein deprivation. This cell loss in the hippocampus proper, at this point of time, is a consequence of neuronal degeneration alone, as the process of cell acquisition of both CA1 and CA3 pyramidal cells is accomplished before birth (Bayer1980). Therefore, the results may indicate an induction of neuronal degeneration as a result of adult protein deficiency. This study also demonstrated that rehabilitation from malnutrition does not lead to improvement in the morphological alterations induced by malnutrition. This also confirms the irreversibility of these malnutritional insults on the adult brain. Although there are no reports suggesting a direct role of adult protein deficiency in spatial memory function, the above mentioned correlation between protein deficiency and hippocampal defects can be extrapolated to establish a link between protein deficiency and hippocampus-dependant spatial memory function. The direct role of late protein deficiency in spatial memory function needs to be further investigated.

Women of reproductive age, and children, are at high risk for iron deficiency. While the effects of iron deficiency on mental function in children are well recognized, not much is known about how an iron shortage affects the adult brain. A number of investigators reported that iron deficiency anemia had a great influence on cognitive functions in infants and children. However, similar studies in adults are few and also controversial. Studies carried out on human subjects shows that reduced brain iron level or anemia in females induces attention deficits and learning and memory impairments (Murray-Kolb and Beard 2007). A study carried out by Khedr et al. on 28 young adults showed the possible influence of iron deficiency anemia and iron supplementation on cognitive function and intelligence. The patients in their study demonstrated lower scores on different cognitive tests like MMSE, WMS-R, and WAIS-R. Prolongation of ERPs and reduction in their amplitude were also seen. These performances however improved following 3 months of supplementation. There are quite a few reports suggesting the important role of iron in the normal functioning of the brain at any time in life, and several reports strongly suggest a link between ID and spatial learning and memory. However, not much data are available demonstrating the role of adult iron deficiency in spatial learning. Little evidence for this comes from the human studies, but more animal studies are needed to establish and confirm the role of adult iron deficiency, if any, in spatial learning and memory function.

The other malnutritional deficiencies known to affect the spatial memory function and hippocampus include vitamin A deficiency and folate deficiency.

Several animal studies have shown that vitamin-A plays a key role in brain development. Vitamin A deficiency exerts its effect on memory functions through retinoic acid hyposignaling (Lane and Bailey 2005; Bremner and McCaffery 2008). Long-term synaptic plasticity in hippocampal formation requires retinoids. Hypofunction of retinoid signaling is implicated in spatial memory dysfunction (Cocco et al. 2002). These types of effects can be reversed by either retinoid or vitamin-A supplementation. Long-term vitamin A deficiency is shown to decrease neurogenesis and leads to memory deficits. These effects were shown to be reversed with RA (retinoic acid) treatment which could be brought about by an upregulation of retinoid-mediated molecular events. Several reports suggest that the effects of vitamin A deficiency at the level of hippoccampal neurogenesis are reversible and that RA treatment also helps in the maintenance of the hippocampal plasticity and function.

Folic acid is another important nutrient whose deficiency has been associated with neurological diseases and mood disorders (D'Anci and Rosenberg 2004). A study which tested the effect of folate deficiency on mice lacking uracil DNA glycosylase (*Ung_/_*) versus wild-type controls showed a clear effect on spatial learning. A hippocampus-dependant spatial learning task in the Morris water maze showed that escape latency and path length was significantly affected in folate-deficient mice. The same study also reported repression of neurogenesis in hippocampal progenitors following folate deficiency (Kronenberg et al. 2008). There is also increasing evidence of the beneficial effect of folate in protection against Alzheimer's disease and cognitive decline with age (Seshadri et al. 2002; Nurk et al. 2005).

146.5.2.1 Nutritional Deficiencies, Spatial Memory Function, and the Aging Brain

The relationship between nutrition and its brain effects become prominent during aging. The aging brain is vulnerable to various factors including malnutritional insults. A sharp decline in food intake accompanied by a slowdown in metabolism during aging contributes significantly to these effects. In addition to hampering cell function, this even weakens the cells' defenses against harmful free radicals, and also impedes the ability to grow new cells. Brain cells and neurons get affected due to free radicals generated through oxidation. All these reasons make the aging brain highly vulnerable to nutritional insults. Since these changes occur in almost all regions of the brain including the hippocampus it is possible that this in turn may contribute to memory loss.

Cognitive decline and memory loss are an inseparable part of natural aging process. So long as memory loss is not as serious as senile dementia or Alzheimer's disease, minor lapse of memory is nothing to worry about. Nutritional deficiencies contribute significantly to both general memory loss as a function of aging and more serious version of memory loss as seen in Alzheimer's disease.

As discussed, the effect of both prenatal and adult protein malnutrition or undernutrition on the brain includes a variety of dysfunctions. The hippocampus is one of the more severely affected brain compartments. Changes in the hippocampus include altered density of various important cell types, namely dentate granule or CA3 pyramidal cells. In addition there is also a reduction in dendritic spine density (Andrade et al. 1995). At the functional level, there seems to be a specific reduction of working memory checked on radial arm maze (Ranade et al. 2008). Since all these structural and functional deficits are manifested even as a function of normal aging, this decrement would be still stronger in aging brains subjected to protein malnutrition. Whether these age-dependant deficits are indirectly an effect of malnutrition by virtue of reduced food intake or not is debatable. Due to lack of experimental evidence, the effect of undernutrition or protein deficiency on the aging brain is purely speculative and needs to be studied in detail. There is growing interest in the role of nutrition in aging diseases such as dementia, in particular sporadic or late-onset Alzheimer's disease. Alzheimer's disease is the most prevalent form of dementia, characterized by significant memory loss. The nutritional deficiencies shown in Alzheimer's patients include a relative shortage of specific macro- and micronutrients. These include omega-3 fatty acids, several B-vitamins, and antioxidants such as vitamins E and C (Bourre 2004). Certain in vitro and in vivo studies also support the idea that nutritional components can compensate for specific defects of neurodegenerative disorders.

The role of iron deficiency in certain neurodegenerative disorders is also speculative at this point in time. The brain regions which accumulate iron in these disorders are the same as those compromised in early iron deficiency. The important questions that come up are: Does early life exposure to iron deficiency make one more prone to neurodegenerative disorders like Alzheimer's disease? If so, does this happen because the profile of iron-metabolizing proteins in the brain of these individuals is altered due to early iron deficiency? Also are these effects aggravated due to iron deficiency during aging? This is an idea that definitely needs to be explored in detail and supported by experimental observations.

The role of zinc deficiency is also suggested in the deterioration of learning and memory in senescence-accelerated mice. The report by Saito et al. (2000) suggests that age-dependent deficiencies of Zn in synaptic vesicles of the mossy fiber pathway induced by low expression of ZnT3 causes glutamatergic excitotoxicity in the hippocampal neurons and the deterioration of learning and memory in SAMP10 (Saito et al. 2000). An unbalanced copper metabolism and homeostasis (due to dietary deficiency) could also be linked to Alzheimer's disease.

Bourre explains the detailed role of different micronutrients on the aging brain (Bourre 2008). Vitamin B9 is known to preserve memory during aging. Vitamin B12 delays the onset of signs of dementia if administered in a precise clinical time window. Poor folate status is associated with cognitive decline and dementia in older adults.

Effects of malnutritional insults on the developing and adult brains are well known. These effects just become more pronounced on the aging brain. These effects need to be demonstrated empirically.

146.6 Applications to the Other Areas of Health and Disease

There is a strong requirement for efforts to be directed towards demonstrating the causal relationship of nutritional deficiencies and spatial memory dysfunction. A greater number of studies are needed to be carried out to demonstrate the specific involvement of a particular type of malnutritional deficiency on specific temporal domain of spatial memory function in detail. Studies which address the involvement of specific components of spatial memory function (either spatial or mnemonic) in overall compromised spatial memory dysfunction following malnutritional insults are also required to be carried out. This type of research will not only help delineate the mechanisms underlying spatial memory dysfunction but will also help us design new intervention strategies.

The information obtained from the above mentioned studies will have many added advantages and will also provide important insights into other areas of research.

A clearer and detailed understanding of the mechanisms involved in spatial memory function is valuable information that can be obtained from such studies, along with a better understanding of spatial memory function per se. The findings of these studies will help researchers link the behavior of an individual with the structural correlates of that particular behavior. This could be achieved by studying the affected brain area in detail at all levels of organization viz. structural, cellular, biochemical, and electrophysiological, and its behavioral manifestation. These studies will also offer valuable information about structural and functional development of the brain in general.

Deficiencies of certain nutrients are implicated in some neurodegenerative and psychiatric disorders. A detailed study in this context will help in finding a progression pattern of some of these disorders and may even shed some light on the detailed mechanisms involved in it. Various intervention strategies can be designed based on this knowledge. The studies will also suggest the critical period of vulnerability of the aging brain to various other insults and mechanisms involved. The mechanisms involved in brain aging can also be studied in detail by using such studies.

Thus, studying malnutritional insults with respect to spatial memory dysfunction will have several other added advantages and provide valuable information in other areas of research.

The age old saying, "You are what you eat," seems quite true even in the modern world. The advancement in techniques, expanding horizons of knowledge, availability of information put together also confirm that you are what you eat. Diet has a very strong influence not only on one's health but also on the outcome of disorders and diseases.

The nervous system is one of the systems that is highly vulnerable to nutritional insults. The effect of malnutrition on behavior and cognition are not usually life threatening but are still serious enough to demand special attention. Memory dysfunction is an issue of great concern. The types of behavioral or cognitive defects induced by malnutrition include reduced ability to learn certain tasks or inability to adapt to changes or inability to retain acquired information. Such defects do not allow an individual to make optimum use of one's own capability and to be the best that one can be in a demanding society. These types of defects deal mostly with "quality of life" issues.

The problem of fetal and neonatal malnutritional deficiencies is grimmer and also long lasting. It is almost the entire future generation which is at stake for suboptimal cognitive performance for the rest of their lives.

The increasing incidence of neurodegenerative and psychiatric disorders suggest a role of lifestyle changes due to modernization. The most obvious yet underrated factor influencing cognitive decline is the role of nutrition. Quite a few of these disorders have memory dysfunction as one of the important characteristics. Although normal decline and impairment in cognitive abilities as a function of aging is very common, increasing incidences of neurodegenerative disorders are alarming and may be blamed on unhealthy eating habits. The above discussion strongly confirms the role of nutrition as an important epigenetic factor influencing cognition and behavior.

The optimum physical, chemical, and physiological development of the brain and consequent behavior is the right of every individual irrespective of their social and/or economic background. Optimum nutrition should therefore be provided to each and every individual to ensure normal and healthy brain development. It is also imperative to employ multiple strategies at various levels to overcome the defects induced by malnutrition. Thus, a combination of economic, educational, behavioral, political, social, therapeutic, and rehabilitation strategies should be used to deal with this widespread and serious issue.

Summary Points

- Optimum nutrition is an essential factor that ensures normal structural and functional development of the brain. A change in even a single constituent of the diet can have a huge yet very specific effect on brain structure and function.
- Nutritional deficiencies affect development and maintenance of the central nervous system.
- Spatial memory function, which is a crucial function of the brain, is also compromised by nutritional deficiencies.
- Spatial memory is a memory of space around one. Spatial memory function involves processes like acquiring knowledge about the space around and retaining it for subsequent use.
- Early age nutritional deficiencies have more severe and long-lasting effects on spatial memory function as compared to late age nutritional deficiencies. The effects of fetal or neonatal nutritional deficiencies are irreversible.
- Although the adult brain is also vulnerable to nutritional insults the defects are mostly reversible at least up to a certain extent.
- Different types of nutritional deficiencies affect different domains of memory function, e.g., Protein deficiency selectively affects working memory, whereas iron deficiency affects reference memory leaving all other memory functions intact.
- Although a strong corelational link between nutritional deficiencies and spatial memory dysfunction is very well established, a causal link between the two needs to be demonstrated by suggesting a biologically plausible mechanism supported by well-designed experiments.

Definitions

Malnutrition: Reduction or complete absence of one or more food constituents in the diet.
Undernutrition: Reduction in total dietary intake or inadequate calorie intake.
Macronutrient deficiency: Reduction or complete absence of one or more macronutrients (e.g., protein or fatty acids) from the diet.
Micronutrient deficiency: Reduction or complete absence of one or more micronutrients (e.g., vitamins, minerals) from the diet.
Spatial memory: Memory of the space around an individual.
Spatial learning: The process of acquisition of information about the space around the individual.
Prenatal: Time period before birth, i.e., during pregnancy or gestation.
Postnatal: Time period just after birth, i.e., during lactation.
Perinatal: Time period covering both prenatal and postnatal periods.

Key Features of Spatial Memory Function

1. A balanced diet is important for the development and maintenance of a healthy nervous system. Imbalance in nutrition can affect various brain functions.
2. Spatial memory function refers to acquiring knowledge about the space around the individual, storing it, and retrieving it for subsequent use.
3. The hippocampus is the brain region important for spatial memory function.
4. Diet has a profound effect on spatial memory function. Any deviation from a balanced diet induces structural or functional defects either in the hippocampus or spatial memory function.
5. Human and animal studies contribute a lot to understanding the mechanisms involved in spatial memory dysfunction.
6. The effects of an imbalanced diet on the developing hippocampus are severe and long lasting.
7. The adult and aging hippocampus is also vulnerable to malnutritional insults.
8. More studies are required for a better understanding of spatial memory dysfunction. The findings of these studies will help design better interventional therapies for reversing these defects.

Acknowledgment I would like to express my sincere thanks to Dr. Pierre Gressens and Dr. Shyamala Mani for critically reviewing earlier versions of this manuscript. I would also like to acknowledge the valuable suggestions and comments from my colleagues Niranjan Kambi, Parthiv Haldipur, and Shashank Tandon. I express my gratitude to Alok Gupta, Chinmoyee Maharana, and Leslee Lazar for the images.

References

Ahmed MG, Bedi KS, Warren MA, Kamel MM J Comp Neurol. 1987;263:146–58.
Altman J, Bayer SA J Comp Neurol. 1990;301:365–81.
Andrade JP, Cadete-Leite A, Madeira MD, Paula-Barbosa MM Exp Neurol. 1991:119–24.
Andrade JP, Madeira MD, Paula-Barbosa MM J Anat. 1995;187:379–93.
Arnold AE, Pinkham SM, Votolato N J Child Adolesc Psycho Pharma. 2000;10:110–7.
Austin KB, Bronzino J, Morgane PJ Brain Res. 1986;394:267–73.
Barnes RH, Cunnold SR, Robert R, Zimmerman RR, Simmons H, Mcleod RB, Krook L J Nutri. 1966;89:399–410.
Bayer SA. J Comp Neurol. 1980;190:87–114.

Beard JL, Connor JR, Jones BC Nutr Rev. 1993;51:157–70.

Becker A, Eyles DW, McGrath JJ, Grecksch G Behav Brain Res. 2005;161:306–12.

Bourre JM. J Nutr Health Aging. 2004;8:163–74.

Bourre JM. J Nutr Health Aging. 2006;10:377–85.

Bremner JD, McCaffery P Biol Psychiatry. 2008;32:315–31.

Bronzino J, Austin-LaFrance RJ, Morgane PJ Brain Res. 1991;515:45–50.

Campbell LF, Bedi KS Physiol Behav. 1989;45:883–90.

Carlson SE, Werkman SH, Peeples JM, Wilson WM Eur J Clin Nutr. 1994;48:S27–S30.

Carlson ES, Tkac I, Magid R, O'Connor MB, Andrews NC, Schallart T, Gunshin H, Georgieff MK, Petryk A J Nutr. 2009;139:672–9.

Cocco S, Diaz G, Stancampiano R, Diana A, Carta M Neuroscience. 2002;115:475–82.

Connan, F, Murphy F, Connor S, Rich P, Murphy T, Bara-Carill N, Landau S, Krljes S, Ng V, Williams S Psychia Res. 2006;146:117–25.

D' Anci KE, Rosenberg IH Curr Opin Clin Nutr Metab Care. 2004;7:659–64.

Diaz-Cintra S, Iaz-Cintra L, Cintra A, Galvan A, Aguilar A, Kemper T, Morgane PJ J Comp Neurol. 1991;36:310–56.

de Regnier RA, Nelson CA, Thomas K, Wewerka S, Georgieff MK. J Pediatr. 2000;137:777–84.

deUngria M, Rao R, Wobken JD, Luciana M, Nelson CA, Georgieff MK Pediatr Res. 2000;48:169–76.

Felt BT, Lozoff B J Nutr. 1996;126:693–701.

Frankland PW, Bontempi B Nat Rev Neurosci. 2005;6:119–30.

Galler JR. Ambulatory Child Health. 2001;7:85–95.

Halas ES, Sandstead HH Pediatric Res. 1975;9:94–7.

Halas ES, Hanlon MJ, Sandstead HH Nature. 1975;257:221–2.

Halas ES, Burger PA, Sandstead HH Anim Learn Behav. 1980;8:152–8.

Halas ES, Hunt CD, Eberhardt MJ Physiol Behav. 1985;37:451–8.

Jordan, TC, Cane SE, Howells KF Dev Psychobiol. 1981;14:317–25.

Jordan, TC, Howells KF, McNaughton N, Heatlie PL Res Exp Med. 1982; 180:201–7.

Jorgenson LA, Wobken JD, Georgieff MK Dev Neurosci. 2003;25:412–20.

Jorgenson LA, Sun M, O'Connor M, Georgieff MK Hippocampus. 2005;15:1094–1102.

Khedr E, Hamed SA, Elbeih E, El-shereef H, Ahmad Y, Ahmed S Euro Arch Psych Clinic Neuroscience. 2008;258:489–96.

Kronenberg G, Harms C, Sobo RW, Cardozo-Pelaez F, Linhart H, Winter B, Balkaya M, Gertz K, Gay SB, Cox D, Eckart S, Ahmadi M, Juckel G, Kempermann G, Hellweg R, Sohr R, Hörtnagl H, Wilson SH, Jaenisch R, Endres M J Neuroscience. 2008;28:7219–30.

Lane MA, Bailey SJ Prog Neurobiol. 2005;75:275–93.

Larkin EC, Rao GA. In: Dobbing J., editor. Brain, behavior and iron in the infant diet. London: Springer. pp. 43–63.

Lewis PD, Patel AJ, Balazs R Brain Res. 1979;168:186–9.

Lozoff B. Pediatr Res. 2000;48:137–9.

Lozoff B, Brittenham GM, Wolf AW, McClish DK, Kuhnert PM, Jimenez E Pediatrics. 1987;79:981–95.

Lynch A, Smart JL, Dobbing J Brain Res. 1975;83:249–59.

Meck WH, Smith RA, Williams CL Dev Psychobiol. 1988;21:339–53.

Morris RG, Garrud P, Rawlins JN, O'Keefe J. Nature. 1982;297:681–3.

Murray-Kolb LE, Beard JL Am J Clin Nutr. 2007;85(3):778–87

Neuringer MWE, Connor DS, Lin LB, Luck S Proc Natl Acad Sci. 1986;83:4021–5.

Noback CR, Eisenman LM Anat Rec. 1981;201:67–73.

Nurk E, Refsum H, Tell GS, Engedal K, Vollset SE, Ueland PM, Nygaard HA, Smith AD Ann Neurol. 2005;58:847–57.

O'Keefe J, Nadel L. The hippocampus as a cognitive map. London: Oxford UP; 1978.

Olton DS, Samuelson RJ J Expert Psychol Animal Behav Processes. 1976;2:97–116.

Paula-Barbosa MM, Andrade JP, Azevedo FP, Madeira MD, Alavs MC Soc Neurosci Abs. 1988;14: 368.

Paula-Barbosa MM, Andrade JP, Castedo JL, Azevdo FP, Cames I, Volk B Expt Neurol. 1989;103:186–93.

Pollit E. Am J Clin Nutr. 1989;50:666–7.

Ranade SC, Rose AJ, Rao M, Gallego J, Gressens P, Mani S Neuroscience. 2008;152:859–66.

Rao R, Tkac I, Townsend EL, Gruetter R, Georgieff MK J Nutr. 2003;133:3215–21.

Rice D, Barone S Jr. Environ Health Perspect. 2000;108:511–33.

Saito T, Takahashi K, Nakagawa N, Hosokawa T, Kurasaki M, Yamanoshita O, Yamamoto Y, Sasaki H, Nagashima K, Fujita H Biochem Biophys Res Commun. 2000;279:505–11.

Schenk F, Brandner C Psycobiol. 1995;23:302–13.

Seshadri S, Beiser A, Selhub J, Jacques PF, Rosenberg IH, D'Agostino RB, Wilson PW, Wolf PA N Engl J Med. 2002;346:476–83.

Siddappa AM, Georgieff MK, Wewerka S, Worwa C, Nelson CA, de regnier RA. Pediatr Res. 2004;55:1034–41.

Smithells RW, Sheppard S, Schorah CJ Arch Child Dis. 1976;51:944–50.

Strupp BJ, Levitsky DA J Nutr. 1995;125:2221S–32S.

Tonkiss J, Galler JR Brain Res. 1990; 40:95–107.

Tran PV, Carlson ES, Stephanie JB, Fretham TB, Georgieff MK. J Nutr. 2008;138:1267–71.

Uauy TDG, Birch E, Birch JE, Tyson A, Hoffman DR Pediatr Res. 1990;28:485–92.

Valadares CT, Almeida SDS Nutr Neurosci. 2005;8:39–47.

Van Gelder NM. Microsc Electron Biol Cel. 1984;8:227–43.

Vendite D, Wofchuk S, Souza D J Nutr. 1985;115:1418–24.

Walter T, de Andraca I, Chadud P, Perales CG Pediatrics. 1989;84:7–17.

Witter MP, Amaral DG J Comp Neurol. 1991;307:437–59.

Yanai S, Okaichi Y, Okaichi H Neurobiol Aging. 2004;25:325–32.

Chapter 147
Arguments for a Relationship Between Malnutrition and Epilepsy

Sabrina Crepin, Bertrand Godet, Pierre-Marie Preux, and Jean-Claude Desport

Abbreviations

BMI   Body mass index
CNS   Central nervous system
CSF   Cerebral spinal fluid
GABA   Gamma amino butyric acid
NMDA   *N*-Methyl-d-aspartate
PEM   Protein-energy malnutrition
PTZ   Pentylenetetrazole
PWE   People with epilepsy

147.1 Introduction

Malnutrition is a serious public-health problem. Approximately one billion people, essentially from developing countries, are affected by malnutrition (Elia et al. 2005). In developed countries, the prevalence of malnutrition is estimated around 5% of the 15 years and older population (Charles and Basdevant 2006). The term malnutrition usually refers both to undernutrition and overnutrition. Here, we will use the term malnutrition only for undernutrition. Malnutrition can be divided into two types: protein-energy malnutrition (PEM) and micronutrient deficiencies. Malnutrition produces adverse functional effects such as loss of muscle mass or alteration of the immune system, increasing the risk of infections that have clinical and public-health consequences or more typical diseases for micronutrients deficiencies (Stratton et al. 2003).

Epilepsy is a neurological disorder that affects 50 million people throughout the world. According to the epidemiological definition from the International League against Epilepsy (ILAE), it is characterized by the occurrence of at least two unprovoked seizures spaced over 24 h (ILAE 1993). An epileptic seizure is a transient occurrence of signs and/or symptoms due to abnormal excessive and synchronous neuronal activity in the brain (Table 147.1). This activity depends on membrane potential regulated by neurotransmitters, voltage-gated ion channels, and gap junctions. Synaptic transmission

S. Crepin (✉)
Service de Toxicologie et Pharmacologie - Pharmacovigilance, Centre Hospitalier Universitaire,
F-87042 Limoges, France
e-mail: sabrina.crepin@chu-limoges.fr

V.R. Preedy et al. (eds.), *Handbook of Behavior, Food and Nutrition*,
DOI 10.1007/978-0-387-92271-3_147, © Springer Science+Business Media, LLC 2011

Table 147.1 Key facts of epilepsy

- Epilepsy is a common chronic neurological disorder characterized by recurrent unprovoked seizures (at least two unprovoked seizures spaced over 24 h). It affects people whatever their age
- A seizure consists in the transient occurrence of signs and/or symptoms due to abnormal excessive and synchronous neuronal discharge in the brain. It can manifest as an alteration in mental state, tonic or clonic movements, convulsions, and various other psychic symptoms. Seizures can occur even in people who do not have epilepsy
- There are different types of epileptic seizures depending on the area affected by the seizures (generalized or focal), and the associated signs and the syndromes
- Epilepsy has many possible causes, including prenatal injuries, infectious diseases, head trauma, and abnormal brain development. In many cases, this cause is unknown.
- About 50 million people suffer from epilepsy all around the word, but about 80% of PWE are found in developing regions
- Drug-resistant epilepsy concerns 20–30% of PWE. This term is used when seizure control is not possible after 2 years, despite the use of at least two antiepileptic drugs from different pharmacological profiles adapted to the epileptic syndrome in a compliant patient
- PWE and their families can suffer from stigma and discrimination in many parts of the world. Stigma is a large part of the burden carried by individuals and occurs more often in developing countries

This table lists the key facts of epilepsy with regard to epidemiologic data, causes, mechanisms, and different types of seizures

is inhibited or excited according to the type of neurotransmitter, respectively gamma amino butyric acid (GABA) or glutamate. Epileptogenesis implies a local or diffuse modification of these mechanisms which are responsible for a loss of balance between GABA and glutamate. Seizure types are first organized according to whether the source of the seizure within the brain is localized (partial or focal onset seizures) or distributed (generalized seizures). The hippocampus plays a major role in partial temporal epilepsy. In these epilepsies, hippocampal modifications appear after an initial brain injury and then a latent period corresponding to epileptogenesis during which many changes occur. The limited nature of the hippocampus, the reproducibility of its reorganization during epileptogenesis made it as a preferred structure for the study of experimental models of epilepsy in animals and humans.

A relationship between nutritional status and epilepsy has been suspected for a long time. In this chapter, we will highlight the different interactions between malnutrition and epilepsy (Fig. 147.1).

Almost 1,000 years ago, Avicenna recommended that people with epilepsy (PWE) avoid excessive eating, sheep meat, fish, onion, garlic, celery, cauliflower, and carrots (Asadi-Pooya and Ghaffari 2004). Several studies examine the relationship between malnutrition and epilepsy in humans (Hackett et al. 1997; Pal 1999; Nkwetngam Ndam 2004; Bertoli et al. 2006; Crépin et al. 2007; Volpe et al. 2007). The main results are summarized in Table 147.2. The studies were carried out essentially in developing countries and the results are divergent, in part due to methodological differences. But, in case-control studies with enough power, a link between malnutrition and epilepsy is found (Hackett et al. 1997; Crépin et al. 2007; Volpe et al. 2007). Prevalence of malnutrition in epilepsy in developing areas like Africa is high: 22.1% in a recent Benin study (West Africa) regardless of age (vs. 9.2% for the population without epilepsy, $p < 0.001$) (Crépin et al. 2007). Significant differences in consumption of cereals, tubers, vegetables, fish/meat and sweets, and several sociocultural factors (food taboos, stigmatization, etc.) are reported between PWE and controls (Table 147.3) (Crépin et al. 2007). In India, only one of two studies shows a link between epilepsy and body mass index (BMI) (Hackett et al. 1997; Pal. 1999). Two other studies performed in Italy and the United States, in children with refractory epilepsy, show existence of a risk of malnutrition, but no studies have been performed in non-drug-resistant PWE from developed

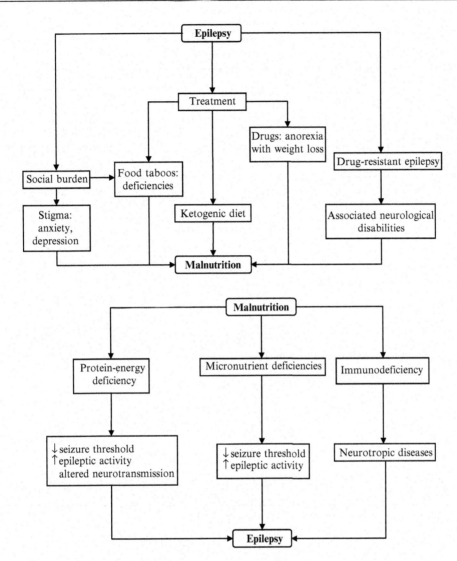

Fig. 147.1 Key facts of relationship between malnutrition and epilepsy. Links between epilepsy and malnutrition are bidirectional. Epilepsy can be responsible for the occurrence of malnutrition because of antiepileptic drugs (anorexic effect), food taboos (depending on the area in the world), and depression due to stigma. In the particular case of drug-resistance epilepsy, PWE can have other neurological disabilities (chewing problems, behavior problems or cerebral palsy, for example). Malnutrition is responsible for protein-energy malnutrition, micronutrient deficiencies, and immunodeficiency. Mechanisms implicated are decrease of seizure threshold, altered neurotransmission or increase of sensibility to infectious diseases as neurotropic diseases. In developed countries, we can speculate that malnutrition is unlikely lead to epilepsy whereas in developed countries the causal relationship is more likely. However, the relationship "epilepsy → malnutrition" is possible in any part of the world

countries. Many studies were performed in animals. The aim of these studies was to bring an assessment of the eventual role of malnutrition in seizure onset by exploring different avenues such as protein or micronutrient deficiencies, but in fact, there are two coexisting hypotheses to explain a link between malnutrition and epilepsy: on the one hand, malnutrition may contribute to the onset of epilepsy or at least seizures and on the other hand, epilepsy could be responsible for malnutrition.

Table 147.2 Studies about malnutrition and epilepsy performed in humans

Place	Study design	population	Age of subjects (years)	Results
Benin (Crépin et al. 2007)	Case-control study	131 PWE 262 controls	All ages	Risk of malnutrition higher for PWE (OR = 2.9, p = 0.0006)
Benin (Nkwetngam Ndam. 2004)	Case-control study	39 PWE 39 controls	All ages	No link between malnutrition and epilepsy (p > 0.05, lack of power)
Inde (Hackett et al. 1997)	Case-control study	26 PWE 1,146 controls	8–12	Mean BMI lower in PWE (OR = 0.74; p = 0.023)
Inde (Pal 1999)	Case-control study	61 PWE 59 controls	2–18	No link between BMI and epilepsy (OR = 31.3; p > 0.05, lack of power)
USA (Volpe et al. 2007)	Case-control study	43 PWE National Health and nutrition examination	1–9	Significant lower intakes for total energy and macro and micronutrients in children with drug-resistant epilepsy (p < 0.05)
Italy (Bertoli et al. 2006)	Cross-sectional study	17 PWE Standard chart	3–16	40% of children with drug-resistant epilepsy malnourished and 24% wasted (p < 0.05); unbalanced dietary intakes

Several studies concerning malnutrition and epilepsy are available. Most of them were performed in developing countries (4/6). Results are divergent because of methodological differences or lack of power. In case-control studies with enough power, malnutrition and epilepsy are linked

PWE people with epilepsy, *OR* odds ratio, *BMI* body mass index

Table 147.3 Factors linked with epilepsy in an African case-control study (Crépin et al. 2007)

Factors	Ajusted odds ratio (95% CI)	p
Mid arm upper circumference per unit	0.7 [0.6–0.9]	0.0020
Third party answering the questionnaire Yes (/no)	16.8 [3.1–90.3]	0.0010
Second occupation No (/yes)	7.1 [2.3–22.3]	0.0008
Cereal consumption ≤1 time/day (/>1 time/day)	4.2 [1.8–10.0]	0.0010
Tooth decay Yes (/no)	2.9 [1.1–7.3]	0.0280
Food taboos Yes (/no)	25.0 [8.3–100.0]	<0.0001
Number of meals/day <3 (/≥3)	4.2 [1.6–10.9]	0.0037

In this case-control study performed in an African country, seven factors are significantly linked to epilepsy. These factors can be gathered in nutritional status factors (mid arm upper circumference, tooth decay), food consumption (cereal consumption, number of meal/day) or social factors (food taboos, second occupation, third party answering the questionnaire). Cases were people with epilepsy (PWE) and controls were people without epilepsy. In African countries, PWE don't usually answer directly to questionnaire or participate to study, a member of the family acts as a third party. It's one of the signs of stigma

CI confident interval

147.2 Effects of Malnutrition in Epilepsy

147.2.1 Protein-Energy Malnutrition

147.2.1.1 Protein Deficiency

Studies on animals show that if malnutrition is not considered a direct cause of epilepsy, it seems to favor the onset of epilepsy or seizures by various nutritional deficiencies. In rats, brain development occurs during the first 3 weeks of life. So, if this hypothesis is extrapolated to humans, it would mean that malnutrition during childhood could predispose someone to epilepsy. In humans, from the prenatal period to third year of life is a time when the central nervous system (CNS) develops, and this is considered a sensitive period depending, in part, on protein, energy, and micronutrient availability. Malnutrition at this time adversely affects the developing brain in numerous ways, largely depending on its timing in relation to various developmental events in the brain and, to a lesser extent, on the type and severity of the deprivation. Many of the effects of prenatal malnutrition are permanent (Morgane et al. 2002). In animals, neuro-anatomical studies provide, for many years, evidences that the hippocampus and cortex are adversely affected by early malnutrition, which exerts its effects not only during the so-called brain growth spurt, but also during early organizational processes such as neurogenesis, cell migration, and differentiation in the cortex and hippocampus. Even if most of nutrients affect brain maturation, proteins seem to be the most important (Morgane et al. 2002; Georgieff 2007). In order to study the effect of malnutrition in the brain, the hippocampal neuronal model is widely used, particularly a study of the dentate gyrus, primarily because its anatomy and physiology are well-known and, secondly, because of its ideal internal geometry to study neuronal organization, reproducibility of the experiments, and its role in epilepsy. Stern et al. show that protein malnutrition during development leads to enhanced seizure susceptibility in adult rats reared on a diet containing inadequate protein levels (decreased seizure threshold and increased epileptic activity) (Stern et al. 1974). This effect is partially abrogated by restoring adequate dietary protein levels in adulthood, and seems to be specific to the type of stimulation used to induce experimental seizures (Forbes et al. 1978). Palencia et al. use a rat model of chronic malnutrition to study the possible influence of malnutrition at late stages of brain development with experimental seizures induced by pentylenetetrazole (PTZ), a $GABA_A$ receptor antagonist (Palencia et al. 1996). In this study, corn tortilla is the only solid food used. The dose of PTZ required to produce seizures is reduced in malnourished rats. This malnutrition model was used because corn and corn derivatives represent the most common food sources of undernourished people from Latin America. Histological studies of the brain show atrophic neurons especially in the hippocampus, cerebellar cortex, and cerebral cortex. In contrast with other studies, Nunes et al. find that malnourished neonatal rats (during the breast-feeding period) are not different from well-nourished rats in terms of flurothyl seizure susceptibility at postnatal day 15 or behavioral manifestations of seizures. But histological assessment shows that flurothyl-induced status epilepticus increases the expression of new cells in the dentate gyrus of malnourished immature rats compared to well-nourished rats; these results may be explained by a cumulative toxicity of malnutrition and status epilepticus (Nunes et al. 2000). However, the pathological function of these new cells has not been clearly established yet.

Protein malnutrition can affect cholinergic, GABAergic, serotoninergic, and glutaminergic transmission. Andrade and Paula-Barbosa randomly assign 2-month-old rats to three groups: (i) malnourished rats fed with an 8% low-protein diet for 12 months; (ii) recovery rats fed like the previous group for 6 months and then switched to a 17% protein standard laboratory diet for a further 6 months; and (iii) controls rats fed for 12 months with the standard laboratory diet (Andrade and

Paula-Barbosa 1996). Prolonged malnutrition lead to a substantial but reversible reduction in the cholinergic innervations of the hippocampal formation which could be explained by a lack of trophic factors, decreased synthesis, availability, and delivery of ordinarily existing neurotrophic substances or an altered ability of neurons to react to these factors. They also show irreversible loss of hippocampal cholinergic and GABAergic neurons.

We are also confronted with the problem of the mechanism leading to epilepsy from extrapolation of effects on hippocampal structures to more global alterations of the CNS explaining different types of epilepsy. Moreover, alterations of the hippocampal area play a key role in some focal epilepsy.

147.2.1.2 Neurotransmitters

Brain cells need certain amino acids and micronutrients to function normally. Several amino acids act as neurotransmitter precursors, such as tryptophan (for serotonin), and some neurotransmitters have amino acid bases, such as GABA or glutamate. Wood et al. show that malnourished rats have lower GABA concentrations in cerebral spinal fluid (CSF) than controls (Wood et al. 1979). For Steiger et al., modifications in $GABA_A$ receptors (variation of affinity or allosteric interactions between benzodiazepines and GABA receptors) are found in rats receiving a low-protein diet during gestation (Steiger et al. 2003). Schweigert et al. find that prenatal and postnatal protein-malnourished rats are more sensitive to picrotoxin ($GABA_A$ receptors antagonist) but there is no difference for quinolinic acid, which has an excitatory effect on neurons as N-methyl-d-aspartate (NMDA) receptor agonist. The authors also note an increase in GABA uptake in the hippocampus. In malnourished humans, GABA level is only measured in blood. The findings are contradictory. For Smith et al., this level is lower than in well-nourished humans (Smith et al. 1974) while for Agarwal et al., it is increased (Agarwal et al. 1981). When brain GABA concentration is increased by administration of antiepileptic drugs, blood and CSF GABA concentrations are also increased. But if GABA plasma concentration decreases no one knows whether CSF and brain GABA concentration is decreased as well.

Another hypothesis concerning the effects of changing cerebral concentration of GABA would be excitatory properties in connection with high intracellular concentration of chloride ($[Cl^-]_i$) due to modification of chloride transporter expression, as shown physiologically during the fetal stages and also in temporal epilepsy hippocampal pyramidal cells (Ben-Ari 2002).

We can speculate that chronic malnutrition in human induces alterations in the brain that decrease seizure threshold, facilitating epileptogenesis that occurs after cerebral injuries or disorders that are prevalent in inhabitants of developing areas.

147.2.2 Immunodeficiency

It is known that malnutrition is a major cause of immunodeficiency (Lesourd and Mazari 1997). PEM is associated with impairment of cell-mediated immunity, phagocyte function, complement system, secretory immunoglobin-A antibody concentration, and cytokine secretion. In tropical areas, poor sanitation and contaminated food or water contribute to alter immunocompetency and to increase risk of infections, especially intestinal infections, which themselves can lead to malabsorption and raise needs in order to adapt immune responses. Malnourished people are more vulnerable to infections, as for example infections known to be epilepsy risk factors, such as neurotropic viruses or cysticercosis, etc. One has to know that neurocysticercosis is the most frequent infectious cause of epilepsy in developing countries (Preux and Druet-Cabanac 2005). Single nutrient deficiencies are also responsible for altered immune responses. This is observed even when the deficiency is mild. Zinc, copper, vitamins A, C, E, and B6 have important influences on immune responses (Lesourd and Mazari 1997).

147.2.3 Micronutrient Deficiencies

Malnutrition can be responsible for electrolyte deficiencies (calcium, magnesium, sodium, phosphorus, etc.), vitamin deficiencies (B1, B6, B12, D) or other elements (zinc or selenium). CNS homeostasis is essential for brain function. Micronutrient deficiencies can have direct or indirect effects on neuronal excitability and may facilitate epileptic activity (Table 147.4). Seizures can occur following hyponatremia, hypocalcemia, hypomagnesemia, or hypophosphatemia. There are usually tonic-clonic seizures but focal seizures are also possible (Castilla-Guerra et al. 2006). Electrolyte lab tests are recommended especially after a first seizure. Several seizure cases due to hyponatremia have been reported. A retrospective survey carried out in an American emergency department shows that hyponatremia (<126 mmol/L) is responsible for seizure occurrence in 56% of less than 2-year-old children and in 70% of children younger than 6 months old when there are no other obvious causes of seizure (Farrar et al. 1995). Seizures can be explained by a decrease in extracellular osmolality responsible for an osmotic gradient and water entry into cells. Several case-reports of seizures associated with hypocalcemia (essentially the neonatal stage, people with hypoparathyroidism or vitamin D deficiency) or hypomagnesemia are also reported (Leaver et al. 1987; Bushinsky and Monk 1998). In slices of human epileptogenic neocortex, a decrease in extracellular magnesium concentration always induces epileptiform discharges by eliminating its blocking effect on NMDA receptors (Avoli et al. 1991). Hypophosphatemia is a well known and possible cause of seizure during the refeeding

Table 147.4 Micronutrients deficiencies and seizure

Deficiencies	Hypotheses
Electrolytes	
Calcium (Bushinsky and Monk 1998)	Neuronal hyperexcitability
Sodium (Farrar et al. 1995; Castilla-Guerra et al. 2006)	Cerebral hypo-osmolality
Magnesium (Leaver et al. 1987; Avoli et al. 1991)	Neuronal excitability modulator
	Disinhibition of the complex sodium-channel- glutamate receptor NMDA-type
	Neuromodulation
Phosphorus (Sobotka 2004)	Unknown
Vitamins	
Vitamin B1 (Keyser and De Bruijn 2001)	Increase of irritative activity in predisposed people
Vitamin B6 (Kretsch et al. 1991)	Decrease of threshold seizure
Vitamin B12 (Biancheri et al. 2001)	Increase of glutamate sensitivity
Vitamine D (Johnson and Willis 2003)	Associated with consequences of calcium deficiency
Trace elements	
Zinc (Takeda 2000)	Genetic susceptibility
	Increase of cortical hyperexcitability
	Neuromodulation
Selenium (Schweizer et al. 2004)	Antioxidant effect

Micronutrient deficiency is a possible cause of seizures. Different types of micronutrients are involved (trace elements, vitamins, and electrolytes). Mechanisms implicated are various and depend on micronutrients. These data are essentially based on animal studies or human case series

syndrome (Sobotka 2004). The role of vitamin deficiencies in seizures has also been reported but mainly on case-reports (Keyser and De Bruijn 1991; Kretsch et al. 1991; Biancheri et al. 2001; Johnson and Willis 2003). For zinc and selenium, neurological effects have been studied in animal models (Takeda 2000; Schweizer et al. 2004). The hypothalamus contains high zinc levels, and is sensitive to deficiency. At a neuronal level, zinc acts as a neurotransmitter in glutaminergic and GABAergic transmission by decreasing the extracellular glutamate concentration and increasing the extracellular concentration of GABA. As selenium is an essential part of glutathione peroxidase involved in antioxidant defence, selenium deficiency can be implicated in oxidative stress (Schweizer et al. 2004). Oxidative stress seems to be implicated in occurrence of seizures. Animal models indicate that occurrence of seizures can increase the content of reactive oxygen species and superoxide generation in the brain. But also, free radicals can induce seizure activity by direct inactivation of glutamine synthase resulting in an abnormal build up of glutamate or inhibition of glutamic acid decarboxylase activity leading to a decrease of GABA. In a study performed in humans, the antioxidant status in the blood of PWE is low compared to controls (lower plasma concentration of vitamins A and C, erythrocyte glutathione reductase and high lipid peroxidation and hemolysis). This status is improved after antiepileptic treatment. Seizure activity may act directly on oxidant blood concentration and antioxidant may be useful to counteract the effect of free radicals (Sudha et al. 2001).

147.3 Effects of Epilepsy on Nutritional Status

147.3.1 Sociocultural Issues

Epilepsy is not only a clinical disorder but also a social label, especially, but not only, for PWE from developing countries. In developing countries, epilepsy is often wrongly considered a contagious disease, the transmission to bystanders being done through saliva, urine, feces, or flatus emitted during a seizure. This situation leads to a restriction on the normal life style and activities, stigma, and then social rejection (Nubukpo et al. 2003). Most African communities still view epilepsy as possession by the Devil or as a witchcraft act. As a consequence of these traditional beliefs, PWE are treated as outcasts. They can be excluded from their family, and not allowed to attend school. It can also be more difficult for them to get married. Seizure occurrence, as well as social rejection, can be responsible for anxiety, decreased food intake, and long-term malnutrition. Nubukpo et al. find that PWE are more anxious or depressed than people without epilepsy (Nubukpo et al. 2004). In developing countries, they have more food-related difficulties than controls: they frequently have fewer than three meals/day, consume cereals less often, and need family help more often (Crépin et al. 2007). Therefore, their nutritional status is worse than that of the control group.

In such countries, beliefs also dictate what PWE may eat. Indeed, food taboos can sometimes be the basis of epilepsy treatment. Nubukpo et al. report that food taboos is found in 63.9% of Benin PWE and 44.2% of Togolese PWE (Nubukpo et al. 2003). In another study performed in Benin, 64% of PWE have food taboos versus 22% for controls (Crépin et al. 2007). In France, food taboos are found in up to 19.5% of a studied population and in the United States, 6% of adults with epilepsy report food as a precipitating factor of seizure (Nubukpo et al. 2003; Asadi-Pooya and Sperling 2007). Eviction can include salty and/or spicy food, sweets, oil but also boiled meat or gummy sauces (with mucilaginous plants such as okra) depending on cultural beliefs and personal experiences (Asadi-Pooya and Sperling 2007; Crépin et al. 2007). If abstinence from certain foods is used, it is because they are considered as responsible for seizure occurrence or saliva secretion during seizures and, in this way, can facilitate "the transmission" of the disease. For Asadi-Pooya and Ghaffari, 55.2% of parents of Iranian children with epilepsy think that there is a relationship between consumption of certain foods and seizure occurrence (Asadi-Pooya and Ghaffari 2004). In addition, this opinion is held by 58.4% of Iranian nurses and physicians (Asadi-Pooya and Hossein-Zade 2005). Almost 50% of the health care professionals and 31.2% of the family of children with epilepsy have experiences with seizure in their PWE after consumption of specific food (dairy products, sour food like vinegar, pepper, meat/fish, vegetables, or fruits) (Asadi-Pooya and Ghaffari 2004; Asadi-Pooya and Hossein-Zade 2005).

147.3.2 Specific Aspects of Drug-Resistant Epilepsy

Growth retardation is reported of children with epilepsy and this could be more prevalent in children with drug-resistant epilepsy. Several factors could explain this: frequent seizures and long post-ictal periods may lead to reduced times of alertness and may lead to decrease in total energy intake.

Two recent studies performed in developed countries suggest that drug resistance in children with epilepsy may favor malnutrition (Bertoli et al. 2006; Volpe et al. 2007). In Italy, 7 children from a cohort of 17 children with drug-resistant epilepsy are malnourished (weight < 80% compared with the reference weight for age) (Bertoli et al. 2006). Children with more severe neurological impairment have the lowest amount of fat-free mass and are hypercatabolic. In the United States, children with drug-resistant epilepsy were compared to healthy children of the same age from the National Health and Nutrition Examination Survey 2001–2002 and Dietary Reference Intakes (Volpe et al. 2007). Energy intake and macronutrients are substantially lower in the children with intractable epilepsy. About 47% of children have significantly lower intakes of total energy, protein, carbohydrate, fat, dietary fibers, certain vitamins, and trace elements compared with recommendations for sedentary healthy children. Drug-resistant epilepsy can be associated with several disabilities including metabolic diseases or cerebral palsy. However, in these two studies, all children for Bertoli et al. (2006) and 53% for Volpe et al. (2007) are at least mildly mentally retarded and, consequently, the risk of malnutrition seems to be partially linked to disabilities related to epilepsy (chewing and swallowing difficulties, anorexia, etc.).

147.3.3 Antiepileptic Treatment

Epilepsy is usually treated with drugs, but traditional treatments in developing countries and specific diets are also used. Because of cultural practices and limited access to medical care, traditional therapies are frequently used in developing countries. In Malawi, for example, treatments are often based on emetic and/or purgative preparations because Malawi people think that epilepsy originates from the stomach where insects can trigger seizures with their movements (Bernet-Bernady et al. 1997). Vomiting and diarrhea due to this type of treatment with long-term use may lead to various deficiencies and weight loss.

Numerous articles deal with the effect of antiepileptic drugs on weight: some can decrease bodyweight and others can increase it or are neutral on weight (Table 147.5). Topiramate, felbamate, zonisamide, and stiripentol induce weight loss due to loss of appetite (Biton 2003; Ben-Menachem 2007). Topiramate is one of the antiepileptics the most associated with weight loss. Weight loss depends on BMI (patients with a higher baseline BMI are more likely to lose weight), gender (females

Table 147.5 Effect of antiepileptic drugs on weight (Chiron et al. 2000; Biton 2003; Ben-Menachem 2007)

Weight gain	No effect	Weight loss
Carbamazepin	Lamotrigine	Felbamate
Oxcarbazepine	Levetiracetam	Topiramate
Gabapentine	Phenytoin	Zonisamide
Pregabalin	Tiagabine	Stiripentol
Sodium valproate	Lacosamide	
Vigabatrin		

Antiepileptic drugs are now known to have an effect on weight. This effect depends on the drug but also on risk factors linked to people with epilepsy (basal body mass index, sex…). The loss of weight is usually due to an anorexic effect of the drugs

are more likely to lose weight) and daily dose (>200 mg/J). Felbamate also significantly reduces the weight of PWE by 15–75%, with some losing up to 4% of their body weight within 6 months (Ben-Menachem 2007). Weight loss with zonisamide is reported in several clinical trials: almost 22% of PWE lose at least 2.3 kg versus 10.5% of PWE using placebo (Ben-Menachem 2007). Stiripentol is also responsible for weight loss: 7% versus 1% in placebo group (Chiron et al. 2000). Antiepileptic drugs can also be responsible for micronutrient deficiencies, such as that of vitamin D with phenytoin or phenobarbital, or taurine deficiency which seems to be responsible for the retinal toxicity of vigabatrin (Gissel et al. 2007; Jammoul et al. 2009). Even if in this chapter we only focus on undernutrition, some antiepileptic drugs can, in contrast, be responsible for an increase of weight. The most well known weight-increasing drugs are: valproate, gabapentine, pregabalin (Biton 2003; Ben-Menachem 2007). Phenytoin, tiagabin, lamotrigine, and lacosamide are themselves considered weight-neutral antiepileptic drugs (Biton 2003; Ben-Menachem 2007).

Dietary therapies are another option in epilepsy treatment. A ketogenic diet is the most often used, but it is not the only one (a modified Atkins diet with high fat, high protein, low carbohydrate, could be used, for example). A ketogenic diet is usually proposed for the treatment of children with drug-resistant epilepsy. It is a strict high fat, adequate protein, and low carbohydrate diet (Fig. 147.2). It decreases seizure frequency in more than 50% of children on the diet. After almost one century of use, the mechanism involved in the clinical efficacy of this treatment is still not clearly understood (Fig. 147.3). The pH hypothesis is based on the idea that the ketogenic diet makes the blood (and brain) slightly acidic because of the production of ketone bodies (acetoacetate, beta-hydroxybutyrate, and acetone). The pH change would be responsible for the antiepileptic effect. In the metabolic hypothesis, a ketogenic diet makes the brain switch from a glucose-based metabolism to a ketone-based metabolism. The antiepileptic effect is due to ketone bodies being more energetic than glucose. or an increase in mitochondrial number, and a decrease in availability of fast energy (glucose) necessary for the seizure. In the amino acid theory, the neurotransmitter balance is modified with an increased production of GABA. In the ketone hypothesis, ketone bodies themselves have antiepileptic properties. A ketogenic diet is efficient in many seizure types and epilepsy syndromes, especially in children who extract and utilize ketone bodies from blood more efficiently than older PWE (Kossoff and Rho 2009). The efficacy appears quickly in the first week of diet. It allows a decrease in seizure severity or duration and increases seizure threshold. In addition to the immediate effect of ketogenic diet, it could have long-term benefits with neuroprotective or antiepileptogenic effects. However, ketone bodies also have anorexigenic properties and other adverse effects as diarrhea and vomiting and can be responsible for growth retardation or weight loss especially in the youngest (Vining et al. 2002). Like the ketogenic diet, a calorie-restricted diet seems to be effective,

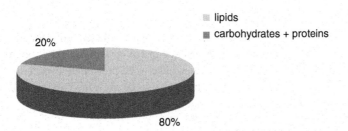

Fig. 147.2 Composition of ketogenic diet. A ketogenic diet is a high fat, adequate protein, and low carbohydrate diet. The ratio of lipid to nonlipid is usually 4:1 with a minimum of 1 mg/kg/day of proteins and a limited intake of carbohydrates (10–15 g/day). Vitamin supplementation is necessary. A nutritionally complete powdered product is available

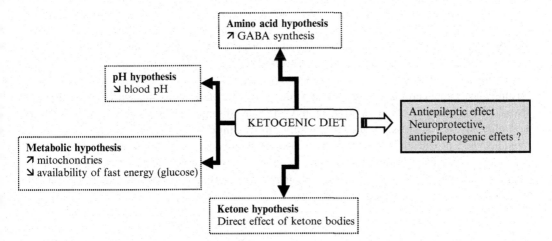

Fig. 147.3 Mechanisms of ketogenic diet. A ketogenic diet, used in drug-resistant epilepsy, is one of the possible treatments in epilepsy. It consists in a strict high fat, adequate protein, and low carbohydrates diet resulting in a production of ketone bodies (acetoacetate, beta-hydroxybutyrate, and acetone). The ketogenic diet has at least an antiepileptic effect and probably neuroprotective and antiepileptogenic effects

on rodent models, in the decrease of seizure susceptibility by reducing the brain glycolytic energy (Greene et al. 2001). It leads to a global decrease in calorie intake without modification of proportions between different food groups and so differs from acute fasting and starvation. A calorie-restricted diet seems to have an additive effect when associated with a ketogenic diet in rodents, but this possible diet therapy has not been yet formally tried on PWE.

147.4 Conclusion

Links between malnutrition and epilepsy are complex. Malnutrition, via different mechanisms, could favor seizure onset and, perhaps, epilepsy. Conversely, epilepsy has consequences on the nutritional status of PWE because of sociocultural factors, severity of epilepsy, or antiepileptic treatments. Consequently, nutritional assessment of PWE appears to be important, as well at the first examination as during the follow-up. The use of simple tools as BMI or body weight variations measurement can be adequate. A better understanding of interactions between malnutrition and epilepsy might prevent the genesis of certain types of epilepsy, especially in developing countries, and improve control of the consequences of epilepsy on nutritional status. Indeed, nutritional interventional studies to determine the best way to limit the occurrence of epilepsy or malnutrition in PWE are lacking. In the mean time, PEM and nutrient deficiencies have to be prevented, especially during pregnancy and childhood. Antiepileptic adverse effects have also to be prevented and treated. Global programs to fight against food taboos and stigmas are necessary.

147.5 Applications to Others Areas of Health and Disease

Neurological disorders are multifactorial. In developing countries, the risk factors for these disorders are numerous and could often interact, as is the case, for example, for infectious diseases, nutrition, and epilepsy. In some African countries, acute or subacute spastic paraparesis and degenerative neuropathy are linked to cyanide intoxication of dietary origin (consumption of large amount of cassava containing cyanogens) (Osuntokun and Monekosso 1969). So the knowledge and the monitoring of nutritional status of people could help to better prevent the occurrence of disorders or to manage existing ones. Other chronic neurological disorders have nutritional consequences, as in Alzheimer's disease. Weight loss is a common problem in Alzheimer's disease and it is associated with mortality, morbidity, disease progression, and poor quality of life (Smith and Greenwood 2008). Malnutrition could also be a prognostic factor in other diseases as in amyotrophic lateral sclerosis (Desport et al. 1999). The mechanisms by which nutrition and epilepsy interact could help to understand the physiopathological mechanisms of morbidity in other diseases, leading to better comprehension and, therefore to improved global public health.

Summary Points

- Malnutrition and epilepsy are two major public health issues. About 800 million people are malnourished and 50 million people have epilepsy all around the world. Both are much more prevalent in developing countries than in developed countries. About 90% of PWE live in developing countries.
- Malnutrition and epilepsy are linked in a two-way relationship. Malnutrition can probably cause seizure and epilepsy can, in turn, lead to malnutrition.
- Malnutrition corresponds to an imbalance between dietary needs and allowance. It can be subdivided in two types: PEM and micronutrient deficiencies.
- Epilepsy is a common chronic neurological disorder characterized by recurrent unprovoked seizures (at least two unprovoked seizures spaced over 24 h).
- Protein and nutrient deficiencies are probably the two most important deficiencies implicated in the occurrence of seizure and epilepsy.
- Protein deficiency acts on epilepsy in numerous ways: decrease of seizure threshold, increase epileptic activity, affecting neurotransmission or inducing the occurrence of atrophic neurons. It can also have an indirect effect by inducing the occurrence of neurotropic infectious diseases.
- Central nervous system homeostasis is essential for brain function. Micronutrient deficiency plays a role in neuronal and epileptic activity.
- Electrolyte lab test is necessary, especially after a first seizure.
- The period between conception to first years of life is considered a sensitive period for the brain. Malnutrition during this period can be responsible for damages.

- Epilepsy occurs essentially in developing countries, where, because of sociocultural issues, it is responsible for malnutrition. Stigma and food taboos are in part responsible for it.
- Food taboos concern various types of food groups as meat/fish, mucilaginous plants, oil, sweets, and vegetables.
- Antiepileptic drugs can be responsible for malnutrition. The nutritional status of PWE on antiepileptic therapies should be monitored.
- Ketogenic diets have proved to be efficacious as treatment for epilepsy. The exact mechanisms, however, remain unknown.

Key Terms

Malnutrition: corresponds to an imbalance between dietary needs and allowance. It can be subdivided in two types: protein-energy malnutrition (PEM) and micronutrient deficiencies.

Protein-energy malnutrition: corresponds to an inadequate protein intake. It is responsible for two types of malnutrition: kwashiorkor and marasmus.

Micronutrient deficiency: concerns deficiency of one of several essential nutrients required for normal body functioning as vitamins, electrolytes, or dietary minerals.

Epilepsy: is a common chronic neurological disorder characterized by recurrent unprovoked seizures (at least two unprovoked seizures spaced over 24 h).

A seizure: consists in the transient occurrence of signs and/or symptoms due to abnormal excessive and synchronous neuronal discharge in the brain.

Drug-resistant epilepsy: corresponds to the lack of control of the disease after 2 years of treatment, despite the use of at least two antiepileptic drugs from different pharmacological profiles adapted to the epileptic syndrome in a compliant patient.

A ketogenic diet: is one of the possible treatments for epilepsy. It's used when drug-resistance is established. It consists in a very strict high lipid diet.

Stigma in epilepsy: it is a mark of shame or discredit, a stain, and an identifying mark or characteristic.

References

Agarwal KN, Bhatia BD, Batta RK, Singla PN, Shankar R. Am J Clin Nutr. 1981;34:924–7.
Andrade JP, Paula-Barbosa MM. Neurosci Lett. 1996;211:211–5.
Asadi-Pooya AA, Ghaffari A. Epilepsy Behav. 2004;5:945–8.
Asadi-Pooya AA, Hossein-Zade A. Epilepsy Behav. 2005;6:604–6.
Asadi-Pooya AA, Sperling MR. Epilepsy Behav. 2007;11:450–3.
Avoli M, Drapeau C, Louvel J, Pumain R, Olivier A, Villemure JG. Ann Neurol. 1991;30:589–96.
Ben-Ari Y. Nat Rev Neurosci. 2002;3:728–39.
Ben-Menachem E. Epilepsia 2007;48(Suppl 9):42–5.
Bernet-Bernady P, Tabo A, Druet-Cabanac M, Poumale F, Ndoma V, Lao H, Bouteille B, Dumas M, Preux PM. Med Trop (Mars). 1997;57:407–11.
Bertoli S, Cardinali S, Veggiotti P, Trentani C, Testolin G, Tagliabue A. Nutr J. 2006;5:14.
Biancheri R, Cerone R, Schiaffino MC, Caruso U, Veneselli E, Perrone MV, Rossi A, Gatti R. Neuropediatrics 2001;32:14–22.
Biton V. CNS Drugs. 2003;17:781–91.
Bushinsky DA, Monk RD. Lancet 1998;352:306–11.
Castilla-Guerra L, del Carmen Fernández-Moreno M, López-Chozas J, Fernández-Bolaños R. Epilepsia 2006;47:1990–8.
Charles M-A, Basdevant A. Obépi, enquête épidémiologique nationale sur le surpoids et l'obésité. Une enquête INSERM, TNS Healthcare SOFRES, Roche. 2006;1–54. doi: http://www.roche.fr/gear/contents/servlet/staticfilesServlet?type=data&communityId=re719001&id=static/attachedfile/re7300002/re72700003/AttachedFile_04700.pdf

Chiron C, Marchand MC, Tran A, Rey E, d'Athis P, Vincent J, Dulac O, Pons G. Lancet 2000;356:1638–42.

Crépin S, Houinato D, Nawana B, Avode GD, Preux PM, Desport JC. Epilepsia 2007;48:1926–33.

Desport JC, Preux PM, Truong TC, Vallat JM, Sautereau D, Couratier P. Neurology 1999;53:1059–63.

Elia M, Zellipour L, Stratton RJ. Clin Nutr. 2005;24:867–84.

Farrar HC, Chande VT, Fitzpatrick DF, Shema SJ. Ann Emerg Med. 1995;26:42–8.

Forbes WB, Stern WC, Tracy CA, Resnick O, Morgane PJ. Exp Neurol. 1978;62:475–81.

Georgieff MK. Am J Clin Nutr. 2007; 85: 614S–20S.

Gissel T, Poulsen CS, Vestergaard P. Expert Opin Drug Saf. 2007;6:267–78.

Greene A, Todorova M, McGowan R, Seyfried T. Epilepsia 2001;42:1371–8.

Hackett RJ, Hackett L, Bhakta P. Acta Paediatr. 1997;86:1257–60.

ILAE. Epilepsia 1993;34:592–6.

Jammoul F, Wang Q, Nabbout R, Coriat C, Duboc A, Simonutti M, Dubus E, Craft CM, Ye W, Collins SD, Dulac O, Chiron C, Sahel JA, Picaud S. Ann Neurol. 2009;65:98–107.

Johnson GH, Willis F. Med J Aust. 2003;178:467; discussion 467–8.

Keyser A, De Bruijn S. Eur Neurol. 1991;31:121–5.

Kossoff EH, Rho JM. Neurotherapeutics 2009;6:406–14.

Kretsch MJ, Sauberlich HE, Newbrun E. Am J Clin Nutr. 1991;53:1266–74.

Leaver DD, Parkinson GB, Schneider KM. Clin Exp Pharmacol Physiol. 1987;14:361–70.

Lesourd BM, Mazari L. Clin Nutr. 1997;16(Suppl 1):37–46.

Morgane PJ, Mokler DJ, Galler JR. Neurosci Biobehav Rev. 2002;26:471–83.

Nkwetngam Ndam M. Epilepsie et statut nutritionnel dans la commune de Djidja-Département du Zou au Bénin [Thèse]. Bénin, université d'Abomey-Calavi. 2004:1–74.

Nubukpo P, Preux PM, Clement JP, Houinato D, Tuillas M, Aubreton C, Radji A, Grunitzky EK, Avode G, Tapie P. Med Trop (Mars). 2003;63:143–50.

Nubukpo P, Preux PM, Houinato D, Radji A, Grunitzky EK, Avode G, Clement JP. Epilepsy Behav. 2004;5:722–7.

Nunes ML, Liptakova S, Veliskova J, Sperber EF, Moshe SL. Epilepsia 2000;41(Suppl 6):S48–52.

Osuntokun BO, Monekosso GL. Br Med J. 1969;3:178–9.

Pal DK. Neurology 1999;53:2058–63.

Palencia G, Calvillo M, Sotelo J. Epilepsia 1996;37:583–6.

Preux PM, Druet-Cabanac M. Lancet Neurol. 2005;4:21–31.

Schweizer U, Brauer AU, Kohrle J, Nitsch R, Savaskan NE. Brain Res Brain Res Rev. 2004;45:164–78.

Smith KL, Greenwood CE. J Nutr Elder. 2008;27:381–403.

Smith SR, Pozefsky T, Chhetri MK. Metabolism 1974;23:603–18.

Sobotka L. In: Sobotka L, editor. Basics in clinical nutrition. Prague: Galen; 2004. p. 288–91.

Steiger JL, Alexander MJ, Galler JR, Farb DH, Russek SJ. Neuroreport 2003;14:1731–5.

Stern WC, Forbes WB, Resnick O, Morgane PJ. Brain Res. 1974;79:375–84.

Stratton R, Green C, Elia M. Cambridge, MA: CABI; 2003. p. 824.

Sudha K, Rao AV, Rao A. Clin Chim Acta. 2001;303:19–24.

Takeda A. Brain Res Brain Res Rev. 2000;34:137–48.

Vining EP, Pyzik P, McGrogan J, Hladky H, Anand A, Kriegler S, Freeman JM. Dev Med Child Neurol. 2002;44:796–802.

Volpe SL, Schall JI, Gallagher PR, Stallings VA, Bergqvist AG. J Am Diet Assoc. 2007;107:1014–8.

Wood JH, Hare TA, Glaeser BS, Brooks BR, Ballenger JC, Post RM. Brain Research Bulletin. 1979;4:707.

Chapter 148
Cortical Spreading Depression: A Model for Studying Brain Consequences of Malnutrition

Rubem Carlos Araújo Guedes

Abbreviations

CNS	Central nervous system
CSD	Cortical spreading depression
EEG	Electroencephalogram
DC	Direct-current
GABA	Gamma-amino butyric acid
REM-sleep	Rapid-eye-movement sleep

148.1 Introduction: Malnutrition and Its Neurological Consequences

In the last decades of the twentieth century, the nutritional scenario in the world was characterized by a situation in which, due to the limited economic possibility of buying nutritionally adequate foods (which have higher costs than poor-quality foods), a large part of the human population was susceptible to the impact of inadequate feeding (Morgane et al. 1978). This situation still affects a considerable number of children, with an important influence on the morbidity and mortality indexes. In Brazil, as well in other developing countries, the poorest part of the population now experiences what has been called a rapid "nutritional transition," characterized by a simultaneous decrease of the prevalence of severe malnutrition and an increase of overnutrition (Monteiro et al. 2004). This nutritional transition has been accompanied by a diminution in the incidence of infectious and parasitic diseases and an increment of nontransmissible chronic diseases affecting homeostatic processes of the cardiovascular and renal systems, among others (Boubred et al. 2007; Ginter and Simko 2009; Popkin et al. 2001). However, the neurological impact of such conditions has not been the object of much investigation. Both the economic and social costs of that scenario are considerable, with regard to the health assistance required to be given to surviving individuals (Popkin et al. 2001). Considering the public health point of view, this situation can be characterized as a matter of great concern.

R.C.A. Guedes (✉)
Departamento de Nutrição, Universidade Federal de Pernambuco, BR-50670901, Recife, PE, Brazil
e-mail: rguedes@ufpe.br; rc.guedes@terra.com.br

V.R. Preedy et al. (eds.), *Handbook of Behavior, Food and Nutrition*,
DOI 10.1007/978-0-387-92271-3_148, © Springer Science+Business Media, LLC 2011

The biochemical and morphological organization of the brain can be disrupted by the dietary deficiency of one or more nutrients, especially if this deficiency occurs early in life, during the so-called "brain growth spurt" period (Grantham-McGregor 1995). Nutrition-dependent alterations in brain development and organization are usually followed by deleterious repercussions on its function and these can be more or less severe, depending on the intensity and duration of the nutritional disturbances (Morgane et al. 1978). The neural analysis of sensory information and perception, as well as the efficient production and control of motor activity, are basic neural functions that can be impaired by nutritional inadequacies. Malnutrition-induced neural impairment can also affect more complex brain functions such as those involving learning, memory, consciousness, cognition, and emotion. Such disturbances can sometimes also result in permanent effects in the nervous system, with the establishment of more or less disabling diseases (Grantham-McGregor 1995). All these social- and biological-related factors illustrate the great importance of studying the effects of malnutrition on the brain. Further, experimental evidence indicates that excessive food intake too can interfere with brain development and function (Davidowa et al. 2003). The systematic investigation of this condition started to increase in the last decade. These facts have motivated a number of clinical and experimental research laboratories to study the effects of early malnutrition on the developing and adult central nervous system, resulting in a considerable amount of data. In this chapter we present experimental results on the brain electrophysiological phenomenon known as "cortical spreading depression" (CSD), and demonstrate how CSD can be used in studies comparing their features in malnourished and well-nourished rats. In addition, the CSD effects of nutritional factors are confronted with those of non-nutritional variables.

148.2 Influence of Nutrition on the Electrical Activity of the Normal Brain

The brain exerts its diverse functions basically by producing electrical signals, which constitute the so-called electrical activity of the brain. This activity can be recorded in humans and in laboratory animals by different techniques and can thus provide valuable information about brain function. For this purpose, one of the most used techniques is the electroencephalogram (EEG), which consists in recording the differences of electrical potential between one or several pairs of electrodes placed at distinct regions on the skin over the skull. As a noninvasive technique, the EEG is extensively used in human patients to help in the diagnosis of certain neurological diseases. The initial human EEG studies (in the 1940–1950s) employed trained observers, who performed a visual analysis of the EEG tracings in order to detect and define normal and pathological EEG patterns. Using this technique, Nelson and Dean (1959) have studied 46 malnourished African children and found abnormal EEG discharges in 36% of the cases, localized predominantly at the temporal region, suggesting an enhancement of the cerebral excitability as also observed in human cases of epilepsy. It must be pointed out, however, that although visual examination of the EEG can be useful for qualitative analysis, it always contains an unavoidable subjectivity. Therefore, it is very difficult to adequately analyze quantitative parameters such as frequency and amplitude of the EEG waves by visual inspection (Morgane et al. 1978). This task was later properly achieved in the 1970s by employing computation science techniques, which allowed the use of spectral analysis and fast Fourier transform algorithms to quantify EEG features (see Morgane et al. 1978). This enabled studying the ontogeny of EEG patterns both in children (Schulte and Bell 1973) and in developing laboratory animals (Gramsbergen 1976). In the malnourished rat, the main EEG disturbance was characterized by an increased power in the theta range of frequencies (Morgane et al. 1978; Cintra et al. 2002).

The hypothesis that malnourished humans would be more prone to epilepsy, as compared with well-nourished controls, is supported by some of the above EEG findings. However, studies on this subject involving human beings are very few and are not yet enough to definitely confirm the causal relationship between malnutrition and proneness to develop epilepsy (Hackett and Iype 2001). The acceptance of this hypothesis in humans requires further extensive investigations, as are already available in laboratory animals. In rats, under conditions of early nutritional imbalance, some brain electrophysiological alterations suggest disturbances in processes related to neural excitability. This includes a lower threshold to experimentally induced seizures (Palencia et al. 1996).

The evidence indicating nutrition-related changes in neural excitability, demonstrated by electro-physiological techniques, prompted us to investigate such changes by using, as a model, the phenom-enon known as CSD as a result of brain electrical activity, and this is presented in the next section.

148.3 What is "Cortical Spreading Depression" of Electrical Activity?

In 1944, a young Brazilian PhD student at Harvard University, USA, described a new electrophysio-logical phenomenon in the anesthetized rabbit brain. The phenomenon was denominated "spreading depression" of the cerebral cortex activity (Leão 1944). Cortical spreading depression (CSD) was then described as being a "wave-like" response, produced as a consequence of electrical, chemical, or mechanical stimulation of one point of the cortical surface. The response consisted in a reduction (depression) of the spontaneous and evoked electrical activity of the stimulated point of the cerebral cortex. From that point, CSD concentrically propagated to remote cortical regions, while the eliciting point started to recover; it is thus a propagating and reversible phenomenon, which was later shown to be accompanied by a reversible negative slow potential change (also called DC-potential change) of the EEG-depressed tissue surface (Leão 1947). This negative slow potential change reaches maxi-mum values after 1–2 min of onset, ranging in the rat from −5 to −20 mV and being completely reverted after a few minutes (Fig. 148.1). It can be measured, with a DC-coupled amplifier, against a remote point that presents an invariant potential, as, for example, the nasal bones. An average recov-ery time of about 5–10 min are usually required for the depressed cortical area to completely restore the predepression EEG pattern and the baseline DC level. The CSD slow potential change has an "all-or-none" feature, which makes it very useful to calculate the CSD velocity of propagation.

Some important key features of CSD are presented in Table 148.1.

In contrast to the propagation velocity of neuronal action potential (in the order of meters per second), the velocity with which CSD propagates is considerably lower, ranging from 2 to 5 mm/min in all vertebrate species so far studied (Guedes 2005). The remarkably slow CSD propagation veloc-ity is compatible with a humoral mechanism of propagation rather than an ion-based mechanism, as in the action potential. It is widely accepted that CSD propagation would be based on one or more chemical factors that would be released from the neural cells under CSD (Martins-Ferreira et al. 1974). These factors, once in the "extracellular milieu," would "contaminate" the neighbor cells, which would become depressed and would also release the postulated CSD factors, generating a feedback loop that would maintain the CSD propagation in an auto-regenerative mode. A complete knowledge of CSD mechanisms has not yet been achieved, despite a very extensive body of informa-tion on CSD phenomenology that has been accumulated during the 65 years elapsed from the time of the initial description of CSD.

Three relevant human diseases are currently postulated to have some relationship to CSD, in terms of sharing at least some common mechanisms: migraine (Eikermann-Haerter et al. 2009; Lehmenkühler et al. 1993), epilepsy (Fabricius et al. 2008; Gorji and Speckmann 2004; Guedes et al. 2009; Leão 1944, 1972), and brain ischemia (Dohmen et al. 2008; Pezzini et al. 2009). This deserves some comments, considering that CSD has already been demonstrated in the human brain (Dohmen et al. 2008; Fabricius et al. 2008; Gorji and Speckmann 2004).

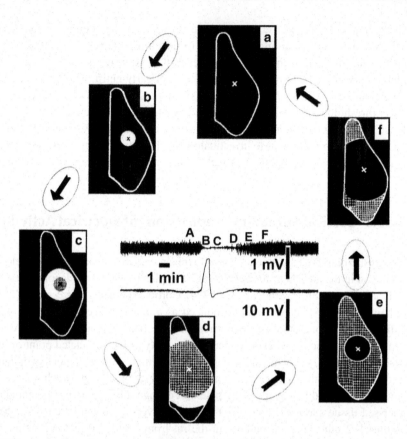

Fig. 148.1 Cycle of reversible electrophysiological events that occur during cortical spreading depression. Sequence of steps (A to F) that characterize the "cortical spreading depression cycle" in the rat cerebral cortex. In A, the normal cortical tissue is stimulated at the point marked with an "x" and one CSD episode is originated at this point. The white circle in B denotes the initially depressed area, from which CSD concentrically propagates to the entire cortex (steps C and D).The black circle in E indicates the area initially recovered after CSD. The recovery process then gradually attains remote areas (step F) and finally the entire cortex comes back to the pre-CSD condition, as in A. The square-lined area represents the post-CSD cortical *refractoriness* before full recovery. The central inset shows the electrocorticogram and the slow potential change of CSD (respectively upper and lower traces). The time-points corresponding to the conditions of the steps A to F are marked in the electrocorticogram with the respective letters]

Experimental evidence suggests that, under normal conditions, the neural tissue presents a certain degree of resistance to CSD propagation (Guedes 2005; Guedes and Do Carmo 1980). This resistance can increase or decrease as a result of experimental treatments, leading the brain to propagate CSD respectively with lower or higher velocities (Guedes 2005). In animals, the calculation of the CSD velocity of propagation along the tissue is an easy and useful way of estimating the brain's susceptibility to CSD. Therefore, animal studies under experimental conditions that either enhance or impair the brain's ability to initiate and propagate CSD may be helpful to understand both the CSD phenomenon and related diseases.

The appearance of epileptiform EEG waves during CSD at the time when spontaneous activity is depressed (Leão 1944; Guedes and Do Carmo 1980) led to the postulation of the "CSD–epilepsy link" (Leão 1944, 1972). The association between CSD and migraine has gained support from studies showing CSD-dependent brain vascular changes (Lehmenkühler et al. 1993), as well as from investigations on genetically modified animals (mouse models of familial hemiplegic migraine) showing genetic and hormonal modulation of CSD (Eikermann-Haerter et al. 2009). Data from

Table 148.1 Key features of relevant aspects of CSD

Aspect	Feature	Remarks
CNS cellular organization	Needs a minimal population of cell bodies for CSD to be generated and propagated	CSD is a "cell population", or "cooperative" phenomenon
Eliciting stimulus	Any kind of sudden energy variation (electrical, chemical, mechanical, etc.)	Eliciting stimulus does not need to be specific
Tissue condition after CSD	The depressed region recovers its electrical activity 5–10 min after depression.	It is a fully reversible phenomenon
Brain functional limits	CSD propagates equally from a sensory to a motor area and vice-versa	No evident relationship with regional functional limits
Phylogenetic aspects	Observed in all animal species so far studied, including the human species	CSD seems to be a very general phenomenon of the CNS
Velocity of propagation	In the order of a few mm/min	A paradoxically very slow propagating phenomenon (mm/min) in a tissue where action potentials propagate very fast (m/s)
Neocortical mammal structure	CSD propagates more easily in lisencephalic than in gyrencephalic brains	Cortical structural organization influences CSD propagation features.
Is CSD a physiological or a pathological phenomenon?	Some CSD features are found in certain neurological diseases	Understanding CSD mechanisms could help in understanding the mechanisms of some neurological diseases.

experimental models of brain ischemia, as well as from human ischemic patients, led also to the postulation of an important role for CSD in the physiopathology of brain ischemic disease (Dohmen et al. 2008; Pezzini et al. 2009). The following physiologic processes have been often postulated as possibly influencing CSD generation and propagation: (1) homeostasis of certain extracellular ions (Guedes and Do Carmo 1980), (2) homeostasis of free radicals produced in the nervous tissue (El-Bachá et al. 1998; Abadie-Guedes et al. 2008), and (3) neurotransmitter-dependent mechanisms (Gorelova et al. 1987; Amâncio-dos-Santos et al. 2006). These are neural processes that can be affected by nutritional and also by non-nutritional factors during brain development.

148.4 Nutritional and Non-nutritional Factors Influencing CSD Propagation

In early malnourished rats (Fig. 148.2), data from our laboratory have demonstrated a facilitation of CSD propagation, as judged by the higher CSD velocities, compared to well-nourished controls.

The maternal protein content of diet seemed to play an important role in determining the CSD effect in offspring: protein supplementation of the maternal diet abolished this effect provided the protein used in the supplementation was of high quality (casein). However, when the deficient diet was supplemented with low-quality protein (of vegetable origin), the CSD effect was not abolished (Andrade et al. 1990).

Considering that within the brain growth spurt period, the maximal intensity of various developmental processes (as, for example, neurogenesis, myelination, and gliogenesis) occurs at distinct time-points in different brain areas, we investigated if short episodes of maternal malnutrition, acting

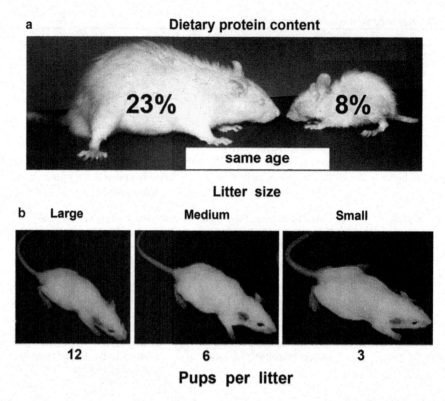

Fig. 148.2 Impact of malnutrition and "overnutrition" on body dimensions. Photographs illustrating the physical aspect of malnourished, normally nourished (control) and "overnourished" rats. In part A, (adult animals) a case of severe malnutrition is confronted with a control rat. In this case, severe malnutrition was provoked by feeding a low-protein diet (containing 8% of protein, instead of the 23% of the control diet) during the whole life. The three young animals in part B (30 days-old) were suckled in litters of different sizes, classified as large, medium, and small-size litters, containing respectively 12, 6, and 3 pups. These three lactation conditions originate pups with moderate-malnutrition (*left*), normal nutrition (*middle*), and with moderate-overnutrition (*right*), respectively. The three pictures of part B were taken under the same magnification. Note the changes in the head size, which indicates alteration in brain size]

at a certain time point within the lactation period, could affect CSD in the progeny. We demonstrated that even a 7-day period of maternal malnutrition within the lactation period was sufficient to significantly enhance CSD propagation in offspring. This effect was shown to be long-lasting, since it was still detected when the pups became adults (Rocha-de-Melo and Guedes 1997). Moreover, the effect was more conspicuous when malnutrition was induced at the late phase of lactation – the third suckling-week, as compared to the groups malnourished in the two earlier weeks (Fig. 148.3), suggesting that with regard to the nutritional effects on CSD propagation, the brain developmental events occurring in this late phase of lactation would have a greater importance.

The mechanism by which early malnutrition results in enhanced CSD incidence and propagation still deserves detailed clarification. In the rat, malnutrition has been shown to reduce brain glutamate uptake (Feoli et al. 2006) and to increase the enzyme glutamic acid decarboxylase (Diaz-Cintra et al. 2007). Both conditions might in all probability increase the brain extracellular glutamate, which would facilitate CSD propagation (Peeters et al. 2007; Tottene et al. 2009).

Three malnutrition-induced brain alterations, however, have been considered as probably involved in the CSD effects found in malnourished animals: (1) reduction in the brain myelin content, (2) impairment of glial function, and (3) increase in the cell packing density with reduction of the

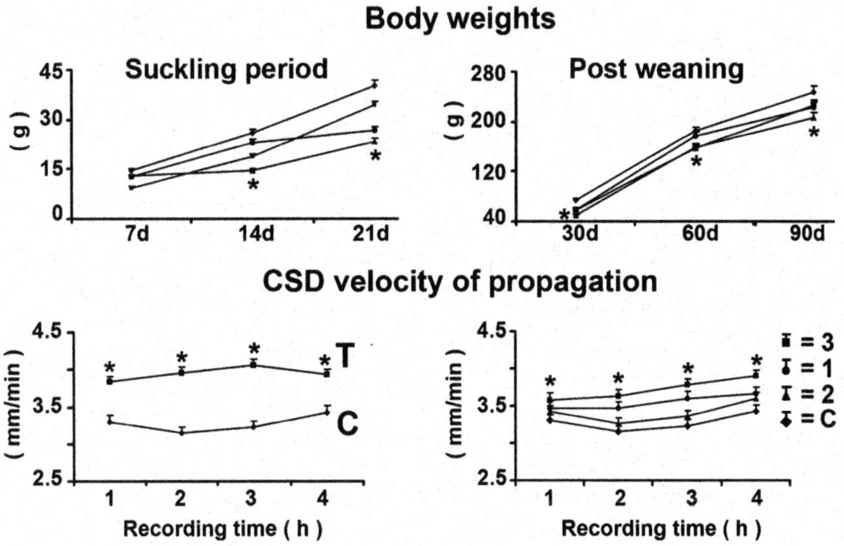

Fig. 148.3 Effect of short episodes of early malnutrition on body weight and CSD propagation. Mean ± SEM of body weights (two *upper panels*) and CSD velocities (*lower panel*) of rats suckled by dams fed a low-protein diet (with 8% protein) for a small period (7 days), during the first (*ball-symbol*; n = 13), second (*triangle-symbol*; n = 17), or third (*square-symbol*; n = 15) week of lactation. The control group (C; *diamond-symbol*; n = 19) received a standard chow-diet with 23% protein. In the lower-left panel, the T group (n = 17) was malnourished during the total lactation period (3 weeks). Note in the lower-right panel the greatest increase in CSD velocity in the group malnourished during the third week of lactation]

extracellular space. Brain myelin has been considered as an obstacle to the humoral propagation of CSD; thus, the less myelin in the brain, the fewer obstacles to CSD propagation (De Luca et al. 1977). Glial impairment has also been demonstrated to facilitate CSD (Largo et al. 1997). Finally, compared with the well-nourished condition, the early-malnourished brain has reduced size and mass, with smaller cells packed in a denser manner and with a reduced extracellular space volume. Since a larger extracellular space volume in the brain hinders CSD elicitation and propagation (Lehmenkühler et al. 1993; Richter et al. 2003), the higher cell packing density and the smaller extracellular space volume, found in the malnourished brain, is thought to favor CSD propagation.

In contrast to malnutrition, the influence of early overnutrition on brain development and function had been almost not investigated at that time (Davidowa et al. 2003), and only a single short report was available concerning the effects of overnutrition on CSD (De Luca et al. 1977). To address this issue, we then used a simple and interesting method to positively influence the nutritional status of the pups during the lactation period. This method consists in diminishing the litter-size (i.e., reducing the number of pups to be suckled by a single dam), and inducing in the newborns a moderate degree of overnutrition (Davidowa et al. 2003). Considering that early malnutrition had facilitated CSD (Rocha-de-Melo and Guedes 1997), we hypothesized that the brain developmental influence of the favorable lactation condition (pups reared in small litters, with only three pups) on the CSD would be to impair CSD propagation, as compared to the control-size litter (six pups). By the same logic, the prediction was made that rat-pups suckled in litters much larger than the controls (litters with 12 pups instead of 6 as in the control) would display higher CSD propagation velocities, as this suckling condition induces a moderate degree of malnutrition; this has indeed been demonstrated (Rocha-de-Melo et al. 2006), and is here illustrated in Fig. 148.4.

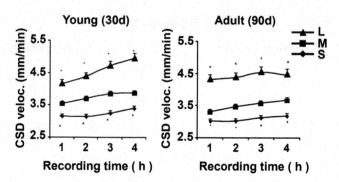

Fig. 148.4 CSD effect of suckling rat-pups in litters of different sizes. Mean ± SEM CSD velocities of propagation in the cortical surface of young (30 days old; *left panel*; $n = 54$) and adult rats (90 days old; *right panel*; $n = 48$) that have been reared, during the suckling period, in large (L; $n = 21$ and 13 rats for the 30-day and 90-day old groups, respectively), medium (M; $n = 18$ and 17 rats) and small litters (S; $n = 15$ and 18 rats). The L, M, and S litters were composed respectively by 12, 6, and 3 pups. The asterisks indicate that the extreme groups (L and S) display CSD velocities of propagation significantly different from the age-matched control (M) group

Another interesting set of results came from testing how certain molecules of metabolic importance for the brain, like glucose, or pharmacological compounds with unequivocal effectiveness in influencing brain function, like the GABAergic compound diazepam, could influence CSD propagation, and how malnutrition would interfere with this possible effect. Data indicated that hyperglycemia reduces whereas diazepam and insulin-induced hypoglycemia facilitates CSD propagation. However, those effects were not found in rats that were previously malnourished (Guedes et al. 1992; Ximenes-da-Silva and Guedes 1991). In contrast, two other drugs that have an impairing action on CSD, the selective serotonin reuptake inhibitor fluoxetine and the cholinergic agonist pilocarpine produced in the malnourished brain respectively a more intense (Vasconcelos et al. 2004) and an equal (Amâncio-dos-Santos et al. 2006) CSD effect as compared to the well-nourished brain. Taken together, these experimental data suggest that malnutrition-induced changes in the brain responsiveness to pharmacological agents may vary depending on the neurotransmitter system under investigation. Concerning CSD, it appears for instance that, in contrast to the serotoninergic system, the responsiveness of the GABAergic and cholinergic systems were respectively decreased and increased by the nutritional deficiency imposed early in life on the malnourished rats. This raises some concerns, regarding the human use of therapeutical drugs acting specifically on a certain neurotransmitter system: if the above-described experimental observations were also to reflect what happens in the human brain, then this would imply that different classes of therapeutically employed drugs (as, for example, anti-epileptics and anti-migraine drugs) could present distinct degrees of effectiveness, eventually depending on the early nutritional condition of the patients. The medical implication would be a strong recommendation for the clinical investigation of this possibility in the human being.

Besides nutritional and the pharmacological variables, other clinically important hormonal and environmental factors have also been studied in several laboratories including ours regarding their significant influence on the brain's ability to generate and propagate CSD. Some of these factors were found to enhance CSD propagation, whereas some others impaired it. Conditions such as extracellular ionic alterations (Guedes and Do Carmo 1980), deprivation of REM sleep (Guedes and Vasconcelos 2008; Vasconcelos et al. 2004), ethanol consumption (Bezerra et al. 2005; Abadie-Guedes et al. 2008), treatment with gliotoxic drugs (Largo et al. 1997), genetic "knockin" manipulation in mice (insertion of the human hemiplegic familiar migraine gene; Eikermann-Haerter et al. 2009), and toxic and autoimmune induced cortical demyelination (Merkler et al. 2009) are some of the studied situations which enhance the CSD phenomenon. A summary of the studied conditions that enhance CSD is presented in Table 148.2.

Table 148.2 Experimental studies under some clinically important conditions that enhance CSD propagation. Pertinent bibliography is also provided

Conditions That Facilitate CSD			
Animal	Reference	Condition	Effect
Rabbit	Guedes and Do Carmo (1980)	Low extracellular chloride (by gastric washing with distilled water)	Increased CSD propagation and EEG epileptiform activity; appearance of a second SD in the opposite hemisphere
Rat	Rocha-de-Melo et al. (2006)	Malnutrition early in life	CSD velocities higher than in well-nourished controls
Rat	Guedes and Vasconcelos (2008)	Deprivation of REM sleep (water-tank technique)	Increased CSD velocities, as compared with nondeprived or pseudodeprived controls.
Rat	Costa-Cruz and Guedes (2001)	Hypoglycemia [by (1) insulin or (2) food restriction + insulin]	CSD velocities higher than in normoglycemic rats
Rat	Guedes et al. (1992)	Increase of the GABAergic activity by diazepam	Higher CSD velocities after diazepam as compared with predrug values
Rat	Bezerra et al. (2005)	Administration of ethanol per gavage	Ethanol facilitated CSD as compared to water-treated or naïve controls.
Rat	El-Bachá et al. (1998)	Dietary deprivation of antioxidant vitamins	Higher CSD velocities; increased CSD-eliciting action of photoactivated riboflavin
Rat	Maia et al (2009)	Early in life treatment with l-arginine, per gavage	L-Arginine facilitates CSD as compared to water-treated or naïve controls.
Rat	Farias-Santos et al. (2009)	Daily sessions of heat exposure early in life	Increase in CSD propagation as compared to controls
Rat	Largo et al. (1997)	Treatment with the gliotoxic drug fluorocitrate	Glial impairment increased CSD propagation
Rat	Fregni et al. (2005)	1 and 20 Hz cortical electrical stimulation, 2x/d, for 2 days	Increase of CSD propagation measured 1 and 15 days after electrical stimulation.
Mouse	Eikermann-Haerter et al. (2009)	Genetic ("knockin") manipulation inserting the hemiplegic familiar migraine gene	Increased SD frequency and propagation speed; enhanced corticostriatal propagation
Mouse	Merkler et al. (2009)	Hypomyelination by dietary treatment with cuprizone	Accelerated CSD propagation, reverted after switching mice to the normal diet
Rat	Tenorio et al. (2009)	Unilateral early vibrissae removal	Facilitation of CSD propagation in well-nourished and malnourished rats.

CSD impairment has also been found in animals submitted to propylthiouracil-induced hypothyroidism (Guedes and Pereira-da-Silva 1993), aging (Guedes et al. 1996), peripheral electrical (Monte-Silva et al. 2007) or environmental stimulation (Santos-Monteiro et al. 2000), antioxidants (Bezerra et al. 2005; Abadie-Guedes et al. 2008), hypermyelination, (Merkler et al. 2009), and genetical proneness to audiogenic epilepsy (Guedes et al. 2009), among other conditions (Table 148.3).

148.5   Applications to Other Areas of Health and Disease

As an "excitable tissue," one of the main physiological properties of the nervous system is that it is capable of generating electrical activity and, through this activity, to execute its normal actions, including the highly complex ones. This is the main reason for using electrophysiologically based

Table 148.3 Conditions of clinical relevance, which have been shown to impair CSD propagation. For detailed information, bibliographic reference is provided

Animal	Reference	Condition	Effect
Conditions That Antagonize CSD			
Rat	Guedes et al. (1989)	Dietary treatment with lithium	Lower CSD velocities compared with controls
Rat	Costa-Cruz and Guedes (2001); Costa-Cruz et al., (2006)	Hyperglycemia (acute and chronic)	Lower CSD velocities compared with controls
Rat	Guedes and Barreto (1992)	Anesthetics	Lower CSD velocities under anesthesia, compared to waking state in the same rat.
Rat	Guedes and Pereira-da-Silva (1993)	Early hypothyroidism (by PTU)	Reduced CSD velocities in PTU-treated rats, compared with saline-treated controls
Gerbil and Rat	Guedes et al. (1996)	Aging	Inverse correlation between age and CSD velocity that is reduced by dietary antioxidant vitamin deficiency
Rat	Santos-Monteiro et al. (2000);Monte-Silva et al (2007)	Early peripheral electrical or environmental stimulation	Reduced CSD velocities compared with nonstimulated controls
Gerbil and Rat	Guedes et al. (1987)	Treatment with the opioid antagonist naloxone	Naloxone antagonizes CSD incidence and propagation
Rat	Guedes et al. (1988)	Topical cortical application of excitatory amino acid antagonists	MK-801 antagonizes CSD propagation.
Rat	Guedes et al. (2002); Amâncio-dos-Santos et al. (2006)	Pharmacological increase of brain serotonin activity	D-Fenfluramine, citalopram, and fluoxetine antagonize CSD propagation
Rat	Guedes and Cavalheiro (1997); Guedes and Vasconcelos (2008)	Single injection of convulsing and subconvulsing dose of pilocarpine	Dose-dependent blocking of CSD propagation.
Rat	Bezerra et al. (2005); Abadie-Guedes et al. (2008)	Treatment with antioxidants, per gavage	Both shrimp carotenoids and pure astaxanthin reduce CSD propagation in ethanol-treated rats.
Mouse	Merkler et al. (2009)	Hypermyelination (transgenic mice)	Lower CSD velocities in the hypermyelinated mice, compared to the wildtype controls
Rat	Guedes et al. (2009)	Genetically prone to audiogenic epilepsy	Gender-dependent impairment of CSD

animal models such as the present one that utilizes the CSD phenomenon in order to get information on normal brain function. These models could also help us to understand how the brain's physiology is altered under nutritional and non-nutritional conditions like those discussed here. In this chapter, we have presented CSD electrophysiological data from both laboratory animals and humans, documenting the importance and usefulness of this phenomenon in studying the nervous system. In the rat, brain structural and functional maturation is programmed to occur mostly during the lactation period. The malnutrition-induced brain alterations during this period probably resulted from the decreased number and/or size of cell elements, as well as from alterations in the events that cause neuronal maturation. Processes such as cell migration, dendrite development, synapse formation, and myelination are certainly implicated in the neurophysiological alterations found when malnutrition occurs early in life (Morgane et al. 1978). This period of intense formation of synapses can be considered equivalent to the human synaptogenic stage, which starts at the third trimester of prenatal development and continues during the first year of child life (Morgane et al. 1978). The well-grounded extrapolation of data from one species (rat) to the other (humans) is a task that, despite some attempts, still needs to be further achieved and the increasing use of the here-described models and techniques is strongly desirable, as a supporting means to clarify the relationship between diet, nutrition, and neural development and function.

In the current world scenario of nutritional transition, experienced by a considerable part of the human population, it can be concluded that the electrophysiological analysis of CSD features constitutes a valuable experimental instrument to investigate the functional brain effects of different unfavorable nutritional as well as non-nutritional conditions that are often stressing and energy-demanding for the developing brain.

Since all the factors presented above in the Tables 148.2 and 148.3 are of clinical relevance, and also considering that they are known to affect the mammalian brain development and function, it is reasonable to assume that knowing the mechanisms by which they affect CSD propagation may shed light on the role of such factors in important human diseases, such as ischemia, migraine, and epilepsy. Furthermore, the complete understanding of CSD generation and propagation mechanisms might be very helpful in developing better treatment of those human neurological diseases.

Summary Points

- The malnourished organism suffers developmental and physiological alterations consequent to insufficient food intake during a certain period of its life. Depending on the intensity and duration of malnutrition, the physiological alterations can become permanent, usually with *neurological disturbances* involving sensory-motor activity, learning, memory, consciousness, cognition and emotion.
- Some data suggest that *malnourished humans would have higher propensity to epilepsy*, as compared with well-nourished controls, but further studies are needed to definitely confirm the causal relationship between malnutrition and proneness to develop the epileptic phenomenon.
- Animal studies under conditions that either enhance or impair the brain ability to initiate and propagate "Cortical Spreading Depression" (CSD) are helpful to understand both the CSD phenomenon and the human neurological diseases related to them, such as brain ischemia, migraine, and epilepsy.
- Besides malnutrition, *excessive food intake* early in life also affects the brain's ability to produce and propagate cortical spreading depression. This raises some concerns about the *impact of obesity on brain development and function*.
- If the findings in laboratory animals reflect what happens in the human brain, then this would imply that different classes of therapeutically employed drugs (as, for example, anti-epileptics and anti-migraine drugs) could present distinct degrees of effectiveness depending on the early nutritional condition of the patients.

Acknowledgments   The author is Research Fellow from the Brazilian Research Council (CNPq – No. 302565/2007–8) and thanks the Brazilian agencies CAPES, FINEP/IBN-Net (No. 01.06.0842-00) and CT-CNPq/MS-SCTIE-DECIT (no. 17/2006) for their financial support.

Definitions and Explanations of Key Terms

Nutritional transition: It is the expression used to define the current epidemiological situation of a great part of the human population, mainly in developing countries. This epidemiological situation comprises an increasing human contingent with obesity, associated to a decreasing number of malnourished persons *in the same population.*

Electroencephalogram (EEG): It is the recording of the spontaneous brain electrical activity that all living mammals present, even when they sleep. This activity can be electronically recorded in chart-paper, ink-writer machines, or digitally in computer-based devices.

Epilepsy: It is a neurological disease resulting from an exacerbated and uncontrolled activity of a certain neuronal population in the brain. The main clinical signs of a generalized epileptic seizure are loss of consciousness and exacerbated and uncontrolled muscle contractions (motor seizure).

Cortical spreading depression (CSD): It is a reversible brain phenomenon provoked by an adequate stimulation of a point of the brain tissue. Current knowledge of the phenomenon leads to the postulation of a link between CSD and human neurological diseases like epilepsy, migraine, and brain ischemia.

Fast Fourier Transform: It is a mathematical technique that employs an algorithm to decompose a sequence of values into components of different frequencies. It is used to decompose the "spectrum of EEG-waves" into its distinct component frequencies, enabling the detection of nutrition-related alterations in one or more of such frequencies.

Extracellular milieu: It is the environment outside the cells. This environment is occupied by the extracellular fluid, the composition of which includes metabolites, ions, proteins, and many other substances that might affect cellular function. These substances are provided by the foods that we daily eat.

GABAergic compound: It is a substance that favors, promotes, or facilitates action, in the neurons or glial cells, of the neurotransmitter gamma-amino butyric acid (GABA). This neurotransmitter is believed to be inhibitory in the mammalian central nervous system.

Knockin mouse: It is a genetically modified animal, in the genome of which a gene has been inserted. The animal then expresses the characteristics coded by that gene (for example, a certain disease). The opposite genetic manipulation (deletion of a gene) originates the "knockout" mouse.

References

Abadie-Guedes R, Santos SD, Cahú TB, Guedes RCA, Bezerra RS. Alcohol Clin Exp Res. 2008;32:1417–21.

Amâncio-dos-Santos A, Pinheiro PCF, Lima DSC, Ozias MG, Oliveira MB, Guimarães NX, Guedes RCA. Exp Neurol. 2006;200:275–82.

Andrade AFD, Guedes RCA, Teodósio NR. Braz J Med Biol Res. 1990;23:889–93.

Bezerra RS, Abadie-Guedes R, Melo FRM, Paiva AMA, Amâncio-dos-Santos A, Guedes RCA. Neurosci Lett. 2005;391:51–5.

Boubred F, Buffat C, Feuerstein JM, Daniel L, Tsimaratos M, Oliver C, Lelièvre-Pégorier M, Simeoni U. Am J Physiol Renal Physiol. 2007;293:F1944–9.

Cintra L, Durán P, Angel-Guevara M, Aguilar A, Castañón-Cervantes O. Nutr Neurosci. 2002;5:91–101.

Costa-Cruz RRG, Guedes RCA. Neurosci Lett. 2001;303:177–80.

Davidowa H, Li Y, Plagemann A. Eur J Neurosci. 2003;18:613–21.

De Luca B, Cioffi LA, Bures J. Activ Nerv Sup. 1977;19:130–1.

Díaz-Cintra S, González-Maciel A, Morales MA, Aguilar A, Cintra L, Prado-Alcalá RA. Exp Neurol. 2007;208:47–53.

Dohmen C, Sakowitz OW, Fabricius M, Bosche B, Reithmeier T, Ernestus RI, Brinker G, Dreier JP, Woitzik J, Strong AJ, Graf R. Ann Neurol. 2008;63:720–8.

Eikermann-Haerter K, Dileköz E, Kudo C, Savitz SI, Waeber C, Baum MJ, Ferrari MD, van den Maagdenberg AM, Moskowitz MA, Ayata C. J Clin Invest. 2009;119:99–109.

El-Bachá RS, Lima-Filho JL, Guedes RCA. Nutr Neurosci. 1998;1:205–12.

Fabricius M, Fuhr S, Willumsen L, Dreier JP, Bhatia R, Boutelle MG, Hartings JA, Bullock R, Strong AJ, Lauritzen M. Clin Neurophysiol. 2008;119:1973–84.

Farias-Santos RC, Lira MCA, Pereira DES et al. Neurosci Lett. 2009;454:218–22.

Feoli AM, Siqueira I, Almeida LM, Tramontina AC, Battu C, Wofchuk ST, Gottfried C, Perry ML, Gonçalves CA. J Nutr. 2006;136:2357–61.

Fregni, F, Monte-Silva, KK, Oliveira, MB et al. Eur J Neurosci. 2005;21:2278–84.

Ginter E, Simko V. Bratisl Med J. 2009;109:224–30.

Gorelova NA, Koroleva VI, Amemori T, Pavlík V, Bur s J. Electroencephalogr Clin Neurophysiol. 1987;66:440–7.

Gorji A, Speckmann EJ. Eur J Neurosci. 2004;19:3371–4.

Gramsbergen A. Brain Res. 1976;105:287–308.

Grantham-McGregor S. J Nutr. 1995;125:2233S–8S.

Guedes RCA, Amorim LF, Medeiros MC et al. Braz J Med Biol Res. 1989;22:923–5.

Guedes RCA, Azeredo FAM, Hicks TP et al. Exp Brain Res. 1987;69:113–8.

Guedes RCA, Andrade AFD, Cavalheiro EA et al. In: Cavalheiro EA, Lehman J, Turski L, editors. Frontiers in excitatory amino acid research. New York: Alan R. Liss. Inc.; 1988. p.667–670.

Guedes RCA, Barreto, Braz J Med Biol Res. 1992;25:393–7.

Guedes RCA, Cavalheiro, Epil Res. 1997;27:33–40.

Guedes RCA, Amancio-dos-Santos A, Manhães-de-Castro R et al. Nutr Neurosci. 2002;5:115–23.

Guedes RCA. In: Liebermann H, Kanarek R, Prasad C, editors. Nutritional neurosciences: overview of an emerging field. New York: CRC Press, 2005. p. 39–54.

Guedes RCA, Cabral-Filho JE, Teodósio NR. In: Do Carmo RJ, editor. Spreading depression. Berlin: Springer; 1992. p. 17–26.

Guedes RCA, Amorim LF, Teodósio NR. Braz J Med Biol Res. 1996;29:1407–12.

Guedes RCA, Do Carmo RJ. Exp Brain Res. 1980;39:341–9.

Guedes RCA, Oliveira JAC, Amâncio-dos-Santos A, García-Cairasco N. Epilep Res. 2009;83:207–14.

Guedes RCA, Pereira-da-Silva MS. Braz J Med Biol Res. 1993;26:1123–8.

Guedes RCA, Vasconcelos CAC. Neurosci Lett. 2008;442:118–22.

Hackett R, Iype T. Seizure. 2001;10:554–8.

Largo C, Ibarz JM, Herreras O. J Neurophysiol. 1997;78:295–307.

Leão AAP. J Neurophysiol. 1944;7:359–90.

Leão AAP. J Neurophysiol. 1947;10:409–14.

Leão, AAP. In: Purpura DP, Penry K, Tower DB, Woodbury DM, Walter RD, editors. Experimental models of epilepsy. New York: Raven Press; 1972. p. 173–195.

Lehmenkühler A, Grotemeyer KH, Tegtmeier F. Migraine: basic mechanisms and treatment. Munich: Urban and Schwarzenberg; 1993.

Maia LMSS, Amancio-dos-Santos A, Duda-de-Oliveira D et al. Nutr Neurosci. 2009;12:73–80.

Martins-Ferreira H, Oliveira Castro G, Stuchiner CJ, Rodrigues PS. J Neurophysiol. 1974;37:785–91.

Merkler D, Klinker F, Jürgens T, Glaser R, Paulus W, Brinkmann BG, Sereda M, Guedes RCA, Brück W, Liebetanz D. Ann Neurol. 2009;66:355–65.

Monte-Silva KK, Assis FLN, Leal GMA, Guedes RCA. Nutr Neurosci. 2007;10:187–194.

Monteiro CA, Conde WL, Popkin BM. Am J Public Health. 2004;94:433–4.

Morgane PJ, Miller M, Kemper T, Stern W, Forbes W, Hall R, Bronzino J, Kissane J, Hawrylewicz E, Resnick O. Neurosci Biobehav Rev. 1978;2:137–230.

Nelson GK, Dean RF. Bull World Health Org. 1959;21:779–82.

Palencia G, Calvillo M, Sotelo J. Epilepsia. 1996;37:583–6.

Peeters M, Gunthorpe MJ, Strijbos PJ, Goldsmith P, Upton N, James MF. J Pharmacol Exp Ther. 2007;321:564–72.

Pezzini A, Del Zotto E, Giossi A, Volonghi I, Grassi M, Padovani A. Curr Mol Med. 2009;9:215–26.

Popkin BM, Horton S, Kim S, Mahal A, Shuigao J. Nutr Rev. 2001;59:379–90.

Richter F, Rupprecht S, Lehmenkühler A, Schaible HG. J Neurophysiol. 2003;90:2163–70.

Rocha-de-Melo AP, Guedes RCA. Braz J Med Biol Res. 1997;30:663–70.

Rocha-de-Melo AP, Cavalcanti JB, Barros AS, Guedes RCA. Nutr Neurosci. 2006;9:155–60.

Santos-Monteiro JS, Teodósio NRT, Guedes RCA. Nutr Neurosci. 2000;3 (1):29–40.

Schulte FJ, Bell EF. Neuropäd. 1973;4:30–45.

Tenorio AS, Oliveira IDVA, Guedes RCA et al. Int J Dev Neurosci. 2009;27:431–7.

Tottene A, Conti R, Fabbro A, Vecchia D, Shapovalova M, Santello M, van den Maagdenberg AM, Ferrari MD, Pietrobon D. Neuron. 2009;61:762–73.

Vasconcelos CAC, Oliveira JAF, Costa LAO, Guedes RCA. Nutr Neurosci. 2004;7:163–70.

Ximenes-da-Silva A, Guedes RCA. Braz J Med Biol Res. 1991;24:1277–81.

Chapter 149
Dietary Zinc and the Brain

Mohammad Tariqur Rahman

Abbreviations

AD	Alzheimer's disease
AMPA	α-amino-3-hydroxy-5-methyl-4-isoxazole propionic acid
ATP/ADP	Adenosine tri/di phosphate
BBB	Blood brain barrier
CSF	Cerebrospinal fluid
CNS	Central nervous system
ECF	Extracellular fluid
ER	Endoplasmic reticulum
MAPK	Mitogen activated protein kinase
MT	Metallothionein
RDA	Recommended daily allowance
UIL	Upper intake level
VGCC	Voltage-gated Ca^{2+} channels
(S)VZ	(Sub)Ventricular zone
ZIP	Zn^{2+} importing proteins
[Zn]	Concentration of Zn
ZnT	Zn transporter

149.1 Introduction

The physiological importance of zinc (Zn) was first recognized in 1940 when the Zn-containing enzyme, carbonic anhydrase, was described (Keilin and Mann 1940). Eventually, Zn was recognized as an 'essential' trace element found widely distributed in all human organs and tissues and required for the structure and functions of many cellular proteins (Table 149.1). Today, the importance of Zn in human health is well documented (Frederickson et al. 2005; Maret and Sandstead 2008). In the brain, Zn plays important roles both in its development and function.

M.T. Rahman (✉)
Department of Biomedical Science, Kulliyyah of Science, International Islamic
University Malaysia (IIUM), Jalan Istana, Bandar Indera Mahkota, 25200 Kuantan, Malaysia
e-mail: tarique@iiu.edu.my; m.tariqur.rahman@gmail.com

V.R. Preedy et al. (eds.), *Handbook of Behavior, Food and Nutrition*,
DOI 10.1007/978-0-387-92271-3_149, © Springer Science+Business Media, LLC 2011

Table 149.1 Key facts on zinc

Chemistry and physical properties
- Discovery: German chemist Andreas Sigismund Marggraf (1746) is normally given credit for discovering pure metallic Zn.
- Avaialability: the 24th most abundant element on the Earth's crust
- Empirical formula: Zn
- Position in the periodic table: 1st element in group 12
- Number of stable isotopes: five
- Atomic number: 30
- Atomic weight: 65.39 g

Uses
- Zinc plating for corrosion-resistance (e.g. on steel).
- Zinc alloys such as brass (alloy of zinc and copper) is used in batteries.
- Zinc chloride in deodorants
- Zinc pyrithione in shampoos
- Zinc sulfide in luminescent paints
- Zinc-carbonate, Zn-gluconate as dietary supplements

Biological importance
- Considered an essential mineral
- Structural component of many enzymes such as alcohol dehydrogenase in humans or other biomolecules important in cellular and molecular processes such as Zn finger transcription factors.
- Half of the total body's Zn is present in muscle. Other major organs of the body that contain zn includes bones, skin, kidneys, testes, and prostate glands
- Zinc deficiency causes growth retardation, delayed sexual maturation, infection susceptibility, and diarrhea, etc.
- Zinc excess is associated with ataxia, lethargy, and copper and iron deficiency.

This table includes the key facts on Zn including its chemical properties, uses, and biological importance

Zinc metalloproteins are the major (~80%) reservoir of the total brain Zn while the rest is free Zn^{2+} and are histochemically detectable by Timm's sulfide-silver staining method (Frederickson and Danscher 1990). In the brain, Zn is relatively concentrated in the hippocampus and amygdala (Takeda et al. 2004). Both regions are enriched with histochemically reactive Zn^{2+} which predominantly exists in the presynaptic vesicles. Zinc homeostasis in the brain is maintained by the blood brain barrier system and is not easily disrupted by dietary Zn deficiency. Nevertheless, histochemically detectable Zn in hippocampus are susceptible to dietary Zn deficiency.

Most of the cells in the human body including neuron maintain Zn homeostasis through the regulated expression of proteins for Zn- import, export, and sequestration. Specific Zn transporters are used in certain tissues and their expression may vary with dietary Zn status and time (Dufner-Beattie et al. 2003; Kelleher and Lonnerdal 2003). Thus Zn homeostatic mechanisms appear to be tissue specific.The mechanism of exact regulation of Zn uptake from extracellular fluids (ECF) into neurons and glial cells, however, is not completely known.

Large numbers of the world's population, an estimated total of about 50%, are at risk of Zn deficiency (Brown et al. 2001). Zinc deficiency in children is a nutritional and health concern in both developing and developed countries (Black 1998; Bryan et al. 2004). Zinc deficiency results in decrease in extracellular [Zn] in the hippocampus which subsequently causes abnormal glucocorticoid secretion from the adrenal cortex. As the hippocampus is enriched with glucocorticoid receptors, the abnormal glucocorticoid secretion alters its function. Abnormal glucocorticoid secretion in Zn deficiency is associated with neuropsychological symptoms affecting cognitive performance and aggravated glutamate excitotoxicity. The decrease in Zn^{2+} pool in the peripheral tissue in Zn deficiency can also change glucocorticoid action by triggering abnormal glucocorticoid secretion.

Alterations in Zn homeostasis in the brain is observed in Parkinson's and Alzheimer's disease (AD) as well as in transient forebrain ischemia, seizures, and traumatic brain injury. There is much evidence to show that amyloid-beta deposition in AD is induced by Zn (see review Mocchegiani et al. 2005). An elevated concentration of Zn or an excess of Zn in the brain might play a role in such pathological conditions. Indeed the exact neuropathological mechanism of either the elevated level of Zn^{2+} or its deficiency has not been completely resolved (Colvin et al. 2003; Sensi et al. 2009).

This chapter will elaborate on the physiological importance of dietary Zn in the brain. Emphasis will be given to the mechanism of Zn homeostasis, the role of dietary Zn in brain development, and the consequences of Zn excess and/or Zn deficiency in brain pathology.

149.2 Dietary Sources of Zn and Its Bioavailability

The richest food sources of Zn (Table 149.2) are sea foods (shellfish, shrimp, lobster, crab-meat), organs and flesh of mammals and fowls (liver, meat), whole grain cereals, and some beans (Brown and Begin 1993). The total Zn content of the diet and its bioavailability, solubility in particular, in the intestinal lumen determines the amount of Zn absorbed and which can be utilized or metabolized in different organs. This also is influenced by the chemical form of Zn and the presence or absence of specific enhancers or inhibitors of Zn absorption. Amino acids such as cysteine and histidine can increase the solubility of Zn. However, some proteins such as casein have an inhibitory effect on Zn absorption. Myoinositol hexaphosphate (phytate) reduces Zn bioavailability (Soto-Quintana et al. 2003), and therefore oils, fats, and sugar are not considered good sources of Zn. Meal proteins have a positive effect on Zn absorption. In humans without excessive intake of Zn, the body burden half-time of absorbed Zn has been observed in the range between 162–500 days. After parenteral administration, half-times of Zn may vary within the range of about 100–500 days (see review Lowe et al. 2009). In spite of its great importance in human health, the amount of zinc in the diet, however, needs to be maintained properly (Table 149.3).

149.3 Blood Brain Barrier and Permeability of Zn in Brain

Both the supply of the required nutrients for proper functioning of the brain and the control of harmful substances present in the bloodstream so as to prevent them from entering the brain are done by the specialized system of capillary endothelial cells of the blood brain barrier (BBB). The transport

Table 149.2 Zinc in human diet (From Brown and Begin 1993)

Category of foods	Example of edibles
Major dietary source of Zn	
Sea foods	flesh of shellfish, shrimp, lobster, crab
Organs and flesh of mammals and fowls	liver, meat, or muscle
Whole grain cereals, vegetables	chickpeas, kidney beans, almonds
Dairy products	yogurt, milk, cheese
Inhibitors of Zn absorption	Casein
Protein	Plant oil
Oils or fats	Sugar
Carbohydrate	

Zinc is available in various food and food products. This table includes a partial list of the dietary sources of Zn. The amount of Zn, however, may vary depending on type and species

Table 149.3 Recommended daily allowance (RDA) and upper intake levels (UIL) for human Zn consumption (From Institute of Medicine, Food and Nutrition Board. Washington, DC: National Academy Press, 2001)

Age	For male RDA/UIL	For female RDA/UIL	In pregnancy RDA/UIL	During lactation RDA/UIL
0–6 months	2 mg/4 mg	2 mg/4 mg		
7–12 months	3 mg/5 mg	3 mg/5 mg		
1–3 years	3 mg/7 mg	3 mg/7 mg		
4–8 years	5 mg/12 mg	5 mg/12 mg		
9–13 years	8 mg/23 mg	8 mg/23 mg		
14-18 years	11 mg/34 mg	9 mg/34 mg	13 mg/34 mg	14 mg/34 mg
19+ years	11 mg/40 mg	8 mg/40 mg	11 mg/40 mg	12 mg/40 mg

Both the recommended amount of dietary Zn or Zn supplement and upper tolerable levels vary depending on age, gender, or stage of growth and development. This table includes the amount of Zn recommended for daily consumption and the maximum or upper tolerable limit (UIL) for different ages or conditions to maintain optimum health

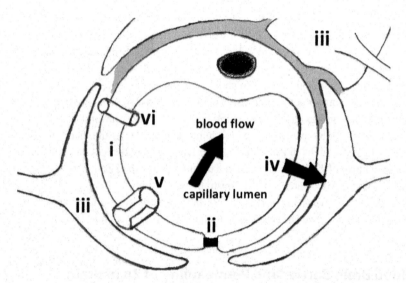

Fig. 149.1 The blood-brain barrier controls the exchange of ions including zinc, amino acids, peptides, and other substances between blood and brain. At the brain blood capillaries, the endothelium cells (i) are joined together at their edges by tight junctions (ii),which prevent water-soluble substances in the blood to enter the CSF. Most of the areas of the blood capillaries are enclosed by the astrocyte's "end-feet" (iii). Thus water-soluble substances can cross the BBB by passing directly through the walls of the cerebral capillaries made up of a lipid/protein bilayer. Fat-soluble molecules, including O_2 and CO_2, anesthetics and alcohol can pass straight through the lipids in the capillary walls (iv). Ions and amino acids can pass through using carrier proteins such as zinc import proteins (v), ion channels or pumps (vi) (Modified from Springer Image library accessed on 01 January, 2010 from http://www.springerimages.com/Images/Pharmacy/1-10.1208_s12248-008-9018-7-0)

of Zn into the brain parenchyma occurs via the BBB system (Kahn 2005). Entry of Zn into the brain is allowed through different kinds of proteins and channels on the BBB (Fig. 149.1). In other words the BBB system provides a strict regulation on Zn homeostasis in the brain and is not easily disrupted by dietary Zn (Franklin et al. 1992).

The presence of specific Zn transport sites on the brain capillary endothelial cells (Buxani-Rice et al. 1994) confirms the important regulatory role of the BBB in brain Zn homeostasis. The BBB-mediated control of Zn homeostasis in the brain is also supported by the enhanced transport of Zn across the BBB, as shown by an in vitro model of the BBB that was exposed to Zn-deficient conditions. The rate of Zn transport across the in vitro BBB model constructed using cultured porcine brain capillary endothelial cells on porous membrane was observed to be slower when [Zn] was below 7 μmol/L and faster when it was above 30 μmol zinc/L (Lehmann et al. 2002). Notably, the zinc transport process is highly selective for Zn since none of the analogous minerals could effectively compete with zinc; besides, the zinc transfer process does not require much energy. Furthermore, metabolic inhibitors also do not influence the transport rate (Bobilya et al. 2008).

In order to maintain Zn homeostasis, brain capillary endothelial cells respond to changes in Zn status, increasing the uptake of Zn in the presence of low [Zn] in the blood and decreasing it in the presence of high [Zn] in the blood (Lehmann et al. 2002). Following its uptake, Zn can be transferred freely through the CSF and the brain ECF compartments. The reduced amount of histochemically reactive Zn in Zn deficiency suggests its reduced uptake in Zn deficiency (Takeda 2001).

149.4 Homeostasis of Zn in the Brain and Dietary Influence

The variation in the amount of Zn in different regions of the mammalian central nervous system (CNS) varies over about a fivefold range, with lower amounts generally in white matter (26–40 ppm in cortical white matter) and higher amounts in grey matter (60–90 ppm in cortical grey matter). On an average, the estimated amount of Zn in one gram of wet brain tissue is about 10μg corresponding to an average total intracellular [Zn] of about 150μM. This concentration is about 10-fold more than the serum [Zn]. On the regional distribution within the brain, the estimated total [Zn] in the hippocampus is more than 200 μM (see review Takeda and Tamano 2009), considered the highest compared to any other region (Frederickson et al. 2005). Notably, hippocampal [Zn] can be decreased significantly in dietary Zn deficiency. Among the other regions, the amygdala and neocortex contain the highest amount of Zn (Fig. 149.2).

In the ECF of the brain, Zn is either bound to low molecular weight ligands such as metalloproteins, or stay as free Zn^{2+} (see review Takeda and Tamano 2009). In the ECF, the estimated total [Zn] and

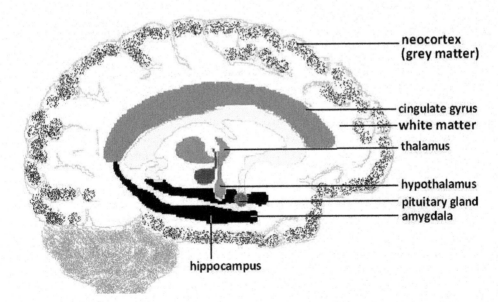

Fig. 149.2 Human brain-zinc map. The hippocampus belongs to the limbic system containing the highest concentration of zinc in the brain (*dark black area*). Other regions of the brain that contain relatively higher amount of Zn is the amygdala (*dark black area*) and grey matter neocortex (*black dotted area*)

free [Zn^{2+}] are 0.15–1 µM (Hershey et al. 1983; Weiss et al. 2000) and ~5–20 µM (Frederickson et al. 2006) respectively. About 80% of the total brain Zn is bound with Zn metalloproteins while the rest is histochemically detectable using Timm's sulfide-silver staining method (Frederickson and Danscher 1990). This is based on the observation that the removal of Zn transporter protein results in a 20% reduction of the total amount of Zn in the brain (Cole et al. 1999).

Within the brain, both the extracellualr and intracellular Zn are exchangeble. Extracellular Zn^{2+} in the brain may change because of its release from cells (Frederickson 1989; Qian and Noebels 2005), while changes in intracellular Zn^{2+} may result from oxidative stress (Frazzini et al. 2006). The concentration of rapidly exchangeable cytosolic free Zn^{2+} is estimated in the subnanomolar level. Such dynamic changes in Zn^{2+} gradients and the availability of specific Zn^{2+} binding domains suggest the importance of Zn^{2+} ions as signaling molecules. However, the signaling effects of Zn^{2+} may be mediated by intracellular or extracellular Zn^{2+} (Sensi et al. 1997).

In Zn deficiency, the level of serum Zn decreases which in turn leads to a decrease in CSF Zn. Although one week of Zn deprivation in young rats can decrease serum Zn level about 50% compared to control animals, a significant change (decrease) in extracellular Zn in the hippocampus is observed only after 4 weeks of Zn deprivation. Histochemically reactive Zn (Timm's stain) also decreases after 4 weeks of Zn deprivation. Thus only a prolonged period of Zn deficiency (4 weeks in contrast to 1 week) can cause a decrease in hippocampal Zn. Notably, extracellular Zn may lead to the decrease in histochemically reactive Zn. Extracellular Zn is also responsive to dietary Zn deficiency in other regions such as the amygdala, followed by a decrease in histochemically reactive Zn (Takeda and Tamano 2009).

The protein-bound Zn in intracellular compartments of the brain, on the other hand, may be resistant to Zn deficiency. It is possible that the response of hippocampal Zn to dietary Zn deficiency reflects that of peripheral Zn since the decrease in serum Zn may lead to the reduction of Zn^{2+} pool in peripheral tissues. It is possible that insufficient Zn^{2+} signaling in peripheral tissues is associated with activation of the hypothalamo-pituitary-adrenocortical system in Zn deficiency (Takeda and Tamano 2009).

149.5 Transport and Homeostasis of Zn in Neuron and Dietary Influence

Cells in different parts of the brain have different amounts of Zn which in turn contributes to the variable amount of Zn in different brain areas. The free [Zn^{2+}] in the cytosol from cultured neurons is estimated at subnanomolar (Weiss et al. 2000). However, Zn content in the synaptic vesicles of some neurons in the forebrain is found to be approximately >1 mM (Frederickson et al. 2005). Although intraneuronal cytosolic Zn^{2+} is in the subnanomolar or picomolar range, it is estimated to rise to micromolar levels in the proximity of axon terminals following release from synaptic vesicles that contain Zn^{2+} at millimolar range (Frederickson et al. 2005). This is most likely also the case in other intracellular compartments such as mitochondria, vesicles, and lysosomes that can take up cytosolic Zn^{2+} (Sensi et al. 2003; Colvin et al. 2006; Hwang et al. 2008; Dittmer et al. 2009).

Neurons that contain free Zn^{2+} in the vesicles of their presynaptic boutons are present both in forebrain areas (such as hippocampus, amygdala, and neocortex) and other areas of the brain (Fig. 149.2). Those neurons in the forebrain area are a subgroup of excitatory glutamatergic (or gluzinergic) neurons and in other areas they are termed Zn-enriched neurons (Frederickson and Danscher et al. 1990). Since the distribution of these neurons within the brain is not uniform, Zn distribution in the brain is also not uniform.

The exact mechanism that regulates Zn uptake from the ECF into neurons and glial cells is still not completely known. Most of the cells maintain Zn homeostasis through the regulated expression of proteins for Zn import, export, and sequestration (Table 149.4). Furthermore, Zn homeostatic

Table 149.4 Zn^{2+} transport and storage in neurons

Zn transporter(s) or storage protein	Important features
VGCCs and Ca^{2+}/Zn^{2+}-permeable AMPA receptors	Located at the plasma membrane the main routes Zn^{2+} entry into neurons
ZnT1	Located at the plasma membrane controls Zn^{2+} efflux interacts with the L-type VGCC that regulates Ca^{2+} and Zn^{2+} influx.
ZnT3	Located at the synaptic vesicles
ZnT5, ZnT6, ZnT7	Located at the golgi apparatus
ZnT5, ZnT6, ZnT7	Located at the lysozome
The Na^s/Zn^{2+} exchanger	Moves Zn^{2+} in or out of neurons depending on the Na^+ gradient
ZIP	H^+- or HCO_3-Zn^{2+} co-transporters and facilitates Zn^{2+} influx.
Ca^{2+} uniporter	Located at mitochondria
MT (MT-III)	Major Zn^{2+}-homeostatic proteins in neurons

AMPA, α-amino-3-hydroxy-5-methyl-4-isoxazole propionic acid; MT, metallothionein VGCCs, voltage-gated Ca^{2+} channels; ZIP, Zinc importing protein
This table summarizes the list of major zinc transporters involved in supply and homeostasis of zinc in neurons (for detail see Ohana et al. 2009)

mechanisms appear to be tissue specific. Specific Zn transporters are used in certain tissues and its expression varies with dietary Zn status and time (Dufner-Beattie et al. 2003; Kelleher and Lonnerdal 2003). A number of Zn^{2+} transporters (ZnTs), Zn^{2+}-importing proteins (ZIPs), and buffering proteins such as the metallothioneins (MT) bind cytosolic Zn^{2+} and mediate the complex intraneuronal cytosolic Zn^{2+} homeostasis. In addition, specific gated Zn-permeable membrane-spanning channels, such as voltage-gated L-type Ca^{2+} channels, Na^+/Zn^{2+} exchangers, N-methyl-D-aspartate (NMDA) receptor gated channels, and Ca^{2+} permeable AMPA/kainate channels can also mediate the neuronal uptake of Zn. Zinc transporter proteins too regulate the efflux of Zn from neurons as well as vesicular Zn uptake. Transporters of the Zip family, which are the main membrane Zn uptake transporters, also seem to be involved in this process (reviewed in Ohana et al. 2009).

ZnTs mediate Zn^{2+} transport from the cytosol to the lumen of intracellular organelles or out of the cell. There are at least ten members of the ZnT family, most of which are ubiquitously expressed, except ZnT3 which is neuron specific and present on synaptic glutamatergic vesicles. With the exception of ZnT1, ZnTs are present on intracellular organelles such as the Golgi and the secretory vesicles of many organs (Table 149.4). Zinc Transporter 1 is expressed, synaptically and extrasynaptically, on the plasma membrane of neurons and glia. Other ZnT family members, ZnT2, ZnT4, ZnT5, and ZnT6, are also expressed in several brain regions (reviewed in Sensi et al. 2009) such as in the hippocampus, cortex, and olfactory bulb (Lee et al. 2003), and in certain cerebellar GABAergic and dopaminergic neurons (Ruiz et al. 2004). Zin Transporter 7, which probably facilitates Zn^{2+} transport from the cytoplasm into the Golgi apparatus, is moderately expressed in the brain and ZnT2, ZnT5, and ZnT6, which are associated with vesicular Zn uptake and Zn efflux in many organs, should similarly play a minor role in the brain.

149.6 Biochemistry of Zn Binding with Proteins in Brain

The knowledge of the biochemical importance of Zn dates back to 1940 with the discovery of the Zn-containing enzyme, *carbonic anhydrase*, now known to contain 1 gram atom of the metal per mole (Keilin and Mann1940). Subsequently, more than 300 such Zn containing proteins with catalytic, structural, and other functional roles have been described. This number is more than that of any other transition or Group IIB metal (Vallee and Falchuk 1993) that is involved in biomolecules. Specific binding sites for Zn^{2+} are present on numerous proteins, including Zn^{2+} fingers on transcription factors that bind it with high affinity, and metallothioneins, from which the Zn^{2+} is easily dissociable.

Zinc binds to many proteins involved in gene regulation. The Zn finger proteins as transcription factor, Zn twists in steroid receptors, and Zn clusters in the galactose metabolism activator are well known examples. Other metalloproteins tightly binding Zn include the RING finger protein family (Freemont 1993), the tumour suppressor p53, the human growth hormone-prolactin receptor complex, and metallothionein proteins (Ebadi 1986; Vallee and Falchuk 1993). Zinc also stabilizes the 3D structure of superoxide dismutase (Salguerio et al. 2007). A partial list of Zn finger transcription factors present in different areas and types of cells in the brain is given in Table 149.5. In the brain, Zn is structurally important for reelin, a large secreted protein, implicated in the cortical development of the mammalian brain. A 2.0-Å crystal structure from the fifth and sixth reelin repeats fragment revealed the presence of Zn^{2+} bound to them (Yasui et al. 2007).

The biochemical importance of Zn lies in its role as catalytic, coactive (or co-catalytic), structural (Vallee and Falchuk 1993; MacDonald 2000), and intracellular signaling factor such as the regulation of

Table 149.5 Zinc finger transcription factors in the brain

Transcription factor	Expression site and/or function
ATBF1	• Protein is highly expressed in the midbrain and diencephalon • mRNA is highly expressed in the brainstem, mostly in embryo and neonatal brain, postmitotic neurons in the brainstem • Expression is transient and weak in the precursor cells at early neurogenesis. • Expression decreases postnatally, but remains in mature neurons • Regulation of neuronal cell maturation or region-specific central nervous system differentiation
Bcl11A/Evi9/CTIP1	• Bcl11A-S/Evi9c is widely expressed in different regions of the rat brain • Bcl11A-L/Evi9a is expressed in the cerebral cortex, hippocampus, and olfactory bulb
DRRF (Sp1 family of transcription factors)	• Highly expressed in the neural ectoderm and neural groove • Moderately expressed in the mesoderm and endoderm at the early embryonic stage. • Highest DRRF mRNA levels in olfactory bulb and tubercle, nucleus accumbens, striatum, hippocampus, amygdala, and frontal cortex. • Regulates dopaminergic neurotransmission
Egr3	• Expressed in cortex and colocalized with zif268. • Important in defining long-term, neuroplastic responses.
FOG-2	• Expressed in developing and adult heart, brain, and testis • Important cofactor for GATA-mediated transcriptional activation in cardiac and neural cell lineages.
Ik-1 and Ik-2	• Positive regulators of enkephalin gene expression in the developing striatum • Participate in regulating enkephalinergic differentiation
Lot1	• High in cerebellar granule cells, a neuronal population undergoing postnatal neurogenesis
MOK2	• *PAX3* and *IRBP* (interphotoreceptor retinoid-binding protein) genes are two potentially important target genes for the MOK2 protein.
NSM1(IA-1)	• In mouse brain, *Insm1* is strongly expressed for 2 weeks after birth but shows little or no expression thereafter. • During embryo development Cbl-associated protein may enter the nucleus through its own nuclear localization signal or by binding to INSM1.

(continued)

Table 149.5 (continued)

Transcription factor	Expression site and/or function
Plag1, Plag-l2	• In the CNS and PNS • In olfactory and neuroendocrine lineages. • Might control cell fate and proliferation decisions in the developing nervous system (Oncogenes)
REST/NRSF/XBR	• Highest levels in the neurons of hippocampus, pons/medulla, and midbrain • A negative regulator rather than a transcriptional silencer of neuronal gene expression and counteracts with positive regulators to modulate target gene expression quantitatively in different cell types, including neurons.
RP58	• mRNA at E 10 in the neuroepithelium, and subsequently in the VZ of the cerebral cortex in the E12 embryo. • Strong expression in the preplate in the cerebral cortex from this stage onward. High levels of expression continue to be detected in the cortical plate and SVZ of the neocortex, hippocampus, and parts of the amygdala
Sp8	• Expressed in neurogenic regions, which gives rise to olfactory bulb interneurons at embryonic and postnatal time points and remains expressed in the calretinin-expressing and GABAcrgic/nondopaminergic interneurons of the glomerular layer. • Contributes to olfactory bulb interneuron diversity by regulating the survival, migration, and molecular specification of neuroblasts/interneurons.
Wt1	• The developing olfactory epithelium
Zac1(Plag family)	• Abundantly expressed in many neuroepithelia during early brain development • Regulates both apoptosis and cell cycle arrest (tumor suppressors)
Zfp423	• Expressed within the cerebellum, both in ventricular and external germinal zones. • Loss of Zfp423 results in diminished proliferation by granule cell precursors in the external germinal layer, especially near the midline, and abnormal differentiation and migration of ventricular zone-derived neurons and Bergmann glia
Zic1–5	• Precursor cells of the granule neuron and the neurons in cerebellar nuclei • Neurulation, neuronal differentiation, neural crest specification, the establishment of left-right asymmetry, and regulation of cell proliferation
Zif268 (Egr1)	• Zif268 is constitutively expressed in several parts including the temporal lobe. • Zif268 regulates neurological genes and cellular growth and proliferation genes. • Expressed in mammalian neurons during visual and fear learning, as well as in song learning in birds. • Expressed in response to cellular growth and proliferation signals by enhancing the expression of TGFβ1
ZNF536	• Most abundant in the developing central nervous system and dorsal root ganglia and localized in the cerebral cortex, hippocampus, and hypothalamic area. • Negatively regulates neuron differentiation.

This table includes a partial list of Zn finger transcription factors expressed in different sites and/or cells of the brain. Related functions of the respective transcription factors at the expression site are listed as well

cell proliferation (Hershfinkel et al. 2007). The catalytic roles of Zn include participating in the transformation of substrates by facilitating the formation of OH^- at neutral pH, or through Lewis acid catalysis. The structural role of Zn is mostly in stabilizing active tertiary peptide conformation. Notably, Zn^{2+} interacts strongly with electronegative sulfur, nitrogen, and oxygen moieties in multiple coordination geometries, and yet unlike Fe or Cu, it is not redox active under physiological conditions and thus does not promote the formation of toxic free radicals. As an extracellular signal factor Zn is involved in synaptic neurotransmission (Frederickson 1989; Vallee and Falchuk 1993). It is generally accepted that an increase in free intracellular Zn^{2+} is associated with cell death. For example, release of intracellular Zn^{2+}, triggered by formation of reactive oxygen species or by nitrosilation, induces proapoptotic molecules, e.g., p38, and activation of K^+ channels leading to cell death (McLaughlin et al. 2001; Pal et al. 2003).

149.7 The Developing Brain and Zn Status in Diet

The impact of Zn supplementation or a Zn-deficient human diet on brain development and function has not been consistent. Various dimensions of research design and a broad range of subjects varying in racial background, age, and food habits might have contributed to the observed inconsistency. However, a growing number of studies have shown the influence of maternal Zn on fetal growth and development (Goldenberg et al. 1995; Georgieff 2007; Cole and Lifshitz 2008). Daily Zn supplementation in women with relatively low plasma [Zn] in early pregnancy is associated with greater infant birth weights and head circumferences, with the effect occurring predominantly in women with a body mass index less than 26 kg/m^2 (Goldenberg et al. 1995). Very low birth weight of Canadian infants scored improved motor development when given Zn supplement (Friel et al. 1993) while low birth weight infants in Brazil (Ashworth et al. 1998) and older infants and toddlers in Guatemala (Bentley et al. 1997) and India (Sazawal et al. 1996) did not show changes in motor development. However, Zn supplementation to Zn-deficient mothers is important for proper brain development in neonates (Gibson 1994; Georgieff 2007). An adequate Zn nurture is essential for optimal neurological development (Takeda 2001; Prasad 1997). Additional Zn intake during pregnancy results in increased neuronal proliferation in the ventricular zone of the developing brain (Azman et al. 2009). Regular consumption of more than the recommended intake, on the other hand, can have adverse effects (Ronowska et al. 2007).

149.8 Neurogenesis and Zn Supplement

Neurogenesis is a process to generate postmitoitc neuronal and glial cells from neuroepithelial stem cells. Proliferation, cell-cycle arrest, differentiation, migration, and the natural developmental death of neural precursors are well coordinated during neurogenesis (Moskowitz and Lo 2003). Optimal development of the brain depends on strict co-ordination of these events during neurogenesis. Various cell-cycle genes and transcription factors including Zn transcription factors expressed in neurons (Table 149.5) govern neurogenesis, which also determines the correct positional identity of the neural cells from the stem/progenitor cells (Araujo et al. 1990; Edenfeld et al. 2002). In most brain regions, the generation and proliferation of neurons is normally restricted to a discrete developmental period with exceptions for the regions such as hippocampus, dentate gyrus, and the subventricular zone (SVZ) of several species (Caviness 1973; Gueneau et al. 1982; Cameron et al. 1993; Kuhn et al. 1996; Gould et al. 1998; Eriksson et al. 1998; Doetsch et al. 1999), and almost all neurons are generated before early postnatal life and are generally not replaced with new ones (Rakic 1982). The ventricular zone (VZ) is the major site of proliferation and presumably produces all the cell types. A second proliferative zone, namely SVZ, also contributes large numbers of neurons to the developing cortex (Nowakowski and Rakic 1981). In addition, granule neurons are generated throughout life from a population of continuously dividing progenitor cells residing in the subgranular zone of the dentate gyrus in the rodent brain (Stanfield and Trice 1988; Kuhn et al. 1996).

In neuronal cells, Zn deficiency induces oxidative stress, alters the normal structure and dynamics of the cytoskeleton, affects the modulation of several transcription factors and induces a decreased cell proliferation and increased apoptotic death. Thus, Zn deficiency affects critical developmental events of neurogenesis (reviewed by Mackenzie et al. 2007; Nakashima and Dyck 2009). Zinc supplement on the other hand results in increased number of proliferating neurons in the VZ of the developing neocortex. This was observed in the mouse pups delivered by the mother given oral Zn supplement in drinking water during pregnancy (Azman et al. 2009). Notably, Zn is involved in activation of enzyme systems that influence cell division and proliferation (Varrault et al. 1998; MacDonald 2000; Valente et al. 2005; Ronowska et al. 2007). During DNA synthesis, Zn affects thymidine kinase, the activity of which increases dramatically during the G1 and early S phases of the cell cycle. Zinc also influences the hormonal regulation of cell division. Insulin-like growth factor-I and the pituitary growth hormone axis are responsive to Zn status (Root et al. 1979; Roth et al. 1994).

149.9 Neuronal Apoptosis and Zn Deficiency

Zn deficiency was found to increase the expression of Zn transporters in the brain, which facilitates increased brain Zn uptake and results in the conservation of brain Zn during Zn deficiency (Chowanadisai et al. 2005). In neuronal cells, Zn deficiency induces oxidative stress, alters the normal structure and dynamics of the cytoskeleton, affects several transcription factors, and results in decreased cell proliferation and increased apoptosis. These closely associated events affect neuronal function and critical developmental events of neurogenesis when Zn availability decreases (Mackenzie et al. 2007).

In human neuronal cell model IMR-32 cells, a decrease in cellular Zn triggers mitogen-activated protein kinases (MAPKs) both in H_2O_2-independent and dependent manner. Cells grown in low Zn-containing media showed increased cell oxidants and H_2O_2 release, increased c-Jun N-terminal kinase (JNK) and p38 activation, high nuclear activator protein-1 (AP-1)-DNA binding activity, and AP-1-dependent gene expression. Increase in cellular H_2O_2 can trigger the activation of JNK and p38, leading to AP-1 activation, events that are not involved in Zn deficiency-induced apoptosis (Zago et al. 2005).

149.10 Zinc Deficiency or Excess and Brain Pathology

The homeostasis of the free Zn^{2+} pool and the mechanisms involved in controlling that homeostasis are pivotal for proper brain physiology. Acute human dietary deficiency is accompanied by CNS related Zn-reversible symptoms such as anorexia, smell and taste dysfunction, emotional and cognitive disturbances, and loss of coordination (Fig. 149.3) (Ashworth et al. 1998; Bhatnagar and Taneja 2001). Perhaps this is because Zn as a neuromodulator at excitatory synapses plays an important role in stress response and in the functionality of Zn-dependent enzymes contributing to maintaining brain compensatory capacity. Dietary Zn deficiency was also reported to affect learning and memory. Deficiency in Zn is also associated with attention deficiency/hyperactivity disorder. Age-related decline in brain functions and impaired cognitive performances could be related to dysfunctions affecting the intracellular Zn^{2+} availability (Golub et al. 1995; Takeda 2000; Takeda et al. 2008).

Zn deficiency causes abnormal glucocorticoid secretion from the adrenal cortex, which is observed prior to the decrease in extracellular [Zn] in the hippocampus. The functions of glucocorticoid receptor-rich hippocampus are changed by abnormal glucocorticoid secretion that in turn aggravates glutamate excitotoxicity in neurological diseases. Thus Zn deficiency elicits neuropsychological symptoms and affects cognitive performance (Fig. 149.3). It is possible that the decrease in Zn^{2+} pool in the peripheral tissues triggers abnormal glucocorticoid secretion. In other words, the decrease in Zn^{2+} pool may cooperate with glucocorticoid action in Zn deficiency.

Again, elevated [Zn] or Zn excess in the brain has a profound negative effect on neurological cells, which are highly susceptible to extremes in extracellular [Zn]. The exact neuropathological mechanism of elevated level of Zn^{2+} is still unclear; however, it is found to be related to the progression

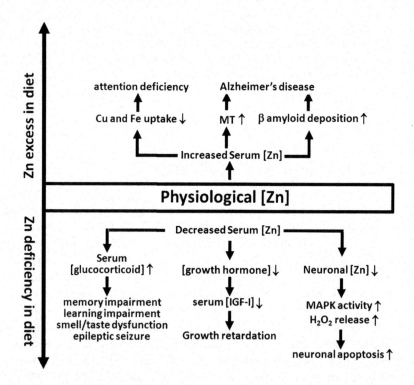

Fig. 149.3 Possible pathological consequences of dietary Zn-deficient or Zn-excess condition. In dietary Zn deficiency, serum [Zn] can be decreased leading to either increased serum glucocorticoid concentration or decreased growth hormone concentration or intracellular [Zn]. These conditions in turn may result in cognitive disturbances such as memory or learning impairment, growth retardation or neuronal apoptosis, respectively. In dietary Zn-excess condition, increased serum [Zn] can lead to decreased uptake of Cu and Fe in different organs, including the brain, or increased depositing of beta amyloid in the brain. *IGF* Insulin like growth factors I, *MAPK* mitogen activated protein kinase, ↓ decrease, increase

of AD and other neuropathologies (reviewed by Sensi et al. 2009). There is considerable evidence that amyloid-beta deposition in AD is induced by Zn, but the exact mechanism is still unclear (reviewd by Mocchegiani et al. 2005; Barnham and Bush 2008). An increased expression of MT-I and MT-II, and in some cases of MT-III (also known to be a growth inhibitory factor), is causally linked to such phenomena (Fig. 149.3). However, the protective roles of these proteins at a young age to maintain brain physiology and their functional ability in aging are not consistent. Alterations in Zn homeostasis have also been reported in Parkinson's disease as well as in transient forebrain ischemia, seizures, and traumatic brain injury. The altered Zn nutritional status of individuals with Down's Syndrome contributes to clinical complications that usually appear with their aging (Lima et al. 2010). Again, Zn metabolism is altered in the presence of Down's Syndrome (Licastro et al. 2001). Zinc supplement in diets has been tried to improve the patient's health albeit with conflicting results (Bucci et al. 2001; Blair et al. 2008).

149.11 Applications to Other Areas of Health and Disease

The importance of Zn in the biological system is remarkable and versatile. Zinc plays a pivotal role in gene expression involving cellular growth and differentiation; yet, unlike other transitional metals, it does not cause any oxidative damage (Berg and Shi 1996). Enough is now known about the clinical and public health importance of Zn in human health and diseases. Community Zn supplementation programs among children in developing countries proved to have had a significant effect on the reduction of pneumonia (Bhutta et al. 1999). Zinc supplement has been beneficial for diarrhea prevention and childhood morbidity and mortality. Other than the brain (CNS), the epidermal, gastrointestinal, immune, skeletal, and reproductive systems are known to be affected clinically by severe Zn deficiency (Solomons 1998; Hambidge et al. 1986).

Summary Points

- The total Zn content of the diet and its bioavailability, especially its solubility in the intestinal lumen, determine the amount of absorbed Zn to be utilized or metabolized in the different organs including the brain.
- In the brain, Zn concentration is highest in the hippocampus which can decrease significantly in dietary Zn deficiency.
- The blood brain barrier system provides strict regulation on Zn homeostasis in the brain and is not easily influenced by dietary Zn.
- Zinc homeostasis is maintained through the regulated expression of proteins for Zn import, export, and sequestration.
- A multitude of Zn^{2+} transporters (ZnTs), Zn^{2+}-importing proteins (ZIPs), and buffering proteins such as the metallothioneins (MT) bind cytosolic Zn^{2+} and mediate the complex intraneuronal cytosolic free Zn^{2+} homeostasis.
- A number of Zn transcription factors are expressed in nerve cells and in different areas of the brain regulating genes involved in proliferation, differentiation, migration, and apoptosis of neurons and other cells of the brain.
- As an extracellular signal factor Zn is involved in synaptic neurotransmission.
- Additional Zn intake during pregnancy can increase neuronal proliferation at the ventricular zone of the developing brain.
- In neuronal cells, Zn deficiency induces oxidative stress, alters the normal structure and dynamics of the cytoskeleton, affects the modulation of transcription factors AP-1, NF-betaB, and NFAT and induces decreased cell proliferation and increased apoptotic death.
- Acute human dietary deficiency is accompanied by symptoms such as anorexia, smell and taste dysfunction, emotional and cognitive disturbances, and loss of coordination. Dietary Zn deficiency also has been reported to affect brain functions, including learning and memory defects.

Key Terms

Apoptosis: A form of cell death (or cell suicide) in which a programmed sequence of events leads to the elimination of cells without leaving or releasing harmful substances into the surrounding area of the dying cell(s). Apoptosis also refers to the structural changes that the cells undergo before the programmed death. Apoptosis is crucial in developing and maintaining health by eliminating old, unnecessary, and unhealthy cells. Hyperactivation and inactivation of apoptosis may result in pathological conditions. Hyperactivation may kill too many cells and inflict grave tissue damage, leading to such neurodegenerative disorders as Alzheimer's, Huntington's, and Parkinson's diseases.

Astrocyte: Astrocytes (collectively known as astroglia) are characteristic star-shaped glial cells in the CNS. Three forms of astrocytes exist in the CNS: *fibrous* (located in white matter and that physically connect the cells to the outside of the capillary wall when they are in close proximity to them), *protoplasmic* (found in grey matter tissue; they possess a larger quantity of organelles and exhibit short and highly branched cellular processes), and *radial* (disposed in a plane perpendicular to the axis of ventricles). Their functions include: biochemical support to the endothelial cells at the BBB, controlling of nutrient supply to the nervous tissue, maintenance of extracellular ion balance, and aiding in repair mechanisms of the brain and spinal cord injuries.

Blood brain barrier (BBB): The BBB is a protective network of blood vessels that filters blood flowing to the brain and separates circulating blood and cerebrospinal fluid (CSF) maintained by the choroid plexus in the CNS. Endothelial cells of the blood vessels restrict the diffusion of microscopic objects (e.g. bacteria) and large or hydrophilic molecules into the CSF, while allowing the diffusion of small hydrophobic molecules (O_2, hormones, CO_2).

Central nervous system (CNS): The CNS is one of the two major divisions of the nervous system and consists of the brain and the spinal cord. The CNS connects to sensory organs (such as the eye and ear) and other organs of the body, muscles, blood vessels, and glands through the peripheral nervous system. The CNS consists of the brain in the cranial cavity and the spinal cord in the spinal cavity.

Hippocampus: The hippocampus is named for its shape like a seahorse (From the Greek *hippos* = horse and *kampos* = a sea monster). It is a closely associated, paired structure with mirror-image halves in the left and right sides of the brain. In humans and other primates, the hippocampus is located inside the medial temporal lobe, beneath the cortical surface. The hippocampus is part of the olfactory cortex essential to the sense of smell and also helps to regulate emotion and memory. Hippocampus also plays important roles in long-term memory and spatial navigation.

Homeostasis: (from Greek: *homoios*, "similar"; and *histēmi*, "standing still"). Generally refers to the property of a system, either open or closed, that regulates its internal environment and tends to maintain a stable, constant condition. When applied to living organisms, homeostasis refers to a property of cells, tissues, and organisms that allow the maintenance and regulation of the stability and constancy needed to function properly and is maintained by the constant adjustment of biochemical and physiological pathways.

Metallothionein (MT): Metallothionein is a family of cysteine-rich, low molecular weight (3.5–14 kDa) proteins. The thiol group of MT contains cysteine residues, which represent ~20–30% of its total amino acidic residues. Both essential (such as Zn, copper, selenium) and toxic (such as cadmium, mercury, silver, arsenic) heavy metals can bind the thiol groups through the cysteine residues. MT has high affinity for Zn (1.4×10^{-13} M). There are four major isoforms (MT-I, MT-II, MT-III, MT-IV) expressed primarily in the liver and kidneys. MT expression is also evident in other tissues and organs such as blood, skin, and heart. In the brain, MT-III is known as the growth inhibitory factor. Expression of MT in different organs and tissues depends on the availability of the dietary minerals, such as Zn, copper, and selenium, and the amino acids histidine and cysteine. MT distributes intracellular Zn as Zn undergoes rapid inter- and intracluster exchange.

Neurogenesis: The process by which new nerve cells are generated i.e., production of new neurons, astrocytes, glia, and other neural lineages from undifferentiated neural progenitor or stem cells. Neurogenesis is most active during prenatal development and inactive in most areas of the adult brain.

Neuron: Neurons are cells in the nervous system including the brain, spinal cord (vertebrate), the ventral nerve cord (invertebrate), and the peripheral nerves that process and transmit information by electrochemical signaling. A typical neuron has a cell body (soma), branching processes specialized to receive incoming signals (dendrites), and a single process (axon) that carries electrical signals away from the neuron toward other neurons or effectors. Electrical signals carried by axons are action potentials. Different types of neurons are named after their specialized structure and functions: for example, *sensory neurons* respond to touch, sound, light, and numerous other stimuli affecting cells of the sensory organs that then send signals to the spinal cord and brain; *motor neurons* receive signals from the brain and spinal cord and cause muscle contractions and affect glands; *interneurons* connect neurons to other neurons within the same region of the brain or spinal cord.

Dopaminergic neuron: Neurons that produce dopamine, a neurotransmitter produced in several areas of the brain, including the substantia nigra and the ventral tegmental area in either vertebrates or invertebrates. Dopamine is a neurohormone released by the hypothalamus mainly to inhibit the release of prolactin from the anterior lobe of the pituitary.

GABAergic neuron: Neurons that produce γ-aminobutyric acid (GABA), the chief inhibitory neurotransmitter in the mammalian CNS. It plays an important role in regulating neuronal excitability throughout the nervous system. In humans, GABA is directly responsible for the regulation of muscle tone. GABA acts at inhibitory synapses in the brain by binding to specific transmembrane receptors in the plasma membrane of both pre- and postsynaptic neuronal processes. This binding causes the opening of ion channels to allow the flow of either Cl^- ions into the cell or K^+ out of the cell. Two general classes of GABA receptor are known: $GABA_A$ in which the receptor is part of a ligand-gated ion channel complex, and $GABA_B$ metabotropic receptors, which are G protein-coupled receptors that open or close ion channels via intermediaries.

Reelin: Reelin is a protein expressed in different tissues of the body including brain, spinal cord, and blood. In the developing brain it helps to regulate neuronal migration and positioning. In the adult brain, it modulates synaptic plasticity by enhancing the induction and maintenance of long-term potentiation. It also stimulates dendrite and dendritic spine development and regulates the continuing migration of neuroblasts generated in adult neurogenesis sites like subventricular and subgranular zones.

Subventricular zone (SVZ): The subventricular zone is a paired brain structure situated throughout the lateral walls of the lateral ventricles. Along with the subgranular zone of the dentate gyrus, the SVZ serves as a source of neural stem cells in the process of neurogenesis. It harbors the largest population of proliferating cells in the adult brain of rodents, monkeys, and humans.

Synaptic vesicle: Synaptic vesicles or neurotransmitter vesicles are 40–100 nanometers in diameter, and made up of a lipid bilayer, store various neurotransmitters (NT) that are released at the synapse for synaptic transmission. The release of NTs is regulated by a voltage-dependent Ca^+ channel. At synapses, the junctional complexes between presynaptic membranes (synaptic knobs) and postsynaptic membranes (receptor surfaces of recipient neurons or effectors), synaptic transmission process signal transfer (communicate) from one neuron (affector) to other neurons (effectors).

Zinc finger transcription factor: Zinc finger transcription factors are the DNA-binding proteins, containing Zn finger domain. Zinc fingers are small protein domains, folds of which are stabilized by one or more Zn^{2+}. They coordinate Zn^{2+} with a combination of cysteine and histidine residues. Different families of Zn finger proteins can bind DNA, RNA, proteins or small molecules involved in transcription, nucleic acid polymerization, and histones.

Acknowledgments Author is grateful to Fawzia Malik and Noor Lide Abu Kassim for their all out support during the manuscript preparation. Special thanks to Rahela Zaman for helping with the drawing of the figures.

References

Araujo DM, Chabot JG, Quirion R. Int Rev Neurobiol. 1990;32:141–74.
Ashworth A, Morris SS, Lira PI, Grantham-McGregor SM. Eur J Clin Nutr. 1998;52:223–7.
Azman MS, Wan Saudi WS, Ilhami M, Mutalib MS, Rahman MT. Nutr Neurosci. 2009;12:9–12.
Barnham KJ, Bush AI. Curr Opin Chem Biol. 2008;12:222–8.
Berg JM, Shi Y. Science. 1996;271:1081–5.
Bentley ME, Caulfield LE, Ram M, Santizo MC, Hurtado E, Rivera JA, Ruel MT, Brown KH. J Nutr. 1997;127:1333–8.
Bhatnagar S, Taneja S. Br J Nutr. 2001;85:S139–45.
Bhutta ZA, Black RE, Brown KH, et al. J Pediatr. 1999;135:689–97.
Black MM. Am J Clin Nutr. 1998;68:464S–9S.
Blair CK, Roesler M, Xie Y, Gamis AS, Olshan AF, Heerema NA, Robison LL, Ross JA. Paediatr Perinat Epidemiol. 2008;22:288–95.
Bobilya DJ, Gauthier NA, Karki S, Olley BJ, Thomas WK. Longitudinal changes in Zn transport kinetics, metallothionein and Zn transporter expression in a blood -brain barrier model in response to a moderately excessive Zn environment. J Nutr Biochem. 2008.;19:129–37
Brown KH, Bégin F. J Pediatr Gastroenterol Nutr. 1993;17:132–8.
Brown KH, Wuehler SE, Peerson JM. Food Nutr Bull. 2001;22:113–25.
Bryan J, Osendarp S, Hughes D, Calvaresi E, Baghurst K, van Klinken JW. Nutr Rev. 2004;62:295–306.
Bucci I, Napolitano G, Giuliani C, et al. Biol Trace Elem Res. 2001;82:273–5.
Buxani-Rice S, Ueda F, Bradbury MWB. J Neurochem. 1994;62:665–72.
Cameron HA, Woolley CS, McEwen BS, Gould E. Neurosci. 1993;56:337–44.
Caviness VS. J Comp Neurol. 1973;151:113–20.
Chowanadisai W, Kelleher SL, Lönnerdal B. J Nutr. 2005;135:1002–7.
Cole CR, Lifshitz F. Pediatr Endocrinol Rev. 2008;5:889–96.
Cole TB, Wenzel HJ, Kafer KE, Schwartzkroin PA, Palmiter RD. Proc Natl Acad Sci USA. 1999;96:1716–21.
Colvin RA, Laskowski M, Fontaine CP. Brain Res. 2006;1085:1–10.
Colvin RA, Fontaine CP, Laskowski M, Thomas D. Eur J Pharmacol. 2003;479:171–85.
Dittmer PJ, Miranda JG, Gorski JA, Palmer AE. J Biol Chem. 2009;284:16289–97.
Doetsch F, Caille I, Lim DA, Garcia-Verdugo JM, Alvarez-Buylla A. Cell. 1999;97:703–16.
Dufner-Beattie J, Wang F, Kuo Y, Gitschier J, Eide D, Andrews G. J Biol Chem. 2003;278:33474–81.
Ebadi M. Biol. Trace Elem Res. 1986;11:101–16.
Edenfeld G, Pielage J, Klambt C. Curr Opin Genet Dev. 2002;12:473–7.
Eriksson PS, Perfilieva E, Björk-Eriksson T, Alborn AM, Nordborg C, Peterson DA, Gage FH. Nat Med. 1998;4:1313–7.
Freemont PS. Ann N Y Acad Sci. 1993;684:174–92.
Franklin PA, Pullen RGL, Hall GH. Neurochem Res. 1992;17:767–1.
Frazzini V, Rockabrand E, Mocchegiani E, Sensi SL. Biogerontology. 2006;7:307–14.
Frederickson CJ, Giblin LJ, Krezel A, et al. Exp Neurol. 2006;198:285–93.
Frederickson CJ, Koh JY, Bush AI. Nat Rev Neurosci. 2005;6:449–62.
Frederickson CJ. Int Rev Neurobiol. 1989;31:145–238.
Frederickson CJ, Danscher G. Prog Brain Res. 1990;83:71–84.
Friel JK, Andrews WL, Matthew JD et al. J Pediatr Gastroenterol Nutr. 1993;17:97–104.
Georgieff MK. Am J Clin Nutr. 2007;85:614S–20S.
Gibson RS. Nutr Res Rev. 1994;7:151–73.
Goldenberg RL, Tamura T, Neggers Y, Copper RL, Johnston KE, DuBard MB, Hauth JC. J Am Med Assoc. 1995;274:463–8.
Golub MS, Keen CL, Gershwin ME, Hendrickx AG. J Nutr. 1995;125:2263–71.
Gould E, Tanapat P, McEwen BS, Flugge G, Fuchs E. Proc Natl Acad Sci USA. 1998;95:3168–71.
Gueneau G, Privat A, Drouet J, Court L. Dev Neurosci. 1982;5:345–58.
Hambidge KM, Casey CE, Krebs NF. Zinc. In: Metz W, editor. Trace elements in human and animal nutrition. New York: Academic Press; 1986. p. 1–37.
Hershey CO, Hershey LA, Varnes A, Vibhakar SD, Lavin P, Strain WH. Neurol. 1983;33:1350–3.
Hershfinkel M, Silverman W, Sekler I. Mol Med. 2007;13:331–6.
Hwang JJ, Lee SJ, Kim TY, Cho JH, Koh JY. J Neurosci. 2008;28:3114–22.

Keilin D, Mann T. Biochem J. 1940;34:1163–76.

Khan E. Br J Nurs. 2005;14:509–13

Kelleher S, Lonnerdal B. J Nutr. 2003;133:3378–85.

Kuhn HG, Dickinson-Anson H, Gage FH. J Neurosci. 1996;16:2027–33.

Lee JY, Kim JH, Palmiter RD, Koh JY. Exp Neurol. 2003;184:337–47.

Lehmann H, Brothwell B, Volak L, Bobilya D. J Nutr. 2002;132:2763–8.

Licastro F, Mariani RA, Faldella G, Carpenè E, Guidicini G, Rangoni A, Grilli T, Bazzocchi G. Brain Res Bull. 2001;55:313–7.

Lima AS, Cardoso BR, Cozzolino SF. Biol Trace Elem Res. Nutritional status of zinc in children with Down syndrome. 2010;133:20–8.

Lowe NM, Fekete K, Decsi T. Am J Clin Nutr. 2009;89:2040S–51S.

MacDonald RS. J Nutr. 2000;130:1500S–8S.

Mackenzie GG, Zago MP, Aimo L, Oteiza PI. IUBMB Life. 2007;59:299–307.

Maret W, Sandstead HH. Exp Gerontol. 2008;43:378–81.

McLaughlin B, Pal S, Tran MP, Parsons AA, Barone FC, Erhardt JA, Aizenman E. J Neurosci. 2001;21:3303–11.

Mocchegiani E, Bertoni-Freddari C, Marcellini F, Malavolta M. Prog Neurobiol. 2005;75:367–90.

Moskowitz MA, Lo EH. 2003;34:324–6.

Nakashima AS, Dyck RH. Brain Res Rev. 2009;59:347–73.

Nowakowski RS, Rakic P. J Comp Neurol. 1981;196:129–54.

Ohana E, Hoch E, Keasar C, Kambe T, Yifrach O, Hershfinkel M, Sekler I. Biol Chem. 2009;284:17677–86.

Pal S, Hartnett KA, Nerbonne JM, Levitan ES, Aizenman E. Neurochem Int. 2003;52:241–6.

Prasad AS. In: Connor JR, editor. Metals and oxidative damage in neurological disorders. New York: Plenum Press; 1997. p. 95–111.

Qian J, Noebels JL. J Physiol. 2005;566: 747–758

Rakic P. Neurosci Res Prog Bull. 1982;20:439–51.

Ronowska A, Gul-Hinc S, Bielarczyk H, Pawelczyk T, Szutowicz A. J Neurochem. 2007;103:972–83.

Root AW, Duckett G, Sweetland M, Reiter EO. J Nutr. 1979;109:958–64.

Roth HP, Kirchgessner M. Horm Metab Res. 1994;26:404–8.

Ruiz A, Walker MC, Fabian-Fine R, Kullmann DM. J Neurophysiol. 2004;91:1091–6.

Salgueiro MJ, Zubillaga M, Lysionek A et al. Nutr Res. 2007;20:737–55.

Sazawal S, Bentley M, Black RE, Dhingra P, George S, Bhan MK. Pediatrics. 1996;98:1132–7.

Sensi SL, Paoletti P, Bush AI, Sekler I. Nat Rev Neurosci. 2009;10:780–91.

Sensi SL, Ton-That D, Sullivan PG, Jonas EA, Gee KR, Kaczmarek LK, Weiss JH. Proc Natl Acad Sci USA. 2003;100:6157–62.

Sensi SL, Canzoniero LMT, Yu SP, Ying HS, Koh JY, Kerchner GA, Choi DW. J Neurosci. 1997;15:9554–64.

Solomons NW. Nutr Rev. 1998;56:280–1.

Soto-Quintana M, Alvarez-Nava F, Rojas-Atencio A, Granadillo V, Fernández D, Ocando A, López E, Fulcado W, et al. Invest Clin. 2003;44:51–60.

Stanfield BB, Trice JE. Exp Brain Res. 1988;72:399–406.

Takeda A, Kanno S, Sakurada N, Ando M, Oku N. J Neurosci Res. 2008;86:2906–11.

Takeda A. BioMetals. 2001;14:343–52.

Takeda A. Brain Res Rev. 2000;34:137–48.

Takeda A, Tamano H. Brain Res Rev. 2009;62:33–44.

Takeda A, Minami A, Seki Y, Oku N. J Neurosci Res. 2004;75:225–9.

Valente T, Junyent F, Auladell C. Dev Dyn. 2005;233:667–79.

Vallee BL, Falchuk KH. Physiol Rev. 1993;73:79–118.

Varrault A, Ciani E, Apiou F, Bilanges B, Hoffmann A, Pantaloni C, Bockaert J, Spengler D, Journot L. Proc Natl Acad Sci USA. 1998;95:8835–40.

Weiss JH, Sensi SL, Koh JY. Trends Pharmacol Sci. 2000;21:395–401.

Yasui N, Nogi T, Kitao T, Nakano Y, Hattori M, Takagi J. Proc Natl Acad Sci USA. 2007;104:9988–93.

Zago MP, Mackenzie GG, Adamo AM, Keen CL, Oteiza PI. Antioxid Redox Signal. 2005;7:1773–82.

Chapter 150
Dietary Copper and the Brain

Helma Antony and Ian G. Macreadie

Abbreviations

Aβ	β-Amyloid Protein
AD	Alzheimer's Disease
AI	Daily Adequate Intake
ALS	Amyotrophic Lateral Sclerosis
APP	Amyloid Precursor Protein
ATP	Adenosine Tri-Phosphate
BACE	Beta-Site APP Cleaving Enzyme
BBB	Blood–Brain–Barrier
BSE	Bovine Spongiform Encephalopathy
CJD	Creutzfeldt-Jacob Disease
CSF	CerebroSpinal Fluid
Cu	Copper
CWD	Chronic Wasting Disease
EC	Enzyme Commission number
ETIC	Endemic Tyrolean Infantile Cirrhosis
Fe	Iron
HD	Huntington Disease
ICC	Indian Childhood Cirrhosis
ICT	Idiopathic Copper Toxicosis
OHS	Occipital Horn Syndrome
PD	Parkinson's Disease
RDA	Recommended Dietary Allowance
ROS	Reactive Oxygen Species
SOD	Superoxide Dismutase
TSE	Transmissible Spongiform Encephalopathy
UL	Daily tolerable Upper intake Level

I.G. Macreadie (✉)
Bio21 Institute, University of Melbourne, 30 Flemington Road, Melbourne, VIC 3010, Australia
e-mail: ian.macreadie@gmail.com

V.R. Preedy et al. (eds.), *Handbook of Behavior, Food and Nutrition*,
DOI 10.1007/978-0-387-92271-3_150, © Springer Science+Business Media, LLC 2011

150.1 Introduction

Copper is essential for life. It is vitally important for the body as it forms a critical component of various fundamental enzymes in the cells. These cuproenzymes (see Table 150.1) are absolutely dependent on copper for its enzymatic activity. At the molecular level, copper is required as a catalytic cofactor or prosthetic group for these metalloenzymes. The cuproenzymes include cytochrome oxidase (EC 1.9.3.1), superoxide dismutase (EC 1.13.11.11), tryptophan-2,3-dioxygenase (EC 1.13.11.11), lysine oxidase (EC 1.4.3.12), monoamine oxidase (EC 1.4.3.4), tyrosinase (EC 1.14.18.1), and dopamine-β-hydroxylase (EC 1.14.17.1).

In humans, these enzymes are required in various organs or sites and indeed some are essential in all cells. Cuproenzymes like cytochrome oxidase are an essential component of cellular respiration and are required in all cells. Other cuproenzymes are involved in iron oxidation, connective tissue formation, nerve cell function, hormone production, and pigmentation (Table 150.1). Cuproenzymes are also important for the synthesis, development and normal functioning of several physiological systems like hemopoietic, cardiovascular, nervous, skeletal, reproductive, and integumentary systems. In addition, copper plays a role as a free metal ion in some nonenzymatic activities like angiogenesis, nerve myelination, and endorphin action.

150.2 Copper in the Diet

Given that copper is essential for normal health, the dietary intake of copper is important. However, increased copper levels in the body can lead to toxicosis resulting in serious consequences (see below). Hence, it is important to consume safe and adequate amounts of copper. The previous recommended dietary allowance (RDA) of 1.5–3.0 mg of copper/day has now been reduced to 0.9 mg/day for adult men and women and 1.0–1.3 mg/day for pregnant and lactating women. For infants up to 1 year old, the daily adequate intake (AI) level is 0.2–0.22 mg/day. To avoid copper toxicity from excessive dietary intake, it is desirable not to exceed the tolerable upper intake level (UL). The UL of copper for adults is 10 mg/day. A comprehensive list of specific AIs, RDAs, and ULs for all ages can be found in Table 150.2 (Klevay 2005).

Table 150.1 Copper-containing proteins (Balamurugan and Schaffner 2006; Zatta and Frank 2007)

Enzymes/Proteins	Function
Cytochrome c oxidase	Energy production (electron transport chain)
Superoxide dismutase (Cu–Zn–SOD)	Protection against free radical damage
Lysyl oxidase	Strengthening connective tissue (cross-linking of collagen and elastin)
Dopamine β mono-oxygenase	Neurotransmission (catecholamine formation)
Peptidyl α amidating mono-oxygenase	Neurotransmission (pituitary peptide hormone maturation)
Amine oxidase	Hormone removal
Mono-oxygenase	Melanin formation
Ascorbate oxidase	Oxidation of ascorbate
Ceruloplasmin	Copper and iron transport (oxidation of Fe^{2+} to Fe^{3+})
Galactose oxidase	Oxidation of primary alcohols to aldehydes
Tyrosinase	Pigmentation (oxidation of phenols)

Enzymes and proteins that require copper and their biological functions are listed

Table 150.2   Dietary copper (Klevay 2005)

Age group	AI	RDA (in mg)	UL (in mg)
Infants			
0–6 months	0.20 mg or 30 µg/kg		
7–12 months	0.22 mg or 24 µg/kg		
Children			
1–3 years		0.34	1.00
4–8 years		0.44	3.00
9–13 years		0.70	5.00
Adolescents			
14–18 years		0.89	8.00
Adults			
19–70 years		0.90	10.00
Pregnant women		1.00	8.00
Lactating mothers		1.30	8.00–10.00

Recommended levels for safe and adequate copper nutrition for the different age groups are listed

AI daily Adequate Intake, *RDA* Recommended Dietary Allowance, *UL* daily tolerable Upper intake Level

150.2.1 Dietary Sources of Copper

Figure 150.1 shows some of the dietary sources of copper. High-copper containing foods such as nuts (0.2–0.5 mg/tablespoon), seeds, seafood – particularly shell fish, lobster, etc. (1.0–3.7 mg/serving), organ meats – like liver (3.8 mg/serving of beef liver) and legumes (0.2 mg/serving) are good dietary sources of copper. Substantial amounts of copper are also present in whole grains, grain products, and chocolates. Other foods like tea, milk, chicken, and potatoes contain low levels of copper. Cooking in copper vessels and drinking water from copper pipes may also offer trace amounts of copper via leaching.

150.2.2 Factors Affecting Copper Nutrition

Adequate copper nutrition also depends on the bioavailability of copper in foods and the influence of other dietary components or nutrient partners. In spite of the higher copper content of vegetarian diets compared to nonvegetarian diet, copper is less efficiently absorbed from a vegetarian diet (Hunt and Vanderpool 2001). Nevertheless, total apparent copper absorption is greater in vegetarians owing to the greater copper content of the vegetarian diet (Hunt and Vanderpool 2001). There are several other factors that affect the intestinal absorption of copper and its bioavailability. Physical and chemical food processing treatments often alter the mineral content of foods (Wapnir 1998). Long-term cooking can reduce the copper content of food considerably. Dietary components like ascorbic acid (vitamin C), zinc, calcium, molybdenum, ferrous iron, stannous tin, etc. are found to reduce copper absorption due to their copper antagonistic, chelating or copper-binding nature; whereas sodium is found to enhance copper absorption (Wapnir 1998). It has also been observed that an increased consumption of saturated and trans fats along with increased copper diet can accelerate brain aging and deteriorate cognitive function (Morris et al. 2006).

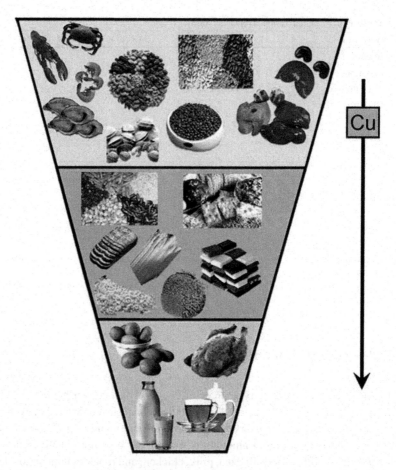

Fig. 150.1 Dietary sources of copper. Copper-containing foods are shown in decreasing order of their copper content. Foods in the upper row are rich in copper, while those in middle row contain substantial amounts of copper. Foods in the bottom row contain low levels of copper

150.3 Physiology of Copper

The physiology of copper involving its dietary intake, absorption, distribution to various tissues, and organs and its excretion is summarized in Fig. 150.2.

150.3.1 Absorption of Copper

Dietary copper uptake has been reviewed by (Linder and Hazegh-Agam 1996). Copper absorption occurs primarily via the brush border cells of the small intestine into interstitial fluid and blood (Linder and Hazegh-Agam 1996), where the copper binds to plasma proteins that carry copper. A small fraction of copper absorbed by the stomach is nutritionally insignificant (Wapnir 1998). Thus the primary site of copper absorption is considered to be the small intestine. At the level of the whole person, it is desirable for copper levels to be neither increased nor decreased. About 4 mg of copper excreted into the bile each day is mostly reabsorbed by the intestines, which in combination with dietary absorption of 0.6–1.5 mg copper, leads to a relatively constant level in the body.

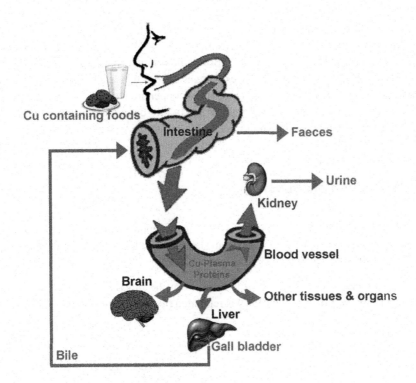

Fig. 150.2 Pathway of copper in the body. The main organs involved in copper uptake, absorption, and excretion are shown

150.3.2 Copper Transport

Copper in blood is transported in a protein-bound form to all tissues and organs (Fig. 150.2). Radiolabeled copper studies have shown that labeled copper disappeared from plasma within 2 h (Weiss and Linder 1985). The plasma-protein carriers of copper are ceruloplasmin, albumin, transcuprein, and some low molecular weight small peptides and amino acids. Of these, ceruloplasmin constitutes the nonexchangeable pool while the rest binds copper in a removable fashion to facilitate easy exchange with tissues.

(i) *Ceruloplasmin* – The major copper binding protein in blood is ceruloplasmin, which is synthesized in the liver where it binds copper. Almost 90% of the serum copper is bound to ceruloplasmin, but it is not utilized for copper transport as the bound copper is in a nonexchangeable form. Ceruloplasmin is a multicopper oxidase that requires copper for its function in the iron transport system. Ceruloplasmin oxidizes Fe^{2+} to Fe^{3+}, which then is bound by transferrin for transport. The equivalent protein in yeast is Fet3, a protein that also functions as a multicopper oxidase (see Table 150.1) (Askwith et al. 1994; de Silva et al. 1997; De Silva et al. 1995; Yuan et al. 1995). People with a total deficiency of ceruloplasmin (aceruloplasminemia) have an iron metabolism disorder and midlife dementia (Harris et al. 1995).

(ii) *Albumin* – Albumin is one of the most abundant plasma proteins. Although albumin can carry ~40 mg copper per litre of blood, it usually carries less than 1% of this amount at a time. Albumin binds copper with high-affinity via three amino acid residues at its N-terminus (Linder 2002).

(iii) *Transcuprein* – Transcuprein is a macroglobulin and is another high-affinity copper carrier found in the serum of mammals, including humans, rats, and dogs (Liu et al. 2007; Hyun and Filippich 2004; Linder 2002; Montaser et al. 1992). Both albumin and transcuprein carries 12% each of the total plasma copper and also rapidly exchanges copper with each other (Linder 2002).

(iv) *Low molecular weight fraction* – Trace amounts of copper are found bound to small peptides and amino acids in blood (Linder 2002). They are less tightly bound and increase copper content in blood directly after a meal (Zatta and Frank 2007).

150.3.3 Distribution of Copper

A healthy man of 70 kg is estimated to contain 110 mg of copper, which is constituted by 10 mg in the liver, 8.8 mg in brain, 6 mg in blood, 26 mg in skeletal muscles, and 46 mg in skeleton and bone marrow (see Fig. 150.3) (Linder et al. 1998).

(i) *Copper in the brain* – Copper enters the brain from the bloodstream as free Cu ions via the blood–brain–barrier (BBB) and the entry is regulated by the blood-CSF barrier (Choi and Zheng

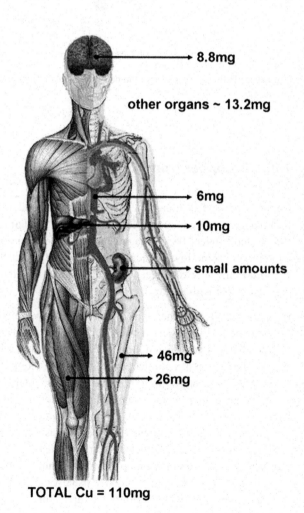

Fig. 150.3 Regional distribution of copper in the human body. Distribution of absorbed copper in different organs of the body is shown. Units are expressed in mg and the amounts are based on a healthy man with a total copper of 110 mg (Source of values: Linder et al. 1998)

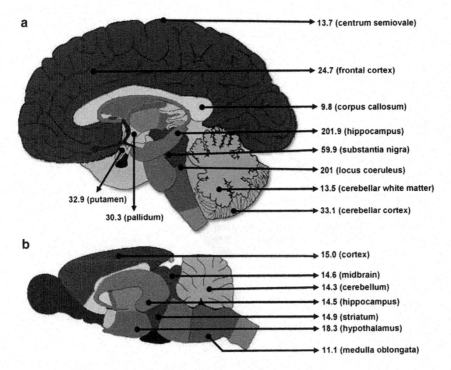

Fig. 150.4 Regional distribution of copper in the brain. Distribution of copper in different regions of (**a**) human brain and (**b**) rat brain are shown. Units are expressed as μg/g dry weight (Source of values: Prohaska 1987)

2009). While the brain contains greater amounts of copper than the blood, the concentration varies between different regions of the brain depending on age, species, environment, and genetics (see Fig. 150.4) (Zatta and Frank 2007). Compared to other animal species, the human brain has the highest copper content (Zatta and Frank 2007). The highest metal ion concentration in the adult human brain is found in substantia nigra, nucleus dentatus, putamen, and nucleus caudatus (reviewed by Speziali and Orvini 2003).

(ii) *Copper in other organs* – Most of the absorbed copper is mainly transported to the liver via enterohepatic circulation and some to the kidneys via systemic circulation. Radiolabelled copper studies show that 40% of the absorbed copper localizes in the liver by 6 h of ingestion (Weiss and Linder 1985). Though only a small amount of copper is taken to the kidneys in normal conditions, excess dietary intake can result in high levels of copper in kidneys and urine.

150.4 Copper in Cells

At the cellular level, much has been learned about the destiny of copper through basic studies of yeast genetics and cell biology. Yeast has been ideal for such studies because it is the best understood eukaryote and because it is readily genetic manipulated. In addition, gene knockouts are available for all yeast genes enabling easy and direct study of their functions. The high-level of similarity and homology between yeast and human genes aids functional identification and also often allows human gene complementation to be achieved. In the case of copper, it appears that both yeast and humans share the same pathway for the destiny of copper (shown in Fig. 150.5). The human proteins involved

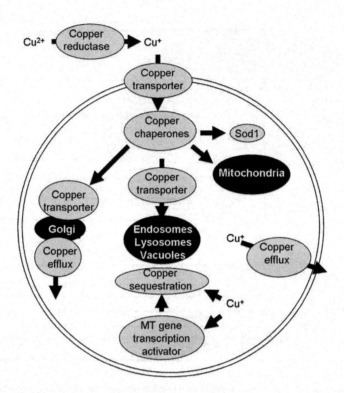

Fig. 150.5 Schematic representation of the cellular destiny of copper in eukaryotes (adapted from Macreadie 2007). The shaded ellipses represent the classes of proteins described in Table 150.3. Exogenous Cu^{2+} is reduced by a copper reductase to Cu^+ which can be transported into the cell by a membrane-spanning copper transporter. Specific chaperones carry Cu^+ to specific locations, including to Sod1, the mitochondrion and the *trans*-Golgi network. Another copper transporter delivers Cu^+ to late endosomes and lysosomes in mammals, or vacuoles in yeast. Efflux pumps and metallothionein remove or sequester excess copper. Levels of metallothionein are tightly controlled at the transcription level by a copper-sensing transcription factor that is itself a copper apothionein

in the intracellular handling of copper and the yeast equivalent proteins are summarized in Table 150.3. Several human diseases involving copper metabolism (e.g., Menkes and Wilson's disease), have also greatly aided in understanding the copper metabolism. The sections below examine copper homeostasis and the fate of copper at the cellular level.

150.4.1 Cellular Copper Homeostasis

Copper homeostasis is critical for the well-being of all organisms. Although copper is essential for the survival of many enzymes and biochemical processes that are dependent on copper for activity, excess free copper can lead to cellular toxicity. Copper toxicity is mainly brought about by the generation of aggressive free radicals via the Fenton reaction catalyzed by copper and the structural disruption of proteins via the ectopic binding of copper (Balamurugan and Schaffner 2006). Hence, all organisms, from bacteria to yeast to humans, possess complex pathways and regulatory mechanisms to control cellular uptake, transport, distribution, detoxification, and efflux of copper in order to maintain cellular homeostasis of copper (further explained below).

Table 150.3 Copper proteins in the cell (Macreadie 2007)

Function	Human proteins	Yeast proteins
Cu reduction	Steap1, Steap2, Steap3, Steap4	Fre1, Fre2
Multicopper oxidase/ Fe transport	Ceruloplasmin, Hephaestin	Fet3
Cu uptake	hCtr1, hCtr2 (late endosomes, lyzosomes)	Ctr1, Ctr3, Ctr2 (vacuoles)
Cu chaperone	Atox1, formerly called Hah1 ($\to$ ATP7A and ATP7B)	Atx1 ($\to$ Ccc2 $\to$ Fet3)
	Ccs1 ($\to$ Sod1)	Ccs1 ($\to$ Sod1)
	Cox17 ($\to$ Sco1 and Cox11)	Cox17 ($\to$ Sco1 $\to$ Cox11)
	Sco1 ($\to$ Cco)	Sco1 ($\to$ Cox2)
	Cox11 ($\to$ Cco)	Cox11 ($\to$ Cox1)
Internal Cu transport/efflux	Atp7A ($\to$ secretory pathway)	Ccc2
	Atp7B ($\to$ ceruloplasmin)	Ccc2
Cu sequestration	Metallothioneins	Metallothioneins
MT transcription factor	Mtf-1	Ace1

Major human and yeast proteins involved in copper homeostasis are listed
The arrows indicate the transfer of copper and its target proteins

150.4.2 Cellular Copper Uptake

The handling of copper in eukaryotic cells is depicted in Fig. 150.5. In the diet, copper occurs in its most oxidized form (Cu^{2+}) and requires reduction by a cell-derived copper reductase (to Cu^+) to enable transport into cells. In yeast the copper transporters, Ctr1 and Ctr2, utilize the same metalloreductase, Fre1 (Rees and Thiele 2007) which is also a ferric reductase. Another ferric reductase, Fre2, appears to have an equivalent role to Fre1. The human counterparts of Fre1, the Steap proteins, function as both cupric and ferric reductases (Ohgami et al. 2006).

The transport of copper through the plasma membrane requires a membrane-localized copper transporter which delivers the Cu^+ to a copper chaperone. In yeast, this transport occurs through a high affinity copper transporter Ctr1 (Dancis et al. 1994a, b). Human equivalents of Ctr1 and hCtr1 were identified by yeast complementation studies (Zhou and Gitschier 1997). Yeast with a defective *ctr1* gene exhibited defects in respiratory growth, iron transport, and Sod1p, all of which were rescued by the human gene, hCtr1. The overproduction of hCtr1 led to copper overload (Zhou and Gitschier 1997). A similarity search of the human proteome identified additional gene, hCtr2 (Zhou and Gitschier 1997), that is expressed in late endosomes and lyzosomes where it facilitates cellular copper uptake (van den Berghe et al. 2007). An equivalent copper transporter in yeast, Ctr2, is found exclusively on the vacuolar membrane where it controls vacuolar copper levels (Kampfenkel et al. 1995; Rees et al. 2004). It appears that Ctr2 is a nonessential vacuolar copper transporter (Portnoy et al. 2001).

150.4.3 Metallochaperones for Copper Trafficking

Unlike chaperones, metallochaperones (e.g., copper chaperones) do not facilitate protein folding. Instead, they protect the cell by binding copper with high affinity and deliver it to specific target proteins within the cell. Each copper chaperone is highly specific for its ultimate destination. Functional identification of the copper chaperones, or metallochaperones, was first made in yeast. Later studies indicated that copper chaperones were conserved from yeast to humans as three functional groups depending on their ultimate destination (reviewed by Balamurugan and Schaffner

2006). Ccs1 chaperones copper to the eukaryotic antioxidant enzyme, Cu/Zn superoxide dismutase (Sod1) in the cytosol (Culotta et al. 1997); while three copper chaperones, Cox17, Cox11 and Sco1, works together to deliver copper to cytochrome *c* oxidase (Cco) in the mitochondria (Glerum et al. 1996; Amaravadi et al. 1997; Horng et al. 2004). Atx1 is the chaperone responsible for delivering copper to the secretory pathway for cuproenzymes at the cell surface or for release (Klomp et al. 1997; Lin et al. 1997; Pufahl et al. 1997). In the Golgi, the copper from Atx1 is utilized by the copper-transporting ATPases, ATP7A and ATP7B in humans and Ccc2 in yeast. Though only yeast chaperones have been mainly cited above, the human homologs of these chaperones are described in Table 150.3.

150.4.4 Internal Copper Efflux

Internal copper efflux is accomplished by ATP-dependent transporters of the ATP7 family, also known as P-type ATPases. Insights on cellular copper efflux in humans are mainly derived from studies of Menkes disease and Wilson's disease, the two major genetically-inherited disorders of copper homeostasis (further detailed under "copper-associated diseases" below). Human cells contain two isoforms of ATPases: ATP7A (or MNK transporter) that is expressed in the mucosal cells of intestinal epithelium and most other tissues other than liver, and ATP7B (or WND transporter) which is primarily expressed in liver and certain areas of the brain (Linder 2002; Balamurugan and Schaffner 2006). Both ATPases contain six copper binding sites at the N-terminus (Zatta and Frank 2007) and are functionally stimulated by copper for trafficking (Balamurugan and Schaffner 2006). At normal or low copper, ATP7A delivers intracellular copper to enzymes in the *trans*-Golgi network (Yamaguchi-Iwai et al. 1996) but at high copper levels, ATP7A moves to the plasma membrane to perform copper efflux (Petris et al. 1996). ATP7A also plays an important role in systemic copper absorption, reabsorption of copper in kidneys and adequate copper supply to the brain (reviewed by Balamurugan and Schaffner 2006). ATP7B is functionally related to ATP7A and they also share 54% sequence similarity. At normal or low copper, ATP7B is found only in the liver where it delivers intracellular copper to apoceruloplasmin in the *trans*-Golgi network (Yamaguchi-Iwai et al. 1996); but at high copper levels, ATP7B moves copper to vesicles for delivery to the biliary caniliculus, performing copper efflux into the bile for excretion (Petris et al. 1996). Yeast cells have an equivalent pump, Ccc2, which facilitates cation transport, including copper (Yuan et al. 1995). Ccc2 is also an ATPase and it translocates copper into the trans-Golgi vesicles, where copper is then packed into the multicopper containing protein ferroxidase Fet3 (Arnesano et al. 2001).

150.4.5 Copper Sequestration and Detoxification

Since excess and free copper are toxic to cells, it is imperative that cellular mechanisms exist to sequester free intracellular copper. Healthy yeast cells maintain free copper levels at less than one free copper ion per cell (Rae et al. 1999).

Metallothioneins (also known as copper scavengers) are the cellular copper binding proteins that provide significant protection against elevated copper levels. Yeast metallothionein (Karin et al. 1984; Winge et al. 1985) is highly regulated by Ace1, a constitutively produced transcriptional activator of the yeast metallothionein gene (Buchman et al. 1989; Szczypka and Thiele

1989). In the presence of copper, Ace1 binds copper and activates transcription. In the converse situation of copper starvation, another yeast transcription factor, Mac1 acts as an intramolecular autoinhibitory domain. In human cells, heavy metal load and copper excess is handled by the transcription factor, MTF1. MTF1 is the functional analog of yeast Ace1; but they are neither related to each other nor similar in their binding sites (reviewed by Balamurugan and Schaffner 2006). In the absence of metallothionein, superoxide dismutase (SOD) plays a major protective role against copper toxicity. It is significant that some cases of amyotrophic lateral sclerosis (ALS) have defects in Cu–Zn SOD, suggesting some linkage between this form of motor neurone disease and copper metabolism. Despite the capacity of metallothioneins to store copper, they cannot perform copper efflux. For pumping out excess copper, cells depend on the afore-mentioned ATPases.

150.5 Copper-Associated Diseases

Deficient or excess copper can lead to serious disorders in many organs of the body, including brain. Depending on the origin, human disorders associated with copper can be classified into three: hereditary, chronic deficiency, and overload.

150.5.1 Hereditary Copper Diseases

Menkes disease and Wilson's disease are the two major genetically-inherited disorders of copper homeostasis resulting from mutations in the copper transporters, ATP7A (MNK transporter) and ATP7B (WND transporter) respectively. Menkes disease, an X-linked recessive disorder, is effectively a copper deficiency disease that presents with growth failure, skeletal defects, degeneration of the central nervous system, and early death (Danks 1995). Contradictorily, despite the copper deficiency in Menkes disease, the kidneys and intestinal epithelial cells in affected individuals accumulate copper, owing to the defect in copper efflux (Mercer 2001). On the other hand, Wilson's disease, an autosomal recessive disorder, is effectively a copper toxicosis disease that presents with copper accumulation in the liver and brain, leading to liver cirrhosis and neurological problems including behavioral disturbances and movement disorders. Menkes and Wilson's disease are similar in that they utilize a similar pump, but they use it in different tissues. The MNK transporter (ATP7A) is also known to be involved in placental copper transfer. Hence, abnormal gestational development and copper-deficient phenotype in fetus and newborn is observed in Menkes disease (Linder 2002). In contrast, Wilson's disease occurs only gradually after birth. Occipital Horn Syndrome (OHS), an X-linked connective tissue disorder, is a mild variant of Menkes disease caused by mutations in the Menkes gene ATP7A and presents with mild neurological disease (Mercer 2001). Another hereditary copper-associated disease is aceruloplasminemia which is caused by mutations in the ceruloplasmin gene, but it manifests as an iron accumulation disorder and does not affect copper metabolism probably due to the presence of other plasma-protein carriers for copper (Mercer 2001; Linder 2002).

Menkes disease can be treated by administering copper histidine, but success rates depend on residual Menkes protein activity. In Wilsons's diseases, treatment by Cu-chelation therapy or use of oral zinc (to reduce copper absorption from diet) is promising if disease is diagnosed prior to irreversible tissue damage (Mercer 2001).

150.5.2 Copper Deficiency Diseases

Clinical copper deficiency is rare in adults (Mercer 2001), but it can occur due to genetic predisposition, malnutrition, marginal intake of copper, reduced bioavailability (caused by excess consumption of zinc, molybdenum, chelating agents, compounds that interfere with copper absorption, etc.), patients with gastrointestinal disorders or surgical treatment such as removal/bypass of a large portion of intestine, peritoneal dialysis, etc. (Zatta and Frank 2007). At the molecular level, copper deficiency reduces the activity of SOD and other components of the oxidant defense system resulting in increased lipid peroxidation and oxidative damage to DNA and proteins (Uriu-Adams and Keen 2005). Deficiency of copper also affects the function of cuproenzymes, thereby leading to anemia, neutropenia, changes in ossification, and elevated plasma cholesterol (Zatta and Frank 2007). Severe cases display seizures. In the brain, deficiency of bioavailable copper plays a major role in the pathogenesis of many neurodegenerative diseases like Prion disease, Alzheimer's disease (AD), Huntington disease (HD), Parkinson's disease (PD), etc. (further explained in "role of copper in neurological diseases" below).

150.5.3 Copper Toxicosis

As mentioned earlier, increased amounts of copper can cause excessive oxidative stress and significant tissue damage. The oxidative stress is a consequence of the redox reactivity of copper via the Fenton reaction, i.e. production of free radicals by catalysing the reaction between superoxide anion and hydrogen peroxide. Tissue damage is caused by the structural disruption of proteins by copper and also as a result of oxidative stress (Uriu-Adams and Keen 2005). Copper toxicosis can occur as a result of copper poisoning, increased dietary intake or genetic defects. Copper poisoning reports indicate instances of accidental or deliberate ingestion of beverages contaminated with copper. Symptoms in these cases progress from abdominal pain, nausea, vomiting, headache, lethargy and diarrhea to tachycardia, respiratory difficulties, hemolytic anemia, gastrointestinal bleeding, liver and kidney failure, finally resulting in death (Hyun and Filippich 2004). Genetic copper toxicity disorders include Wilson's disease, Idiopathic copper toxicosis (ICT), Indian childhood cirrhosis (ICC), and endemic Tyrolean infantile cirrhosis (ETIC), all of which have an autosomal recessive mode of inheritance (Mercer 2001; Hyun and Filippich 2004; Balamurugan and Schaffner 2006). ICT, ICC, and ETIC are all fatal hepatic diseases. Copper contaminated milk feeds have been implicated in ICC and ETIC (Hyun and Filippich 2004; Balamurugan and Schaffner 2006). Copper toxicosis also contributes toward some neurodegenerative diseases like ALS and Creutzfeldt-Jakob disease (CJD) (Uriu-Adams and Keen 2005). In liver, copper accumulation can also occur as a consequence of chronic cholestatic liver diseases like primary biliary cirrhosis and chronic hepatitis.

150.5.4 Other Diseases Associated with Copper

Although metallic copper is insoluble, inhalation of copper dust from industrial processes can cause "copper fever" that presents with sweetish taste in mouth, dry throat, burning eyes, followed by severe headache, leukocytosis, fatigue, and catarrhic symptoms (Balamurugan and Schaffner 2006). Altered copper metabolism has also been reported in inflammation, infection, and cancer (reviewed by Linder 2002).

Key Points of Copper

- A number of essential enzymes in the cell require copper for their normal function.
- Copper is a trace element that is essential for life.
- Too little or too much is bad, but exquisite handling at the level of the cell and organs, ensures the desired homeostasis.
- We require less than 1 mg of copper per day.

150.6 Copper and the Brain

Copper contributes positively to brain development and function. Besides cytochrome c oxidase, which is essential for energy generation in brain, copper is utilized by dopamine β mono-oxygenase and peptidyl α amidating mono-oxygenase, both of which are important for the biosynthesis of neurotransmitters. Transport of copper across the BBB and distribution within the brain is regulated by ATP7A, the mutation of which leads to severe deficiency of copper in the brain. Bioavailability of copper is also important for normal functioning of the brain. While chronically high or low copper levels lead to major abnormalities such as Menkes or Wilson's disease, some evidence suggest that even more subtle changes in copper homeostasis have an impact on the brain, leading to some of the major late onset neurological diseases. However, more work is required to decipher the exact mechanisms of these relationships.

150.6.1 Role of Copper in Neurological Diseases

PD is the second most common neurodegenerative disorder after Alzheimer's disease, affecting both men and women over 50. PD is characterized by abnormalities of movement, such as tremor, muscular rigidity, and postural instability brought about by the degeneration of neurons in a region of the brain that controls movement. Copper affects the oligomerization of α-synuclein (Paik et al. 1999), a key protein implicated in PD. Furthermore, dopamine that is strongly associated with PD may become more toxic when it interacts with copper (Paris et al. 2001; Snyder and Friedman 1998; Spencer et al. 1994).

Prions are infectious protein particles involved in transmissible spongiform encephalopathies (TSEs), which includes CJD, scrapie, chronic wasting disease (CWD), and bovine spongiform encephalopathy (BSE). These fatal neurodegenerative diseases are caused by the misfolding of cellular prion protein PrP^c to the infective disease causing isoform, PrP^{sc}. Brain copper has been reported to be low in TSEs (reviewed by Legleiter et al. 2007). Furthermore, some studies indicate that human prions have copper binding sites (Brown et al. 1997; Hornshaw et al. 1995). It is speculated that the binding of copper to PrP^c may serve to stabilize the protein and allow normal function (Legleiter et al. 2007). However, this requires further research.

ALS is a progressive neurodegenerative disease that affects upper and lower motor neurons resulting in muscle weakness and atrophy. Death due to respiratory failure occurs within a short time from the onset of symptoms. The familial form of ALS is found to have a mutation in Cu–Zn SOD gene. Though one group has reported severe copper depletion of spinal cord in copper-deficient SOD, contradictory results have been reported by others (reviewed by Zatta and Frank 2007). Hence, further investigation is warranted to understand the molecular mechanism.

HD is another progressive neurodegenerative disease characterized by glutamine expansion within the N-terminus of huntingtin protein. Affected individuals undergo progressive motor, cognitive, and psychiatric deterioration. HD brain has shown an accumulation of copper and iron in the striatum (Dexter et al. 1991). Recent studies indicate a pro-oxidant interaction between copper and huntington protein (Fox et al. 2007).

150.6.2 Copper and Alzheimer's Disease

AD is a fatal and highly debilitating progressive mental disorder that generally affects people over 65 or as young as 40–50 years. It is the most prevalent form of dementia and is characterized by severe cognitive impairment due to degeneration of brain cells that handle speech, memory, and thought. The most important protein implicated in AD is the Alzheimer's Precursor Protein (APP) from which the Aβ peptide, or β-amyloid is derived. APP has two copper binding sites, including one in the Aβ peptide sequence (Atwood et al. 1998; Hesse et al. 1994). In transgenic mice, the overexpression of APP appeared to reduce levels of copper in brains (Bayer et al. 2003; Maynard et al. 2002; Phinney et al. 2003) suggestive of APP being a copper transporter (White et al. 1998). Although APP has no yeast equivalent, it performed copper efflux in yeast (Treiber et al. 2004) as it does in brains. Two other proteins, Aplp1 and Aplp2, may also perform copper efflux since they have copper binding domains and structural similarity (Hesse et al. 1994; White et al. 1998, 1999a, b).

APP is unique among the APP/Aplp1/Aplp2 family because it is cleaved by the BACE protease (Vassar et al. 1999) and γ secretase protease to produce Aβ. Aβ exhibits neurotoxicity and is a major component of the extracellular Aβ plaques associated with AD. The extracellular plaques are a reservoir for a number of metals, including copper, and it is has been considered that the copper in these plaques may be available for the production of reactive oxygen species (ROS) which could cause neuronal loss and brain damage (Bush 2000). However, in view of the overall decline in copper levels as brains age, the alternate possibility of a build up of Aβ causing a copper shortfall, should also be considered.

150.6.3 Manipulation of Brain Copper Levels

The possibility of manipulating neuronal copper levels may lead to rational approaches to the treatment of neurological diseases. Clioquinol, a metal chelating compound, and some related compounds represent some of the most promising drugs that have been trialled to date. Clioquinol reduces plaque in mouse AD models and it appears to alter copper levels (Cherny et al. 2001). In a treatment of APP 750[SL] transgenic mice, clioquinol was shown to improve survival (Schafer et al. 2007). While clioquinol reduced serum copper levels from around 800 to around 500 µg/l, even with added copper in the diet, brain copper significantly increased, from 3.9 to 4.2 µg/g with added dietary copper. The treated mice also exhibited normal survival and improved memory, suggesting that clioquinol enabled brain copper levels to increase, and this in turn gave the positive benefit. Clioquinol also increased copper levels in yeast producing APP (Treiber et al. 2004).

Interesting results from Sparks and Schreurs show that in cholesterol-fed rabbits, increased copper led to increased deposits of Alzheimer's Aβ brain plaque (Sparks and Schreurs 2003). Plaques were induced at levels of 0.12 ppm copper in drinking water (much lower than the levels of 1.3 ppm permitted by water supply agencies). We suggest that conversely, lower cholesterol levels could lead to lower copper levels, reducing Aβ plaques. Interestingly the statins, blockbuster cholesterol-lowering drugs, appear to be the best drug to lower the incidence of AD. One particular statin, simvastatin, is unique with respect to reducing AD (Wolozin et al. 2007). Unlike many other statins, simvastatin is lipophilic and crosses the blood–brain–barrier (BBB), so it may be expected that simvastatin would reduce cholesterol synthesis in the brain.

Finally, vaccine approaches may have some merit in animal models of AD by clearing Aβ plaque. Whether this affects brain copper has not been considered but presumably metals associated with the plaque would be removed along with plaque.

It is clear that much is now known about copper homeostasis, but there is still some way to go before we conquer neurological diseases that involve copper. It is likely that an increased understanding of copper homeostasis may help in unravelling the many important neurological diseases involving copper metabolism.

Key Points of Copper in Brain

- Copper contributes positively to brain development and function.
- Most of the major neurological disorders are due to the disruption of copper homeostasis caused by abnormal copper interactions or irregular copper metabolism.
- Manipulation of brain copper levels with compounds like clioquinol or statins could be a rational solution.

150.7 Applications to Other Areas of Health and Disease

The importance of copper in nutrition and copper homeostasis has been emphasized in this chapter. This knowledge has implications for the animal husbandry, crop management, biological control strategies, and possibly the treatment of human diseases. For example, upsetting the copper homeostasis by increasing copper levels is a strategy in antifungal control in agriculture, where copper sulphate can be applied to prevent the growth of mould, mildew, and rust fungus in crops. Likewise copper sulphate performs effectively as an algaecide in domestic swimming pools. The converse strategy, lowering copper levels, may also be a strategy to consider for impeding cell growth. Specific copper chelators such as bathocuproine sulphate can effectively inhibit the growth of cells.

Copper-deficiency in soils may also adversely affect agricultural outputs. In Australia, copper deficient soils were associated with lower wool yields in sheep. Recognizing the deficiency of copper and other trace elements in many soils have led to remedial practices such as the use of salt licks.

Detailed knowledge of copper homeostasis also provides the insights required in engineering super microbes that may help in bioremediation. For example, copper is a significant pollutant at mining sites and its removal requires novel strategies such as organisms that have increased ability to sequester copper. Metallothioneins are not limited to copper sequestration; they can sequester other metals as well.

Potentially copper homeostasis could also be altered to control cell proliferative diseases; however, lack of specificity is likely to be an issue.

Summary Points

- Copper is essential for all cells. Depletion of copper leads to loss of growth and survival.
- Copper is a cofactor for a number of cuproenzymes involved in diverse reactions.
- Excess copper can be toxic. Thus all biological systems have complex mechanisms to maintain correct copper levels.

- The fate of copper, its roles, and its biological functions has been strongly supported by studies in yeast.
- The brain may be very sensitive to copper levels which change with aging.
- Copper is a significant factor in neurodegenerative diseases, including Alzheimer's Disease.

Definitions and Explanations

Bioavailability: The amount of substance that is absorbed by the body and becomes available at the site of biological activity.

Blood–brain–barrier: A membrane barrier that separates many compounds from the brain, including various drugs, biochemicals, and macromolecules.

Copper Efflux: Outward flow of copper from the cell in the event of excess copper.

Cuproenzymes: Enzymes that require copper for their normal function.

Homeostasis: The maintenance of a constant state. Cells require homeostasis for survival, as well as for growth.

Statins: The world's largest selling prescription drugs. Although prescribed for lowering cholesterol levels they also lower the incidence of AD and PD.

Yeast studies: The yeast Saccharomyces cerevisiae is a model organism for human studies. Resources pertaining to the yeast genome can be found at www.yeastgenome.org.

References

Amaravadi R, Glerum DM, Tzagoloff A. Hum Genet. 1997;99:329–33.

Arnesano F, Banci I, Bertini F, Cantini F, Ciofi-Baffoni S, Huffman DL, O'Halloran TV. J Biol Chem. 2001;276:41365–76.

Askwith C, Eide D, Van Ho A, Bernard PS, Li L, Davis-Kaplan S, Sipe DM, Kaplan J. Cell. 1994;76:403–10.

Atwood CS, Moir RD, Huang X, Scarpa RC, Bacarra NM, Romano DM, Hartshorn MA, Tanzi RE, Bush AI. J Biol Chem. 1998;273:12817–26.

Balamurugan K, Schaffner W. Biochim Biophys Acta. 2006;1763:737–46.

Bayer TA, Schafer S, Simons A, Kemmling A, Kamer T, Tepest R, Eckert A, Schussel K, Eikenberg O, Sturchler-Pierrat C, Abramowski D, Staufenbiel M, Multhaup G. Proc Natl Acad Sci USA. 2003;100:14187–92.

Brown DR, Qin K, Herms JW, Madlung A, Manson J, Strome R, Fraser PE, Kruck T, von Bohlen A, Schulz-Schaeffer W, Giese A, Westaway D, Kretzschmar H. Nature. 1997;390:684–7

Buchman C, Skroch P, Welch J, Fogel S, Karin M. Mol Cell Biol. 1989;9:4091–5.

Bush AI. Curr Opin Chem Biol. 2000;4:184–91.

Cherny RA, Atwood CS, Xilinas ME, Gray DN, Jones WD, McLean CA, Barnham KJ, Volitakis I, Fraser FW, Kim Y, Huang X, Goldstein LE, Moir RD, Lim JT, Beyreuther K, Zheng H, Tanzi RE, Masters CL, Bush AI. Neuron. 2001;30:665–76.

Choi BS, Zheng W. Brain Res. 2009;1248:14–21.

Culotta VC, Klomp LW, Strain J, Casareno RL, Krems B, Gitlin JD. J Biol Chem. 1997;272:23469–72.

Danks DM. In: Scriver CR, Beaudet AL, Sly WM, Valle D, editors. The metabolic and molecular basis of inherited disease. McGraw-Hill: New York; 1995. pp. 2211–35.

Dancis A, Haile D, Yuan DS, Klausner RD. J Biol Chem. 1994a;269:25660–7.

Dancis A, Yuan DS, Haile D, Askwith C, Eide D, Moehle C, Kaplan J, Klausner RD. Cell. 1994b;76:393–402.

de Silva D, Davis-Kaplan S, Fergestad J, Kaplan J. J Biol Chem. 1997;272:14208–13.

De Silva DM, Askwith CC, Eide D, Kaplan J. J Biol Chem. 1995;270:1098–101.

Dexter DT, Carayon A, Javoy-Agid F, Agid Y, Wells FR, Daniel SE, Lees AJ, Jenner P, Marsden CD. Brain. 1991;114:1953–75.

Fox JH, Kama JA, Lieberman G, Chopra R, Dorsey K, Chopra V, Volitakis I, Cherny RA, Bush AI, Hersch S. PloS One. 2007;2:e334 1–12.

Glerum DM, Shtanko A, Tzagoloff A. J Biol Chem. 1996;271:14504–9.

Harris ZL, Takahashi Y, Miyajima H, Serizawa M, MacGillivray RT, Gitlin JD. Proc Natl Acad Sci USA. 1995;92:2539–43.

Hesse L, Beher D, Masters CL, Multhaup G. FEBS Lett. 1994;349:109–16.

Horng YC, Cobine PA, Maxfield AB, Carr HS, Winge DR. J Biol Chem. 2004;279:35334–40.

Hornshaw MP, McDermott JR, Candy JM. Biochem Biophys Res Commun. 1995;207:621–9.

Hunt JR, Vanderpool RA. Am J Clin Nutr. 2001;74:803–7.

Hyun C, Filippich LJ. J Exp Anim Sci. 2004;43:39–64.

Kampfenkel K, Kushnir S, Babiychuk E, Inze D, Van Montagu M. J Biol Chem. 1995;270:28479–86.

Karin M, Najarian R, Haslinger A, Valenzuela P, Welch J, Fogel S. Proc Natl Acad Sci USA. 1984;81:337–41.

Klevay LM. In: Coates PM, Blackman MR, Cragg GM, Levine M, Moss J, White JD, editors. Encyclopedia of dietary supplements. Marcel Dekker: USA; 2005. pp. 133–41.

Klomp LW, Lin SJ, Yuan DS, Klausner RD, Culotta VC, Gitlin JD. J Biol Chem. 1997;272:9221–6.

Legleiter LR, Ahola JK, Engle TE, Spears JW. Biochem Biophys Res Commun. 2007;352:884–8.

Lin SJ, Pufahl RA, Dancis A, O'Halloran TV, Culotta VC. J Biol Chem. 1997;272:9215–20.

Linder MC. In: Massaro EJ, editor. Handbook of copper pharmacology and toxicology. Humana Press: New Jersey; 2002. pp. 3–32.

Linder MC, Hazegh-Agam M. Am J Clin Nutr. 1996;63:797S–811S.

Linder MC, Wooten L, Cerveza P, Cotton S, Shulze S, Lomeli N. Am J Clin Nutr. 1998;67:965S–71S.

Liu N, Lo LS, Askary SH, Jones L, Kidane TZ, Trang T, Nguyen M, Goforth J, Chu YH, Vivas E, Tsai M, Westbrook T, Linder MC. J Nutr Biochem. 2007;18:597–608.

Macreadie IG. Eur Biophys J. 2007;37:295–300.

Maynard CJ, Cappai R, Volitakis I, Cherny RA, White AR, Beyreuther K, Masters CL, Bush AI, Li QX. J Biol Chem. 2002;277:44670–76.

Mercer JFB. Trends Mol Med. 2001;7:64–9.

Montaser A, Tetreault C, Linder M. PSEBM. 1992;200:321–9.

Morris MC, Evans DA, Tangney CC, Bienias JL, Schneider JA, Wilson RS, Scherr PA. Arch Neurol. 2006;63:1085–8.

Ohgami RS, Campagna DR, McDonald A, Fleming MD. Blood. 2006;108:1388–94.

Paik SR, Shin HJ, Lee JH, Chang CS, Kim J. Biochem J. 1999;340:821–8.

Paris I, Dagnino-Subiabre A, Marcelain K, Bennett LB, Caviedes P, Caviedes R, Azar CO, Segura-Aguilar J. J Neurochem. 2001;77:519–29.

Petris MJ, Mercer JF, Culvenor JG, Lockhart P, Gleeson PA, Camakaris J. EMBO J. 1996;15:6084–95.

Phinney AL, Drisaldi B, Schmidt SD, Lugowski S, Coronado V, Liang Y, Horne P, Yang J, Sekoulidis J, Coomaraswamy J, Chishti MA, Cox DW, Mathews PM, Nixon RA, Carlson GA, St George-Hyslop P, Westaway D. Proc Natl Acad Sci USA. 2003;100:14193–8.

Portnoy ME, Schmidt PJ, Rogers RS, Culotta VC. Mol Genet Genomics. 2001;265:873–82.

Prohaska JR. Physiol Rev. 1987;67:858–901.

Pufahl RA, Singer CP, Peariso KL, Lin SJ, Schmidt PJ, Fahrni CJ, Culotta VC, Penner-Hahn JE, O'Halloran TV. Science. 1997;278:853–6.

Rae TD, Schmidt PJ, Pufahl RA, Culotta VC, O'Halloran TV. Science. 1999;284:805–8.

Rees EM, Thiele DJ. J Biol Chem. 2007;282:21629–38.

Rees EM, Lee J, Thiele DJ. J Biol Chem. 2004;279:54221–9.

Schafer S, Pajonk FG, Multhaup G, Bayer TA. J Mol Med. 2007;85:405–13.

Snyder RD, Friedman MB. Mutat Res. 1998;405:1–8.

Sparks DL, Schreurs BG. Proc Natl Acad Sci USA. 2003;100:11065–9.

Spencer JP, Jenner A, Aruoma OI, Evans PJ, Kaur H, Dexter DT, Jenner P, Lees AJ, Marsden DC, Halliwell B. FEBS Lett. 1994;353:246–50.

Speziali M, Orvini E. In: Zatta P, editor. Metal ions and neurodegenerative disorders. World Sci: London; 2003. pp. 15–65.

Szczypka MS, Thiele DJ. Mol Cell Biol. 1989;9:421–9.

Treiber C, Simons A, Strauss M, Hafner M, Cappai R, Bayer TA, Multhaup G. J Biol Chem. 2004;279:51958–64.

Uriu-Adams JY, Keen CL. Mol Aspect Med. 2005;26:268–98.

van den Berghe PV, Folmer DE, Malingre HE, van Beurden E, Klomp AE, van de Sluis B, Merkx M, Berger R, Klomp LW. Biochem J. 2007;407:49–59.

Vassar R, Bennett BD, Babu-Khan S, Kahn S, Mendiaz EA, Denis P, Teplow DB, Ross S, Amarante P, Loeloff R, Luo Y, Fisher S, Fuller J, Edenson S, Lile J, Jarosinski MA, Biere AL, Curran E, Burgess T, Louis JC, Collins F, Treanor J, Rogers G, Citron M. Science. 1999;286:735–41.

Wapnir RA. Am J Clin Nutr. 1998;67:1054S–60S.

Weiss KC, Linder MC. Am J Physiol. 1985;249:E77–E88.

White AR, Zheng H, Galatis D, Maher F, Hesse L, Multhaup G, Beyreuther K, Masters CL, Cappai R. J Neurosci. 1998;18:6207–17.

White AR, Multhaup G, Maher F, Bellingham S, Camakaris J, Zheng H, Bush AI, Beyreuther K, Masters CL, Cappai R. J Neurosci. 1999a;19:9170–9.

White AR, Reyes R, Mercer JF, Camakaris J, Zheng H, Bush AI, Multhaup G, Beyreuther K, Masters CL, Cappai R. Brain Res. 1999b;842:439–44.

Winge DR, Nielson KB, Gray WR, Hamer DH. J Biol Chem. 1985;260:14464–70.

Wolozin B, Wang SW, Li N-C, Lee A, Lee TA, Kazis LE. BMC Med. 2007;5:20 doi:10.1186/1741-7015-5-20.

Yamaguchi-Iwai Y, Stearman R, Dancis A, Klausner RD. EMBO J. 1996;15:3377–84.

Yuan DS, Stearman R, Dancis A, Dunn T, Beeler T, Klausner RD. Proc Natl Acad Sci USA. 1995;92:2632–6.

Zatta P, Frank A. Brain Res Rev. 2007;54:19–33.

Zhou B, Gitschier J. Proc Natl Acad Sci USA. 1997;94:7481–6.

Chapter 151
Fetal–Neonatal Iron Deficiency Affects Neurotrophic Factor Expression, Neural Differentiation, and Neuroplasticity in the Rat Hippocampus

Michael K. Georgieff and Phu V. Tran

Abbreviations

BDNF	Brain-Derived Neurotrophic Factor
CNTF	Ciliary Neurotrophic Factor
Dcx	Doublecortin
Dusp4	Dual Specificity Phosphatase 4
Egr1 and 2	Early-Growth-Response-Gene 1 and 2
EGF	Epidermal Growth Factor
ERK1 and 2	Extracellular-Signal Regulated Kinase 1 and 2
FID	Formerly Iron-Deficient
GDNF	Glial-Derived Neurotrophic Factor
Hif1α	Hypoxia Inducible Factor 1α
HMGCR	3-Hydroxy-3-Methylglutaryl Coenzyme A Reductase
ID	Iron-Deficient
IS	Iron-Sufficient
LTP	Long-Term Potentiation
Mbp	Myelin Basic Protein
mTOR	Mammalian Target of Rapamycin
NGF	Nerve Growth Factor
p75^{NTR}	Neurotrophic Receptor p75
P	Postnatal Day
PARV	Parvalbumin
qPCR	Quantitative RT-PCR
TrkB	Tyrosine-Receptor Kinase B
TUNEL	TdT-Mediated biotin-dUTP Nick End Labeling

M.K. Georgieff (✉)
Department of Pediatrics, Neonatology Division & Center for Neurobehavioral
Development, School of Medicine, University of Minnesota, 420 Delaware St. SE,
MMC 39 (for mail), D-136 Mayo Building (for courier), Minneapolis, MN 55455, USA
e-mail: georg001@umn.edu

V.R. Preedy et al. (eds.), *Handbook of Behavior, Food and Nutrition*,
DOI 10.1007/978-0-387-92271-3_151, © Springer Science+Business Media, LLC 2011

151.1 Introduction

151.1.1 Fetal and Neonatal Iron Deficiency Impairs Cognitive Development

Iron deficiency is one of the foremost early-life micronutrient deficiencies, affecting approximately 30–50% of preschool age children and pregnant women worldwide (WHO 2008). Late gestational and neonatal (perinatal) iron deficiency arises from four common maternal gestational conditions: severe iron deficiency anemia (IDA), placental vascular insufficiency resulting from maternal hypertension, diabetes mellitus, and cigarette smoking (Chockalingam et al. 1987; Petry et al. 1992; Sweet et al. 2001). The adverse neurobehavioral effects of early-life iron deficiency in humans and animal models are considerable and long-lasting (Lozoff and Georgieff 2006). For example, iron-deficient (ID) human newborns exhibit deficits in cognitive development that last beyond the period of iron deficiency (Nelson et al. 2000; Siddappa et al. 2004; Riggins et al. 2009). While certain developmental deficits recover with iron treatment, cognitive deficits following neonatal and early postnatal iron deficiency in humans persist up to 10 years after iron treatment (Tamura et al. 2002; Lozoff et al. 2006). Fetal and neonatal ID rodents and monkeys showed similar adverse neurobehavioral effects (Golub et al. 2006; Felt et al. 2006; Schmidt et al. 2007). The potential neural basis of these cognitive deficits continues to be an active research area; however, these effects imply an impaired hippocampus, a brain region responsible for learning and memory.

151.1.2 Fetal–Neonatal Iron Deficiency Alters Hippocampal Structure, Function, and Gene Expression in the Rat Model

In rats, fetal–neonatal iron deficiency resulted in abnormal hippocampal CA1 dendritic structure, impaired synaptic transmission, and increased susceptibility to deleterious infarction (Jorgenson et al. 2003, 2005; Rao et al., 2007). These findings support the hypothesis of an abnormal hippocampus in ID rats. The possibility of early-life ID leading to dysregulation of genes necessary for proper hippocampal development was investigated with a microarray mRNA profiling analysis (Carlson et al. 2007). This work identified alterations in salient molecular pathways involved in neuronal differentiation with most notably the Alzheimer-related gene network centered on amyloid precursor protein and the mammalian target of rapamycin (mTOR) pathway (Carlson et al. 2007, 2008). The amyloid precursor protein gene network has been implicated in cytoskeletal remodeling, cell motility and growth cone formation during hippocampal development (Guenette et al. 2006; Ikin et al. 2007). The mTOR pathway integrates external stimuli such as nutrients and growth factors and gene expression necessary for the synaptic maturation and plasticity in the hippocampus (Tang et al. 2002; Schratt et al. 2004).

151.1.3 Neurotrophic Factors Mediate Hippocampal Development and Function

Neurotrophic factors such as nerve growth factor (NGF) and brain-derived neurotrophic factor (BDNF) regulate multiple aspects of neuronal differentiation and plasticity in the hippocampus (Hennigan et al. 2007). Fetal and neonatal environments affect the expression of these neurotrophic factors. For example, an enriched environment has beneficial effects on hippocampal function and is accompanied by increased NGF and BDNF levels, whereas an adverse environment impairs memory function and lowers NGF and BDNF expression (Pham et al. 2002; Branchi et al. 2004). In addition, neural activity such as induction of long-term potentiation (LTP), a cellular phenomenon associated with memory formation, in the rodent hippocampus rapidly increases NGF and BDNF mRNA levels (Patterson et al. 1992; McAllister et al. 1999).

The role of BDNF in mediating hippocampal function is well established, as exemplified by deficits of learning and memory in rodents with BDNF suppression or gene targeted-deletion (Korte et al. 1995; Heldt et al. 2007). BDNF is a complex gene with multiple mRNA variants containing a common protein-encoding region (Timmusk et al. 1993). BDNF signaling is mediated by tyrosine-receptor kinase B (TrkB) and p75 neurotrophic receptor (p75^{NTR}) (Chao 2003). Full-length TrkB (TrkB$_{FL}$) contains the intracellular kinase signaling domain, while several short (truncated) isoforms (TrkB$_S$) lack this signaling domain (Klein et al. 1990). The p75^{NTR} is a low affinity receptor that binds promiscuously to BDNF as well as other known neurotrophic factors. BDNF binding of TrkB promotes neurite outgrowth and synaptic plasticity in part through regulation of activity-dependent immediate early genes c-fos, early-growth-response-gene 1 and 2 (Egr1 and Egr2) (Alder et al. 2003; Calella et al. 2007). In contrast, BDNF binding of p75^{NTR} reduces neurite outgrowth and mediates long-term depression (Woo et al. 2005; Zagrebelsky et al. 2005).

151.1.4 Fetal–Neonatal Iron Deficiency and Hippocampal Expression of Neurotrophic Factors

The effects of fetal–neonatal iron deficiency on the expression of neurotrophic growth factors critical for hippocampal neurogenesis, differentiation and plasticity have remained unresolved. However, the abnormal hippocampal dendritic morphology and impaired neurotransmission observed in fetal–neonatal ID rats led to the hypothesis that iron deficiency would result in dysregulation of neurotrophic factors involved in hippocampal differentiation and neuroplasticity. Moreover, the persistent deficits of hippocampal-dependent tasks in formerly iron-deficient (FID) rats, that were ID during fetal–neonatal period (Felt et al. 2006; Schmidt et al. 2007), imply a long-lasting change in regulation of neurotrophic factors including BDNF. Indeed, we found evidence of diminished BDNF signaling during and after a period of iron deficiency in the rat hippocampus (Tran et al. 2008, 2009).

151.2 Fetal–Neonatal IDA Acutely Alters Expression of Neurotrophic Factors and Delays Hippocampal Neuron Differentiation

151.2.1 Increased Expression of Neurotrophic Factors During Peak Normal Neuronal Differentiation in Rat Hippocampus

Differentiation of hippocampal neurons occurs rapidly during P15 and P30 in rats (Pokorny and Yamamoto 1981; Steward and Falk 1991) with a corresponding increase in iron uptake (Siddappa et al. 2002). Quantitative measurement (real-time PCR) of messenger RNA (mRNA) for ciliary neurotrophic factor (CNTF), epithelial growth factor (EGF), glial-derived neurotrophic factor (GDNF),

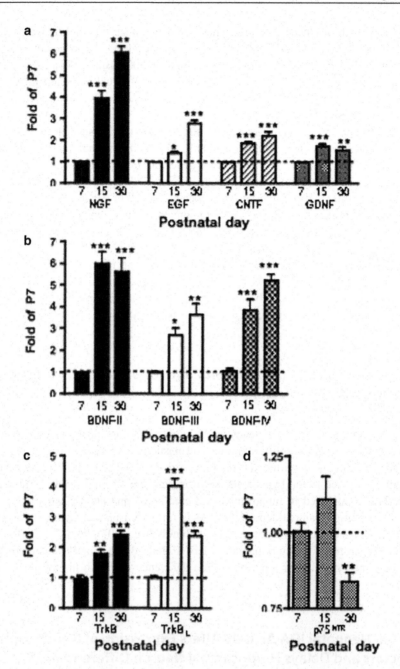

Fig. 151.1 Expression of neurotrophic factor mRNA levels at P7, P15, and P30 in the male rat hippocampus. Levels of messenger RNA (mRNA) were compared to P7, demonstrating the developmental expression of neurotrophic factors. (**a**) Nerve growth factor (NGF), EGF, CNTF, and glial-derived neurotrophic factor (GDNF), (**b**) BDNF -II, -III, and -IV, (**c**) total TrkB and TrkB full-length (TrkB$_L$), and (**d**) p75 neurotrophic receptor (p75^{NTR}). Values are means ± SEM, $n = 4–6$. Asterisks denote P-values as follows: *$P < 0.05$, **$P < 0.01$, ***$P < 0.001$ (Modified and printed with permission from American Society for Nutrition)

and NGF showed higher levels at P15 and P30 compared to P7 (Fig. 151.1a). Likewise, BDNF-II, III and IV transcripts were greater at P15 and P30 compared to P7, with BDNF-II mRNA being at a negligible level compared to BDNF-III and IV in the developing rat hippocampus (Fig. 151.1b). Similar findings were also observed for BDNF receptors, TrkB and p75^{NTR} (Fig. 151.1c). Taken together, peak expression of NGFs and their cognate receptors occurs during periods of rapid differentiation in the rat hippocampus (Tran et al. 2008). These findings are consistent with the role of neurotrophic factors in promoting neuronal differentiation and dendritic outgrowth.

151.2.2 Increased EGF, GDNF, NGF and p75^{NTR}, and Deceased BDNF Expression During Fetal–Neonatal ID in the Hippocampus

While CNTF levels were unaffected, levels of EGF, GDNF and NGF were greater in the ID compared to IS rats at P15 (Table 151.2). In contrast, iron deficiency decreased BDNF transcripts across development with a significant reduction of BDNF-III at P7 and BDNF-IV at P7 and P15 (Table 151.2). The difference was less significant between groups at P30, suggesting a normalization of expression with iron therapy. Despite lower BDNF levels, expression of its high affinity receptor TrkB was similar between ID and IS groups, suggesting an absence of an expected compensatory upregulation (Table 151.2). However, iron deficiency increased p75^{NTR} levels at P7 and P15. Collectively, iron deficiency dysregulates neurotrophic factors and associated receptors during the period of iron deficiency (Tran et al. 2008).

The reduced BDNF during periods of neural proliferation and differentiation (P7 and P15) may account for the 14% reduction in hippocampal size (Rao and Georgieff, unpublished data) and abnormal CA1 dendritic structure in older FID rats (Jorgenson et al. 2003). The effect of iron deficiency on proliferation and cell number remains unresolved with preliminary findings of increased neuronal turnover in a late gestational embryonic ID hippocampus (Lehman and Georgieff, unpublished data). Increased EGF, GDNF, NGF, and p75^{NTR} expression in the ID hippocampus suggest utilization of alternate pathways to compensate for the lower BDNF expression. Upregulation of EGF might facilitate neurogenesis and differentiation in ID hippocampus (Wong and Guillaud 2004). Likewise, GDNF could synergize with BDNF to promote neuronal survival (Erickson et al. 2001), minimizing the adverse effects of reduced BDNF. It is worthwhile to note that both EGF and GDNF mediate astrocyte proliferation and differentiation (Wong and Guillaud 2004; Chen et al. 2005). The effects of fetal–neonatal iron deficiency on astroglia development have not been fully investigated, albeit metabolomic evidence suggests increased astroglia in the ID hippocampus (Rao et al. 2003). Increased EGF and GDNF levels may affect the astroglia number as well as regulation of glutamine synthase activity (Yamada et al. 1997), in line with increased glutamine levels observed in the ID hippocampus (Rao et al. 2003). However, it is less clear what effects increased NGF and p75^{NTR} may have in the ID hippocampus. ProNGF/p75^{NTR} signaling induces neuronal apoptosis contrasting the survival effect of the mature-NGF/TrkA sig-

Table 151.1   Key facts of neurotrophic factors

1. A family of proteins classically includes nerve growth factor (NGF), BDNF, neurotrophin-3 (NT-3), and neurotrophin-4/5 (NT-4/5). These factors each bind a specific tyrosine receptor kinase (Trk) with high affinity (i.e. NGF/TrkA, BDNF/TrkB, NT-3, 4/TrkC). All bind p75 receptor with low affinity.

2. The non-classical members of neurotrophic factors include glial-derived neurotrophic factor (GDNF), CNTF, cardiotrophin-1 (CT-1), interleukin-6 (IL-6), and leukemia inhibitory factor (LIF). With the exception of GDNF, which initiates intracellular signaling by binding to the RET receptor tyrosine kinase, other factors bind and signal via G-protein coupled receptor (GPR130).

3. The role of neurotrophic factors is to regulate differentiation, growth, survival, and plasticity of both central and peripheral nervous systems.

This table describes general key facts of neurotrophic factors and their receptors. The binding of the neurotrophic factor to its cognate receptor initiates a signaling cascade that results in increased transcription and/or translation of downstream effectors

Table 151.2 Comparison of neurotrophic factor and receptor expression in the developing IS and ID rat hippocampus (Modified and printed with permission from American Society for Nutrition)

| | P7 | | P15 | | P30 | | 2-Way ANOVA P-values | | |
| | IS | ID | IS | ID | IS | ID | | | |
Transcript	Fold of P7 IS						Iron status	Postnatal age	Interaction
CNTF	1.0±0.0[a]	1.3±0.1	1.9±0.1[b]	2.1±0.2	2.2±0.2[b]	2.2±0.2	0.11	<0.01	0.65
GDNF	1.0±0.0[a]	1.8±0.1*	1.7±0.1[b]	2.4±0.2*	1.5±0.2[b]	1.6±0.2	<0.01	<0.01	0.01
EGF	1.0±0.1[a]	1.2±0.1	1.4±0.2[b]	2.2±0.2*	2.8±0.33[c]	2.9±0.4	<0.01	<0.01	<0.01
NGF	1.0±0.0[a]	1.0±0.1	3.8±0.4[b]	5.2±0.5*	5.8±0.3[c]	6.5±0.3	<0.01	<0.01	0.07
BDNF-III	1.0±0.1[a]	0.6±0.0*	1.3±0.0[b]	1.1±0.1	1.3±0.1[b]	1.0±0.0	<0.01	<0.01	0.13
BDNF-IV	1.0±0.1[a]	0.6±0.1*	1.7±0.1[b]	1.1±0.1*	1.5±0.2[b]	1.1±0.1*	<0.01	<0.01	0.96
TrkB	1.0±0.1[a]	1.0±0.0	2.3±0.3[b]	2.2±0.3	3.0±0.2[c]	2.8±0.3	0.38	<0.01	0.91
TrkB$_L$	1.0±0.0[a]	1.2±0.1	2.5±0.3[b]	2.3±0.2	2.4±0.2[b]	2.9±0.2	0.22	<0.01	0.14
p75	1.0±0.0[a]	1.6±0.2*	1.1±0.1[a]	1.9±0.1*	0.8±0.0[a]	0.9±0.1	<0.01	<0.01	<0.01

Levels of transcript (messenger RNA) for relevant neurotrophic factors and BDNF receptors were compared between iron-sufficient (IS) control and iron-deficient (ID) hippocampi. Data were standardized to P7 value to demonstrate changes in transcript level across postnatal ages. Values are means ± SEM, $n = 4$–6. Means in a row without a common letter differ, $P < 0.05$ (a < b < c). *Asterisk denotes the difference from IS at a time, $P < 0.05$ Post-hoc Bonferroni corrected t-test

naling (Friedman 2000; Lee et al. 2001). Elevated NGF and p75^{NTR} transcripts in the ID hippocampus would have predicted an increase in neuronal apoptosis. However, the observed reduction in apoptosis in postnatal ID hippocampus (Tran et al. 2008) suggests that increased NGF and p75^{NTR} likely have a survival effect as seen in other studies (Bui et al. 2002; Culmsee et al. 2002). In addition, p75^{NTR} is known to promote high-affinity ligand/receptor binding (e.g., BDNF/TrkB) and ligand/receptor retrograde transport (Chao 2003). The upregulation of p75^{NTR} might act in a compensatory manner to promote BDNF/TrkB signaling, facilitating synaptic formation and LTP (Minichiello et al. 2002).

151.2.3 Reduced Doublecortin (Dcx) Expression is Associated with Delayed NeuN-Nuclear Accumulation in the Developing ID Hippocampus

The persistently immature form of electrophysiology (Jorgenson et al. 2005) combined with reduced NMDAR (NR2B) expression (Jorgenson and Georgieff, unpublished data) suggest an abnormal development of hippocampal glutamatergic neurotransmission in fetal–neonatal ID rats. Consistent with this effect, the level of Dcx, a microtubule-associated protein expressed in differentiating neurons (Francis et al. 1999), was reduced by 40% in the ID hippocampus at P15 (Fig. 151.2a). Dcx localization was similar in P15 IS and ID hippocampi with prominent expression in the dentate gyrus proper (Fig. 151.2b). ID rats also showed a failure of NeuN, a nuclear neuronal marker, localization to the nucleus of pyramidal neurons by P30 as seen in IS rats (Fig. 151.2c,d) (Tran et al. 2008). These findings imply a delay of neuronal maturation in the ID hippocampus during a period of rapid differentiation. Based on the increase demand of iron uptake during this developmental period (Siddappa et al. 2002), we propose that iron deficiency results in deferment of neuronal differentiation, perhaps leading to an extension of this rapid growth period, until sufficient iron replenishment. This developmental brake hypothesis is in agreement with the observed NeuN-nuclear localization in the hippocampus of iron-repleted P65 rats (Fig. 151.2e,f).

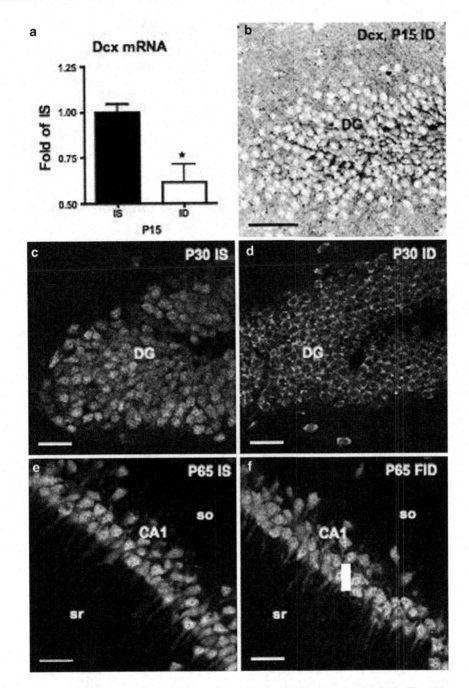

Fig. 151.2 Reduced P15 doublecortin (Dcx) expression and abnormal NeuN localization in the ID rat hippocampus. (**a**) Expression of a neuronal differentiation marker, doublecortin (Dcx), showed a significant reduction in the postnatal day (P)15 ID hippocampus compared to the IS control. Values are means ± SEM, $n = 4$–6. *$P < 0.05$, Mann-Whitney U-test. (**b**) Localization of Dcx protein in the dentate gyrus (DG) of the P15 ID rat. There was no apparent difference in Dcx localization between the IS and ID hippocampus. (**c–d**) NeuN staining in the dentate gyrus of P30 IS (**c**) and ID (**d**) hippocampi. Note the absence of NeuN in nuclei of ID neurons. Similar observations were seen in CA1 and CA3 hippocampus (data not shown). (**e–f**) NeuN staining in CA1 of P65 IS and FID rats. Note the presence of NeuN in cell nucleus. Scale bar = 50 μm

151.3 Long-Term Reduction of BDNF Activity in Adult Rats That Experienced Iron Deficiency During Fetal–Neonatal Period

The etiology of long-term the learning impairment seen in fetal and neonatal ID humans and rodent models remain largely unknown. The possibility of long-term dysregulation of neurotrophic factors and their downstream targets that regulate a cascade of molecular mediators of synaptic plasticity in FID rats was investigated (Tran et al. 2009).

151.3.1 Decreased Hippocampal BDNF and TrkB Expression in P65 FID Rats

Levels of p75[NTR], CNTF, CTGF, EGF, GDNF, and NGF were not different between the always IS control and FID P65 rats. However, P65 FID rats had lower levels of BDNF and its high affinity receptor TrkB (Fig. 151.3). Interestingly, truncated TrkB (TrkB$_S$) is expressed at a higher level than TkB$_{FL}$ in the control hippocampus, but not in the FID hippocampus at P65 (Fig. 151.3d). This finding

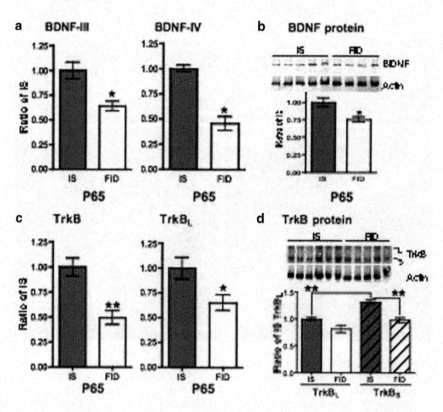

Fig. 151.3 Reduced BDNF and TrkB expression in the P65 FID hippocampus. Hippocampal expression of BDNF and TrkB receptor were compared between the control (always IS) and the formerly iron-deficient (FID) rats. Data were normalized to IS control. FID rats showed a reduced expression of BDNF and its cognate receptor TrkB. BDNF mRNA (**a**) and protein (**b**). TrkB mRNA (**c**) and protein (**d**). Values are means ± SEM, $n = 4$–6. *$P < 0.05$ and **$P < 0.01$, Mann-Whitney U-test (Modified and printed with permission from Wolters Kluwer Health)

suggests that the P65 FID hippocampus retains immature characteristics compared to the IS control hippocampus (Silhol et al. 2008). Despite having limited signaling capability, $TrkB_S$ has been implicated to negatively affect BDNF/TrkB signaling (Eide et al. 1996; Pillai and Mahadik 2008). Thus, the lower level of $TrkB_S$ in the FID hippocampus might have a compensatory effect by increasing the signaling capability of the available full-length receptor. Even with lower levels of BDNF and TrkB expressions, protein localization appeared similar in the hippocampus of both groups (Tran et al. 2009). While further ultrastructural analysis of protein localization is needed to ascertain these findings, preliminarily they imply an overall lower BDNF signaling in the hippocampus of FID rats without compromising their localization. The specific reduction of BDNF expression in FID rats suggests a more permanent change in its regulation induced by early iron deficiency. The precise mechanism awaits further investigation. One possibility may involve epigenetic modification (e.g., DNA methylation) at the BDNF gene, which was hypermethylated in rats exposed to adverse early-life environment (Roth et al. 2009).

151.3.2 Reduced Hippocampal Expression of BDNF-Activity Dependent Gene Cascades

In the postnatal brain, BDNF regulates neuronal HMGCR, the rate-limiting enzyme in cholesterol synthesis that facilitates synaptic vesicle formation (Suzuki et al. 2007). Consistent with lower BDNF activity, the level of HMGCR was decreased in P65 FID hippocampus (Fig. 151.4a), suggesting that vesicle formation may be compromised (Tran et al. 2009). Combined with a lower level of synaptobrevin I (Carlson et al. 2007), a protein involved in vesicle fusion (Schiavo et al. 1997), this finding may underlie the impaired paired-pulse facilitation and reduced synaptic efficacy seen in adult hippocampal slice preparations following recovery from fetal–neonatal iron deficiency (Jorgenson et al. 2005). Paired-pulse facilitation and LTP are important indices of neuroelectrophysiologic events during neurotransmission and LTP is widely accepted as a cellular substrate for learning and memory (Malenka 2003).

BDNF also induces the expression of c-fos, Egr1, and Egr2, which are activity-dependent immediate early transcription factors that facilitate LTP in the hippocampus (Alder et al. 2003; Rossler and Thiel 2004). Expression of these genes was also decreased in FID rats (Fig. 151.4b–d) (Tran et al. 2009). Lower c-fos expression may not only lead to a reduction in expression of genes necessary for LTP (Miyamoto 2006) but may also contribute to further reduction of BDNF expression (Dong et al. 2006), thereby leading to lesser plasticity in the hippocampus of FID rats. As expected, reduced expression of Egr1 was accompanied by lower expression of its known target genes, hif1α and Dusp4 (Berasi et al. 2006; Sperandio et al. 2009), in the hippocampus of FID rats (Fig. 151.5a,b) (Tran et al. 2009). Hif1α is an oxidative-state-dependent transcription factor that regulates chemokine (C-X-C motif) ligand 12 (Cxcl12), an important modulator of synaptic formation (Klein and Rubin 2004). Cxcl12 mRNA expression is reduced in FID rats (Carlson et al. 2007). Combined with similar long-term reductions in post-synaptic density 95 (PSD95) and calmodulin-dependent kinase IIα (CamKIIα), these changes may account for the abnormal apical dendritic length and branching in FID hippocampal neurons (Jorgenson et al. 2003; Carlson et al. 2007). DUSP4 (protein) is a dual specificity phosphatase targeting phosphorylated extracellular signal-regulated kinases 1 and 2 (ERK1 and ERK2), factors phosphorylated during formation of memory (Guan and Butch 1995; Kelly et al. 2003). Reduction of DUSP4 activity and the consequential increased level of phosphorylated ERK1/2 in FID compared to IS rats (Fig. 151.5c) could further contribute to impaired synaptic

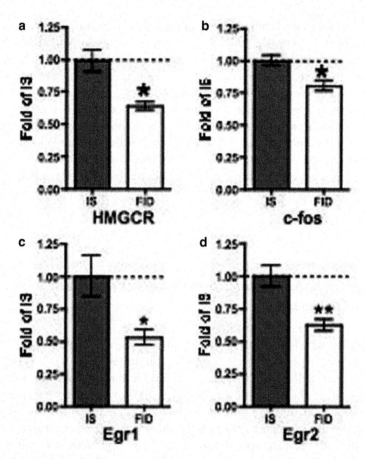

Fig. 151.4 Reduced expression of BDNF activity-dependent genes in the P65 FID hippocampus. Hippocampal expression of (**a**) HMGCR, (**b**) c-fos, (**c**) Egr1, and (**d**) Egr2 were compared between the IS control and the FID rats. FID rats showed a lower expression of these factors, consistent with a decrease in BDNF signaling. Values are means ± SEM, $n = 4-6$. *$P < 0.05$, **$P < 0.01$ Mann-Whitney U-test (Modified and printed with permission from Wolters Kluwer Health)

plasticity by dampening neuronal responsiveness to stimulation (Tran et al. 2009). Alternatively, sustained phosphorylation of ERK1/2 may reflect the compensatory state of the already lowered neural plasticity in FID rats. Reduced Egr2 expression resulted in lower expression of its target genes (Fig. 151.5d,e) (Tran et al. 2009), insulin-like growth factor 2 (IGF-II) and myelin basic protein (Mbp) (Gillian and Svaren 2004; Jang et al. 2006), which are important for myelin health and glial contributions to plasticity. In the adult brain, IGF-II is expressed in astroglia (Rotwein et al. 1988) and regulates myelin associated protein genes (Ye et al. 2002). Mbp is a complex gene with multiple splice variants, encoding a major component of the myelin sheath of oligodendrocytes. Decreased IGF-II and Mbp expression together may contribute to the impairment of myelination and the compromised neural transmission seen in the P65 FID hippocampus (Jorgenson et al. 2005). While whole brain Mbp expression is acutely reduced during iron deficiency (Beard et al. 2003; Clardy et al. 2006), these findings in the hippocampus of FID animals provide evidence for a long-term effect of fetal–neonatal iron deficiency on the health and function of astrocytes and oligodendrocytes.

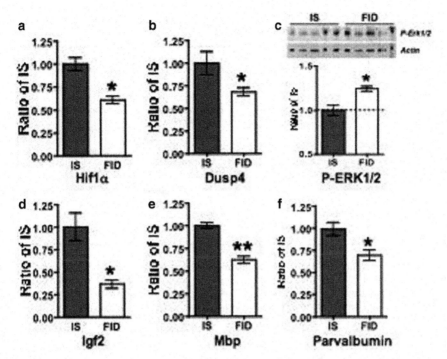

Fig. 151.5 Reduced expression of Egr1- and Egr2-target genes and parvalbumin in the P65 FID hippocampus. Assessment of Egr1 target, Hif1a (**a**) and Dusp4 (**b**), showed a lower expression in FID rats. (**c**) The increase of phosphorylated-ERK1/2 (P-ERK1/2) suggests a decrease in Dusp4 activity because Dusp4 converts P-ERK1/2 to ERK1/2. Lower transcript levels of Egr2 target, Igf2 (**d**) and Mbp (**e**), indicate a decrease in Egr2 transcriptional activity in FID rats. Together with Igf2 and Mbp, reduced parvalbumin expression (**f**) suggests impaired astroglia function in FID rats. Values are means ± SEM, $n = 4$–6. $*P < 0.05$ and $**P < 0.01$, Mann-Whitney U-test (Modified and printed with permission from Wolters Kluwer Health)

BDNF also mediates interneuron differentiation in rodent hippocampus (Marty et al. 1996; Grosse et al. 2005). More research is needed to determine comprehensively the effect of early-life iron deficiency on interneuron development. However, mRNA level of parvalbumin (PARV), a calcium-binding protein expressed in a subset of interneurons, was lower in the FID rat hippocampus (Fig. 151.5f). Whether the lower parvalbumin transcript in the FID hippocampus reflects a decrease in gene expression or a fewer number of PARV-positive (+) cells remain to be determined. It is unclear if lower BDNF expression would lead to a decrease in PARV+ cell number. Study of BDNF knock-out mice suggested a decrease of hippocampal PARV+ cell (Grosse et al. 2005); however, exogenous administration of BDNF showed no such effect in cultured rat hippocampal slice preparations (Marty et al. 1996). Nonetheless, lower parvalbumin expression might contribute to impaired plasticity in the FID rat by reducing synaptic efficacy (Jiang et al. 2004).

In summary, these findings reveal an overall diminished BDNF-mediated neural development and plasticity during and beyond iron deficiency periods. We propose that this specific effect may serve as molecular basis for the electrophysiological, morphological, and ultimately behavioral abnormalities that persist beyond the period of fetal–neonatal iron deficiency (Fig. 151.6) (Lozoff et al. 2006).

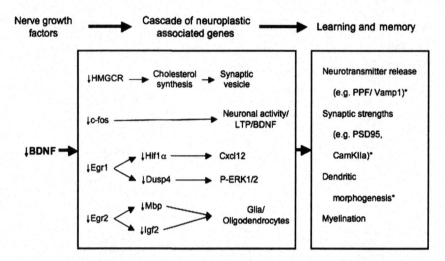

Fig. 151.6 Proposed mechanism. A possible molecular mechanism underlying a reduced BDNF activity leading to decreased neuroplasticity in FID rats. BDNF signaling regulates a cascade of factors that modulate neural plasticity, a basis of learning and memory. *Asterisk denotes previously altered factors contributing to lower synaptic plasticity (Modified and printed with permission from Wolters Kluwer Health)

151.4 Applications to Other Areas of Health and Disease

Fetal–neonatal iron deficiency is a common clinical sequela in offspring of pregnancies complicated by maternal diabetes mellitus, maternal hypertension causing intrauterine growth restriction (IUGR), maternal smoking, and severe maternal anemia. These risk groups are characterized by poorer long-term neurodevelopmental outcomes particularly in the cognitive domain suggesting that the developmental trajectory of neural circuits that support these behaviors are compromised. Long-term compromise in spite of prompt neonatal iron treatment suggests the possibility of long-term changes in regulation of the salient genes, perhaps by epigenetic mechanisms.

The lower BDNF activity induced by fetal–neonatal iron deficiency during periods of rapid neural differentiation may underlie the delay of neuronal differentiation in the developing ID hippocampus. It may also serve as the molecular basis for the morphologic and functional abnormalities seen during the period of iron deficiency. Whether these alterations are consequences of the deficit of neuronal iron or to other confounding factors in this anemia model, such as hypoxia at systemic and/or cellular levels, remain unresolved. IUGR models are also characterized by both hypoxia and iron deficiency, however, our ID model differed in terms of compensatory expression of TrkB receptor. Whereas a pig model of chronic placental insufficiency showed an obligatory increase of TrkB expression due to lower BDNF expression (Dieni and Rees 2005), we did not find such effect in ID rats. Thus, difference in TrkB finding may be attributed to the effect of ID rather than hypoxia. Despite an absence of upregulation, a greater $TrkB_L$/BDNF ratio suggests an increased availability of this TrkB isoform for BDNF binding in the ID hippocampus. This finding may be important in terms of understanding the early antecedents of adult neurological disorders characterized by reduced hippocampal function or early hippocampal degeneration. For example, Alzheimer and Parkinson's diseases are characterized by reduction of BDNF levels without compensatory increases in TrkB expression (Siegel and Chauhan 2000). The altered expression of genes involved in the pathogenesis of Alzheimer's disease as well as an increased susceptibility of brain injury in this same model supports this possibility (Carlson et al. 2007, 2008; Rao et al. 2007).

The long-term dysregulation of BDNF suggests that iron treatment alone is insufficient to attenuate the effects of iron deficiency during sensitive periods of hippocampal development, providing a role for iron in long-term programming of hippocampal BDNF. The underpinning mechanisms of this long-term effect are unknown but may be similar to those involved in the developmental origins of health and disease (Gluckman et al. 2008), including epigenetic modifications. This possibility is supported by a recent report of early-life negligence resulted in long-term down regulation of BDNF that is associated with hypermethylation of its regulatory region (Roth et al. 2009). Our results also emphasize the concept that provision of nutrients alone is inadequate to maintain optimal brain function. We propose that proper regulation of growth factors is also essential to ensure optimal utilization of nutrients. Long-term dysregulation of these growth factors may thus account for persistent abnormal function despite nutrient repletion.

In summary, our findings provide insights into a possible molecular mechanism underpinning acute and long-term cognitive deficits in fetal–neonatal iron deficiency model (Fig. 151.7). Further research is needed to determine precisely how iron regulates the expression of BDNF and its downstream effectors. While the long-term effect may be accounted by potential epigenetic modification (i.e., DNA methylation), the acute effect remains virtually unknown. We speculate that iron may have a direct role in modulating the binding of transcriptional machinery/complex at the BDNF regulatory region (Tsuji et al. 1999; Wong et al. 2005). Our data suggest that interventions that enhance BDNF activity such as exercise or selective serotonin reuptake inhibitors (Russo-Neustadt et al. 2000) may be useful as therapeutic approaches to treat long-term effects of fetal–neonatal iron deficiency, complementing iron therapy.

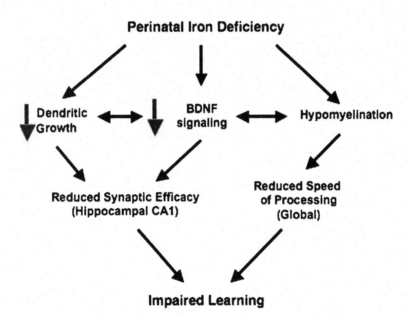

Fig. 151.7 Proposed working hypothesis. A proposed model accounting for learning impairments induced by fetal–neonatal iron deficiency. BDNF signaling affects both neuronal maturation (e.g., dendritic growth) and myelination. In turn, these processes alter synaptic efficacy and speed of neurotransmission, which ultimately contribute to learning impairments

Summary Points

- Peak expression of neurotrophic factors and their cognate receptors occurs during periods of rapid differentiation in the rat hippocampus are consistent with the role of neurotrophic factors in promoting neuronal differentiation and dendritic outgrowth.
- Fetal–neonatal iron deficiency dysregulates neurotrophic factors with specific reduction of BDNF and is associated with a delay of neuronal maturation during a period of rapid differentiation, which may reflect an extension of this rapid growth period in ID hippocampus.
- The specific reduction of BDNF expression in formerly-iron-deficient (FID) rats that were ID during early life suggests a more permanent change in its regulation. A possible underlying mechanism may involve epigenetic modification (e.g., DNA methylation) at the BDNF gene.
- Despite an absence of compensatory upregulation, an increased TrkB$_L$/BDNF ratio may maximize available BDNF signaling in the ID hippocampus. This may be important in terms of understanding the early antecedents of adult neurological disorders (e.g., Alzheimer and Parkinson's diseases) characterized by reduced BDNF and hippocampal function or early hippocampal degeneration.
- The overall diminished BDNF activity accompanied by reduced expression of a cascade of downstream factors during and beyond iron deficiency periods may serve as molecular basis for the electrophysiological, morphological, and ultimately behavioral abnormalities that persist beyond the period of fetal–neonatal iron deficiency.
- The long-term dysregulation of BDNF suggests that iron treatment alone is insufficient to attenuate the effects of iron deficiency during sensitive periods of hippocampal development, emphasizing the concept that the provision of nutrients and proper regulation of growth factors are essential to ensure optimal utilization of nutrients for brain function.

Definitions and Explanations of Key Terms

BDNF: A member of neurotrophic factors that plays critical roles in mediating neuronal proliferation, differentiation, and survival.

Dendritogenesis: A process of neural differentiation in which dendrite grows and branches into a complex pattern specifically unique to each neuronal type.

FID rats: Refers to rats that experienced iron deficiency during fetal–neonatal period, but are no longer bodily or brain ID.

Hippocampus: A brain region responsible for learning and memory that is classically organized into three subregions: CA1, CA3, and dentate gyrus.

LTP: A sustained electrophysiological activity resulting from a long-term increase of synaptic strength between two neurons, which is widely accepted as a cellular form of memory formation.

Microarray gene expression analysis: A molecular genetic technique that simultaneously assesses expression levels of thousands of genes.

Neural plasticity (neuroplasticity): The ability of neuron to adapt to its environment by altering its intracellular properties.

Quantitative (real-time) PCR: A molecular technique to measure levels of gene expression by simultaneously amplify and monitor RNA/cDNA per each thermocycle over the course of the polymerase chain reaction (PCR).

Key Points

1. Fetal–neonatal iron deficiency and cognitive development – Fetal–neonatal iron deficiency is a common clinical sequela in offspring of pregnancies complicated by maternal diabetes mellitus, maternal hypertension causing intrauterine growth restriction (IUGR), maternal smoking, and severe maternal anemia. These risk groups are characterized by poorer long-term neurodevelopmental outcomes particularly in the cognitive domain suggesting that the developmental trajectory of neural circuits that support these behaviors are compromised. According to a recent W.H.O estimate (2003), the prevalence of IDA among pregnant women and preschool age children ranges between 30% and 50% of global population worldwide.
2. Fetal–neonatal iron deficiency reduces BDNF expression and signaling – Early life iron deficiency diminishes acute as well as long-term BDNF-mediated neural development and plasticity. In turn, expression of molecular factors downstream of BDNF signaling is reduced, contributing to decreased neural maturation and plasticity. These effects may serve as molecular bases for the electrophysiological, morphological, and ultimately behavioral abnormalities during and beyond the period of fetal–neonatal iron deficiency.

Acknowledgments We apologize that we were unable to cite all relevant works in this article to due space constraint. We thank Heather McLaughlin for editorial assistance. This work is supported by NICHD RO1 HD29421 to MKG and NIMH Training grant T32MH073129 to PVT.

References

Alder J, Thakker-Varia S, Bangasser DA, Kuroiwa M, Plummer MR, Shors TJ, Black IB. J Neurosci. 2003;23:10800–8.

Beard JL, Wiesinger JA, Connor JR. Dev Neurosci. 2003;25:308–15.

Berasi SP, Huard C, Li D, Shih HH, Sun Y, Zhong W, Paulsen JE, Brown EL, Gimeno RE, Martinez RV. J Biol Chem. 2006;281:27167–77.

Branchi I, Francia N, Alleva E. Behav Pharmacol. 2004;15:353–62.

Bui NT, Konig HG, Culmsee C, Bauerbach E, Poppe M, Krieglstein J, Prehn JH. J Neurochem. 2002;81:594–605.

Calella AM, Nerlov C, Lopez RG, Sciarretta C, von Bohlen und Halbach O, Bereshchenko O, Minichiello L. Neural Dev. 2007;2:4.

Carlson ES, Stead JD, Neal CR, Petryk A, Georgieff MK. Hippocampus. 2007;17:679–91.

Carlson ES, Magid R, Petryk A, Georgieff MK. Brain Res. 2008;1237C:75–83.

Chao MV. Nat Rev Neurosci. 2003;4:299–309.

Chen Y, Ai Y, Slevin JR, Maley BE, Gash DM. Exp Neurol. 2005;196:87–95.

Chockalingam UM, Murphy E, Ophoven JC, Weisdorf SA, Georgieff MK. J Pediatr. 1987;111:283–6.

Clardy SL, Wang X, Zhao W, Liu W, Chase GA, Beard JL, True Felt B, Connor JR. J Neural Transm Suppl. 2006;173–96.

Culmsee C, Gerling N, Lehmann M, Nikolova-Karakashian M, Prehn JH, Mattson MP, Krieglstein J. Neuroscience. 2002;115:1089–108.

Dieni S, Rees S. Exp Neurol. 2005;192:265–73.

Dong M, Wu Y, Fan Y, Xu M, Zhang J. Neurosci Lett. 2006;400:177–80.

Eide FF, Vining ER, Eide BL, Zang K, Wang XY, Reichardt LF. J Neurosci. 1996;16:3123–9.

Erickson JT, Brosenitsch TA, Katz DM. J Neurosci. 2001;21:581–9.

Felt BT, Beard JL, Schallert T, Shao J, Aldridge JW, Connor JR, Georgieff MK, Lozoff B. Behav Brain Res. 2006;171:261–70.

Francis F, Koulakoff A, Boucher D, Chafey P, Schaar B, Vinet MC, Friocourt G, McDonnell N, Reiner O, Kahn A, McConnell SK, Berwald-Netter Y, Denoulet P, Chelly J. Neuron. 1999;23:247–56.

Friedman WJ. J Neurosci. 2000;20:6340–6.

Gillian AL, Svaren J. J Biol Chem. 2004;279:9056–63.

Gluckman PD, Hanson MA, Cooper C, Thornburg KL. N Engl J Med. 2008;359:61–73.

Golub MS, Hogrefe CE, Germann SL, Capitanio JP, Lozoff B. Neurotoxicol Teratol. 2006;28:3–17.
Grosse G, Djalali S, Deng DR, Holtje M, Hinz B, Schwartzkopff K, Cygon M, Rothe T, Stroh T, Hellweg R, Ahnert-
    Hilger G, Hortnag H. Brain Res Dev Brain Res. 2005;156:111–26.
Guan KL, Butch E. J Biol Chem. 1995;270:7197–203.
Guenette S, Chang Y, Hiesberger T, Richardson JA, Eckman CB, Eckman EA, Hammer RE, Herz J. EMBO J.
    2006;25:420–31.
Heldt SA, Stanek L, Chhatwal JP, Ressler KJ. Mol Psychiatry. 2007;12:656–70.
Hennigan A, O'Callaghan RM, Kelly AM. Biochem Soc Trans. 2007;35:424–7.
Ikin AF, Sabo SL, Lanier LM, Buxbaum JD. Mol Cell Neurosci. 2007;35:57–63.
Jang SW, LeBlanc SE, Roopra A, Wrabetz L, Svaren J. J Neurochem. 2006;98:1678–87.
Jiang B, Kitamura A, Yasuda H, Sohya K, Maruyama A, Yanagawa Y, Obata K, Tsumoto T. Eur J Neurosci.
    2004;20:709–18.
Jorgenson LA, Wobken JD, Georgieff MK. Dev Neurosci. 2003;25:412–20.
Jorgenson LA, Sun M, O'Connor M, Georgieff MK. Hippocampus. 2005;15:1094–102.
Kelly A, Laroche S, Davis S. J Neurosci. 2003;23:5354–60.
Klein R, Conway D, Parada LF, Barbacid M. Cell. 1990;61:647–56.
Klein RS, Rubin JB. Trends Immunol. 2004;25:306–14.
Korte M, Carroll P, Wolf E, Brem G, Thoenen H, Bonhoeffer T. Proc Natl Acad Sci U S A. 1995;92:8856–60.
Lee R, Kermani P, Teng KK, Hempstead BL. Science. 2001;294:1945–8.
Lozoff B, Georgieff MK. Semin Pediatr Neurol. 2006;13:158–65.
Lozoff B, Beard J, Connor J, Barbara F, Georgieff M, Schallert T. Nutr Rev. 2006;64:S34–S91.
Malenka RC. Nat Rev Neurosci. 2003;4:923–6.
Marty S, Carroll P, Cellerino A, Castren E, Staiger V, Thoenen H, Lindholm D. J Neurosci. 1996;16:675–87.
McAllister AK, Katz LC, Lo DC. Annu Rev Neurosci. 1999;22:295–318.
Minichiello L, Calella AM, Medina DL, Bonhoeffer T, Klein R, Korte M. Neuron. 2002;36:121–37.
Miyamoto E. J Pharmacol Sci. 2006;100:433–42.
Nelson CA, Wewerka S, Thomas KM, Tribby-Walbridge S, deRegnier R, Georgieff M. Behav Neurosci. 2000;114:950–6.
Patterson SL, Grover LM, Schwartzkroin PA, Bothwell M. Neuron. 1992;9:1081–8.
Petry CD, Eaton MA, Wobken JD, Mills MM, Johnson DE, Georgieff MK. J Pediatr. 1992;121:109–14.
Pham TM, Winblad B, Granholm AC, Mohammed AH. Pharmacol Biochem Behav. 2002;73:167–75.
Pillai A, Mahadik SP. Schizophr Res. 2008;100:325–33.
Pokorny J, Yamamoto T. Brain Res Bull. 1981;7:113–20.
Rao R, Tkac I, Townsend EL, Gruetter R, Georgieff MK. J Nutr. 2003;133:3215–21.
Rao R, Tkac I, Townsend EL, Ennis K, Gruetter R, Georgieff MK. J Cereb Blood Flow Metab. 2007;27:729–40.
Riggins T, Miller NC, Bauer PJ, Georgieff MK, Nelson CA. Dev Sci. 2009;12:209–19.
Rossler OG, Thiel G. Am J Physiol Cell Physiol. 2004;286:C1118–29.
Roth TL, Lubin FD, Funk AJ, Sweatt JD. Biol Psychiatry. 2009;65:760–9.
Rotwein P, Burgess SK, Milbrandt JD, Krause JE. Proc Natl Acad Sci U S A. 1988;85:265–9.
Russo-Neustadt AA, Beard RC, Huang YM, Cotman CW. Neuroscience. 2000;101:305–12.
Schmidt AT, Waldow KJ, Grove WM, Salinas JA, Georgieff MK. Behav Neurosci. 2007;121:475–82.
Schratt GM, Nigh EA, Chen WG, Hu L, Greenberg ME. J Neurosci. 2004;24:7366–77.
Schiavo G, Stenbeck G, Rothman JE, Sollner TH. Proc Natl Acad Sci USA. 1997;94:997–1001.
Siddappa AJ, Rao RB, Wobken JD, Leibold EA, Connor JR, Georgieff MK. J Neurosci Res. 2002;68:761–75.
Siddappa AM, Georgieff MK, Wewerka S, Worwa C, Nelson CA, Deregnier RA. Pediatr Res. 2004;55:1034–41.
Siegel GJ, Chauhan NB. Brain Res Rev. 2000;33:199–227.
Silhol M, Arancibia S, Perrin D, Maurice T, Alliot J, Tapia-Arancibia L. Rejuvenation Res. 2008;11:1031–40.
Sperandio S, Fortin J, Sasik R, Robitaille L, Corbeil J, de Belle I. Mol Carcinog. 2009;48:38–44.
Steward O, Falk PM. J Comp Neurol. 1991;314:545–57.
Suzuki S, Kiyosue K, Hazama S, Ogura A, Kashihara M, Hara T, Koshimizu H, Kojima M. J Neurosci. 2007;27:
    6417–27.
Sweet DG, Savage G, Tubman TR, Lappin TR, Halliday HL. Arch Dis Child Fetal Neonatal Ed. 2001;84:F40–3.
Tamura T, Goldenberg RL, Hou J, Johnston KE, Cliver SP, Ramey SL, Nelson KG. J Pediatr. 2002;140:165–70.
Tang SJ, Reis G, Kang H, Gingras AC, Sonenberg N, Schuman EM. Proc Natl Acad Sci U S A. 2002;99:467–72.
Timmusk T, Palm K, Metsis M, Reintam T, Paalme V, Saarma M, Persson H. Neuron. 1993;10:475–89.
Tran PV, Carlson ES, Fretham SJB, Georgieff MK. J Nutr. 2008;138:2495–501.
Tran PV, Fretham SJ, Carlson ES, Georgieff MK. Pediatr Res. 2009;65:493–8.
Tsuji Y, Moran E, Torti SV, Torti FM. J Biol Chem. 1999;274:7501–7.
WHO. Micronutrient deficiencies. 2008. http://www.who.int/nutrition/topics/ida/en/index.html

Wong K, Sharma A, Awasthi S, Matlock EF, Rogers L, Van Lint C, Skiest DJ, Burns DK, Harrod R. J Biol Chem. 2005;280:9390–9.

Wong RW, Guillaud L. Cytokine Growth Factor Rev. 2004;15:147–56.

Woo NH, Teng HK, Siao CJ, Chiaruttini C, Pang PT, Milner TA, Hempstead BL, Lu B. Nat Neurosci. 2005;8:1069–77.

Yamada M, Ikeuchi T, Hatanaka H. Prog Neurobiol. 1997;51:19–37.

Ye P, Li L, Richards RG, DiAugustine RP, D'Ercole AJ. J Neurosci. 2002;22:6041–51.

Zagrebelsky M, Holz A, Dechant G, Barde YA, Bonhoeffer T, Korte M. J Neurosci. 2005;25:9989–99.

Chapter 152
Iodine and Brain Metabolism

R.H. Verheesen and C.M. Schweitzer

Abbreviations

T4	3′,5′,3,5-tetraiodo-l-thyronine or thyroxine
T3	3′,3,5-triiodo-l-thyronine or triiodothyronine
MIT	Monoiodotyrosine
DIT	Diiodotyrosine
NIS	Sodium iodide symporter
DEHAL1	Iodotyrosine dehalogenases
TH	Tyrosine hydroxylase
RDA	Recommended daily allowances
TSH	Thyrotropin
NOS	Nitric oxide synthase
Pts	6-pyruvoyltetrahydropterin synthase
WHO	World Health Organization
ICCIDD	International Council for the Control of Iodine Deficiency Disorders
UI	Urinary iodine
ADHD	Attention deficit hyperactivity disorder

152.1 Introduction

The role of iodine in brain metabolism and development has been recognized since the first half of the twentieth century. Its ability to prevent and even cure goiter was described in 1918 by Marine et al. (Marine and Kimball 1990). Soon afterwards, substantial evidence arose for its role in preventing cretinism and the deterioration of brain development (Table 152.1). It is estimated that 5–30% of the people suffering from iodine deficiency eventually suffer from neurological impairment. The latest reports on iodine deficiency published by WHO (Benoist de et al. 2004; Andersson et al. 2007). make it clear that 2 billion people continue to suffer from iodine deficiency, with Europe having the biggest proportion of people who are iodine-deficient (Andersson et al. 2007) (Table 152.2).

R.H. Verheesen (✉)
Regionaal Reuma Centrum Z.O. Brabant, Máxima Medisch Centrum, Ds. Th. Fliednerstraat 1, 5631
BM Eindhoven, The Netherlands
e-mail: rh.verheesen@mmc.nl; rhverheesen@onsbrabantnet.nl

V.R. Preedy et al. (eds.), *Handbook of Behavior, Food and Nutrition*,
DOI 10.1007/978-0-387-92271-3_152, © Springer Science+Business Media, LLC 2011

Table 152.1 Spectrum of iodine deficiency disorders (From Andersson et al. 2007; Hetzel 1983; Stanbury et al. 1998; Laurberg et al. 2000)

Fetus	Abortions
	Stillbirths
	Congenital anomalies
	Increased perinatal mortality
	Endemic cretinism
Neonate	Neonatal hypothyroidism
	Endemic mental retardation
	Increased susceptibility of the thyroid gland to nuclear radiation
Child and adolescent	Goitre
	(Subclinical) hypothyroidism
	(Subclinical) hyperthyroidism
	Impaired mental function
	Retarded physical development
	Increased susceptibility of the thyroid gland to nuclear radiation
Adult	Goitre with its complications
	Hypothyroidism
	Impaired mental function
	Spontaneous hyperthyroidism in the elderly
	Iodine-induced hyperthyroidism
	Increased susceptibility of the thyroid gland to nuclear radiation

Effects of iodine deficiency not only a fetus-related health problem

Table 152.2 Proportion of population, and number of individuals with insufficient iodine intake in school-age children (6-12 years), and in the general population (all age groups) by WHO region, 2003

	Insufficient iodine intake (UI <100 µg/l)			
	School-age children		General population	
WHO region[a]	Proportion (%)	Total number (millions)[b]	Proportion (%)	Total number (millions)[b]
Africa	42.3	49.5	42.6	260.3
Americas	10.1	10.0	9.8	75.1
South-East Asia	39.9	95.6	39.8	624.0
Europe	59.9	42.2	56.9	435.5
Eastern Mediterranean	55.4	40.2	54.1	228.5
Western Pacific	26.2	48.0	24.0	365.3
Total	36.5	285.4	35.2	1988.7

[a]192 WHO Member States
[b]Based on population estimates in the year 2002

Thus far, iodine and its relation to brain development have been considered from a thyroid hormone point of view. Despite research during the last 40 years in this area several questions still wait for answers. In this chapter we provide a different point of view and relate iodine deficiency to the basic nutrients that are involved in iodine and thyroid metabolism. We focus on iodine, selenium, tyrosine, and vitamin D and point out their interactive relationships. By looking at the same problem from a different point of view new research and solutions could arise.

Iodine is available in the soil and recently the iodine cycle has been described in more detail. This availability in soil is probably reduced in countries with a young geographical background and in areas suffering from the latest ice age, repeated flooding, and elevated regions subject to glaciations and higher rainfalls.

152.2 Iodine and the Thyroid Hormone

152.2.1 Thyroid Hormone

Iodine is known for its role in the production of thyroid hormones. The thyroid hormone consists of two tyrosine molecules and four or three iodine molecules. The brain is known for its selectivity for thyroxin. After uptake in the brain, thyroxin is deiodinized by selenium-dependent selenodeiodinase enzymes (Kvicala and Zamrazil 2003; Kohrle 2005; Beckett and Arthur 2005).

The thyroid hormone is not only a source of iodine and tyrosine but is also a source of 3-iodothyronamines, their deiodinated products (Scanlan et al. 2004; Scanlan 2009). It is known that these 3-iodothyronamines are trace amines that overlap with classical biogenic amines, such as catecholamines and serotonin. They are capable of increasing catecholamine release.

Theoretically, this could mean that the production of 3-iodothyronamines will lead to a greater availability of the classical catecholamine. In that respect, iodine is necessary for the production of these 3-iodothyronamines and/or the binding of tyrosine.

152.2.2 Deiodination

Deiodination is a process in which deiodination enzymes are involved (Table 152.3 Iodine and brain development, Berber and Morales). As mentioned above, it is clear that the first deiodination is performed by selenium-dependent selenodeiodinase enzymes (Kohrle 2005; Beckett and Arthur 2005). These enzymes are influenced by the availability of thyroxine and triiodothyronine. In case of iodine

Table 152.3 Benefits from iodine supplementation programs (From Andersson et al. 2007; Hetzel and Maberly 1986; Levin 1987; Levin et al. 1993)

Physiologic benefits		Benefits to society
Humans	Reductions in:	• Higher work output
	• Mental deficiency	• Reduced costs of medical and custodial care
	• Deafmutism	• Reduced educational costs (because of less absenteeism and grade repetition)
	• Spastic diplegia	
	• Squint	
	• Dwarfism	
	• Motor deficiency	
	• Goitre	
	• Birth defects	
Livestock	Increases in:	Higher output of meat and other animal products and hence:
	• Live births	• Profits
	• Weight and meat yield	• Higher work output of animals
	• Strength for work	
	• Health (less deformity)	
	• Wool coat in sheep	

Beneficial effects of iodine supplementation. Important are the effects for society as well. Noteworthy is the beneficial effect on the livestock; certainly in developing countries an important additional effect if supplementation is extended to livestock.

deficiency there are several up- and downregulating mechanisms. By increasing selenodeiodinase proteins in the brain it is, at least in the earlier stage, relatively protected from the lower T4 production (Obregon et al. 2005).

However, in the last few years it has become clear that other deiodinase proteins play an important role in the deiodination of diiodotyrosine (DIT) and monoiodotyrosine (MIT). These iodotyrosine dehalogenases (DEHAL1) have been studied only in relation to the deiodination of MIT and DIT in the thyroid. However, several studies show that their presence is not limited to the thyroid but can be found in human kidney, trachea, liver, and colon. The enzymatic deiodination is a reductive process leading to the formation of iodine and tyrosine, increasing both levels. Tyrosine itself is a known inhibitor of the process (Gnidehou et al. 2004). Since the research on the expression of the DEHAL1 in several tissues is very young it cannot be excluded that DEHAL1 is expressed in the (developing) brain. During metamorphosis in frogs, the presence of the DEHAL1 has been described in the olfactory epithelium, the nucleus infundibularis ventralis, the ventricular lining, cerebellum, in the pituitary gland, and in the mucus glands of skin (Gaupale et al. 2009). The same expression could be possible in the developing fetus. Neither studies on the effects of iodine deficiency on the expression of the gene, nor studies on the influence of iodine deficiency on the activity of the enzyme itself have been performed.

By this two-step deiodination, not only 3-iodothyronamines are formed but delivery of iodine and tyrosine into the tissues is provided as well. It is known that tyrosine is the precursor of dopamine and adrenalin, both highly important in the development and metabolism of the brain. Thyroid hormones may therefore be seen as a targeted on-demand system for catecholamine metabolism by increasing their release and also by providing the precursor itself.

152.2.3 Sodium Iodine Symporter (NIS)

In the last 10 years much research has been done on iodine uptake. The presence of the NIS was revealed in 1996. Since its discovery, many researches have been performed, predominantly related to medication development. Some interesting observations have been made. First of all, the distribution pattern of the NIS reveals that NIS is not located in the brain. Most of the NIS is present in tissues that have a direct contact to the outside world, such as the skin, salivary glands, and the stomach (Levy et al. 1998; Riesco-Eizaguirre and Santisteban 2006). Given the known interaction between bacteria and viruses and iodine it could provide a first line of defense against microorganisms. It is unlikely that the NIS is not present in the brain given the dependency of the development of the brain on iodine. Moreover, iodine uptake has been demonstrated in the ventricle system and choroid plexus, although the precise effect on the concentration of iodine in the cerebrospinal fluid and the brain tissues has not been studied thus far (Welch 1962). It could mean we have to look at the role of iodine from another perspective. By looking at iodine from a thyroid point of view we neglect the role of iodine uptake in the choroid plexus, but also the possible role of tyrosine and 3-iodothyronamines.

The NIS has also been located in the kidney, in Henle's loop. Even more important is the fact that the uptake of iodine in the kidney is dependent on the plasma sodium concentration (Spitzweg et al. 2001) (Fig. 152.1). Furthermore, the NIS could be blocked by thiocyanate and perchlorate (Fig. 152.2), the first present in cigarettes (Sande van et al. 2003; Groef de et al. 2006). This could mean that in case of strict sodium restriction or presence of per- or thiocyanate, iodine reabsorption could be impaired, leading to a high iodine excretion in the urine, but to a low presence in the body. This has implications for the availability of iodine during pregnancy and the development of the child in the smoking mother. Smoking is

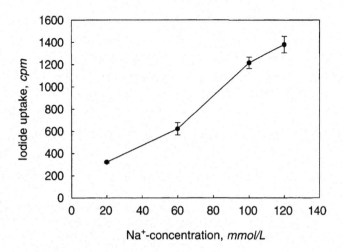

Fig. 152.1 Sodium dependency of iodide uptake by human kidney cells. Sodium dependency of iodide uptake by human kidney cells. Optimal iodide uptake is related to higher sodium levels in the kidney. The relationship with sodium restriction diets has not been investigated thus far, but could attribute to iodine deficiency (From Spitzweg et al. 2001)

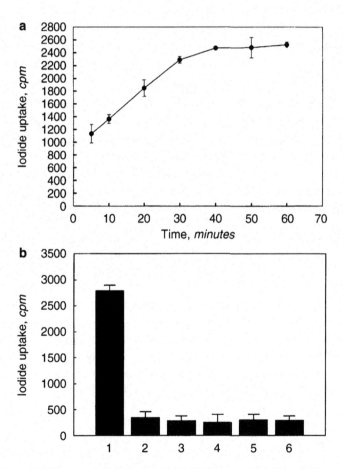

Fig. 152.2 Time course of iodine uptake by kidney cells and influence of perchlorate. Figure a shows that iodide uptake by human kidney cells is rapid and reaches maximum levels after 40 min. This is in line with the rapid iodide uptake in the stomach. Perchlorate inhibits iodide uptake by a factor of eight as can be seen in figure b. Lane 1 is normal uptake by kidney cells, lane 2 represents the same kidney cells incubated with 10 μmol/L perchlorate. Lane 3–6 are control cell lines known not to be able to take up iodine. This observation is in line with another study, which shows a similar inhibitory pattern in case of thiocyanate, abundantly present in cigarettes (From Spitzweg et al. 2001)

known to increase stillbirths, slower fetal growth, and infertility and could have a negative effect on intelligence capabilities. It may be hypothesized that these effects can be deduced to iodine deficiency.

152.2.4 Keypoints of Iodine Uptake by Sodium Iodide Symporter

- Iodine uptake takes place by the NIS. Its presence is not limited to the thyroid but widely distributed throughout the body.
- This observation should lead to reconsidering the recommended daily allowances (RDA), a line of thought consistent with the grounds to change the vitamin D RDA.
- Iodine uptake is negatively influenced by low sodium concentration, perchlorate, and thiocyanate. Because thiocyanate is present in cigarettes, smokers are more at risk for iodine deficiency.

152.3 Iodine and Diseases

152.3.1 Cretinism

The most dramatic effect of iodine repletion is the disappearance of cretinism and the neurological impairments in severe iodine deficiency. Before the introduction of iodine it was considered to be a disease without understanding of the mechanism. Even today the role of iodine in the development of cretinism is not fully explained. Most research concerns the measurable changes in behavior or development but not the unraveling of the mechanism itself.

The clinical manifestation depends on the degree of iodine deficiency and varies widely. Early clinical recognition is made by subnormal temperature, slow heart rate, wide fontanelles, dwarfism, and submature and sluggish behavior. Other signs include slow dentition, slow reaction time, constipation, dystonia, thick tongue and skin, and a delay in sexual development.

One of the most striking pathophysiological discrepancies is the fact that in observed cretinism there is no difference in urinary iodine excretion when compared to individuals in the same region. Moreover, a clear relationship between mental retardation and thyroid hormone levels does not seem to be present.

In the previous century some aspects of the mechanisms involved in iodine deficiency have become more apparent. In case of iodine deficiency, selenodeiodinase enzymes in the brain are upregulated, and the brain is protected against the lower production of thyroxin. The fetus is protected by upregulation of the NIS in the placenta and thus the embryo is protected at the cost of the mother. After birth too the child is protected by upregulation of the NIS in the breast in case of breastfeeding. Of course this protection is not present in the case of baby formula being used.

So it could be possible that other factors are contributing to the development of cretinism. As mentioned above, with thyroxin, tyrosine and 3-iodothyronamine are also delivered to the brain. In the process of dopamine formation out of tyrosine, tyrosine hydroxylase (TH) is the most rate-limiting step. Its activity is upregulated by vitamin D and vitamin A (Puchacz et al. 1996; Jeong et al. 2006; Gelain et al. 2007). In research we have to take other known cofactors into account, especially if it concerns widespread deficiencies, such as that of vitamin D.

If tyrosine is influencing the development of cretinism and neurological deterioration there should be clinical overlap with tyrosine–dopamine-related deficiency disorders.

152.3.2 Attention Deficit Hyperactivity Disorder (ADHD)

Recently, Vermiglio et al. showed that mothers with iodine deficiency had a greater chance that their offspring would get ADHD (Vermiglio et al. 2004). Given the fact that during pregnancy there is an upregulation of the NIS in the placenta, it is logical to suppose that the child is protected from the mother's deficiency. It would also mean that the mother will become more deficient post partum. Not only the child's iodine but also the recirculating iodine pool from the child will vanish. Given the child's protection for iodine deficiency by the upregulating NIS it is more logical to suppose that the real ADHD development takes place after birth at the moment the child starts to eat the same (iodine deficient) food the whole family takes. Just as was the case with cretinism, it is highly questionable if syndromes like ADHD have a genetic base or are just micronutrient (and thereby family) related, with the highest impact during childhood and adolescence.

It is known that iodine deficiency leads to less development of intelligence capabilities. Given the reports it could mean a decrease of IQ of 10–15 points (Bautista et al. 1982; Tiwari et al. 1996; Briel van den et al. 2000; Andersson et al. 2007). Even more important are the observed changes in social behavior (Table 152.3). Several studies point out that iodine repletion leads to a more social behavior, higher working capacity. and higher initiative level (Tiwari et al. 1996; Briel van den et al. 2000; Andersson et al. 2007).

152.4 The Role of Iodine in Brain Metabolism

Despite the fact that much literature does not concern the physiological mechanism itself we now try to explain the role of iodine. One should realize that some parts are hypothetical.

Iodine is known to be a potent antioxidant (Polley 1971; Kupper et al. 2008). It is the most simple antioxidant compared to the vitamins we know. It finds its way into the brain mostly by T4, but also by iodine uptake in the choroid plexus. Given the fact that the thyroid increases the production of T3 during iodine deficiency at the cost of T4 it means a lower iodine influx in the brain. This lower influx is counteracted by increasing the selenodeiodinase proteins.

As pointed out above, the role of iodine on the brain has thus far been discussed from the thyroid hormone perspective. It is difficult to distinguish between effects of iodine and the thyroid hormone and between thyroid hormone and tyrosine effects. In this respect, it is impossible to unravel the underlying physiological processes that account for the beneficial effects of iodine and/or tyrosine or thyroid hormones.

152.4.1 Tyrosine Effects

Studying the role of the thyroid hormone one must account for the effects of its deiodinization metabolites, iodine, 3-iodothyronamine, and tyrosine. In earlier days, thyroid hormone was, at least in part, considered a tyrosine delivery hormone. However, the idea was finally rejected based on the observation that tyrosine was widely available in the proteins present in all tissues.

It can be questioned whether that rejection was evidence-based. The fact that tyrosine is available in proteins does not have to mean that there is no need for a second delivery system. It can be even quite advantageous to have a second system, especially as we know that tyrosine is the precursor of dopamine and (nor) adrenaline. These are short-lived monoamines that have to be instantly available on several demands from several tissues. So next to a basal slowly adapting system provided for by proteins, which cannot react to individual tissue demands, it could be very ingenious to have a second swift acting system.

In this respect, it is known that the deiodination time for T4 is longer than for T3. This could explain the greater metabolic effects of T3 compared to T4. Second, the system is a post translation system and thereby a quickly adapting system. Third, by having several deiodination products, there is a buffer level within the cells, all with their own deiodination response times. T4 is slower deiodinated than T3, which in turn is slower deiodinated than DIT, which at its turn is slower deiodinated than MIT. It is even known that these products themselves can influence the thyroid-stimulating hormone (TSH) and TH (Nakano and Danowski 1959; Lutsky and Zenker 1968; Groot de and Jaksina 1969). In this way, there is an intelligent regulating system, which is not only regulated by T4 or T3 but also by its other metabolic products, next to the effectors themselves such as dopamine and adrenaline. The final metabolic reaction will depend on the total product of stimulatory and inhibitory signals.

There are not many publications about the role of tyrosine and the development of the brain. However, as being the precursor of dopamine and the amino acid thyroid hormones are made of, it could play a crucial role in brain development.

152.4.2 Tetrahydrobiopterin Deficiency

Tetrahydrobiopterin (BH4) is a crucial cofactor in the biosynthesis of catecholamines. It is encoded by the 6-pyruvoyltetrahydropterin (Pts) synthase gene. Pts knockout mice die after birth, although they develop with normal morphology in utero. However, when the mice are fed BH4, L-Dopa, and 5-hydroxyptryptophan, they survive. The mice were sacrificed and studied at 6 weeks. Qualitative characteristics showed dwarf mice with reduced activity, dystonia, tremor, no signs of sexual maturation, hair loss, and hypothermia (Elzaouk et al. 2003). These characteristics show great overlap with the clinical features of cretinism and interestingly develop after birth. Chemical analysis showed normal serotonin and phenylalanine levels as well as normal nitric oxide synthase activity in the brain. However, the dopamine levels in the brain appeared to be only 3% of normal.

152.4.3 Tyrosine Hydroxylase Deficiency

TH is a rate-limiting enzyme involved in the synthesis of dopamine out of tyrosine. TH deficiency is a relatively rare disorder, with the severest form called infantile parkinsonism, which is mostly related to an insufficient dopamine metabolism. In the case of enzyme deficiency, the development of the syndrome is faster than in the case of a nutrient-related insufficiency, because of the compensating mechanisms occurring in the latter. Clinical symptoms of TH deficiency are lack of motion, dystonia, irritability, lack of speaking development, decreased intellectual development, low body temperature, and constipation (Eiduson 1971; Eisenhofer et al. 2003; Giovanniello et al. 2007). As with cretinism, the clinical presentation can vary greatly but there is some striking overlap with the clinical pattern of cretinism.

Given the fact that TH plays a crucial role in dopamine and adrenaline synthesis, the factors that are known to influence this enzyme have to be taken into account if we study the effects of iodine deficiency on brain development. Vitamin D is known to increase TH and vitamin D deficiency is widespread. It therefore could negatively affect the fetus if the mother is severely vitamin D deficient. Of course it will also have a negative effect on the development of the child after birth although most countries advice vitamin D supplementation, but only until the third year. Given the new insights in vitamin D, optimal levels of vitamin D supplementation are a point of discussion nowadays (Puchacz et al. 1996; Holick 2007).

152.5 Micronutrients Contributing to Iodine Deficiency

In short, the interactions between the nutrients known for their role in the iodine–tyrosine metabolism have to be mentioned. Even the earliest study on iodine and goiter by Marine et al. showed only a 60% positive effect. In those days, other nutritional influences were not known, but might account for the 40% nonresponders. The role of those other nutrients follows in brief.

Iron is crucial in the forming and functioning of peroxidases, in this case thyroid peroxidase. Thyroid peroxidase is crucial for the iodination of tyrosine (Zimmermann and Kohrle 2002).

Vitamin A is known to play an important role in the uptake of iodine by the NIS. It is known to be capable of increasing this uptake (Schmutzler 2001; Zimmermann et al. 2007).

Selenium is necessary for the formation and functioning of selenodeiodinase, which is essential for the deiodination of the thyroid hormones. It is advised not to start supplementation of selenium in case of iodine deficiency, since it can worsen or cause hypothyroidism. Nevertheless, it is widely used, not only in reform stores but also in the animal food industry. This could be harmful and give rise to increasing thyroid problems in countries with iodine deficiency. But even in countries considered to be iodine sufficient a negative effect can be expected since a median urinary iodine excretion of 100 microgram per liter could still mean a large proportion of the population being iodine deficient (Zimmermann et al. 2008).

Finally, tyrosine itself is essential for an optimal metabolism, being the precursor of catecholamines and crucial for thyroid hormone synthesis. Several studies mention the relationship between tyrosine levels and thyroid functioning (Melmon et al. 1964; Malamos et al. 1966; Tahara et al. 1988). Optimal nutrition levels are not known.

Also, vitamin D could influence thyroid functioning. Although not widely studied, a few studies showed an interaction between vitamin D and thyroid hormones levels (Zofkova et al. 1981; Smith et al. 1989). The exact mechanism is unknown but could be related to the influence of vitamin D on TH. However, other influencing factors such as deiodinase upregulation should be studied.

In conclusion, it is clear that in our search for an optimal iodine-related metabolism all known other factors have to be taken into account as well (Verheesen and Schweitzer 2009).

152.5.1 Keypoints of Tyrosine Metabolism in Relation to Diseases

- Mono- and diiodotyrosine are reduced by iodotyrosine dehalogenases to iodine and tyrosine. Iodotyrosine dehalogenases are widely distributed. In developing frogs they are upregulated in the brain. Other animals have not been investigated.
- Dopamine deficiency diseases are related to a clinical picture with great similarity to cretinism.

- ADHD is treated with dopamine increasing medication. Instead of increasing dopamine by block-ing its conversion, deficiency of nutrients such as iodine, tyrosine, and vitamin D leading to lower dopamine production capabilities should be investigated.

152.6 Alternative Solutions to Fight Iodine Deficiency

More than 90 years after the discovery of iodine as an essential mineral in the prevention of cretinism and hypothyroidism, 2 billion people still suffer from iodine deficiency. It is hard to believe that the strategy followed thus far will finally lead to eradication of iodine deficiency, especially if we take into account the numerous programs that have been implemented and billions of dollars that have been spent in the last decades.

Given the fact that iodine is naturally taken up by animals and plants it would be logical to increase iodine content in the soil (Steinnes 2009). Thereby it enters the natural food chain and increases the recirculation of iodine. This could lead to various profitable effects.

First, it is a far more natural way to provide enough iodine in the food chain and we are no longer dependent on one single iodine source, as in iodized salt. This single route prevention strategy is very vulnerable and depends largely on diet choices and requires a continuous very active policy. When the complete food chain is soaked with iodine many alternatives are present even when people choose to eat a very invariable diet.

Second, it has been proven that organic selenium gives rise to fewer side effects than inor-ganic selenium and that inorganic selenium can easily be transformed into organic selenium by plants (Broadley et al. 2006). The same phenomenon could be true for iodine. Iodine is organi-cally bound to tyrosine, its natural partner, as is the case of iodine in seaweed. Deiodinase activ-ity has to be present to release this bounded iodine. Furthermore, the conversion of MIT and DIT into tyrosine and iodine is inhibited by the product tyrosine itself (Gnidehou et al. 2004),thereby reducing overdose and side effects. On the other hand, the presence of thyroid antibodies could very well be related to other contributing micronutrients, especially selenium deficiency (Xu et al. 2006; Duntas 2008). Before addressing iodine as the main cause of side effects, other factors have to be taken into account and need further investigation. In this respect, organic iodine in the form of iodotyrosine or diiodotyrosine could also be an attractive bio-marker for individual longstanding iodine status, since it represents net iodine uptake. Measuring iodotyrosine or diiodotyrosine means that factors negatively influencing iodine uptake by the NIS have been taken into account. This is in contrast to the situation where iodine excretion in the urine is established.

Despite several reports from the WHO about increasing iodine deficiency levels, especially in developed countries, politics either do not or are slow in responding. Most countries do not follow the advice of the WHO concerning iodine supplementation in case of pregnancy and breastfeeding. Even recent advice reports from health care government agencies do not include this 6-year-old WHO directive (Health Council of the Netherlands 2008). Moreover, these countries also do not implement the directives on monitoring iodine supplementation. The case becomes worse if we are aware of the limitations of the population indicator used to define iodine sufficiency. Although some countries are regarded as iodine sufficient, up to 50% of their population can, in fact, be regarded as iodine insufficient (Zimmermann et al. 2008; Verheesen and Schweitzer 2008). However, most of these countries interpret sufficient as no deficiency at all and are not motivated to erase iodine defi-ciency completely. A better way to present deficiency data is by showing prevalence figures, even if they are estimated statistically. For instance, 10% of a population being deficient sounds like a good achievement, but if it means that still 27 million people are suffering from iodine deficiency (USA) it sounds like work needs to be done (Benoist de et al. 2004).

In this chapter, we chose to look at iodine and the brain from an unconventional point of view. By doing this we might find new solutions for old unresolved problems and physiological and medical questions. By studying how to nurture nature we could find a way to prevent or even change the course of diseases and syndromes without changing nature itself, and without gene therapy or by medication alone.

152.6.1 Keypoints of Alternative Strategies on Solving Iodine Deficiency

- Given the large number of children affected, the pregnancy and lactation supplementation directive from WHO should be implemented by all countries who signed the United Nations-sponsored "Declaration for the Survival, Protection and Development of Children" in 1990, before 2012.
- New iodine supplementation strategies must be considered, such as enrichment of soil.
- Iodotyrosine or diiodotyrosine could be attractive biomarkers for the individual longstanding iodine status.

152.7 Application to Other Areas of Health and Disease

Deficiencies are, even in developed countries, still widespread. History has taught us that solving severe deficiency leads to solving diseases that were thought to be heritable and untreatable, like cretinism. It showed us that genetic polymorphism is not to be blamed for diseases but environmental factors are the cause. Also mild deficiency will lead to related health problems, although not as obvious as in severe deficiencies. Iodine deficiency is by far the most widespread deficiency worldwide. It will lead to unbalanced thyroid metabolism, which theoretically, depending on the genetic polymorphism, can cause related health problems such as hypercholesterolemia, heart disease, infertility, depression, and health problems related to a disturbed tyrosine or iodine metabolism. Before changing the genetic blueprint we have to study the influence of nutrients on the expression of genes and finally diseases.

152.8 Conclusions

Based on the literature available on the role of iodine and tyrosine on the development and metabolism of the brain, several conclusions can be drawn, although some could be seen as hypothetical until more specific research on the topic is undertaken.

It is remarkable that in the case of the Pts knockout mice, the development of the fetus in utero is normal and problems begin only after birth. It could be assumed that during pregnancy the maternal delivery of catecholamines and iodine is more essential than the producing possibilities of the fetus. This could have consequences for the way we look at iodine deficiency disorders and their development. In contrast to the assumption nowadays, developmental problems could occur mainly after birth.

As with the knockout mice this could mean that the developmental disorders could very well be reduced by providing adequate levels of the required tyrosine, iodine or thyroxin. This is in line with

Table 152.4 Proportion of population, and number of estimated individuals with insufficient iodine intake in school-age children (6–12 years) and in the general population (all are groups) in Europe,[a] 2004

Insufficient iodine intake (UI <100 mg/l)			
School-age children		General population	
Prevalence (%)[a]	Total number (millions)[b]	Prevalence (%)[a]	Total number (millions)[b]
47.8	24.9	46.1	272

[a]Based on data from 40 countries

[b]Based on population estimates in the year 2002

the observations that iodine supplementation can improve the deteriorated intelligence and social behavior because of iodine deficiency. Furthermore, it is in line with the observation of the upregulated NIS in the placenta and in the breast feeding breast, the first one to prevent fetal deficiency at the cost of the mother, the second to provide optimal iodine nutrition after birth, again at the cost of the mother.

In the case of ADHD, the most effective medicine is methylphenidate. As stated, it is known to increase dopamine levels in the brain. Instead of focusing on ways to increase dopamine levels by blocking its degradation, one should focus on the possibility that essential elements in the synthesis of dopamine are lacking. Several micronutrients need to be investigated. Given the widely distributed deficiency, iodine is the most important one to investigate. In addition, the following also have to be investigated: tyrosine as being the precursor, vitamin D as being a stimulator of TH, tetrahydrobiopterin as being the cofactor for biosynthesis, vitamin A as being a second stimulator of TH, and selenium as being essential for the deiodination of thyroxin by selenodeiodinases. Since studies never focus on these specific micronutrients, no literature is available on the presence of deficiencies, let alone combinations of even very mild deficiencies that could become more relevant because of their combined existence (Verheesen and Schweitzer 2009).

The sodium symporter in the brain has not been studied, so no data are available on its presence in the various parts of the brain. Furthermore, no data are available on the effects of iodine deficiency at the NIS level. We know, however, that the distribution of the selenodeiodinases differs significantly throughout the body.

Finally, the most important concern is the fact that today iodine deficiency is still widespread. The fact that countries are characterized as developed does not guarantee that iodine deficiency has been solved, as the latest report on Europe shows (Table 152.4). Governments not only need to sign declarations, but need to execute them with the greatest efforts possible. Given the few experts involved in specific deficiencies, governments need to be willing to request for expertise from the WHO or International Council for the Control of Iodine Deficiency (ICCIDD) when they formulate and publish national guidelines. An authorization for the guidelines by the very few experts in cooperation with the leading authorities like the WHO or ICCIDD would be even more preferable. Unfortunately, national politics are very protective and have not reached that level of openness yet.

By studying the effect of iodine on the development and metabolism of the brain only as part of the thyroid hormone we could very well be missing the real effectors, tyrosine and iodine. In addition, interacting nutritional factors could be missed and not studied in relationship to each other.

Summary Points

- Iodine deficiency is the most widespread micronutrient deficiency worldwide since 1918, with 2 billion people affected anno 2007.
- To make governments better aware of the extent of the problem, the estimated number of individuals affected should be the first priority and not the overall classification based on the median urinary iodine excretion.
- Europe has the largest proportion of people affected of all WHO regions; South East Asia has the highest absolute number of individuals affected of all WHO regions.
- A biomarker for the longstanding individual iodine status is crucial to present solid prevalence data. Iodo- or diiodotyrosine could be attractive candidates since they represent the iodine level after uptake by the NIS.
- In our understanding of the physiological mechanisms of iodine deficiency, other micronutrients have to be taken into account. Most relevant nutrients are vitamin A, selenium, tyrosine, and vitamin D.
- To eliminate iodine deficiency after 90 years it is important to search for other strategies. The most logical strategy is to enrich the soil with iodine.
- To understand the side effects of iodine other contributors, especially selenium, need to be investigated since it is known for lowering thyroid peroxidase antibodies.

Explanation of Key Terms

Iodine: Member of the halogens, soluble in water, with the greatest concentrations in seawater. Seaweed and some plants are known for their high uptake of iodine.

Iodine deficiency: Iodine deficiency is characterized by a median urinary iodine excretion less than 100 microgram per liter. Goiter and elevated TSH should be regarded as a sign for longstanding inadequate iodine intake.

Deiodination: Deiodinaton of thyroid hormones is regulated by three selenodeiodinase isoforms. Deiodination of mono- and diiodotyrosine takes place by iodotyrosine dehalogenase, which is upregulated in the brain of developing frogs. In humans, selenodeiodinase and iodotyrosine dehalogenase are widely distributed.

Cretinism: Cretinism is the most severe clinical feature of iodine deficiency or congenital hypothyroidism. It leads to seriously impaired physical growth and mental development.

Sodium Iodide Symporter: The sodium iodide symporter is widely distributed throughout the body and not limited to the thyroid. In pregnancy and lactation, it is upregulated in the uterus and breasts. Iodine uptake is inhibited by perchlorate and thiocynate, next to the other halogens, bromide, and fluoride.

References

Andersson M, Benoist de B, Darnton-Hill I, Delange F. Iodine deficiency in Europe: a continuing public health problem. Geneva: World Health Organisation; 2007.

Bautista A, Barker PA, Dunn JT, Sanchez M, Kaiser DL. Am J Clin Nutr. 1982;35:127–34.

Beckett GJ, Arthur JR. J Endocrinol. 2005;184:455–65.

Benoist de B, Andersson M, Egli I, Takkouche B, Allen H. Iodine status worldwide: WHO Global Database on Iodine Deficiency. Geneva: World Health Organisation; 2004.

Briel van den T, West CE, Bleichrodt N, Vijver van de F, Ategbo EA, Hautvast JG. Am J Clin Nutr. 2000;72:1179–85.
Broadley MR, White PJ, Bryson RJ, Meacham MC, Bowen HC, Johnson SE, Hawkesford MJ, McGrath SP, Zhao FJ, Breward N, Harriman M, Tucker M. P Nutr Soc. 2006;65:169–81.
Duntas LH. Nat Clin Pract Endoc. 2008;4:454–60.
Eiduson S. UCLA Forum Med Sci. 1971;14:391–418.
Eisenhofer G, Tian H, Holmes C, Matsunaga J, Roffler-Tarlov S, Hearing VJ. FASEB J. 2003;17:1248–55.
Elzaouk L, Leimbacher W, Turri M, Ledermann B, Burki K, Blau N, Thony B. J Biol Chem. 2003;278:28303–11.
Gaupale TC, Mathi AA, Ravikumar A, Bhargava SY. Ann NY Acad Sci. 2009;1163:402–6.
Gelain DP, Moreira JC, Bevilaqua LR, Dickson PW, Dunkley PR. J Neurochem. 2007;103:2369–79.
Giovanniello T, Leuzzi V, Carducci C, Carducci C, Sabato ML, Artiola C, Santagata S, Pozzessere S, Antonozzi I. Neuropediatrics. 2007;38:213–5.
Gnidehou S, Caillou B, Talbot M, Ohayon R, Kaniewski J, Noel-Hudson MS, Morand S, Agnangji D, Sezan A, Courtin F, Virion A, Dupuy C. FASEB J. 2004;18:1574–6.
Groef de B, Decallonne BR, Geyten van der S, Darras VM, Bouillon R. Eur J Endocrinol. 2006;155:17–25.
Groot de LJ, Jaksina S. J Lab Clin Med. 1969;74:257–64.
Health Council of the Netherlands. Towards maintaining an optimal iodine intake. The Hague: Health Council of the Netherlands; 2008.
Hetzel B. Lancet. 1983;2:1126–9.
Hetzel B, Maberly G. In: Mertz C, editor. Trace elements in human and animal nutrition. New York: Academic Press; 1986. p. 139–208.
Holick MF. N Engl J Med. 2007;357:266–81.
Jeong H, Kim MS, Kim SW, Kim KS, Seol W. J Neurochem. 2006;98:386–94.
Kohrle J. Thyroid. 2005;15:841–53.
Kupper FC, Carpenter LJ, McFiggans GB, Palmer CJ, Waite TJ, Boneberg EM, Woitsch S, Weiller M, Abela R, Grolimund D, Potin P, Butler A, Luther GW, III, Kroneck PM, Meyer-Klaucke W, Feiters MC. Proc Natl Acad Sci USA. 2008;105:6954–8.
Kvicala J, Zamrazil V. Cent Eur J Public Health. 2003;11:107–13.
Laurberg P, Nohr SB, Pedersen KM, Hreidarsson AB, Andersen S, Bulow P, I, Knudsen N, Perrild H, Jorgensen T, Ovesen L. Thyroid. 2000;10:951–63.
Levin HM. In: Hetzel B, Dunn J, Stanbury J, editors. The prevention and control of iodine deficiency disorders. New York: Elsevier; 1987. p. 195–208.
Levin H, Pollitt E, Galloway R, McGuire J. In: Jamison D, editor. Disease control priorities in developing countries. New York: Oxford University Press; 1993. p. 421–451.
Levy O, Vieja de la V, Carrasco N. J Bioenerg Biomembr. 1998;30:195–206.
Lutsky BN, Zenker N. J Med Chem. 1968;11:1241–2.
Malamos B, Miras CJ, Karli-Samouilidou JN, Koutras DA. J Endocrinol. 1966;35:223–8.
Marine D, Kimball OP. J Lab Clin Med. 1990;115:128–36.
Melmon K, Rivlin R, Oates J, Sjoerdsma A. J Clin Endocr Metab. 1964;24:691–8.
Nakano M, Danowski T. Endocrinology. 1959;65:889–901.
Obregon MJ, Escobar del Rey F, Morreale de Escobar G. Thyroid. 2005;15:917–29.
Polley MJ. J Immunol. 1971;107:1493–5.
Puchacz E, Stumpf WE, Stachowiak EK, Stachowiak MK. Brain Res. 1996;36:193–6.
Riesco-Eizaguirre G, Santisteban P. Eur J Endocrinol. 2006;155:495–512.
Sande van J, Massart C, Beauwens R, Schoutens A, Costagliola S, Dumont JE, Wolff J. Endocrinology. 2003;144: 247–52.
Scanlan TS. Endocrinology. 2009;150:1108–11.
Scanlan TS, Suchland KL, Hart ME, Chiellini G, Huang Y, Kruzich PJ, Frascarelli S, Crossley DA, Bunzow JR, Ronca-Testoni S, Lin ET, Hatton D, Zucchi R, Grandy DK. Nat Med. 2004;10:638–42.
Schmutzler C. Exp Clin Endocr Diab. 2001;109:41–4.
Smith MA, McHenry C, Oslapas R, Hofmann C, Hessel P, Paloyan E. Surgery. 1989;106:987–91.
Spitzweg C, Dutton CM, Castro MR, Bergert ER, Goellner JR, Heufelder AE, Morris JC. Kidney Int. 2001;59: 1013–23.
Stanbury JB, Ermans AE, Bourdoux P, Todd C, Oken E, Tonglet R, Vidor G, Braverman LE, Medeiros-Neto G. Thyroid. 1998;8:83–100.
Steinnes E. Environ Geochem Health. 2009;31:523–35.
Tahara Y, Hirota M, Shima K, Kozu S, Ikegami H, Tanaka A, Kumahara Y, Amino N, Hayashizaki S, Miyai K. Metabolism. 1988;37:9–14.
Tiwari BD, Godbole MM, Chattopadhyay N, Mandal A, Mithal A. Am J Clin Nutr. 1996;63:782–6.
Verheesen RH, Schweitzer CM. Med Hypotheses. 2008;71:645–8.

Verheesen RH, Schweitzer CM Med Hypotheses. 2009;73:498–502.

Vermiglio F, Lo P, V, Moleti M, Sidoti M, Tortorella G, Scaffidi G, Castagna MG, Mattina F, Violi MA, Crisa A, Artemisia A, Trimarchi F. J Clin Endocr Metab. 2004;89:6054–60.

Welch K. Am J Physiol. 1962;202:757–60.

Xu J, Yang XF, Guo HL, Hou XH, Liu LG, Sun XF. Biol Trace Elem Res. 2006;111:229–38.

Zimmermann MB, Jooste PL, Mabapa NS, Schoeman S, Biebinger R, Mushaphi LF, Mbhenyane X. Am J Clin Nutr. 2007;86:1040–4.

Zimmermann MB, Jooste PL, Pandav CS. Lancet. 2008;372:1251–62.

Zimmermann MB, Kohrle J. Thyroid. 2002;12:867–78.

Zofkova I, Blahos J, Bednar J. Endokrinologie. 1981;78:118–20.

Chapter 153
Riboflavin Deficiency, Brain Function, and Health

Rita Sinigaglia-Coimbra, Antonio Carlos Lopes, and Cicero G. Coimbra

Abbreviations

BBB	Brain-blood barrier
BH4	Tetrahydrobiopterin
CADCase/CSADCase	Cysteine and sulfinic acid decarboxylase
CBS	Cystathionine β-synthase
cGMP	Cyclic guanosine monophosphate
CL	Cystathionine-γ-lyase, or cystathionase
CNS	Central nervous system
CO	Carbon monoxide
CSF	Cerebrospinal fluid
EGRAC	Erythrocyte glutathione reductase activation coefficient
eNOS	Endothelial nitric oxide synthase
FAD	Flavin adenine dinucleotide
FMN	Flavin mononucleotide
GABA	γ-aminobutyric acid
GAD	Glutamic acid decarboxylase
γ-GCS	γ-glutamylcysteine synthetase
GMP	Guanosine monophosphate
GR	Glutathione reductase
GSH	Reduced glutathione
GSSG	Oxidized glutathione
GSTs	Glutathione S-transferases
H_2S	Hydrogen sulphide
HO	Heme oxygenase
HPLC	High-performance liquid chromatography
iNOS	Inducible nitric oxide synthase
MADD	Multiple acyl coenzyme A dehydrogenase deficiency
MPTP	1-methyl-4-phenyl-1,2,3,6-tetrahydropyridine
MS	Methionine synthase

C.G. Coimbra (✉)
Laboratory of Clinical and Experimental Pathophysiology, Department of Neurology and Neurosurgery,
Federal University of São Paulo (UNIFESP), São Paulo SP BRAZIL
e-mail: coimbracg.nexp@epm.br

V.R. Preedy et al. (eds.), *Handbook of Behavior, Food and Nutrition*,
DOI 10.1007/978-0-387-92271-3_153, © Springer Science+Business Media, LLC 2011

MTHFR	Methylenetetrahydrofolate reductase
NADPH	Nicotinamide adenine dinucleotide phosphate
nNOS	Neuronal nitric oxide synthase
NO	Nitric oxide
NOS	Nitric oxide synthase
PD	Parkinson's disease
PLP	Pyridoxal-5′-phosphate
PPO	Pyridoxine(pyridoxamine)-5′-phosphate oxidase
Rbf	Riboflavin
SHMT	Hydroxymethyltransferase
VDR	Vitamin D receptor

153.1 Introduction

Vitamin B2 (Rbf) is an essential micronutrient playing a key role in energy production (Hendler and Rorvik 2008). The active forms FAD and FMN act as either coenzymes or prosthetic groups in a wide diversity of biochemical reactions. Rbf deficiency has been also related to developmental abnormalities, altered iron status (ferritin iron mobilization, iron absorption and loss), cancer, visual abnormalities, neurodegeneration, and high plasma homocysteine (Powers 2003).

Nevertheless, clinical and experimental evidence compiled in this chapter support the view that the significance of Rbf deficiency for the pathophysiology and treatment of human diseases (of CNS disorders in particular) has been largely underestimated. First, current views merely consider low vitamin B2 status as a component of multiple vitamin deficiencies associated with malnutrition related to either poverty or alcoholism, because Rbf and other vitamins of the B complex share similar food sources such as whole grains, leafy green vegetables, eggs, meat, and milk (Powers 2003). Allegedly, deficiency of vitamin B2 could not occur as an isolated nutritional disorder, and the clinical consequences of multiple nutrient deficiencies would inevitably veil the specific manifestations of restricted availability of Rbf active metabolites.

Second, such views neglect the epidemiological studies by Anderson and coworkers who provided direct evidence showing that a substantial part of the world population (10–15%) carries an inherited restriction of Rbf absorption. Such restricted absorption is only balanced with a relatively high dose of Rbf (Anderson et al. 1994) repeated three to four times a day to stabilize circulating levels within the normal range throughout the 24 h (Coimbra and Junqueira 2003), suggesting increased urinary loss due to limited tubular reabsorption of Rbf from glomerular filtrate. The fundamental importance of these findings for human pathologies has been long neglected, possibly for being initially confined to the literature related to the epidemiology of malaria, against which Rbf deficiency seems to provide resistance. The data reviewed here suggest that a critical pathophysiologic role for Rbf deficiency is clearly feasible and likely, and worth research attention, particularly due to immediate implications in the prevention and therapeutic control of a wide range of prevalent human disorders like Parkinson's disease, arterial hypertension, fetal malformation and spontaneous abortion, migraine, and the full range of autoimmune diseases.

Third, a single inherited polymorphic gene disturbing cellular uptake of Rbf could explain all data related to poor absorption at the proximal ileum, low transport into red blood cells, and reduced reabsorption by proximal tubules. Anderson and coworkers provided evidence showing that the highly prevalent low vitamin B2 status is genetically determined, and suggested a polymorphic flavokinase, which catalyzes the conversion of Rbf to FMN, as a possible inherited feature responsible for the impaired cellular uptake and trafficking of Rbf (Anderson et al. 1994). Regardless of whether or not Rbf phosphorylation is the metabolic step to blame, the polymorphic gene involved may simultaneously affect the homeostatic system reported by Spector (1980), which privileges the brain tissue with normal vitamin B2 concentrations during severe systemic deficiency. Due to the evident pathophysiologic relevance of disrupted Rbf homeostatic mechanisms in the CNS, neurologic disorders are particularly likely to develop in genetically affected individuals. Conversely, experimental attempts to replicate human neurologic disease requiring disruption of CNS mechanisms of vitamin B2 homeostasis by submitting genetically intact animals to dietary Rbf restriction may comprehensibly fail (DalPai et al. 2007).

Fourth, a wide range of metabolic pathways requires other essential micronutrients that are dependent on Rbf status, including vitamins B6 (PLP), B9 (folate), B12, and D3, which are similarly involved in numerous additional metabolic routes. Some other pathways (such as NO synthesis, HO activity, and the activity of the whole cytochrome P-450 enzyme superfamily) are doubly dependent on vitamin B2, for requiring both flavin active forms (FMN and FAD) for constant switching of critical heme enzymes to the reduced state. Furthermore, heme synthesis and degradation are also primarily or secondarily dependent on vitamin B2 status. The metabolic interdependency of these bioactive molecules significantly amplifies the spectrum of pathophysiologic phenomena potentially related to vitamin B2 deficiency, while creating direct and indirect pathways and positive feedback loops that further enhance several disease mechanisms.

153.2 Riboflavin and Its Bioactive Forms – FAD and FMN

Rbf is a water soluble light sensitive vitamin chemically named 7,8-dimethyl-10-(1′-d-ribityl-isoalloxazine), molecular formula: $C_{17}H_{20}N_4O_6$, and molecular weight: 376.4 Da (Hendler and Rorvik 2008). Originally isolated from milk in the ninth century by Wynter Blyth as a bright yellow pigment, Rbf was later recognized as a member of the vitamin B complex. Richard Kuhn in Heidelberg (1934) and Paul Karrer in Zurich (1935) almost concurrently succeeded in determining the chemical structure, and the name "riboflavin" was given to replace the variety of previous names. Soon after, Hugo Theorell (1937) and Otto Warburg and Walter Christian (1938) identified the two Rbf active forms, FMN and FAD, respectively (Massey 2000) (Fig. 153.1).

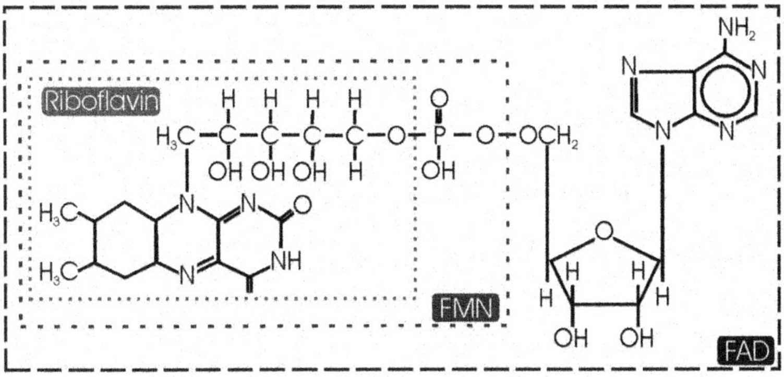

Fig. 153.1 Structure of riboflavin and its bioactive forms. Riboflavin, also known as vitamin B2, is the core of its bioactive forms – flavin mononucleotide (*FMN*) and flavin adenine dinucleotide (*FAD*). It contains a so-called "flavin ring system," an isoalloxazine ring methylated at the 7 and 8 positions, having also a d-ribityl moiety at the position 10. FMN is generated by phosphorilation at the 5′ position of ribityl group, and the addition of adenosine-5′-monophosphate yields the second bioactive form, the FAD.

153.3 Sources, Dietary Requirements, and Pharmacokinetics

Humans are not able to synthesize Rbf, and must thus obtain the vitamin from their diet. Dietary vitamin B2 is scarcely available as free Rbf, but rather mostly as FAD and FMN integrated into proteins (flavoproteins). The dietary sources of vitamin B2 are similar to those of other B vitamins. The main specific sources are milk and dairy products, which contribute to 51% of the overall intake in preschool children, 35% in schoolchildren, 27% in adults, and 36% in the elderly (Powers 2003). To a lesser extent, meat, green vegetables, and grains are also good sources of vitamin B2. UV light exposure is the most important factor impairing the bioavailability of vitamin B2 (Foraker et al. 2003).

The daily intake recommended by the World Health Organization varies from 0.3 mg for infants to 1.3 mg for adult males, being the highest requirements reserved for pregnant and lactating women (up to 1.6 mg/day). However, those recommendations do not take into account the possibility of hereditary malabsorption that may affect an average of 10–15% of the general population as suggested by Anderson and coworkers (1994), nor pathological conditions like celiac disease, malignancy or resection of the small bowel (WHO/FAO 2009). The maximal amount of Rbf that can be absorbed from a single dose is 27 mg (Zempleni 1996), which represents approximately 20 times the recommended daily dose. Therefore, humans tolerate large doses (multiple grams) given orally without toxicity – limited intestinal absorption affords protection at high intakes (Bates 1997).

The dietary bioactive forms of the vitamin (FMN and FAD) undergo hydrolysis to Rbf for absorption. Enterocytes at the proximal ileum can take up only free Rbf, which is rapidly absorbed (1.4–2.0 h) and further metabolized by specific enzymes. FAD-pyrophosphatase converts FAD to FMN, and FMN-phosphatase converts FMN to Rbf. Once within the intracellular compartment, Rbf accumulates in tissues after the resynthesis of FMN and FAD. Rbf flavokinase turns Rbf into FMN, and the enzyme FAD synthetase converts FMN to FAD (Rivlin and Pinto 2001). Intracellular FMN is either converted to FAD or integrated to flavoenzymes as a prosthetic group (covalent bounds), while FAD is mainly (covalently) incorporated into apo-flavoenzymes. Interestingly, thyroid and adrenal hormones regulate the consecutive conversions of Rbf to FMN and FMN to FAD, as well as the covalent binding of flavins to their apo-flavoenzymes (Zempleni et al. 1996).

Rbf absorption occurs through two distinct mechanisms: (1) active transport, which is dominant under low or physiologic concentrations of Rbf within the proximal ileum, and (2) passive diffusion, which becomes prominent at intraluminal Rbf concentrations above the physiological range. In addition, Ca^{++}/calmodulin, protein kinase A and G may regulate Rbf absorption (Foraker et al. 2003). The role of binding proteins in Rbf absorption and transport requires further investigation (Fig. 153.2). Several drugs (including psychotropic agents, antidepressants, chemotherapeutic and antimalarial medicines) may reduce Rbf absorption by impairing Rbf conversion into bioactive forms. It is worth noticing that all these drugs share structural similarities to Rbf. Alcohol may also impair Rbf utilization due to inhibition of both digestive and absorptive processes (Pinto et al. 1987).

Mammals have a variety of tissular and circulating Rbf binding-proteins, including albumin, immunoglobulins, and pregnancy-specific Rbf-binding proteins and Rbf kinase (White and Merril 1988), all of them endowed with high potential clinical significance. The literature has scarce information about Rbf homeostasis in the brain. Spector (1980) showed that Rbf rapidly crosses the rabbit BBB and accumulates in the brain tissue by a saturable system after phosphorylation. CSF Rbf either accumulates in brain cells or crosses the choroid plexus into the blood by a saturable, probenecid-sensitive mechanism. Rbf excretion is mainly renal, and several flavin metabolites are detectable in the urine (Zempleni et al. 1996). Further studies should address the identification of proteins

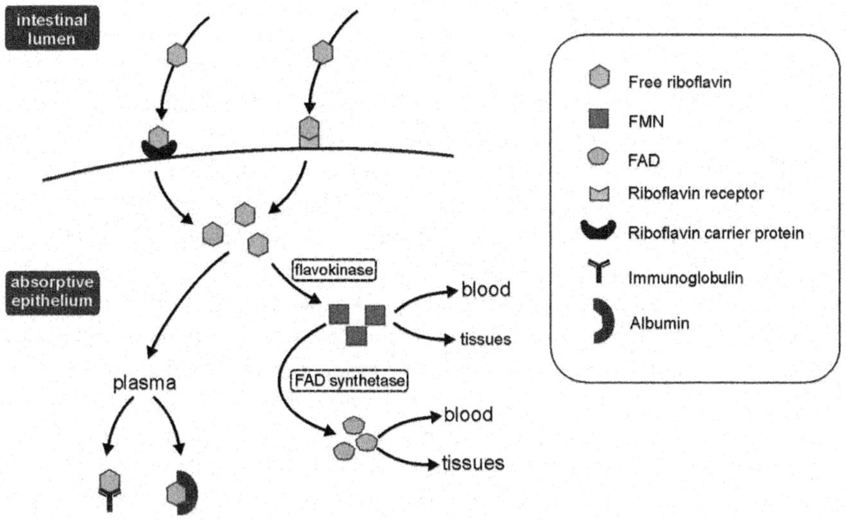

Fig. 153.2 Riboflavin absorption at the proximal ileum. Free riboflavin can be uptaken by either a receptor or a carrier protein. After uptake, riboflavin may have two possible fates: (**a**) phosphorylation to FMN by flavokinase, and then converted to FAD by FAD synthase, or (**b**) transportation to plasma. Note that small amounts of FMN may be found in blood and scarcely in tissues, while FAD is the most abundant bioactive form of vitamin B2 in blood and tissues. Part of free riboflavin is transported through the cell into the bloodstream in the unphosphorylated form, and then bound to riboflavin-binding proteins, such as albumin and immunoglobulins. *FMN* flavin mononucleotide, *FAD* flavin adenine dinucleotide

(and related gene polymorphisms) involved in uptake, trafficking, and cellular homeostasis of Rbf in humans, including at the levels of renal tubules and the BBB (Foraker et al. 2003).

153.4 Vitamin B2 Status Assessment

Although all forms of vitamin B2 (free Rbf, FMN, and FAD) are present in measurable concentrations, FAD is the main form of the vitamin found in tissues and whole blood (Powers 1999) and is therefore, most representative of total body flavin content. Although HPLC with fluorometric detection may accurately detect FAD, a functional test (EGRAC) is the method of choice for assessment of vitamin B2 status (Powers 1999). EGRAC measures saturation of the enzyme GR with its coenzyme (FAD). When vitamin B2 stores are significantly low, the addition of FAD to a sample of erythrocytes in vitro produces a percentage increase in measured enzyme activity (activity coefficient) that exceeds 15–20% (EGRAC = 1.15–1.20, respectively). Therefore, EGRAC is the ratio between enzyme activity determined with and without the addition of FAD. The larger the increase in EGRAC noted after the addition of FAD in vitro, the greater the degree of unsaturation of the apoenzyme with its cofactor and the more severe the deficiency of vitamin B2. The loss of erythrocyte FAD at an early stage in vitamin B2 deficiency makes EGRAC a sensitive method for the diagnosis of vitamin B2 deficiency (Bates 1993). EGRAC is an index independent of any uncontrolled denominator, and hence is robust as well as sensitive in practice (Bates 1987). Following blood-sampling, 31.5–84.8% of plasma FAD is hydrolyzed to FMN within 10–40 mm at 37°C (Zempleni et al. 1996). Therefore, blood should be immediately processed after sampling, and erythrocytes stored at 4.0°C for early EGRAC assessment.

153.5 Riboflavin Functions

Many key enzymes require FAD and/or FMN to catalyze a wide range of different types of reactions, particularly oxidation–reduction reactions, dehydrogenation, and oxidative decarboxylation. Most importantly, FAD and/or FMN is involved in the respiratory chain, lipid metabolism, the cytochrome P-450 system, and drug metabolism. Monoamine oxidase, sarcosine dehydrogenase, and succinate dehydrogenase are flavoproteins. Vitamin B2 also plays a role in the metabolism of essential fatty acids in brain lipids (Ogunleye and Odutuga 1989).

Complexes I and II are respectively FMN- and FAD-dependent (Nelson and Cox 2009), while flavoproteins are also responsible for oxygen reduction to hydrogen peroxide (Rivlin and Pinto 2001). Upon reduced vitamin B2 bioavailability, ATP production is selectively preserved, while the less critical FAD- or FMN-dependent metabolic pathways are impaired (Anderson et al. 1994).

Another critical feature is the influence of vitamin B2 on the glutathione system. Glutathione is a tripeptide occurring in reduced (GSH) and oxidized (GSSG) states. GSH is the major endogenous cellular antioxidant, which not only directly neutralizes free radicals, but also deactivates hydrogen peroxide molecules that result from the action of superoxide dismutase on superoxide ions. GSH is the most abundant form of glutathione under physiological conditions, and increased GSSG-to-GSH ratio becomes evident under oxidative stress. Following inactivation of free radicals or peroxides, GSH is regenerated from GSSG by the FAD-containing enzyme GSSG reductase (Hustad et al. 2002) (Fig. 153.3).

The two alternative pathways of deoxynucleotide synthesis primarily or secondarily require FAD at the expense either of FAD or GSH, respectively (Nelson and Cox 2009) (Fig.153.4), and decreased bioavailability of vitamin B2 should therefore affect DNA synthesis. Not surprisingly, the activity of the glutathione system affects the pathophysiology of cancer, regulation of apoptosis, and DNA repair (Hall 1999; Berwick and Vineis 2000; Locigno and Castronovo 2001). Vitamin B2 deficiency may affect the mitochondrial pool of GSH which in turn may affect the activities of the flavoenzymes NADPH-cytochrome P-450 reductase and NADPH-cytochrome b reductase (Hustad et al. 2002).

The GSTs comprise a super family of multifunctional enzymes widely expressed in mammalian tissue cytosols and membranes that play a pivotal role in electrophile detoxification, while protecting cells from the consequences of oxidative stress. They catalyze the conjugation of GSH with a wide

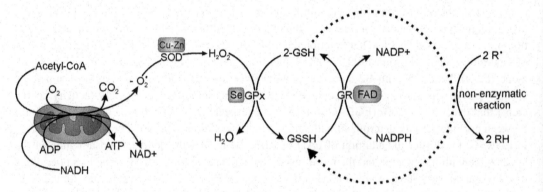

Fig. 153.3 The role of FAD on the glutathione antioxidation system. Glutathione peroxidase (*GPx*) neutralize free radicals and peroxides. The FAD-dependent enzyme glutathione redutase (*GR*) regenerates oxidized (*GSSG*) to reduced (*GSH*) glutathione. *FAD* flavin adenine dinucleotide, *SOD* superoxide dismutase, *NAD+* oxidized nicotinamide adenine dinucleotide, *NADH* reduced nicotinamide adenine dinucleotide, *NADP+* oxidized nicotinamide adenine dinucleotide phosphate, *NADPH* reduced nicotinamide adenine dinucleotide phosphate, *ADP* adenosine diphosphate, *ATP* adenosine triphosphate

Fig. 153.4 The role of riboflavin bioactive forms (FAD and FMN) on the cytochrome P-450 system. The microsomal cytochrome P450 receives electrons from a FAD- and FMN-containing enzyme – the NADPH-dependent cytochrome P450 reductase, where both FMN and FAD operate as prosthetic groups. *FAD* flavin adenine dinucleotide, *FMN* flavin monophosphate, *NADPH* nicotinamide adenine dinucleotide phosphate, *NADP+* nicotinamide adenine dinucleotide phosphate

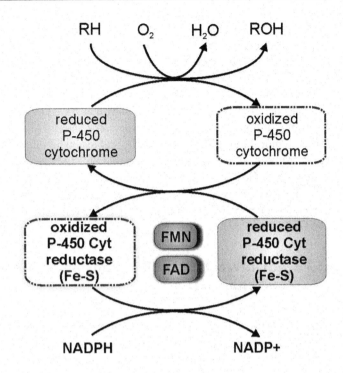

variety of exogenous and endogenous chemicals with electrophilic functional groups (e.g., products of oxidative stress, oxidized DNA and lipid molecules, environmental pollutants, xenobiotics, and carcinogens). By neutralizing the electrophilic sites, the process prevents these products from attacking macromolecules and renders them more water-soluble (Parl 2005). The impairment of GR activity by abnormally low vitamin B2 status should plausibly limit the availability of GSH required for GST activity, thereby increasing the oxidative stress.

The cytochrome P-450 is a superfamily of hemeproteins (comprising 57 human genes) that catalyze the oxidation of a wide array of lipophilic compounds such as drugs and carcinogens or endogenous compounds such as prostaglandins, fatty acids, and steroids (Nebert and Russell 2002). The microsomal cytochrome P-450 receives electrons from a FAD- and FMN-containing enzyme – the NADPH-dependent cytochrome P-450 reductase, where both FMN and FAD operate as prosthetic groups (Wang et al. 1997) (Fig. 153.4). Therefore, the whole spectrum of cytochrome P-450 reactions is impaired with vitamin B2 deficiency. That includes the metabolism of drugs, foreign chemicals (carcinogens as well), arachidonic acid and eicosanoids, cholesterol metabolism and bile acid biosynthesis, steroid synthesis and metabolism, vitamin D3 metabolism, retinoic acid hydroxylation, and the activity of other enzymes of unknown function (Nebert and Russell 2002).

The microsomal NADPH-dependent cytochrome P-450 reductase is also required to provide the reducing equivalent necessary for heme oxidation through the HO enzymatic activity (Maines 1997). HO is the only enzyme that can degrade heme (iron protoporphyrin-IX, hemin) to biliverdin, free iron, and CO. Maintaining cellular heme homeostasis, HO protects tissues against hemin-triggered oxidative stress, thereby limiting damage in diverse in vitro and in vivo models of cellular and tissue injuries. HO consists of two major isozymes: the inducible HO-1, known as heat shock protein-32 (HSP-32), and the constitutively expressed HO-2, which is highly concentrated in the brain and testes. HO-1 under basal conditions is barely detectable in the brain, but is induced in numerous conditions, such as hyperthermia, Alzheimer disease, transient and global ischemia, and subarachnoid hemorrhage (reviewed by Kim et al. 2005). By impairing the activity of the biflavin

(FMN- and FAD-dependent) enzyme NADPH-cytochrome P-450 reductase, vitamin B2 deficiency may conceivably compromise HO-dependent cytoprotective effects.

To date, tens of thousands of publications and three Nobel Laureates have unveiled and emphasized the fundamental biological importance of NO for both normal cellular and whole body physiology, and also in the pathology of many diseases, especially those related to inflammation and long term degenerative disorders. Enzymes known as NO synthases (without ATP utilization) synthesize NO from l-arginine in mammalian tissues. The activity of the three isoenzymes (eNOS, iNOS, and nNOS) requires l-arginine and NADPH, and results in the formation of citrulline and NO. NO synthesis requires not only these substrates but also the presence of calmodulin, as well as four other coenzymes/cofactors: BH4, NADPH and, particularly relevant for this discussion, the active flavins FMN and FAD (Bruckdorfer 2005). Vitamin B2 deficiency therefore, may affect the whole spectrum of metabolic pathways, physiologic and pathophysiologic phenomena related to NO.

153.6 Rbf Interactions with Pyridoxine, Folic Acid, Cobalamin, and Vitamin D

FMN and/or FAD are required for maintenance of pyridoxine (vitamin B6), folic acid (vitamin B9), and cobalamin (vitamin B12) statuses, so that vitamin B2 deficiency may lead to secondary impairment of all B6-, B9-, and B12-dependant enzyme activities. Such metabolic relationships largely amplify the spectrum of pathophysiologic implications and diseases potentially related to vitamin B2 deficiency. They provide likely explanations for the relation of vitamin B2 availability to plasma homocysteine levels, which is associated with cardiovascular disease, pregnancy complications, and cognitive impairment (Hustad et al. 2000; Skoupy et al. 2002).

A number of folate-dependent pathways related to methionine and nucleotide biosynthesis explain how folic acid may prevent neural tube and other birth defects like spina bifida, lower homocysteine and risk of cardiovascular disease, prevent several types of cancer, dementia, affective disorders, Down's syndrome, and serious conditions affecting pregnancy outcome. FAD is the cofactor for MTHFR (Fig. 153.5), which catalyzes the formation of 5-methyltetrahydrofolate – a methyl donor for homocysteine remethylation. The MTHFR C677T (cytidine to thymidine substitution at position 677) polymorphism causes alanine to be replaced by valine in the catalytic domain. This genotypic alteration affects the FAD binding and destabilizes the quaternary structure of the enzyme, making it thermolabile with approximately half-normal activity (Joshi et al. 2009), and increasing total plasma homocysteine concentrations, particularly in association with low folate status (Moat et al. 2003). Therefore, low vitamin B2 status should further impair folate-dependent pathways in individuals carrying MTHFR polymorphisms and potentiates this and other genetic susceptibilities to folic acid deficiency. Folate-dependent key physiologic roles potentially impaired in vitamin B2 deficiency, include maintenance and repair of the genome, regulation of gene expression, amino-acid metabolism, neurotransmitter synthesis, and the formation of myelin (Djukic 2007).

FMN serves as a cofactor for PPO, which catalyzes the terminal and rate-limiting step of the biosynthesis of PLP (the biologically active form of vitamin B6) from pyridoxine, the main dietary and therapeutic form of vitamin B6 (Powers 2003). PLP is a coenzyme in the catabolism of carbohydrates, fats, and proteins, and in the synthesis of hormones, red blood cells, neurotransmitters, and enzymes. PLP is a coenzyme for more than 100 enzymes involved in amino acid metabolism, including aminotransferases, decarboxylases, racemases, and dehydratases. PLP is a coenzyme for CBS (unique in having both PLP and heme as cofactors) and CL, the two enzymes involved in the transsulfuration pathway from homocysteine to cysteine (Fig. 153.5).

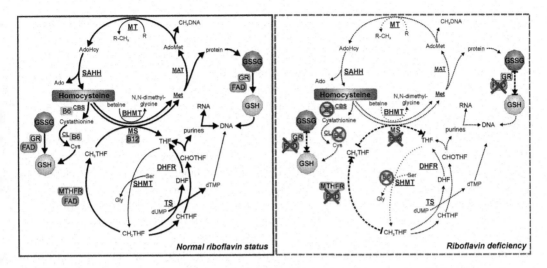

Fig. 153.5 FAD interactions with pyridoxine, folic acid, cobalamin. For maintenance of normal metabolism (*left panel*), the folic acid/methylcobalamin cycle needs FAD as a coenzyme for methylenetetrahydrofolate reductase (*MTHFR*) and methionine synthase (*MS*) activities. The synthesis of pyridoxal 5'-phosphate (PLP, the active form of vitamin B6) from pyridox(am)ine 5'-phosphate requires FMN, while serine hydroxymethyltransferase (*SHMT*), cystathionine-γ-lyase (*CL*, cystathionase) and cystathionine β synthase (*CBS*) are PLP-dependent enzymes and therefore, secondarily depend on FMN. Glutathione reductase (*GR*) activity requires FAD, while cysteine synthesis from homocysteine requires the consecutive activities of two PLP enzymes (CL and CBS). Hence, the levels of reduced glutathione (*GSH*, an antioxidant molecule with multiple essential metabolic functions) are doubly dependent on vitamin B2 status. The role of GSH in deoxynucleotide production (required for DNA synthesis) is explained in Fig. 153.7 and text. Upon vitamin B2 deficiency (*right panel*) all B6-, B9-, and B12-dependent enzyme activities may be impaired. "X" and "X inside the circle" respectively indicate enzyme activities primarily and secondarily inhibited under low vitamin B2 status (secondary to low PLP or methylcobalamin availability). Associated reductions of FMN-dependent SHMT activity, DNA methylation (CH₃DNA), deoxynucleotide production, and purine synthesis contribute to impairment of DNA repairing mechanisms under low vitamin B2 status. *GSSG* oxidized glutathione, *MT* metallothionein, *AdoHcy* adenosylhomocysteine, *SAHH* S-adenosyl homocysteine hydrolase, *Ado* adenosine, *BHMT* betaine-homocysteine methyltransferases, *Met* methionine, *MAT* methionine adenosyltransferase, *AdoMet* S-adenosyl-methionine, *MS* methionine synthase, *DHFR* dihydrofolate reductase, *TS* thymidylate synthase, *DHF* dihydrofolate, *CHTHF* methenyltetrahydrofolate, *CHOTHF* formyl tetrahydrofolate, *THF* tetrahydrofolate, *dUMP* deoxyuridine monophosphate, *dTMP* deoxythymidine monophosphate, *CH₃DNA* methylated DNA

PLP is also a coenzyme for δ-aminolevulinate synthase – the rate-limiting step in the biosynthesis of heme, which is incorporated as a prosthetic group to a wide variety of proteins with biologically diverse critical functions. Heme proteins include:

(a) Oxygen transport and storage proteins – hemoglobin and myoglobin;
(b) Heme redox enzymes – the cytochrome P-450 superfamily; peroxidases, catalases, and catalase-peroxidases; the dioxygenases indoleamine 2,3-dioxygenase and tryptophan 2,3-dioxygenase; the three NOS isoforms;
(c) Electron transfer proteins – cytochromes b and c;
(d) Heme sensor proteins – heme-responsive heme sensor proteins, such as the HRI system which regulates the translation of genes required for globin synthesis in red blood cells; gas-responsive heme sensor proteins such as guanylate cyclases.

The classical clinical symptoms of B6 deficiency are seborrheic dermatitis, microcytic anemia, epileptiform convulsions, insomnia, depression, and confusion (Mooney et al. 2009). By limiting the conversion of pyridox(am)ine 5'-phosphate to PLP, vitamin B2 deficiency may impair the whole wide range of PLP-dependent vital metabolic pathways (Fig. 153.5).

The enzyme MS (also known as methionine synthase reductase), which converts homocysteine to methionine, is dependent on 5-methyltetrahydrofolate as a methyl donor and on vitamin B-12 (as methylcobalamin). Vitamin B-12 plays an essential role in the methyl transfer reaction by acting as an intermediate methyl carrier between methyltetrahydrofolate and homocysteine. MS also contains both FMN and FAD as coenzymes, which are essential for maintenance of proper redox state of cobalt ions in the methylcobalamin molecule, thereby preventing inactivation of the enzyme (Olteanu and Banerjee 2001) (Fig. 153.5).

The dependency of vitamins B6, B12, and folate on FAD and/or FMN availability largely amplifies the metabolic importance of vitamin B2. For instance, Rbf deficiency may both limit the activation of vitamin B6 to PLP and inactivate methylcobalamin. Metabolic derangement of methionine and folate metabolism in this circumstance may result not only primarily from reduced MTHFR and SHMT activities, but also from oxidation of methylcobalamin secondary to Rbf deficiency.

Likewise, rather than solely resulting from decreased coenzymes (FMN and FAD) required for NOS activity, diminished NO synthesis and reduced NO-mediated biological effects in vitamin B2 deficiency may also be secondary to low PLP production by FMN-dependent PPO, which limits the synthesis of prosthetic heme to be incorporated during the assembly of NOS isoenzymes and GC (Fig. 153.6). Similarly, oxidative stress in vitamin B2 deficiency would not merely result from decreased GSH regeneration from GSSG by the FAD-dependent enzyme GSSG reductase: decreased prosthetic heme incorporation during the assembly of catalases may further aggravate oxidative stress.

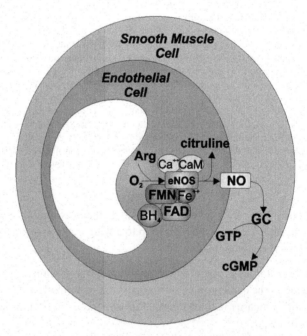

Fig. 153.6 The importance of vitamin B2 for NO production. Dependency of endothelium-derived nitric oxide (*NO*) function on vitamin B2 status. Endothelial nitric oxide synthase (*eNOS*) activity requires both active forms of vitamin B2, flavin adenine dinucleotide (*FAD*), and flavin mononucleotide (*FMN*). The vasodilatatoy effect of NO depends on guanylate cyclase (*GC*) for cGMP synthesis within smooth muscle cells. Both eNOS and GC are hemeproteins, and prosthetic heme synthesis requires the activity of pyridoxal 5′-phosphate (*PLP*)-dependent δ-aminolevulinate synthase. The synthesis of PLP (the active form of vitamin B6) from pyridox(am)ine 5′-phosphate requires FMN. Therefore, vitamin B2 deficiency may impair the vasodilatatoy effect of NO at multiple biochemical steps, including depressed eNOS activity and low availability of prosthetic heme for posttranslational incorporation into the expressed proteins eNOS and GC. *Arg* arginine, O_2 oxygen, *Fe*++ ferrous iron, *Ca*++*CaM* calcium/calmodulin complex, *BH4* tetrahydrobiopterin, *GTP* guanosine triphosphate, *cGMP* cyclic guanosine monophosphate

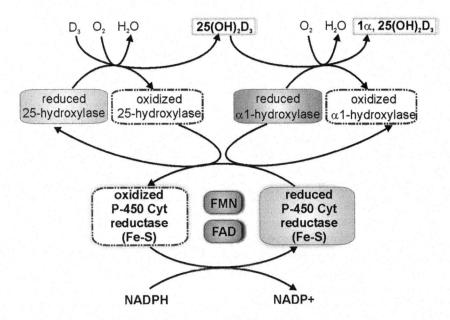

Fig. 153.7 FAD and FMN interactions with vitamin D. The deficiency of vitamin B2 bioactive forms may secondarily affect the activity of vitamin D hydroxylases. Note that enzymes 25-hydroxylase and 1α-hydroxylase are members of the cytochrome P-450 superfamily and require the activity of the flavo-enzyme NADPH-dependent cytochrome P450 reductase. *FAD* flavin adenine dinucleotide, *FMN* flavin monophosphate, *NADPH* reduced nicotinamide adenine dinucleotide phosphate, *NADP⁺* oxidized nicotinamide adenine dinucleotide phosphate

In addition, vitamin B2 deficiency may significantly affect the activity of vitamin D hydroxylases. The enzymes 25-hydroxylase and 1α-hydroxylase are members of cytochrome P-450 superfamily. The consecutive syntheses of 25(OH)D3 (calcidiol) from cholecalciferol and 1α,25(OH)2D3 (calcitriol, the active form of Vitamin D) from calcidiol are expected to be reduced vitamin B2 deficiency. This may occur because of both decreased prosthetic heme incorporation (secondary to reduced heme synthesis due to low PLP production) to hydroxylases and limited prosthetic FMN/FAD incorporation to NADPH-dependent cytochrome P-450 reductase (Fig. 153.7).

153.7 Deficiency Consequences in Both Human and Experimental Studies

Rather than restricted to developing countries, vitamin B2 deficiency may be widespread in industrialized countries as well, where it affects both the elderly and young adults rather than occurring only in patients suffering from chronic conditions such as celiac disease, cancer, and alcoholism (Powers 2003). The importance of the work by Anderson and associates – showing that low vitamin B2 status may result from defective absorption in a relatively large number of otherwise well-nourished individuals – cannot be overemphasized. In spite of an adequate dietary intake, 10–15% of the inhabitants of London and Florence showed a low activation coefficient of two vitamin B2-dependent enzymes – GR and PPO. High doses of Rbf (24–30 mg/day for 5–8 weeks) corrected the activity of both enzymes in the affected individuals. The dependency of both FMN and FAD levels on Rbf absorption, and the normalization of the activities of both FMN- and FAD-dependent enzymes only at a high Rbf intake, taken together, are consistent with the expression of polymorphic genes related to Rbf absorption such as the flavokinase gene. The similar number of persons affected in different ethnic groups

(10–15%) indicates that these percentages may be representative of the world prevalence of genetic polymorphisms impairing Rbf absorption in the proximal ileum (Anderson et al. 1994).

Normal vitamin B2 body homeostasis also depends on a renal saturable uptake system that reabsorbs almost all the filtered micronutrient in the proximal tubule epithelial cells (Jusko and Levy 1970). Moreover, maintenance of normal EGRAC levels in vitamin B2 deficiency unrelated to dietary restriction requires the administration of high doses of Rbf at least three times a day (Coimbra and Junqueira 2003). This finding suggests an increased urinary loss of vitamin B2 in the affected individuals, implying a general impairment of uptake, trafficking, and cellular homeostasis of Rbf. In other words, a single genetic polymorphism may cause widespread changes in Rbf transport in several cell types, and underlie both malabsorption of Rbf by proximal ileum cells and impaired Rbf uptake from glomerular filtrate by proximal tubule cells. This issue has major implications for neurologic disorders as explained ahead.

The classical signs of vitamin B2 deficiency are cheilosis, angular stomatitis, glossitis, seborrheic dermatitis (Hendler and Rorvik 2008), and cataract (Powers 2003). Experimental studies in vitamin B2 deprivation in rats demonstrated disruption of iron metabolism (Powers 2003). Other studies on vitamin B2 deprivation during fetal development showed a reduction of the terminal electron transport system, increased fetal mortality and decreased fetal growth, mental retardation, and complete cessation of growth (Bates 1997; Powers 2003).

153.8 Vitamin B2 Deficiency and Neurological Diseases

The wide array of metabolic functions of FMN and FAD and their interactions with pyridoxine, folic acid, cobalamin, and vitamin D exceedingly amplify the range of human diseases potentially associated with Rbf deficiency. Additionally, the high prevalence of Rbf deficiency (probably secondary to polymorphisms of genes related to uptake, trafficking, and cellular homeostasis of vitamin B2 in humans) highly emphasizes the pathophysiologic and epidemiologic relevance of the issue.

The issues related to a highly prevalent genetic mechanism impairing cellular trafficking of Rbf in multiple tissues, possibly involving the flavokinase gene (Anderson et al. 1994), are particularly relevant for the CNS. A very efficient homeostatic system for Rbf renders the brain tissue privileged in circumstances of low dietary Rbf availability in genetically normal individuals, so that the total CNS content of vitamin B2 is preserved in contrast to other tissues (Spector 1980). The concentrations of total Rbf in plasma, CSF, and brain were 0.2, 0.1, and 8.8 2 M, respectively, in genetically normal adult rabbits (Spector 1980). Conceivably, polymorphisms of genes related to cellular uptake mechanisms may also impair the transport of Rbf across the choroid plexus epithelial cells, the main transport locus of the blood-cerebrospinal fluid barrier (Spector and Johanson 2006), thereby disrupting the activity of those powerful homeostatic mechanisms.

153.8.1 Parkinson´s Disease

Genetically impaired CNS Rbf homeostasis may underlie the predisposition to PD by enabling the activity of pathophysiologic mechanisms related to degeneration of dopaminergic nigral cells (Coimbra and Junqueira 2003). These homeostatic mechanisms would be intact in genetically normal rats and prevent the activity of similar pathophysiologic phenomena in the experimental setting (DalPai et al. 2007).

Several pathophysiologic issues related to PD may be related to disturbed Rbf homeostasis in the CNS. GSH depletion – considered an early key event in the pathogenesis of PD (Jenner et al. 1992; Schulz et al. 2000) may occur as a consequence of impaired FAD-dependent GR activity. Because humans lack efficient iron excretory mechanisms, iron excess is dealt with by increasing the synthesis of the iron-storage protein ferritin (Casey et al. 1988). Disturbed systemic (Logroscino et al. 1997) and brain (Dexter et al. 1990) iron metabolism has been reported in PD, suggesting that a selective decrease in the levels of ferritin may result in an increase in intracellular free iron, thereby enhancing free radical production (Mann et al. 1994). Indeed, vitamin B2 deficiency in rodents is associated with low circulating iron concentrations, increased iron turnover, and excretion into the intestinal lumen, which may occur in response to impaired ferritin synthesis (Powers 2003). Therefore, the consistent finding of an abnormal Rbf status in PD (Coimbra and Junqueira 2003), may help to explain the disturbed iron metabolism found in PD patients, with the underlying mechanisms possibly involving (1) impaired hemin catabolism by HO secondary to low activity of FMN- and FAD-dependent cytochrome P-450 reductase, and (2) reduced neuronal ferritin synthesis. Free iron concentrations in the cytosol increase due to impaired ferritin synthesis and/or reduced hemin catabolism associated with hydrogen peroxide accumulation due to glutathione depletion, thereby triggering the Fenton reaction, and ultimately leading to the selective formation of the potent neurotoxin 6(OH)DA in dopaminergic neurons.

Moreover, because FAD is required in both alternative pathways of deoxynucleotide synthesis (Nelson and Cox 2009) (Fig. 153.8), DNA repair and replication are expected to be disturbed by decreased Rbf bioavailability, and abnormal Rbf status may also explain the cumulative mitochondrial DNA mutations reported in PD (Di Monte 1991). In addition to mitochondrial DNA mutations, the reduced bioavailability of FMN and/or FAD required for the activity of mitochondrial complexes I and II, respectively, may further explain the impaired oxidative metabolism of PD patients (Schapira et al. 1990; Mytilineou et al. 1994; Mizuno et al. 1994).

Emotional stress may cause PD (Smith et al. 2002; Sipetic-Grujicicl et al. 2007) in individuals turned susceptible to stress-induced nigral degeneration by polymorphic genes that disturb cellular uptake and trafficking of Rbf and affect the homeostatic preservation of the vitamin stores in the CNS. Excessive dopamine concentrations in nigral cells under prolonged stressful situations (Kim et al. 2005) may cause accumulation of dopamine-derived salsolinol (Naoi et al. 2002), a potent endogenous aromatic heterocyclic amine similar to MPTP (Speciale 2002) capable of covalent binding to DNA (DNA adduct formation) and inducing degeneration of nigral cells. Additionally, exogenous aromatic heterocyclic amines absorbed from ingested meat cooked at high temperatures may contribute to Parkinsonian neurodegeneration (Collins and Neafsey 2002). Both the synthesis and catabolism of heterocyclic amines require the participation of cytochrome P-450 enzymes (Sinha and Caporaso 1997). The metabolism of (endogenous or exogenous) heterocyclic amines by cytochrome P-450 enzymes is secondarily altered in vitamin B2 deficiency due to impairment of NADPH-cytochrome P-450 reductase. Simultaneously, the vulnerability of the nervous tissue to DNA adduct formation is increased due to this and other FMN of FAD-dependent metabolic pathways, such as impaired mitochondrial DNA repair (Figs. 153.5 and 153.8), low GSH levels (Fig. 153.3), and diminished local synthesis of calcitriol (Fig. 153.7).

153.8.2 Migraine

Endothelial NO production has been implicated in the pathophysiology of migraine. This short-lived free radical is responsible for cerebral blood vessel relaxation activating guanylate cyclase and increasing cGMP in smooth muscle (reviewed by Murad 2008). Migraine-like headache is induced

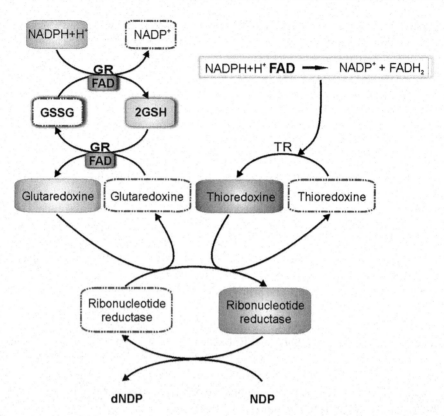

Fig. 153.8 The role of FAD in deoxynucleotide biosynthesis. *NADPH* reduced nicotinamide adenine dinucleotide phosphate, *NADP+* oxidized nicotinamide adenine dinucleotide, *FAD* flavin adenine dinucleotide, *GR* glutathione reductase, *GSH* reduced glutathione, *GSSG* oxidized glutathione, *dNDP* deoxyribonucleoside diphosphate, *NDP* ribonucleoside diphosphate

by i.v. infusions of glyceryl trinitrate (an exogenous NO donor) and histamine (which liberates NO from the vascular endothelium). Furthermore, the i.v. infusion of eNOS inhibitors effectively controls migraine attacks. These data suggest that the release of NO from blood vessels, perivascular nerve endings or from brain tissue may trigger spontaneous migraine. By reacting with superoxide, NO forms peroxynitrite, which is a highly reactive free radical that exerts noxious effects on tissues. Following interaction with superoxide, NO may cause the headache through variations of cerebral blood flow (Olesen 2008).

The synthesis of guanylate cyclase requires the incorporation of prosthetic heme, while the production of heme depends on the availability of PLP (from FMN-dependent PPO) for δ-aminolevulinate synthase activity, as mentioned elsewhere. Therefore, both adequate synthesis of NO by FMN/FAD-dependent eNOS and the triggering of intracellular signaling events by NO ultimately rely on normal vitamin B2 status. On the other hand, abnormally low vitamin B2 status with secondary impairment of GR activity should limit the availability of GSH required for elimination of peroxides, direct inactivation of reactive oxygen species, and activity of GSTs. Therefore, increased production and decreased inactivation of reactive molecules, with the consequent increase in peroxynitrite formation may enable the variations of cerebral blood flow that underlie migraine attacks. The polymorphisms of enzymes involved in FAD-dependent metabolic pathways (GSTs) and polymorphic flavo-enzymes (C677T mutation of MTHFR), respectively, correlate with susceptibility to migraine with (Kowa et al. 2000) and without (Kusumi et al. 2003) aura, supporting the relevance of vitamin B2 status for the pathophysiology of migraine.

Accordingly, several studies, including randomized control trials demonstrate that high-dose (200–400 mg) Rbf taken once a day is a well-tolerated, effective, and low-cost prophylactic treatment in children, adolescents, and adults suffering from migraine (Schoenen et al. 1998; Boehnke et al. 2004; MacLennan et al. 2008; Condo et al. 2009). Current views regard the benefits of Rbf in migraine prophylaxis as the result of a pharmacological effect, due to the high doses employed. However, the authors have not assessed the pretreatment status of vitamin B2 nor taken into consideration the seminal series of studies by Anderson and coworkers (1994) who have demonstrated a high prevalence of genetically determined Rbf malabsorption in the general population. As reviewed above, Rbf deficiency facilitates multiple pathophysiologic mechanisms of migraine; conceivably, migraine and Rbf malabsorption (with disruption of the homeostatic system for CNS flavin content) may be co-morbid conditions in a potentially large number of individuals. Furthermore, the authors have neither considered that a single dose of 27 mg saturates absorptive mechanisms, so that any excess to that dose is not actually absorbed (Zempleni 1996). Multiple daily doses of Rbf may be required for a steadily normal status of vitamin B2 (Coimbra and Junqueira 2003) that may conceivably occur in a potentially large number of migraine sufferers who could concomitantly bear genetically disturbed flavin uptake by renal proximal tubule cells increasing urinary loss of vitamin B2. A therapeutic paradigm rationalized according to current knowledge of the altered vitamin B2 dynamics may enhance the effectiveness of Rbf therapy not only in migraine prophylaxis, but also in other disorders potentially related to that genetically determined and highly prevalent metabolic defect.

153.8.3 Multiple Sclerosis, Guillain-Barré Syndrome, Myasthenia, and Other Autoimmune Disorders

Vitamin D activation requires two sequential biosynthetic steps (25-hydroxylation in hepatocytes and 1α-hydroxylation in immune cell) by mitochondrial/microsomal cytochrome P-450 enzymes, respectively 25-hydroxylases (CYP2R1, CYP27A1) and 1alpha-hydroxylase (CYP27b), yielding calcitriol, which plays a central role in maintaining immune tolerance. Vitamin D-induced immune tolerance is therefore, critically dependent on vitamin B2 status, as the activities of all cytochrome P-450 super family members require continuous restoration of their prosthetic heme to the reduced state by FAD- and FMN-containing, NADPH-dependent cytochrome P450 reductase (Wang et al. 1997) (Fig. 153.7).

During the last decades, epidemiologic studies unequivocally demonstrated a strong negative correlation between the prevalence of autoimmune diseases and the bioavailability of vitamin D, from either consumption of fish oil or sunshine exposure. Both experimental and clinical data provide evidence that the concentration of circulating 25(OH)D3 (calcidiol), which best reflects vitamin D status, critically affects the outcome of autoimmune diseases such as multiple sclerosis, systemic lupus erythematosus, rheumatoid arthritis, insulin-dependent diabetes mellitus, and inflammatory bowel disease (Correale et al. 2009; Cutolo 2009).

The active form of vitamin D (calcitriol) synthesized from circulating calcidiol by the enzyme 1alpha-hydroxylase within the immune cells maintains immunologic tolerance to self-antigens upon interaction with nuclear VDR (Bikle 2009). The expression of 1alpha-hydroxylase and VDR has been described in dendritic cells, macrophages, B cells, and activated T cells, which are, therefore, both producers and targets of calcitriol. Calcitriol changes the phenotype and the activity of the very calcitriol-producing cell (autocrine effect) and the nearby cells (paracrine effect), thereby effectively inducing tolerance to auto-antigens without causing significant immune-suppression or endocrine effects (hypercalcemia and/or hypercalciuria) (Vieth 2004).

Predisposition to autoimmune diseases due to low sunlight exposure and poor ingestion of fish oil is conceivably more prominent in individuals bearing 1alpha-hydroxylase or VDR gene polymorphisms, which respectively impair the efficiency of the enzyme and/or the affinity of VDR for its agonist (calcitriol). Accordingly, the development of auto-immune pathology related to polymorphic changes of 1alpha-hydroxylase (Pani et al. 2002) or VDR (Smolders et al. 2009), and both polymorphisms of the VDR (Smolders et al. 2009) and vitamin D metabolite levels (Smolders et al. 2008) have been linked to multiple sclerosis susceptibility and disability.

Conceivably, the administration of cholecalciferol in doses much higher than those currently recommended has a remarkable therapeutic potential in multiple sclerosis (Vieth 2004; Kimball et al. 2007; Niino et al. 2008). High levels of calcidiol may compensate for the higher Michaelis–Menten constant of a polymorphic 1alpha-hydroxylase. Similarly, a high calcidiol-to-calcitriol conversion rate provided by the effect of optimized substrate provision (to a genetically normal 1alpha-hydroxylase within the immune cells) may increase intracellular ligand levels and counteract the low binding affinity of a polymorphic VDR. However, the effect of high-dose cholecalciferol therapy in either of these circumstances may be significantly compromised by low FMN and FAD incorporation to NADPH-dependent cytochrome P-450 reductase in altered vitamin B2 status.

A low vitamin B2 status may significantly impair vitamin D metabolism for two reasons: (1) the two sequential steps of calcitriol biosynthesis require the activity of the NADPH-dependent cytochrome P-450 reductase, which (2) is doubly dependent on vitamin B2 as it uses the two active flavins (FMN and FAD) as prosthetic groups. In addition, vitamin B2 deficiency may further dysregulate the immune system by at least two other ways. First, the immune function seems to be exquisitely sensitive to changes in the intracellular GSH:GSSG ratio (Fidelus and Tsan 1987; Droge and Breitkreutz 2000), and low availability of FAD diminishes both GR activity and intracellular concentration of GSH, while increasing GSSG levels. Second, a wealth of evidence now supports the existence of extra-adrenal production of corticosteroids, particularly in the cardiovascular system and CNS, where the full array of enzymes required for the de novo synthesis of corticosteroids from cholesterol has been identified (Davies and MacKenzie 2003). The synthesis of endogenous steroids requires the activity of cytochrome P-450 enzymes (Nebert and Russell 2002), and therefore, altered vitamin B2 status could credibly favor local inflammatory and autoimmune responses in these sites.

Vitamin B2 and vitamin D statuses may similarly affect other autoimmune neurological disorders, including Guillain-Barré syndrome (acute inflammatory demyelinating polyradiculoneuropathy), myasthenia, and optic neuritis. These disorders may also respond to therapy with high doses of cholecalciferol and Rbf for the same reasons exposed here.

153.8.4 Neurodegenerative Disorders and Cell Death

Inherited low vitamin B2 status and related disruption of Rbf homeostasis in the CNS feasibly favor cell death in neurodegenerative disorders by a number of mechanisms leading to a decline in GSH/GSSG ratio (Bains and Shaw 1997). One is increased conversion of GSH to GSSG by oxidative stress (overproduction of reactive species of both oxygen and nitrogen) secondary to impairment of mitochondrial function related to low availability of FMN and FAD. Another mechanism is decreased GSH synthesis: the availability of cysteine to γ-GCS activity is the rate-limiting factor in GSH formation, and cysteine synthesis from S-adenosylhomocysteine is impaired in low Rbf status due to decreased PLP supply. A third mechanism is decreased reduction of GSSG to GSH by FAD-dependent GR. GSH depletion and post-translational modifications of proteins through glutathionylation mediate apoptotic cell death triggered by a wide variety of stimuli including activation of death receptors, oxidative stress, environmental agents, and cytotoxic drugs (Franco and Cidlowski 2009). Accordingly, disturbed NO (peroxynitrite formation from superoxide and NO) and GSH metabolism may be involved in both necrotic and apoptotic phenomena related to Parkinson's disease, Alzheimer's disease, Huntington's disease, amyotrophic lateral sclerosis, multiple sclerosis, and brain ischemia (Guix et al. 2005).

Within the CNS, both microglia and neurons express 1alpha-hydroxylase and VDR, while VDR is also expressed by astrocytes and oligodendrocytes. Besides tolerance to neural auto-antigens, the local bioactivation of calcidiol into calcitriol provides a myriad of critical autocrine and paracrine benefits in the developing as well adult CNS. These include neuroprotective (through antioxidative mechanisms, neuronal calcium regulation, neuro-immunomodulation, enhanced nerve conduction and detoxification mechanisms), and neuroregenerative effects (neurogenesis stimulation, neurotrophin biosynthesis, myelination) (Garcion et al. 2002; Buell and Dawson-Hughes 2008).

Current knowledge indicates that progesterone synthesis occurs in the brain, for the brain, by neurons and glial cells in the central and peripheral nervous system of both male and female individuals. Progesterone has anticonvulsant actions, enhances mitochondrial function, neurogenesis and regeneration, promotes myelin repair, protects or reconstructs the BBB, downregulates inflammatory cascades, and limits cellular necrosis and apoptosis (reviewed by Brinton et al. 2008). According to the mechanisms explained elsewhere, a low vitamin B2 status associated with genetically determined disruption of Rbf homeostasis in the CNS may significantly impair the synthesis of calcitriol, progesterone, and other steroids in the nervous tissue.

153.8.5 Brain Ischemia and Traumatic Brain Injury

Enhanced lipolytic activity secondary to intracellular calcium overload during brain ischemia removes considerable amounts of arachidonic acid from membrane phospholipids. Reperfusion of the ischemic tissue restores oxygen supply required for the activity by the arachidonate oxygenase (prostaglandin synthetase) system, generating a sudden burst of free radical formation followed by postischemic inflammation-induced iNOS expression, with continuous production of reactive species of oxygen and nitrogen. The results include peroxidation of cellular membranes, oxidative damage to proteins and nucleic acids. The so-called "reperfusion injury" affects mitochondrial respiratory enzyme complexes and mitochondrial DNA with subsequent defects in oxidative phosphorylation, impaired ATP production, and sustained mitochondrial generation of reactive species at a rate sufficient to escape endogenous antioxidant defenses. Subsequently, peroxynitrite and hydroxyl radical production resulting from the combined effects of disturbed electron transport in the mitochondrial respiratory chain, active inflammatory processes, and failure of antioxidant defenses create a vicious cycle by further damaging lipids, nucleic acids, and proteins. This scenario of pathophysiologic events ultimately results in both necrotic and apoptotic cell death.

Conceivably, ischemia/reperfusion creates a potentially unmatched demand for numerous FNM- and/or FAD-dependent metabolic processes, including DNA resynthesis and replication (mitochondrial DNA repair), GST-mediated detoxification of oxidized DNA and lipid molecules, maintenance of the GSSG-GSH antioxidant cycle, reactions requiring NADPH-dependent cytochrome P450 reductase activity (catabolism of arachidonic acid and eicosanoids, heme degradation by HO, synthesis of steroid molecules endowed with neuroprotective and neurodegenerative actions like calcitriol and progesterone), eNOS and nNOS activities. A higher supply of vitamin B2 active forms (FMN and FAD, respectively required by complexes I and II) may plausibly improve the activity of the electron transport chain, reducing the electron leakage and the formation of superoxide ions. Preservation of GSH levels may prevent apoptotic cell death (Franco and Cidlowski 2009).

The metabolic dependency of PLP, folate, and methylcobalamin on FMN and/or FAD availability unveils other neuroprotective and neurodegenerative enzyme activities indirectly dependent on vitamin B2 status. Rbf administration may optimize PLP synthesis and the activity of several PLP-dependent enzymes is of potential benefit in ischemia/reperfusion. The synthesis of l-cysteine by γ-GCS increases the availability of l-cysteine for GSH synthesis (Griffith 1999), thereby enhancing antioxidant defenses and antagonizing apoptosis. Rbf administration may facilitate amino acid, protein, and nucleic acid synthesis by increasing PLP availability. The PLP-dependent activity of δ-aminolevulinate synthase allows the biosynthesis of prosthetic heme required for de novo synthesis of HO, cytochrome P-450 superfamily, electron transfer proteins (cytochromes b and c), peroxidases, catalases, iNOS and nNOS isoforms, and guanylate cyclases, thus further enhancing antioxidant defenses, decreasing free radical production, and opposing necrotic and apoptotic pathophysiologic events. Enhancement folic acid cycle (Fig. 153.5) by Rbf administration may optimize the methylation of phospholipids, proteins, DNA, RNA, and other small molecules and critically improve cell survival in ischemia/reperfusion.

Accordingly, Rbf protects the brain tissue against brain ischemia (Betz et al. 1994) and traumatic brain injury (Hoane et al. 2005). The proposed mechanism of action is the intracellular formation of dihydroriboflavin from administered Rbf by a NADPH-dependent flavin reductase, first detected in erythrocytes 75 years ago. Dihydroriboflavin quickly reduces Fe(IV)O and Fe(V)O oxidation states of hemeproteins (implicated in tissue damage associated with ischemia and reperfusion) to Fe(III)O thus protecting cells from oxidative injury (Hultquist et al. 1993). Due to the wide range of FMN- and or FAD-dependent metabolic processes required for cell survival after ischemia/reperfusion, the protective effect of Rbf administration is not likely to be exclusively determined by increased dihydroriboflavin synthesis. Conceivably, individuals with inherited low vitamin B2 status associated with disruption of brain Rbf homeostasis may be particularly vulnerable to reperfusion injury of the nervous tissue.

153.8.6 Epilepsy and Antiepileptic Therapy

Some epileptic disorders are responsive to specific vitamins like pyridoxine and folic acid derivatives (Wolf et al. 2005). The administration PLP may result in better seizure control than pyridoxine in vitamin B6-responsive epilepsy (Hoffmann et al. 2007). PLP plays a key role in the synthesis of many neurotransmitters, particularly biogenic amines like dopamine and serotonin, and in the decarboxylation of the dominant excitatory neurotransmitter glutamate to the major inhibitory transmitter GABA in the mammalian CNS (Jansonius 1998) by serving as a coenzyme for the rate-limiting enzyme GAD (Fricke et al. 2007). Patients with an autosomal recessive defect of GAD have an imbalance of the neurotransmitters glutamate and GABA (Gospe 1998). Accordingly, GAD-knockout mice show decreased GABA transmission and increased seizure susceptibility (Asada et al. 1997); low vitamin B6 status in genetically normal humans is associated with a lowered seizure threshold (Apeland et al. 2003). Conceivably, a decreased activity of PPO (the FMN-dependent, PLP synthesizing enzyme) or abnormalities of folate metabolism may facilitate seizures. Thus, a low vitamin B2 status reduces FMN availability, which may destabilize neuronal excitability by impairing GABA synthesis.

The active form of vitamin D (calcitriol) also plays an anticonvulsant role in the brain (Siegel et al. 1984; Kalueff et al. 2005). A reduced FMN and FAD availability and incorporation to NADPH-dependent cytochrome P450 reductase may impair the hydroxylations of vitamin D to calcitriol in the brain tissue, thereby lowering the threshold for epileptic seizures.

Similarly, a number of folate-dependent metabolic roles may influence neuronal excitability, and a specific epileptic disorder responds to folic acid derivatives (Wolf et al. 2005). Folate-dependent mechanisms possibly involved in stabilization of neuronal activity include biosynthesis of the neurotransmitters serotonin, catecholamines, and melatonin (Djukic 2007), and the regulation of homocysteine concentrations (Fig. 153.5). The main route of catabolism of homocysteine is through conversion to cystathionine, catalyzed by a PLP-dependent enzyme (CBS). Cystathionine is converted to cysteine and cysteine is oxidized to cysteine sulfinic acid and subsequently, to cysteic acid. Cysteine sulfinic acid and cysteic acid are decarboxylated to hypotaurine and taurine, respectively, by another PLP-dependent enzyme (CADCase/CSADCase). The oxidation products of homocysteine (homocysteine sulfinic acid and homocysteic acid) and cysteine (cysteine sulfinic acid and cysteic acid) are excitatory sulfur amino acids and may act as excitatory neurotransmitters, whereas taurine and hypotaurine (decarboxylation products of cysteic acid and cysteine sulfinic acid) may act as inhibitory transmitters (Santhosh-Kumar et al. 1994). As discussed elsewhere, vitamin B2 deficiency impairs folate (and methylcobalamin) cycle and PLP synthesis. Vitamin B2 deficiency is expected to increase homocysteine-derived excitatory sulfur amino acids while decreasing the levels of inhibitory transmitters, hypotaurine and taurine. The result is a shift in excitatory–inhibitory balance toward a lower threshold for epileptic seizures (Fig. 153.9).

The dependency of vitamins D3 (Fig. 153.7) B6, B12, and folate on FAD and/or FMN availability (Fig. 153.5) therefore, indicates that vitamin B2 deficiency may be epileptogenic. Accordingly, high doses of Rbf abolish epileptic activities in MADD (Kmoch et al. 1995) and high prevalence of low vitamin B2 status is found in association with preeclampsia (Wacker et al. 2000) which may evolve to eclamptic convulsive seizures. The large prevalences of epilepsy (Sander 2003) and Rbf malabsorption (Anderson et al. 1994) suggest that uptake, trafficking, and cellular homeostasis of Rbf in the brain tissue may be disturbed in a significant number of epileptic individuals, and may contribute for a lower threshold for epileptic seizures (Fig. 153.9).

Taken together these data support the need for adequate diagnosis and treatment of all these vitamin deficiencies in epileptic patients to optimize seizure control. In contrast, antiepileptic drug therapy is associated with hyperhomocysteinemia (Schwaninger et al. 1999; Apeland et al. 2003) and

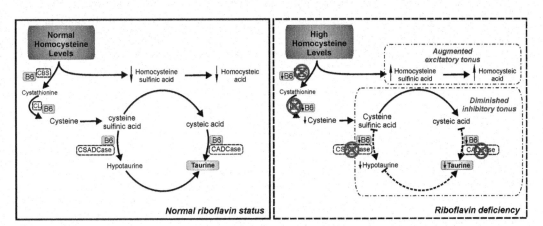

Fig. 153.9 The role of vitamin B2 status on seizure control in epileptic patients. *Left panel*: normal neuronal excitability is observed when enough flavin monophosphate is available for pyridoxal 5′-phosphate (PLP, the active form of vitamin B6) synthesis by pyridox(am)ine 5′-phosphate oxidase. *Right panel*: reduced epileptic threshold for epileptic seizures in low vitamin B2 status due to both increased levels of excitatory compounds and decreased levels of inhibitory neurotransmitters (hypotaurine and taurine). "X inside the circle" indicate enzyme activities secondarily inhibited under low vitamin B2 status (primarily due to low PLP availability). *CL* cystathionine-γ-lyase, *CBS* cystathionine β-synthase, *CADCase/CSADCase* cysteine and sulfinic acid decarboxylase

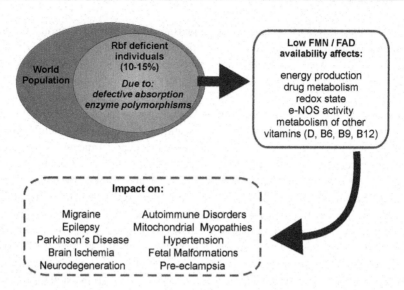

Fig. 153.10 Key facts of riboflavin. Key facts about the impact of riboflavin deficiency on human health. Riboflavin is an essential micronutrient playing a critical role in myriad of biological phenomena, including energy production, DNA replication and repair, nitric oxide synthesis, necrosis and apoptosis, drug metabolism, and antioxidant defense systems. The potential relevance of Rbf status for the pathophysiology, prevention, and treatment of a wide range of human diseases has been largely underestimated

multiple vitamin deficiencies, including those of vitamins B1, B2, B6, B12, C, D, E, beta-carotene, biotin, and folate (Krause et al. 1988; Apeland et al. 2003; Aslan et al. 2008; Nettekoven et al. 2008). Whether these metabolic changes are related to the epileptic condition or represent a pharmacologic side effect is unknown. Discussions on the relevance of vitamin supplementation to patients on anti-epileptic therapy have been usually limited to the preventive context of decreasing the risks of cardiovascular disease and birth defects (Apeland et al. 2002). Only pyridoxine supplementation for enhancing seizure control has been (barely) considered in patients on antiepileptic therapy. However, the metabolic interdependency among these vitamins, as well as their key neurophysiologic roles strongly indicate that untreated multiple vitamin deficiencies may significantly hamper the very antiepileptic effect of these drugs, leading to poor seizure control (apparent drug-resistant epilepsy) and avoidable polytherapy (Fig. 153.10).

Summary Points

- Vitamin B2 directly or indirectly participates in a much wider range of metabolic pathways than usually considered in human physiology; often the same biologic function involves FMN and/or FAD in more than one of its regulatory and integrative steps.
- The high prevalence of genetic polymorphisms related to absorption and cellular trafficking of Rbf, particularly considering the primary and secondary participation of FMN and FAD in a large number of regulatory and metabolic networks highly emphasizes the pathophysiological significance and potential therapeutic/preventive implications of unrecognized deficiency of this micronutrient.
- The interactions between the genetically determined low Rbf status and another highly prevalent inherited metabolic change – the MTHFR mutation restrictive of FAD binding (C677T) – may be of clinical relevance, since high-dose Rbf therapy may plausibly minimize the metabolic effects of that particular MTHFR polymorphism.

- The concrete possibility of a highly prevalent genetically determined disruption of Rbf homeostasis in the CNS makes the nervous tissue particularly prone to Rbf deficiency and raises higher potentially significant implications for prevention and therapy of neurologic disorders in comparison to systemic diseases.
- According to experimental evidence of benefits of Rbf treatment in models of tissue injury, the pathophysiology of cellular damage seem to set up localized higher demands for FMN and FAD required for upregulation of antioxidant, antiapoptotic and proregenerative processes dependent on Rbf metabolism.
- Future research should address the potential association between genetically determined Rbf malabsorption and disorders like migraine, neurodegenerative and autoimmune diseases, as well as in several other neurologic and systemic conditions pathophysiologically related to disturbed metabolism of lipids, amino acids, DNA, cytochrome P-450, NO, vitamin D3, HO and homocysteine metabolism;
- Whenever such association is demonstrated, further studies should investigate the dynamics (including CSF distribution) and therapeutic potential of high-dose Rbf administration in affected individuals, as well as the expression of polymorphic genes related to cellular uptake and trafficking of Rbf at the terminal ileum, proximal renal tubules, and CNS.
- Following the demonstration of low vitamin B2 status (altered EGRAC) associated with a normal dietary Rbf content, a paradigm of 30 mg three to four times a day required for maintenance of normal EGRAC throughout the 24-h period should be considered in future clinical trials aimed at investigating the therapeutic value of Rbf status normalization.

Definition Terms

Enzymes are proteins that catalyze chemical reactions in virtually all biochemical processes, requiring a substrate molecule for conversion into a product.

Cofactor is a nonproteic component that is necessary for the enzyme activity. It can be categorized into a coenzyme or prosthetic group.

Coenzyme is a cofactor of organic nature not covalently bound to the enzyme. Many coenzymes are vitamin derivatives, such as FMN and FAD.

Heme is a prosthetic group, usually an iron-containing heteroclyclic ring, the porphyrin.

Heme oxigenase is an enzyme that catalyzes the degradation of heme group, producing biliverdin, iron, and carbon monoxide.

Prosthetic group is a cofactor covalently bounded to the enzyme. It may be of organic nature, such as vitamins, or inorganic nature, like metal ions.

Synthetases are enzymes that catalyze the linkage of two molecules by using the energy derived from the ATP hydrolysis. The International Union of Biochemistry now classifies them as type 6 enzymes (ligases).

Synthases are enzymes that do not use energy from nucleoside triphosphates, differently from synthetases (see above). The Joint Commission on Biochemical Nomenclature (JCBN) dictates that the term 'synthase' may be applied to any enzyme that catalyzes synthesis (whether or not it uses nucleoside triphosphates), whereas 'synthetase' is to be used synonymously with ligase.

Microsomes are vesicles only formed from the endoplasmic reticulum in laboratory preparations for studying the metabolism of some compounds and drug interactions.

Acknowlegments The authors acknowledge the support of Brazilian governmental funding agencies FAPESP, CAPES, CNPq.

References

Anderson BB, Scattoni M, Perry GM, Galvan P, Giuberti M, Buonocore G, Vullo C. Am J Hum Genet. 1994;55:975–80.

Anderson B, Vullo C. Gut. 1994:35:1487–89

Apeland T, Mansoor MA, Pentieva K, McNulty H, Strandjord RE. Clin Chem. 2003;49:1005–8.

Asada H, Kawamura Y, Maruyama K, Kume H, Ding R, Ji FY, Kanbara N, Kuzume H, Sanbo M, Yagi T, Obata K. Biochem Biophys Res Commun. 1997;229:891–5.

Aslan K, Bozdemir H, Unsal C, Guvenc B. J Lab Hematol. 2008;30:26–35.

Bains JS, Shaw CA. Brain Res Brain Res Rev. 1997;25:335–58.

Bates CJ. World Rev Nutr Diet, Riboflavin deficiency. 1987;50:215–65.

Bates CJ, Riboflavin C. Int J Vitam Nutr Res. 1993;63:274–7.

Berwick M, Vineis P. J Natl Cancer Inst. 2000;92:874–97.

Bikle DD. Curr Osteoporos Rep. 2009;7:58–63.

Boehnke C, Reuter U, Flach U, Schuh-Hofer S, Einhaupl KM, Arnold G. Eur J Neurol. 2004;11:475–7.

Brinton RD, Thompson RF, Foy MR, Baudry M, Wang J, Finch CE, Morgan TE, Pike CJ, Mack WJ, Stanczyk FZ, Nilsen J. Front Neuroendocrinol. 2008;29:313–39.

Bruckdorfer R. Mol Aspects Med. 2005;26:3–31.

Buell JS, Dawson-Hughes B. Mol Aspects Med. 2008;29:415–22.

Casey JL, Hentze MW, Koeller DM, Caughman SW, Rouault TA, Klausner RD, Harford JB. Science. 1988;240:924–8.

Coimbra CG, Junqueira VBC. Braz J Med Biol Res. 2003;36:1409–17.

Collins MA, Neafsey EJ. Neurotoxicol Teratol. 2002;24:571–7.

Condo M, Posar A, Arbizzani A, Parmeggiani A. J Headache Pain. 2009;10:361–5.

Correale J, Ysrraelit MC, Gaitan MI. Brain. 2009;132:1146–60.

Cutolo M. Rheumatology. 2009;48:210–2.

DalPai J, Borges AA, Grassl C, Favero LA, Xavier GF, Junqueira VBC, Lopes AC, Coimbra CG, Sinigaglia-Coimbra R. Curr Top Nutr Res. 2007;5:149–55.

Davies E, MacKenzie SM. Clin Exp Pharmacol Physiol. 2003;30:437–45.

Dexter DT, Carayon A, Vidailhet M, Ruberg M, Agid F, Agid Y, Lees AJ, Wells FR, Jenner P, Marsden CD. J Neurochem. 1990;55:16–20.

Di Monte DA. Neurology. 1991;41:38–42.

Djukic A. Pediatr Neurol. 2007;37:387–97.

Droge W, Breitkreutz R. Proc Nutr Soc. 2000;59:595–600.

Fidelus RK, Tsan MF. Immunology. 1987;61:503–8.

Foraker AB, Khantwal CM, Swaan PW. Adv Drug Deliv Rev. 2003;55:1467–83.

Franco R, Cidlowski JA. Cell Death Differ.2009;16:1303–14.

Fricke MN, Jones-Davis DM, Mathews GC. J Neurochem. 2007;102:1895–1904.

Garcion E, Wion-Barbot N, Montero-Menei CN, Berger F, Wion D. Trends Endocrinol Metab. 2002;13:100–5.

Gospe SM Jr (1998) J. Pediatr. 132: 919–923

Griffith OW. Free Radic Biol Med. 1999;27:922–35.

Guix FX, Uribesalgo I, Coma M, Munoz FJ. Prog Neurobiol. 2005;76:126–52.

Hall AG. Eur J Clin Invest. 1999;29:238–45.

Hendler SS, Rorvik D. In: Hendler SS, Rorvik D, editors. PDR for nutritional supplements. Montvale: Thomson Reuters; 2008. p. 547–553.

Hoane MR, Wolyniak JG, Akstulewicz SL. J Neurotrauma. 2005;22:1112–22.

Hoffmann GF, Schmitt B, Windfuhr M, Wagner N, Strehl H, Bagci S, Franz AR, Mills PB, Clayton PT, Baumgartner MR, Steinmann B, Bast T, Wolf NI, Zschocke J. J Inherit Metab Dis. 2007;30:96–9.

Hultquist DE, Xu F, Quandt KS, Shlafer M, Mack CP, Till GO, Seekamp A, Betz AL, Ennis SR. Am J Hematol. 1993;42:13–8.

Hustad S, McKinley MC, McNulty H, Schneede J, Strain JJ, Scott JM, Ueland PM. Clin Chem. 2002;48:1571–7.

Hustad S, Ueland PM, Vollset SE, Zhang Y, Bjørke-Monsen AL, Schneede J. Clin Chem. 2000;46:1065–71.

Jansonius JN. Curr Opin Struct Biol. 1998;8:759–69.

Jenner P, Dexter DT, Sian J, Schapira AHV, Marsden CD. Ann Neurol. 1992;32:S82–7.

Joshi G, Pradhan S, Mittal B. J Neurol Sci. 2009;277:133–7.

Jusko WJ, Levy G. J Pharm Sci. 1970;59:765–72.

Kalueff AV, Minasyan A, Tuohimaa P. Brain Res Bull. 2005;67:156–60.
Kim ST, Choi JH, Chang JW, Kim SW, Hwang O. J Neurochem. 2005;95:89–98.
Kimball SM, Ursell MR, O'Connor P, Vieth R. Am J Clin Nutr. 2007;86:645–51.
Kmoch S, Zeman J, Hrebicek M, Ryba L, Kristensen MJ, Gregersen N. J Inherit Metab Dis. 1995;18:227–9.
Kowa H, Yasui K, Takeshima T, Urakami K, Sakai F, Nakashima K. Am J Med Genet. 2000; 96:762–4.
Krause KH, Bonjour JP, Berlit P, Kynast G, Schmidt-Gayk H, Schellenberg B. Drug Nutr Interact. 1988;5:317–43.
Kusumi M, Ishizaki K, Kowa H, Adachi Y, Takeshima T, Sakai F, Nakashima K. Eur Neurol. 2003;49:218–22.
Locigno R, Castronovo V. Int J Oncol. 2001;19:221–36.
Logroscino G, Marder K, Graziano J, Freyer G, Slavkovich V, LoIacono N, Cote L, Mayeux R. Neurology. 1997;49:714–7.
MacLennan SC, Wade FM, Forrest KM, Ratanayake PD, Fagan E, Antony J. J Child Neurol. 2008;23:1300–4.
Maines MD. Annu Rev Pharmacol Toxicol. 1997;37:517–54.
Mann VM, Cooper JM, Daniel SE, Srai K, Jenner P, Marsden CD, Schapira AH. Ann Neurol. 1994;36:876–81.
Massey V. Biochem Soc Trans. 2000;28:283–96.
Mizuno Y, Matuda S, Yoshino H, Mori H, Hattori N, Ikebe S. Ann Neurol. 1994;35:204–10.
Moat SJ, Ashfield-Watt PAL, Powers HJ, Newcombe RG, McDowell IFW. Clin Chem 2003;49:295–302.
Mooney S, Leuendorf JE, Hendrickson C, Hellmann H. Molecules. 2009;14:329–351.
Murad F. Can J Ophthalmol. 2008;43:291–4.
Mytilineou C, Werner P, Molinari S, Di Rocco A, Cohen G, Yahr MD. J Neural Transm Park Dis Dement Sect. 1994;8:223–8.
Naoi M, Maruyama W, Akao Y, Yi H. Neurotoxicol Teratol. 2002;24:579–91.
Nebert DW, Russell DW. Lancet. 2002;360:1155–62.
Nelson DL, Cox MM. In: Lehninger principles of biochemistry. New York: Worth Publishers; 2009. Chapters 8 and 13.
Niino M, Fukazawa T, Kikuchi S, Sasaki H. Curr Med Chem. 2008;15:499–505.
Ogunleye AJ, Odutuga AA. J Nutr Sci Vitaminol. 1989;35:193–7.
Olesen J. Pharmacol Ther. 2008;120:157–71.
Olteanu H, Banerjee R. J Biol Chem. 2001;276:35558–63.
Pani MA, Regulla K, Segni M, Krause M, Hofmann S, Hufner M, Herwig J, Pasquino AM, Usadel KH, Badenhoop K. Eur J Endocrinol. 2002;146:777–81.
Parl FF. Cancer Lett. 2005;221:123–9.
Pinto J, Huang YP, Rivlin RS. J Clin Invest. 1987;79:1343–51.
Powers HJ. Proc Nutr Soc. 1999;58:435–40.
Powers HJ. Am J Clin Nutr. 2003;77:1352–60.
Rivlin RS, Pinto JT. In: Rucker RB, Suttie JW, McCormick DB, Machlin LJ, editors. Handbook of vitamins. New York: Marcel Dekker; 2001. p. 255–274.
Sander JW. Curr Opin Neurol. 2003;16:165–70.
Santhosh-Kumar CR, Hassell KL, Deutsch JC, Kolhouse JF. Med Hypotheses. 1994;43:239–44.
Schapira AH, Cooper JM, Dexter D, Clark JB, Jenner P, Marsden CD. J Neurochem. 1990;54:823–7.
Schoenen J, Jacquy J, Lenaerts M. Neurology. 1998;50:466–70.
Schulz JB, Lindenau J, Seyfried J, Dichgans J. Eur J Biochem. 2000;267:4904–11.
Schwaninger M, Ringleb P, Winter R, Kohl B, Fiehn W, Rieser PA, Walter-Sack I. Epilepsia. 1999;40:345–50.
Siegel A, Malkowitz L, Moskovits MJ, Christakos S. Brain Res. 1984;298:125–9.
Sinha R, Caporaso N. Ann Epidemiol. 1997;7:350–6.
Sipetic-Grujicicl S, Vlajinac H, Maksiniovic J, Marinkovic J, Dzoljic E, Ratkov I, Kostic V. Parkinsonism Relat Disord. 2007;13:S35.
Skoupy S, Fodinger M, Veitl M, Perschl A, Puttinger H, Rohrer C, Schindler K, Vychytil A, Horl WH, Sunder-Plassmann G. J Am Soc Nephrol. 2002;13:1331–7.
Smith AD, Castro SL, Zigmond MJ. Physiol Behav. 2002;77:527–31.
Smolders J, Menheere P, Kessels A, Damoiseaux J, Hupperts R. Mult Scler. 2008;14:1220–4.
Smolders J, Peelen E, Thewissen M, Menheere P, Cohen Tervaert JW, Hupperts R, Damoiseaux J. Autoimmun Rev. 2009;8:621–6.
Speciale SG. Neurotoxicol Teratol. 2002;24:607–20.
Spector R. J Clin Invest. 1980;66:821–31.
Spector R, Johanson C. Pharm Res. 2006; 23:2515–24.
Vieth R. J Steroid Biochem Mol Biol. 2004;89–90:575–9.
Wacker J, Fruhauf J, Schulz M, Chiwora FM, Volz J, Becker K. Obstet Gynecol. 2000;96:38–44.
Wang M, Roberts DL, Paschke R, Shea TM, Masters BSS, Kim JJP. Proc Natl Acad Sci USA. 1997;94:8411–6.
White HB, Merril Jr AH. Ann Rev Nutr. 1988;8:279–99.
WHO – World Health Organization/FAO – Food and Agriculture Organization of the United Nations. Vitamin and mineral requirements in human nutrition. 2009.
Wolf NI, Bast T, Surtees R. Epileptic Disord. 2005;7:67–81.
Zempleni J, Galloway JR, McCormick DB. Am J Clin Nutr. 1996;63:54–66.

Chapter 154
Brain Mechanisms Involved in the Detection and Adaptation to Lysine Deficiency

Takashi Kondoh and Kunio Torii

Abbreviations

LHA	Lateral hypothalamic area
MSG	Monosodium L-glutamate
PEP	Purified egg protein
TVX	Subdiaphragmatic total vagotomy
VMH	Ventromedial nucleus of the hypothalamus

154.1 Introduction

Essential amino acids, such as L-lysine, cannot be produced by the body, and must therefore be obtained from diet in order to support growth, reproduction, and, ultimately, survival. Deficiency of a specific essential amino acid represents a relevant model to describe the overall adaptive changes in ingestive behaviors resulting from nutrient deficiency. Lysine deficiency is, arguably, one of the best models to study the adaptive changes in behavior that take place during specific nutrient deficiencies (Table 154.1). For example, while lysine is the limiting amino acid in proteins found in feed grains (Torii et al. 1987), it is not a direct precursor of any neurotransmitter in the brain. Lysine levels both in the blood and cerebrospinal fluid are high among 20 amino acids (Nishimura et al. 1995). The risk of lysine deficiency is high in low socioeconomic human populations who depend predominantly on wheat for their protein supply (Young and Pellett 1990). Rats fed a bread-based, lysine-impoverished diet based on wheat gluten, show low weight gain, reduced appetite, nervousness, and ingestion of their own body hair (Culik and Rosenberg 1958). However, rats fed lysine-supplemented bread do not show any of the above signs, and grow normally. In humans, negative nitrogen balance by consumption of wheat gluten is also observed (Bricker et al. 1945).

Deficiency of an essential amino acid affects both appetite and taste preferences for other amino acids and NaCl. Rats in nutritionally well-balanced conditions normally display strong preferences for monosodium L-glutamate (MSG; an umami substance) and L-arginine solutions (Torii et al. 1987). However, inducing states of lysine deficiency will result in concomitant abnormal patterns in both body physiology and taste preferences. In fact, when rats are restricted to a lysine-deficient diet, lysine levels in both plasma and brain decline (Mori et al. 1991a), since lysine concentrations in

K. Torii (✉)
Institute of Life Sciences, Ajinomoto Co., Inc., Suzuki-cho 1-1, Kawasaki-ku, Kawasaki 210-8681, Japan
e-mail: kunio_torii@ajinomoto.com

V.R. Preedy et al. (eds.), *Handbook of Behavior, Food and Nutrition*,
DOI 10.1007/978-0-387-92271-3_154, © Springer Science+Business Media, LLC 2011

Table 154.1 Key features of L-lysine

1. Lysine is a basic and essential amino acid with bitter taste quality.
2. Among 20 amino acids, lysine levels in the blood and cerebrospinal fluid are high.
3. Lysine is not a direct precursor of any neurotransmitter in the brain.
4. Lysine is the first limiting amino acid in proteins of some feed grains (wheat and corn).
5. Substantial risk of lysine deficiency exists in low socioeconomic human populations who consume wheat or corn as a major protein supply.
6. Characteristic symptoms of lysine (or an essential amino acid) deficiency are reduced appetite, low weight gain, and nervousness.
7. Replete of missing nutrient will cause rapid recovery from these symptoms.

This table lists the key facts of lysine in our body or in food

plasma directly reflect the lysine content in the diet (Mori et al. 1991a). Under lysine deficiency, food intake and growth are depressed, a physiological pattern that is accompanied by increased preferences for NaCl in detriment of MSG or arginine (Torii et al. 1987). However, when offered a lysine solution, which is bitter and hence normally aversive to animals, lysine-deficient rats will robustly drink the solution, resulting in normalization of food intake levels and growth (Tabuchi et al. 1991; Torii et al. 1987, 1996). In this repleting process, their initial preference for NaCl changes towards MSG as in nondeficient rats. As the immediate licking responses to lysine solution in brief (10 s)-access tests do not increase during lysine deficiency (Markison et al. 1999), the preference for the missing amino acid appears to be learned rather than innate. In other words, learning a positive association between the taste of lysine (conditioned stimulus) and its repleting, postingestional consequences (unconditioned stimulus) is required before a lysine-deficient animal will engage in adaptive increases in lysine intake. However, the sensing mechanisms involved in detecting the deficient nutrient and the brain mechanisms regulating adaptive preferences remain poorly understood.

This review describes our current knowledge on the peripheral sensing sites, signaling pathways, and primary brain areas regulating adaptation to nutrient deficiency. We focus on lysine deficiency since this constitutes a functional working model of essential amino acid deficiency.

154.2 Changes in Food Intake, Weight Gain, and Taste Preference During Protein Deficiency

Before discussing overall changes occur during lysine deficiency, we would like to describe what happens during protein deficiency. Protein is a macronutrient essential for growth, reproduction and survival. Protein is involved not only for muscle contraction but also for numerous physiological functions since they form the constitutive material of receptors, ion channels, transporters, enzymes, immunoproteins, and transcription factors.

During low protein intake starvation, body nitrogen concentration declines to negative levels (Harper 1974). During fasting, body protein breaks down into amino acids that are used to produce energy as a replacement for glucose (Harper 1974). A characteristic symptom of Kwashiokor disease is hypoproteinemia, due to fasting-induced malnutrition; recovery takes place immediately upon treatment with a high-protein diet (Rosenberg and Rohdenburg 1952). Rats offered a low or no-protein diet show reduced food intake and reduced body weight (Mori et al. 1991a) (Fig. 154.1). Considering data from body weight measurements, the minimum percentage of protein content in diet required for normal growth in young growing rats is estimated to be 12.5% (Mori et al. 1991a) in the case of purified egg protein (PEP), an ideal protein source associated with highly efficient nitrogen storage (Forbes et al. 1958). In fact, in the choice experiments involving low (5% PEP) and

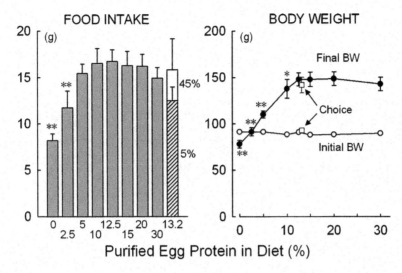

Fig. 154.1 Mean daily food intake and body weight (BW) changes in rats fed diets with various protein levels for 1 week. Rats at 4 weeks of age were fed a diet containing purified egg protein (PEP) at levels between 0% and 30%, or given a choice between 5% PEP and 45% PEP diets. Results are expressed as mean ± SD, $n = 8$. $^{*}P < 0.05$ and $^{**}P < 0.01$, significance compared to rats fed 20% PEP diet (control) by ANOVA followed by Dunnet's test (Reprinted from Mori et al. 1991a. With permission)

high (45% PEP) protein diets, rats tend to ingest an average of 13.2% protein content, very close to the 12.5% minimal estimate, a pattern associated with normal growth (Mori et al. 1991a).

Preferences for amino acid and NaCl solutions are also related to protein nutrition (Fig. 154.2). When dietary protein levels are normal, preference for umami taste substances such as MSG is high, suggesting that umami taste is a marker of protein ingestion (Torii et al. 1987). In contrast, preference for NaCl and glycine increases under severe protein deficiency, possibly reflecting negative nitrogen balance in the body. Glycine is effective in ameliorating low nitrogen levels under protein deficiency, suggesting a sparing effect on endogenous protein degradation (Torii et al. 1987). Therefore, preferences for certain amino acids (e.g., MSG and glycine) and NaCl depend on protein nutrition.

154.3 Lysine Deficiency and Lysine Levels in the Plasma and Brain

Some protein-rich foods contain low levels of certain amino acids. For example, wheat gluten contains low levels of lysine and methionine (20% and 17%, respectively), and corn zein is low in lysine and tryptophan (0.7% and 15%, respectively) compared to PEP (Table 154.2). Wheat flour is a major supply of plant protein for humans, and gluten is the major protein in the wheat. These proteins have been used to investigate animal ingestive behaviors associated with protein or amino acid deficiency.

Since feeding of crystalline amino acid mixture-based diets readily suppress further food intake, the protein component of a lysine-deficient diet is obtained from wheat gluten fortified with crystalline essential amino acids excluding lysine (Table 154.3). Control diets ("lysine-sufficient" diets) are fortified with crystalline lysine (L-lysine HCl). Different amounts of glutamine are added to the diets to make them isonitrogenous to a 20% PEP diet (Mori et al. 1991a). Since wheat gluten contains 20% of the total lysine levels found in PEP, a lysine-deficient diet should have 20% of the lysine levels of a control diet, rather than 0% (unless stated otherwise). This level of lysine (20% of control) is required to maintain homeostasis and avoid negative nitrogen balance in experimental animals (Torii et al. 1987).

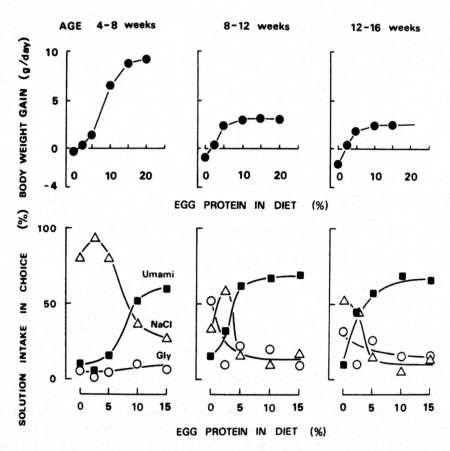

Fig. 154.2 Body weight gain (*upper*) and taste preference (*lower*) in rats fed diets with various protein levels and at various ages. Rats at 4, 8, and 12 weeks of age were fed diets containing purified egg protein at levels between 0% and 15% for 4 weeks. Averaged values of daily weight gain and percentage intake of each solution [NaCl, glycine (Gly), and umami] are shown, $n = 8$ (Reprinted from Torii et al. 1987. With permission)

The diurnal patterns of lysine concentrations in the plasma and brain are quite comparable to each other. In lysine-repleted (control) rats, lysine levels in plasma and brain are stable throughout the day (Mori et al. 1991a). In lysine-deficient rats, however, both plasma and brain lysine levels decline dramatically following onset of feeding (mainly during the dark phase since rats are nocturnal animals), but return to control levels by the end of the light phase (Fig. 154.3). During the dark phase, plasma lysine declines to near zero, but brain lysine declines to approximately one-third of control levels. Recovery of lysine levels during the light phase may reflect degradation of body proteins in order to supply amino acids to the body, especially to the brain. In fact, lysine concentrations in plasma reflect dietary lysine levels (Mori et al. 1991a) (Fig. 154.4).

154.4 Changes in Taste Preferences During Lysine Deficiency

When rats are offered diets deficient in or containing imbalanced levels of amino acids, food intake is remarkably depressed (Harper et al. 1970), followed by an attempt by animals to change their dietary source (Inoue et al. 1995). Under states of amino acid deficiency, the dietary restricted amino acid, rather than protein content, can act as the dietary stimulus to control food selection.

Table 154.2 L-Amino acid composition of whole egg protein (PEP), wheat gluten, and corn zein (Reprinted with modification from Torii et al. 1987. With permission)

L-amino acid	Concentration (% of 16 g nitrogen)		
	PEP	Wheat gluten	Corn zein
Essential amino acids			
Lysine	7.39	1.48	0.05
Methionine	3.30	0.56	1.62
Tryptophan	1.44	0.77	0.21
Phyenlyalanine	5.66	4.87	7.47
Isoleucine	5.72	3.23	3.91
Leucine	9.71	6.71	21.85
Valine	6.61	3.53	3.69
Threonine	4.83	2.46	2.81
Histidine	2.41	1.90	1.23
Nonessential amino acids			
Glutamic acid	12.84	33.58	23.81
Aspartic acid	10.08	3.13	5.70
Arginine	7.04	3.27	1.31
Serine	7.76	4.87	5.48
Alanine	6.05	2.50	10.98
Glycine	3.53	3.31	1.18
Proline	4.28	13.95	1.15
Tyrosine	4.05	3.09	5.17
Cysteine	2.30	2.82	0.34

Each protein sample was hydrolyzed and assayed for amino acid content by an automatic amino acid analyzer (micro-Kjeldahl method)

Table 154.3 Composition of lysine-sufficient (control) and lysine-deficient diets (Reprinted from Torii et al. 1987. With permission)

Composition	Experimental diets	
	Control	Lysine-deficient
Wheat gluten	24.35	24.35
L-Lysine HCl	1.35	–
L-Glutamine	0.68	1.76
L-Amino acid mixture	3.72	3.72
Corn starch	55.69	55.96
Mineral mixture	4.00	4.00
Vitamin mixture	1.00	1.00
Choline chloride	0.20	0.20
Vitamin E	0.01	0.01
Cellulose powder	4.00	4.00
Corn oil	5.00	5.00
Total	100	100
L-Lysine content in diet (%, w/w)	1.35	0.27

Each protein sample was hydrolyzed and assayed for amino acid content by an automatic amino acid analyzer (micro-Kjeldahl method). Values are shown as % of weight in each diet

Lysine deficiency drastically changes the behavioral response of rats to lysine solutions from aversion to attraction. When rats are given a lysine-deficient diet, they will select the lysine solution out of various other sapid solutions (Mori et al. 1991a; Tabuchi et al. 1991; Torii et al. 1987).

DIURNAL VARIATION OF LYSINE

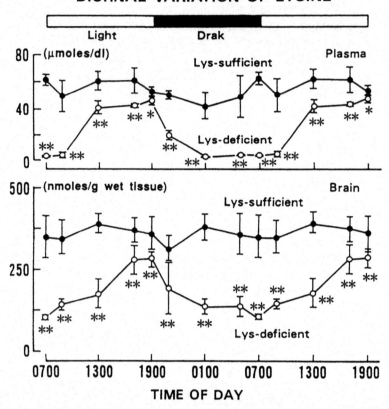

Fig. 154.3 Diurnal variation of lysine concentration in the plasma (*upper*) and brain (*lower*) under lysine-sufficient (control) and lysine-deficient conditions in rats. (**a**), in control, lysine levels in blood and brain are stable within a day. During lysine deficiency, however, lysine levels in both plasma and brain are reduced during dark period (feeding period). Lysine solution was not supplied in this experiment. Lysine concentration was assayed using an automated amino acid analyzer after deproteinization by sulfosalicylic acid. Results are expressed as mean ± SD, $n = 5$. [*]$P < 0.05$ and [**]$P < 0.01$, significance compared to control by Student's t-test (Reprinted from Mori et al. 1991a. With permission)

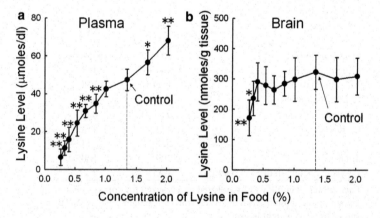

Fig. 154.4 Lysine levels in the plasma (**a**) and brain (**b**) in rats fed diets with various lysine levels. Rats at 4 weeks of age were given free access to a diet with various levels of lysine from deficiency to excess, equivalent to a lysine composition in 4–30% purified egg protein (PEP), for 8 weeks. The diet containing 1.35% lysine (equivalent to the lysine content in 20% PEP) was employed as control. Lysine solution was not supplied in this experiment. Results are expressed as mean ± SD, $n = 6$. [*]$P < 0.05$ and [**]$P < 0.01$, significance compared to control by ANOVA followed by Dunnet's test (Reprinted from Mori et al. 1991a. With permission)

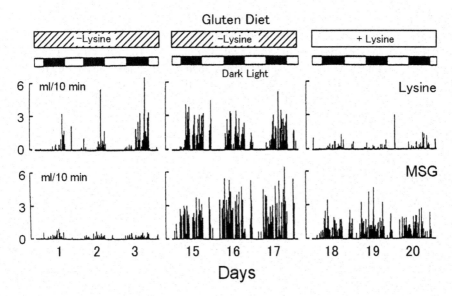

Fig. 154.5 Preference for lysine solution appears during lysine deficiency. *Upper*, intake (mL/10 min) of 0.4 M lysine solution; *Lower*, intake (mL/10 min) of monosodium L-glutamate (MSG) solution. Rats were offered lysine-deficient (– Lysine) or lysine-sufficient (+ Lysine) diets. Preference for lysine solution increased gradually during lysine deficiency and reduced rapidly after recovery from deficiency. Preference for MSG solution also appeared only when nutritive conditions are well-balanced (Reprinted from Mori et al. 1991a. With permission)

Preference for lysine solutions increase gradually during lysine deficiency and is rapidly reduced after repletion (Fig. 154.5). Preferences for MSG solution also appear only when nutritive conditions are well-balanced. Rats fed a tryptophan-deficient diet also prefer a tryptophan solution (bitter) over a saccharin solution (sweet), a choice that ameliorates their state (Mori et al. 1991b). The increased preference for a deficient nutrient is commonly observed when rats are given a diet deficient in one of the other essential amino acids (Mori et al. 1991a). These adaptive behavioral changes are considered to be learned preferences (Gietzen et al. 1992; Markison et al. 1999; Naito-Hoopes et al. 1993). In fact, lysine deficiency in rats does not seem to enhance the "palatability" of lysine as assessed by licking responses including lick rate, bout size and bout number (Markison et al. 2000). In contrast, increases in acceptance (i.e., reduction in aversion) to lysine solution are reported in lysine-deficient mice (Ninomiya et al. 1994b).

154.5 Peripheral Mechanisms

The detection of deficiency in amino acid levels will take place only after digestion of protein. Absorption of amino acids also plays an important role in sensing the levels of a deficient nutrient. Nutritional stimuli in the gut elicit hormonal release into the circulation as well as vagal activation, which are key components of the gut-brain communication. For detection of chemical compounds, specific receptors and neural coding mechanisms may exist in the gastrointestinal tract and hepato-portal region. Integration of postingestive consequences with oronasal sensory stimuli (e.g., taste, odor, and texture) occurs in the brain. Both peripheral and central mechanisms are involved in the responses observed during amino acid deficiency (Hawkins et al. 1994; Tabuchi et al. 1991).

In what follows, we describe the elevated serum levels of inhibin, a heterodimeric protein composed of α and β-subunits and a member of the transforming growth factor-β (TGF-β) superfamily, and increases in the sensitivity of hepatic vagal efferent fibers 100-fold during lysine deficiency. Behavioral aversion threshold to lysine solutions also increases 100-fold. Sensitivity of taste nerves, however, does not change under the same condition. Furthermore, in the transection of peripheral nerves, we describe the contributions of the taste and vagus nerves to the adaptive behavioral changes induced by lysine deficiency.

154.5.1 Humoral Factors

It is possible that different neurotrophic or neuromodulatory factors are released in the systemic circulation during lysine deficiency resulting in changes in sensitivity to the deficient nutrient and/or in adaptive responses. There are a number of bioactive candidates that may act at concentrations too low to be detected by most available methods. One very sensitive assay, able to detect a number of humoral factors at the femtomolar concentration range, makes use of Hydra Japonica (hydra) (Hanai 1981). Tentacle ball formation is a sign of feeding behavior in the hydra under various levels of S-methylglutathione, and inhibition of this behavior can be differentially and quantitatively observed when certain humoral factors are present along with the feeding stimulus (Hanai 1981).

Rats fed a protein-restricted diet overnight show elevated serum levels of activin A (Torii et al. 1993), a homodimeric protein composed of two inhibin β_A-subunits and a member of the TGF-β superfamily. In contrast, inhibin is increased during lysine deficiency while activin A-like activity in the serum is severely suppressed. Inhibin has opposing biological effects to activin by competing with activin for binding with its receptors and/or binding to inhibin-specific receptors (Robertson et al. 2004). Results from additional assays, i.e., radioimmunoassays for inhibin and an erythroid differentiation assay for activin A, also confirmed the release of inhibin during lysine deficiency (Torii et al. 1996). These results suggest that activin A levels in the blood plays a role in alerting the brain of amino acid imbalance, and might subsequently induce an adaptive response aimed at reversing amino acid imbalances.

154.5.2 Taste Nerve

Neurophysiological studies have shown that the chorda tympani and glossopharyngeal nerves considerably differ in their responses to various taste stimuli. For example, bitter-tasting substances, such as quinine, sucrose octaacetate, and some essential amino acids (tryptophan, phenylalanine, and histidine), elicit greater responses in the glossopharyngeal nerve compared to the chorda tympani (Ninomiya et al. 1993; Shingai and Beidler 1985). The glossopharyngeal nerve also shows greater responses to MSG, an umami substance (Ninomiya et al. 1993), suggesting that the glossopharyngeal nerve carries the main taste inputs regarding both behaviorally aversive and nutritionally important substances present in food (Ninomiya et al. 1994b).

In mice, behavioral aversion thresholds to lysine solution, which is bitter and normally aversive for animals, increase approximately 100-fold during lysine deficiency compared to the control in brief (10 s) acceptance tests (Ninomiya et al. 1994b). Licking responses to other essential amino acids (phenylalanine, leucine), quinine, and various other taste substances do not change during lysine deficiency. The increase in acceptability to lysine induced by deficiency is also observed after

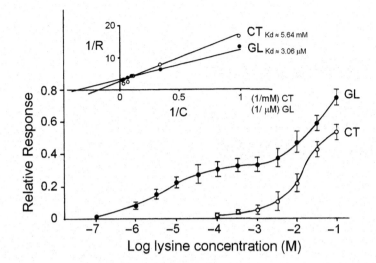

Fig. 154.6 Concentration-response relationships for lysine in the chorda tympani (CT) and glossopharyngeal (GL) nerves, and their double reciprocal plots in mice. The vertical axis represents relative responses to 0.1 M NH$_4$Cl as the standard stimulus. C, concentration of lysine (in mM for CT and in μM for GL). R, relative response. Results are expressed as mean ± SD, n = 8-10 (Reprinted from Ninomiya et al. 1994a. With permission)

transection of the chorda tympani while it disappears after bilateral transections of the glossopharyngeal nerve. These results suggest that taste information conveyed via the glossopharyngeal nerve plays a major role on an increase in hedonic value of lysine solution.

Neural responses to lysine are relatively larger in the glossopharyngeal nerve compared to the chorda tympani in control mice (Ninomiya et al. 1994a) (Fig. 154.6). The neural threshold for detection of a lysine solution is 2.5 log units lower in the glossopharyngeal nerve (~1.0 μM) than in the chorda tympani (~300 μM). An analysis of concentration-response relationships suggest a possibility that there are two different receptors (high- and low-affinity types) for lysine, each showing a different dissociation constant. The posterior region of the tongue would express both types, while the anterior region would express only the low-affinity type (Ninomiya et al. 1994a). Interestingly, lysine deficiency hardly affects the neural thresholds of both chorda tympani and glossopharyngeal nerves to lysine (see discussion in Ninomiya et al. 1994b), suggesting that the increased acceptance to lysine during lysine deficiency is primary mediated by the brain not by alteration of peripheral taste information.

In contrast to mice data mentioned above, rats show behavioral changes for lysine ingestion only over mM concentration range (Pritchard et al. 1982) and data from transection of taste nerves in rats point to a relatively more important role for the chorda tympani than the glossopharyngeal nerve in selecting lysine solutions during lysine deficiency (Tabuchi et al. 1996). Further studies are required to clarify the roles of these primary taste nerves in increasing preferences for deficient amino acids.

154.5.3 Vagus Nerve

The vagus nerve innervates major portions of the gastrointestinal system and is important in the control of feeding. As lysine in food normally exists in a protein-bound form, it is reasonable to assume that a peripheral lysine sensor that monitors free lysine levels following protein digestion exist in the

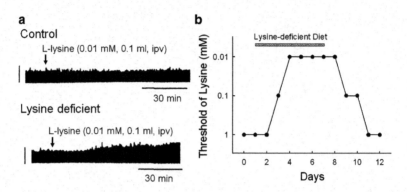

Fig. 154.7 Responses of hepatic vagal afferent fibers to lysine (**a**) and the chronological changes in lysine sensitivity (**b**) in control and during lysine deficiency. (**a**) Administration of L-lysine solution (0.01 mM, 0.1 mL) in the portal vein (ipv) increases the firing rate of the hepatic vagal afferents during lysine deficiency but not in control. Vertical bar, 60 spikes/5 s. (**b**) The threshold (the least effective concentration) of lysine changes 100-fold within 4 days both during lysine deficiency and recovery, each period from deficiency. Each data correspond to observation from one rat (Reprinted from Torii and Niijima 2001. With permission)

luminal side of gastrointestinal tract, the hepatoportal region, or in the systemic circulation. The hepatoportal region is an appropriate area for detecting amino acid levels, and abdominal vagal afferents may provide the brain with information about the current levels of dietary amino acids. Accordingly, sensitivity of hepatic vagal afferents to intraportal administrations of lysine increases 100-fold during lysine deficiency compared to control states: the lowest effective concentration of lysine to evoke hepatic vagal activity is 1 mM during lysine repletion and 0.01 mM during lysine deficiency in rats (Torii and Niijima 2001) (Fig. 154.7). Sensitivity to other L-amino acids (L-alanine and L-leucine) and D-lysine remains unchanged. To reach maximum sensitivity to lysine, 4 days of lysine restriction are required (Torii and Niijima 2001). These results indicate the existence of putative lysine sensors in the hepatoportal region that contribute to maintain amino acid homeostasis.

Recently, a receptor for basic amino acids, namely "GPRC6A" (G-protein-coupled receptor, family C, group 6, subtype A), was found in the brain and peripheral organs such as kidney, skeletal muscle, testis, and white cells (Wellendorph et al. 2004). The receptor is also evident in the mesenteric arteries (Harno et al. 2008). The receptor may contribute monitoring of lysine levels in the blood and brain. However, GPRC6A responds not only to lysine, but is a broadly-tuned sensor of other basic amino acids such as arginine, citrulline, and ornithine with EC_{50} values in the range 20–100 µM (Wellendorph et al. 2005). If there are other types of basic amino acid receptors with different ligand specificity, combination of these putative receptors may enable to monitor the lysine levels in our body.

The enhanced sensitivity of hepatic vagal afferents contributes in the identification of the deficient nutrient, and to alter preferences towards enhancing selective intake of foods containing the deficient nutrients, which prevents malnutrition and anorexia.

154.5.4 Effects of Vagotomy on Food Intake and Food Selection

The abdominal vagotomy, especially the transection of the hepatic branch, attenuates anorexia induced by an amino acid (threonine) imbalanced diet (Dixon et al. 2000), suggesting an involvement of the vagus nerve in detecting peripheral nutritional signals. To investigate the primary sensing site for lysine, Inoue et al. (1995) studied the effects of continuous lysine infusions via the intragastric, intraperitoneal, and intracerebroventricular routes on dietary choice. Rats were given a food choice between a lysine-deficient and a protein-free diet. Previous to lysine infusions, they consumed consistently more of the protein-free compared to the lysine-deficient diet (approximately 70% versus 30% in preference, respectively). After lysine infusions via either intragastric or intraperitoneal routes, ingestion of the lysine-deficient diet increased while the intracerebroventricular infusions, within the physiological range, failed to affect food choice. Hepatic vagotomy delayed the increased preference for the lysine-deficient diet in rats injected with lysine intraperitoneally. These results implicate postabsorptive mechanisms (but not the cerebrospinal fluid) in sensing a deficient amino acid, and suggest the involvement of the hepatic vagal afferents in this sensing pathway.

154.6 Brain Mechanisms

154.6.1 Neuronal Activity in the Lateral Hypothalamic Area

The lateral hypothalamic area (LHA) is one of the most important central structures involved in feeding and drinking behaviors (Oomura 1980). LHA neurons receive information from various exogenous (visual, auditory, olfactory, and gustatory) and endogenous inputs (Ono et al. 1985; Nakamura et al. 1989; Nishino et al. 1988; Oomura et al. 1980), which are important factors regulating the ingestion and rejection of foods and fluids. Some LHA neurons respond during feeding and gustatory stimulation, and the ingestion responses are modulated by food palatability, deprivation, and satiation (Fukuda et al. 1986; Aou et al. 1991). Accordingly, it is reasonable to hypothesize that the LHA may control the selection of amino acids and NaCl under different nutritive conditions.

To evaluate the role of the LHA in the regulation of preference for amino acids and NaCl, single neuronal activity from the LHA was recorded during cue tone presentation and subsequent ingestion of various amino acids and NaCl solutions in both control and lysine-deficient rats (Tabuchi et al. 1991). Generally, LHA neurons do not discriminate between sapid solutions during ingestion. However, "MSG (umami)-specific" neurons that respond only during licking of a MSG solution are found only in control rats, whereas "lysine-specific" neurons that respond only during licking of a lysine solution were found only in lysine-deficient animals (Tabuchi et al. 1991) (Fig. 154.8). Although it is difficult to determine whether MSG-specific neurons are the same as lysine-specific neurons, these neural responses appear to be related to behavioral preferences; MSG is the most preferred solution in control and lysine is the most preferred one in lysine-deficient rats (Torii et al. 1987). Moreover, both MSG and lysine-specific neurons are localized mainly in the dorsal and lateral part of the LHA (Tabuchi et al. 1991), where gustatory pathways are traced via the pontine taste area in rats (Norgren et al. 1976). It is plausible that some LHA neurons might be related to positive reinforcement such as "satisfaction", when rats ingest a solution that is metabolically necessary for the body. These data suggest that plastic changes in neuronal responses do occur, at least in the LHA, to promote ingestion of required nutrients. The LHA may be the primary site regulating the increased preferences for deficient amino acids.

154.6.2 Microinjection in the Lateral Hypothalamic Area

Lysine levels in the brain, as well as in the blood, decreases a few hours after ingestion of a lysine-deficient diet (Mori et al. 1991a). Neurons in the LHA are more responsive to iontophoretically applied amino acids (i.e., extracellular environment) than those in thalamus or zona incerta (Wayner

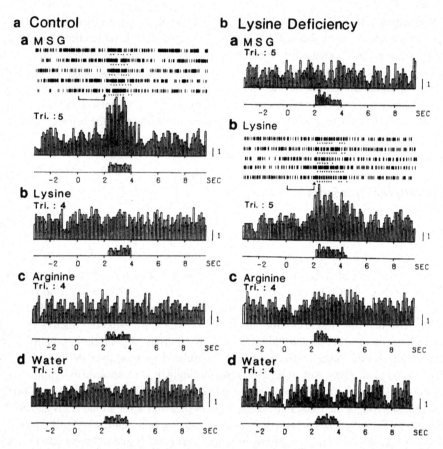

Fig. 154.8 Two examples of taste specific neurons in the lateral hypothalamic area, responding only to monosodium L-glutamate (MSG) in control (**a**) and to lysine during lysine deficiency (**b**). Rats were trained to lick solutions for 2 s licking period (2.0–4.0 s) after the end of each 2 s cue tone period (0.0–2.0 s). The neuron in (**a**) is excited during licking of MSG solution but not for any other solutions. In (**b**), the neuron is excited during licking of lysine solution but not for any other solutions. Neuronal responses to MSG in control (Aa) and to lysine during lysine deficiency (Bb) are shown by raster display (*bars*). Small dots, lick signals. Horizontal brackets, cue tone period. Arrow heads, presentation of drinking tube for licking. In each pair of averaged histograms: upper, neuronal responses; lower, lick signals; Tri, trial number. Calibration of 1 impulse per bin (100 ms) are shown at right of each upper histogram (Reprinted from Tabuchi et al. 1991. With permission)

et al. 1975). Microinjection of balanced solutions of amino acid mixture directly into the dorsolateral perifornical hypothalamus inhibited feeding in rats (Panksepp and Booth 1971). These data suggest that the LHA may be involved in the detection and recognition of deficient nutrients.

Intakes of lysine-deficient and nonprotein diets induce the release of the growth factors inhibin and activin, respectively, in the systemic circulation (Torii et al. 1993). These indicate that ingestion of lysine-deficient or nonprotein diets cause changes in blood (and possibly brain) levels of physiological factors, including inhibin and activin. These factors may be involved in the plasticity of LHA neurons regarding their responses to deficient amino acids. In addition to these peripheral changes, the β_A subunit of activin and inhibin (Torii et al. 1993) and activin receptors (Funaba et al. 1997) has been immunolocalized in a variety of brain regions including the LHA.

To investigate the roles of LHA on ingestive behavior of a deficient nutrient, rats were trained to press a bar to obtain small (50 mg) pellets of a complete diet (Hawkins et al. 1994, 1995, 1998). Rats given a lysine-deficient diet maintained a high rate of bar pressing. This behavior is reduced by (1) ad

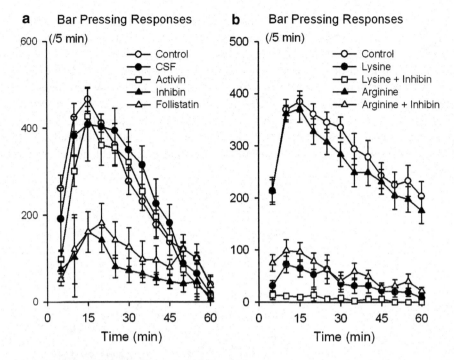

Fig. 154.9 Bar pressing behavior of lysine-deficient rats to receive complete diet (lysine-containing diet). Continuous infusions of inhibin ($P < 0.001$), follistatin ($P < 0.01$) or lysine ($P < 0.01$) into the lateral hypothalamic area reduces bar pressing behavior, while infusions of artificial cerebrospinal fluid (CSF), activin A or arginine have no effects. Results are expressed as mean ± SEM, $n = 9$ (Reprinted from Hawkins et al. 1995. With permission)

libitum access to a lysine solution, (2) intraperitoneal injections of lysine 2 h before the test session, (3) continuous infusion of a lysine solution into the LHA, (4) continuous infusion of inhibin or follistatin (activin inhibitors) into the LHA (Fig. 154.9), or (5) continuous infusion of activin antiserum into the LHA. Interestingly, infusions of lysine, inhibin, follistatin, or activin antiserum into the LHA do not ameliorate the reduced consumption of a lysine-deficient diet, suggesting the presence of different mechanisms involved in anorexia and in the preference for the missing amino acid. Neither the voluntary consumption of other solutions nor the continuous infusion of other amino acids or activin into the LHA suppressed bar-pressing behaviors. Although LHA lysine infusion decreases consumption of a concurrently available lysine solution, inhibin infusion does not change ad libitum lysine consumption. These results indicate that inhibin may work in the LHA to inhibit bar pressing to obtain a complete diet via mechanisms other than sensing lysine deficiency.

154.6.3 Norepinephrine Release in the Hypothalamus

Hypothalamic norepinephrine is involved in regulation of food intake (Bray 1993). Lysine is not a precursor of norepinephrine and does not affect norepinephrine synthesis. In control rats, norepinephrine release in the ventromedial nucleus of the hypothalamus (VMH) shows a diurnal pattern, with the lowest levels measured at the onset of the dark phase (Smriga et al. 2000a). This circadian release of norepinephrine is depressed during early lysine deficiency and ingestion of lysine solution restores the circadian pattern of norepinephrine release.

In longitudinal measurements, norepinephrine release in the VMH significantly declines within the first 24 h after the introduction of a lysine deficient diet, and the reduction of norepinephrine release persists throughout the lysine deficiency period i.e., 1 week (Smriga et al. 2000b) (Fig. 154.10). When the lysine-sufficient diet is offered, the reduced norepinephrine levels recover rapidly. The pattern of norepinephrine release is parallel to the suppression of food intake. In threonine deficient rats, increases in norepinephrine levels in homogenized VMH tissue have been reported (Gietzen et al. 1998). This increase can be attributed to reduced release of norepinephrine. Since no changes in norepinephrine release were observed in the LHA (Smriga et al. 2000b), reduced norepinephrine release in the VMH appears to be involved in both the initiation and the regulation of anorexia during lysine deficiency.

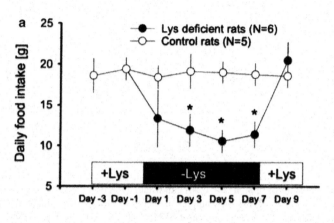

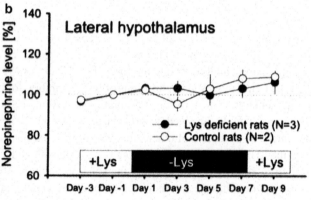

Fig. 154.10 Daily food intake (**a**), and norepineph-rine release in the lateral hypothalamus (**b**) and medial hypothalamus (**c**) in rats fed lysine-deficient diet for 1 week (Day 0–7). Dietary lysine status is illustrated in each lower part of panel. +Lys, lysine-sufficient (control) diet; –Lys, lysine-deficient diet. Results are shown as percent differences from basal levels that were measured just before the introduction of lysine-deficient diet (Day -1). *$P < 0.05$, significance compared to control rats by Student's t-test (Reprinted from Smriga et al. 2000b. With permission)

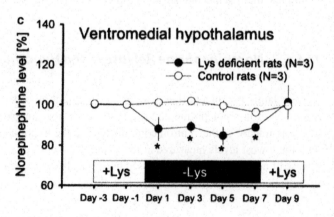

154.6.4 Lysine Preference and Reward Circuits

The dopaminergic neurons in the ventral tegmental area have a crucial role in regulating behavioral responses to natural rewards such as sweet solutions, as well as artificial rewards such as drugs of abuse. However, lesions of the ventral tegmental area dopaminergic neurons by microinjection of 6-hydroxydopamine (a selective neurotoxin for dopaminergic neurons) do not interfere with enhanced preference for lysine during lysine deficiency, whereas the preference for sucrose is largely reduced (Shibata et al. 2009). Preferences for umami (MSG and 5'-ribonucleotides) and NaCl solutions are also unaffected by ventral tegmental area lesions. These results suggest that preferences for essential amino acids, umami, and NaCl, but not sweet, solutions operate through reward circuits that are independent of ventral tegmental area dopaminergic neurons. Contribution of dopaminergic neurons from other brain areas and the identification of the reward circuits regulating preferences for deficient nutrient must be clarified in future experiments.

154.7 Applications to Other Areas of Health and Disease

Essential amino acids are absolutely necessary for growth, reproduction, and survival. Since lysine is the limiting amino acid in proteins of some feed grains (wheat and corn), lysine deficiency is commonly found in human populations living in developing areas, where staple diet is based on such grains. Characteristic symptoms of essential amino acid deficiency include reduced appetite, low weight gain, and nervousness. Repletion of the missing nutrients will result in rapid attenuation of these symptoms. Supplementation of deficient nutrients in food is one reasonable treatment or preventive measure against nutrient deficiency. The further clarification of the mechanisms involved in the adaptation to and recovery from nutrient deficiency may provide us with significant information on how to improve the quality of our dietary choices.

Summary Points

- Lysine is a basic and essential amino acid with a bitter taste quality.
- Lysine is present at low levels in proteins found in some feed grains (wheat and corn), and hence a substantial risk of lysine deficiency exists in low socioeconomic human populations who depend predominantly on such grains for their protein supply.
- Lysine is not linked directly to the synthesis of any neurotransmitter in the brain.
- Lysine deficiency can be induced in animals upon presentation of a lysine-deficient diet.
- During lysine deficiency, lysine levels in the blood and brain decline.
- During lysine deficiency, food intake and weight gain are suppressed.
- Lysine-deficient animals display increased preferences for lysine solutions, and the consumption of which results in normalization of food intake and growth.
- During lysine deficiency, blood levels of inhibin are increased and activin A-like activity are severely suppressed.
- During lysine deficiency, aversion thresholds for lysine, but not for other bitter solutions, increase 100-fold.
- During lysine deficiency, sensitivity of primary taste nerves to lysine does not change, while the sensitivity of the hepatic vagal afferents to intraportal lysine increases 100-fold within just 4 days.
- During lysine deficiency, some LHA neurons specifically respond to the ingestion of lysine.

- Microinjection of lysine, or an activin inhibitor (inhibin, follistatin, or activin antiserum), into the LHA suppresses bar pressing behaviors to obtain lysine-containing food.
- During lysine deficiency, norepinephrine release is decreased in the VMH but does not change in the LHA.
- Lesions of the ventral tegmental area dopaminergic neurons (a reward circuit) do not interfere with enhanced preference for lysine during lysine deficiency.
- These findings indicate that signals conveyed by vagal hepatic afferent fibers play an important role in the detection of a deficient nutrient. Taste information is important in the expression of taste-guided behaviors upon association of taste information with the metabolic effects of lysine.
- Brain circuits including the lateral and medial nuclei of the hypothalamus integrate neural and humoral inputs, and regulate taste preferences for deficient nutrients. The reward circuit of the ventral tegmental area is not involved in the development of lysine preferences during lysine deficiency.

Definitions and Explanations of Key Terms

Activin: A gonadal hormone composed of two inhibin beta subunits ($\beta_A\beta_A$, $\beta_A\beta_B$, or $\beta_B\beta_B$) and belongs to the transforming growth factor-β (TGF-β) superfamily. Activin is produced in the gonads, pituitary gland, placenta, and other organs and has multiple functions including secretion of follicle-stimulating hormone and regulation of erythrocyte differentiation.

Follistatin: A monomeric autocrine glycoprotein that binds directly to both activin and inhibin through the common β subunit. Follistatin is produced by folliculostellate cells of the anterior pituitary and inhibits follicle-stimulating hormone secretion. Its primary function is binding and bioneutralization of members of the TGF-β superfamily, with primary focus on activin.

Homeostasis: Conditions under which the internal environment in the body is maintained within a stable level. Homeostasis is very important for animals to live well in a healthy condition and its disturbance may cause illness.

Inhibin: A gonadal glycoprotein closely related activin, composed of α and β subunits. Inhibin has opposing biological effects to activin such as inhibition of follicle-stimulating hormone synthesis and inhibition of gonadotropin-releasing hormone release in the pituitary gland. Inhibin is considered to compete with activin for activin receptors and/or binding to inhibin specific receptors.

Lateral hypothalamic area (LHA): One of the most important central structures involved in feeding and drinking behavior (also known as the feeding center). LHA neurons receive information from various exogenous (visual, auditory, olfactory, and gustatory) and endogenous inputs, which are important determinant for ingestion or rejection of foods and fluids, and appropriate autonomic responses.

L-Lysine: A basic and essential amino acid with bitter taste quality. Since lysine content in the wheat and corn is very low, people who eat wheat or corn as a staple food are susceptible to lysine deficiency. Lysine is not linked to levels of any neurotransmitter in the brain and hence lysine deficiency is considered as one of the best models for investigating mechanisms of nutrient deficiency.

Monosodium L-glutamate (MSG): A sodium salt of L-glutamic acid. Glutamate has multi-function involvement in perception of umami taste, intermediary metabolism, and excitatory neurotransmission. In addition, it plays important roles in activation of gut–brain axis and regulation of energy homeostasis. Several types of glutamate receptors (ionotropic and metabotropic receptors) are expressed in the body.

Vagus nerve: The Xth cranial nerve that innervates the larynx, heart, lungs, and visceral organs. It consists of both afferent and efferent fibers at the abdominal levels. Several stimuli such as mechanical pressure, temperature, osmotic pressure, and chemicals alter afferent activity of the vagus nerve.

Ventral tegmental area: An area in the midbrain implicated in drug and natural reward circuitry, motivation, cognition, drug addiction, and several psychiatric disorders. Dopaminergic cell bodies originate and their two primary efferent projections are the mesocortical (innervates the prefrontal and insular cortices) and mesolimbic (innervates septum, hippocampus, amygdala, and nucleus accumbens) pathways.

Ventromedial nucleus of the hypothalamus (VMH): A nucleus in the hypothalamus most commonly associated with satiety (also known as the satiety center). Early studies showed that VMH lesions caused overeating and obesity in animals.

Acknowledgments We thank Dr. Ivan E. de Araujo (The John B. Pierce laboratory and Yale University School of Medicine, New Heaven, CT) for the valuable comments on the manuscript. Our research work cited frequently on this manuscript was supported by the Japan Science and Technology Agency (JST) and by research groups of Torii Nutrient-stasis Project (1990–1996) on the Exploratory Research for Advanced Technology (ERATO).

References

Aou S, Takaki A, Karádi Z, Hori T, Nishino H, Oomura Y. Brain Res Bull. 1991;27:451–5.
Bray GA. Brain Res Bull. 1993;32:537–41.
Bricker M, Mitchell HH, Kinsman GM. J Nutr. 1945;30:269–83.
Culik R, Rosenberg HR. Food Technol. 1958;12:169–74.
Dixon KD, Williams FE, Wiggins RL, Pavelka J, Lucente J, Bellinger LL, Gietzen DW. Am J Physiol Regul Integr Comp Physiol. 2000;279:R997–1009.
Forbes RM, Vaughan L, Yohe M. J Nutr. 1958;64:291–302.
Fukuda M, Ono T, Nishino H, Sasaki K. Brain Res. 1986;374:249–59.
Funaba M, Murata T, Fujimura H, Murata E, Abe M, Torii K. J Neuroendocrinol. 1997;9:105–11.
Gietzen DW, McArthur LH, Theisen JC, Rogers QR. Physiol Behav. 1992;51:909–14.
Gietzen DW, Erecius LF, Rogers QR. J Nutr. 1998;128:771–81.
Hanai K. J Comp Physiol. 1981;144:503–8.
Harno E, Edwards G, Geraghty AR, Ward DT, Dodd RH, Dauban P, Faure H, Ruat M, Weston AH. Cell calcium. 2008;44:210–9.
Harper AE. In: Henry Brown AB, editor. Protein nutrition. Springfield: Charles Thomas; 1974. p. 130–79.
Harper AE, Benevenga NJ, Wohlhueter RM. Physiol Rev. 1970;50:428–558.
Hawkins RL, Inoue M, Mori M, Torii K. Physiol Behav. 1994;56:1061–8.
Hawkins RL, Inoue M, Mori M, Torii K. Brain Res. 1995;704:1–9.
Hawkins RL, Murata T, Inoue M, Mori M, Torii K. Proc Soc Exp Biol Med. 1998;219:149–53.
Inoue M, Funaba M, Hawkins RL, Mori M, Torii K. Physiol Behav.1995;58:379–85.
Markison S, Gietzen DW, Spector AC. J Nutr. 1999;129:1604–12.
Markison S, Thompson BL, Smith JC, Spector AC. J Nutr. 2000;130:1320–8.
Mori M, Kawada T, Ono T, Torii K. Physiol Behav. 1991a;49:987–95.
Mori M, Kawada T, Torii K. Brain Res Bull. 1991b;27:417–22.
Naito-Hoopes M, McArthur LH, Gietzen DW, Rogers QR. Physiol Behav. 1993;53:485–94.
Nakamura K, Ono T, Tamura R, Indo M, Takashima Y, Kawasaki M. Brain Res. 1989;491:15–32.
Ninomiya Y, Kajiura H, Mochizuki K. Neurosci Lett. 1993;163:197–200.
Ninomiya Y, Kajiura H, Ishibashi T, Imai Y. Chem Senses. 1994a;19:617–26.
Ninomiya Y, Kajiura H, Naito Y, Mochizuki K, Katsukawa H, Torii K. Physiol Behav. 1994b;56:1179–84.
Nishimura F, Nishihara M, Mori M, Torii K, Takahashi M. Brain Res. 1995;691:217–22.
Nishino H, Oomura Y, Karádi Z, Aou S, Lénárd L, Kai Y, Fukuda A, Ito C, Min BI, Salaman CP. Brain Res Bull. 1988;20:839–45.

Norgren R. J Comp Neurol. 1976;166:17–30.

Ono T, Sasaki K, Nakamura K, Norgren R. Brain Res. 1985;327:303–6.

Oomura Y. In: Morgane PJ, Panksepp J, editors. Handbook of the hypothalamus: physiology of the hypothalamus, vol. 2. New York: Marcel Dekker; 1980. p. 557–620.

Panksepp J, Booth DA. Nature 1971;233:341–2.

Pritchard TC, Scott TR. Brain Res. 1982;253:81–92.

Robertson DM, Burger HG, Fuller PJ. Endocr Relat Cancer. 2004;11:35–49.

Rosenberg HR, Rohdenburg EL. Arch Biochem. 1952;37:461–8.

Shibata R, Kameishi M, Kondoh T, Torii K. Physiol Behav. 2009;96:667–74.

Shingai T, Beidler LM. Brain Res. 1985;335:245–9.

Smriga M, Mori M, Torii K. J Nutr. 2000a;130:1641–3.

Smriga M, Murakami H, Mori M, Torii K. Biofactors 200b;12:137–42.

Tabuchi E, Ono T, Nishijo H, Torii K. Physiol Behav. 1991;49:951–64.

Tabuchi E, Uwano T, Kondoh T, Ono T, Torii K. Brain Res. 1996;739:139–55.

Torii K, Niijima. Physiol Behav. 2001;72:685–90.

Torii K, Mimura T, Yugari Y. In: Kawamura Y, Kare MR, editors. Umami: a basic taste. New York: Marcel Dekker; 1987. p. 513–63.

Torii K, Hanai K, Oosawa K, Funaba M, Okiyama A, Mori M, Murata T, Takahashi M. Physiol Behav. 1993;54:459–66.

Torii K, Yokawa T, Tabuchi E, Murata T, Hawkins RL, Mori M, Kondoh T, Takezawa M, Ono T. In: Ono T, McNaughton BL, Molotchnikoff S, Rolls ET, Nishijo H, editors. Perception, memory and emotion: frontiers in neuroscience. Oxford: Elsevier Science; 1996. p. 467–78.

Wayner MJ, Ono T, DeYound A, Barone FC. Pharmacol Biochem Behav. 1975;3(1 Suppl):85–90.

Wellendorph P, Bräuner-Osborne H. Gene 2004;335:37–46.

Wellendorph P, Hansen KB, Balsgaard A, Greenwood JR, Egebjerg J, Bräuner-Osborne H. Mol Pharmacol. 2005;67:589–97.

Young VR, Pellet PL. Food Nutr Bull. 1990;12:289–300.

Part XXV
Anorexia Nervosa

Chapter 155
Genotypes and Phenotypes of Anorexia Nervosa

Janet Treasure, Natalie Kanakam, and Christine-Johanna Macare

Abbreviations

5HT	5-hydroxytryptamine
ACC:	Anterior cingulate cortex
AN	Anorexia nervosa
AN-R	Anorexia nervosa restricting subtype
AN-BP	Anorexia nervosa binge-purge subtype
ASD	Autistic spectrum disorders
DSM IV	Diagnostic and Statistical Manual of Mental Disorders, 4th edition
BDNF	Brain-derived neurotrophic factor
BMI	Body mass index
BN	Bulimia nervosa
COMT	Catechol-O-methlytransferase
CSF	Cerebrospinal fluid
CT studies	Computed tomography studies
CT	Constitutionally thin
DA	Dopamine
ED	Eating disorders
EDNOS	Eating disorder not otherwise specified
fMRI	Functional magnetic resonance imaging
HTR1D	Serotonin 1D receptor.
ICD-10	International Statistical Classification of Diseases and Related Health Problems 10th Revision
NICE	National Institute for Clinical Excellence

J. Treasure (✉)
Institute of Psychiatry, King's College London, London, United Kingdom
and
Department of Academic Psychiatry, Eating Disorder Research Unit, Guy's Hospital, Bermondsey Wing, SE1 9RT, London, United Kingdom
e-mail: Janet.Treasure@iop.kcl.ac.uk

V.R. Preedy et al. (eds.), *Handbook of Behavior, Food and Nutrition*,
DOI 10.1007/978-0-387-92271-3_155, © Springer Science+Business Media, LLC 2011

OA	Object Assembly subtest
OCD	Obsessive compulsive disorder
OCPD	Obsessive compulsive personality disorders
QTL	Quantitative trait linkage
PYY	PeptideYY
SNP	Single nucleoid polymorphisms
WAIS	Wechsler Adult Intelligence Scale
WCC	Weak Central Coherence

155.1 Introduction

This chapter aims to discuss individual characteristics such as genotypes and intermediate phenotypes that increase the susceptibility to developing Anorexia Nervosa (AN). First, clinically specified phenotypes of anorexia nervosa will be outlined and the difficulties in diagnosis will be discussed. A summary of the literature relating to possible intermediate phenotypes, biomarkers, and endophenotypes relevant to AN follows. Subsequently, the methodological issues in the search for AN genotypes will be presented. Finally, the implication of these findings for health and treatments will be suggested.

155.1.1 Diagnostic Criteria

Anorexia Nervosa was first described by Gull (1873). The current DSM classification includes the following symptoms (Table 155.1):

There are two subtypes of AN: restricting (AN-R) and binge-purge type (AN-BP). The restricting subtype is characterized by behaviors of extreme and prolonged fasting and restraint. The binge-purge subtype is also defined by prolonged fasting although it is punctuated by episodes of overeating followed by behaviors to compensate for weight gain such as self-induced vomiting; the misuse of laxatives, diuretics, or enemas; and exercise.

155.1.2 Epidemiology

The onset of AN is usually reported in puberty and females are more likely to be affected than males (APA 2000). The likelihood of being diagnosed with AN at least once during lifetime is estimated at

Table 155.1 DSM IV diagnostic criteria for AN (APA 2000)

DSM IV criteria for anorexia nervosa
• Severe weight loss and maintenance of that under 85% of the expected
• Intense fear of weight gain
• Distortion of body image and overemphasis on weight as an index for self-evaluation
• Amenorrhea

These diagnostic criteria must be satisfied for AN diagnosis. At present, diagnosis is based on its visible phenotypes.

approximately 1% (Hudson et al. 2007). The annual incidence of new AN cases presenting to primary care is given in 8 out of 100,000 individuals (Hoek and van Hoeken 2003).

155.1.3 Prognosis

Mortality in AN is increased (standard mortality ratio of 6.2–10.5 (Birmingham et al. 2005; Papadopoulos et al. 2009; Lowe et al. 2001); and life expectancy reduced by 25 years for females who have suffered from AN since the age of 15 (Harbottle et al. 2008). The outcome for AN patients is poor, with only half recovering, approximately 6–10% developing a chronic condition (Berkman et al. 2007; Lowe et al. 2001), and up to 25% having poor psychosocial functioning (Wentz et al. 2009).

155.1.4 Chronic Disability

People with AN have a diminished quality of life (Mond et al. 2005). Eating disorders were placed fourth in terms of burden of disease (years of life lost through death or disability) in women aged 15–24 years (Mathers et al. 1999) with both physical and psychological comorbidity. Education in terms of attendance at school is disrupted (Byford et al. 2007). Moreover vocational functioning is impaired: 21% of cases still rely on state benefits 10–15 years after the onset of the illness (Hjern et al. 2006). Social isolation is common; social communication skills are poor (Takahashi et al. 2006) and social networks are small (Tiller et al. 1997). The costs of these disabilities are high (Su and Birmingham 2003).

155.1.5 Diagnostic Difficulties

The nosological status of the current DSM IV diagnostic criteria has been questioned (Hebebrand et al. 2004). A substantial number of patients change diagnosis over time. As many as 55% of patients who initially suffer with restrictive AN (AN-R) subsequently develop AN-BP, bulimia nervosa or eating disorder not otherwise specified (Eddy et al. 2008).

Some patients do not present with all the symptoms necessary for a diagnosis of AN according to DSM IV criteria or ICD criteria. The ICD operationalized the weight threshold as a Body Mass Index (BMI, weight in kg/height in m) below 17.5. Regular menses may occur below this threshold and medication or the contraceptive pill may make amenorrhea an unreliable diagnostic marker. Furthermore, a subgroup of patients do not fulfill the criterion of having a fear of weight gain or a distorted body image (Strober et al. 1999). Comorbidity with other psychiatric disorders can make diagnosis on the basis of phenotypes challenging. As weight loss increases, patients often present with a variety of mood and anxiety disorders. For instance, 30% of AN patients meet the criteria for Obsessive Compulsive Disorder (OCD). Also a subgroup has characteristics associated with the Autistic Spectrum Disorders (ASD). Gillberg and colleagues described 20% with an empathy disorder and social disturbances (1994). These features were predictive of poor psychosocial outcome over time (Rastam et al. 2003). Intermediate phenotypes or biomarkers may be more stable over time than illness phenotypes.

155.2 Biomarkers and Endophenotypes

Increasingly, there is an interest in intermediate phenotypes such as biomarkers (biological marker) and endophenotypes as a means to describe and identify an illness. Biomarkers are underlying cognitive or behavioral traits that are associated with a disorder, but not part of their visible presentation. They can be state or trait related. Biomarkers have a number of different applications such as being antecedent, screening, diagnostic, prognostic, or stratification markers (Ritsner and Gottesman 2009). One valuable kind of biomarker is that of an endophenotype: a heritable trait biomarker that falls on the pathway between behavior and biology (phenotype and genotype). Gottesman and Gould (2003) have defined specific criteria to be fulfilled for an endophenotype status (Table 155.2):

Although the endophenotype and biomarker concepts have been used interchangeably in the literature, Gottesman and Gould (2003) use the former when there are some signs of heritability, and biomarkers when the trait does not fulfill the criteria of genetic underpinnings. It is hoped that endophenotypes will provide a more direct association with the genotype than the phenotypes of AN (see Fig. 155.1). Recent reviews have included the concept of endophenotypes in discussions of ED etiology (Treasure et al. 2007).

Table 155.2 Endophenotype criteria (Gottesman and Gould 2003)

Endophenotype criteria

- Association with the illness in the population
- Heritability
- State-independence
- Cosegregation with the illness in families
- Presence in unaffected relatives at a higher level than in the general population

Endophenotypes are heritable trait biomarkers. The above criteria must be satisfied for the trait to be classified as an endophenotype.

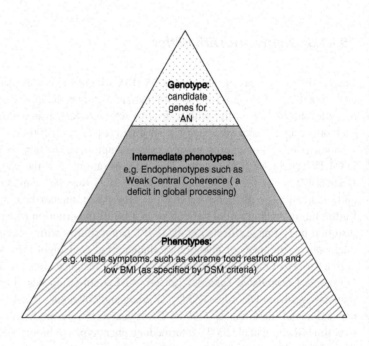

Fig. 155.1 Pathway between genotype and phenotype. Intermediate phenotypes lie on the pathway between candidate genes that make an individual susceptible to anorexia nervosa (*AN*) and its visible symptoms. Potential biomarkers and endophenotypes are more directly associated with AN etiology. For example, endophenotypes such as "weak central coherence" (which refers to deficits in global processing) may be involved in causing and maintaining visible symptoms such as the inability to see the adverse consequences of extreme food restriction on physical health

It is hoped that research to establish characteristics as intermediate phenotypes of AN will lead to a more biologically based system of classification and a more accurate understanding of causation, pathophysiology, prognosis, and treatment.

155.2.1 Distinguishing Biomarkers Associated with the Illness from Secondary Consequences of Starvation

The search for suitable biological markers in AN is complex since starvation and impaired nutrition, core elements of the disorder, have a profoundly disrupting effect on both the psychology and physiology of the individual. This causes a proliferation of biological abnormalities in the acute state. One way of trying to distinguish between the consequences of starvation and features that suggest an underlying biological vulnerability is to examine people after weight recovery. This in itself is not without problems; for example, how does one define recovery? Is it important to have a minimal duration of recovery? Is the abnormality a risk factor or a scar from the illness? Some risk factors may only occur in the context of environmental or developmental risk factors and may remain hidden. Despite these difficulties several groups have undertaken studies of biomarkers in patients after recovery. Fewer studies have taken the next step which is to examine whether the biomarkers represent a familial and genetic vulnerability.

155.3 Introduction to the Concept of Biomarkers

At present, evidence-based relevant biomarkers include (a) altered serotonin function (Kaye 2008); (b) opioid alterations (Kaye et al. 1982); (c) dopamine disturbances (Frank et al. 2005); (d) variant hormonal profiles (Germain et al. 2007); (e) alterations in brain structure (Gagel 1953; van den Eynde and Treasure 2008; Martin 1958; Roser et al. 1999); and neuropsychological endophenotypes such as (f) difficulties in set-shifting (Roberts et al. 2007; Tchanturia et al. 2004); (g) weak central coherence (Lopez et al. 2008b); and (h) social cognitive deficits (Gillberg et al. 1994).

155.3.1 Serotonin

There is growing evidence that a disturbance in serotonin function may be a biomarker involved in the etiology and pathogenesis of AN (Kaye 2008). 5HT1A receptors are increased especially in the acute state but also after recovery (Bailer et al. 2005a, b, 2007; Galusca et al. 2008), particularly in the prefrontal areas (associated with regulatory control) and the mesial temporal/subgenual areas (associated with reward). 5HT receptors in the striatum are increased in the restricting form of anorexia nervosa after recovery whereas they appear to be decreased in the binge-purge form (Bailer et al. 2004). In summary, people with eating disorders have key abnormalities in 5HT function in both the hedonic and the regulatory regions of the brain.

Dysregulation of these emotional and reward pathways not only impacts upon feeding but also contributes to a dysphoric temperament with symptoms of anxiety, obsessionality, and inhibition.

Indeed Walter Kaye has developed a hypothesis which states that, restricting food can become powerfully reinforcing since it reduces the availability of plasma tryptophan, which is a rate-limiting step in the production of 5HT. The reduced functional activity of 5HT is thought to reduce anxiety, which is in itself reinforcing (2008).

In support of this theory, positive correlations between anxiety measures used to assess harm avoidance and 5-HT2a binding have been shown in the temporal cortex (Bailer et al. 2004) and the supragenual cingulate, frontal, and parietal brain regions of recovered AN patients. This is regardless of any abnormality in overall 5-HT2a receptor activity (Bailer et al. 2007).

155.3.2 BDNF

Brain derived neurotrophic factor (BDNF), a protein, has been shown to regulate the serotonergic neurotransmitter system. BDNF is also present in the hypothalamic nuclei that are associated with weight regulation (Pelleymounter et al. 1995). Research has shown that BDNF levels are significantly decreased in people with anorexia nervosa in comparison to healthy controls (Monteleone et al. 2004) and persists into recovery (Nakazato et al. 2006).

155.3.3 Opioid

The opioidergic neurotransmitter system is also associated with regulating feeding behavior. It is thought to be implicated in the "liking" aspects of food intake and may mediate the rewarding aspects of food. Blockade of opioid receptors in rats using the opioid antagonist, naloxone, decreases consumption of more preferred and palatable foods (Glass et al. 1996). In AN higher levels of cerebrospinal fluid activity was found in those who were severely underweight in comparison to those with AN who were weight recovered, suggesting that it may be related to BMI (Kaye et al. 1982).

155.3.4 Dopamine

Dopamine-related disturbances has been related to a number of symptoms encountered in AN, such as amenorrhea, obsessive compulsive traits, hyperactivity, and weight loss (Kaye et al. 2004). This potential biomarker may also contribute to feeding behavior and to the generally anhedonic temperament in AN. Dopamine DA is a key neurochemical in the hedonic system For example, the presentation of palatable foods to fasting humans is associated with an increase in DA in the dorsal striatum (Volkow et al. 2002). Furthermore the amount of dopamine released is correlated with the amount of pleasure experienced when eating (Small et al. 2003).

Frank and colleagues (2005) demonstrated higher dopamine D2/D3 receptor binding in recovered AN subjects in the anteroventral striatum, suggesting either decreased intrasynaptic dopamine concentration or increased D2/D3 receptor density or affinity to be present in AN. This abnormality of dopamine in the hedonic system might be associated with the altered response to reward seen in AN (difficulties in differentiating between positive and negative feedback) (Wagner et al. 2007).

Moreover, in the AN group, dopamine binding potential in the dorsal caudate and dorsal putamen correlated positively with harm avoidance. This observation supports the view that the dopamine abnormalities in AN might contribute to the characteristic harm avoidance or increased physical activity (Frank et al. 2005).

155.3.5 Hormones

AN is associated with many abnormalities in the hormonal profile. Adiponectin and leptin are produced by adipose tissue and are involved in energy metabolism. Serum leptin levels were found to be severely decreased in restricting anorexics and only moderately decreased in purging anorexics. Furthermore, compared to controls, circulating levels of adiponectin were increased by 53% in purging anorexics and by 96% in restricting anorexics (Liu et al. 2008).

Other orexogenic and anorexogenic hormones which regulate appetite have been found to be important biomarkers that distinguish between AN and people who are constitutionally thin (CT). Orexogenic hormones such as ghrelin which is known to initiate appetite was found to be significantly higher in those that were CT than in people with AN. Anorexogenic hormones including PeptideYY and leptin were significantly lower in people with anorexia nervosa than in CT subjects. Interestingly, GLP-1 concentrations were significantly higher in AN than in CT subjects (Germain et al. 2007).

155.3.6 Brain Structure

Structural and metabolic changes occur in the brain during the acute phase of AN. The most consistent alteration is the reduction in brain mass. This was first suggested by postmortem findings of reduced cerebral mass with prominent sulci and small gyri (Gagel 1953; van den Eynde and Treasure 2008; Martin 1958) and later confirmed in vivo in several CT studies that additionally demonstrated enlarged ventricles (Dolan et al. 1988; Krieg et al. 1989; Palazidou et al.1990). For the most part, brain mass is restored with weight gain (Castro-Fornieles et al. 2009; McCormick et al. 2008).

155.4 Neuropsychological Endophenotypes

155.4.1 Cognitive Biomarkers

A number of cognitive deficits have been observed in AN. In particular, executive function is disrupted in the acute phase of ED. For example, Jones and collegues (1991) reported mild cognitive impairments in the domains of focusing/execution, memory, and verbal and visuospatial processing. However, most of these deficits were not present in weight recovered AN participants. Set-shifting deficits and weak central coherence are of interest in that they are associated with obsessive compulsive traits which are present before and after the acute illness phase.

155.4.2 Set Shifting

Set-shifting is one of the main aspects of executive functioning and refers to the ability to be flexible with one's mindset in adapting to new task demands or changes in situations (Miyake et al. 2000). A series of studies using a variety of neuropsychological tasks to measure this concept found that people with AN have difficulties in set-shifting in the acute state (Anderluh et al. 2003; Tchanturia et al. 2001, 2002). A meta-analytic systematic review of the literature confirmed this impairment in cognitive flexibility which was present in the various eating disorder subgroups (Roberts et al. 2007).

Women recovered from AN also demonstrate impairment in set-shifting ability but with reduced effect sizes (Tchanturia et al. 2004; Roberts et al. 2007). Examples of effect sizes across a range of set shifting tasks are shown in Table 155.3. Problems with set-shifting were also seen in the sisters of individuals with ED (Holliday et al. 2005).

Results from these studies suggest that executive function as marked by poor cognitive flexibility may be a state independent trait in some cases but that this difficulty is exaggerated during the illness phase. It does not appear to be simply a consequence of malnutrition alone since other aspects of eating disorder psychopathology such as depression and anxiety also have an impact. The limitation of a cross-sectional design to address state-independence is noted. As the recovered group had managed to overcome their AN, it is possible that they represent a different cohort than those with chronic, persistent AN.

Poor set-shifting may represent a prognostic biomarker of AN and be involved in the maintenance of the illness. Cognitive remediation therapy which addressed this deficit has been tested and proved effective (Tchanturia et al. 2006). Replication of these studies with larger samples is required as well as genetic examination to complete the exploration as to whether poor set shifting might meet the criteria for an endophenotype of some forms of ED.

155.4.3 Weak Central Coherence

Weak central coherence is another neuropsychological trait of interest because of its association with OCPD and the autistic spectrum of disorders. Central coherence is the natural cognitive

Table 155.3 Effect sizes (Cohen's d)* for neuropsychological tasks relating to set-shifting in AN

Task	Current AN	Recovered AN	Time	Repeat
Set-shifting				
TMT-B	0.8	0.5	5	Yes-2
WCST	0.6	0.4	10	No
Brixton	0.2	0.3	5	Yes-2
CatBat	0.6	0.4	3	No
Haptic	1.2	0.9	5	No

TMT-B (Trail Making Task, Trial B); WCST (Wisconsin Card Sorting Test); Time (Time taken in minutes to administer each task); Repeat (Can the task be repeated?); Yes, Yes-2 (have 2 versions of the task), No, ? (unsure if task can be repeated); The effect size in the table represent the mean of the published studies.
*Cohen's d effect sizes are understood as follows: 0 to <0.15 – negligible; >0.15–0.40 – small; >0.40–0.75 – medium; >0.75–1.10 – large; >1.10 – huge.

style of most people in adult life, and is defined as the skill of integrating large amounts of incoming information into context, gestalt, and meaning (Frith 1989). The opposite tendency, weak central coherence, is characterized by a tendency to process information in parts (detail) rather than as a whole, with relative difficulty in global or integrative processing (Happe and Booth 2008).Weak central coherence is a key component of the cognitive style in autistic spectrum disorders (ASD) (Happe and Booth 2008; Happe and Frith 2006) and has also been found in their first-degree relatives (Smalley and Asarnov 1990; Happe et al. 2001; Baron-Cohen and Hammer 1997).

Initial findings which suggested that this trait was associated with ED were found in Gillberg and collaborators' longitudinal study (1996). This cohort of early onset cases of AN were found to be persistently impaired over time on the Object Assembly subtest (OA) from WAIS. This test requires the ability to integrate pieces of information into a whole, to construct a familiar object (Gillberg et al. 1996, 2007). They also found that a subgroup of people with AN who met the criteria for ASD also had a cognitive profile resembling that found in ASD. Although the authors initially hypothesized that the poor performance in the OA was due to poor abstract thinking (Gillberg et al. 1996), they later associated their findings with weak central coherence (Gillberg et al. 2007). Our group has furthered the investigation of the weak central coherence hypothesis in people with ED with a systematic, hypothesis driven approach using a battery of tests used to measure central coherence. It was found that weak central coherence may be a feature of AN since there is superiority in tasks that require detail processing (e.g., Group/Embedded Figures and Matching Familiar Figures) and a weakness in tests that require a global strategy such as the Sentence Completion and Homograph Reading Tasks, the Rey-Osterrieth Complex Figure, and OA (Lopez et al. 2008a, b, c; Southgate et al. 2008) (see Table 155.4). A recent systematic review of the literature found some evidence supporting this account particularly for decreased global processing (Lopez et al. 2008a).

This trait has been reported also to be present in women in recovered state, with medium effect sizes for global integration and large for detail focused processing. A recent study of our group has

Table 155.4 Effect sizes (Cohen's d)* for neuropsychological tasks relating to weak central coherence in AN

Task	Current AN	Recovered AN	Time	Repeat
Central coherence				
D-EFT	0.5	1.0	10	Yes-2
D-GEFT	0.8		15	?
D-BD	0.0	0.2	10	?
D-MFFT	0.9		10	No
G-Rey CC	0.9	0.6	5	Yes-2
G-OA	0.6	0.6	15	No
G-Frag. Pic	1.7		10	Yes-2
G-SCT	0.7	1.2	10	No
H-HRT	0.0	0.4	10	No

EFT (Embedded Figures Task); BD (Block Design); MFFT (Efficiency Matching Familiar Figures Test); Rey CC (Rey Central Coherence Index); OA (Object Assembly); Frag. Pic. (Fragmented Pictures Task); SCT (Total Score in Sentence Completion Task); HRT (Total Score in Homograph Reading Task); Time (Time taken in minutes to administer each task); Repeat (Can the task be repeated?); Yes, Yes-2 (have 2 versions of the task), No, ? (unsure if task can be repeated). The effect size in the table represent the mean of the published studies.

*Cohen's d effect sizes are understood as follows: 0 to <0.15 – negligible; >0.15–0.40 – small; >0.40–0.75 – medium; >0.75–1.10 – large; >1.10 – huge.

J. Treasure et al.

found that weak central coherence is also present in the healthy sisters of those with AN. Using the Group Embedded Figure Test and the Rey-Osterreith Complex figure copy (central coherence index), it was found that like their AN sisters, 30 healthy sisters displayed a more detail focused processing style on both.

Thus weak central coherence appears to be a trait associated with AN. Enhanced detail function is present even in the acute phase of the illness and superiority in this skill is similar in size to that seen in cases of Asperger's Syndrome. Global integration appears to be weakened in the acute phase of the illness and deficits in this are less apparent after recovery. Thus the imbalance between local and global functioning and weak central coherence is most marked during the acute phase. This biomarker may be involved in maintaining maladaptive behaviors so that they are unable to see the "bigger picture" and ignore the severe consequences of applying a detailed thinking style to the laws of thermodynamics has on their health in terms of weight loss.

155.4.4 Social Cognition

Social cognition refers to those complex cognitive processes involved in attuning behavior to that of other people (Adolphs 1999). The study by Gillberg and colleagues suggested that a subgroup of early onset cases of AN have empathy deficits similar to those found in ASD and this was associated with poor outcome in AN (Gillberg et al. 1994). A recent review has summarized the evidence for problems in this area (Zucker et al. 2007). Traits of emotional dysregulation, social inhibition, and compulsivity are found in acute AN and persist with recovery, although to a milder degree (Holliday et al. 2006).

Women with acute AN appear to be impaired in visual and verbal recognition of emotions (Zonnevijlle-Bendek et al. 2002, 2004; Kucharska-Pietura et al. 2004). This contrasts with normal self-reported levels of empathic response (Hambrook et al. 2008). A study in our unit that administered tasks developed in the field of ASD to women with acute AN (e.g., Reading the Mind in the Voice, Films, Eyes) found large effects in all of the task domains suggesting greater difficulties in the acute state relative to a healthy comparison group (see Table 155.5). However, the deficits in the tasks particularly related to theory of mind (voice and film) were not present in people who had recovered from the illness. Our group has found that in the acute illness state, women with AN have an attentional bias to threatening social stimuli using the E-Stroop paradigm. This appears to be present albeit in an attenuated form in people recovered from the illness.

These findings suggest that emotional recognition problems which may be associated with a tendency to avoid threatening stimuli may be trait abnormality in AN whereas poor Theory of Mind is

Table 155.5 Effect sizes (Cohen's *d*) for neuropsychological tasks relating social cognition in AN

Social cognition	Current AN	Time
RMI eyes	1.1	10
RMI voice	0.8	10
RMI film	0.8	10
E-Stroop	1.6	10

RMI (Reading the Mind in the Eyes; Voice and Films); E-Stroop (Emotional Stroop Task); Time (Time taken in minutes to administer each task)

more of a state effect. Poor regulation of emotional and social stimuli possibly contributes to both causal and perpetuating factors. This has implications for the development of novel approaches to treatment.

155.4.5 Genotypes

Cultural, social, and interpersonal elements have been well recognized as having etiological significance in AN. However, increasingly, the pathogenesis of AN is investigated by looking at familial and genetic patterns. Twin studies have estimated the heritability of AN around 56% (Bulik et al. 2006). In general, relatives of those with AN have a tenfold increased risk to develop AN (Strober et al. 2000; Lilenfeld et al. 1998). These results indicate that AN has a genetic component, which makes it reasonable to go one step further and identify genes that might be involved in AN (Table 155.6).

One approach to discover genetic loci are genome-wide studies wherein large regions are mapped which then can be scrutinized further using candidate gene approaches. No previous knowledge on the genes involved in the disorder are required (Winchester and Collier 2003). Linkage studies aim to identify the genomic regions that might harbor predisposing factors for the disorder. For complex disorders such as AN, nonparametric (i.e., model-free) methods are used so that no knowledge on the mode of inheritance is needed. It is assumed that risk alleles and marker alleles will be inherited more frequently in affected relatives than expected by chance alone. The pattern of inheritance is usually compared within families with affected family members (Winchester and Collier 2003). Having identified a region, it is possible to narrow down the search space for potential candidate genes (Bulik et al. 2007). The advantage of genome-wide linkage studies is that genes with a small effect on a trait can be identified and therefore this approach offers a potential tool in investigating genes involved in complex disorders (Winchester and Collier 2003). Grice and colleagues (2002) examined the linkage of the gene coding for serotonin in families wherein two siblings were affected by an eating disorder. They found modest evidence for a linkage at marker D4S2367 and D1S3721 at chromosome 1 in a "pure" AN restricting subsample. Linkage analysis on a sample of binge-purge and restricting AN patients provided evidence for a smaller linkage peak at marker D1S3721 at chromosome 1. However, as acknowledged by the authors, these linkage peaks might also represent false positives, as the genetic makeup of AN might be composed of a large number of interacting

Table 155.6 Methodology to identify genotypes

Methodology for investigating disorder relevant genes	
Approach	Candidate gene studies
	Genome wide studies
Methodology	Linkage mapping
	Association
Types of samples	Family trios
	Case control

Relevant genes can be studied using two main approaches: candidate gene studies and genome wide studies. Within these approaches linkage or association can be studied. Types of sample include family trios, wherein families with one affected member are studied, and case-control studies wherein affected cases and matched controls are used.

loci, with each locus contributing a small effect to susceptibility, which are difficult to localize with linkage analysis (Grice et al. 2002).

In contrast to linkage studies, association studies focus on population frequency of susceptibility genes rather than heritance pattern of markers. Two types of samples are used: case control and family trios. In case control studies, affected individuals are matched and compared to healthy controls. Here, the aim is to examine patterns of differences in allelic frequency with differences in disease frequency. In family trio samples, these measures are compared within one family (i.e., mother, father, and affected child). Genes associated with key putative neuronal pathways have been examined (Bulik et al. 2007). In the following section: serotonin, dopamine, opioid systems, and the brain-derived neurotrophic factor will be discussed.

155.4.6 Serotonin

Chromosome 1 was examined closely by Bergen and colleagues(2003) who focused on region 1p36.3–34.4 and examined genes that were suggested to code for the serotonin 1D receptor. Additional evidence for the implication of a gene coding for serotonin at rs674386 SNP in AN was found (Bergen et al. 2003). Brown and colleagues (2007) reported an association between a gene encoding for HTR1D at marker rs674386 and AN. Moreover, evidence was given for an association between the restricting subtype with marker rs856510 (Brown et al. 2007). The latter results however have to be replicated in an independent sample.

Focusing on the 2A receptor, Gorwood and colleagues (2002) reviewed the evidence for an association between the rs6311 polymorphism of the HTR2A gene. Ricca and colleagues (Ricca et al. 2002) examined the −1438 G/A polymorphism, which has been located in the regions of the 5-HT2A receptor gene and has been linked to AN. In particular, an over-representation of the A allele and the AA genotypes have been documented in ANR (and BN) patients as compared to healthy controls. Interestingly, this pattern of results did not emerge in AN-BP patients who showed a similar allelic frequency as the control group (Ricca et al. 2002). Devlin and colleagues (2002) also focused on the HTR2A gene in AN patients and compared linkage of this gene in 196 families with an individual suffering from AN. This group has identified 3 regions on chromosomes 1, 2, and 12, suggestive of a linkage (markers D1S1660, DS1790 and D13S894).

The general picture with genes involved in serotonin functioning linked to AN is unclear. Overall, studies investigating genes involved in the serotonin system have been hampered by low power and a lack of replication in independent samples. Therefore, results should be interpreted with caution and replication in larger, independent samples is awaited.

155.4.7 Dopamine

The genetic basis underlying dopamine dysfunction has been examined. Gabrovsek and colleagues (2004), for instance, looked at a gene that encodes catechol-O-methlytransferase (COMT), which metabolizes more than 60% of dopamine especially in frontal areas. Results yielded no evidence for an association between the Val158 allele of the COMT gene and AN. The D2 receptor has been implicated in altered reward, affect, decision-making, executive control, stereotypic motor activity and decreased food ingestion in AN patients (Kaye 2008). An association was found for the rs1800497 and the rs6278 polymorphism, both polymorphisms in the gene encoding for D2 receptor, and the binge-purge subtype of AN (Bergen et al. 2005). Overall, evidence for genes involved in encoding the dopamine system involved in AN is sparse and further methodologically sound evidence is needed to draw conclusions.

155.4.8 Opioids

Bergen and colleagues (2003) examined delta opioid receptor loci in the 1p33–36 region and reported evidence for an association at 3 SNPs (8214T4C, 23340A4G, 47821A4G) for AN patients. However, as acknowledged by the authors, replications in a larger sample are needed as the current sample ($N = 191$) was underpowered. Further examination of the implication of the gene encoding for OPRD1 was added by Brown and colleagues (2007) who examined the impact of the two candidate genes previously identified by Bergen and colleagues (2003) in a case control study of AN patients. Using different SNPs than Bergen and colleagues (2003) this group found evidence for marker rs56356 with AN. Further analyses revealed a higher frequency of the C,T genotype in AN-R as compared to AN-BP patients. Patients suffering from the binge-eating/purging subtype presented with this genotype at a lower rate than controls. It was therefore tentatively suggested that this locus not only compromises susceptibility towards AN but might differentiate even between subtypes (Brown et al. 2007). Yet, it has to be kept in mind that power in this study varied between 0.63 and 0.99.

155.4.9 Brain-derived Neurotrophic Factor

Evidence for a susceptibility gene for brain-derived neurotrophic factor (BDNF) related to AN has been found. It has been suggested that this gene predisposes to AN through its impact on affective symptoms (Ribases et al. 2005). Associations have been found between the Met 66 allele, AN-R, and minimum BMI and replicated in 359 family trios.

155.5 Conclusion

Progress towards revealing potential biomarkers in AN has considerably advanced in the last decade. The search for potential genotypes, biomarkers, and endophenotypes in AN has revealed a number of features that are present in the acute state, some of which persist into recovery. The main findings in this direction highlight the involvement of altered neurotransmitters systems particularly those relating to serotonin, dopamine, BDNF, and the opiates. In addition, cognitive information processing anomalies such as weak set-shifting and central coherence may be biomarkers. The talent for perceiving detail forms part of the endophenotype in some cases of AN. Problems with executive function may arise as a secondary consequence of the illness. Difficulties in emotional recognition and avoidance of threat may be part of the trait biomarkers associated with anxiety in some cases of anorexia nervosa. Problems with social cognition with impairments in the theory of mind tasks may arise as a consequence of the illness. The trait biomarkers may be part of the causal process that leads to the development of an eating disorder. Also in conjunction with state related markers these can form part of the maintaining processes that cause eating disorders to be stuck and less easy to recover from the longer they persist. Thus, biomarkers have implications for the prognosis of the illness. Furthermore biomarkers can inform treatment strategies (emotional, social, and cognitive remediation skills) that may reduce the duration of the illness and improve outcome. It is hoped that a deeper understanding of AN based on biomarkers and the search for endophenotypes will improve awareness, early intervention, and make for better prognosis in the long term.

155.6 Applications to Other Areas of Health and Disease

Food is one of the several natural rewards amongst others, such as sex, fluid, and social affiliation. There is evidence that the brain systems which modulate these natural rewards are also used in the processing of other rewards, such as money and material assets. Interactions between these different forms of reward can occur. Therefore, investigation into the addictive nature of extreme food restriction may inform research into other addictive behaviors.

The reward system is comprised of dopamine, opioid, and cannabinoid signaling (Cota et al. 2006). Extreme food restriction or dieting can disrupt the systems that underlie appetite motivation, increasing the reinforcing aspects of food (Epstein et al. 2003). Furthermore overactivation of the homeostatic system by extreme hunger may result in problems with regulating eating such as binge eating, emotional eating, and reduction in metabolic rate, making weight gain more likely (Lowe and Levine 2005). It may be argued that a greater understanding of AN etiology in terms of a disrupted reward system may facilitate research into the binge eating seen in bulimia nervosa and obesity.

Substance abuse disorders may also be informed by research into the reward system since this may rely on the same neuronal pathways as eating (Cota et al. 2006). Chronic food deprivation increases reward to all addictive drugs (Carr 2002). Furthermore, both eating and drugs such as cocaine and amphetamines have the same effect of increasing dopamine in the reward system (Hernandez and Hoebel 1988).

Current research findings on genotypes and phenotypes of AN can be applied to other areas of health and disease. The aforementioned serotonin and dopamine systems are known to be involved in other mental disorders such as depression and schizophrenia. Furthermore, genomic variation studies which reveal risk alleles for AN might inform other pathologies that are comorbid with AN, such as depression, anxiety disorders, and in particular obsessive compulsive disorder.

As yet clear recommendations for the effective treatment of AN have not been established. The National Institute for Clinical Excellence (NICE) guidelines state that AN patients should be treated on an outpatients basis and emphasize the combination of re-feeding with psychosocial interventions in AN, but do not specify a treatment for AN. Gaining more knowledge of the neurobiological mechanisms and genotypes is essential when designing new therapies for AN and all types of eating disorders. Treatment which addresses the stable traits of AN such as weak set-shifting and central coherence have been pioneered by our group. Cognitive remediation therapy has been developed as a pre-therapy intervention for in-patients to moderate information processing biases by strengthening flexibility in daily activities and eating rituals. This has been shown to improve the outcome of subsequent therapy interventions (Tchanturia et al. 2006; Davies and Tchanturia 2005).

Summary Points

- Diagnostic difficulties: Given the difficulties with diagnostic categories (Anderluh et al. 2009) attention should be directed toward identifying core stable traits. This will facilitate diagnosis, the creation of more accurate models of AN etiology, and enhance the search for more effective treatments.
- Biomarkers and endophenotypes: Biomarkers are traits associated with the disorder, but not part of their visible presentation. They can be state- or trait-related and may be used for screening, diagnostic, prognostic, or stratification markers. One valuable type is that of an endophenotype; a heritable trait biomarker.
- Serotonin, dopamine, and neuropsychological traits such as weak central coherence and set-shifting have been researched as potential biomarkers and endophenotypes of AN.
- Genotypes are defined as the genetic makeup of an individual. It can be described in terms of the combination of alleles at a particular locus. The locus is determined using association or linkage studies.
- Several loci have been identified and relate to serotonergic, dopaminergic, opioid, and BDNF systems. However, further research is awaited since current studies are subject to methodological limitations.

Definitions and Explanations

Anorexia nervosa: The term derives from the Greek word an-orexis which can be translated as "without appetite." The term "nervosa" is of Latin origin and indicates that the lack of food intake is due to a nervous constitution. Anorexia nervosa is one type of eating disorder that is a psychiatric illness. Individuals with this diagnosis control their body weight and often present with severe weight loss, an intense fear of weight gain, distortion of body image, and amenorrhea.

Genotypes: They contain an individual's genetic information in the form of a pair of genes.

Endophenotype: A valuable kind of biomarker is that of an endophenotype; a heritable trait biomarker that falls on the pathway between behavior and biology (phenotype and genotype). Gottesman and Gould (2003) have defined specific endophenotype criteria which include: (1) association with the illness in the population, (2) heritability, (3) state-independence, (4) cosegregation with the illness in families and (5) presence in unaffected relatives at a higher level than in the general population.

Biomarkers: They are underlying cognitive or behavioral traits associated with a disorder, but not part of their visible presentation. They can be state- or trait-related, and have a number of different applications such as being antecedent, screening, diagnostic, prognostic, or stratification markers (Ritsner and Gottesman 2009). The term biomarker is used when the trait does not fulfill the criteria of genetic underpinnings.

Phenotypes: They are the observable symptoms of a psychiatric illness, such as behavior. The AN phenotype involves a range of symptoms characterized by a disturbance of body (or self) image associated with extreme behaviors to control weight (e.g., fasting) and underweight BMI.

Key Facts of Diagnostic Difficulties in Anorexia Nervosa

1. The nosological status of the current DSM IV diagnostic criteria is suggested to lack an empirical basis. Some patients do not present with all the symptoms required for a clinical AN diagnosis. Furthermore, a substantive number of AN patients switch between diagnostic categories over the course of the illness.
2. Intermediate phenotypes such as biomarkers and endophenotypes may represent more stable characteristics of AN than illness phenotypes.
3. The search for intermediate phenotypes may lead to a more biologically based system of classification and a more accurate understanding of causation, pathophysiology, prognosis, and treatment.

Key Features of Endophenotypes and Biomarkers

1. Biomarkers are underlying cognitive or behavioral traits that are associated with a disorder, but not part of their visible presentation.
2. One valuable kind of biomarker is that of an endophenotype.
3. Gottesman and Gould (2003) use the term "endophenotype" when there are some signs of heritability, and biomarkers when the trait does not fulfill the criteria of genetic underpinnings.

Key Facts of Genotypes

1. To identify genetic loci involved in a disorder, linkage and association approaches can be used.
2. A large number of genetic loci are supposed to be involved in AN, each of which is suggested to express a small effect in the occurrence of the disorder.
3. Genetic loci relating to serotonergic, dopaminergic, and opioid systems and BDNF have been investigated in AN.
4. Research into AN genotypes should address the methodological limitations, such as population stratification and low sample sizes, which may distort results.

References

Adolphs R. Trends Cogn Sci. 1999;3:469–79.
American Psychiatric Association. Diagnostic and statistical manual of mental disorders (4th ed., text rev.). Washington, DC: Author 2000.
Anderluh M, Tchanturia K, Rabe-Hesketh S, Al E. Am J Psychiatry. 2003;160:242–7.
Anderluh M, Tchanturia K, Rabe-Hesketh S, Collier D, Teasure J. Psychol Med. 2009;39:105–14.
Bailer U, Frank G, Henry S, Al E. Arch Gen Psychiatry. 2005a;62:1032–41.

Bailer UF, Frank GK, Henry SE, Al E. Psychopharmacology (Berlin). 2005b;195:315–24.

Bailer UF, Price JC, Meltzer CC, Al E. Neuropsychopharmacology. 2004;29:1143–55.

Baron-Cohen S, Hammer J. J Cogn Neurosci. 1997;9:548–54.

Bergen AW, Van Den Bree MBM, Yeager M, Welch R, Ganjei JK, Haque K, Bacanu S, Berrettini WH, Grice DE, Goldman D, Bulik CM, Klump K, Fichter M, Halmi K, Kaplan A, Strober M, Treasure J, Woodside B, Kaye WH. Mol Psychiatry. 2003;8:397–406.

Bergen AW, Yeager M, Welch RA, Haque K, Ganjei JK, Van Den Bree MB, Mazzanti C, Nardi I, Fichter MM, Halmi KA, Kaplan AS, Strober M, Treasure J, Woodside DB, Bulik CM, Bacanu SA, Devlin B, Berrettini WH, Goldman D, Kaye WH. Neuropsychopharmacology. 2005;30:1703–10.

Berkman ND, Lohr KN, Bulik CM. Int J Eat Disord. 2007;40:293–309.

Birmingham CL, Su J, Hlynsky JA, Goldner EM, Gao M. Int J Eat Disord. 2005;38:143–6.

Brown KM, Bujac SR, Mann ET, Campbell DA, Stubbins MJ, Blundell JE. Biol Psychiatry. 2007;61:367–73.

Bulik CM, Slof-Op't Landt MC, Van Furth EF, Sullivan PF. Annu Rev Nutr. 2007;27:263–75.

Bulik CM, Sullivan PF, Tozzi F, Furberg H, Lichtenstein P, Pedersen NL. Arch Gen Psychiatry. 2006;63:305–12.

Byford S, Barrett B, Roberts C, Clark A, Edwards V, Smethurst N, Gowers SG. Br J Psychiatry. 2007;191:436–40.

Carr KD. Physiol Behav. 2002;76:353–64.

Castro-Fornieles J, Bargallo N, Lazaro L, EA. J Psychiatr Res. 2009;43:331–40. Epub 2008.

Cota D, Tschop MH, Horvath TL, Levine AS. Brain Res Rev. 2006;51:85–107.

Davies H, Tchanturia K. Eur Eat Disord Rev. 2005;13:311–6.

Devlin B, Bacanu SA, Klump KL, Bulik CM, Fichter MM, Halmi KA, Kaplan AS, Strober M, Treasure J, Woodside DB, Berrettini WH, Kaye WH. Hum Mol Genet. 2002;11:689–96.

Dolan RJ, Mitchell J, Wakeling A. Psychol Med. 1988;18:349–53.

Eddy KT, Dorer DL, Franko DL, Tahilani K, Thompson-Brenner H, Herzog DB. Am J Psychiatry. 2008;165:245–50.

Epstein LH, Truesdale R, Wojcik A, Paluch RA, Raynor HA. Physiol Behav. 2003;78:221–7.

Frank G, Bailer U, Henry S, Al E. Biol Psychiatry. 2005;58:908–12.

Frith U. Autism: explaining the enigma, Cambridge: Blackwell Science; 1989.

Gabrovsek M, Brecelj-Anderluh M, Bellodi L, Cellini E, Di Bella D, Estivill X, Fernandez-Aranda F, Freeman B, Geller F, Gratacos M, Haigh R, Hebebrand J, Hinney A, Holliday J, Hu X, Karwautz A, Nacmias B, Ribases M, Remschmidt H, Komel R, Sorbi S, Tomori M, Treasure J, Wagner G, Zhao J, Collier DA. Am J Med Genet Part B Neuropsychiatr Genet. 2004;124B:68–72.

Gagel O, Magersucht. vol. 5. Berlin: Springer. 1953.

Galusca B, Costes N, Zito NG, Peyron R, Bossu C, Lang F, Le Bars D, Estour B. Biol Psychiatry. 2008;64:1009–13.

Germain N, Galusca B, Le Roux CW, Bossu C, Ghatei MA, Lang F, Bloom SR, Estour B. Am J Clin Nutr. 2007;85:967–71.

Gillberg C, Rastam M, Gillberg C. Am Acad Child Adolesc Psychiatry. 1994;33:729–39.

Gillberg I, Rastam M, Wentz E, Al E. J Clin Exp Neuropsychol. 2007;29:170–8.

Gillberg IC, Gillberg C, Rastam M, Johansson M. Compr Psychiatry. 1996;37:23–30.

Glass MJ, Grace M, Cleary JP, Billington CJ, Levine AS. Am J Physiol Regul Integr Comp Physiol. 1996;271: 217–21.

Gorwood P, Ades J, Bellodi L, Cellini E, Collier DA, Di Bella D, Di Bernardo M, Estivill X, Fernandez-Aranda F, Gratacos M, Hebebrand J, Hinney A, Hu X, Karwautz A, Kipman A, Mouren-Simeoni MC, Nacmias B, Ribases M, Remschmidt H, Ricca V, Rotella CM, Sorbi S, Treasure J. Mol Psychiatry. 2002;7:90–4.

Gottesman IL, Gould TD. Am J Psychiatry. 2003;160:636–45.

Grice DE, Halmi KA, Fichter MM, Strober M, Woodside DB, Treasure JT, Kaplan AS, Magistretti PJ, Goldman D, Bulik CM, Kaye WH, Berrettini WH. Am J Hum Genet. 2002;70:787–92.

Hambrook D, Tchanturia K, Schmidt U, Al E. Br J Clin Psychol. 2008;47:335–9.

Happe F, Briskman J, Frith U. J Child Psychol Psychiatry Allied Disciplines. 2001;42:299–307.

Happe F, Frith U. J Autism Dev Disord. 2006;36:5–25.

Happe FG, Booth RD. Q J Exp Psychol. 2008;61:50–63.

Harbottle EJ, Birmingham CL, Sayani F. Eat Weight Disord. 2008;13:e32–4.

Hebebrand J, Casper R, Treasure J, Schweiger U. J Neural Transm. 2004;111:827–40.

Hernandez L, Hoebel BG. Life Sci. 1988;42:1705–12.

Hjern A, Lindberg L, Lindblad F. Br J Psychiatry. 2006;189:428–32.

Hoek HW, Van Hoeken D. Int J Eat Disord. 2003;34:383–96.

Holliday J, Tchanturia K, Landau S, Collier DA, Treasure J. Am J Psychiatry. 2005;162:2269–75.

Holliday J, Uher R, Landau S, Collier D, Treasure J. J Pers Disord. 2006;20:417–30.

Hudson JI, Hiripi E, Pope HG, Jr., Kessler RC. Biol Psychiatry. 2007;61:348–58.

Jones BP, Duncan CC, Brouwers P, Mirsky AF. J Clin Exp Neuropsychol. 1991;13:711–28.

Kaye W. Physiol Behav. 2008;94:121–35.

Kaye W, Strober M, Jimerson D. The neurobiology of eating disorders. In: Charney, DS, Nestler EJ, editors. The neurobiology of mental illness. New York: Oxford Press; 2004.

Kaye WH, Pickar D, Naber D, Ebert MH. Am J Psychiatry. 1982;139:643–5.

Krieg JC, Lauer C, Leinsinger G, Al E. Biol Psychiatry. 1989;25:1041–8.

Kucharska-Pietura K, Nikolaou V, Masiak M, Al E. Int J Eat Disord. 2004;35:42–7.

Lilenfeld LR, Kaye WH, Greeno CG, Merikangas KR, Plotnicov K, Pollice C, Rao R, Strober M, Bulik CM, Nagy L. Arch Gen Psychiatry. 1998;55:603–10.

Liu P, Jiang Y, Chen C, Chang C, Lee T, Sun HS, Chuang L. Twin Res Hum Genet. 2008;11:495–504.

Lopez C, Tchanturia K, Stahl D, Al E. Psychol Med; 2008a;37:1075–84.

Lopez C, Tchanturia K, Stahl D, Al E. Int J Eat Disord. 2008b;41:143–52.

Lopez C, Tchanturia K, Stahl D, Al E. J Clin Exp Neuropsychol. 2008c;4:1–9.

Lowe B, Zipfel S, Buchholz C, Dupont Y, Reas DL, Herzog W. Psychol Med. 2001;31:881–90.

Lowe ML, Levine AS. Obes Res. 2005;13:797–806.

Martin F. Acta Neurol Belg. 1958;52:816–30.

Mathers C, Vos T, Stevenson C. MJA. 1999;172:592–6.

Mccormick LM, Keel PK, Brumm MC, Al E. Int J Eat Disord. 2008;41:602–10.

Miyake A, Friedman NP, Emerson MJ, Witzki AH, Howerter A. Cogn Psychol. 2000;41:49–100.

Mond JM, Hay PJ, Rodgers B, Owen C, Beumont PJ. Qual Life Res. 2005;14:171–8.

Monteleone P, Tortorella A, Martiadis V, Serritella C, Fuschino A, Maj M. Psychosom Med. 2004;66:744–8.

Nakazato M, Hashimoto K, Yoshimura K, Haluzik T, Shimizu E, Iyo M. Prog Neuropsychopharmacol Biol Psychiatry. 2006;30:1117–21.

Palazidou E, Robinson P, Lishman WA. Psychol Med. 1990;20:521–7.

Papadopoulos FC, Ekbom A, Brandt L, Ekselius L. Br J Psychiatry. 2009;194:10–7.

Pelleymounter MA, Culbert MJ, Wellman CL. Exp Neurol. 1995;131:229–38.

Rastam M, Gillberg C, Wentz E. Eur Child Adolesc Psychiatry. 2003;12 (Suppl 1):I78–90.

Ribases M, Gratacos M, Fernandez-Aranda F, Bellodi L, Boni C, Anderluh M, Cavallini MC, Cellini E, Di Bella D, Erzegovesi S, Foulon C, Gabrovsek M, Gorwood P, Hebebrand J, Hinney A, Holliday J, Hu X, Karwautz A, Kipman A, Komel R, Nacmias B, Remschmidt H, Ricca V, Sorbi S, Tomori M, Wagner G, Treasure J, Collier DA, Estivill X. Eur J Hum Genet. 2005;13:428–34.

Ricca V, Nacmias B, Cellini E, Di Bernardo M, Rotella CM, Sorbi S. Neurosci Lett. 2002;323:105–8.

Ritsner MS, Gottesman IL. Where do we stand in the quest for Neuropsychiatric Biomarkers and Endophenotypes and what next? In Ritsner MS, editor. The handbook of neuropsychiatric biomarkers, endophenotypes and genes. Berlin: Springer; 2009.

Roberts ME, Tchanturia K, Stahl D, Al E. Psychol Med. 2007;37:1075–84.

Roser W, Bubl R, Buergin D, Al E. Int J Eat Disord. 1999;26:119–36.

Small DM, Jones-Gotman M, Daghera A. NeuroImage. 2003;19:1709–15.

Smalley S, Asarnov R. J Autism Dev Disord. 1990;20:271–8.

Southgate L, Tchanturia K, Treasure J. Psychiatry Res. 2008;160:221–7.

Strober M, Freeman R, Lampert C, Diamond J, Kaye W. Am J Psychiatry. 2000;157:393–401.

Strober M, Freeman R, Morrell W. Int J Eat Disord. 1999;25:135–42.

Su JC, Birmingham CL. Eat Weight Disord. 2003;8:76–9.

Takahashi M, Tanaka K, Miyaoka H. Psychiatry Clin Neurosci. 2006;60:211–8.

Tchanturia K, Morris R, Anderluh M, Al E. J Psychiatr Res. 2004;38:545–52.

Tchanturia K, Morris R, Surguladze S, Al E. Eat Weight Disord. 2002;7:312–5.

Tchanturia K, Serpell L, Troop N, Al E. J Behav Ther Exp Psychiatry. 2001;32:107–15.

Tchanturia K, Whitney J, Treasure J. Weight Eat Disord. 2006;11:112–7.

Tiller JM, Sloane G, Schmidt U, Troop N, Power M, Treasure JL. Int J Eat Disord. 1997;21:31–8.

Treasure J, Lopez C, Roberts M. Pediatric Health. 2007;1:171–81.

van den Eynde F, Treasure J. Child Adolesc Psychiatric Clin N Am. 2008;18:95–115.

Volkow ND, Wang G-J, Fowler JS, Logan J, JayneM, Franceschi D, Wong C, Gatley SJ, Gifford AN, Ding Y-S, Pappas N. Synapse. 2002;44:175–80.

Wagner A, Aizenstein H, Venkatraman VK, Fudge J, May C, Mazurkewicz L, Frank GK, Bailer U, Fischer L, Nguyen L, Carter C, Putnam K, Kaye WH. Am J Psychiatry. 2007;164:1842–9.

Wentz E, Gillberg C, Anckarsater H, Gillberg C, Rastam M. Br J Psychiatry. 2009;194:168–74.

Winchester E, Collier D. Genetic aetiology of eating disorders and obesity. In Treasure J, Schmidt U, Van Furth E, editors. Handbook of eating disorders. Chichester: John Wiley & Sons; 2003.

Zonnevijlle-Bendek M, Van Goozen S, Cohen-Kettenis P, Al E. Eur Child Adolesc Psychiatry. 2002;11:38–42.

Zonnevijlle-Bendek MJ, Van Goozen S, Cohen-Kettenis P, Al E. Depress Anxiety. 2004;19:35–42.

Zucker NL, Losh M, Bulik CM, Labar KS, Piven J, Pelphrey KA. Psychol Bull. 2007;133:976–1006.

Chapter 156
Metabolic Consequences in Anorexia Nervosa

Daniel Rigaud and Marie-Claude Brindisi

Abbreviations

ACTH	Adrenocorticotropic hormone
AN	Anorexia nervosa
BMI	Body mass index
CETP	Cholesterol ester transfer protein
DIT	Diet-induced thermogenesis
ED	Eating disorder
EE	Energy expenditure
EEPA	Energy expenditure linked to physical activity
EETR	Energy expended for thermoregulation
FFM	Fat free mass
HDL-C	High density lipoprotein cholesterol
IGF1	Insulin like growth factor 1
LDL-C	Low density lipoprotein cholesterol
REE	Resting energy expenditure
TSH	Thyroid stimulating hormone
VLDL-C	Very low density lipoprotein cholesterol

156.1 Introduction

Anorexia nervosa (AN) is a chronic disease which affects eating behavior and has severe health consequences (Rigaud 2003). It is the psychiatric disease with the highest mortality rate in such young women (15–35 years old). It is the rarest, but the most severe eating disorder (ED). AN is a complex disease that includes mental, genetic, behavioral, and somatic factors. Metabolic and energetic adjustments take place in the wake of the restrictive diet and malnutrition, and the mechanisms involved in these adjustments are beginning to be understood. In this chapter, impact on energy of AN will be developed. All the components of the energy expenditure (EE) will be detailed: resting energy

D. Rigaud (✉)
Department of Endocrinology and Nutrition, CHU Le Bocage
(Dijon University Hospital), BP 77908, 21079 Dijon Cedex, France
e-mail: daniel.rigaud@chu-dijon.fr

V.R. Preedy et al. (eds.), *Handbook of Behavior, Food and Nutrition*,
DOI 10.1007/978-0-387-92271-3_156, © Springer Science+Business Media, LLC 2011

expenditure (REE); diet-induced thermogenesis (DIT); EE linked to physical activity; thermoregulation. Then, we will pay attention to the metabolism of the different energetic substrates (protein, carbohydrates, lipids) in AN. The evolution of the body mass will be detailed, as will the physical activity and other abnormal behaviors (smoking, obsessive compulsive disorder, compulsive food intake, and bulimic crises) observed in AN. Then, we will detail the hormonal changes due to ED.

Anorexia nervosa is associated with a weight loss of more than 15% of previous weight, low weight (body mass index or BMI < 18.5 kg/m²), impaired body image, amenorrhea, and, above all, an intense fear of gaining weight (Rigaud 2003). More than 90% of the patients see themselves as fat, even though they know they are thin. In AN, there is a voluntary restriction in fat and protein intake (Rigaud 2003). In most of the chronic cases, it is not true anorexia, i.e. a decrease in hunger feeling. On the contrary, there is a strong will to decrease food consumption because of an overpowering need to slim. In AN, the fear of gaining weight, the fear of not being able to stop the increase in body weight, and the fear of eating too much are foremost in the minds of patients.

Two clinical types of AN are described (Rigaud 2003):one is called the restrictive type and the other the binge eating type with vomiting. In the restrictive type, patients lose weight by reducing food intake and, in 50–60% of the cases, by developing hyperactivity. In the second form, patients can't bear losing control, and because they are afraid of gaining weight, they cause themselves to vomit. If they cannot vomit or lose enough weight (5–10% of cases), they use laxatives and diuretic drugs. The binge-eating/purging type represents 30–40% of AN.

Females account for 95% of cases of AN patients, of whom 75–80% are under 25 years old and 20–25% are 20–30 years old (Rigaud 2003).

Anxiety is frequent in AN. In more than 60–70% of the cases, anxiety contributes to the evolution of the disease. In around one patient in five, anxiety is a pre-existing trait of the ED. Finally, a depressive state is often seen: in one case in seven, a depressive state precedes AN; and in one case in four, a depressive state is the price to pay for going to recovery.

156.1.1 Impact on Energy: Energy Expenditure (EE) *(Table 156.1)*

Two periods are seen in AN: A restrictive period (fasting state) when high energy foods are low or absent from the patient's diet; a refeeding and/or binge-eating period, where an excessive increase in food consumption is noted, either related to binge eating episodes and/or to hypercaloric diet medically prescribed. In terms of energy metabolism, these two periods are associated with very different profiles in the four components of EE (Rigaud and Melchior 1992): REE, DIT, EE related to physical activity, and thermoregulation.

1. REE is low during the fasting state (Melchior et al. 1989; Vaisman et al. 1991; Obarzanek et al. 1994; Platte et al. 1994; Scalfi et al. 2001; Forman-Hoffman et al. 2006; Konrad et al. 2007). It is around 80–88% of normal levels when the BMI is between 16 and 18 kg/m², and it can be around 60–65% of normal levels if the BMI is under 12 kg/m². In AN, the ratio of REE to lean mass is approximately 7–14% lower (extreme values, in 87 patients) than in same-age, same-sex controls with the same lean body mass (Van Wymelbeke et al. 2004). During this chronic fasting state, the calculation of REE is as follows: weight (kg) × 0.90 (lean mass) × 28 kcal/day. When the BMI is under 10 kg/m² (ultimate phase of the disease), the REE can increase, almost exclusively by the oxidation of the proteins, because of a lack of usable fatty substances (Rigaud et al. 2000). An increase in REE follows the start of refeeding: An increase in REE from 12% to 20% (Rigaud et al. 2000; Van Wymelbeke et al. 2004) within the first days of starting renutrition is seen, long

Table 156.1   Key facts of energy expenditure

Energy expenditure	Is the amount of energy, measured in calories, that a person uses (e.g. during a particular activity). The energy expenditure (EE) of a man or woman over a whole day is often divided into different components, which can be individually determined. These are: resting energy expenditure (REE), diet-induced thermogenesis (DIT), physical activity (PA), and thermoregulation
Resting energy expenditure	Is the minimum amount of energy that a body requires when lying in physiological and mental rest
Diet-induced thermogenesis (DIT):	Also called postprandial thermogenesis or the thermic effect of food. This is the amount of energy utilised in the digestion, absorption, and transportation of nutrients.
Energy expenditure linked to physical activity (PA):	Is the most variable component of EE in humans. It includes the additional EE above resting metabolic rate and DIT due to muscular activity and comprises minor physical movement (such as shivering and fidgeting) as well as purposeful gross muscular work or physical exercise.
Thermoregulation	Is the ability of an organism to keep its body temperature within certain boundaries.

Key facts of EE with its different components and their definitions: Resting energy expenditure, diet-induced thermogenesis (DIT), EE linked to physical activity (PA), and thermoregulation

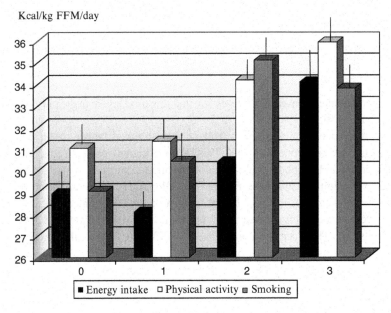

Fig. 156.1   Resting energy expenditure (REE) and level of energy intake, physical activity, and smoking. This figure shows the increase in REE according to the levels of energy intake (food intake), physical activity, and smoking behavior. When there is an increase in these factors, the REE increases too. *FFM* fat-free mass

■ *For energy intake:*"0" = before renutrition (energy intake = 830 kcal/day), "1" to "3" = during refeeding; "1" = for patients having energy intake between 1.1 and 1.3 × REE; "2" = for patients having energy intake between 1.3 and 1.8 × REE; "3" = for patients having energy intake higher than 1.8 × REE

□ *For physical activity:*"0" = none; "1" = 1 to 2 h/day; "2" = 2 to 3 h/day; "3" = >3 h/day

▨ *For smoking:*"0" = none; "1" = 1 to 5 cig/day; "2" = 6 to 10 cig/day; "3" = >10 cig/day

time before any significant increase in fat-free mass (Obarzanek et al. 1994; Platte et al. 1994; Van Wymelbeke et al. 2004; Winter et al. 2005; Konrad et al. 2007). Four factors were described to be associated with this increase in REE: smoking, having a high level of physical hyperactivity,

Fig. 156.2 Resting energy expenditure (REE) and levels of anxiety and depressed state. Level of anxiety and depressive state: 0 = none; 1 = a little; 2 = much; 3 = very much. *FFM* fat-free mass. This figure shows that when anxiety increases, there is an increase in REE, unlike depression. Indeed, when depressive state increases, we can observe a decrease in REE

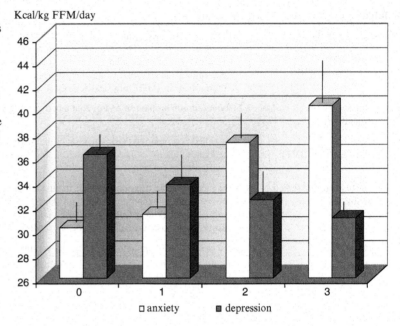

anxiety, and food intake. Conversely, depression and low food intake in the previous days decrease it (Figs. 156.1 and 156.2).

2. Diet-induced thermogenesis: A high level of DIT is observed before renutrition, compared to normal subjects (Moukaddem et al. 1997). This DIT still increases at the eighth day of renutrition, before any increase in lean body mass. In a double-blind experimental study, a 300- or 700-kcal load was given through a gastric tube. Before renutrition, DIT accounted for 36% of the 300 kcal and 26% of the 700 kcal. At the eighth day of renutrition, DIT accounted for 52% and 39% of the 300 and 700 kcal, respectively (for normal females: it was 14% and 16% for 300- and 700-kcal-loads, respectively). This increase correlates with different factors: the energy content of the meal, the fear of gaining weight, anxiety, and digestion disorders (Rigaud et al. 2007). This profile persists during renutrition; it disappears once normal weight has been reached and anxiety has disappeared. The increase in DIT during renutrition is due to the increase in food intake, and, first of all, protein intake (Fig. 156.3).

3. The EE linked to physical activity is low before renutrition (fasting period). It increases rapidly during renutrition, but it is no higher than in normal subjects with the same fat-free mass and the same level of physical activity (Rigaud et al. 1997). In fact, the increase is due to the increase in physical activity during renutrition (Kaye et al. 1988; Casper et al. 1991; Birmingham et al. 2005).Two causes explain this, a good and a bad one. The good one is that, when a severely malnourished patient is on refeeding program, his activity increases, although it was very low before refeeding. Such a behavior is seen, for example, in patients suffering from cystic fibrosis. The bad reason in AN patients is excessive exercising. Indeed, because of the fear of gaining weight, some patients engage in physical hyperactivity, and thus, largely increase their EE. This explains, in part, the slow rate of weight gain in AN (Walker et al. 1979; Dempsey et al. 1984; Leonard et al. 1996; Bossu et al. 2007). Moreover, obsessive compulsive disorders may increase EE significantly.

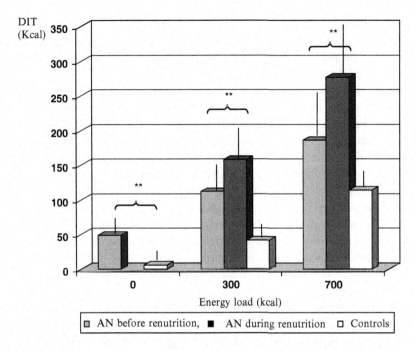

Fig. 156.3 Diet-induced thermogenesis (DIT) and energy load before and during renutrition. This study shows the increase in diet-induced thermogenesis according to the energy load before and during renutrition in 15 AN patients vs. 15 age-matched healthy women (controls). The period of renutrition corresponds to the eighth day of a renutrition program with input > 2,200 kcal/day. Loads are given in double blind manner by a nasogastric tube (0, 300 and 700 kcal in random order). This figure shows that diet-induced thermogenesis increases with the level of intragastric load

4. Energy expended for thermoregulation (EETR): it is at a low level before renutrition (fasting phase), but it increases rapidly with renutrition. Two causes explain this: the increase in thyroid hormone secretion (free T3 and T4) as soon as food intake is higher than energy needs. The increase in plasma T3 and T4 levels are noted only after the third week of renutrition. But the increase in secretion probably starts earlier, and could be responsible for the increase in REE (Onur et al. 2005). The second reason is that the body cannot store the energy (because of a lack of adipose tissue) when the fat mass is too low. This problem disappears during renutrition, well before a normal weight is reached.

156.2 Metabolism of Energetic Substrates

1. Protein metabolism: during the fasting period, a deep decrease in protein catabolism is observed, with very low nitrogen and urea 24-h urinary outputs: in 118 AN patients with a BMI of 13.4 ± 1.5 kg/m^2, the urinary nitrogen loss was 4.9 ± 0.6 g/24 h and the fecal nitrogen loss was 0.29 ± 0.6 g/24 h. This decrease in catabolism is an adaptive response to malnutrition and is due to the decrease in food intake and in hepatic and muscle protein synthesis. It does not exist during renutrition and recovery (Gniuli et al. 2001). This very low catabolism explains why markers of nutritional protein synthesized in the liver remain at a normal level for a long time (until a BMI of 12 kg/m^2 has been reached). In our study (Rigaud et al. 1989), patients with decreased plasma concentrations

of albumin, pre-albumin (transthyretin) and transferrin were AN patients with a BMI below 12 kg/m^2, or with an associated infectious or inflammatory disease. Moreover, the amino-acids from muscle catabolism might be used for the hepatic synthesis. Indeed, in AN, muscle mass decreases as quickly as body weight (see below).

2. Metabolism of carbohydrates: during the fasting period, low serum glucose, insulin, and C peptide levels are observed. Hypoglycemia (< 3.6 mmol/L) is found in 28% of AN patients (cohort of 487 patients hospitalized in our nutrition department, unpublished data). At the beginning of renutrition, insulin sensitivity, measured by the glycemia/insulinemia ratio is nearly always high. A decrease in fasting and postprandial serum glucose level can be observed during the first 2 weeks of renutrition. However, insulin resistance has been found during renutrition, when intakes are higher than energy needs. After a glucose load, the area under the insulin curve was reduced (3.2 ± 0.6 nmol/L/5 h in 14 AN patients and 49.6 ± 2.7 nmol/l/5 h in 12 normal patients), glucose oxidation was increased (646 ± 84 μmol/L/min vs. 368 ± 62 μmol/L/min in normal subjects), and lipid oxidation was decreased (16 ± 34 μmol/L/min, vs. 351 ± 57 μmol/L/min) (as measured by calorimetry and urinary nitrogen). Gniuli et al. found similar results (2001). This abnormal profile disappears with renutrition, well before the recovery of a normal weight.

3. Plasma lipids and lipoprotein metabolism: lipid oxidation is reduced during the fasting period. However, REE mostly depends on lipid metabolism. Lipids contribute to 22% of the REE, proteins to 16% and carbohydrates to 62% in AN (14 patients), versus 54% (lipids), 16% (proteins) and 30% (carbohydrates) in 12 normal subjects. On average, the fasting respiratory quotient is higher during fasting phase of the disease, in severely malnourished patients than in normal subjects (in 118 patients with BMI = 13.4 ± 1.5 kg/m^2, the respiratory quotient was 0.78 in AN patients vs. 0.71 in normal patients) (Russell et al. 2001). The reason is the increase in protein and carbohydrate oxidation, above all during renutrition. Concerning plasma lipoproteins, a decrease in cholesterol and total triglycerides is often observed (Jaguenaud et al. 1989). But, hypercholesterolemia is observed in one case in six (Rigaud et al. 2009): in 120 AN patients, a total cholesterolemia > 270 mg/100 mL was observed in 18% of cases. Low density lipoprotein-cholesterol (LDL-C), apo B, high density lipoprotein-cholesterol (HDL-C) and apo A1 levels were higher in the AN patients. Cholesterol ester transfer protein (CETP) activity is high during fasting periods in AN, partly explaining the increase in LDL-C (Ohwada et al. 2006); only denutrition and a decrease in apolipoprotein synthesis can counteract this (Jaguenaud et al. 1989). Triglycerides, which are normally low in malnutrition cases, are high in 15% of AN cases, because of a lack of lipoprotein lipase.

156.2.1 Evolution of Body Mass

AN patients want to lose fat mass, but the loss of fat-free mass and muscle mass is high (Dempsey et al. 1984; Obarzanek et al. 1994; Forman-Hoffman et al. 2006), which disturbs muscle functions (Rigaud et al. 1988; Murciano et al. 1994; Polito et al. 2000; Cuerda et al. 2007). The AN patients loss similar percentage of body weight and fat-free mass (a 15% body weight loss corresponds to a 15% fat-free mass loss). In AN patients, the fat mass represents 20–25% of body weight at the beginning of the disease and only 7–8% when their BMI is 12–14 kg/m^2. A decrease in cerebral grey mass and white mass are observed in AN, probably because of malnutrition. Under a BMI of 15 kg/m^2, hydro-sodium retention appears, with edema of the lower limbs during renutrition. This leads to excessive weight gain, which is independent of the food intake, if a salted diet is prescribed. So, a low-salt diet is necessary as soon as BMI is under 15 kg/m^2.

156.2.2 Physical Activity

Physical hyperactivity is frequent in EDs, and particularly in AN patients (Rigaud 2003). It is observed in 35–85% of the patients. In our cohort of 487 patients followed for 10 years, physical hyperactivity was quoted in 68% of the patients with the restrictive type, and in 52% of the bulimic ones (unpublished data).

The restrictive diet and the physical hyperactivity increase each other. The activity-based anorexic rat is a very interesting model (Hillebrand et al. 2005). This model has been developed by several teams, with similar results. In this model, four groups of rats are compared: the first control group includes rats that eat normally and are put in individual cages where they can engage in limited activity. The second group has the same diet (20–21g/day) but they can go on a wheel as often as they wish. The third control group is on a low-calorie diet (–25% of the previous intake), and their cages are standard. In the experimental group, the rats receive a low-calorie diet (15–16 g of food) and can use the wheel as much as they want to. Rats eating normal diet and allowing going to the wheel increase their physical activity during few days, then less and less. Rats on a restrictive diet in standard cage do not develop physical hyperactivity. Rats on sliming diet allowed to go on the wheel, use it more often each day, and curiously decrease their restricted food intake. They lose more weight than any other rat. A recent study using a quite different model found similar results (Martin et al. 2007): when male and female rats are put on a low-calorie diet; the females lose their menstruation, take on a male hormonal profile and lose weight faster, have more stress, and engage in more physical activity than do males. So, in rats, the female predisposition to AN is seen, without the need for psychological mechanisms (which, however, does not exclude them).

156.2.3 Other Behavioral Consequences

Smoking: there is a relationship between smoking and EDs. Generally speaking, binge eating and bulimic patients smoke more and are more often dependent on tobacco (addiction), than normal subjects and restrictive AN patients. This is also true in the bulimic form of AN (binge-eating, vomiting, and low BMI). Conversely, restrictive AN patients smoke less and are less dependent on tobacco than normal subjects of the same age and sex.

Obsessive compulsive disorder: Obsessive compulsive disorder may have an effect on daily EE for two reasons: by the physical activity that they often impose (obsessive compulsive disorder for housework, cleaning, washing hands, etc.) and by the anxiety, which is often associated (obsessive-compulsive disorder patients are very frequently anxious). It must be remembered that physical hyperactivity can be considered as an obsessive compulsive disorder at least in some eating-disorder patients.

Compulsive food intake and bulimic crises: In AN patients, true bulimia is 80–100 times more frequent than compulsion without vomiting (Rigaud 2003). Bulimia means there at least two episodes a week of compulsive food intakes, without pleasure or hunger, ending with vomiting. Bulimia is six times more frequent in AN patients than in nonanorexic women. It's hard to assess the precise risk of developing bulimic crises (binge-eating/purging episodes) in AN. Such crises occurred in 25–45% of AN patients. In our statistics (unpublished data), 31% of our 487 patients followed-up for more than 10 years developed binge-eating/purging episodes within the first 2 years. If no such crisis or vomiting is noted during the two first years, the risk of developing chronic bulimia is ten times less (4% of cases) than it is if patients exhibit such crises (36%). Almost 20–30% of the AN patients of the bulimic type do develop normal-weight chronic bulimia nervosa. On the contrary, evolution from bulimia nervosa towards the pure restrictive form of AN is very rare (6% of cases).

There are three explanations for going from the pure restrictive form to binge-eating/purging episodes: (1) frustration due to chronic food deprivation, in patients who keep the sensation of hunger and desire to eat; (2) Chronic energy deficit and various nutritional deficiencies, which lead patients to "need to eat" to avoid death; (3) An on-off response in such patients who deny the hedonic value of any sweet and savory foods. So in AN patients, cognitive restriction could be responsible for similar consequences that what is seen in obese patients on very restrictive low-calorie diet for a long time.

156.2.4 Hormonal Component

1. **Thyroid hormones**: Plasma concentrations are low during fasting; this is called the "low T3 syndrome". Thyroid hormones increase during renutrition and return to the normal level in 3–4 weeks. Normal levels of thyroid stimulating hormone (TSH) are restored at about the same time (Onur et al. 2005).
2. **Cortisol and adrenomedulla hormones**: During fasting, plasma cortisol and free urinary cortisol are often increased. Adrenocorticotropic hormone (ACTH) is high too. Physiological stress linked to the fatal risk of denutrition can explain this increase in cortisol. But physical hyperactivity increases both cortisol and ACTH. When the BMI is below 15 kg/m^2, hyperaldosteronism due to denutrition is observed.
3. **Leptin:** Leptin is reduced in AN (Polito et al. 2000; Satoh et al. 2003; Haas et al. 2005). This decrease correlates with the BMI, and may be responsible for reduced REE. But this leptin related decrease can be avoided by renutrition, because REE increases before any increase in fat mass, while leptin does not increase. When the BMI is above 18 kg/m^2, leptin increases and menstruation starts again.
4. **Adiponectin**: This is often high in AN (Pannacciulli et al. 2003). It could contribute to the increase in energy metabolism during renutrition.
5. **Ghrelin and PYY**: Their roles in EE regulation have been mentioned, but are still unclear (Misra et al. 2006).
6. **Catecholamines:** A high level of catecholamines has been found, but the results are inconsistent. They could be responsible for the increase in REE, postprandial EE, and EE linked to physical activity (Rigaud et al. 2007).

156.3 Conclusion

Understanding of the energy and metabolism components of AN and their evolution during refeeding are increasing. AN seems to be a metabolic and psycho-behavioral syndrome in which the different elements work together to perpetuate the disease. The body has a remarkable capacity to adapt to chronic fasting, but also wastes energy as soon as the patient starts eating again to build up body weight. These mechanisms of adaptation to fasting are partly known: decrease in leptin and thyroid hormone secretion, increase in cortisol secretion, reduction of the cardiac rhythm, reduction

Table 156.2 Evolution of energy needs, before and during renutrition according to the physical activity of the patient

Energy expenditure components	Restrictive AN	Restrictive + physical hyperactivity AN	Stable AN	Stable AN + physical hyperactivity	AN during renutrition	AN during renutrition plus hyperactivity
REE	924	1023	1089	1188	1353	1517
DIT	180	180	442	442	616	616
EEPA	180	260	190	280	210	290
EETR	20	20	35	35	50	55
EE weight gain	0	0	0	0	700	700
Total	**1305**	**1483**	**1756**	**1945**	**2929**	**3178**

This table describes the necessary Kcalories for a 36-kg AN patient of 1.70 m (BMI = 12.4 kg/m²), 92% of fat-free mass (33 kg), who wants to reach a weight of 48 kg, with 86% (41 kg) of lean mass, on the measured basis of a supplement of 700 kcal/day to have a weight gain of 100 g/day. The AN patient is able to not lose weight, eating 1,300 kcal/day (for 36 kg), and she is able to not gain weight eating 1,950 kcal/day if she engages in moderate activity. In order to gain 100 g/day at 48 kg, she will need 3,200 kcal/day

AN anorexia nervosa, *REE* resting energy expenditure, *DIT* diet-induced thermogenesis, *EEPA* energy expenditure linked to physical activity, *EETR* energy expended for thermoregulation

in the body temperature, in association with a state of depression. Mechanisms involved in the increase in EE are better known too: increase in lean mass, increase in metabolic activities linked to the high energy content of meals and increased physical activity. Nearly all of the abnormalities described above are the consequences of the disease and do not seem to play a direct role in the physiopathology.

156.4 Applications to Other Areas of Health and Disease

Knowledge of the evolution of EE and its different components in AN patients will help to understand the mechanisms involved in weight gain in this disease (Table 156.2). REE should be used to know the level of food intake required to obtain the desired weight gain. For example, one can analyze the body weight gain on the basis of the need of 700 kcal/day above the daily total EE to obtain a weight gain of 100 g/day.

The measure of the EE at rest and after physical activity will be useful for a cognitive behavioral therapy. Indeed, one of the bases of the cognitive therapy is the understanding of the body's needs. The aim of this approach is to reassure AN patients and help physicians to prescribe more scientifically based therapy.

Summary Points

- In anorexia nervosa (AN), weight loss and malnutrition trigger a cascade of metabolic, hormonal, and behavioral consequences.
- A considerable decrease in energy expenditure (EE) is observed during fasting states of the disease, but refeeding and weight gain induce a marked increase in EE, including an increase in resting EE, in DIT, and in EE related to physical activity.

Definitions of Key Terms

Anorexia nervosa: Anorexia nervosa (AN) is a psychiatric diagnosis that describes an ED characterized by low body weight and body image distortion with an obsessive fear of gaining weight.

Fat-free mass: Fat-free mass is comprised of the nonfat components of the human body. Skeletal muscle, bone, and water are all examples of fat-free mass.

Body mass index (BMI): Body Mass Index is a standardized ratio of weight to height, and is often used as a general indicator of health. BMI can be calculated by dividing weight (in kilograms) by the square of height (in meters). A BMI between 18.5 and 24.9 is considered normal for most adults.

Obsessive compulsive disorder: Is a mental disorder characterized by intrusive thoughts that produce anxiety, by repetitive behaviors aimed at reducing anxiety, or by combinations of such thoughts (obsessions) and behaviors (compulsions).

Binge eating: Is a pattern of disordered eating which consists of episodes of uncontrollable overeating. It is sometimes as a symptom of binge ED. During such binges, a person rapidly consumes an excessive amount of food.

- There is a dramatic fall in protein catabolism and in glucose disposal during the fasting stages of the disease. Lipid oxidation is reduced too. During renutrition, these profiles become normal a long time before normalization of body weight.
- The loss of fat-free mass and muscle mass is high, which disturbs muscle functions.
- Physical hyperactivity is frequent in EDs, and particularly in AN patients.
- Hormonal disturbances are observed: Low T3 syndrome, increased plasma cortisol, reduced leptin level, high adiponectin level, high level of catecholamines.

References

Birmingham CL, Hlynsky J, Whiteside L, Geller J. Eat Weight Disord. 2005;10:6–9.
Bossu C, Galusca B, Normand S, Germain N, Collet P, Frere D, Lang F, Laville M, Estour B. Am J Physiol Endocrinol Metab. 2007;292:E132–7.
Casper RC, Schoeller DA, Kushner R, Hnilicka J, Gold ST. Am J Clin Nutr. 1991;53:1143–50.
Cuerda C, Ruiz A, Velasco C, Camblor M, García-Peris P. Clin Nutr. 2007;26:100–106.
Dempsey DT, Crosby LO, Pertschuk MJ, Feurer ID, Buzby GP, Mullen JL. Am J Clin Nutr. 1984;39:236–42.
Forman-Hoffman VL, Ruffin T, Schultz SK. Ann Clin Psychiatry. 2006;18:123–7.
Gniuli D, Liverani E, Capristo E, Greco AV, Mingrone G. Metabolism 2001;50:876–81.
Haas V, Onur S, Paul T, Nutzinger DO, Bosy-Westphal A, Hauer M, Brabant G, Klein H, Müller MJ. Am J Clin Nutr. 2005;81:889–96.
Hillebrand JJ, Koeners MP, de Rijke CE, Kas MJ, Adan RA. Biol Psychiatry. 2005;58:165–71.
Jaguenaud P, Malon D, Cosnes J, Réveillard V, Apfelbaum M, Rigaud D. Cah Nutr Diét. 1996;31:45–51.
Kaye WH, Gwirtsman HE, Obarzanek E, George DT. Am J Clin Nutr. 1988;47:987–94.
Konrad KK, Carels RA, Garner DM. Eat Weight Disord. 2007;12:20–26.
Léonard T, Foulon C, Samuel-Lajeunesse B, Melchior JC, Rigaud D. Appetite 1996;27:223–33.
Martin B, Pearson M, Kebejian L, Golden E, Keselman A, Bender M, Carlson O, Egan J, Ladenheim B, Cadet JL, Becker KG, Wood W, Duffy K, Vinayakumar P, Maudsley S, Mattson MP. Endocrinology 2007;148(9):4318–33.
Melchior JC, Rigaud D, Rozen R, Malon D, Apfelbaum M. Eur J Clin Nutr. 1989;43:793–9.
Misra M, Miller KK, Tsai P, Gallagher K, Lin A, Lee N, Herzog DB, Klibanski A. J Clin Endocrinol Metab. 2006;91:1027–33.

Moukaddem M, Boulier A, Apfelbaum M, Rigaud D. Am J Clin Nutr. 1997;66:133–40.

Murciano D, Rigaud D, Pingleton S, Armengaud MH, Melchior JC, Aubier M. Am J Respir Crit care Med. 1994;150:1569–74.

Obarzanek E, Lesem MD, Jimerson DC. Am J Clin Nutr. 1994;60(5):666–75.

Ohwada R, Hotta M, Oikawa S, Takano K. Int J Eat Disord. 2006;39:598–601.

Onur S, Haas V, Bosy-Westphal A, Hauer M, Paul T, Nutzinger D, Klein H, Müller MJ. Eur J Endocrinol. 2005;152:179–84.

Pannacciulli N, Vettor R, Milan G, Granzotto M, Catucci A, Federspil G, De Giacomo P, Giorgino R, De Pergola G. J Clin Endocrinol Metab. 2003;88:1748–52.

Platte P, Pirke KM, Trimborn P, Pietsch K, Krieg JC, Fichter MM. Int J Eat Disord. 1994;16(1):45–52.

Polito A, Fabbri A, Ferro-Luzzi A, Cuzzolaro M, Censi L, Ciarapica D, Fabbrini E, Giannini D. Am J Clin Nutr. 2000;71(6):1495–502.

Rigaud D. In: Marabout, editor. Les troubles du comportement alimentaire. Paris; 2003.

Rigaud D, Melchior JC. In: Lavoisier, editors. Paris: Ed Med Intern; 1992. p. 69–132.

Rigaud D, Bedig G, Merrouche M, Vulpillat M, Apfelbaum M. Dig Dis Sci. 1988;33:919–25.

Rigaud D, Sogni P, Hammel P, Melchior JC, Rozen R, Labarre C, Mignon M, Apfelbaum M. Ann Med Intern. 1989;140:86–90.

Rigaud D, Cohen B, Melchior JC, Moukaddem M, Reveillard V, Apfelbaum M. Am J Clin Nutr. 1997;65:1845–51.

Rigaud D, Hassid J, Meulemans A, Poupard AT, Boulier B. Am J Clin Nutr. 2000;72:355–62.

Rigaud D, Colas-Linhart N, Verges B, Petiet A, Moukkaddem M, Van Wymelbeke V, Brondel L. J Clin Endocrinol Metab. 2007;92(5):1623–9.

Rigaud D, Tallonneau I, Vergès B. Diabetes Metab. 2009;35:57–63.

Russell J, Baur LA, Beumont PJ, Byrnes S, Gross G, Touyz S, Abraham S, Zipfel S. Psychoneuroendocrinology 2001;26(1):51–63.

Satoh Y, Shimizu T, Lee T, Nishizawa K, Iijima M, Yamashiro Y. Int J Eat Disord. 2003;34(1):156–61.

Scalfi L, Marra M, De filippo E, Caso G, Pasanisi F, Contaldo F. Int J Obes Relat Metab Disord. 2001;25:359–64.

Vaisman N, Rossi MF, Corey M, Clarke R, Goldberg E, Pencharz PB. Eur J Clin Nutr. 1991;45:527–37.

Van Wymelbeke V, Brondel L, Brun JM, Rigaud D. Am J Clin Nutr. 2004;80:1469–77.

Walker J, Roberts SL, Halmi KA, Goldberg SC. Am J Clin Nutr. 1979;32:1396–1400.

Winter TA, O'Keefe SJ, Callanan M, Marks T. J Parenter Enteral Nutr. 2005;29:221–8.

Chapter 157
Application of Personal Construct Theory to Understanding and Treating Anorexia Nervosa

Malgorzata Starzomska and Marek Smulczyk

Abbreviations

DSM	Diagnostic and statistical manual of mental disorders
DSM-IV-TR	Diagnostic and statistical manual of mental disorders, Fourth edition, Text revision
PCP	Personal construct psychotheraphy

157.1 Introduction

Anorexia nervosa is a serious, chronic illness with significant morbidity and mortality for most patients (Kaplan 2002). This condition continues to be poorly understood and is rather mysterious (Schmidt and Treasure 2006). To be diagnosed as having anorexia nervosa according to the DSM-IV-TR (2000), a person must display: (1) Refusal to maintain body weight at or above a minimally normal weight for age and height (e.g., weight loss leading to maintenance of body weight less than 85% of that expected; or failure to make expected weight gain during the period of growth, leading to body weight less than 85% of that expected); (2) Intense fear of gaining weight or becoming fat; (3) Disturbance in the way in which one's body weight or shape is experienced, undue influence of body weight or shape on self-evaluation, or denial of the seriousness of the current low body weight; (4) In postmenarcheal, pre-menopausal females (women who have had their first menstrual period but have not yet gone through menopause), amenorrhea (the absence of at least three consecutive menstrual cycles). Anorexia nervosa is seen by clinicians as one of the most frustrating and undisciplinable forms of psychopathology (Blank and Latzer 2004) because of the anorectic's apparent stubbornness in the face of impending death which blocks all attempts to help her (Lemma-Wright 1994). It is no wonder that anorectic patients have retained the reputation of being difficult to help or treat. This is the most difficult problem for clinicians who try to help anorectics. Their resistance to treatment and denial of illness seem to result from the fact that anorexia nervosa provides the afflicted person with a sense of identity. Many scientists assume that anorexia nervosa is caused by impairment of healthful identity develop-

M. Starzomska (✉)
The Maria Grzegorzewska Academy of Special Education, Institute of Applied Psychology,
40 Szczesliwicka Street, 02-353 Warsaw, Poland
e-mail: eltram@life.pl

V.R. Preedy et al. (eds.), *Handbook of Behavior, Food and Nutrition*,
DOI 10.1007/978-0-387-92271-3_157, © Springer Science+Business Media, LLC 2011

ment and failure to establish a self-definition (Stein and Corte 2007). It is highly probable that controlling and perfectionistic parents can be held responsible for impairment in the development of an independent sense of one's self as well as hindrance of autonomy (Stein and Corte 2007). Such adolescents often seek self-definition in the ability to control their body weight (Stein and Corte 2007) because this way they try to counterbalance the lack of clear identity and the accompanying feeling of impotence (Stein and Corte 2007). Thus anorexia nervosa seems to be the result of maladaptive coping with the absence of an authentic self (Stein and Corte 2007) and the search for a new, ideal identity. As a consequence, such persons begin to define their self through self-starvation (Lemma-Wright 1994) and success can be easily quantified in lost pounds, which offers immediate gratification and may explain why anorectics find it difficult to abandon weight loss (Lemma-Wright 1994). This problem is easy to notice in the following statement of a former anorectic: 'When I looked at myself in the mirror I saw someone beautiful; I saw myself ... the clearer the outline of my skeleton became, the more I felt my true self to be emerging (...). Without anorexia I should have been a nothing' (Lemma-Wright 1994, p. 40). Clearly, such identity, which is also called thin (Fransella and Button 1983) or anorectic (Wojciechowska 2000), is maladaptative (Wojciechowska 2000) but for the anorectic it is highly desirable because her beliefs about weight and shape are viewed as being specifically relevant for her (Vandereycken 2006). This phenomenon, which is typical only of anorexia nervosa and refers to the sense experienced by many patients that anorexia nervosa is their identity (Tan et al. 2003a), is called egosyntonicity and it is deemed to be the condition's core feature (Crisp 2006). This specific state is very difficult to change because self-starvation can be very empowering – it offers a sense of accomplishment and self-control as well as fulfilment of the need to make autonomous decisions (Lemma-Wright 1994). Thus, anorexia nervosa is highly valued by people who suffer from it. Notably, afflicted patients sometimes call the disorder their friend (Serpell et al. 1999). It is highly probable that anorectic symptoms are maintained by beliefs about the positive function of the illness for the person (Schmidt and Treasure 2006) and that the egosyntonic nature of anorexia nervosa may be responsible for the chronicity of this condition.

157.2   Egosyntonicity Within a Cognitive Model of Anorexia Nervosa

The egosyntonicity of anorexia nervosa can be well explained and understood within a cognitive model of anorexia nervosa. Central to all cognitive theories of eating disorders is the hypothesis that beliefs and expectancies pertaining to body size and eating are biased in favor of selectively processing information related to fatness/thinness, dieting, and control of food intake or body weight. According to this hypothesis, the anorectic's beliefs and values should be treated as implicit rules which affect the way she assesses her experience of herself and her world as well as the meaning she associates with it (Lemma-Wright 1994). Thus, the primary disorder in anorexia is distortion of the individual's perception of shape and weight (Lemma-Wright 1994), and self-starvation seems to be secondary to the individual's overvalued ideas. Recently, controlled investigations of the predictions of cognitive theories of eating disorders have yielded empirical support for these theories. Vitusek and Hollon (1990) argue that the core psychopathology of anorexia nervosa results from highly organized cognitive structures that unite views of the self with beliefs about weight. These weight-related self-schemas may exert automatic effects on the processing of information and may also help to account for the clinical observation that patients frequently regard their symptoms as egosyntonic. Stein and Corte (2007) found that anorectic patients had fewer positive and more negative and highly interrelated self-schemas compared to controls and that their self-concept was associated with pathological eating- and weight-related attitudes and behaviors. The anorectic person is continuously under the influence of her maladaptative self-constructs that are very difficult to change. She believes that without these schemas she would lose herself because they seemingly create her sense of identity. Studies conducted by cognitive researchers have clearly revealed that egosyntonicity of anorexia can be understood in terms of cognitive self-structures which are predominantly negative and very persistent.

157.3 Egosyntonicity Within an Existential Model of Anorexia Nervosa

Some researchers underline that the most important task in the psychotherapy of anorexia nervosa is to understand the anorectic's worldview. This term was proposed by Binswanger who described various aspects of so-called being-in-the-world. This theory has its roots in the existential psychotherapeutic literature which was preoccupied with emphasizing the importance of understanding the client's experience and herself in the world (Lemma-Wright 1994).

According to existential psychologists, although the anorectic's choice not to eat sometimes leads to death, it is the search for another life, a pursuit of attaining internally what cannot be accomplished or managed in the outer world (Lemma-Wright 1994). The anorectic's worldview seems to be dominated by control. Without control, she would be without a self, thus her unfailing perseverance essentially turns her life into a self-starvation project (Lemma-Wright 1994). Thus, according to the existentialists, anorexia nervosa is a specific solution to psychic pain. It is very important to note that existential clinicians are quite sceptical of diagnoses, for example DSM diagnoses, in general, and the diagnosis of anorexia nervosa in particular. Their primary concern is not whether the diagnosis exists but how it is used. For them, the question of so-called cure in anorexia is a controversial issue when the most important criterion appears to be weight gain. According to the existentialists, the individual who cannot find any other way of being-in-the-world than living a life of self-starvation is not necessarily cured when she starts to eat again. In our attempts to help the anorectic achieve this, we may well benefit from reminding ourselves that, as Joseph Conrad claimed, the question is not how to get cured but how to live (Lemma-Wright 1994).

Undoubtedly, the existentialists' most important contribution to the understanding of anorexia is their critical analysis of refeeding (treated as an element of behavioral therapy) in the case of this condition.

157.4 Similarities Between Cognitive and Existential Approaches to Anorexia Nervosa

Both cognitive and existential models seem to explain the meaning of self and especially its disturbances in the etiology and maintenance of anorexia nervosa. While cognitive researchers focus on the specific maladaptive self-schemas of anorectics, existentialists focus on their worldview but both groups despair that biological therapies of anorexia are insufficient and may even have paradoxical effects because they ignore the most important feature of the disorder, namely self-disturbances. Both cognitive and existential theories strive to understand the meaning of personal identity in anorectic patients. Vitousek and colleagues (1991), cognitive researchers, explain the reasons for therapeutic difficulties during anorexia nervosa treatment partly from an existential perspective: eating disorder patients, notably anorectics, are notorious for their secrecy, making it difficult to establish communication based on mutual trust and openness. They do so by concealing their behavior, feelings, and experiences, and especially by denying that they are ill (Vitousek et al. 1991). The authors review traditional methods of entering or reconstructing the private experience and overcoming or correcting

Table 157.1 Similarities between cognitive and existential approaches to anorexia nervosa

Understanding anorexia nervosa	
In cognitive approaches	In existential approaches
Both underline that anorectics in particular are notoriously protective of their private experience.	
Both seem to explain the meaning of self and especially its disturbances in the etiology and maintenance of anorexia nervosa	
Both despair that biological therapies of anorexia are insufficient, and even have paradoxical effects, because they ignore the most important feature of the disorder, namely self-disturbances.	

Both cognitive and existential approaches adopt a similar stance with respect to anorexia nervosa in that they emphasize the importance of private experience and self-disturbance in the etiology, maintenance, and treatment of this condition

the denial of the anorectic individual but they suggest that these methods which rely on clinical intuition, patients' testimony, and direct confrontation are likely to result in a combined perspective of clinician-researchers and their subjects (1991) so they propose a variety of alternative methods of reducing denial and distortion in patients' self-report that may prove to be more useful. Surprisingly, their terminology (internal world, private experience, etc.) is partly existential (Table 157.1).

157.5 George Kelly – Cognitivist or Existentialist?

Interestingly enough, one of the most well-known cognitive researchers, George Kelly, whose Personal Construct Theory has been successfully applied to anorexia nervosa, has been deemed an existentialist by some. Although Kelly was sceptical of phenomenology per se because of its introspective idealism and lack of clear theory and rigorous methodology and experimentation, he was convinced, just like the phenomenologists, that to understand behavior one needs to understand how a person construes reality: how he or she understands it, perceives it, and that this is more important than knowing what that reality truly is. In fact, he pointed out that everyone's view – even the hard-core scientist's – is just that: a view. This is exactly the meaning of the phenomenologist's basic principle, known as intentionality. Although Kelly's theory may sound very cognitive, with its emphasis on constructs and constructions, Kelly himself disliked being called a cognitive theorist. He maintained that his theory included the more traditional ideas of perception, behavior, and emotion. According to Boeree (2006) it is yet to be seen whether Kelly will be remembered as a phenomenologist or a cognitivist. Nevertheless it must be underlined that there are aspects of Kelly's theory that are in contradiction to phenomenology. First, Kelly was a true theory-builder whereas existential researchers tend to avoid theory. Second, he had high hopes for a rigorous methodology for psychology (Boeree 2006). Most existential researchers are much more sceptical about experimentation.

157.6 A Personal Construct Theory Framework

Personal Construct Psychology is a theory of personality developed by George Kelly in the 1950s. Kelly called his theory and philosophy constructive alternativism. His idea was that although there is only one true reality, reality is always experienced from one or another perspective, namely each person perceives the world from his/her own, completely unique vantage point. According to Kelly, people develop internal models of reality, which he called constructs, in order to understand and explain the world around them in the same way as scientists develop theories (Kelly 1955; Hall Lindzey and Campbell 2004). Therefore, all people can be called scientists because they have constructions of their reality. Like scientists, they have theories and they improve their understanding of reality on the basis of their experiences and, like scientists, they adjust their theories to fit the facts. Constructs are usually defined by words but they can sometimes be nonverbal and very difficult to explain (http://changingminds.org/explanations/theories/personal_construct.htm).

According to Kelly, we store experience in the form of personal, usually bipolar constructs. Where there is thin, there must be fat, where there is good, there must be bad, etc. If everyone were fat, then fat would become meaningless or identical in meaning to everyone. Some people must be skinny in order for fat to have any meaning, and vice versa.

157.7 Roots and Core of Psychopathology and Psychotherapy in Personal Construct Theory

Kelly believed that a psychological disorder was any personal construction which was used repeatedly in spite of consistent invalidation. The behaviors and thoughts which occur in depression, paranoia, schizophrenia, addictions, eating disorders, and so on are examples. Such people cannot learn new ways of relating to the world. They are full of anxiety and/or hostility and other negative feelings (Kelly 1955; Hall et al. 2004).

The main method that Kellian psychotherapists use to diagnose and treat patients with various disorders or psychological problems is the repertory grid interview. Kelly derived this technique from his theory to help patients uncover their own constructs with minimal intervention or interpretation by the therapist and to reconstruct them (Kelly 1955; Hall et al. 2004; http://en.wikipedia.org/wiki/Personal_construct_psychology). In other words, Kellian psychotherapy gets the client to see things in a different way, from a new perspective. It has the following goals: to open people up to alternatives, help them to discover their freedom, and allow them to live up to their potentials (Boeree 2006). This is a noninvasive approach to psychotherapy (Kelly 1955; Hall et al. 2004). The UK Council for Psychotherapy, a regulatory body, classifies PCP therapy under Experiential Constructivism.

157.8 Repertory Grid Presentation

To create their own repertory grid (Table 157.2), patients must first name a set of ten to twenty people, called elements, likely to be of some importance in their lives. In therapy, these people are named in response to certain suggestive categories, such as "my mother," "my father," etc. Second, the therapist (or researcher) must pick out three of these at a time, and ask the patient to tell her/him which of two are similar and which one is different. Then the therapist must ask the patient to give her/him something to call the similarity and the difference. The similarity label is called the similarity pole, and the difference is called the contrast pole. Together they make up one of the constructs applied in social relations. If, for example, a girl says that both she and her mother are nervous people but her father is very calm, then nervous is the similarity pole and calm the contrast pole

Table 157.2 Elements used by 20 anorectics in Button's study

Elements 1–10	Subject's personal elements
Element 11	Me now
Element 12	Me if I was overweight
Element 13	Me as I was one year ago
Element 14	Me as I will be one year ahead
Element 15	Patient's consultant psychiatrist
Element 16	Me at the weight I would prefer to be
Element 17	Me at the sort of weight I imagine the treatment team wants me to be
Element 18	Me at what most people would call a normal weight for me
Element 19	Me as I would ideally like to be
Element 20	Me at the thinnest I've been
Element 21	Me at the heaviest I've been
Element 22	Father – if not included in the subject's personal elements
Element 23	Mother – if not included in the subject's personal elements

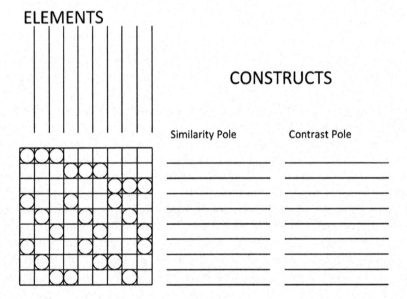

Fig. 157.1 A blank rep grid. The blank rep grid has two components, namely: elements (which correspond to important persons in one's life) and constructs (which correspond to both similarity and contrast between the elements) (Reprinted from Boeree 2006 [Online]. Available at: http://webspace.ship.edu/cgboer/kelly.html [accessed 1 June 2009]. With permission)

of the construct nervous–calm. The patient and therapist continue in this fashion, with different combinations of three, until about 20 (but sometimes fewer) contrasts are listed. The therapist, but especially the researcher, may perform certain statistical operations on the completed chart (Kelly 1955; Hall et al. 2004). The rep grid itself is a matrix where the rows represent the discovered constructs, the columns represent the elements, and cells indicate (numerically) the position of each element within each construct (Fig. 157.1). Software is available to produce several reports and graphs from these grids. In diagnostic and self-discovery applications, the therapist may encourage the patient to use constructs that refer to people's behaviors and personalities and, if necessary, to the self (Kelly 1955; Hall et al. 2004).

In therapy, the rep grid gives the therapist and client a picture of the client's view of reality that can be discussed and worked with. The rep grid is a unique test in that the client is invited to change his or her mind about it at any time. Neither is it assumed to be a complete picture of the person's mental state. It is what it is: a diagnostic tool.

Noteworthy, in research, therapists and researchers use a number of computer programs that enable measurement of the distances between constructs or elements. Thus it is possible to get a picture, created by the subjects themselves, of their world-views. It is also possible to compare the views of several people, for example a person's world-view, before and after training or therapy. Such comparisons were made in the studies described in this article (Boeree 2006).

The rep grid is an exciting tool, a creative combination of the subjective and objective side of personality research. It could be said that this technique is very attractive not only for cognitive researchers but also, due to its sensitivity to subjectivity, for methodologically oriented existentialists (Boeree 2006).

157.9 Application of Kellian Theory to Egosyntonic Aspects of Anorexia Nervosa

In 1980 Button (cited in Fransella and Button 1983) conducted a study in which he used the rep grid method. He asked 20 anorectic patients to rate 23 elements in terms of 21 constructs on a 7-point scale. It must be underlined that the constructs and elements were both specific to the individual (named: personal) and supplied by the experimenter (Tables 157.3 and 157.4).

Table 157.3 Constructs used by 20 anorectics in Button's study (Reprinted from Fransella and Button 1983. With permission)

Constructs 1–12	Subject's personal constructs
Construct 13	Very thin–very fat
Construct 14	Attractive–unattractive
Construct 15	Sexually attractive–sexually unattractive
Construct 16	Anorectic–nonanorectic
Construct 17	Eats normally–doesn't eat normally
Construct 18	Needs medical help–doesn't need medical help
Construct 19	Doesn't need psychiatric help–needs psychiatric help
Construct 20	Not physically ill–physically ill
Construct 21	Mentally ill–not mentally ill

Button construed his rep grid on the basis of the answers of 20 anorectic patients whom he asked to rate 23 elements in terms of 21 constructs on a 7-point scale. Both constructs and elements were specific to the individual (he called them personal) and supplied by the experimenter

Table 157.4 Effects of the anorectic's (thin) self construal on treatment results in Button's study

The more extremely the self (especially ideal, anorectic, thin self) was construed, the poorer the treatment outcome. The more fixed patients' views of themselves, the more resistant they were to permanent weight change.

At first follow-up a more extreme view of the self at treatment team weight and at normal weight was associated with good outcome. It therefore appears that weight maintenance after discharge is associated with the patient having a reasonably clear idea of what it means to be normal in terms of weight.

Between first and second follow-up the most significant finding was that a decrease in meaningfulness of the construct fat–thin was associated with good weight maintenance. This suggests that an important goal of therapy is to help anorectics find ways of construing themselves other than in terms of weight or fatness.

Button demonstrated that treatment outcome depends on the importance of the fat–thin construct for the anorexic patient

Results, as in the former study conducted by Fransella and Crisp in 1979, showed no evidence of denial of illness among these patients: intercorrelations between the construct anorectic–nonanorectic (its "anorectic" end) and remaining constructs supplied by the experimenter that could be named "illness" constructs (the following ends: very thin, needs medical help, mentally ill) were positive and very high, ranging between 0.95 and 0.63. Intercorrelations between the "not anorectic" end of the construct anorectic–nonanorectic and such ends of "illness" constructs as: attractive, sexually attractive, eats normally, doesn't need psychiatric help, not physically ill were negative and very high, ranging between 0.98 and 0.74. Analysis of the results showed that the present "thin self" (me now) is seen as undesirable and the "normal weight self" as desirable.

Interestingly, Button decided to take the analysis one step further by scrutinizing the relationships between the "self" elements only in terms of the personal (specific to the individual) constructs because he wanted to establish whether the dispersion of elements was simply a function of the particular constructs supplied by the experimenter (constructs 13–21, Table 157.4). Analysis of data using the same elements (Table 157.3) but different constructs (constructs 1–12, Table 157.4) revealed very similar relationships between the aforementioned elements when all constructs were used, namely self now (element 11) was not ideal (element 19) and thin (element 20), but it also revealed a new, astonishing result (compared with the analysis using all constructs), namely there was an interesting relationship between ideal self (element 19), self at treatment team, weight and self at normal weight (personal elements); ideal self was not self at treatment team and self at normal weight (Figs. 157.2 and 157.3). This

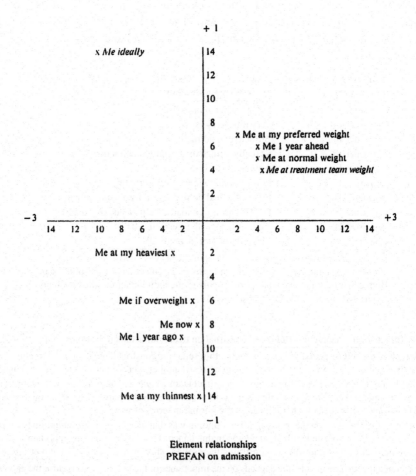

Fig. 157.2 Plot of "Self" Elements in terms of their loadings on components1 and 2 for a group of 20 anorectic patients

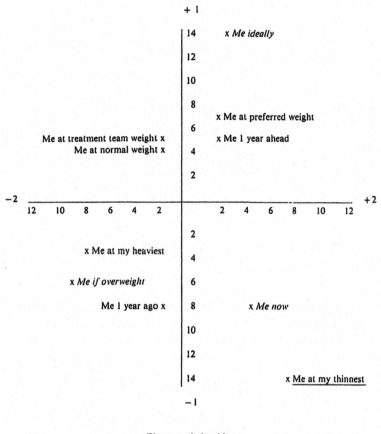

Element relationships
PREFAN on admission

Fig. 157.3 Plot of "Self" Elements in terms of their loadings on components 1 and 3 for a group of 20 anorectc patients. Interestingly, Button decided to scrutinize the relationships between the "self" elements only in terms of the personal (specific to the individual) constructs because he wanted to establish whether the dispersion of elements was simply a function of the particular constructs supplied by the experimenter (constructs 13–21, Table 157.4). This analysis of group data using identical elements but different constructs can be performed using Slater's PREFAN program. Analysis of data using the same elements (Table 157.3) but different constructs (constructs 1–12, Table 157.4) revealed very similar relationships between the aforementioned elements when all constructs were used, namely self now (element 11) was not ideal (element 19) and thin (element 20) (Fig. 157.2), but it also revealed a new, astonishing result (compared with the analysis using all constructs), namely there was an interesting relationship between ideal self (element 19), self at treatment team, and self at normal weight (personal elements); ideal self was not self at treatment (Fig. 157.3) (Reprinted from Fransella and Button 1983. With permission)

implies that ideal self is probably closer to thin self than to medically treated self at normal weight. According to Button, this result may be a possible source of insight into the anorectic's dilemma – wanting to gain weight and be normal while at the same time sensing that this is not viable for her.

157.10 Egosyntonicity of Anorexia in the Light of Results of the Study

Disclosure of this specific ambivalence (ideal self is in contradiction to self at treatment team and self at normal weight) provides us with a real and reliable picture of anorexia: this is a condition which is inextricably linked with sense of identity, namely an anorectic person must be anorectic (i.e., thin) in order to preserve a sense of identity (Lemma-Wright 1994) and to preserve its egosyntonic symptomatology (Vandereycken 2006). Clearly, in addition to having an anorectic (thin) self, the afflicted person also has other selves (for example, self at normal weight) but the anorectic (thin) self seems to dominate. This is why anorectics are so reluctant to accept treatment, even when they are very low in weight and at significant risk to themselves (Tan et al. 2003b). Using Kellian terms it could be said that an anorectic person is caught with her constructs down and her anxiety involves anticipations of great changes in her core (Kelly's term) constructs (interestingly, Crisp described egosyntonicity as a core feature) (1990). It is therefore understandable that she does not want to get rid of her anorexia because it constitutes her most important construct: anorectic, i.e., thin–nonanorectic, i.e., fat. Button's findings confirm that egosyntonicity (craving for an anorectic, thin identity) is the most important feature of anorexia and it is impossible to understand this condition without this phenomenon which scientists, clinicians, and lawyers dealing with capacity problems must take into account.

157.11 Effects of the Anorectic's (Thin) Self-Construal on Treatment Results

Button (1980, cited in Fransella and Button 1983) also intended to explore the effects of self-construal, in the sense of relationships between elements within specific constructs, on treatment results measured by weight maintenance. His analyses revealed that:

- The more extremely the self (especially ideal, anorectic, thin self) was construed, the poorer the outcome of treatment. The more fixed patients' views of themselves, the more resistant they were to permanent weight change.
- At first follow-up a more extreme view of the self at treatment team weight and at normal weight was associated with good outcome. It therefore appears that weight maintenance after discharge is associated with the patient having a reasonably clear idea of what it means to be normal in terms of weight.
- Between first and second follow-up the most significant finding was that a decrease in meaningfulness of the construct fat–thin was associated with good weight maintenance. This suggests that an important goal of therapy is to help anorectics find ways of construing themselves other than in terms of weight or fatness.

One statistically significant relationship of some interest was found between change in construal from time of admission to time of discharge and poor clinical outcome; this was an increase in meaningfulness of being anorectic compared with being normal weight. It was as if the girls who failed to maintain their weight came to see themselves more clearly as anorectic while in hospital. Therefore, how patients see themselves in relation to their disorder at the onset of treatment has prognostic significance. For anorectics, the more meaningful the self in relation to weight, the poorer the clinical outcome (Fransella and Button 1983). These results show that our self-image affects our behavior and may influence our proneness to change (Fransella and Button 1983) (Table 157.5).

157.12 Applications to Other Areas of Health and Disease

Results of studies on self-construal in anorexia nervosa within Personal Construct Theory may be applied to other mental disorders, or simply to problems which seem to be connected with the sense of identity. It is worth mentioning patients with anxiety disorders whose anxiety concerns a specific

Table 157.5 Key points concerning application of Personal Construct Theory to understanding and treating anorexia nervosa

Resistance to treatment and denial of illness in anorexia nervosa seem to result from the fact that anorexia nervosa provides the afflicted person with a sense of identity which is named egosyntonicity.
Personal Construct Psychology provides us with a very useful tool with which to study the egosyntonicity of anorexia nervosa, the rep grid. Studies which have used this technique show that the way patients see themselves in relation to their disorder at the onset of treatment has prognostic significance. For anorectics, the more meaningful the self in relation to weight, the poorer the clinical outcome.
Analyzing personal constructs of anorectic patients and attempts to find ways of construing themselves other than in terms of objects of fear or problems can literally change their life into easier to bear and even very successful.
Resistance to treatment and denial of illness in anorexia nervosa seem to result from the egosyntonicity of this condition, and Personal Construct Psychology provides us with a very useful tool with which to study the egosyntonicity of anorexia nervosa, the rep grid. Studies using this method have shown that the main aim in treating anorexics should be to help them find ways of construing themselves other than in terms of fatness

area of life or persons but who are not mentally disordered, only distressed about, for example, stuttering. When analyzing their personal constructs and attempts to find ways of construing themselves other than in terms of objects of fear or problems, they can literally change their life, making it easier to bear or even very successful.

157.13 Conclusion

Thanks to Button who explored various self elements, especially in anorectics, i.e., thin constructs, it is possible to understand what the term egosyntonic really means. Anorexia with its main symptom, thinness, is inseparably linked with sense of identity. As a consequence, an anorectic person is scared of life without her disorder and this phenomenon seems to be responsible for her denial of illness and resistance to treatment. It is noteworthy that both cognitive and existential models seem to explain the importance of the self and especially its disturbances in the etiology and maintenance of anorexia nervosa and both models try to explain the sense of personal identity in anorectic patients. Although some researchers stress the importance of the sense of identity in the course of anorexia nervosa, biological (mainly refeeding) and behavioral therapeutic programs are still in common use. The results of the studies presented show that the most important aim in the therapy of anorectics should be to help them find a way of self-realization that does not involve self-starvation (and sometimes death). Existential and cognitive researchers and therapists manifest considerable consensus in their analyses of this phenomenon. This aim is very ambitious and very difficult to achieve but undoubtedly worth the effort.

Summary Points

1. Anorexia nervosa is a serious, chronic illness with significant morbidity and mortality. This condition continues to be poorly understood and rather mysterious and is also seen by clinicians to be one of the most frustrating forms of psychopathology because of the anorectic's apparent stubbornness in the face of impending death which blocks all attempts to help her.
2. Resistance to treatment and denial of illness seem to result from the fact that anorexia nervosa provides the afflicted person with a sense of identity called egosyntonicity.
3. Paradoxically, both cognitive and existential models seem to explain the meaning of self and especially its disturbances in the etiology and maintenance of anorexia nervosa and both attempt to understand anorectic patients' sense of personal identity.

4. Personal Construct Psychology provides us with a very useful tool with which to study the ego-syntonicity of anorexia nervosa, the rep grid.
5. Studies which have used this technique show that the way patients see themselves in relation to their disorder at the onset of treatment has prognostic significance. In anorectics, the more meaningful the self is in relation to weight, the poorer the clinical outcome.

Definitions and Explanations of Key Terms

Anorexia nervosa: A serious psychiatric disorder characterized by distorted body image which triggers intensive self-starvation and – as a consequence – significantly diminished body weight. The very essence of this eating disorder is categorical refusal to change in conjunction with profound denial of illness.

Cognitive theories of eating disorders: Theories according to which beliefs and expectancies pertaining to body size and eating are biased in favor of selective processing of information related to fatness/thinness, dieting, and control of food intake or body weight.

Egosyntonicity: A phenomenon present in very few disorders, whose main feature is that the afflicted person derives a sense of identity from the disorder.

Personal construct theory: A theory of personality developed by George Kelly in the 1950s, based on constructive alternativism, that is, on the idea that although there is only one true reality, reality is always experienced from one perspective or another.

The repertory grid interview: The main method used by Kelly and designed on the basis of Personal Construct Theory.

Acknowledgments Malgorzata Starzomska and Marek Smulczyk are very greateful to Professor Melena Yanet Grzegorzewska klarkowske for her invaluable assistance.

References

Blank S, Latzer Y. Am J Family Therapy. 2004;32:43–54.

Boeree CG. George Kelly [Online]. Available at: http://webspace.ship.edu/cgboer/kelly.html [Accessed 1 June 2009]; 2006

Crisp A. Eur Eat Disord Rev. 2006;14:189–202.

Diagnostic and Statistical Manual of Mental Disorders. Fourth Edition. Text Revision (DSM-IV-TR). Washington, DC: American Psychiatric Association; 2000.

Fransella F, Button E. In: Darby PL, Garner DM, Garfinkel PE, Coscina DV, editors. Anorexia nervosa. Recent developments in research.New York: Alan Liss; 1983. pp. 107–16.

Hall CS, Lindzey G, Campbell J. Theories of personality.Oshawa: Crystal Dreams; 2004.

Kaplan AS. Can J Psychiatry. 2002;47:235–42.

Kelly GA. The psychology of personal constructs.New York: Norton; 1955.

Lemma-Wright AL. Starving to live. The paradox of anorexia nervosa. London: Central Book; 1994.

Personal Construct Theory [Online]. Available at: http://changingminds.org/explanations/theories/personal_construct.htm [Accessed 1 June 2009]

Personal Construct Theory [Onlin]. Available at: http://en.wikipedia.org/wiki/Personal_construct_psychology [Accessed 1 June 2009]

Schmidt U, Treasure J. Br J Clin Psychol. 2006;45:343–66.

Serpell L, Treasure J, Teasdale J, Sullivan V. Int J Eat Disord. 1999;25:177–86.

Stein K, Corte C. Eur Eat Disord Rev. 2007;15:58–69.

Tan J, Hope T, Steward A. Int J Law Psychiatry. 2003a;26:533–48.

Tan J, Hope T, Steward A, Fitzpatrick R. Int J Law Psychiatry. 2003b;26:627–45.
Vandereycken W. Eur Eat Disord Rev. 2006;14:341–51.
Vitousek KB, Hollon SD. Cogn Ther Res. 1990;14:191–214.
Vitousek KB, Daly J, Heiser C. Int J Eat Disord. 1991;10:647–66.
Wojciechowska I. In: Sucha ska A, editor. Podmiotowe i społeczno-kulturowe uwarunkowania anoreksji [The subjective and socio-cultural determinants of anorexia]. Wydawnictwo Fundacji Humaniora, Poznań; 2000. pp. 77–124.
Kelly GA. The psychology of personal constructs. New York: Norton; 1955.

Chapter 158
Comorbidity in Anorexic Adolescents: Assessment Through ASEBA System and Semistructured Interviews

Filippo Muratori, Valentina Viglione, Chiara Montalto, and Sandra Maestro

Abbreviations

AN	Anorexia Nervosa
ASEBA	Achenbach System of Empirically Based Assessment
BAI	Beck Anxiety Inventory
BDI	Beck Depression Inventory
BMI	Body Mass Index
CBCL	Child Behavior CheckList
CDI	Children's Depression Inventory
CDRS-R	Children's Depression Rating Scale Revised
DICA	Diagnostic Interview for Children and Adolescents
DSM	Diagnostic and Statistical Manual of Mental Disorders
EAT-26	Eating Attitude Test
ED	Eating Disorders
EDI-3	Eating Disorder Inventory
EXT	Externalizing
HDRS	Hamilton Depression Rating Scale
INT	Internalizing
K-SADS	Schedule for Affective Disorders and Schizophrenia for School Aged Children
MASC	Multidimensional Anxiety Scale for Children
OCD	Obsessive Compulsive Disorder
OCPD	Obsessive-Compulsive Personality Disorder
PARS	Pediatric Anxiety Rating Scale
PD	Personality Disorders
SCID-I	Structured Clinical Interview for Axis I
SCID-II	Structured Clinical Interview for Axis II
SIAB-EX	Structured Interview for Anorexic and Bulimic Disorders-Expert Form
STAI	State-Trait Anxiety Inventory
TP	Total Problem
Y-BOCS	Yale-Brown Obsessive Compulsive Scale
YSR	Youth Self-Report

F. Muratori (✉)
Division of Child Neuropsichiatry, Stella Maris Scientific Institute, University
of Pisa, IRCCS Stella Maris, Via dei Giacinti, 2-56018 Calambrone, Pisa, Italy
e-mail: filippo.muratori@inpe.unipi.it

V.R. Preedy et al. (eds.), *Handbook of Behavior, Food and Nutrition*,
DOI 10.1007/978-0-387-92271-3_158, © Springer Science+Business Media, LLC 2011

158.1 Introduction

It is well established that individuals with eating disorders (ED) have a high rate of Axis I psychiatric comorbidity, particularly depressive and anxiety disorders broadly termed as internalizing conditions. The association between Axis II personality disorders (PD) and ED is also frequent with a prevalence of cluster C and B. Accompanying Axis I and Axis II diagnoses play an important role in the outcome of ED and in the planning of therapeutic interventions.

Although psychiatric disorders are common in ED, current literature shows an overlapping of data. In fact, many studies do not consistently consider the distinction between different types of ED; considering ED as a whole, additional axis I disorders were found in 86% by Lewinsohn et al. (2000) and Cotrufo et al. (1998), in 73% by Salbach-Andrae et al. (2008), in 74% by Milos et al. (2004), in 58% by Zaider et al. (2000), in 43% by Kennedy et al. (1994), in 66% by Geist et al. (1998). All these studies found a higher comorbidity in the binge-purging subtype than in the restricting subtype. As regards Axis II disorders, incidence varies from 90% in the study by Piran et al. (1988), to 84% by Grilo et al. (1996), and to 68% in the sample studied by Milos et al. (2004), where a prevalence of cluster C was found.

Secondly, many of these studies have examined comorbidity without considering limited ranges of age. Encompassing adolescent, young adult, and adult patients creates a loophole in the research on the specific psychiatric comorbidity of ED during adolescence when the disorder does not last for many years.

158.2 Depressive Comorbidity in Adolescent Eating Disorders

A wide range of depressive symptoms such as depressed mood, low self-esteem, and social withdrawal are very frequent in anorexic adolescents. Literature data report up to 80% of anorexic samples with a depressive disorder, especially during the acute phase of illness: depressive symptoms were found in 86% by Rastam (1992), in 62% by Smith and Steiner (1992), in 60% by Salbach-Andrae et al. (2008), in 56% by Fosson et al. (1987), and in 46% by North and Gowers (1999) and Saccomani et al. (1998). Lilenfeld et al. (1998) found high multiple lifetime comorbidity with significant differences with a control group. Herzog et al. (1992b) investigated current and lifetime comorbidity and found current comorbidity on axis I in 73% of the restricting subtype. In the study by Heebink et al. (1995), a lower level of depression and anxiety was found in younger restricting patients than in older patients.

Data on the incidence of suicide and suicidal attempts in adolescent samples are lacking (Herpertz-Dahlmann 2008); however, this varies from 10% to 20% in anorexic patients, especially combined with major depression (Bulik et al. 2008; Franko et al. 2006). In particular, in the sample studied by Bulik, around 17% of AN patients (mean age: 30 years) attempted suicide, this being significantly more evident in the purging or binging subtype.

To explain this high comorbidity between AN and depressive symptoms, some authors consider AN as a particular form of mood disorder (Alessi et al. 1989; Cooper et al. 2002; Levy and Dixon 1985). Similarly, Mouren-Simeoni MC et al. (1993), in describing a prepubertal anorexic sample, reported an association with depressive symptoms in 85% of subjects and considered prepubertal AN as a depressive equivalent. In a more recent study, Chen et al. (2009) found that dietary restraint and depressive symptoms combined at age 10 and became a risk factor for binge-eating at ages 12–14. Moreover, "dietary-depressive" subtypes (with a greater negative effect) compared to "dietary" subtypes (with dietary restraint only) had considerably greater eating disorder behaviors. Presnell et al. (2009) revealed that depressive and bulimic symptoms contributed reciprocally to each other. In particular, they examined the reciprocal relations between the two disorders over an 8-year period, and concluded that depressive symptoms predicted increase in bulimic symptoms while bulimic symptoms predicted increase in depressive symptoms.

Other authors consider depressive symptoms as a result of a prolonged state of starvation with neuroendocrine and serotoninergic alterations (Couturier 2004).

158.3   Anxiety Comorbidity in Adolescent Eating Disorders

Anxiety disorders such as social phobia, obsessive-compulsive disorder (OCD), panic disorder, general anxiety disorder are common both in adult and juvenile anorexic samples with percentages ranging from 7% to 65% (Herzog et al. 1992b; Kaye et al. 2004). In the adolescent sample studied by Salbach-Andrae et al. (2008), anxiety disorders without OCD followed by OCD occurred in 26% and 17% respectively. Moreover, the category containing anxiety disorders without OCD was three times likely to co-occur with the AN binge eating and purging type than with the AN restrictive type. In the study by Godart et al. (2000), the most frequent lifetime anxiety disorder in its adolescent sample was social phobia (55%) followed by simple phobia (45%). In anorexic patients, food-related obsessive-compulsive symptoms arise, especially during the acute phase, such as cutting food into a certain number of pieces, counting calories, preparing meals, and setting the table in the same way. However, real OCD comorbidity with additional thought and behavior is often signaled in anorexic samples with a range from 17% to 40% (Kaye et al. 2004; Salbach-Andrae et al. 2008) and with frequent childhood onset preceding the onset of AN. Furthermore, anorexic patients show rigidity and perfectionism which are considered risk factors for obsessive disorders.

Finally, the majority of studies report the onset of anxiety disorders before the onset of an ED, supporting the possibility that anxious symptoms are a vulnerability factor for developing AN. This temporal correlation between anxiety disorders and AN has significant implications for course and treatment. In particular, since social preoccupations are very frequent in anorexic patients, many authors propose social competence training during treatment (Herpertz-Dahlmann 2008).

158.4   Personality Disorders in Adolescent Eating Disorders

The frequent association between personality traits and disorders (both in acute phase and during recovery) and ED is well described in literature. Above all, perfectionism, rigidity, and obsessiveness (cluster C) seem to be prevalent personality traits in restrictive AN patients. In the study by Thornton (Thornton and Russell 1997), 34% of an AN sample met criteria for obsessive-compulsive personality disorder (OCPD; Cluster C); Wonderlich et al. (1990) also found 60% prevalence of OCPD in 46 women with restricting subtype. Impulsivity, emotional liability, and self-aggressiveness (cluster B, Borderline Personality Disorder) are more evident in the binge eating/purging subtype of AN.

The incidence seems to decrease with the state of ED severity; for example in the study conducted by Herzog et al. (1992a), the incidence of PD in a sample of 210 nonsevere outpatients with ED was only 27%. Recent research (Thompson-Brenner et al. 2008) on ED during adolescence confirmed the results of several studies carried out on ED in adults (Claes et al. 2006; Holliday et al. 2006). Three personality subtypes were found: a high-functioning, an undercontrolled, and an avoidant/depressed group. In particular, the high-functioning/perfectionist group showed negative associations with comorbidity and positive associations with treatment response. The Emotionally Dysregulated group was associated with externalizing Axis I and Cluster B Axis II disorders, poor school functioning, and adverse events in childhood. The Avoidant/Depressed group showed specific associations with internalizing Axis I disorders and Cluster A Axis II disorders, and poor peer relationships.

158.5 Assessment of Comorbidity in Adolescent Eating Disorders

The accurate assessment of internalizing and externalizing symptoms is a key aspect in adolescent eating disorders, where there is a tendency to deny not only anorexic behavior, but also anxiety and depression, which is very common in AN psychopathology (Viglione et al. 2006).

It is exactly for this reason that assessment with anorexic adolescent patients should be performed by a child psychiatrist having extensive experience with adolescents and sufficiently trained in psychological assessment, use of standardized measures, developmental psychology, and adolescent eating disorders. The assessment should be conducted in an office or other site where confidentiality can be ensured and where the adolescent can feel comfortable and safe. The validity of the information provided by the youth may depend on the setting and on the level of trust between the adolescent and the assessor. During the first interviews, both with the adolescent and with the parents, information should be collected on the history of eating disorders and mental health, with a focus on depression, suicidal ideation or attempts, anxiety disorders, and behavioral disorders (aggressiveness toward self and others, impulsivity, etc.); family history and school history, including academic, behavioral performance, and peer relationships.

The use of instruments is evidently required to perform standardized assessment, that is to say, to systematically, and as coherently as possible, explore the psychopathology so as to receive answers from the patients and their parents and to compare them. Psychiatric assessment instruments enable exploration of the psychopathological entity and provide a quantitative assessment in terms of severity or frequency.

The presence of comorbidity in ED is usually assessed with structured or semistructured clinical interviews, self-report questionnaires, and checklists. Nevertheless, in a recent critical review (Godart et al. 2007) it is observed that diagnostic instruments were not used in earlier studies and that, in later studies, those used varied with differences in diagnostic procedures.

The instruments more frequently used in literature to explore comorbidity in ED are: the Structured Clinical Interview for Axis I (SCID-I, Williams et al. 1992) and the Structured Clinical Interview for Axis II (SCID-II, Skodol et al. 1988) for Axis I and II diagnosis; the Hamilton Depression Rating Scale (HDRS, Williams 1988) and the Beck Depression Inventory (BDI Beck et al. 1996) for depression symptomatology; the Yale-Brown Obsessive Compulsive Scale (Y-BOCS Goodman et al. 1989), the Beck Anxiety Inventory (BAI Beck et al. 1988) and the State-Trait Anxiety Inventory (STAI Spielberger et al. 1970) for anxiety symptoms.

Studies dealing with adolescent samples make use of several specific instruments such as the Child Behavior Checklist (CBCL, Achenbach 1991) for the general psychopathology; the Schedule for Affective Disorders and Schizophrenia for School Aged Children (K-SADS, Chambers et al. 1985) or the Diagnostic interview for children and adolescents (DICA Reich 2000) for Axis I diagnosis; the Multidimensional Anxiety Scale for Children (MASC, March et al. 1999) or the Pediatric Anxiety Rating Scale (PARS, The Research Units on Pediatric Psychopharmacology anxiety study group 2002) for anxiety; the Children's Depression Inventory (CDI, Kovacs 1985) or the Children's Depression Rating Scale – Revised (CDRS – R, Overholser et al. 1995) for depression.

Table 158.1   IRCCS-Stella Maris Eating Disorder Assessment Protocol used at admission in the ED Unit

ED diagnosis	Comorbidity	Family assessment
Anamnestic interview	Kiddie-SADS (Axis I)	Family interview
Kiddie-SADS	SCID- II (Axis-II)	SCL-90
EAT-26;ChEAT	CBCL and YSR	PBI
EDI-3		
BS		
SIAB-EX		

The diagnostic instruments that we selected consider the specificity of the disorder in the young age of our patients

Kiddie-SADS Schedule for Affective Disorders and Schizophrenia for School Aged Children, *EAT-26* Eating Attitude Test (*ChEAT* Children version), *EDI-3* Eating Disorder Inventory, *BS* Binge Scale, *SIAB-EX* Structured Interview for Anorexic and Bulimic Disorders-Expert Form, *SCID-II* Structured Clinical Interview for Axis II, *CBCL* Child Behavior CheckList; *YSR* Youth Self Report, *PBI* Parental Bonding Instrument

The assessment protocol used in the Eating Disorder Program at the Stella Maris Scientific Institute was elaborated by considering the type of patients and, above all, the clinical features of the eating disorders, and the patients' young age. It is composed of: the Schedule for Affective Disorders and Schizophrenia for School Aged Children (K-SADS) for ED diagnosis and Axis I comorbidity; the Structured Clinical Interview for DSM-IV Axis II Disorders (SCID-II) for Axis II comorbidity; the Achenbach System of Empirically Based Assessment (ASEBA), in particular, the Child Behavior CheckList (CBCL) and Youth Self Report (YSR, Achenbach 1990) for general psychopathology. Naturally, instruments for assessing eating disorders are also used (EDI-3; EAT-26; SIAB-EX; Table 158.1).

158.5.1 Psychopathological Assessment Using the ASEBA System

To verify if psychopathology in adolescent anorexia is as frequent as in older samples, we assessed a sample of 43 anorexic adolescents referred to the Eating Disorder Program at the Stella Maris Scientific Institute with a mean age at admission of 14.9 (range from 10.7 to 17.8 years) and with a mean duration of illness prior to admission of 13 months (Muratori et al. 2004).

ED diagnosis and psychiatric assessment were carried out by an independent trained child psychiatrist who interviewed the child and the parents separately, using the Schedule for Affective Disorders and Schizophrenia for School Aged Children (K-SADS). The K-SADS belongs to the category of clinical diagnostic interviews which – although long – are very useful instruments (Table 158.2).

They may only be used by trained child psychiatrists and explore Axis I diagnosis (some of them also Axis II), allowing the psychiatrist to formulate diagnosis. They envisage a first nonstructured part (10–20 min) and a second semistructured part (40–60 min) during which the child psychiatrist conducts the interview according to a predefined layout. In particular, the K-SADS is a semistructured psychiatric interview based upon the diagnostic criteria of DSM-IV (Chambers et al. 1985; APA 1994) which is used to asses current and past episodes of psychopathology in children and adolescents. The K-SADS is administered by interviewing the parent(s), the child, and finally achieving summary ratings which include all sources of information (parent, child, school, etc.). At the start of the interview (first part), it is important to establish an empathic relationship, to explain the purpose of the interview, and inform the patient on the obligation of professional secrecy. Generally, if the patient is a preadolescent we interview the parents first and then the patient; instead, if the patient is an adolescent, it is important to start with the patient. In the case of discrepancies between

Table 158.2 Criteria for diagnosing adolescents anorexic syndrome (DSMIV)

Anorexia nervosa (full syndrome)

1. Refusal to maintain body weight above minimal normal weight for age and height (body weight less than 85% of the expected) or failure to achieve expected weight gain during period of growth
2. Intense fear of gaining weight or becoming fat, even though underweight
3. Disturbance in the way in which one's body weight or shape is experienced or denial of the seriousness of the current low body weight
4. In postmenarcheal femeles, amenorrhea of at least three consecutive menstrual cycles

Specify if Restricting subtype or Binge Eating/purging subtype

Eating disorders not otherwise specified (partial syndrome)

Eating disorders that do not meet the criteria for a AN full syndrome, for example:

1. AN criteria are met but the individual has regular menses
2. AN criteria are met except that, despite significant weight loss, the individual's current weight is in the normal range
3. Regular use of inappropriate compensatory behavior by an individual of normal body weight after eating small amounts of food

EDNOS diagnosis (partial syndromes) is very frequent in adolescent samples; furthermore, in these syndromes psychopathological and physical conditions are very serious and require a multidimensional treatment

AN anorexia nervosa

Table 158.3 Key features of Achenbach System of Emirically Based Assessment (ASEBA)

1. ASEBA gives a dimensional description of psychiatric symptomatology by elaborating an individualized profile in the various areas taken into consideration.
2. ASEBA allows psychopathological assessment by using several information sources. In fact, it may be filled in by the parents (CBCL), the youth (YSR) or the teachers (TRF: Teaching Report Form)
3. The checklist forms that are more extensively used to obtain standardized reports of child and adolescent behavior are Child Behaviour CheckList (CBCL) and Youth Self Report (YSR).
4. They contain 118 item behavioral scales which allow evaluation of a total problem score (TP), eight syndromes (withdrawn, anxious/depressed, somatic complaints, social problems, thought problems, attention problems, delinquent behavior, aggressive behavior) and two broadband groups of syndromes designated as internalizing (INT) and externalizing (EXT).
5. The last version also includes DSM-oriented scales.
6. In clinical activities, ASEBA is useful for diagnosis and for the treatment follow-up. A cut-off distinguishing clinical from non-clinical cases is defined.

In the ASEBA checklists filled in by anorexic patients and by their parents the anxious-depressed symptomatology is very evident and may cause great disturbances

parents' and child's reports, the most frequent disagreements occur in the items dealing with subjective phenomena where the parent does not know, but the child is very definite about the presence or absence of certain symptoms. This is particularly true for internalizing items such as hopelessness and suicidal ideation. Reliability, validity, administrative characteristics, and use of the K-SADS were recently reviewed (Ambrosini 2000).

Psychopathology was also studied using the Achenbach System of Empirically Based Assessment (ASEBA), in particular the Child Behavior CheckList (CBCL) and Youth Self Report (YSR). ASEBA gathers assessment data through several sources of information (it may be filled in by the parents, youth, or teachers); it provides a dimensional description of symptomatology and elaborates an individualized profile in the various areas taken into consideration. The aim is to reach a diagnostic formulation which is not focused on one or on a few symptoms, but which bears in mind the countless features of the child's/adolescent's life and of his/her complexity (Table 158.3).

The CBCL and YSR are two of the most frequently used empirically-based assessment instruments for obtaining standardized reports of children and adolescent behavior as observed by the parents (CBCL) or self-evaluated (YSR). They contain 118 item behavioral scales which allow the evaluation of a total problem score (TP), eight syndromes (Withdrawn, Anxious/Depressed, Somatic Complaints, Social Problems, Thought Problems, Attention Problems, Delinquent Behavior, Aggressive Behavior) and two broad-band groups of syndromes designated as Internalizing (INT) and Externalizing (EXT). Internalizing score encompasses emotional disorders characterized by inhibition and overcontrol, while Externalizing score indicates the presence of attention, oppositional, antisocial, and aggressive problems. A cut-off to distinguish clinical from nonclinical cases is defined. Good reliability and validity have been reported in literature for both scales (Krol 1990). Only two symptoms of anorexia nervosa are comprised in the CBCL and YSR (no. 24: "Doesn't eat well" and no. 53: "Overeating") but they are not included in any patterns of internalizing or externalizing scales, which is of importance for our study.

Briefly, the results of our study, thanks to the use of the ASEBA, revealed that the pathological mean score on the internalizing CBCL summary scale (parents' evaluation), with 67.4% of subjects within pathological range, is highly consistent with the findings of a prevalence of affective and anxiety disorders in ED, and the percentage of subjects with psychopathological problems associated with ED are parallel to those reported in literature (Braun et al. 1994; Fosson et al. 1987; Halmi et al. 1991; Herzog et al. 1992b; Lilenfeld et al. 1998; Smith et al. 1993; Smith and Steiner 1992). Above all, on the basis of these internalizing and externalizing profiles and on the number of subjects in the clinical range, three types of adolescent anorexia emerged from our study (Fig. 158.1): (1) "normal" anorexia (32.5% of cases) with a nonclinical CBCL profile; (2) pure internalizing anorexia (51.2% of cases) with TP and INT pathological values; and (3) mixed anorexia (16.3%) with TP, INT, and EXT pathological values. Even if both restricting and binge eating/purging subgroups are allocated in each group, the majority of both of them are represented in the pure internalizing group. The small mixed group, featuring a more severe psychopathology, highlights a type of adolescent anorexia characterized by opposition and difficulties in concentration where Internalizing symptoms are also more severe. This latter type is totally different from the pure internalizing type characterized by a lower rate of psychopathological problems and which we could call unipolar. On the basis of these psychopathological findings we could hypothesize a less severe type of ED in binge eating/purging anorexia and a more severe type in restricting anorexia; the identification of these different anorexic disorders could be of particular interest for subtyping eating disorders, for therapeutic decisions and for defining prognostic trajectory.

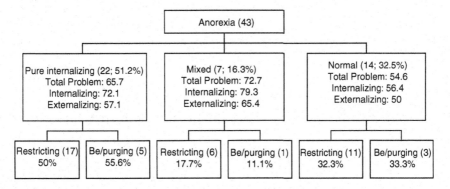

Fig. 158.1 Clinical and psychopathological characteristics at CBCL for the three types of adolescents with anorexia nervosa. The three types of anorexic groups differ on the basis of CBCL score. In fact, in the pure internalizing group, the pathological score is reached on total and internalizing global scales; in the mixed the pathological score is reached on INT and EXT scales, while in the normal group the pathological score is not reached

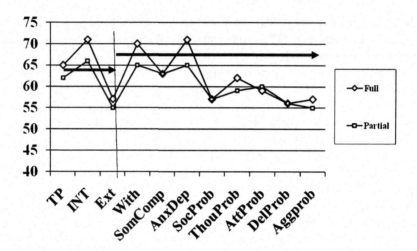

Fig. 158.2 Comparison of pscychopathological asset between full (all criteria of DSM-IV) and partial anorexic adolescent subgroups using CBCL. *Black lines* represent the clinical cutoff for global and syndrome scales. The scores of global and syndrome scales are expressed as mean values. *TP* total problems, *Int* internalizing, *Ext* externalizing, *With* withdrawn, *SomComp* somatic complaints, *AnxDep* anxious/depressed, *SocProb* social problems, *ThougProb* thought problems, *AttProb* attention problems, *Delprob* delinquent problems, *Aggprob* aggressive behavior

By comparing Full versus Partial at CBCL and YSR it is possible to assume a psychopathological continuum between full and partial syndromes, although in full syndromes anxious-depressed and concentration problems combine to represent a more disturbed anorexic adolescent (Fig. 158.2).

When comparing the Restrictive versus the Binge-eating subgroup, higher internalizing psychopathology was found in binge eating/purging subtype only at YSR (no differences at the CBCL), especially for the anxious/depressed subscale. These data seem to describe the binge eating/purging group as a group where self-reported psychopathology is specifically higher compared to that reported by parents. This is probably due to a greater difficulty by the parents in recognizing these disorders in their offspring or due to a particular way of underlining self-symptomatology by the adolescent girls.

To conclude, the use of ASEBA revealed that the amount of psychopathology in anorexia increases over time (higher mean values were found at CBCL and YSR for almost all summary and syndrome scales in the group arrived 12 months after disease onset) and suggests that it could represent a secondary complication of the illness. This finding seems a powerful argument for early intervention in adolescent ED; in fact an ongoing devious pathway can produce negative effects on many domains of functioning.

158.5.2 Psychopathological Assessment Through Semistructured Interviews

Subsequently, we investigated the incidence of personality disorders in a sample of 100 anorexic girls (mean age at admission: 14.4 years). The Kiddie-SADS was used to assess axis I comorbidity, and the SCID-II was used to asses personality disorders (PD). The Structured Clinical Interview for DSM-IV Axis II Disorders (SCID-II) is a semistructured interview for assessing DSM-IV Axis II PD through integration of the personality diagnosis in appendix B of the manual. It consists of a self-report Questionnaire and a semistructured Interview. The Questionnaire comprises 119 items for

Fig. 158.3 Axis I comorbidity in an adolescent anorexic sample using Kiddie-SADS. The anorexic adolescent sample shows a high internalizing symptomatology (depressive and anxiety disorders together: 80%). *MaD* major depression, *MiD* minor depression, *GAD* generalized anxiety disorder, SAD separation anxiety disorder

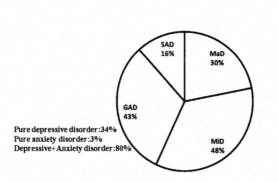

Sample
100 AN ♀
Mean Age: 14.4 ys
Mean BMI:15.6

Pure depressive disorder:34%
Pure anxiety disorder:3%
Depressive+Anxiety disorder:80%

screening the ten DSM-IV PDs, in addition to the Passive-Aggressive and Depressive PDs in Appendix B of the DSM-IV. Since the Questionnaire was created for adults, we adjusted it for use with adolescents: we changed certain items, making them more suitable for the age range (for example, the term "school" was used instead of "job") but without altering their original meaning. The "yes" response to the items of the Questionnaire is reassessed in the Interview through specific questions. The answers to these questions are rated on a four-level scale. PD diagnosis is made when the number of items assessed as present (that is, presenting pathological, persistent, and diffused features) is above the cut-off determined for making diagnosis.

We confirm high axis I comorbidity also in adolescent girls with anorexia, with a prevalence of depressive and anxiety disorders. In particular, acute depressive symptoms are very frequent (Major depression: 30%; Minor Depression: 48%), as also Generalized Anxiety Disorder (43%) and Separation Anxiety Disorder (16%). Furthermore, our study highlights how 34% of the sample had a pure depressive disorder. This percentage rises to 80% if the association between depressive and anxiety disorders (46%) is considered, while only 3% of the sample had at least 1 pure anxiety disorder (Fig. 158.3).

The Kiddie-SADS is a semistructured psychiatric interview in which the items score used for the categorical diagnosis is obtained by posing the same questions separately to both parents and to the children/adolescents. In our case, therefore, the high percentage of internalizing symptoms (and in particular depressive symptoms) is the expression of both parents' and children's combined opinions. The Kiddie-SADS results are in accordance with the previous study based on CBCL and YSR data, and they seem to support the hypothesis that in anorexic girls, depressive disorder and AN are strictly connected, mutually influencing each other. Nevertheless, the high depressive values in our sample may also be considered as an expression of serious clinical and physical conditions since the mean BMI value of the sample was only 15.6.

The association with axis II comorbidity PD is also high, with values similar to those of recent studies (Milos et al. 2004). In fact, 59% of the sample had at least one PD with a prevalence of OCDP (25%) and Borderline PD (22%). It is very interesting to notice that our binge-eating subgroup also presented higher psychopathology values both in axis I and II. In particular, 88% of this subgroup had at least one PD against 53% of the restrictive subgroup, with a significantly higher value for various PDs, especially for Borderline PD (65% vs. 13%), Avoidant PD (35% vs. 11%) and Depressive PD (47% vs. 13%). We also observed that OCPD reached similar values both in the restricting and in the Binge-Eating subgroup, while there are clear differences between the full and the partial subgroup, with higher values in the first case (28% vs. 18%). Accordingly, we may assume that certain personality traits may highly favor the early onset of AN. Specifically, traits such as perfectionism, rigidity, and overcontrol may favor, together with other factors, the complete onset of the anorexic disorder, while traits such as impulsivity and emotional liability may contribute to be a defining AN quality.

158.6 Clinical Implications

It is possible to confirm the importance of psychopathological evaluation in adolescent eating disorders. The prevalence of internalizing conditions, the worst psychopathology in full syndromes and in the binge-eating/purging subtypes deserves attention when establishing treatments. Finally, the increasing psychopathology later on after the onset of the disease is of particular importance for the development of specialized services for adolescents with anorexia nervosa where early interventions, designed to change both medical and psychological issues, could prevent secondary psychopathology.

158.7 Applications to Other Areas of Health and Disease

Psychiatric assessment of adolescent pathologies is an extremely important step in clinical practice. It provides an accurate and prompt diagnosis in an age when comorbidity is extremely frequent. For this reason, a large amount of standardized interviews and self-administered scales have been identified for adolescents, in order to acquire a complete and objective description of clinical picture. Incidentally, the use of such tools is equally diffused in nonpsychiatric populations for the purpose of identifying risk factors. This aspect is particularly evident as far as Eating Disorders are regarded. Some of the tests mentioned, such as the EAT-26 or the CBCL and YSR, are often used for the screening phase in the general population.

Summary Points

• Adolescent anorexia nervosa presents high psychiatric comorbidity, as in adults.
• Depressive disorders (above all, major depression), especially during the acute phase of illness, are the most common axis I comorbidity in adolescent anorexia nervosa.
• Social difficulties as well as generalized and separation anxiety disorders are also frequent in AN.
• Obsessive–compulsive symptoms, not only food related, are often signaled in anorexic samples, with frequent onset during childhood preceding the onset of AN.
• Axis II comorbidity is frequent in adolescent anorexic samples, with a prevalence of Cluster B (especially in the binge-eating subtype) and Cluster C (especially in the restrictive subtype).

Definitions and Explanations of Key Terms

Adolescent Eating Disorders: Anorexia nervosa (AN), bulimia nervosa (BN) and EDNOS (eating disorder not otherwise specified) are all characterized by an excessive concern with weight and shape, accompanied by inadequate and irregular food intake. Many adolescents do not fulfill criteria for AN and BN but for subthreshold eating disorders (EDNOS), which are often as severe as the classical syndromes

Comorbidity: Presence of more than one diagnosis occurring in an individual at the same time. In the ED is a frequent condition that plays an important role as for diagnosis as for outcome and for planning of specific treatments.

Assessment: Evaluation of the patient for the purposes of forming a diagnosis and a treatment plan. It is very important, in clinical work with eating disorder (ED), to have a comprehensive assessment of DSM-IV comorbid disorders.

Internalizing condition: Depressive and anxiety disorders; this is the most frequent comorbidity in adolescent ED.

Personality disorders: An enduring pattern of inner experience and behavior that deviates markedly from the expectations of the culture of the individual who exhibits it. This pattern is manifested in two (or more) of the following areas: cognition, affect, interpersonal functioning, and impulse control. This diagnosis is a very frequent comorbidity in adolescent ED.

Key Points on Comorbidity in Adolescent Anorexic Disorders

High comorbidity of adolescent anorexia nervosa contributes to define specific and well-defined clinical disorders and to make therapeutic decisions more effective.

The Restrictive AN subtype is associated to higher levels of internalizing symptomatology, perfectionism, rigidity and obsessiveness (they frequently describe a Cluster C personality disorder). Impulsivity, emotional liability and self-aggressiveness (which frequently describe a Borderline Personality Disorder) are more evident in the binge eating/purging subtype of AN.

A psychopathological continuum may be assumed between full and partial syndromes.

The anxious-depressed symptomatology may cause greater disturbances in adolescents with anorexia.

The prevalence of internalizing conditions and the worst psychopathology in full syndromes and in the binge-eating/purging subtypes, deserves attention when establishing treatments. The identification of girls with anorexic partial syndrome is an opportunity to intervene at an early stage of the disorder and to improve outcome.

References

Achenbach TM. Manual for the Child behaviour Checklist/4–18 and 1991 profile. Burlington, University of Vermont department of Psychiatry; 1991a.

Achenbach TM. Manual for the Youth self-Report and 1991 profile. Burlington, University of Vermont Department of Psychiatry; 1991b.

Alessi NE, Krahn D, Brehm D, Wittekindt J. J Am Acad Child Adolesc Psychiat. 1989;28:380–4.

Ambrosini PJ. J Am Acad Child Adolesc Psychiat. 2000;39:49–56.

American Psychiatric Association. Diagnostic and statistical manual of mental disorders, 4th ed.Washington, DC: APA; 1994.

Beck AT, Epstein N, Brown G, Steer RA. J Consult Clin Psychol. 1988;56:893–7.

Beck AT, Steer RA, Ball R, Ranieri W. J Pers Assess. 1996;67:588–97.

Braun DL, Sunday SR, Halmi KA. Psychol Med. 1994;24:859–67.

Bulik C, Thornton L, Pinheiro A, Plotnicov K, Klump K, Brandt H, Crawford S, Fichter M. et al. Psychosom Med. 2008;70:378–83.

Chambers WJ, Puig-Antich J, Hirsch M, Paez P, Ambrosini PJ, Tabrizi MA. Arch Gen Psychiat. 1985;42:696–702.

Chen EY, McCloskey MS, Keenan KE. Int J Eating Disord. 2009;42:275–83.

Claes L, Vandereychen W, Luyten P, Soenens B, Pieters G, Vertommen H. J Pers Disord. 2006;20:401–16.

Cooper PJ, Watkins B, Bryant-Waugh R, Lask B. Psychol Med. 2002;32:873–80.

Cotrufo P, Barretta V, Monteleone P. Acta Psychiat Scand. 1998;98:112–5.

Couturier J. Canadian J CME. 2004; February: 81–4.

Fosson A, Knibbs J, Bryant-Waugh R, Lask B. Arch Dis Childhood. 1987;62:114–8.

Franko DL, Keel PK. Clin Psychol Rev. 2006;26:769–82.

Geist R, Davis R, Heinmaa M. Can J Psychiat. 1998;43:507–12.

Godart NT, Flament MF, Lecrubier Y, Jeammet P. Eur Psychiat. 2000;15:38–45.

Godart NT, Perdereau F, Rein Z, Berthoz S, Wallier J, Jeammet Ph, Flament MF. J Affect Disord. 2007;97:37–49.

Goodman WK, Price LH, Rasmussen SA, Mazure C, Fleischman RL, Hill KL, Heninger GR, Charney DS. Arch Gen Psychiat. 1989;46:1006–11.

Grilo CM, Levy KN, Becker DF, Edell WS, McGlashan TH. Psychiat Serv. 1996;47:426–9.

Halmi KA, Eckert E, Marchi P, Sampugnano V, Apple R, Cohen J. Arch Gen Psychiat. 1991;48:712–8.

Heebink DM, Sunday S, Halmi KA. J Am Acad Child Adolesc Psychiat. 1995;34:378–82.

Herpertz-Dahlmann B. Child Adolesc Psychiatric Clin N Am. 2008;18:31–47.

Herzog DB, Keller MB, Lavori PW, Kenny GM, Sacks NR. J Clin Psychiat. 1992a;53:147–52.

Herzog DB, Keller MB, Sacks NR, Yeh CJ, Lavori PW. J Am Acad Child Adolesc Psychiat. 1992b; 31:810–8.

Holliday J, Uher R, Landau S, Collier D, Treasure J. J Pers Disord. 2006;20:417–26.

Kaye WH, Bulik CM, Thornton L, Barbarich N, Masters K. Am J Psychiat. 2004;161:2215–21.

Kennedy SH, Kaplan AS, Garfinkel PE, Rockett W, Toner B, Abbey SE. J Psychosomatic Res. 1994;38:773–82.

Kovacs M. Psychopharmacol Bull. 1985;21:995–8.

Krol NP. J Am Acad Child Adolesc Psychiat. 1990;29:986–7.

Levy AB, Dixon KN. Int J Eating Disord. 1985;4:389–405.

Lewinsohn P, Striegel-Moore R, Seeley J. J Am Acad Child Adolesc Psychiat. 2000;39:1284–92.

Lilenfeld LR, Kaye WH, Greeno CG, Merikangas KR, Plotnicov K, Pollice C. Arch Gen Psychiat. 1998;55:603–10.

March JS, Sullivan K, Parker J. J Anxiety Disord. 1999;13:349–58.

Milos G, Spindler A, Schnyder U. Can J Psychiat. 2004;49:179–84.

Mouren-Simeoni MC, Fontanon M, Bouvard MP, Dugas M. Revue Can. de Psychaitrie. 1993; 38:51–5.

Muratori F, Viglione V, Maestro S, Picchi L. Psychopathology. 2004;37:92–7.

North C, Gowers S. Int J Eating Disord. 1999;26:386–91.

Overholser JC, Brinkman DC, Lehnert KL, Ricciardi AM. J Clin Child Adolesc Psychol. 1995;24:443–52.

Piran N, Lerner P, Garfinkel PE, Kennedy SH, Brouillette C. Int J Eat Disord. 1988;7:589–99.

Presnell K, Stice E, Seidel A, Madeley MC. Clin Psychol Psychother. 2009;16:357–65.

Rastam M. J Am Acad Child Adolesc Psychiat. 1992;31:819–29.

Reich W. J Am Acad Child Adolesc Psychiat. 2000;39:59–66.

Saccomani L, Savoini M, Cirrincione M, Verzellino F, Ravera G. J Psychosomatic Res. 1998; 44:565–71.

Salbach-Andrae H, Lenz K, Simmendinger N, Klinkowski N, Lehmkuhl U, Pfeiffer E. Child Psychiat Hum Dev. 2008;39:261–72.

Skodol AE, Rosnick L, Kellman D, Oldham JM, Hyler SE. Am J Psychiat. 1988;145:1297–9.

Smith C, Steiner H. J Am Acad Child Adolesc Psychiat. 1992;31:841–3.

Smith C, Feldman S, Nasserbakht A, Steiner H. J Am Acad Child Adolesc Psychiat. 1993;32:1237–45.

Spielberger CD, Gorsuch, RL, Lushene RE. Manual for the state-trait anxiety inventory. Palo Alto, CA: Consulting Psychologists Press; 1970.

Thompson-Brenner H, Eddy KT, Satir DA, Boisseau C, Westen D. J Child Psychol Psychiat. 2008;49:170–80.

Thornton C, Russell J. Int J Eat Disord. 1997;21:83–7.

The Research Units on Pediatric Psychopharmacology anxiety study group. J Am Acad Child Adolesc Psychiat. 2002;41:1061–9.

Viglione V, Muratori F, Maestro S, Brunori E, Picchi L. Psychopathology. 2006;39:255–60.

Williams JB. Arch Gen Psychiat. 1988;45:742–7.

Williams JBW, Gibbon M, First MB, Spitzer RL, Davis M, Borus J, Howes MJ, Kane J, Pope HG, Rounsaville B, Wittchen H. Arch Gen Psychiat. 1992;49:630–6.

Wonderlich SA, Swift WJ, Slomik HB, Goodman S. Int J Eat Disord. 1990;9:607–16.

Zaider TI, Johnson JG, Cockell S. Int J Eating Dis. 2000;28:58–67.

Chapter 159
ACTH, Cortisol, Beta Endorphin, Catecholamines, and Serotonin in Anorexia Nervosa: Implications for Behavior

Marie-Claude Brindisi and Daniel Rigaud

Abbreviations

AN	Anorexia nervosa
ACTH	Adrenocorticotropic hormone
CBG	Cortisol binding globulin
5-HIAA	5-hydroxyindolacetic acid
5-HT	5-hydroxytryptamine or Serotonin
CNS	Central nervous system
CRH	Corticotropin-releasing hormone
CSF	Cerebrospinal fluid
DHEA-S	Dehydroepiandrosterone-sulfate
ED	Eating disorder
FFA	Free fatty acid
NE	Norepinephrine
PET	Positron emission tomography
POMC	Proopiomelanocortin
SNS	Sympathetic nervous system
SPECT	Single photon emission computed tomography
SSRIs	Selective serotonin reuptake inhibitors

159.1 Introduction

Anorexia nervosa (AN) is a psychiatric disorder with a current prevalence of 1.5% and a mortality rate of 5–10%. AN is characterized by a dramatic decrease in energy and fat intake and by excessive physical exercise, which together result in physiological, biochemical, and behavioral disturbances. Excessive exercise is present in 40–80% of AN patients. In one-third to one-half of cases, AN patients control their body weight by purging, vomiting, or even laxative abuse, or by using diuretics. Two subtypes of AN have been identified: Restricting-type AN patients lose weight by pure dieting;

M.-C. Brindisi (✉)
Endocrinology and Nutrition Department, CHU le Bocage (Dijon University Hospital),
BP 77908, 21079 Dijon Cedex,
e-mail: marie-claude.brindisi@chu-dijon.fr

V.R. Preedy et al. (eds.), *Handbook of Behavior, Food and Nutrition*,
DOI 10.1007/978-0-387-92271-3_159, © Springer Science+Business Media, LLC 2011

bulimic anorexics also restrict food, but engage in inappropriate episodic compensatory behaviors (binge-purge behavior).

Understanding of how genetic and neurobiologically mediated mechanisms contribute to the likelihood of developing eating disorders (ED) is growing. In this review, we will focus on the role of hormones, above all adrenocorticotropic hormone (ACTH) and cortisol, and neurotransmitter pathways.

159.2 Corticotrope Axis

The adrenal glands of AN patients produce more cortisol in response to ACTH than do those of normal women (Gold et al. 1986). Thus, an increase in 24h-urinary free cortisol (Bliss and Migeon 1957), and a 30% increase in plasma cortisol, with a normal nycthemeral cycle, are observed with normal levels of cortisol-binding globulin (CBG). Most studies have reported maintenance of a plasma cortisol rhythm in AN patients (Boyar et al. 1977). The rhythm of both the free salivary cortisol secretion and the plasma cortisol has been investigated by Putignano et al. (2001). The authors pointed out that the circadian rhythm was maintained in blood and saliva levels, although they reported a "flattening" of the 24-h cortisol concentration curve in AN patients as compared to controls (Putignano et al. 2001). Dos Santos et al hypothesized that this flattened daily curve of cortisol may reflect altered circadian rhythm in some, but not all of the patients included in the analysis (dos Santos et al. 2007). Sensitivity of the corticotrope axis to the inhibitory effect of a free fatty acid load (FFA) is preserved, like in healthy adult subjects (Lanfranco et al. 2006).

Most investigators have attributed the elevated level of plasma cortisol to dysfunctions in hypothalamic mechanisms that control ACTH secretion in AN patients, but the mechanisms involved have not been fully clarified. The elevated serum concentration of cortisol results partly from increased secretion, and partly from increased half-life due to malnutrition and hypometabolism; changes such as a decrease in the metabolic rate of cortisol clearance have been reported too, suggesting a dysfunction in peripheral glucocorticoid metabolism (Vierhapper et al. 1990). A nearly constant finding in AN patients is the response to ACTH, which contrasts with the weakened response to stimulation with corticotropin- releasing hormone (CRH). Moreover, CRH hypersecretion has been observed frequently in AN: patients have a high level of CRH in their cerebrospinal fluid (CSF). Studies on cortisol and ACTH responses to the dexamethasone-suppression test or the response to a competitive glucocorticoid antagonist showed abnormal cortisol suppression and high CRH secretion. Finally, CRH activates the same cerebral area as the one associated with stress and causes anorexia, an increase in motor activity, and a decrease in sexual activity. It appears that these high levels of cortisol and ACTH are secondary to weight loss, since they are normalized by weight gain. Nevertheless, they could also have a pathophysiological role, since in AN patients, low weight is associated with anxiety in 40% of the patients, true anorexia in some patients, and sexual dysfunction in most of them, which may decrease after weight gain. The hypersecretion of CRH, ACTH, and cortisol could be part of a vicious circle in AN patients, by counteracting the need to eat and increasing the risk of binge-eating in malnutrition.

The mechanisms of the flattened cortisol rhythm still need to be elucidated. Besides the effects of the central nervous system (CNS) on the hypothalamic–pituitary–adrenal axis, other factors could be involved, such as reduction in CBG levels due to the low estrogen levels and/or by the malnourished status of these patients (dos Santos et al. 2007).

A high level of cortisol is not associated with an increase in other ACTH-dependent adrenal hormones, such as dehydroepiandrosterone sulfate (DHEA-S). Sirinathsinghji and Mills (1985) demonstrated that in AN patients, hypercortisolism is observed together with a loss of DHEA-S rhythm, and a low DHEA-S level. This situation cannot be explained by the mechanisms involved in the increase in cortisol.

This excess of cortisol could be responsible for lanugo and for the decrease in bone formation, and could also be implicated in the feeling of well-being observed in denutrition. Moreover, the size of the increase in fasting serum cortisol levels is dependent on the severity of the fasting hypoglycemia observed in these patients (Casper 1996).

159.3 Beta-endorphin

The opioid system has a direct influence on eating behavior and motor activity. It certainly plays a role in the ability of predators to catch their prey in the wild: endorphin, secreted with cannabinoids, decreases pursuit-related pain and fatigue. One may suppose that in AN patients the oversecretion of beta-endorphin enables them to deny the seriousness of their malnutrition and to endure the pain and distress related to their disease. Despite some discrepancies among studies, an increase in beta-endorphin activity has been observed in AN patients (Ericsson et al. 1996). Whereas moderately high levels of beta-endorphin stimulate feeding, higher levels allow tolerance to starvation (Hubner 1993).

Feeding blindly by a nasogastric tube induced a dose-dependent decrease in beta-endorphin and a dose-dependent increase in levels of ACTH, cortisol, norepinephrine, and dopamine in hospitalized malnourished AN patients. There was no significant change in these variables in healthy women (Rigaud et al. 2007). The decrease in the level of beta-endorphin could partly explain the abdominal discomfort, the anxiety, and the depressive state after a meal. This could also explain why some AN patients feel the need to engage in physical activity after a meal, because exercise stimulates the release of beta-endorphin. With this drop after a meal, there is a loss of the sensory benefit related to the elevated fasting level of beta-endorphin (Russell et al. 2001).

159.4 Catecholamines

159.4.1 1-Dopamine

Several symptoms of AN, such as excessive exercise, reduction in food intake, and amenorrhea have been attributed to dopamine dysfunction (Barry and Klawans 1976). Most studies have found abnormalities in peripheral and central noradrenergic activity in ill AN patients (Pirke 1996). But the results are inconsistent. For example, homovanillic acid, the major metabolite of dopamine in humans, is decreased in the CSF of AN subjects (Kaye et al. 1984). But Jimerson (1993) found normal CSF levels of dopamine in their AN patients.

By contrast, Barbato et al. (2006) showed significant increase in the eye-blink rate in their AN patients. Such an increase suggests excessive central dopaminergic activity, since the eye-blink rate is a peripheral measure of central dopaminergic activity. Moreover, a trait-related disturbance of dopamine metabolism has been shown to contribute to vulnerability to restricting-type AN (Kaye et al. 1999)

In activity-based anorexia in rats, an animal model mimicking AN, treatment with a dopaminergic antagonist inhibits anorexic behavior (Verhagen et al. 2009). This result suggests that hyperactive behavior and reduced food intake observed in anorexic patients may be treated by dopamine receptor antagonists. Antipsychotics may therefore be considered in the treatment of AN patients, when reducing an important hyperactive behavior is likely to accelerate body weight gain.

159.4.2 2-Norepinephrine

Catecholamines, especially norepinephrine (NE), are the main lipolytic hormones in human. In some studies, based on the levels of NE in plasma, urine or CSF, lower basal sympathetic nervous system (SNS) activity was found in AN patients compared with healthy controls (Pirke 1996). This contrasts with basal NE levels in subcutaneous abdominal adipose tissue which were markedly higher in AN patients than in healthy women, suggesting an increase in SNS activity in this area (Nedvidkova et al. 2004).

159.4.3 Serotonin

Serotonin (5-hydroxytryptamine, 5-HT) is a brain neurotransmitter that plays a key role in satiety (Leibowitz 1990). A lot of data are available concerning serotonin and AN. High serotonin activity could be responsible for anxiety, sleep deprivation, excessive physical exercise, true anorexia (loss of appetite), a feeling of high power, and denial of nervous and physical exhaustion (Capasso et al. 2009). In contrast, depressed serotonin activity could be responsible for a depressive mood and binge eating (symptoms frequently observed after months or years of AN). It is well known that estrogens modulate serotonergic function as well as levels of CRH; this could be why AN often begins after puberty, during late adolescence. A recent review suggested that anorexia is linked to a disturbed serotonin system (Kaye et al. 2005). Low cerebral-spinal fluid levels of the serotonergic metabolite 5-hydroxyindolacetic acid (5-HIAA) have been found in AN patients as compared to healthy women. This low level normalizes after weight gain (Kaye et al. 1988). Whether this is caused by reduction in dietary supplies of the 5-HT synthesizing amino-acid tryptophan, or by other effects of malnutrition on hormonal or neurotransmitter systems remains uncertain.

Altered brain serotonin function thus contributes to the dysregulation of appetite, mood, and impulse control in AN. A trait-related disturbance of 5-HT neuronal modulation precedes the onset of AN and contributes to premorbid symptoms of anxiety, obsessionality, and inhibition (Steiger et al. 2004). Such a dysphoric temperament may involve the inherent dysregulation of emotional and reward pathways which also mediate the hedonic aspects of feeding, thus making these individuals vulnerable to disturbed appetitive behaviors. Restricting food intake may become powerfully reinforced because it provides a temporary respite from a dysphoric mood. Puberty-related female gonadal steroids or age-related changes may exacerbate 5-HT dysregulation. Stress and/or cultural and social pressures may contribute by aggravating an anxious and obsessional temperament. AN patients may discover that reduced dietary intake, by reducing plasma tryptophan availability, is a means by which they can modulate brain 5-HT functional activity and anxiety (Kaye 2008).

Platelet monoamine oxidase activity has been proposed as an index of cerebral serotonin activity. Studies in AN patients have shown contradictory results: in 59 malnourished AN patients, platelet monoamine oxidase activity was similar to that observed in normal women. In contrast, in 35 AN patients who had recovered their normal BMI, it was 20% lower than in normal controls (Ehrlich et al. 2008). Diaz-Marsa et al. (2000) found lower than normal platelet monoamine oxidase activity in their malnourished AN patients. Biederman et al. (1984) hypothesized that this low platelet monoamine oxidase activity could be related to a depressive mood, since they found low levels in their 13 depressive AN patients, and normal levels in their 18 nondepressive AN patients, as compared with 28 matched normal control subjects. Carrasco et al. (2000) reported that this low level was found both in bulimia nervosa patients and in patients with the binge/purging form of AN.

The efficacy of antidepressant medications in the treatment of eating disorders has been tested. Cyproheptatide, a drug with 5-HT properties has been tried to accelerate weight gain in AN. The effect of the drug was quite small (Halmi et al. 1986). Whereas antidepressants have been shown to be effective in patients with bulimia nervosa, initial studies with traditional antidepressant agents in AN patients only showed a limited benefit. Several studies have failed to demonstrate any beneficial effect of including selective serotonin reuptake inhibitors (SSRIs) in the treatment of hospitalized AN patients (Ferguson et al. 1999).

Moreover, AN patients who have recovered their normal weight often have persisting psychological symptoms that are accompanied by a significant risk of recurrent low-weight episodes. This has led to interest in studies on relapse prevention. A clinically-based, prospective, longitudinal, follow-up study failed to show any significant benefit of treatment with fluoxetine (SSRI) (Strober et al. 1997). However, recent data from a double-blind, placebo-controlled trial in weight-restored patients demonstrated that treatment with fluoxetine was associated with a reduced relapse rate and reductions in depression, anxiety, obsessions, and compulsions. This study showed that after 1 year, 10 of 16 subjects treated with fluoxetine remained well while only 3 of 19 subjects who received placebo remained well (Kaye et al. 2001).

Today, new technology using brain imaging with radioligands may lead to a better understanding of brain 5-HT neurotransmitter function and its dynamic relationship with human behavior. Up to now, single photon emission computed tomography (SPECT) and positron emission tomography (PET) studies have been used. The 5-HT2A receptor is of interest because it is thought to be involved in the regulation of feeding, mood, and anxiety, and in the action of antidepressants. Other studies of ill, underweight AN patients, which used SPECT with a 5-HT2A receptor antagonist (Audenaert et al. 2003), found a significant reduction in 5-HT2A receptor activity in the left frontal cortex, the left and right parietal cortex, and the left and right occipital cortex. These studies are consistent in that they report reduced 5-HT2A activity in cortical regions in AN, and the findings are independent of the severity of the illness. These studies raise the possibility that anorexic subtypes may share a disturbance of 5-HT2A receptor activity in the subgenual cingulate, whereas regional differences in 5-HT2A receptor activity may distinguish between ED subgroups after recovery. The subgenual cingulate is thought to play a role in emotional and autonomic responses (Freedman et al. 2000), and a disturbance in this region has been implicated in mood disorders. Mood disturbances are common in individuals with EDs, although there is some controversy as to whether EDs and mood disorders are transmitted from generation to generation independently or together (Lilenfeld et al. 1998). These data raise the possibility that some factor related to subgenual cingulated function, perhaps related to mood and autonomic modulation, creates a predisposition for anorexia.

A chapter of this book is devoted to HT1A receptor images.

159.5 Applications to Other Areas of Health and Disease

AN is a complex disease involving psychological, sociological, and neurobiological components. By understanding these mechanisms, physicians will be able to treat this eating disorder using not only dietetic and psychiatric approaches, but also chemical approaches. Nevertheless, because of the contradictions between studies and the current lack of knowledge, AN is still difficult to treat. Hopefully, as new technologies like imaging (developed in another chapter) become increasingly available, they may open doors to new therapeutic approaches (Table 159.1).

Table 159.1 Key features of biology in anorexia nervosa

1. An excess of cortisol is observed in AN with a normal nycthemeral cycle. A nearly constant finding in AN patients is the normal response to ACTH, which contrasts with the weakened response to stimulation with corticotropin- releasing hormone (CRH).
2. An increase in beta-endorphin activity has been observed in AN patients. During refeeding, there is a decrease in the level of beta-endorphin.
3. Results about catecholamines are inconsistent.
4. Low cerebral-spinal fluid levels of the serotonergic metabolite 5-hydroxyindolacetic acid (5-HIAA) have been found in AN patients as compared to healthy women. This low level normalizes after weight gain.

This table lists the different biological abnormalities observed in anorexia nervosa

Summary Points

- Anorexia nervosa (AN) is a psychiatric diagnosis that describes an eating disorder characterized by low body weight and body image distortion with an obsessive fear of gaining weight.
- AN is a complex disease including social, psychological, and biological factors.
- An excess of cortisol is observed in AN, and could be responsible for lanugo, decrease in bone formation, and in the feeling of well-being observed in denutrition.
- Oversecretion of beta-endorphin enables AN patients to deny the seriousness of their malnutrition and to endure the pain and distress related to their disease.
- Serotonin plays a key role in satiety; however, several studies have failed to demonstrate any beneficial effect of selective serotonin reuptake inhibitors (SSRIs) in the treatment of hospitalized AN patients.
- New technology using brain imaging with radioligands may lead to a better understanding of brain serotonin neurotransmitter function and its dynamic relationship with human behavior.

Definitions of Key Terms

Anorexia nervosa: Anorexia nervosa (AN) is a psychiatric diagnosis that describes an eating disorder characterized by low body weight and body image distortion with an obsessive fear of gaining weight.

Corticotrop axis: Corticotrop axis is the hypothalamic–pituitary–adrenal axis. CRH (Corticotropin-releasing hormone) from the hypothalamus stimulates ACTH (in the pituitary gland) in a pulsatile manner, and ACTH stimulates the secretion of glucocorticoids (cortisol) from the adrenal cortex.

Beta-endorphin: Beta-endorphin is an endogenous opioid peptide neurotransmitter found in the neurons of both the central and peripheral nervous system. It is a peptide 31 amino acids long, resulting from processing of the precursor proopiomelanocortin (POMC).

Catecholamines: Catecholamines are molecules that have a catechol nucleus. They include dopamine, norepinephrine and epinephrine. Epinephrine is synthesized mainly in the adrenal medulla, whereas norepinephrine is found not only in the adrenal medulla but also in the central nervous system and in the peripheral sympathetic nerves. Dopamine, the precursor of norepinephrine, is found in the adrenal medulla and in noradrenergic neurons.

Serotonin: Serotonin is a monoamine neurotransmitter. It is found extensively in the gastrointestinal tract of animals, and about 80–90% of the human body's total serotonin is located in the enterochromaffin cells in the gut, where it is used to regulate intestinal movements. The remainder is synthesized in serotonergic neurons in the central nervous system where it has various functions, including control of appetite, mood, and anger.

References

Audenaert K, Van Laere K, Dumont F, Vervaet M, Goethals I, Slegers G, Mertens J, van Heeringen C, Dierckx RA. J Nucl Med. 2003;44 (2):163–9.

Barbato G, Fichele M, Senatore I, Casiello M, Muscettola G. Psychiatry Res. 2006;142:253–5.

Barry VC, Klawans HL. J Neural Transm. 1976;38:107–22.

Biederman J, Rivinus TM, Herzog DB, Ferber RA, Harper GP, Orsulak PJ, Harmatz JS, Schildkraut JJ. Am J Psychiatry. 1984;141 (10):1244–7.

Bliss EL, Migeon CJ. J Clin Endocrinol Metab. 1957;17:766–76.

Boyar RM, Hellman LD, Roffwarg H, Katz J, Zumoff B, O'Connor J, Bradlow HL, Fukushima DK. N Engl J Med. 1977;296:190–98.

Capasso A, Petrella C, Milano W. Rev Recent Clin Trials. 2009;4:63–9.

Carrasco JL, Díaz-Marsá M, Hollander E, César J, Saiz-Ruiz J. Eur Neuropsychopharmacol. 2000;10 (2):113–7.

Casper RC. Psychiatry Res. 1996;62:85–96.

Díaz-Marsá M, Carrasco JL, Hollander E, César J, Saiz-Ruiz J. Acta Psychiatr Scand. 2000;101 (3):226–30.

dos Santos E, dos Santos J, Ribeiro RP, Rosa E Silva AC, Moreira AC, Silva de Sá MF. J Pediatr Adolesc Gynecol. 2007;20:13–8.

Ehrlich S, Franke L, Schott R, Salbach-Andrae H, Pfeiffer E, Lehmkuhl U, Uebelhack R. Pharmacopsychiatry. 2008;41 (6):226–31.

Ericsson M, Poston WS 2nd, Foreyt JP. Addict Behav. 1996;21 (6):733–43.

Ferguson CP, La Via MC, Crossan PJ, Kaye WH. Int J Eat Disord. 1999;25 (1):11–7.

Freedman LJ, Insel TR, Smith Y. J Comp Neurol. 2000;421:172–88.

Gold PW, Gwirtsman H, Avgerinos PC, Nieman LK, Gallucci WT, Kaye W, Jimerson D, Ebert M, Rittmaster R, Loriaux DL, et al. N Engl J Med. 1986;314:1335.

Halmi KA, Eckert E, LaDu TJ, Cohen J. Arch Gen Psychiatry. 1986;43 (2):177–81.

Hubner HF. In: Hubner HF, editor. Endorphins, eating disorders, and other addictive behaviors. New York: WW Norton & Company; 1993.

Jimerson DC. In: Ferrari E, Brambilla F, Solerte SB, editors. The role of central catecholamine pathways in eating disorders. Primary and secondary eating disorders: a psychonettroendocrine and metabolic approach. Oxford: Pergamon Press; 1993. p. 5944–5952.

Kaye W. Physiol Behav. 2008;94 (1):121–35.

Kaye WH, Ebert MH, Raleigh M, Lake R. Arch Gen Psych. 1984;41:350–5.

Kaye WH, Gwirtsman HE, George DT, Jimerson DC, Ebert MH. Biol Psychiatry. 1988;23:102–5.

Kaye WH, Frank GKW, McConaha C. Neuropsychopharmacology. 1999;21:503–6.

Kaye WH, Nagata T, Weltzin TE, Hsu LK, Sokol MS, McConaha C, Plotnicov KH, Weise J, Deep D. Biol Psychiatry. 2001;49 (7):644–52.

Kaye WH, Frank GK, Bailer UF, Henry SE, Meltzer CC, Price JC, Mathis CA, Wagner A. Physiol Behav. 2005;85 (1):73–81.

Lanfranco F, Gianotti L, Picu A, Giordano R, Daga GA, Mondelli V, Malfi G, Fassino S, Ghigo E, Arvat E. Eur J Endocrinol. 2006;154:731–8.

Leibowitz. SF. Drugs. 1990;39:33–48.

Lilenfeld LR, Kaye WH, Greeno CG, Merikangas KR, Plotnicov K, Pollice C, Rao R, Strober M, Bulik CM, Nagy L. Arch Gen Psychiatry. 1998;55 (7):603–10.

Nedvídková J, Dostálová I, Barták V, Papezov H, Pacák K. Physiol Res. 2004;53 (4):409–13.

Pirke KM. Psychiatry Res. 1996;62:43–9.

Putignano P, Dubini A, Toja P, Invitti C, Bonfanti S, Redaelli G, Zappulli D, Cavagnini F. Eur J Endocrinol. 2001;145:165–71.

Rigaud D, Vergès B, Colas-Linhart N, Petiet A, Moukkaddem M, Van Wymelbeke V, Brondel L. J Clin Endocrinol Metab. 2007;92 (5):1623–9.

Russell J, Baur LA, Beumont PJ, Byrnes S, Gross G, Touyz S, Abraham S, Zipfel S. Psychoneuroendocrinology. 2001;26:51–63.

Sirinathsinghji DJ, Mills IH. Acta Endocrinol. 1985;108:255–61.

Steiger H, Gauvin L, Israel M, Kin NM, Young SN, Roussin J. J Clin Psychiatry. 2004;65 (6):830–7.

Strober M, Freeman R, DeAntonio M, Lampert C, Diamond J. Psychopharmacol Bull. 1997;33 (3):425–31.

Verhagen LAW, Luijendijk MCM, Hillebrand JJG, Adan RAH. Eur Neuropsychopharmacol. 2009;19:153–60.

Vierhapper H, Kiss A, Nowotry P, Wiesnagrotzki S, Monder C, Waldhausl W. Acta Endocrinol. 1990;122:753–8.

Chapter 160
Ethnicity in Bulimia Nervosa and Other Eating Disorders

Athena Robinson and W. Stewart Agras

Keywords Anorexia nervosa • Bulimia nervosa • Binge eating disorder • Obesity • Minorities • Treatment

Abbreviations

BMI   Body mass index
WHO   World Health Organization

160.1 Introduction

Historically, epidemiological studies of eating disorders have focused on white women and girls and relatively little research has been conducted utilizing participants from racial and ethnic minority groups (National Eating Disorder Association (NEDA) 2005). Consequently, eating disorders are often described as affecting primarily white women of high socio-economic classes (American Psychiatric Association 1993; Fairburn and Beglin 1990; Striegel-Moore and Smolak 1996). Thus, research prior to the mid-1990s typically reported that eating disorders were less common among specific minority groups in the United States including blacks, Hispanics, Native Americans, and Asian Americans (Dolan 1991; Hsu 1987; Jones et al. 1980). However, more recent empirical studies suggest that minority populations are substantially affected by disordered eating behaviors (Yanovski 2000, Streigel-Moore et al. 2003; Taylor et al. 2007).

This chapter provides a review of the occurrence of disordered eating among ethnic minority groups for anorexia nervosa, bulimia nervosa, binge eating disorder, overweight and obesity, and dieting and other forms of body disturbance. Discussion of issues related to assessment and access to treatment, and areas for future research are provided.

A. Robinson (✉)
Department of Psychiatry and Behavioral Sciences, Stanford University, School of Medicine, 401 Quarry Road, Stanford, CA 94305-5722
e-mail: athenar@stanford.edu

V.R. Preedy et al. (eds.), *Handbook of Behavior, Food and Nutrition*,
DOI 10.1007/978-0-387-92271-3_160, © Springer Science+Business Media, LLC 2011

Table 160.1 Prevalence rates of anorexia nervosa, bulimia nervosa, binge eating disorder, and any binge eating

Reference	Sample	Lifetime prevalence n (%)			
		Anorexia nervosa	Bulimia nervosa	Binge eating disorder	Any binge eating
Streigel-Moore et al. (2003)	985 white women	15 (1.5)	23 (2.3)	27 (2.7)	–
	1061 black women	0	4 (.4)	15 (1.4)	–
Taylor et al. (2007)	5191 African American and Caribbean Black adults	7 (.17)	79 (1.49)	88 (1.66)	245 (5.08)
	Adolescents[a]	2 (.07)	5 (.40)	4 (.28)	18 (1.56)
Alegria et al. (2007)	2554 Latino adults	2 (.08)	41 (1.61)	49 (1.92)	143 (5.61)
Nicado et al. (2007)	2095 Asian American adults	2 (.08)	23 (1.09)	43 (2.04)	91 (4.35)

This table lists the prevalence rates of anorexia nervosa, bulimia nervosa (BN), binge eating disorder, and binge eating as reported by four recent studies

Rates for Alegria et al. 2007 and Nicado et al. 2007 were calculated by A. Robinson using percentage data provided in manuscripts

–Data not provided by study

[a] Only 12-month prevalence rates for adolescents provided by original paper

160.2 Prevalence Rates

Table 160.1 outlines data from four recent studies that provide prevalence estimates of anorexia nervosa, bulimia nervosa, binge eating disorder, and the presence of any binge eating among whites, blacks, Latinos, and Asian Americans. Taken together these studies suggest, with the exception of anorexia nervosa among blacks, that the rates of disordered eating behaviors among ethnic minorities are substantial.

160.2.1 Anorexia Nervosa

General anorexia nervosa prevalence estimates are approximately 0.3 among young females (Hoek 2006; Hoek and van Hoeken 2003) with crude mortality rates ranging from 5.1% to 7.4% (Herzog et al. 2000; Sullivan 1995; Crow et al. 1999) and relatively poor prognosis (Steinhausen 2002). Key features of anorexia nervosa are outlined in Table 160.2.

Prevalence rates of lifetime criteria for anorexia nervosa among 2,046 young black and white women assessed via telephone and confirmatory in-person diagnostic interviews were reported as 15 (1.5%) and 0 (0%) for white and black women respectively (Striegel-Moore et al. 2003). Another recent study interviewed a nationally representative sample of 5,191 African American and Caribbean black adults and adolescents and found that anorexia nervosa was the rarest eating disorder among African American adults and adolescents and that no single case of anorexia nervosa of at least 12-months in duration was found among Caribbean black adults (Taylor et al. 2007). Other authors echo the rarity of anorexia nervosa among black women (Hoek 2006; Mullholland and Mintz 2001). Results from the National Latino and Asian American Study (NLAAS) indicate that 2 women out of 2,554 Latinos (1,127 male, 1,427 female) met lifetime criteria for anorexia nervosa and none met current criteria for anorexia nervosa or subthreshold anorexia nervosa (Alegria et al. 2007). Lifetime and 12-month prevalence rates of anorexia nervosa among a nationally representative sample of 2,095 Asian Americans (998 male, 1,097 female) were reported as 0.08% and 0.02% for men and women respectively (Nicado et al. 2007).

Table 160.2 Key features of anorexia nervosa

Disorder	Features
Anorexia Nervosa	• Refusal to maintain body weight at or above minimum normal weight for age and height
	• Intense fear of weight gain
	• Disturbance in perception and experience of body weight and/or shape, or denial of the seriousness of low body weight
	• Amenorrhea (the absence of menstruation)

This table lists the key features of anorexia nervosa, including behavioral and cognitive symptoms and physical manifestations. Diagnostic criteria are described fully in the Diagnostic and Statistical Manual of Mental Disorders, 4th ed (DSM IV) (APA 1994)

Table 160.3 Key features of bulimia nervosa

Disorder	Features
Bulimia nervosa	• Recurrent episodes of binge eating
	• Purging behaviors (such as vomiting, laxative abuse, or compulsive exercise) used to control weight and shape
	• Self-evaluation largely based on perceptions of body shape and weight

This table lists the key features of bulimia nervosa including behavioral and cognitive symptoms. Diagnostic criteria are described fully in the Diagnostic and Statistical Manual of Mental Disorders, 4th ed (DSM IV) (APA 1994)

While firm conclusions cannot be drawn regarding the prevalence of anorexia nervosa among ethnic minority groups, data to date suggest that rates of anorexia nervosa are lower among ethnic minority groups than among their white counterparts, and are particularly low among blacks.

160.2.2 Bulimia Nervosa

General prevalence rates of bulimia nervosa have been estimated at 1% among young females (Hoek 2006). Key features of bulimia nervosa are outlined in Table 160.3.

Striegel-Moore and colleagues (2003) reported lifetime prevalence rates for bulimia nervosa among 2,046 young white and black women to be 23 (2.3%) and 4 (0.4%), respectively, and concluded that bulimia nervosa is less common among blacks than white women. Among 4997 African American and Caribbean black adults, 79 (1.49%) and 38 (0.69%) met lifetime and 12-month criteria for bulimia nervosa respectively (Taylor et al. 2007). Rates of bulimia nervosa were significantly lower among black than white college women (Gray et al. 2006) and no cases of bulimia nervosa were found among 421 black college women enrolled at a predominately white public university (Mulholland & Mintz, 2001). Alegria et al. (2007) reported a lifetime and 12-month bulimia nervosa prevalence rate of 0.08% and 0.03% respectively among a sample of 2,554 Latinos. Lifetime and 12-month prevalence rates of bulimia nervosa among 2,095 Asian American adults were 1.09% and 0.36% respectively (Nicado et al. 2007). Women from four ethnic groups (Hispanic, Asian–American, black, white) were equally likely to present behavioral symptoms of bulimia nervosa (Regan and Cachelin 2006). Similarly, a review noted bulimia nervosa rates among white women were not significantly greater than nonwhite women (Wildes et al. 2001).

160.2.3 Binge Eating Disorder

Binge eating disorder impacts approximately 2–5% of the general population (Bruce and Agras 1992) and up to 30% of weight control program participants (Spitzer et al. 1992, 1993). Key features

Table 160.4 Key features of binge eating disorder

Disorder	Features
Binge eating disorder	• Recurrent episodes of binge eating
	• Binge episodes are associated with some of the following: eating much more rapidly than normal, eating until uncomfortably full, eating large amounts of food when not physically hungry, eating alone due to embarrassment over food quantity consumed, and feeling depressed, guilty, or disgusted after eating
	• No purging behavior present

This table lists the key features of binge eating disorder including behavioral and cognitive symptoms. Diagnostic criteria are described fully in the Diagnostic and Statistical Manual of Mental Disorders, eth ed (DSM IV) (APA 1994)

of binge eating disorder are outlined in Table 160.4. The literature is in agreement that binge eating is the most prevalent disordered eating behavior among minority groups. Data from field studies reported comparable rates of binge eating disorder in white and black women (Spitzer et al. 1992, 1993) and some studies suggest that binge eating rates among black women are equal or even more common than among white women (Striegel-Moore and Smolak 2000). Similar lifetime prevalence rates of binge eating were found among adults of three minority groups: African American and Caribbean blacks at 5.08% (Taylor et al. 2007), Latinos at 5.61% (Alegria et al. 2007), and Asian Americans at 4.35% (Nicado et al. 2007).

160.2.4 Applications: Overweight and Obesity

Overweight and obesity are one of the leading causes of morbidity and mortality in the USA (US Department of Health and Human Services 2001) and obesity may be a risk factor for binge eating disorder. These conditions are particularly prevalent among some ethnic minority and immigrant groups in the USA including African–Americans and Hispanics (Centers for Disease Control (CDC) 2003). For example, Mexican American adults have reported higher rates of overweight (11% higher for males; 26% higher for females) and obesity (7% higher for males; 32% higher for females) than non-Hispanic whites. Similarly, Mexican–American adolescents aged 12–19 years reported higher rates of overweight (112% higher for males and 59% higher for females) than non-Hispanic white adolescents. Acculturation to the USA has been identified as a risk factor for obesity-related behaviors, specifically the high frequency of eating fast food and low rates of physical activity among Asian–Americans and Hispanic adolescents (Lauderdale and Rathouz 2000; Unger et al. 2004).

Overweight rates among Asian–Americans are relatively low compared to other ethnic minority groups (Lauderdale and Rathouz 2000). Whereas Asian-Americans have been found to have lower Body Mass Index (BMI), they have a higher percent body fat than whites (Wang et al. 1994). A World Health Organization (WHO) expert consultation recently reviewed evidence suggesting that Asian populations have different associations between BMI, percent body fat, and health risks than European populations and concluded that while the international BMI specifications (<18.50 = underweight, 18.50–24.99 = normal weight, 25.00–29.99 = overweight, and >30.00 = obese; WHO 2000) should be retained, the proportion of Asians with a high risk of type 2 diabetes and cardiovascular disease is substantial at BMIs lower than the existing WHO cut-off point for overweight (WHO Expert Consultation 2004).

Findings from clinic, community, and population-based studies note that binge eating disorder is associated with overweight and obesity (Bruce and Agras 1992; Fairburn et al. 2000; Smith et al. 1998, Spitzer et al. 1992; Striegel-Moore et al. 2000) and the prevalence of binge eating increases with BMI (Telch et al. 1988). Given the high rates of obesity among ethnic minority populations, experts have hypothesized that binge eating or binge eating disorder is a significant concern among these groups (Striegel-Moore and Smolak 2000). Interestingly, a recent study found that despite white women having statistically significant higher rates of binge eating disorder than black women (2.7% vs 1.4%), black women remained significantly more likely than white women to have ever been obese and be currently obese (Striegel-Moore et al. 2003). More data on the association between overweight/obesity and binge eating disorder in minority populations is needed.

160.3 Rates of General Disordered Eating Behaviors

Key features of disordered eating behaviors are outlined in Table 160.5.

160.3.1 Among Minorities

Various studies note the presence of general disordered eating behaviors among minority populations. For example, Hispanics were found to have equal rates of eating disturbances compared to whites, while blacks, Native Americans, and Asian Americans had lower rates than whites (Crago et al. 1996). However, black females in South Africa had higher rates of eating disorder symptoms than white females (Le Grange et al. 1998; Szabo and Hollands 1997). Black college women reported less fear and discouragement concerning food and weight control than white women (Gray et al. 2006). A meta-analytic review, based on data from over 17,000 participants, indicated that as a whole, white women living in Western countries experience greater eating disturbance and body dissatisfaction than nonwhite women (Wildes et al. 2001). However, results suggested that Asian American women report similar and in some cases higher levels of disordered eating than their white counterparts. For example, Asian women, who report weighing significantly less than white women, differ from white women in having higher body dissatisfaction in the magnitude of one-third of a standard deviation.

160.3.2 Among Adolescent Minorities

Research on disordered eating behaviors and dieting among adolescents from minority groups has also challenged preexisting assumptions about the prevalence of such behaviors. Data from the 1998 Minnesota Student Survey indicated that among 9th graders, 56% of girls and 28% of boys report disordered eating behavior (i.e., one or more of the following to lose weight: fasting or skipping meals, diet pills, vomiting, laxatives, and binge eating) and that among both genders, Hispanic and Native American youth reported the highest prevalence of disordered eating (Croll et al. 2002).

Table 160.5 Key features of disordered eating

Disordered eating	• Severe restriction of food intake (may include limiting type, quantity, or frequency of consumption)
	• Compensatory behaviors used to prevent weight gain such as laxative abuse, self-induced vomiting, fasting, diuretics, diet pills, and excessive exercise
	• Intense scrutiny of body (may include repetitively analyzing self in mirrors or pinching of body parts) or purposeful avoidance of seeing body (in mirrors or when changing clothes)
	• Negative feelings about body weight and shape
	• Self-esteem and self-evaluation largely influenced by perception of body weight and shape
	• Exaggerated sense of the importance of weight and shape

This table lists examples of various behavioral and cognitive symptoms of disordered eating

Another study found few differences between ethnic groups among adolescent girls on eating disorder symptoms whereas among boys, black, Native American, Asian/Pacific Islander, and Hispanic boys reported significantly more eating disorder symptoms than white boys (Austin et al. 2008).

Dieting was found to be associated with weight dissatisfaction, perceived overweight status, and low body pride among adolescents of all ethnic groups assessed (Story et al. 1995). Perceived overweight and body dissatisfaction were found to be consistent correlates of dieting and binge eating among white, black, Hispanic, Native American, and Asian American adolescent females (French et al. 1997). Among the leanest 25% of sixth and seventh grade girls, Hispanics and Asians reported significantly more body dissatisfaction than did white girls (Robinson et al. 1996). A survey of 6,504 adolescents indicated that Asians, blacks, Hispanics, and white adolescents all reported attempting to lose weight at similar rates (32.7%, 31.9%, 36.1%, 34.9%, respectively) while 48.1% of Native American adolescents were attempting to lose weight (Kilpatrick et al. 1999).

A recent study examining family adaptability, cohesion, and satisfaction among white and ethnic minority families of adolescents seeking treatment for BN found that there were no significant differences between whites and ethnic minority patients' perceived and ideal levels of family cohesion and adaptability, or level of family functioning (Hoste et al. 2007). Likewise, there were no significant differences between white and ethnic minority parents on these same measures. In fact, both white and ethnic minority patients perceived their families to be less cohesive than did their mothers and fathers and reported lower ideal levels of cohesion than their mothers and fathers.

160.4 Treatment

Primary care physicians play a critical role as a liaison between patients and potential eating disorder treatment. Such practitioners may benefit from being more aware of recent data on the prevalence of disordered eating behaviors among ethnic minority groups and attempt to provide thorough assessments to all suspect eating disorder presentations regardless of ethnic and/or racial backgrounds. In addition, increased knowledge regarding ethnic minorities' differing worldviews, values and beliefs, patterns of acculturation, assimilation, and immigration, effects of oppression, and ethnic identity, as well as naturally occurring individual differences within eating disorder diagnostic classification could serve to augment the physician's cultural sensitivity in assessment of eating disorder symptoms and provision of appropriate treatment referrals (NEDA 2005). A recent study found that ethnic minority patients were less likely to be referred for eating disorder treatment services than white patients although once treatment was offered, treatment type did not differ (Waller et al. 2009). Race-based stereotypes about the frequency of eating disorder among minorities have been found to prevent physician detection of eating disorder symptoms in black girls (Gordon et al. 2006). Data to date suggest the necessity of a re-evaluation of assumptions regarding who is susceptible to disordered eating in order to better ensure that our efforts to combat these issues are inclusive of all (NEDA 2005). In terms of response to treatment, a recent study found that black women, compared to other ethnic groups, demonstrated greater reductions in binge eating when treated with Interpersonal Psychotherapy rather than Cognitive Behavioral Therapy (Chui et al. 2007).

Erroneous assumptions about eating disorder prevalence, cultural influence, course of illness, and access to treatment among minority persons can create referral biases and differences in service availability and access and, consequently, make it more difficult to estimate the true prevalence of eating disorders in these groups (Dolan 1991; Crago et al. 1996). Data are needed to further our understanding about disordered eating behaviors among all ethnic and racial groups in order to prevent bias in assessment, prevention, and intervention endeavors.

160.5 Areas for Further Research

There remain a variety of areas in need of further research regarding disordered eating behaviors among ethnic minorities. First, further research is needed to better understand potential variation of psychosocial risk factors for eating disorders within a minority group. For example, a recent study of Hispanic women including Dominicans, Venezuelans, Columbians, Brazilians, Puerto Ricans, Central Americans, and Mexicans found that Dominicans, Venezuelans, and Columbians had significantly higher total scores on the Psychosocial Risk Factor Questionnaire and Concern subscale than White Non-Hispanics, Central Americans, and Mexicans (George et al. 2007) and that Puerto Ricans had significant higher BMIs and ideal body image scores than Brazilians. Second, additional longitudinal studies among minority groups, perhaps assessing eating disorder symptoms and risk factors within the same cohort over time, may serve to illuminate patterns that may change across the age span. The potential influence of level of acculturation on eating disorder development and maintenance, and the relationship between overweight/obesity and binge eating disorder among various minority groups should be explored further. It is also critical to ascertain variation in minority groups' access and response to eating disorder treatment. Last, consistent use of standardized eating disorder assessment instruments can facilitate cross-study comparisons. Such research will encourage the reexamination of assumptions regarding who is susceptible to disordered eating behaviors in order to better ensure that our prevention and intervention efforts are inclusive of all, regardless of ethnic and/or racial background.

Summary Points

- Data indicate that disordered eating behaviors are notably prevalent among ethnic minorities.
- It can be tentatively concluded that anorexia nervosa is rare among blacks.
- Data are mixed on whether the rates of bulimia nervosa among ethnic minority and white females differ.
- Rates of binge eating among ethnic minorities are higher than other forms of disordered eating.
- There remain a variety of areas in need of further research regarding disordered eating behaviors among ethnic minorities.
- Further studies of eating disturbances among minority groups are needed before firm conclusions can be made about disordered eating prevalence and risk factors in such groups.

Key Terms

Anorexia nervosa: Characterized by severely limiting food intake, refusal to maintain body weight at or above minimum normal weight for age and height, and intense fear of weight gain

Bulimia nervosa: Characterized by binge eating episodes that are followed by compensatory behaviors to prevent weight gain and reduce feelings of distention resulting from the binge episode

Binge eating disorder: Characterized by binge eating episodes without associated compensatory behaviors

Binge eating: Eating episodes defined as

(a) The consumption of an unusually large amount of food within a discrete time period (e.g., eating, within a 2-h time period, an amount of food that is unambiguously large) and

(b) Accompanied by a sense of loss of control over eating (e.g., feeling loss of control over type or quantity of food consumed, or unable to stop the episode from continuing once it has begun).

Purging: Compensatory behavior used to control weight and shape. Examples include laxative abuse, self-induced vomiting, fasting, diuretics, diet pills, and excessive exercise.

Disordered eating behaviors: Weight and shape controlling/influencing behaviors including but not limited to restrictive eating, fasting, excessive dieting and exercise, binge eating, vomiting, and abuse of laxatives, diet pills, diuretics.

Body Mass Index (BMI): A ratio that relates a person's body weight to their height. The ratio is weight (in kilograms) divided by height (in meters squared). Normal weight is defined as having a BMI of 18.5 through 24.9.

Overweight/obesity: Categorization based upon BMI. Overweight and obese are defined as having a BMI of 25.00–29.99 and greater than 30.00, respectively.

Ethnic minority: For the purposes of this chapter, ethnic minority refers to a subgroup of a population defined by ethnicity and/or race such as Asian Americans and Latinos.

Prevalence: A statistical concept which refers to the proportion of individuals in a population having a particular disease at a given time.

References

Alegria M, Woo M, Cao Z, Torres M, Meng X, Striegel-Moore R. Prevalence and correlates of eating disorders in Latinos in the United States. Int J Eating Disord. 2007; 40:S15–21.

American Psychiatric Association. Diagnostic and statistical manual of mental disorders. 4th ed. Washington, DC: Author; 1994.

American Psychiatric Association. Practice guidelines for eating disorders. Am J Psychiatry. 1993;150:212–28.

Austin SB, Ziyadeh NJ, Forman S, Prokop LA, Keliher A, Jacobs D. Screening high school students for eating disorders: results of a national initiative. Prevent Chronic Dis. 2008;5 (4):A114.

Bruce B, Agras WS. Binge eating in females: a population-based investigation. Int J Eating Disord. 1992;12:365–73.

Centers for Disease Control. Health, United States, 2003: table 68. Hyattsville, MD: US. Department of Health and Human Services, CDC, National Center for Health Statistics; 2003. Available at http://www.cdc.gov/nchs/data/hus/tables/2003/03hus068.pdf.

Chui W, Safer DL, Bryson SW, Agras SW, Wilson GT. A comparison of ethnic groups in the treatment of bulimia nervosa. Eating Behav. 2007;8(4):485–91.

Crago M, Shisslak CM, Estes LS. Eating disturbances among American minority groups: a review. Int J Eating Disord. 1996;19 (3):239–48.

Croll J, Neumark-Sztainer D, Story M, Ireland M. Prevalence and risk and protective factors related to disordered eating behavior among adolescents: relationship to gender and ethnicity. J Adolescent Health. 2002;31 (2):166–75.

Crow S, Praus B, Thuras P. Mortality from eating disorders – a 5 to 10 year record linkage study. Int J Eating Disord. 1999;26 (1):97–101.

Dolan B. Cross-cultural aspects of anorexia nervosa and bulimia: a review. Int J Eating Disord. 1991;10:67–8.

Fairburn CG, Beglin SJ. Studies of the epidemiology of bulimia nervosa. American Journal of Psychiatry. 1990;147:401–408.

Fairburn CG, Cooper Z, Doll HA, Norman P, O'Conner M. The natural course of bulimia nervosa and binge eating disorder in young women. Arch Gen Psychiatry. 2000;57:659–65.

French S, Story M, Neumark-Sztainer D, Downess B, Resnick M, Blum R. Ethnic differences in psychosocial and health behavior correlates of dieting, purging, and binge eating in a populations-based sample of adolescent females. Int J Eat Disord. 1997;22 (3):315–22.

Herzog DB, Greenwood DN, Dorer DJ, Flores AT, Ekeblad ER, Richards A, Blais MA, Keller MB. Mortality in eating disorders: a descriptive study. Int J Eating Disord. 2000;28 (1):20–6.

Hoek HW. Incidence, prevalence and mortality of anorexia nervosa and other eating disorders. Curr Opin Psychiatry. 2006;19 (4):389–94.

Hoek HW, van Hoeken D. Review of the prevalence and incidence of eating disorders. Int J Eating Disord. 2003;34 (4):383–96.

Hoste RR, Hewell K, LeGrange D. Family interaction among white and ethnic minority adolescents with bulimia nervosa and their parents. European Eating Disorders Review. 2007;15:152–158.

Hsu LKG. Are the eating disorders becoming more common in Blacks? Int J Eating Disord. 1987;6:113–24.

George VA, Erb AF, Harris CL, Casazza K. Psychosocial risk factors for eating disorders in Hispanic females of diverse ethnic background and non-Hispanic females. Eat Behav. 2007;8:1–9.

Gordon KH, Brattole MM, Wingate LR, Joiner TE. The impact of client race on clinician detection of eating disorders. Behav Ther. 2006;37 (4):319–25.

Gray JJ, Ford K, Kelly LM. The prevalence of bulimia in a black college population. Int J Eat Disord. 2006;6:733–40.

Jones DJ, Fox MM, Babigian HM, Hutton HE. Epidemiology of anorexia nervosa in Monroe County, New York: 1960–1976. Psychosom Med. 1980;42:551–8.

Kilpatrick M, Ohannessian C, Bartholomew J. Adolescent weight management and perceptions: an analysis of the National Longitudinal study of Adolescent Health. J Sch Health. 1999;69:148–52.

Lauderdale DS, Rathouz PJ. Body mass index in a US national sample of Asian Americans: effects of nativity, years since immigration and socioeconomic status. International Journal of Obesity and Related Metabolic Disorders. 2000;24:1188–1194.

Le Grange D, Telch CF, Tibbs K. Eating attitudes and behaviors in 1435 South African Caucasian and non-Caucasian college students. Am J Psychiatry. 1998;155:250–4.

Mullholland AM, Mintz LB. Prevalence of eating disorders among African American women. J Counsel Psychol. 2001;48:111–6.

National Eating Disorder Association. Eating disorders in women of color: explanations and implications. National Eating Disorder Association. 2005: www.nationaleatingdisorders.org

Nicado EG, Hong S, Takeuchi DT. Prevalence and correlates of eating disorders among Asian Americans: results from the National Latino and Asian American Study. Int J Eat Disord. 2007;40:S22–6.

Regan PC, Cachelin FM. Binge eating and purging in a multi-ethnic community sample. International Journal of Eating Disoders. 2006;39:523–526.

Robinson TN, Killen JD, Litt IF, Hammer LD, Wilson DM, Haydel KF, Hayward C, Taylor CB. Ethnicity and body dissatisfaction: are Hispanic and Asian girls at increased risk for eating disorders? J Adolescent Health. 1996;19:384–93.

Smith DE, Marcus MD, Lewis CE, Fitzgibbon M, Schreiner P. Prevalence of binge eating disorder, obesity, and depression in a biracial cohort of young adults. Ann Behav Med. 1998;20:227–32.

Spitzer RL, Devlin MJ, Walsh BT, Hasin D, Wing RR, Marcus MD, Stunkard A, Wadden T, Yanovski S, Agras WS, Nonas C. Binge eating disorder: a multisite field trail of the diagnostic criteria. Int J Eat Disord. 1992; 11:191–203.

Spitzer RL, Yanovski S, Wadden T, Wing R, Marcus MD, Stunkard A, Devlin M, Mitchell J, Hasin D, Horne RL. Binge eating disorder: Its further validation in a multisite study. Int J Eat Disord. 1993;13:137–53.

Steinhausen HC. The outcome of anorexia nervosa in the 20th century. Am J Psychiatry. 2002;159:1284–93.

Story M, French S, Resnick M, Blum R. Ethnic/racial and socioeconomic differences in dieting behaviors and body image perceptions in adolescents. Int J Eat Disord. 1995;18 (2):173–9.

Striegel-Moore R, Dohm FA, Kraemer HC, Taylor CB, Daniels S, Crawford PB, Schreiber GB. Eating disorders in black and white women. Am J Psychiatry. 2003;160:1326–31.

Striegel-Moore R, Smolak L. The role of race in the development of eating deisorders. In: Smolak L, Levine MP, Striegel-Moore R, editors. The developmental psychopathology of eating disorders. Mahwah: Lawrence Erlbaum Associates; 1996.

Striegel-Moore R, Smolak L. The influence of ethnicity on eating disorders in women. In Eisler RM, Hersen M, editors.Handbook of gender, culture, and health. Mahwah: Lawrence Erlbaum Associates; 2000. p. 227–254.

Striegel-Moore RH, Wilfley DE, Pike KM, Dohm FA, Fairburn CG. Recurrent binge eating in Black American women. Arch Fam Med. 2000;9:83–7.

Sullivan PF. Mortality in anorexia nervosa. Am J Psychiatry. 1995;152:1073–4.

Szabo CP, Hollands, C. Factors influencing eating attitudes in secondary girls in South-Africa – a preliminary study. S Afr Med J. 1997;87 (4):531–4.

Taylor JY, Caldwell CH, Baser RE, Faison N, Jackson JS. Prevalence of eating disorders among blacks in the National Survey of American Life. Int J Eat Disord. 2007;40: S10–4.

Telch CF, Agras WS, Rossiter EM. Binge eating increases with increasing adiposity. Int J Eat Disord. 1988;7:115–9.

Unger JB, Reynolds K, Shakib S, Spruijt-Metz D, Sun P, Johnson CA. Acculturation, physical activity, and fast-food consumption among Asian American and Hispanic adolescents. J Community Health. 2004;29:467–81.

US Department of Health and Human Services. The Surgeon General's call to action to prevent and decrease overweight and obesity. Rockville: US Department of Health and Human Services, Public Health Service, Office of the Surgeon General; 2001.

Waller G, Schmidt U, Treasure J, Emanuelli F, Alenya J, Crockett J, Murray K. Ethnic origins of patients attending specialist eating disorders services in a multiethnic urban catchment area in the United Kingdom. Int J Eat Disord. 2009;42:459–463.

Wang J, Thornton JC, Russell M, Burastero S, Heymsfield S, Pierson RN. Asians have lower body mass index (BMI) but higher percent body fat than do whites: Comparisons of anthropometric measures. Am J Clin Nutr. 1994;60:23–8.

Wildes JE, Emery RE, Simons AD. The roles of ethnicity and culture in the development of eating disturbance and body dissatisfaction: A meta-analytic review. Clin Psychol Rev. 2001;21 (4):521–51.

WHO Expert Consultation. Appropriate body-mass index for Asian American populations and its implication for policy intervention strategies. Lancet. 2004;363:157–163.

World Health Organization. Obesity: preventing and managing the global epidemic. Report of a WHO consultation, WHO Technical Report Series 854. Geneva: World Health Organization; 2000.

Yanovski SZ. Eating disorders, race, and mythology. Arch Fam Med. 2000;9:88.

Chapter 161
Dyscontrol in Women with Bulimia Nervosa: Lack of Inhibitory Control over Motor, Cognitive, and Emotional Responses in Women with Bulimia Nervosa

Sonia Rodríguez-Ruiz, Silvia Moreno, M. Carmen Fernández, Antonio Cepeda-Benito, and Jaime Vila

Keywords Bulimia nervosa • Lack of inhibitory control • Sexual behavior • Decision-making • Food craving • Psychophysiological regulation

Abbreviations

AN	Anorexia nervosa
BN	Bulimia nervosa
ANR	Anorexia nervosa restrictive-type
ANBP	Anorexia nervosa binge/purging-type
BNP	Bulimia nervosa purging-type
BNNP	Bulimia nervosa non-purging-type
CDR	Cardiac defense response
DSM IV TR	Diagnostic and Statistical Manual of Mental Disorders, fourth edition
ED	Eating disorders
FCQ-T	Food Craving Questionnaire-Trait
GNG	Go/No-Go task
HRV	Heart rate variability
IAPS	International Affective Picture System
IGT	Iowa Gambling Task
SAM	Self-Assessment Manikin
SMR	Startle motor reflex

161.1 Introduction

The cardinal feature of bulimia nervosa (BN) is bouts of uncontrolled food intake (binges). During bingeing, individuals ingest large amounts of food while experiencing an uncontrollable desire to eat. Individuals with BN tend to be highly concerned or dissatisfied with their body shape and, as a consequence, repeatedly display compensatory behaviors aimed at preventing weight gain. Compensatory behaviors include purging, excessive exercise, dietary restraint, or fasting between periods of binge eating (APA 2000).

S. Rodríguez-Ruiz (✉)
Departamento de Personalidad, Evaluación y Tratamiento Psicológico, Facultad de Psicología, Universidad de Granada, Campus de la Cartuja s/n, 18071, Granada, Spain
e-mail: srruiz@ugr.es

V.R. Preedy et al. (eds.), *Handbook of Behavior, Food and Nutrition*,
DOI 10.1007/978-0-387-92271-3_161, © Springer Science+Business Media, LLC 2011

Individuals with BN are characterized by obsessiveness and perfectionism and by their greater impulsivity in comparison to anorexia nervosa (AN) patients (Fairburn 1995). BN patients also tend to be emotionally unstable, experience strong food cravings (Cepeda-Benito and Gleaves 2001), and be prone to substance abuse, sensation seeking, and antisocial behaviors (Rosval et al. 2006; Ortega-Roldán et al. 2009).

161.2 Loss of Control Over Eating and Sexual Behaviors in Women with Bulimia Nervosa

There are reasons to suspect that BN also has an impact on women's sexuality. First, the biological effects of severe dietary restrictions lead directly to dysfunctions of the reproductive system, affecting secondary sexual characteristics (Pirke 1995). Moreover, it seems plausible that individuals who are not comfortable with their bodies, such as individuals with eating disorders, will have difficulties in deriving pleasure from sexual activity (Wiederman and Pryor 1997). Finally, eating and sexual activity are highly self-reinforcing behaviors controlled by the primary appetitive motivational circuit in the brain: the mesolimbic dopaminergic system (Koch and Schnitzler 1997). This neurophysiological circuit may explain why women with AN seem to be able to go on without food and sex so consistently (Zuckerman 1994), whereas women with BN go through cycles of restriction and loss of control over both appetitive behaviors.

Published empirical research confirms that women with eating disorders (ED) tend to face disorder-specific sexual difficulties throughout their lives (Wiederman and Pryor 1997). Inadequate body weight in women with AN compromises the presence of secondary postpubertal characteristics and leads to a childlike appearance. Women with BN are more dissatisfied with their body image than women with AN, but BN individuals are able to maintain normal body weight and also engage more frequently in sexual activity than women with AN (Cash and Deagle 1996). Compared to controls, women with BN report more sexual activity and more pressure to "perform" sexually (Katzma and Wolchick 1984), as well as greater sexual dissatisfaction. This association between increased sexual activity and sexual dissatisfaction in women with BN seems to parallel their pattern of binge eating and subsequent dysphoria.

Based on clinical observations, several authors have suggested that impulsivity and loss of control seem to be the central clinical features that discriminate between BN and AN (Matsunaga et al. 2000). Zerbe (1993) has speculated that loss of control over eating prompts individuals with BN to attempt, in vain, to gain external approval through promiscuous behavior with new partners (see also Troop 1998). Interested in this hypothesis, we recently tested the extent to which women with BN and healthy controls differed in their reactivity to food images and erotic pictures (Rodríguez et al. 2007a). Women with ($n = 24$) and without ($n = 24$) BN observed a set of food and erotic pictures, together with neutral and unpleasant ones, all selected from the *International Affective Picture System* [IAPS]. Participants rated their feelings while viewing the pictures using the *Self-Assessment Manikin* [SAM] scales: valence (pleasant–unpleasant), arousal (activated–relaxed), and control (dominant–dominated). In comparison to women without BN, women with BN responded to the erotic and food pictures with lower scores in valence and control (see Fig. 161.1). These results suggest that women with BN experience less pleasure and control over both food and sexual impulses than healthy individuals.

The finding by Rodríguez et al. (2007a) of similar reactivity to erotic and food pictures is not surprising given that both eating and sexual behaviors are controlled by the same brain circuit (Bradley and Lang 2007). According to these authors, there are two primary motivational circuits

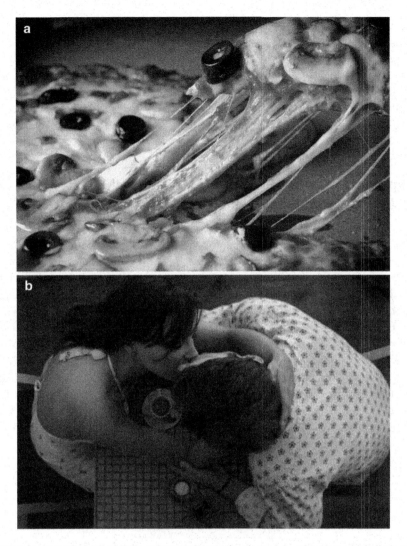

Fig. 161.1 Food and sexual-related stimuli used to test the emotional reactivity of women with bulimia nervosa (*BN*). Food images and erotic stimuli retrieved from the Internet with similar content to the International Affective Picture System (*IAPS*) pictures used in the study of Rodríguez et al. (2007a). Food and erotic pictures were rated by women with bulimia nervosa as less pleasant and controllable than women without bulimia nervosa

in the brain: the appetitive and the defensive. The appetitive circuit is mediated by the mesolimbic dopaminergic system (nucleus accumbens) and its activation is signaled by approach/consumption behaviors. The defensive circuit is mediated by the amygdala and other subcortical areas (e.g., stria terminalis, ventral tegmental area, and paraventricular hypothalamus, among others) and its activation results in avoidance/defense behaviors. For the majority of people, eating and sexuality are two basic gratifying activities that reflect the exclusive activation of appetitive mechanisms. However, sexual and food-related stimuli seem to evoke dyscontrol and negative mood in women with BN, an effect congruent with the simultaneous co-activation of aversive and appetitive motivations (Bradley 2000). Co-activation of both circuits would lead to a typical approach–avoidance conflict, explaining the observed reduction in pleasure and control in both eating and sex observed in individuals with BN.

The dyscontrol hypothesis also predicts that increased sexual activity leads to increased sexual dissatisfaction in women with BN. It has been suggested that individuals with BN use sexual activity instrumentally as a means of obtaining approval (Zerbe 1993) or of assuring continuity in their relationships (Katzma and Wolchick 1984). Some authors consider eating disorders the result of a faulty coping mechanism aimed at resolving unpleasant emotional states (Troop 1998). That is, women with BN may attempt to gain emotional relief and control by bingeing, or becoming sexually promiscuous. However, bingeing, like promiscuity, increases rather than decreases the feelings of dyscontrol and dissatisfaction.

161.3 Impulsivity and Impairment of Decision-making in Women with Bulimia Nervosa

Whereas the cognitive and behavioral symptoms that characterize eating disorders have been researched since the beginning of the nineteenth century, our understanding of the neuropsychological characteristics of individuals with eating disorders is restricted to research conducted mostly over the past two decades. Neuropsychological research in this area aims to explore the possible implication of neural dysfunctions in the etiology of ED (Duchesne et al. 2004). The general symptoms that characterize ED have been associated with damage in the right frontal and parietal lobes. This finding was supported by reports of cerebral hypoperfusion in parietal, temporal, and right frontal lobes of patients with BN purging-type (BNP) and AN restrictive-type (ANR). Images of high-calorie food were associated with anomalous activity in the ventromedial prefrontal cortex and anterior cingulate cortex of patients with BN and AN (Uher et al. 2004). Thus, the presence of functionally altered cortical (cognitive) and subcortical (emotional) areas in the brain are congruent with some of the most frequent problems reported by BN patients: deficits in selective attention and in executive function related to poor inhibitory control (Figs. 161.2 and 161.3).

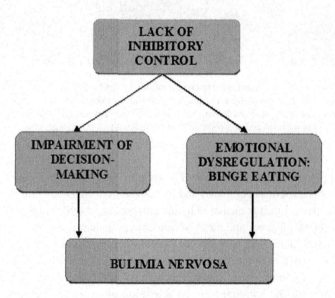

Fig. 161.2 Relationship between impulsivity, decision-making, and emotional dysregulation in bulimia nervosa. The poor inhibitory control shown by bulimia nervosa patients suggests that impulsivity may be a central and distinctive component of the disorder, mediating emotionally guided decision-making and binge eating behavior as demonstrated by Ortega-Roldán et al. (2009)

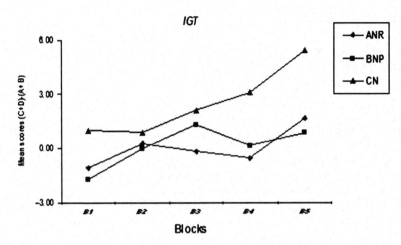

Fig. 161.3 Decision-making impairment in bulimia nervosa. The overall IGT performance of Bulimia Nervosa-Purging patients (*BNP*) was significantly worse than the one of the Anorexia Nervosa-Restrictive patients (*ANR*) or controls, which may be a consequence of their poor learning from rewards and punishments received during the course of the task (Reprinted from Ortega-Roldán et al. 2009. With permission)

The cognitive behavioral model of ED hypothesizes that ED symptoms are precipitated and maintained by maladaptive thoughts and dysfunctional assumptions about food. Research using the emotional *Stroop task* (Black et al. 1997) found higher interference and lower inhibitory control in bulimia and anorexia nervosa participants than in controls when presented words related to food, body shape, and weight (Fassino et al. 2002). Studies using the *Go/No-Go task* (Newman et al, 1985) to examine inhibitory control in ED patients have found greater impulsivity (see Table 161.1) in patients with BN and AN bingeing/purging type (ANBP), compared to patients with AN restrictive-type (ANR), and individuals without ED (Rosval et al. 2006). Finally, studies using the *Iowa Gambling Task* (IGT) (Cavedini et al. 2004; Davis et al. 2004) have found impairment of decision-making function (see Table 161.2) in individuals with AN, BN, and obesity, reflected by their inability to successfully perform the task.

The above findings on impulsivity, a key factor in emotionally triggered binge eating (Nederkoorn et al. 2004), prompted our team to examine the relationships between impulsivity, emotion, and decision-making in women with BN ($n = 14$), ANR ($n = 22$), and controls ($n = 29$) (Ortega-Roldán et al. 2009). Participants carried out two tasks: the IGT and an affective version of the Go/No-Go task. The IGT imitates real-life decision-making by means of a card game that evaluates the capacity to balance immediate rewards with long-term negative consequences. The affective version of the Go/No-Go task is a measure of motor impulsivity, since the participant must inhibit a behavioral response (pressing a key) to affect-related stimuli. Participants also completed a set of questionnaires on cognitive impulsivity, mood state, anxiety, and food craving. The results showed that patients with BN performed considerably worse in the IGT and Go/No-Go task than both AN and control participants. In addition, the results indicated that BN and AN patients performed differently in the Go/No-Go task, with BN participants showing greater cognitive impulsivity, more negative mood, and greater anxiety and food craving than AN participants. The poor inhibitory control shown by BN patients suggests that impulsivity may be a central and distinctive component of the disorder, mediating emotionally guided decision-making and binge eating behavior.

The lower performance in the IGT of BN than AN may be related to the different nature of both disorders. AN individuals may derive strong short-term reinforcement from successfully avoiding food intake, such as a reduction in their fear of becoming fat, at the expense of the long-term negative

Table 161.1 Key features of impulsivity

1. Impulsivity has been defined as the inability to think over when confronting a conflictive situation, resulting in failure to anticipate the consequences of one's actions, a rushed style when making decisions, difficulties in planning one's future behavior, and/or inability to exert self-control
2. Motor (or behavioral) impulsivity has been distinguished from cognitive (or choice) impulsivity
3. Motor impulsivity is equivalent to lack of response inhibition
4. Cognitive impulsivity is considered the inability to weigh the consequences of immediate and future events and, consequently, delay gratification
5. Motor impulsivity has been measured with a variety of instruments such as the Go/No-Go, reversal learning tasks, continuous performance tests, or stop tasks
6. Cognitive impulsivity has been measured using decision-making tasks such as the Iowa Gambling Task
7. Motor impulsivity is associated with impairments to the dorsolateral prefrontal cortex
8. Cognitive impulsivity is associated with impairments to the ventromedial prefrontal cortex

This table lists the key features of impulsivity, including the definition of impulsivity, the differentiation between motor and cognitive impulsivity, the measurement and the location of brain impairments for each type of impulsivity

Table 161.2 Key facts of decision-making

1. The generic structure of decision-making involves three independent processes:
   (a) Appraisal of the stimuli or options
   (b) Selection or execution of an action
   (c) Evaluation of the experience or outcome of the choices that were made
2. Each of these stages may be differentially affected by various psychological and neural factors
3. When pleasurable or aversive events are confronted in one's immediate circumstances, appropriate somatic states are generated via activation of subcortical circuitry, and these emotions are subconsciously remembered for future occurrences of the same stimuli
4. The orbitofrontal cortex, in particular, is critical for activating feelings or emotional states from "thoughts" about rewarding or punishing events that are not currently present in one's environment
5. The behavioral deficits of the impaired decision-making are typically caused by an inability to advantageously assess future consequences
6. Poor decision-making is a core symptom of certain mental health problems such as drug dependence, mania, and some forms of eating disorder

This table lists the key facts of decision-making including the processes involved, the psychological and neural factors that influence these processes, the behavioral deficits of the impaired decision-making, and the affected populations

consequences of their behavior, i.e., severe physical and psychosocial impairments. Similarly, BN individuals appear to succumb to binge and purging impulses, arguably to escape negative emotional states, causing an unhealthy, long-term cycle of extreme dieting, bingeing, and purging.

On the other hand, the results obtained with the *Go/No-Go* task support the hypothesis that patients with BN have greater motor and cognitive impulsivity than patients with AN. Thus, our findings support the notion that lack of impulsivity diagnostically differentiates AN from BN.

161.4 Loss of Control Evoked by Dietary Restraint, Food Craving, and Binge Eating in Women with Bulimia Nervosa

Women with BN not only show risk-behaviors (e.g., multiple sexual relationships) and impulsivity, they also experience very intense food cravings (Fig. 161.4). Craving has been defined as a state of strong desire to consume a given substance. Food craving has been linked to binge eating in women with BN, increased food consumption in restrained eaters, early dropout from weight-loss treatments, overeating in obese individuals, and lifetime prevalence rates of BN (Cepeda-Benito and

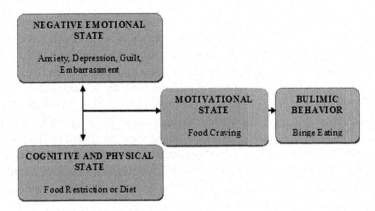

Fig. 161.4 Relationship between emotional states, dietary restraint, and food craving in bulimia nervosa. This model (Moreno et al. 2009a) proposes that a negative emotional state (such as anxiety, depression, guilt, embarrassment...) and a cognitive and physical state (associated with food restriction) are required to provoke a motivational state of food craving. The food craving might be a trigger of the binge eating as a typical behavior of bulimia nervosa patients

Gleaves 2001). The experience of craving has often been conceptualized as an "irresistible demand" for a substance and having a craving equates with losing control over the craved substance (e.g., Gendall et al. 1997).

Researchers have postulated that food craving plays an instrumental role in the development and maintenance of binge-eating behavior (e.g., Heatherton and Polivy 1992). For example, the starvation/dietary restraint model explains that dietary restraint practices produce a state of strong food craving that provokes a loss of control over eating (i.e., binge eating; Cepeda-Benito and Gleaves 2001).

However, it has also been reported that energy deprivation does not always precede food cravings and binge eating (Hill et al. 1991). Specifically, negative emotions such as anger, fear, or sadness have been found to increase binge eating among BN individuals, as well as in people diagnosed with Binge Eating Disorder (Agras and Telch 1998).

BN patients use binge eating to seek relief from their negative moods (anxiety, sadness, boredom...), but overeating also produces negative emotions as a consequence of the recognition of their inability to maintain control over their intake (Cavallo and Pinto 2001). Thus, food deprivation allows BN individuals to escape the negative affect produced by excessive consumption of food, and it may also be a maladaptive response to cope with other negative aspects of their daily lives. From this perspective, dieting may be considered a self-regulatory mechanism to reduce both the negative affect elicited by food intake and the fear of gaining weight (Mann and Ward 2004).

The effects of emotions on eating have been studied extensively, but less research has been conducted on how negative emotions modulate food craving responses as potential mediators of overeating (Waters et al. 2001). In order to better understand the relationship between negative mood and food craving, we asked women with BN ($n = 21$) and healthy controls ($n = 21$) to refrain from eating and drinking (except water) for 20 h (see Moreno et al. 2009a). Participants were asked to complete several self-report measures at different time intervals to assess mood, anxiety, and food craving. After the 20-h fasting period, all participants were allowed to eat as much as they wanted from a breakfast buffet. The number or calories and the portion of carbohydrates, proteins, and fats consumed were estimated for each participant by weighing the food and counting the servings remaining in the buffet.

The results showed that food deprivation increased food cravings in both BN and healthy controls, but that the effect was considerably greater in the BN participants. The results also demonstrated that emotional state and craving fluctuated together throughout the period of deprivation in both groups. Initially, food deprivation increased craving and negative mood in both BN and control participants. However, as the fasting period increased, food craving was associated with higher negative mood and anxiety in healthy individuals, but with improved mood and reduced anxiety in participants with BN. Finally, although BN and healthy participants did not differ in the amount of food consumed, food cravings and caloric intake were positively correlated just in BN participants.

Together, our findings support several hypotheses put forth by numerous authors. The observed increase in craving as a direct result of fasting is congruent with the hypothesis that food deprivation increases the desire to eat and may lead to binge eating (Hill et al. 1991). This conclusion is further strengthened by the finding that craving and food intake were correlated in BN but not in healthy participants. That is, BN patients appeared to be particularly vulnerable to the effects of food cravings on food intake. The observation that prolonged fasting reduced negative emotions in women with bulimia nervosa support our earlier conclusion that women with BN escape negative emotional states through fasting (Mann and Ward 2004).

We also studied the nature of the relationship between dietary restraint and loss of control over eating in AN and BN participants (Moreno et al. 2009b). It was hypothesized that food craving would be highly prevalent in individuals known to have marked tendencies to temporarily restrain their diets but lose control over eating (BN participants), but would be rare in individuals with marked tendencies to restrain food intake but not break their diets (AN participants). Using the Discriminatory Factor Analysis (DFA) on the *Food Craving Questionnaire-Trait* (Cepeda-Benito et al. 2000) to differentiate between women diagnosed with ANR, ANBP, BNP, and BNNP, we found that patients with ED who reported very low levels of food craving were accurately classified as individuals with AN, whereas patients with ED that reported high levels of food craving were accurately classified as individuals with BN (Fig. 161.5).

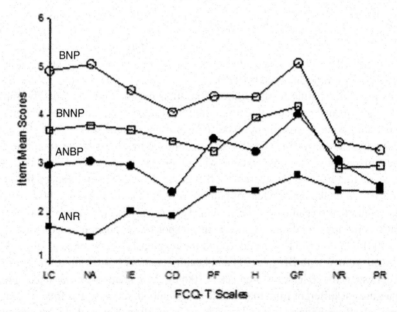

Fig. 161.5 Food Craving Questionnaire-Trait (*FCQ-T*) scales for the different types of Eating Disorders. Mean scores of the nine scales of the Food Craving Questionnaire-Trait (*FCQ-T*) for Anorexia Nervosa-Restrictive (*ANR*), Anorexia Nervosa-Binge/Purging (*ANBP*), Bulimia Nervosa-Non-Purging (*BNNP*), and Bulimia Nervosa-Purging (*BNP*) participants. The order of scale presentation is Lack of Control over Eating (*LC*), Negative Affect (*NA*), Intentions to Eat (*IE*), Cue-Dependent Eating (*CD*), Preoccupation with Food (*PF*), Hunger (*H*), Guilty Feelings (*GF*), Negative Reinforcement (*NR*), and Positive Reinforcement (*PR*). Clearly, ANR patients reported the lowest levels of food cravings across the board, followed in ascending order by ANBP, BNNP, and BNP participants (Reprinted from Moreno et al. 2009b. With permission)

Overall, the above findings suggest that dietary restraint does not lead to food craving in individuals with AN. Food craving is associated with binge eating only in women diagnosed with BN. This result is congruent with the observation by Cepeda-Benito and Gleaves (2001) that a positive association between dietary restraint and food craving is confined to unsuccessful dieters.

161.5   Lack of Inhibitory Control on Physiological and Emotional Processes in Women with Bulimia Nervosa

Heart Rate Variability (HRV) has recently attracted the interest of scientists as an index of autonomic and emotional regulation. Thayer and Lane (2000) proposed a model of neurovisceral integration in which a network of neural structures associated with emotional and autonomic regulation is related to HRV via connections from the prefrontal cortex to the amygdala, and from the amygdala to the sympathetic and parasympathetic innervations of the heart. Numerous authors have found a negative association between vagally-mediated HRV and poor psychological and physiological functioning, including conditions characterized by a lack of impulse control, i.e., cravings (Ingjaldsson et al. 2003; Rodríguez-Ruiz et al. 2009). Experimental data also support a relationship between HRV and emotional regulation. High vagally-mediated HRV has been associated with larger orienting responses but faster habituation to nonthreat stimuli, whereas low HRV has been related to a failure to habituate (hypervigilance) and to greater defensive reactions (Thayer and Lane 2000).

The modulation of defensive reflexes also offers an interesting paradigm to examine autonomic and emotional regulation in BN. The magnitude of defense reflexes, such as the *startle motor reflex* and the *cardiac defense response* elicited by a brief acoustic probe stimulus, is augmented during viewing of unpleasant and threatening pictures and is reduced while viewing pleasant images (see Bradley 2000 and Vila et al. 2007, for review). The phenomenon has been explained, according to the *motivational priming hypothesis* (Lang 1995), as due to the congruence or incongruence between the emotional state induced by the pictures (positive versus negative) and the type of reflex being elicited (appetitive versus defensive): defensive reflexes are augmented if the organism is in a negative emotional state and reduced if the organism is in a positive emotional state.

Several studies have examined the modulation of defensive reflexes in people with eating disorders. Drobes et al. (2001) used this methodology to evaluate the affective state evoked by food stimuli in women who suffer from binge eating. The results showed that women who suffer from binge eating displayed an increased startle reflex when presented with food pictures. Nevertheless, some verbal, behavioral, and psychophysiological responses were consistent with an appetitive motivational reaction to food pictures, while other responses were consistent with a defensive one. Rodríguez et al. (2005) also found that the experience of chocolate craving included both appetitive (inhibition of the cardiac defense) and aversive (potentiation of the startle reflex) components. These findings suggested that the motivational circuits (appetitive and defensive) in women with bulimic symptomatology would be co-activated by food stimuli (Konorski 1967; Lang 1995).

Similarly, Mauler et al. (2006) studied the modulation of the eye-blink startle reflex while viewing food pictures in women without ED and those with BN (both groups under food deprivation and non-deprivation, respectively). Their findings showed a greater magnitude of the startle reflex to food pictures in women suffering from BN. However, food pictures did not elicit greater skin conductance responses in women with BN. These findings suggest that food pictures instead of provoking a typical fear response mediated by the sympathetic nervous system (*flight*) seem to provoke a disgust or anxiety response mediated by the parasympathetic nervous system. In addition, the startle reflex potentiation upon presentation of food pictures in patients with BN was attenuated by food deprivation, a finding also reported by Rodríguez et al. (2007b). Thus, a period of successful food restriction might create a sense of control over food and this may render it less threatening.

Overall, the above findings are congruent with the observation that food deprivation increases craving but reduces negative mood in BN participants (Moreno et al. 2009a). This observation suggests that negative affect primed by food cues might motivate dietary restraint to ameliorate the negative affect associated with food intake in women with BN. It could be argued that individuals with BN make food less threatening by demonstrating control over their consumption through restrained eating.

Nevertheless, it has been reported that the above findings are also modulated by individual differences in emotional regulation indexed by HRV. Rodríguez-Ruiz et al. (under review) found that food cues evoked negative emotional responses, comparable to those elicited by unpleasant stimuli, in deprived individuals with BN and low HRV. Participants with BN and low HRV exhibited a substantial potentiation of their blink response magnitudes to all stimulus categories (see Fig. 161.6),

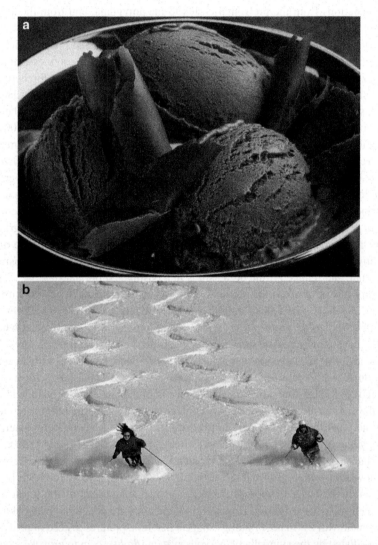

Fig. 161.6 Food, pleasant, neutral, and unpleasant stimuli used to examine the physiological reactivity of women with bulimia nervosa (*BN*). Food, pleasant, neutral, and unpleasant stimuli retrieved from Internet with similar content to the International Affective Picture System (*IAPS*) pictures used in the study of Rodríguez-Ruiz et al. (under review).

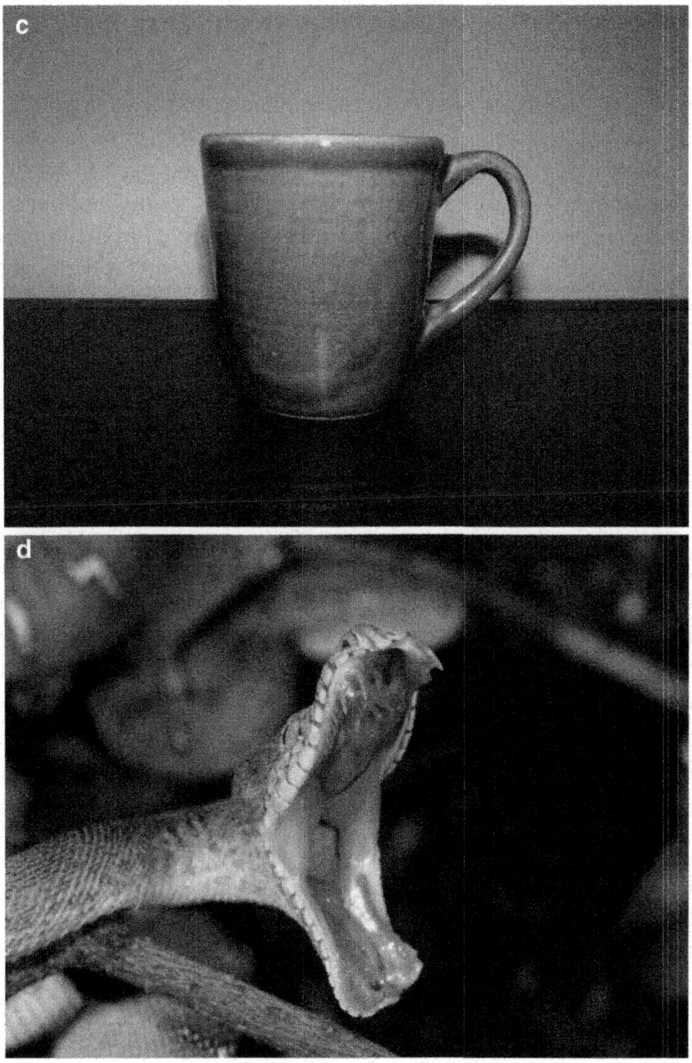

Fig. 161.6 (continued) All pictures provoked in women with bulimia nervosa and low HRV a greater eye-blink startle compared to those with bulimia nervosa and high heart rate variability (*HRV*), although food pictures evoked a blink response almost comparable to the augmentation that could be observed during the viewing of unpleasant emotional stimuli

although food pictures evoked a blink response almost comparable to the augmentation that could be observed during the viewing of unpleasant emotional stimuli. Deprived participants with BN and low HRV also labeled their feelings associated with food cues as more disgusting and uncontrollable than deprived participants with BN and high HRV and control participants.

Thus, our results confirm the inverse association between vagally-mediated HRV and psychological functioning (Thayer and Lane 2000). To sum up, HRV appears to modulate defensive reactions to food in BN individuals, supporting the hypothesis that poor emotional and autonomic regulation plays a role in the observed lack of inhibitory control in BN.

161.6 Applications to Other Areas of Health and Disease

The research reviewed in this chapter has potential applications. For example, IGT could become a useful tool for the assessment and treatment of ED patients. IGT provides an individual profile on the decision-making process of the individual and could be used to enhance the patient's awareness of the nature of his/her disease and improve patients' motivation for treatment compliance. IGT can also serve as a pre- and post-treatment measure to evaluate treatment outcome. IGT may be also useful in the detection of individuals at risk for ED. Finally, the data indirectly support the presence of neurological deficits in ED, with probable involvement of the frontal lobe, indicating that neuropsychological rehabilitation might be an appropriate treatment for these patients.

The clinical implications of the research on dietary restraint, food craving, and emotion in BN are twofold. First, it would be advisable, in the context of cue-exposure therapy, to elicit craving by means of manipulation other than mere food exposure and include strategies to modulate affective states, feelings of control over eating, and motivation to consume or avoid foods. The goal would be to elicit and extinguish the underlying craving factors that are most relevant to bingeing (e.g., negative affect and lack of control). Second, the effectiveness of cue exposure therapy might be increased if exposure is combined with physiological techniques aimed at improving emotional and autonomic regulation in patients with BN, as well as in patients with disorders characterized by lack of control (e.g., drug addiction). A number of nonpharmacological techniques have been used to increase HRV, including breathing training and HRV biofeedback (Lehrer et al. 1999). HRV biofeedback has been proposed as a powerful tool to help individuals learn emotional and autonomic self-regulation skills (Nolan et al. 2005).

Summary Points

- Impulsivity and loss of control seem to be the central clinical features that discriminate between bulimia and anorexia nervosas
- In our studies the women with bulimia nervosa experience lack of pleasure and control over both food-related and sexual impulses
- They showed significant motor impulsivity and an impairment of decision-making abilities based on short-term consequences, more negative mood, anxiety, and food craving than women with anorexia nervosa
- Prolonged fasting increased food craving and reduced negative emotions in women with bulimia nervosa since they escape from negative emotional states by fasting
- The positive association between dietary restraint and food craving is confined to unsuccessful dieters who lose control over eating as do women with bulimia nervosa
- In our studies the women with bulimia nervosa and low heart rate variability labeled their feelings associated with food cues as more disgusting and uncontrollable than women with bulimia nervosa and high heart rate variability
- To be effective, treatment interventions for bulimia nervosa must combine not only behavioral and neuropsychological approaches, but also physiological techniques aimed at improving emotional and autonomic regulation.

Definitions

International Affective Picture System [IAPS]: (Lang et al. 1999). The IAPS is an instrument for the study of emotion in laboratory settings. The IAPS is an instrument under continuous development created by the Center for the Study of Emotion and Attention, under the direction of Professor Peter J. Lang, at the University of Florida. It includes over 800 color photographs, in slide and digitalized format, belonging to different semantic categories: animals, nature scenes, house objects, naked people, erotic couples, human faces, mutilated bodies, weapons, food, sports, etc.

Self-Assessment Manikin [SAM]: (Lang 1980). The SAM is a universally applied instrument consisting of three pictographic nonverbal scales (valence, arousal, and control or dominance). It does not require language and is therefore easy to administer. The instrument provides information for each picture on three general emotional dimensions: valence (pleasant–unpleasant), arousal (activated–relaxed) and control (dominant–dominated).

Stroop task: (Stroop 1935). The Stroop task is a classic experimental paradigm to examine the Stroop interference effect, a measure of word reading's influence upon color naming. The procedure involves naming the color of a color word presented visually using the same or different color. The interference is quantified in terms of increase in reaction time to color naming when noun and presentation color are incongruent compared to the condition, in which they are congruent. The task demands resolution of a conflict between two competing tendencies, that of reading versus naming.

Go/No-Go task [GNG]: (Newman et al. 1985). The GNG is a computerized measure of motor impulsivity in which participants must try to inhibit their responses to certain stimuli, with the number of errors and false alarms indicating motor impulsivity.

Iowa Gambling Task [IGT]: (Bechara et al. 1994). The IGT is a computerized task that imitates a card game and is made up of 100 trials. Participants choose a card from one of four virtual decks (A, B, C, and D). Depending on the deck selected in each trial, the person gains (reward) or loses (punishment) symbolic money. Two of the decks, A and B, generate losses in the long term because, although profits are higher, so too are the losses. The other two decks, C and D, generate a profit in the long-term because the losses are smaller. The IGT score is calculated by subtracting the number of cards selected from decks A and B from the number of cards selected from decks C and D in each of the 5 blocks of 20 trials that comprise the task.

Food Craving Questionnaire-Trait [FCQ-T]: (Cepeda-Benito et al. 2000). The FCQ was created consistent with the theory that food cravings can arise from and be expressed as both physiologically and psychologically mediated processes. Using confirmatory Factor Analyses (CFA), the FCQ-T has yielded excellent fit indices for a nine-factor solution (e.g., Moreno et al. 2009b). The nine factor derived scales of the FCQ-T measure cravings experienced as or associated with: (1) *Positive Reinforcement*; (2) *Negative Reinforcement*; (3) *Cue-dependent Eating*; (4) *Feelings of Hunger*; (5) *Preoccupation with Food*; (6) *Intentions to Eat*; (7) *Lack of Control*; (8) *Negative Affect*; and (9) *Guilty Feelings*. The FCQ-T instructs participants to indicate how frequently each statement "would be true for you in general" using a six point scale that ranges from 1 (*Never or Not Applicable*) to 6 (*Always*). Full-scale and factor-scale totals can be calculated by simply adding the corresponding item scores.

> **Startle motor reflex [SMR]:** (Lang 1995). The SMR is a pattern of motor activation elicited by sudden intense stimulation. The SMR in humans is based on the psychophysiological recording via the electromiography (EMG) of the orbicularis oculi muscle. The pattern and magnitude of the response can be obtained through both raw EMG and filtered EMG.
>
> **Cardiac defense response [CDR]:** (Vila et al. 2007). The CDR is a complex pattern of heart rate changes to an intense acoustic stimulus with accelerative and decelerative components that appear in an alternate sequential order (acceleration–deceleration–acceleration–deceleration) during the 80 s following the presentation of the stimulus.

Acknowledgments The present research was supported by grants from the Spanish Ministry of Science and Technology, the European Union (projects BSO 2001-3015, BSO 2001-3211, and SEJ 2005-06699), and the Junta de Andalucía (research group HUM-388).

References

Agras WS, Telch CF. Behav Ther. 1998;29:491–503.

American Psychiatric Association. Diagnostic and statistical manual of mental disorders. 4th ed. Text revision. Washington, DC: Author; 2000.

Bechara A, Damasio AR, Damasio H, Anderson SW. Cognition. 1994;50:7–15.

Black CM, Wilson GT, Labouvie E, Heffernan K. Int J Eat Disord. 1997;22:329–33.

Bradley MM. In: Cacioppo JT, Tassinary LG, Berntson GG, editors. Handbook of psychophysiology. New York: Cambridge University Press; 2000. p. 602–642.

Bradley MM, Lang PJ. In: Cacioppo JT, Tassinary LG, Berntson GG, editors. Handbook of psychophysiology. 3rd ed. New York: Cambridge University Press; 2007.

Cash TF, Deagle EA. Int J Eat Disord. 1996;22:107–25.

Cavallo DA, Pinto A. Eat Behav. 2001;2:113–27.

Cavedini P, Bassi T, Ubbiali A, Casolari A, Giordani S, Zorzi C, Bellodi S. Psychiatry Res. 2004;127:259–66.

Cepeda-Benito A, Gleaves D. In: Hetherington M, editor. Food cravings and addiction. Leatherhead: Surrey; 2001. p. 3–29.

Cepeda-Benito A, Gleaves DH, Williams TL, Erath ST. Behav Ther. 2000;31:151–73.

Davis C, Levitan RD, Muglia P, Bewell C, Kennedy JL. Obesity Research. 2004;12:929–35.

Drobes DJ, Miller EJ, Hillman CH, Bradley MM, Cuthbert BN, Lang PJ. Biol Psychol. 2001;57:153–77.

Duchesne M, Mattos P, Fontenelle LF, Veiga H, Rizo L, Appolinaro JC. Rev Bras Psiquiatr. 2004;26:107–17.

FairburnCG. In: Brownell KD, Fairburn CG, editors. Eating disorders and obesity: a comprehensive handbook. New York: Guildford Press; 1995.

Fassino S, Pieró A, Daga GA, Leombruni P, Mortara P, Rovera GG. Int J Eat Disord. 2002;31:274–83.

Gendall KA, Joyce PR, Sullivan PF. Appetite. 1997;28:63–72.

Heatherton TF, Polivy J. In: Crowther J, Hobfall SE, Stephens MAP, Tennenbaum DL, editors. The etiology of bulimia: the individual and familial context. Washington, DC: Hemisphere; 1992. p. 135–155.

Hill AJ, Weaver CFL, Blundell JE. Food craving, dietary restraint and mood. Appetite. 1991;17:187–97.

Ingjaldsson JT, Laberg JC, Thayer JF. Biol Psychiatry. 2003;54:1427–36.

Katzma MA, Wolchick SA. J Consult Clin Psychol. 1984;52:423–8.

Koch M, Schnitzler HU. Behav Brain Res. 1997;89:35–49.

Konorski J. Integrative activity of de brain: an interdisciplinary approach. Chicago: University of Chicago Press; 1967.

Lang PJ. In: Sidowski JB, Johnson JH, Williams TA, editors. Technology in mental health care delivery systems. Norwood: Ablex; 1980. p. 119–137.

Lang PJ. Am Psychol. 1995;50:372–85.

Lang PJ, Bradley MM, Cuthbert BN. The international affective picture system: technical manual and affective ratings. Gainesville: The Center for Research in Psychophysiology, University of Florida; 1999.

Lehrer P, Sasaki Y, Saito Y. Psychosom Med. 1999;61:812–21.

Mann T, Ward A. J Abnorm Psychol. 2004;113:90–8.

Matsunaga H, Kiriike N, Iwasaki Y, Miyata A, Matsui T. Int J Eat Disord. 2000;27:348–52.

Mauler BI, Hamm AO, Weike, AI, Tuschen-Caffier B. J Abnorm Psychol. 2006;115:567–79.

Moreno S. Rodríguez-Ruiz S, Fernández-Santaella MC. ?Qué es el ansia por la comida? Manuales Prácticos. Madrid: Pirámide; 2009a.

Moreno S, Warren CW, Rodríguez S, Fernández M.C., Cepeda-Benito A. Appetite. 2009b;52:588–94.

Nederkoorn C, Van Eijs Y, Jansen A. Pers Individ Differ. 2004;37:1651–8.

Newman J, Widom C, Nathan S. J Pers Soc Psychol. 1985;48:1316–27.

Nolan R, Kamath MV, Floras JS, Stanley J, Pang C, Picton P, Young QR. Am Heart J. 2005;149:1137.

Ortega-Roldán B, Rodríguez S, Moreno S, Morandé G, Fernández MC. In: Chambers N, editor. Binge eating: psychological factors, symptoms, and treatment. New York: Novascience; 2009.

Pirke KM. In Brownell KD, Fairburn CG, editors. Eating disorders and obesity: a comprehensive handbook. New York: Guildford Press; 1995.

Rodríguez-Ruiz S, Ruiz-Padial E, Vera MN, Fernández, MC, Anllo-Vento L, Vila J. J Psychophysiol. 2009;23:95–103

Rodríguez-Ruiz S, Moreno S, Guerra PM, Fernández MC, Vila J. J Psychophysiol. [under review].

Rodríguez S, Fernández MC, Cepeda-Benito A, Vila J. Biol Psychol. 2005;70 (1):9–18.

Rodríguez S, Mata JL, Lameiras M, Fernández MC Vila J. Eur Eat Disord Rev. 2007a;15 (3):231–9.

Rodríguez S, Mata JL, Moreno S, Fernández MC, Vila J. Psicothema. 2007b;19:30–6.

Rosval L, Steiger H, Bruce K, Israël M, Richardson J, Aubut M. Int J Eat Disord. 2006;39:590–3.

Stroop JR. J Exp Psychol Gen. 1935;18:643–62.

Thayer JF, Lane RD. J Affect Disord. 2000;61:201–16.

Troop NA. Eur Eat Disord Rev. 1998;6:229–37.

Uher R, Murphy T, Brammer MJ, Dalgleish T, Phillips ML, Ng VW, Andrew CM, Williams SCR, Campbell I, Treasure J. Am J Psychiatry. 2004;161:1238–46.

Vila J, Guerra P, Muñoz MA, Vico C, Viedma MI, Delgado LC, Perakakis P, Kley E, Mata JL, Rodríguez S. Int J Psychophysiol. 2007;66 (3):169–82.

Waters A, Hill A, Waller G. Behav Res Ther. 2001;39:877–86.

Wiederman MW, Pryor T. Int J Eat Disord. 1997;22:395–401.

Zerbe KJ. The body betrayed: Women, eating disorders, and treatment. Washington, DC: American Psychiatric Press; 1993.

Zuckerman M. Behavioral expressions and biosocial bases of sensation seeking. New York: Cambridge University Press; 1994.

Chapter 162
Experiences of Women with Bulimia Nervosa

Abbreviations

CBT   Cognitive behavioral treatment
DBT   Dialectical behavioral treatment
DSM IV TR Diagnostic and Statistical Manual of Mental Disorders, Fourth Edition, Text Revision.
EMDR   Eye movement desensitization and reprocessing

162.1 Introduction

The following chapter reflects qualitative data collected as part of a broader study that sought to understand how college-age women with bulimia nervosa experienced participating in a Mindfulness-Based Eating Disorder Treatment Group (Proulx 2008). In that phenomenological study, six college-age women who met the DSM-IV-TR criteria for bulimia nervosa (APA 2000) were interviewed prior to the group by the researcher. Initial data was collected and self-portraits were completed. Then the participants attended an 8-week mindfulness group designed and facilitated by the researcher. Journal data was collected during the group and the researcher kept notes for each group. When the group was completed, the researcher again interviewed each participant to explore their experience of the group. Final self-portraits were completed at that time. In addition to having bulimia nervosa for several years, participants also had comorbid mood or anxiety disorders and some were taking psychotropic medications. None of the participants met DSM-IV-TR criteria for substance abuse or Dissociative Identity Disorder (Table 162.1).

162.2 Bulimia Nervosa

In response to the cultural idealization of thinness, over 50% of adolescent girls think they are overweight and consequently diet (Fisher et al. 1995). Moreover, 5–10 million adolescent girls and women in the USA are estimated to struggle with eating disorders (National Eating Disorders Association 2006). Bulimia nervosa occurs in 1–4% of American college-age women (APA 2000).

K. Proulx (✉)
Mental Health Services, University of Massachusetts, Hills North, Amherst, MA 01103
e-mail: kproulx@nursing.umass.edu

V.R. Preedy et al. (eds.), *Handbook of Behavior, Food and Nutrition*,
DOI 10.1007/978-0-387-92271-3_162, © Springer Science+Business Media, LLC 2011

Table 162.1 Key features of bulimia nervosa

- Recurrent episodes of binge eating characterized by both:
  1. Eating, in a discrete period of time (e.g., within any 2-h period), an amount of food that is definitely larger than most people would eat during a similar period of time and under similar circumstances
  2. A sense of lack of control over eating during the episode, defined by a feeling that one cannot stop eating or control what or how much one is eating
- Recurrent inappropriate compensatory behavior to prevent weight gain
  1. Self-induced vomiting
  2. Misuse of laxatives, diuretics, enemas, or other medications
  3. Fasting
  4. Excessive exercise
- The binge eating and inappropriate compensatory behavior both occur, on average, at least twice a week for 3 months.
- Self evaluation is unduly influenced by body shape and weight.
- Gradually binge eating becomes a response to emotional upset. It functions to reduce stress and is triggered by such emotions as anxiety, anger, and depression.

This table lists key criteria of bulimia nervosa as identified by the Diagnostic and Statistical Manual of Mental Disorders

Bulimia nervosa typically begins with a fear of weight gain and the need for dieting (Fairburn and Cooper 1982; Pipher 1994). Self-imposed starvation eventually leads to binge eating in 30–50% of patients with anorexia nervosa referred for treatment (Garfinkel et al. 1980; Hsu et al. 1979). The gradual breakdown of self-control and the emergence of binge eating typically occur about 9 months after the initiation of dieting (Garfinkel et al. 1980).

An episode of binge eating is characterized by eating, within a 2-h period of time, an amount of food that is definitely larger than most people would eat during a similar period of time in similar circumstances (APA 2000). Individuals with bulimia nervosa experience a sense of lack of control over their eating during the episode including the feeling either that one cannot stop eating, control how much one is eating, or control the type of foods eaten. Recurrent inappropriate compensatory behaviors include self-induced vomiting, the misuse of laxatives, diuretics, diet pills, medications, fasting, and excessive exercise. Individuals with bulimia nervosa are often normal weight or overweight, making it a hidden disorder.

Gradually, the eating binges get separated from mealtime or desire for food and become more and more a response to emotional upset. Once bulimia is entrenched, it functions to reduce stress and is triggered by such emotions as anxiety, anger, and depression. Over time, the behavior takes on a life of its own where eventually pleasure and normal interpersonal relationships are replaced by compulsion, secrecy, and guilt. According to Bruch (1988), the drive for excessive thinness experienced by young women with bulimia nervosa acts as a "cage" that constricts their psychological growth and the development of a genuine self.

Many women with bulimia nervosa are disconnected from their bodies and feelings, rendering them easily influenced by cultural pressures and peer expectations (Brown and Gilligan 1992; Pipher 1994). These women experience low self-esteem, anxiety, depression, and interpersonal difficulties (Bruch 1988).

162.3 Methodological Considerations

This chapter will focus on the phenomenology of living with bulimia nervosa as it emerged thematically from the qualitative data. Data analysis was completed from a phenomenological, interpretive Hermeneutic perspective (Husserl 1913/1983; Van Manen 1990), which included my own process of self-reflection throughout every aspect of the study (Drew 1999, 2001, 2004). Once the data from the initial assessments, interview transcripts, self portraits, and journals were closely examined and highlighted, common themes were identified and then synthesized into an integrated whole.

162.4 Thematic Analysis of Living with Bulimia Nervosa

This section will present themes that emerged from the data analysis related to the participants' sense of self, coping skills, and interpersonal relationships. The first theme, "Waging War on a Fragile Self," is divided into two major subsections. The first subsection entitled the "Fragile Self" describes how the participants see themselves and reveals the highly judgmental quality of their attitudes towards themselves. The second subsection in this theme entitled "Waging War as a Means of Gaining Control" addresses how the participants try to cope with the day-to-day stress experienced in their lives. Family and cultural influences on identity and women's roles are imbedded within these themes. The names of the six participants: Ana, Kelley, Rena, Sophia, Eva, and Ruth as they appear below are fictitious to preserve their confidentiality.

162.5 Waging War on a Fragile Self

162.5.1 The Fragile Self

Each of the participants identified that their experience of themselves felt fragmented and incongruent. Their sense of self changed in different environments and seemed to vacillate between extremes. They internalized the media images of beauty and strove to achieve this standard of thinness as the most important measure of self worth and success.

Because of their high degree of disconnection from themselves, they were unable to receive accurate feedback from their bodies. They unanimously experienced self-loathing and distorted body perceptions. The commonalities of their experiences related to self are organized as follows: Hiding the truth, Hating myself, Distorting my body, and Keeping me from where I want to be.

162.5.1.1 Hiding the Truth: I Am Not Who I Seem On the Outside

Kelley is a graduate student who has experienced symptoms of bulimia nervosa for approximately 14 years (Fig. 162.1). Her problems with eating and body image began following a motor vehicle accident that immobilized her for several months. She abruptly went from having been very physically active to total inertia and began to gain weight. As she reflects on her first self-portrait in which she drew two separate images of herself, she comments that the two images are "polar opposites of me." "There is the completely horrible, ugly, fat way I feel inside which is also the way I think that other people see me now, and a 19 year old version of me that is thin, pretty, perfect, very put together, and confident."

In her initial self-portrait Kelley draws two completely separate versions of herself reflecting her sense of "being split within myself, like there are multiple versions of me in here."

Rena, a college junior with a performance major, describes herself as being made up of "sunshine and happiness which is the ultimate of what I want from life, as well as fatigue and depression, which

Fig. 162.1 Kelley's self portrait. This figure represents Kelley's first self-portrait. The left image represents the idealized, thin confident self and the right image is the horrible, ugly, fat, totally devalued self

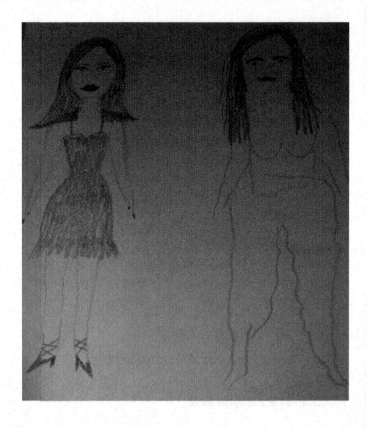

is a plague on my life and not so good." She points out that in her first self-portrait, love was surrounding her but was outside of her. Her focus was on being thin, pretty, and perfect in order to attract the prince who would provide her with love so she could feel sunny and happy evermore.

She was hoping for a man to feed her the love she craved so she could feel good about herself (Fig. 162.2). She believed that in order for any man to love her, she had to be thin and beautiful. When a man would hurt or reject her she would blame herself and think, "What did I do wrong? What's wrong with me? Look at my stomach, that's why it all went wrong."

Before the start of one group, Rena verbally told me she was having a very stressful day and was feeling quite depressed, all the while smiling, laughing, and impeccably dressed and groomed. Her affect and appearance were incongruent with her verbal description of how she was feeling and how she had experienced her day.

Sophia, a graduating senior, has had problems with bulimia nervosa since middle school. She is interested in Buddhism and feminism and so remarks about her "inability to find a middle ground", a topic she has been writing about all semester. She sees herself as "vacillating between extremes and torn between all the dichotomies of life." Sophia approaches every interpersonal situation with pre-planned ideas of "who I think I am and how I think I ought to act or how I've got to be." She adds, "When I am in a room with a bunch of people I would become those people. They envelop me instead of me being able to stay grounded in myself. I don't feel a core self."

Ruth is a junior student experiencing some academic problems this semester due to her mood instability and problems with focus and concentration. Out of all the women, Ruth was the most apprehensive about participating in a group. She had never joined a group before and indicated that her greatest fear was "hearing about my problem coming out of someone else's mouth." Secrets are really important to Ruth, which is why she was so apprehensive about coming to the group. She had

Fig. 162.2 Rena's self
portrait. This figure
represents Rena's first
self-portrait. It depicts her
belief that she must be thin,
pretty, and perfect in order to
attract the prince whose love
would bring her happiness.
She is dependent on external
sources for validation and
love

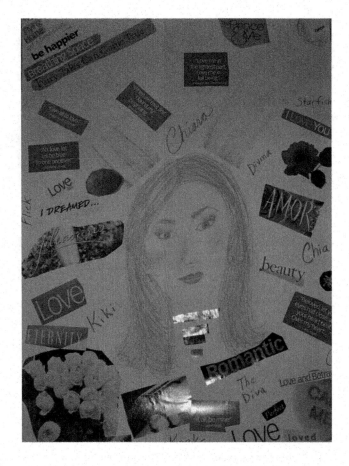

never told anyone about her eating disorder. She was ambivalent about keeping her secrets in that, although her secrets made her feel special, they also kept her separate from others. She worked hard at presenting herself as happy, funny, outgoing, and competent but expressed the following in her journal: "Fucking body. Fucking secrets. DO YOU UNDERSTAND THAT I AM NOT ON THE OUTSIDE THIS PERSON ON PAPER – DO YOU UNDERSTAND? I like who I am on the outside; I love myself. I am a very good person. Nobody knows. My mom knows about my anxiety and depression, but I still have my fucking secrets (bulimia, cutting), even from her."

Ana, a graduate student, who continues to live with her abusive parents admits, "I have to be two different people, like I am one person inside the house with my family but as soon as I step outside the house, I become somebody else, like I have to smile." Ana recognizes that she so urgently wants "approval from authority figures and peers that I won't rock the boat or stir up trouble for fear that people won't respect or like me." The outcome is that she sacrifices getting her needs met or creating authentic connections in her life, especially with herself. She is frustrated with herself, "I need to find myself in me but I don't know how to do that. I don't know how to be happy in myself." With respect to connections with others she describes, "I always tried to hide myself behind my hair…so people wouldn't see my face (Fig. 162.3)."

Eva was an undergraduate freshman and the youngest member of the group with a history of trauma, depression, and bulimia nervosa. She was experiencing significant emotional distress over the first 3 weeks of the group, frequently tearful and, on one occasion, needing to be seen at urgent care at the health service for symptoms of anxiety. Of all the participants, Eva was perhaps the least

Fig. 162.3 Ana's self portrait. This figure represents Ana's first self-portrait. It demonstrates her preoccupation with weight and how her sense of self is totally connected to her external appearance

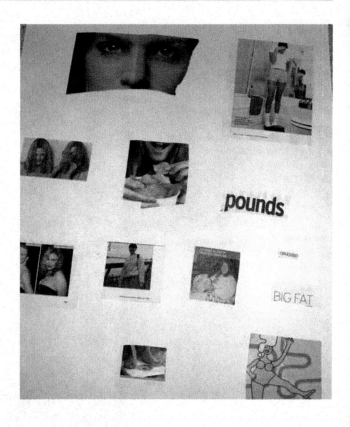

verbal about her experience in the group but as you will see below her initial self-portrait is quite remarkable with respect to the experience of self-fragmentation (Fig. 162.4).

It is evident from Eva's self-portrait that she experienced herself as fragmented, disconnected, and barely held together.

162.5.1.2 Hating Myself

All the participants believed their sense of self worth was entirely contingent on perfectionistic standards of accomplishment and external validation and approval from others. The women were consistently self-critical and judgmental and felt the need to constantly compare themselves to others.

Ruth describes her tendency towards self-criticism, "I'm sooo hard on myself… I bash, I bash, I bash…I'll say, Damn, I should have done that. And then all the would'ves, could'ves, should'ves cross my mind. I am judging myself without even thinking about it."

Eva explains that she is "overly self-critical" and describes "a constant barrage of negative self-talk such as 'You know you're not doing this right'." Or "Why can't I do it correctly?" She adds that if she falls short of her goals or self-expectations, she is "devastated." Her self worth is reliant on her accomplishments, primarily in the academic realm. She is generally unaccepting of her body shape and size and feels self-conscious about her appearance.

Rena was a performer who had several shows at the end of the semester. These were very stressful experiences for her. She shared that she is very critical of her performances so that, even if people she admires complement her, she continues to doubt and degrade her abilities. "I can never say I'm

Fig. 162.4 Eva's self portrait. This figure represents Eva's first self-portrait. It clearly depicts the fragility of Eva's sense of self

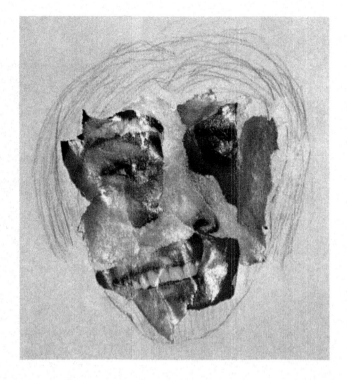

proud of my performance because there's always something wrong with it." She uses words such as "heferly" and "walrus" to describe her body size, even if others reassure her she is attractive.

Both Ruth and Ana had actresses on their original self-portraits reflecting the cultural image of what is valued as real beauty. Actresses in our culture set the standards for beauty and the ideal towards which women should strive. The actresses on their posters (Elizabeth Taylor, Katherine Hepburn, Renee Zellweiger) were thin, beautiful, glamorous women whom Ruth and Ana actually resembled (Fig. 162.5).

162.5.1.3 Distorting the Body

The women objectified their bodies as a "thing" to be "controlled and manipulated". They regarded their bodies as nonself, thereby justifying their regular abuse of their bodies. By placing their highly judgmental focus on their objectified bodies, they were distracted from the painful underlying emotional turmoil they felt powerless to change. As the women strove to meet self-imposed, perfectionistic standards, their level of stress rose, which they then took out on their objectified body, creating a never-ending cycle of self-dissatisfaction, failure, and guilt.

In reflecting on her first self-portrait in which she depicts two distinctly separate selves (Fig. 162.1), Kelley notes that in the right hand self representation,

> I didn't even have a neck because I just did not feel at all connected to my body. I could not feel anything; I was just numb. I perceived it more like the Michelin Tire man, the one that's like a stack of tires, like a snowman. That's kind of how I felt, like a series of ripples of fat stacked together or something. But I was missing any connection between my body and mind.

Kelley remembers that while some people may not like what they see when they look in a mirror, she took it one step further, "When I looked in the mirror I would simply say that isn't me." She totally

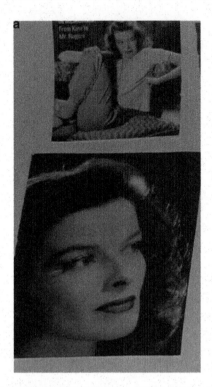

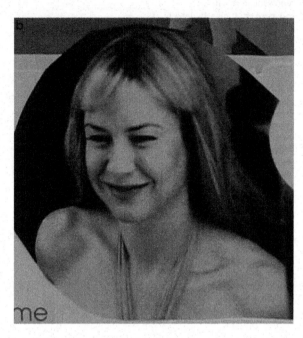

Fig. 162.5 Part of Ruth's self portrait (**a**). Part of Ana's self portrait (**b**). These figures display components of Ruth and Ana's Self-portraits related to their idealization and identification with glamorous movie stars who are held as the standard of beauty in our culture

refused to have a conscious connection with her body. She further illustrates her disconnection from her body by recounting this story, "A couple of years ago I wanted to know what I looked like to other people so I actually took pictures of myself without my head because I didn't want to know that it was me." She adds that she has no pictures of herself after the age of 23.

Following a body scan, Ruth commented that if her stomach could talk with her it would say, "You hurt me with all you put me through." Her response was "You know, I'd think about my stomach as another unit, a thing, not a part of me."

In looking at her first self-portrait (Fig. 162.2), Rena remembers that she deliberately left off her body because "There is so much more I can think and laugh about without having to worry about the thing that's attached to my head." She confesses she had thoughts of "just wanting to get a knife and cutting off her abdomen" she hated it so much.

In exploring with Ana ways that she could begin to nurture herself more she observed,

> I guess I don't recognize my body as being important or valid. I know that my body needs to be taken care of and that it doesn't deserve all the treatment from my parents and myself, its just so much easier for me to be caring to somebody else.

162.5.1.4 Keeping Me from Where I Want To Be

As the participants reflected on their earlier self-portraits, significant insights emerged regarding the depths of their inner emptiness and emotional fragility, inability to tolerate the intensity of their emotions, and unending fears of not being good enough or lovable. Although each of these women was

Fig. 162.6 Part of Ruth's self portrait (**a**). This figure was included in Ruth's initial self-portrait. Ruth felt that her bipolar disorder and intense moods interfered with her ability to reach her full potential and created problems in her relationships

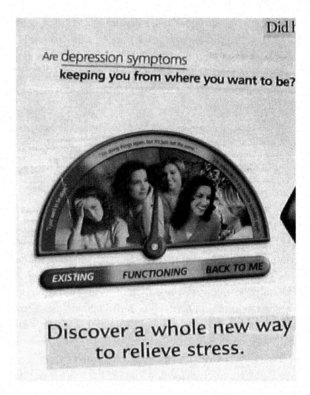

obsessively focusing on body shape and size, controlling all aspects of eating and exercise, they clearly felt out of control and overwhelmed on an emotional level.

The women identified experiencing very intense emotions that were difficult to regulate and that interfered with their functioning at times. Anxiety was a common emotion that frequently escalated to the level of panic. Most of the women had been treated for symptoms of depression. One woman had bipolar disorder. Several women had experienced significant traumatic events in their lives. The angry feelings experienced by the women were primarily viewed as negative and frightening. Participants also identified guilty feelings, for not being good daughters, for displeasing others, or in response to their own anger.

In her initial self-portrait (Fig. 162.6), Ruth poses the question: "Are depression symptoms keeping you from where you want to be?" She worries,

that question will go with me for the rest of my life. Right now it's keeping me from where I want to go. It kept my grandmother from going where she wanted to go. Sometimes I just break down uncontrollably and I can't…I lose all control, and that's really scary. In the past I would take out my anger and frustration on the people closest to me, like my family. I would beat them with words and I felt so bad afterwards.

Eva shared with the group that she has problems managing her anger. When faced with conflict within her family she would become very angry and retreat to her room, slamming the door and turning off communication. During family therapy she learned how to be assertive and has found that helpful. She has had problems with depression since age 16 and there is a maternal family history of depression as well. During the time of the mindfulness group, Eva was having symptoms of panic, which was making it difficult for her to sit through class, thereby interfering with her schoolwork.

Sophia recalls being an angry, difficult child and that she frequently expressed her anger through head-banging behaviors. She first experienced depression as a high school sophomore, which included irritability and self-harming behaviors. She describes being abusive to her boyfriend at the time. In addition, Sophia experiences problems with social anxiety that can culminate in panic attacks. Her mother also has a history of depression and eating disorder. As a result of her experiences within her family and her own depression, anxiety, and bulimia, Sophia had difficulty feeling positive about herself and establishing healthy relationships. She often felt that she lost herself in relationships with others.

> If you threw me in a room with a bunch of people and they were the only people I had to interact with, I am afraid that I would become those people, and that's really scary. Especially when lets say, it's a room full of misogynists, which leaves me hating myself. That's why I fear looking at magazines and stuff like that, because I feel like it will envelop me, instead of me being able to take a position against it.

Rena has experienced symptoms of depression since seventh grade marked by extreme self-criticism and thoughts of hopelessness such as "life is not worth living." She also can become highly anxious and experience panic attacks. Rena's mother and maternal extended family have been treated for depression. Rena recognizes that the level of self-hatred and self-criticism she experiences can have a detrimental effect on her performance and will hinder her career aspirations.

Kelley tracks the onset of her depression to her father's unexpected death by motor vehicle accident. Her father's death was very difficult for Kelley and she continues to harbor guilt feelings. Her anxiety and depression have kept her feeling dependent and inadequate. She admits there is a part of her that is terrified of finishing her degree and beginning a professional career beyond the university. Because of this, she delayed her comprehensive exams and remained in an abusive relationship for quite some time.

Ana experiences intense feelings of grief and sadness for the childhood she did not have within her abusive family. She often blames herself for the abuse and explains,

> I feel like the abuse is my fault, like I haven't been that good to my parents; or like I'm betraying them if I get angry about the way they treat me. The anger goes inside and that's what like goes to the eating and stuff because there's no other place for it. Usually my parents focus their abuse on me and I take some pride in the fact that this protects my two younger brothers; but if my brothers do something really crazy and my parents focus on them, I feel guilty since I'm the oldest and should protect them.

Ana also experiences symptoms of panic when her mother is berating her for long periods of time. She typically turns her emotions against herself rather than externalizing them. She is desperate for approval from others so avoids conflict as much as possible. She has learned to experience pleasure somewhat vicariously by observing others having fun, with little expectation of experiencing happiness for herself.

162.5.2 Waging War as a Means of Gaining Control

This second subsection of the theme describes the strategies used by the participants to cope with stress in their daily lives. Their choice of coping methods is connected to their experience of themselves as described above. Although in the short term the strategies they used helped to lower the intensity of their emotional turmoil, over time these choices perpetuated their sense of fragmentation, ineffectiveness, and lack of control within themselves and within the world. Their experiences are synthesized as follows: Numbing out; Going into Trance; Binging; Purging; Weighing, Measuring and Constantly Comparing; Cutting; and Abusing Alcohol and Pot.

162.5.2.1 Numbing Out

Many of the participants unconsciously used denial rather than face the emotional pain of their situations, particularly in relation to family dysfunction and past trauma. Being aware of and facing

emotional pain is very difficult for all of us, but for the women in this study who experienced a fragmented, inadequate sense of self, it was especially overwhelming.

Sophia experienced a great deal of emotional numbness to create an illusion of calm. She became
aware of this emotional numbness while completing self-awareness assignments in the group.
In attempting to notice pleasant and unpleasant events she recognized that she does not allow herself
to experience any emotions at all. She explained,

> Numbness is not in and of itself a bad thing. It's sort of like a placid thing. It becomes problematic when some-
> thing is being covered up or isn't being handled. Its harder to notice problems when things are placid, so then a
> variety of symptoms may emerge such as anxiety, depression, and bulimia nervosa.

Sophia used a great deal of numbing out to avoid her angry, sad feelings about her family situation.
She did not feel comfortable with those feelings and preferred to feel nothing.

162.5.2.2 Going into Trance

Going into trance is another way that participants unconsciously tried to manage powerful, unpleasant
feelings. When the stress of a situation was sufficiently high, an alternate mode of consciousness
took over to protect them from the painful feelings of their current experience.

In describing her choice of spiral as a representation of herself, Sophia explained, "the spiral
characterizes the experience of a drowning kind of hypnotic thing, like falling into a tunnel, and
where your mind goes away (Fig. 162.7)."

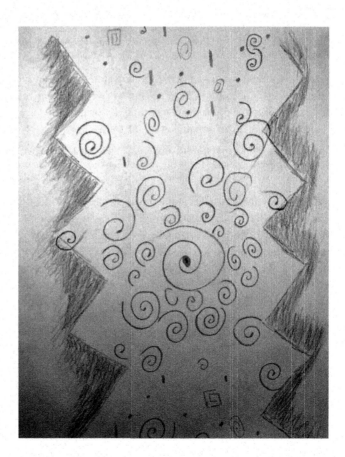

Fig. 162.7 Sophia's self
portrait. This figure
represents Sophia's self-
portrait. She describes that
the spirals represent her
tendency to use dissociation
to cope with stress. Several of
the women describe
dissociation as part of the
binge–purge cycle

In situations where she experiences extreme emotional distress such as when her mother is verbally abusing her or she experiences personal rejection, Ana described the following,

> When I get very wound up there's something inside me that I feel like is not even me, that automatically sets in and I can't stop it. Its like I go into a trance and binging is all I can think about. Nothing's satisfied until the binge is over. The trance takes over and everything else stops.

Ana has not found a way to stop the trance from occurring. Nor has she found anything that soothes her as completely as a binge when she is feeling her worst emotionally.

162.5.2.3 Binging

Several of the participants identified that when they felt stressed, they frequently binged. Binging with food was self-soothing. Binges were frequently anticipated in advance and a great deal of time and energy went into the planning. Social opportunities were passed up if they would interfere with the binge. Guilt and shame commonly followed the binge, triggering the urge to purge or to socially isolate.

Ana has occasional success with delaying the urge to binge but she notes that there are times when she wants to binge and will consciously choose to binge because she has been unable to find anything else that is as self-soothing. She is aware that the urge to binge is associated with stress and remembers that she started eating instead of crying during high school. "My mother was always big on appearances so when I began to wear mascara in high school I stopped crying because I had to look good and crying would cause my mascara to run." Moreover,

> I didn't want my parents to have the satisfaction of seeing me cry. I knew they had control over everything I did and I didn't want them to have control over me too. I guess I always thought of crying as weakness and once my parents knew how to get to me they would use it against me over and over. I didn't want to give them something else to hurt me with. With eating, once I cleaned up all the food, they never noticed.

Ana knows the locations of many grocery stores between school and home. She will buy food in the store and eat it secretly in her car. She worries what her roommate thinks when large quantities of food come into the dorm room and quickly disappear.

Ruth describes the previous week as follows,

> I didn't stop eating and throwing up one after the other. I couldn't sit still, I didn't sit while I ate, I jumped around fidgeting, scrounging around in my cabinets looking for more to eat. Right now, I don't have enough money to eat normally, never mind to binge with. I sneak into the dining halls and go crazy.

When Kelley feels anxious and depressed she goes to fast food restaurants, buys large quantities of fast food, isolates in her apartment, and eats and sleeps for an entire weekend. She will cancel social obligations, not do any work, and stay in bed around the clock. If friends come to her door she won't let them in because all the food wrappers are visible. Other times she will purchase large quantities of food at the grocery store, spread it out on her bed, and eat is as fast as she can. Kelley bakes desserts in large quantities, which she rarely eats but just keeps in her apartment or sends to relatives.

When Sophia feels stressed she isolates in her room and eats large quantities of whatever food is available, although she prefers sugary foods and carbohydrates such as ice cream, cake, or cereal. She eats until she literally feels ill and then stays alone until the gastric symptoms subside. She alternates between the extremes of binging and restricting and struggles to achieve moderation. Sophia shared her story of buying an entire cake for herself in preparation for a binge. She had the bakery write "happy birthday Joe" on the top of the cake so that if she ran into a classmate, she then had a story to hide her true purpose. She remembers occasions even in middle school where she would binge on food on returning home from having been out socially with friends.

162.5.2.4 Purging

Purging refers to the compensatory behaviors participants used to rid their body of the food or calories resulting from a binge. The two main purging behaviors that the women reported using were inducing vomiting or compulsive, rigorous exercise. Each of these will be described below.

162.5.2.5 Vomiting

Each of the participants acknowledged that stress and anxiety led to purging behaviors. Purging generally followed eating, and was not always in response to a binge. Just the sensation of food in the stomach could result in purging. For most participants, vomiting was cyclical in relation to stress levels and could occur following every meal. Following the initial lowering of anxiety that resulted from vomiting, guilt and shame frequently ensued. The women felt isolated by their secret behaviors. For some vomiting could occur spontaneously with minimal or no inducement.

On spring break Ruth went home to visit her family. She and her mother went to a tearoom for lunch and Ruth ate tiny tea sandwiches, scones, and drank tea. She wrote in her journal,

> Such a nice place and what do I do? I got up to the bathroom and threw it up! Then what? The toilet didn't flush the vomit away (which Ruth has perfected over the years). Then I noticed a sign *Antique Plumbing*. Blah, Blah, Shit! What do I do?!!! Panic. People are outside waiting! Waiting! I wait until the water stops hissing and flush a second time but still lettuce is floating on top. I try to sift it out with my fingers, but still a few left. Why didn't I throw up in the garbage? Sometimes I do that. Throw up in paper towel and stick it under wads of used towels. I flush a third time and walk out. Panicky that people next in line will know. Will they say something? My hands are shaking; itty-bitty shakes that rattle my teacup. My chest is aching, pressure.

Ruth has been purging since high school. Her eating symptoms began as restricting (anorexia) but then she switched to binging and purging since the effects of bulimia could be hidden from her mother. Her binging and purging episodes may be correlated with her mood swings. There are stretches of time when she purges multiple times a day at least following every meal alternating with a period of time when she is not binging or purging at all or only a few times per week. Generally if she is eating more than she would like, she will purge. If her eating is restricted, there is less need to purge.

As a performer, there are times when Rena cannot purge since this adversely affects her performance. At times, she has performances daily over the course of a week. She relates that, "As soon as my performances are over, the first thing I do after I eat is just purge." She notes that when she feels very stressed she finds it difficult to tolerate the feeling of food in her stomach. Usually purging will alleviate the feeling and lower her stress. At those times when it is not possible for her to purge, she may then engage in self-mutilation as an alternative means of lowering her stress.

Kelley has purged for so long, it happens reflexively with minimal stimulation. Just brushing her teeth results in vomiting. She has to warn her dentist to use a light touch or she vomits in the chair. Kelley tends to vomit every morning on awakening without any noticeable precipitant. On one occasion she began to wretch in my office while exploring deeply emotional issues related to her fears of taking care of herself as an adult.

162.5.2.6 Exercising

An alternative way to purge is through excessive exercise. The goal is enhanced body shape and lowered weight, rather than health. The workouts have a compulsive, frantic quality to them, so if they are missed or shortened, the women experience feelings of guilt and failure.

Ana exercises excessively and compulsively. Prior to the mindfulness group she was jogging on a treadmill at home for 10 miles or 3 h daily. Occasionally she jogged twice a day. Missing a workout created tremendous guilt and anxiety.

Kelley described herself as "rigid" in regards to her exercise routine. She would not allow herself a day off and would only work out on a certain piece of equipment. If someone else were using the equipment, she would either pressure that individual to give up "my machine" or leave the gym angry and resentful. She could never override her need to go the gym for any reason.

Rena was forcing herself to go to the gym in order to work out at the end of a full day of classes during which time she had only eaten "lightly." She confides, "The exercising I do now is like punishing myself, really it is. I've never really liked going to the gym. I watch the clock and it's just a pain. Even while doing Palates I have to be distracted by music or some kind of dance moves."

Eva historically was a gymnast and was a member of the crew team at school. Practice for crew was daily and entailed hours of grueling exercise and rowing beginning in the early morning hours before dawn. She was used to being very physically active which had reduced her need to restrict or purge. Eva decided to drop crew because playing a sport and academic pressures had overwhelmed her. With less physical activity, her eating and purging markedly increased.

162.5.2.7 Weighing, Measuring, and Constantly Comparing

Each of the participants was obsessively preoccupied with their body shape and size. They compulsively weighed themselves, scrutinized themselves, compared themselves to others, and counted calories and fat content in their diet.

As Rena puts it,

> Beauty, I'm obsessed with beauty and any achievement thereof. That, together with the perfectionist in me, grows eating disorders. I want to be like a Barbie doll but I can't because, even at my thinnest, I have a certain size bone. I wake up in the morning and I'm just like 'Oh gosh you look awful' because I'm expecting to see a size 4 in the mirror, but I'm a size 10 or 12."

She historically has counted carbohydrates, fat, and calories, and measured and weighed herself after grueling exercise workouts.

Kelley is preoccupied with her appearance and weight. She was so unhappy with her body that she would only use the exercise machine at the gym that was located in the corner next to the wall away from the mirrors. That way neither she nor anyone else could see her while she exercised. She tended to weigh herself frequently at home and at the gym and would set specific weight loss goals for herself. Her standard of comparison was her own body image at age 16. She has cycles where she restricts her food intake and exercises regularly alternating with loss of control of her eating resulting in binging and purging.

Sophia reveals that she is really neurotic about her diet.

> If I eat pizza it has to be completely blotted and then I pick half the cheese off. I have so many habits in terms of food. It has to do with the fact that I am not accepting of a certain weight. I chronically buy clothing that is too small for me and then I have nothing nice to wear.

162.5.2.8 Cutting

Sometimes, as an alternative to purging, women in the M-BED Group turned to self-mutilation to reduce intolerable levels of stress and anxiety. While some of the women were continuing to use cutting to lower emotional distress, others had used it in the past, but had stopped.

In her journal, Rena wrote about what these episodes were like for her,

I was feeling tired and weak from a long day of classes, followed by an hour of exercise with nothing to eat. While I was undressing to take a shower, I happened to glance in the mirror and had never looked so disgustingly fat. I freaked out and began to hyperventilate. All I could focus on was my walrus-sized gut. I didn't know what to do. There was nothing in my stomach to throw up, so I cut my wrist. What I really wanted to do was to cut my stomach open and drain out whatever was in there making me fat!!! I HAVE to be thin.

Only a few days later Rena again viewed herself in the mirror and judged herself to be "incredibly, disgustingly fat." She again "freaked out" and began to have a panic attack. She was feeling all alone and unable to accept her body size. She could not throw up because of a performance the following day. All she could think of was to hurt herself. She cut herself with a pair of scissors and with a piece of glass hoping that "draining my blood might make me thinner." She wrote in her journal, "My mind is out of control and I want to destroy all my mirrors and murder any humans who decided thin was desirable."

Sophia had a history of cutting herself in high school but has not had recent self-harming behaviors. Like wise, Ruth had cut her arms between the ages of 12–14 but not recently. In fact, Ruth had an angry reaction to the group's discussion of Rena's cutting behavior. Ruth wrote in her journal "When I hear the mention of cutting I cringe, I feel ill to my stomach." She obsesses about a visible scar on her arm from a time she cut herself at age 14. This scar is very upsetting to her because she feels people who see it know her secret (similar to the lettuce floating in the toilet).

162.5.2.9 Abusing Alcohol and Pot

In another attempt at lowering stress and anxiety, two of the women used marijuana and alcohol to relax and numb intense emotion. Ruth relates that she was a "little pothead" during high school and that now she drinks, "to have fun and to make myself happy." While drinking last year, Ruth had an unwanted sexual experience about which she continues to feel angry and taken advantage of (Fig. 162.8).

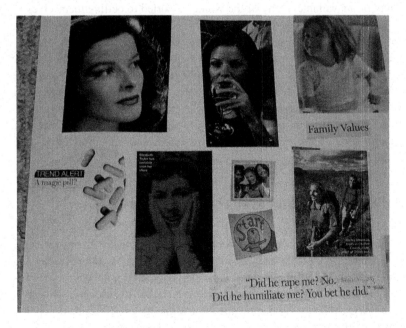

Fig. 162.8 Part of Ruth's self portrait (C). This figure represents a part of Ruth's initial self-portrait. It reveals her tendency to rely on alcohol and drugs to cope with stress. At the bottom, she refers to her unwanted sexual experience and her residual guilt, shame, and anger

Sophia was not very academically motivated when she started college. She was still struggling with depression and ended up partying with drugs and alcohol through freshman year. After counseling and a medical withdrawal in her sophomore year, Sophia stopped using drugs and alcohol, realized she had nothing in common with her old friends, and transferred to a college that could better meet her academic and social needs.

162.6 Implications for Recovery from Bulimia Nervosa

Human vulnerability and suffering is an existential given (Chodron 1997; Clemence 1966; Peck 1978). This human "wound" (Todres 2004), common to us all, can serve as a vehicle for hardening (becoming psychologically defended) and closing off to relational life or softening (remaining vulnerable and open) and extending empathy as the great connector to relational life on behalf of humanity's shared "wound" (Salzberg 1997; Todres 2004; Welwood 2000). It is clear that in response to their human vulnerability, these six women were experiencing extremes in their thoughts, feelings, and behavior. They felt worthless, unlovable, inadequate, powerless, victimized, angry, sad, and numb. They were out of touch with their authentic selves, their bodies, and their personal needs. The women could not trust themselves or others to meet their needs because their needs were perceived as being either too great or altogether unimportant. Because they were so disconnected from their inner selves and because of their underlying, negative beliefs about themselves, the women experienced great difficulty regulating their extreme feelings, causing their behaviors to become out of control. Based on their temperaments, family experiences, and cultural expectations, they developed a belief system that if they achieved the perfect body size and shape, they would be seen as successful and loveable. In response to this belief system, they adopted the coping behaviors of restricting eating, which then progressed to binging and purging. When controlling food and purging activities were insufficient or unavailable, many of the women resorted to cutting themselves to obtain relief from their excruciating feelings and self-loathing. The women's thoughts, feelings, and behaviors were aimed at control, self-sufficiency, and completeness in response to their internal sense of lack of control, dependency, and incompleteness. They had grown to hate their personal experience of vulnerability and human need, closing off to authentic relational life with self and other.

Binging and purging, as private and secret activities, isolated them from others, creating a deep sense of loneliness. The women experienced shame regarding their behaviors, further lowering their self worth. In the mean time, they engaged in a driven and endless pursuit of external achievements, abusive or sexualized relationships, and culturally defined beauty in a futile effort to feel lovable.

162.7 Application for Other Areas of Health and Disease

Bulimia nervosa reflects an underlying disorder of self and, as such, effective treatment requires a trauma-informed, interdisciplinary, integrated approach that restores both physiological and psychological health. Because of the serious medical risks associated with bulimia nervosa, consistent medical and nutritional monitoring and education are central to recovery. Concurrent with these interventions, a phase model of psychotherapeutic treatment is essential that includes cultivating a therapeutic relationship, providing ongoing psychoeducation, building a positive support system, and developing nonharming coping skills. Depending on the severity of the symptoms and the presence of comorbid disorders, additional therapies that may be helpful to the recovery process include mindfulness-based approaches (Proulx 2008), sensorimotor approaches (Ogden et al. 2006), ego state work (Seubert 2008), Eye Movement Desensitization and Reprocessing (EMDR) (Forgash and Copeley 2008; Shapiro 2009), dialectical behavioral treatment (Linehan 1993), and cognitive behavioral treatment (Fairburn et al. 1993). Up to 40% of women with bulimia nervosa do not respond to traditional treatments and symptoms can become chronic with deleterious medical, psychological, and social outcomes (Fairburn et al. 1992; Stice 1999). Bulimia nervosa is a mind-body disorder that responds best to the active collaboration of many healthcare disciplines.

Summary Points

- The women in this study with bulimia nervosa lacked connection with their inner selves as well as their bodies.
- They experienced deep self-loathing and were highly self-critical.
- They sense of lovability became related to the achievement of external, cultural ideals of beauty, thinness, and perfection.
- The symptoms of bulimia, which originated as a way to control body size and shape, became a coping strategy for lowering stress and regulating emotion.
- The addictive coping cycle compounded feelings of shame and guilt and was cloaked in secrecy and isolation.
- In up to 40% of women with bulimia nervosa, the condition can become chronic, with significant medical sequelae.
- To be effective, treatment interventions for bulimia nervosa must not only address health and nutritional concerns, but also the lack of self-connection, self-compassion, and effective coping strategies that are not self-harming.

Definitions

Cognitive behavioral therapy: A therapy developed by Beck that is aimed at changing maladaptive, distorted thoughts and behaviors to lower depression and anxiety. Relaxation and deep breathing exercises are emphasized behaviorally.

Dialectical behavioral treatment: An empirically tested, cognitive-behavioral treatment approach developed by Marsh Linehan to assist individuals with symptoms of borderline personality disorder to improve the quality of their lives by learning how to regulate emotions, tolerate emotional distress, and improve their interpersonal effectiveness.

Ego state therapy: A therapeutic approach developed by Watkins & Watkins that identifies and connects with all parts of the personality for the purpose of relieving symptoms and healing conflicts. Ego states formed in childhood trauma may function maladaptively in present life situations. Ego state therapy helps the healthier, core parts of the self to collaborate with and reparent the immature, wounded parts of the self.

EMDR: Eye Movement Desensitization and Reprocessing is a therapeutic intervention developed by Francine Shapiro that utilizes dual stimulation to activate the information processing system allowing individuals to transform dysfunctionally stored traumatic events into a normal narrative memory that is no longer disturbing.

Hermeneutic phenomenology: a philosophy and qualitative research methodology that attempts to understand the internal world or lived experience of human beings by "going to the things themselves." The researcher approaches the phenomenon with rigorous self- awareness and an open mind in order to more deeply understand and accurately interpret the specific phenomenon. It is based on the beliefs of Husserl, Heidegger, Gadamer, and Merleau-Ponty.

Mindfulness: Paying attention to one's moment-to-moment experience with an attitude of non-judgment. Derived from Buddhist mediation practices and adapted to Western culture as a life style that has been shown to lower stress and depression.

Sensorimotor approaches: Based on the belief that traumatic experience disrupts the body's physiological and emotional regulation, these approaches advocate for working with the body's own defensive systems, autoregulatory patterns, and adaptive responses to promote reconnection with the body.

Acknowledgements In gratitude to the woman whose personal stories are depicted in this chapter. May their courage and honesty inspire other women along their journeys towards recovery.

References

American Psychiatric Association (APA). Diagnostic and statistical manual of mental disorders. 4th ed. Text revision. Washington, DC: Author; 2000.

Brown LM, Gilligan C. Meeting at the crossroads. New York: Ballantine Books; 1992.

Bruch H. Conversations with anorexics. New York: Basic Books; 1988.

Chodron P. When things fall apart: Heart advice for difficult times. Boston: Shambhala Publications; 1997.

Clemence M. AJN. 1966;66:500–5.

Drew N. In: Polifroni EC, Welch M, editors. Perspectives on philosophy of science in nursing: An historical and contemporary anthology. Philadelphia: Lippincott, Williams, & Wilkins; 1999. p. 263–272.

Drew N. ANS. 2001;23:16–31.

Drew N. ANS. 2004;27:215–23.

Fairburn CG, Agras WS, Wilson GT. In: Anderson GH, Kennedy SH, editors. The biology of feast and famine: relevance to eating disorders. San Diego: Academic; 1992. p. 317–340.

Fairburn CG, Cooper PJ. BMJ. 1982;284:1153–5.

Fairburn CG, Marcus MD, Wilson GT. In: Fairburn CG, Wilson GT, editors. Binge eating: nature assessment, and treatment. New York: The Guilford Press; 1993. p. 361–404.

Fisher M, Golden NH, Katzman, DK et al. J Adol Health. 1995;16: 420–37.

Fogash C, Copeley M (eds). Healing the heart of trauma and dissociation with EMDR and ego state therapy. New York: Springer Publishing Company; 2008.

Garfinkel PE, Moldofsky H, Garner DM. Arch Gen Psych. 1980;37:1036–40.

Hsu LKG, Crisp AH, Harding B. Lancet. 1979;i:61–5.

Husserl E. Ideas pertaining to a pure phenomenology and to a phenomenological philosophy, first book (F. Kersten, Trans.). Boston: Kluwer Academic Publishers; 1983. (Original work published 1913)

Linehan M. Cognitive-behavioral treatment of borderline personality. NewYork: Guilford Press; 1993.

National Eating Disorders Association. General eating disorders information: facts for activists. 2006. Retrieved 23 Mar 2006 from http://www.edap.org/p.asp?WebPage_ID=320&Profile_ID=95634.

Ogden P, Minton K, Pain C. Trauma and the body: a sensorimotor approach to psychotherapy. New York: W W Norton; 2006.

Peck MS. The road less traveled. New York: Simon & Schuster; 1978.

Pipher M. Reviving Ophelia: saving the selves of adolescent girls. New York: Ballantine Books; 1994.

Proulx K. Eat Dis. 2008;16:52–72.

Salzberg S. Loving kindness: the revolutionary art of happiness. Boston: Shambhala Publications; 1997.

Seubert A. The courage to feel: a practical guide to the power and freedom of emotional honesty. West Conshohocken: Infinity; 2008.

Shapiro R, editor. EMDR solutions II: for depression, eating disorders, performance and more. New York: WW Norton; 2009.

Stice E. J Clin Psych. 1999;55:675–83.

Todres L. Indo-Pac J Phenomenol. 2004;4:1–12.

Van Manen M. Researching lived experience: human science for an action sensitive pedagogy. Ontario: Althouse Press; 1990.

Welwood J. Toward a psychology of awakening. Boston: Shambhala Publications; 2000.

Chapter 163
The Night Eating Syndrome: An Overview

Jennifer D. Lundgren

Abbreviations

AN	Anorexia Nervosa
BED	Binge Eating Disorder
BN	Bulimia Nervosa
NEDQ	Night Eating Diagnostic Questionnaire
NEQ	Night Eating Questionnaire
NES	Night Eating Syndrome
NESHI	Night Eating Syndrome History and Inventory
SCID	Structured Clinical Interview for the DSM
SRED	Sleep-related Eating Disorder
SSRI	Selective Serotonin Reuptake Inhibitor

163.1 Introduction

Night Eating Syndrome (NES) is a delay in the circadian pattern of food intake, manifested by evening hyperphagia (consuming $\geq 25\%$ of the total daily food intake after the evening meal) and/or nocturnal awakenings accompanied by ingestions of food (O'Reardon et al. 2004). First recognized by Stunkard and colleagues (1955), research on the nosology, etiology, pathophysiology, and treatment of NES has advanced over the past decade. This chapter will provide an overview of NES, including a brief history of its conceptualization over the past 50 years, its prevalence and comorbidity, hypothesized etiology and pathophysiology, its consequences and treatment, and will end with a review of future directions needed to further characterize the nutritional, behavioral, and neurobiological aspects of NES (Table 163.1). Other chapters in this section will review in detail the current status of the neurobiological and neuroendocrine aspects of NES.

J.D. Lundgren (✉)
Department of Psychology, University of Missouri-Kansas City, 4825 Troost Avenue, Ste. 124, Kansas City, Missouri, 64110, USA
e-mail: lundgrenj@umkc.edu

V.R. Preedy et al. (eds.), *Handbook of Behavior, Food and Nutrition*,
DOI 10.1007/978-0-387-92271-3_163, © Springer Science+Business Media, LLC 2011

Table 163.1 Key facts of NES

Diagnosis	NES research diagnostic criteria have been developed and should be used in future studies to diagnose NES
Prevalence and comorbidity	The prevalence of NES in the general population is low (around 1.5%) and increases with adiposity and psychiatric symptoms
Etiology	The etiology of NES is unknown, but likely involves behavioral/functional (i.e., night eating serves to help someone sleep), nutritional, neuroendocrine, and pathophysiological mechanisms
Health implications	Studies of the relationship between NES and obesity are equivocal, although certain populations may be at higher risk for weight gain due to night eating (e.g., those who are already obese or taking weight promoting medications). More research is needed on the health implications of NES
Assessment and treatment	Validated assessment measures and efficacious treatments exist for NES. Individuals with NES should be referred for treatment to a qualified healthcare provider

NES night eating syndrome

Table 163.2 Comparison of 1955 and 1999 NES diagnostic criteria

Symptom domain	1955 NES criteria[a]	1999 NES criteria[b]
Evening hyperphagia	Consumption of large amounts of food in the evening and night; at least 25% of total calories for the day during the period following the evening meal	Evening hyperphagia ≥ 50% of total daily energy after the evening meal
Sleep disturbance	Sleeplessness, at least until midnight, more than half of the time	Awakening at least once a night
Nocturnal ingestions	–	Consumption of snacks during the awakenings
Morning hunger	Morning anorexia with negligible food intake at breakfast	Morning anorexia, even if the person eats breakfast
Duration	–	At least 3 months
Other diagnoses	–	Person cannot receive a diagnosis of NES if they meet criteria for BN or BED

This table compares the 1955 and 1999 proposed diagnostic criteria for NES
NES night eating syndrome, *BED* binge eating disorder, *BN* bulimia nervosa
[a]Criteria cited in Stunkard et al. (1955)
[b]Criteria cited in Birketvedt et al. (1999)

163.2 History of Night Eating Syndrome

NES was first described in 1955 as a disorder of morning anorexia, evening hyperphagia, and insomnia, usually accompanied by depressed mood and stressful life circumstances (Stunkard et al. 1955). Table 163.2 shows the original diagnostic criteria outlined by Stunkard and colleagues (1955).

NES did not receive much research or clinical attention until the 1990s, coinciding with increasing rates of obesity and the search for factors related to excessive weight gain. In 1999, Birketvedt and colleagues added awakenings with ingestions of food (*nocturnal ingestions*), increased the percent of food consumed after the evening meal from 25% to 50% (*evening hyperphagia*), and added duration and rule out criteria to those originally described in 1955 (see Table 163.2 for a comparison of the diagnostic criteria). Additionally, they noted that NES affects both obese and nonobese persons, which is an observation that has become more important as discussions of the clinical significance of NES have ensued.

163.3 Current Conceptualization of NES

As research has advanced our understanding of NES, the diagnostic criteria for NES have continued to evolve, making comparisons across studies difficult. In an effort to move NES research forward based on current research evidence, the First International Night Eating Symposium (April 26, 2008, Minneapolis, MN) was held to reach a consensus on a set of provisional research diagnostic criteria for NES and to discuss a roadmap for future NES research. Approximately 20 researchers in the areas of eating disorders, obesity, and sleep attended the meeting and contributed to the development of the proposed research diagnostic criteria presented in Table 163.3.

These criteria offer the most comprehensive conceptualization of NES to date. The first criterion reflects the notion that NES is at its core a disorder of eating and circadian rhythm. This is manifested by either the consumption of an unusually large percent of the total daily food intake in the evening hours after the evening meal (*evening hyperphagia*) and/or the consumption of food upon awakening in the middle of the night (*nocturnal ingestions*). Figures 163.1 and 163.2 demonstrate the differences in eating patterns of individuals diagnosed with NES compared to weight matched controls.

O'Reardon and colleagues (2004) found that obese persons with NES did not consume significantly more total daily calories than weight matched controls, but they did have a strikingly different circadian pattern of food intake (Fig. 163.1). Weight matched controls showed typical increases in food consumption during the lunch and supper hours, whereas night eaters had a steady food intake that continued until 6:00 a.m. the following morning. There were no significant differences in sleep onset or offset times, indicating that the circadian sleep pattern is not delayed in parallel with the food intake delay, but the night eaters did report significantly more awakenings per night (1.5 vs. 0.5 awakenings).

Table 163.3 2009 Proposed research diagnostic criteria

Symptom domain	Diagnostic criterion
Eating pattern	I. The daily pattern of eating demonstrates a significantly increased intake in the evening and/or night-time, as manifested by one or both of the following: (A) At least 25% of food intake is consumed after the evening meal (B) At least two episodes of nocturnal eating per week
Awareness of eating behavior	II. Awareness and recall of evening and nocturnal eating episodes are present
Associated mood, hunger, and sleep features	III. The clinical picture is characterized by at least three of the following features: (A) Lack of desire to eat in the morning and/or breakfast is omitted on four or more mornings per week (B) Presence of a strong urge to eat between dinner and sleep onset and/or during the night (C) Sleep onset and/or sleep maintenance insomnia are present four or more nights per week (D) Presence of a belief that one must eat in order to initiate or return to sleep (E) Mood is frequently depressed and/or mood worsens in the evening
Distress/impairment in functioning	IV. The disorder is associated with significant distress and/or impairment in functioning
Duration	V. The disordered pattern of eating has been maintained for at least 3 months
Other diagnoses or Medical conditions	VI. The disorder is not secondary to substance abuse or dependence, medical disorder, medication, or another psychiatric disorder

This table shows the 2009 proposed research diagnostic criteria for NES. These criteria are comprehensive and based on more recent research than those presented in 1955 and 1999 (see Table 163.2)

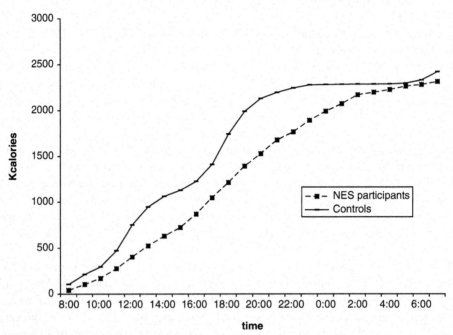

Fig. 163.1 Comparison of 24-h food patterns of obese persons with NES and weight-matched controls. This figure illustrates the significantly different circadian patterns of food intake between obese persons with night eating syndrome and weight matched controls, although the total caloric intake is not significantly different over 24 h (Reprinted with permission)

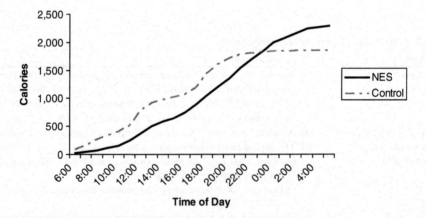

Fig. 163.2 Comparison of 24-h food patterns of non-obese persons with NES and weight-matched controls. This figure illustrates the significantly different circadian pattern of food intake between nonobese persons with night eating syndrome and weight matched controls. Total daily caloric intake is significantly greater for the group with night eating syndrome (Reprinted with permission)

Lundgren and colleagues (2008a) found nearly identical patterns of delayed circadian food intake in nonobese night eaters compared to weight matched controls (Fig. 163.2). Nonobese night eaters, compared to weight matched controls, however did consume significantly more total calories per day (night eater = 2284.5 kcal; control = 1856.2 kcal). Nonobese night eaters had significantly more nocturnal awakenings and ingestions of food than did controls.

Currently, only evening hyperphagia *or* nocturnal ingestions are necessary to meet the first proposed NES diagnostic criterion. This criterion was left intentionally broad because further research is needed clarify the relationship between these two manifestations of the circadian delay of food intake, and because individuals often report both behaviors. For example, Lundgren and colleagues (2008a) found that 84% of nonobese individuals with NES met criteria for both evening hyperphagia *and* nocturnal ingestions of food. In another study of night eating in women diagnosed with bulimia nervosa (BN), however, Lundgren and colleagues (2008b) found that only 14% of BN patients with night eating features reported both behaviors. More research is needed to clarify this core criterion.

The second criterion (Table 163.3), that awareness and recall of evening and nocturnal eating episodes are present, was proposed to differentiate NES from parasomnias such as sleep-related eating disorder (SRED) (Howell et al. 2009). Persons with SRED can consume food in the middle of the night, do so while in a sleep-walking state, and often consume nonfood items. Although persons with NES occasionally report a lack of full awareness with nocturnal ingestions of food, they must report awarness and recall of the nocturnal eating episodes in general.

At least three of five additional features must be present in order for one to receive a diagnosis of NES (Table 163.3). These include a lack of morning hunger or omission of food in the morning, a strong urge to eat either after dinner or upon awakening in the middle of the night, difficulty falling or staying asleep at night, presence of a belief that one must eat in order to return to sleep, and mood that is frequently depressed and that may worsens in the evening hours.

Evidence of problems with morning hunger, morning food omission, and sleep disturbance in individuals with NES is presented in Figs. 163.1 and 163.2. Anecdotal evidence and that collected with self-report instruments, such as the night eating questionnaire (NEQ; Allison et al. 2008) suggest that many persons with NES experience a strong urge to eat after dinner or upon awakeing in the middle of the night. Allison and colleagues (2004) noted several different themes associated with these urges, including cravings for specific foods, anxiety and agitation, distress about sleep disruption, and feeling compelled to eat/needing to feel full to sleep.

Similarly, some persons with NES feel that they must eat in order to fall asleep initially or to fall back asleep after a nocturnal awakening. Again, this is assessed with the NEQ (Allison et al. 2008) and is often described as a function of night eating for some who suffer from NES (Allison et al. 2004).

Night eating syndrome is associated with mood disturbance in some individuals. Stunkard and colleagues (1955) noted this disturbance in their original description of NES and several studies have confirmed that night eaters have high rates of comorbid mood disorders and increased scores on depression measures (Gluck et al. 2001; de Zwaan et al. 2006; Lundgren et al. 2008a). Interestingly, persons with mood disorders are not necessarily at increased risk for NES (Lundgren et al. 2006). A recent SPECT study has provided preliminary evidence that the pathophysiology of NES and MDD is distinct (Lundgren et al. 2009), and will be reviewed in a later chapter.

Finally, the night eating and associated features must cause distress and impairment, be present for at least 3 months, and not be better explained by another psychiatric diagnosis, medical condition, or medication/substance. The conditions which are frequently comorbid with NES, in addition to mood disorders, will be reviewed below.

163.4 Prevalence of NES

The prevalence of NES varies substantially depending on the criteria used to diagnose it and the population under study. To date, no studies have examined the prevalence of NES using the recently proposed research diagnostic criteria (Table 163.3). Studies using previous criteria have provided a general sense of the magnitude of NES in the general population, among obese individuals, and

Table 163.4 Prevalence of NES

Population	Prevalence (%)	Citation
General population	1.5	Rand et al. (1997)
	1.6	Striegel-Moore et al. (2006)
	5.7	Colles et al. (2007)
	2.2–7.1	Lundgren et al. (in press a)
Special populations:		
Weight loss seeking	6	Stunkard et al. (1996)
Bariatric surgery	16	Adami et al. (2002)
Diabetes	9	Allison et al. (2006)
Psychiatric	27	Rand et al. (1997)
	3.8	Allison et al. (2007)
	9.7	Morse et al. (2006)
	12.3	Lundgren et al. (2006)
	25	Lundgren et al. (in press b)

This table shows the prevalence of night eating syndrome in several populations

among other psychiatric populations, such as those with eating disorders and severe mental illness (Table 163.4).

Variability in prevalence is due to differences in assessment measures, diagnostic criteria, and populations.

Prevalence of night eating in the general population has been reported at 1.5% (Rand et al. 1997) to 7.1% (Lundgren et al. 2010a). Prevalence rates in special populations suggest ranges of 6% (Stunkard et al. 1996) to 16% (Adami et al. 2002) in weight loss samples of class I and II obesity. Among bariatric surgery candidates, the range in prospective interview studies is 9% (Allison et al. 2006) to 27% (Rand et al. 1997); Allison and colleagues (2007) found a prevalence of 3.8% among older adults in a large multicenter study of type 2 diabetes (Allison et al. 2007).

Three studies have examined the prevalence of night eating in other psychiatric populations. Lundgren and colleagues (2006) found a prevalence of 12.3% in two university outpatient psychiatric clinics which included patients with a variety of Axis I and Axis II psychiatric disorders. In a sample of weight loss seeking individuals with serious mental illness (schizophrenia, bipolar disorder, and severe major depressive disorders), the prevalence of NES was striking at 25% (Lundgren et al. 2010b). It is unlikely that participants grossly over-reported night eating behavior in this sample, as only 5.9% of participants met the criteria for binge eating disorder (BED) (Lundgren et al. 2010b). Finally, Lundgren, Shapiro, and Bulik (2008b) reported that nearly half of women seeking outpatient treatment for BN reported evening hyperphagia, nocturnal ingestions of food, or both core symptoms of NES. These later prevalence studies suggest that much research on the comorbidity of NES, especially the temporal relationship of night eating to other psychiatric symptoms is needed.

163.5 Comorbidity of NES

163.5.1 Medical Comorbidity

The most commonly studied medical comorbidity of NES is obesity (Stunkard et al. 1955, 1996; Colles et al. 2007; Lundgren et al. 2010a) and early descriptions of NES suggested that it was a pathway to obesity. Andersen and colleagues (2004) found that endorsement of the question "Do you get up at night to eat?" prospectively predicted weight gain among obese women in the Danish MONICA study. Recently, Lundgren and colleagues (2010a) found that nocturnal eating, but not evening hyperphagia, was associated with obesity in a sample of community adults.

Not all studies have supported a relationship between NES and obesity. Using large national databases Striegel-Moore and colleagues (2005, 2006) did not find an increased risk of obesity with night eating; these studies, however, were not designed to assess NES specifically, but were based on 24-h food record data. More recent research, however, has suggested that obesity may only be associated with NES in certain populations. For example, psychiatric outpatients with NES were nearly five times more likely to be obese than the non-night eating outpatients (Lundgren et al. 2006). Discrepancies in studies examining the comorbidity of NES and obesity suggest that more work, using similar diagnostic criteria, is needed to understand the relationship between NES and obesity.

163.5.2 Psychiatric Comorbidity

High rates of psychiatric comorbidity have been noted among persons diagnosed with NES. Lifetime prevalence of Axis I disorders assessed by the Structured Clinical Interview for the DSM (SCID) is high among those with NES. Lundgren and colleagues found that 74% of night eaters, compared with 18% of controls had at least one comorbid Axis I diagnosis (Lundgren et al. 2008a). Mood disorders are common and NES has been related to high rates of lifetime diagnosis for major depressive disorder at 52.6% (Lundgren et al. 2008a), 55.7% (de Zwaan et al. 2006), and 57.1% (Boseck et al. 2007). Lundgren and colleagues (2008a) also found high rates of anxiety disorders among NES patients (47.4%).

Fewer studies have examined the comorbidity of NES among psychiatric samples. Lundgren and colleagues (2006) examined the prevalence of NES in psychiatric outpatients with a variety of diagnoses. In this sample, the only diagnoses to co-occur with NES were current and lifetime histories of substance use disorders. Participants prescribed atypical antipsychotics were more likely to be diagnosed with NES compared to those not prescribed this class of medication, but in this study serious mental illness was not associated with NES. In a follow-up to this study, Lundgren and colleagues (2010b) found that obese adults with serious mental illness who were prescribed psychotropic medications were at risk of NES, with nearly 25% of the sample meeting criteria. Combined, these studies suggest that there is perhaps a synergistic effect of obesity, medication use, and psychiatric symptoms that increase risk of night eating behavior.

The relationship of NES to other eating disorders has also been investigated. The comorbidity of BED and NES ranges from 5% to 20% (Stunkard et al. 1996; Geliebter 2002, Allison et al. 2005b, 2007; Striegel-Moore et al. 2005). Few studies have examined the relationship between NES and anorexia nervosa (AN) or BN. Lundgren and colleagues (2008b) found that 35.5% of women seeking outpatient treatment for BN reported evening hyperphagia of at least 25% of their caloric intake after dinner, and 19.3% reported eating at least half of their intake after dinner. It is unclear, however, whether their reported evening hyperphagia is distinct from evening binge eating episodes. More striking, however, is that 38.7% of the patients with BN reported at least occasional nocturnal ingestions, while 12.9% reported eating during awakenings at least half of the time. More research is needed to clarify the relationship of NES to these other eating disorders.

163.6 Hypothesized Causes of NES and Potential Pathophysiology

The causes of NES are unknown and hypothesized explanations include behavioral/functional (i.e., night eating serves to help someone sleep), nutritional, neuroendocrine, and pathophysiological. From a behavioral level of explanation, the onset of NES is often associated with a life stressor (Allison et al. 2004; Stunkard et al. 2006) and the function of night eating behavior could be to calm someone who experiences difficulty with sleep onset and/or maintenance and help him or her return to sleep. In a review of common thoughts experienced by persons with NES, Allison and colleagues (2004) point out that many people with NES have a core belief that they must eat in order to return to sleep. This explanation is informative for behavioral and cognitive-behavioral treatments for NES, but alone do not explain the development of NES.

Early hypotheses involving nutritional deficits or carbohydrate craving were suggested by Birketvedt and colleagues (1999). They found that the proportion of carbohydrates consumed during night eating episodes was greater than during the day and that the carbohydrate to protein ratio was 7:1 during nocturnal ingestions. More recent data have not supported such differences in the proportion of macronutrient content of foods consumed during the night versus the day (Allison et al. 2005a).

Neuroendocrine and pathophysiological abnormalities have been noted among persons with NES. These will be reviewed in detail in later chapters.

163.7 Consequences and Clinical Significance of NES

Although NES research has progressed significantly in the past decade, there are lingering questions about the consequences of evening and nocturnal eating. Specifically, questions have been raised about its *clinical significance*, given that late evening dinners and midnight snacking are normative in different cultures. The clinical significance of NES has been challenged even more as studies on NES and obesity have been equivocal (see above) and because earlier versions of NES diagnostic criteria did not specify that distress or impairment in functioning due to night eating be present for a diagnosis. The most recently proposed criteria (Table 163.4) have included such specifiers. Other than obesity, the two primary health consequences of NES that have been reported in the literature are diabetic complications and poor oral health.

Morse and colleagues (2006) examined night eating in individuals with Type I and II diabetes. They found that patients with NES were less adherent with their nutrition and exercise plans, as well as glucose monitoring. Night eaters' had higher A1C values and were more likely to have diabetes complications than non-night eaters. No studies have reported the prevalence of metabolic syndrome among persons with NES, and more research is needed to replicate Morse and colleagues' findings.

In a recent study, nocturnal ingestions of food, but not evening hyperphagia, predicted poor oral health on a variety of oral heath indices (Lundgren et al. 2010a). Specifically, nocturnal eating was a significant predictor of the number of missing teeth, periodontal disease, and active tooth decay.

163.8 Assessment and Treatment of NES

Assessment of NES can be aided with the help of self-report inventories, interviews, and food records. A description of common NES assessment measures is presented in Table 163.5. The NEQ (Allison et al. 2008) is a brief self report inventory which assesses the pattern and timing of food

Table 163.5 Commonly used NES assessment measures

Measure	Description
Night Eating Questionnaire (NEQ)	14-item self report inventory which assesses the pattern and timing of food intake, hunger and cravings for food, and mood and sleep difficulties. Administration time is approximately 5 min. Published in Allison et al. (2008)
Night Eating Syndrome History and Inventory (NESHI)	Semi-structured, unpublished interview available from Drs. Albert Stunkard and Kelly Allison at the University of Pennsylvania. This interview assesses current eating behavior, cravings, sleep patterns, and mood, as well as the history and precipitating NES factors. Administration time is approximately 30 min
Night Eating Diagnostic Questionnaire (NEDQ)	Similar to the NEQ, this brief measure provides information on one's eating patterns, sleep, and mood, as well as diet and weight history. It has recently been revised to reflect proposed research diagnostic criteria, and can be obtained from its authors (Gluck et al. 2001). Administration time is approximately 5 min
Food Record	Prospective food records which assess the timing of food intake, type of food consumed, and amount of food consumed and which can be helpful in identifying night eating patterns and in confirming night eating behavior. Week-long food records are preferred as they provide more stable estimates of night eating behavior than 1–2 day records or recalls
Dietary Recall	Dietary recalls assess the timing, type, and amount of food consumed retrospectively and typically focus on the previous 24-h. Recalls can be helpful in assessing very recent night eating behavior, but are less useful than prospective food records at assessing night eating behavior for longer periods of time
Actigraphy	Actigraphy can be used to assess patterns of activity and sleep. Actigraphs can be purchased through commercial suppliers and are useful in research studies to verify nocturnal awakenings

This table shows assessment measures that are available for screening and diagnosing NES
NES night eating syndrome

intake, hunger and cravings for food, and mood and sleep difficulties. The NEQ can be used as a symptom or screening measure, and a score of 30 or greater is suggestive of NES (Allison et al. 2008). The Night Eating Diagnostic Questionnaire (NEDQ) (Gluck et al. 2001) is useful in establishing a diagnosis of NES. It has recently been revised to reflect the proposed NES diagnostic criteria (Table 163.3) and can be obtained from its authors.

For a more thorough assessment of one's current and past night eating patterns, the Night Eating Syndrome History and Inventory (NESHI) can be used. It is an unpublished, semi-structured interview that assesses the current and past symptoms of NES, precipitating factors, familial night eating patterns, and treatment attempts. It can be obtained from its authors, Drs. Kelly Allison and Albert Stunkard at the University of Pennsylvania.

Finally, food and sleep records, dietary recalls, and actigraphy are essential in documenting eating and sleeping patterns in both research and clinical contexts. Food records and sleep records can be used to establish antecedents of night eating and treatment targets. Actigraphy is helpful in verifying nocturnal ingestions of food and in studying sleep/activity patterns.

With the increased research interest in NES over the past decade, several promising therapies have been developed and tested. Three studies have found that the selective serotonin reuptake inhibitor (SSRI), sertraline, significantly reduces evening hyperphagia, night-time awakenings, and nocturnal ingestions of food, as well as body weight (O'Reardon et al. 2004, 2006; Stunkard et al. 2006). These studies were the impetus for examining the role of serotonin transporter in the development and maintenance of NES, which is reviewed in a later chapter.

Cognitive behavioral therapy has also shown promise for treating NES. In a pilot study patients have shown a benefit, including a weight loss of 3 kg for completers, which is comparable to that seen with sertraline (Allison et al. 2010a). The combination of pharmacotherapy and psychotherapy has not been tested; this may prove to be a useful approach in the future.

Investigators have also reported some success with progressive muscle relaxation (Pawlow et al. 2003), paroxetine (Miyaoka et al. 2003), and light therapy (Friedman et al. 2002). Further research is necessary to confirm these findings and to determine whether behavioral weight loss treatment would be effective for reducing weight and NES symptoms.

163.9 Future Directions

As can be concluded from the review of NES above, the research community is just starting to develop a knowledge base of the causes and correlates of NES. Several research initiatives are underway to further characterize NES, including the standardization and testing of the newly proposed NES Research Diagnostic Criteria (Allison et al. 2010b; Table 163.4). As these new criteria are being tested, several aspects of NES are in need of more research, including its health implications, its relationship to other eating disorders, obesity, and sleep disorders, its pathophysiology, and its treatment. Later chapters in this section will review state-of-the-art findings on the neuroendocrine aspects of NES as well as recent research on the potential role of serotonin transporter in its pathophysiology. Significantly more research is needed in these areas as well to further understand and treat NES.

163.10 Applications to Other Areas of Health and Disease

Research on NES has significant implications for other areas of health, including obesity and eating disorders, sleep disorders, metabolic syndrome, and oral heath. As reviewed above, the impact of night eating on obesity has potentially serious consequences for certain populations, especially those with serious mental illness. Given the potential for weight gain that so many antipsychotic medications have, it is crucial to understand why night eating is so prevalent in this population. Similarly, the field is only now beginning to study night eating in the context of other eating disorders. The data reviewed above regarding night eating in women with BN suggests that there is potentially much more overlap between NES and other eating disorders than previously suspected. This has implications for the diagnosis and treatment of not only NES, but of BN and, potentially, AN as well.

Although not reviewed in detail in this chapter, the relationship between NES and sleep disorders is understudied. Both sleep and eating disorder researchers would benefit from improved communication and collaboration when studying night eating. There is likely much that both fields can share with one another to further understand the neurobiology of NES and other eating-related sleep disorders, such as SRED.

Finally, as this chapter points out, much work is needed on further understanding the health implications of NES. Preliminary studies have suggested that NES puts one at increased risk for metabolic disturbance and poor oral health. Future studies are needed to replicate and extend these findings so that they can better inform weight management, endocrine, and dental professionals.

Summary Points

- Night Eating Syndrome (NES) is a disorder of circadian rhythm manifested by the core criteria of evening hyperphagia and/or nocturnal ingestions of food.
- Research diagnostic criteria for NES have recently been proposed and should be tested in future NES research.
- NES is rare among the general population, but its prevalence increases with obesity and among persons with psychiatric symptoms.
- The etiology of NES is unknown, but research on behavioral and neuroendocrine causes, as well as the role of the serotonin system, is underway.
- Assessments and treatments for NES are available and should be disseminated more broadly, despite limitations in known pathophysiology.

Definition of Key Terms

Night eating syndrome: A disorder of the circadian pattern of food intake, manifested by evening hyperphagia and/or nocturnal awakenings accompanied by ingestions of food.

Evening hyperphagia: The consumption of an unusually large amount of food after the evening meal. Current NES diagnostic criteria suggest that the consumption of 25% or more of one's total daily calories after supper constitutes evening hyperphagia.

Nocturnal awakenings: Awakening in the middle of the night after sleep onset.

Nocturnal ingestions of food: Consuming food upon awakening in the middle of the night after sleep onset.

Acknowledgments The author would like to thank Drs. Albert Sunkard, Kelly Allison, and John O'Reardon for their collaboration and mentorship, as well as their many contributions to the NES literature.

References

Adami GF, Campostano A, Marinari GM, Ravera G, Scopinaro N. Nutrition 2002;18:587–9.

Allison KC, Stunkard AJ, Thier SL. Overcoming night eating syndrome: a step-by-step guide to breaking the cycle. Oakland: New Harbinger; 2004.

Allison KC, Ahima RS, O'Reardon JP, Dinges DF, Sharma V, Cummings DE., Heo, M, Martino N, Stunkard AJ. J Clin Endocrinol Metab. 2005a;90:6214–7.

Allison KC, Grilo CM, Masheb RM, Stunkard AJ. J Consult Clin Psychol. 2005b;73:1107–15.

Allison KC, Wadden TA, Sarwer DB, Fabricatore AN, Crerand C, Gibbons L, Stack R, Stunkard AJ, Williams N. Obesity 2006;14:77S–82S.

Allison KC, Crow S, Reeves RR, West DS, Foreyt JP, DiLillo VG, Wadden TA, Jeffery RW, Van Dorsten B, Stunkard AJ, and the Eating Disorders Subgroup of the Look AHEAD Research Group. Obesity 2007;15:1285–91.

Allison KC, Lundgren JD, O Reardon JP, Sarwer DB, Wadden TA, Stunkard AJ. Eat Behav. 2008;9:62–72.

Allison KC, Lundgren JD, O'Reardon JP, Moore RH, Stunkard AJ. Am J Psychotherapy. 2010a;64:94-106.

Allison .C, Lundgren JD, O'Reardon JP, Geliebter A, Gluck M, Vanai P, Mitchell JE, Schenck CH, Howell MJ, Crow SJ, Engel S, Latzer Y, Tzischinsky O, Mahowald MW, Stunkard AJ. 2010b;43:2414–247.

Andersen GS, Stunkard AJ, Sorensen TIA, Pedersen L, Heitman BL. Int J Obesity. 2004;28:1138–43.

Birketvedt G, Florholmen J, Sundsfjord J, Osterud B, Dinges D, Bilker W, Stunkard AJ. JAMA 1999;282:657–63.

Boseck JJ, Engel SG, de Zwaan M, Allison KC, Crosby RD, Mitchell JE. Int J Eat Disord. 2007;40:271–6.

Colles S L, Dixon JB, O'Brien PE. Int J Obesity. 2007;31:1722–30.

de Zwaan M, Roerig DB, Crosby RD, Karaz S, Mitchell JE. Int J Eat Disord. 2006;39:224–32.

Freidman S, Even C, Dardennes R, Guelfi JD. Am J Psychiatry. 2002;159:875–6.

Geliebter A. Appetite 2002;38:1–3.

Gluck M E, Geliebter A, Satov T. Obesity Res. 2001;9:264–7.

Howell M, Crow S, Schenck C. Sleep Med. 2009;13:23–34.

Lundgren JD, Allison KC, Crow S, Berg KC, Galbraith J, Martino NS, O'Reardon JP, Stunkard AJ. Am J Psychiatry. 2006;163:156–8.

Lundgren JD, Allison KC, O'Reardon JP, Stunkard AJ. Eat Beh. 2008a;9:343–51.

Lundgren JD, Shapiro JR, Bulik C. Eat Weight Disord. 2008b;13:171–5.

Lundgren JD, Amsterdam J, Newberg A, Allison KC, Wintering N, Stunkard AJ. Eat Weight Disord. 2009;14:45–50.

Lundgren JD, Smith B, Williams K, Spresser C, Harkins P, Zolton L. General Dentistry. 2010a;58:163.

Lundgren JD, Rempfer MV, Brown CE, Goetz J, Hamera E. Psychiatry Res. 2010b;175: 233–236.

Miyaoka T, Yasukawa R, Tsubouchi K, Miura S, Shimizu Y, Sukegawa T, Maeda T, Mizuno S, Kameda A, Uegaki J, Inagaki T, Horiguchi J. Int Clin Psychopharmacol. 2003;18:175–7.

Morse SA, Ciechanowski PS, Katon WJ, Hirsch IB. Diabetes Care. 2006;29:1800–4.

O'Reardon JP, Stunkard AJ, Allison KC. Int J Eat Disord. 2004;35:16–26.

O'Reardon JP, Ringel BL, Dinges DF, Costello Allison K, Rogers NL, Martino NS, Stunkard AJ. Obes Res. 2004;12:1789–96.

O'Reardon JP, Allison KC, Martino NS, Lundgren JD, Heo M, Stunkard AJ. Am J Psychiatry. 2006;163:893–8.

Pawlow LA, O'Neil PM, Malcolm RJ. Int J Obes Relat Metab Disord. 2003;27:970–8.

Rand CSW, Macgregor MD, Stunkard AJ. Int J Eat Disord. 1997;22:65–9.

Striegel Moore RH, Dohn FA, Hook JM, Schreiber GB, Crawford PB, Daniels SR. Int J Eat Disord. 2005;37:200–6.

Stunkard AJ, Berkowitz R, Wadden T, Tankirut C, Reiss E, Young L. Int J Obes Relat Metab Disord. 1996;20:1–6.

Striegel-Moore RH, Franko DL, Thompson D, Affenito S, Kraemer HC. Obes Res. 2006;14:139–47.

Stunkard AJ, Allison KC, Lundgren JD, Martino NS, Heo M, Etemad B, O'Reardon JP. J Clin Psychiatry. 2006;67:1568–72.

Stunkard AJ, Grace WJ, Wolff HG. Am J Med. 1955;9:78–86.

Part XXVII
Metabolic Syndrome and Non-obese Overweight

Chapter 164
Metabolic Syndrome as a Disorder of the Brain with Its Origins in the Perinatal Period

Undurti N. Das

Abbreviations

PUFAs	Polyunsaturated fatty acids
EFAs	Essential fatty acids
IL	Interleukin
TNF	Tumor necrosis factor
ROS	Reactive oxygen species
NO	Nitric oxide
CRP	C-reactive protein
CHD	Coronary heart disease
NF-κB	Nuclear factor kappaB
IkBα	Inhibitor kappaB alpha
NADPH	Nicotinamide adenine dinucleotide phosphate
G6P	Glucose-6-phosphate
TBSA	Total body surface area
NPY	Neuropeptide Y
AgRP	Agouti-related peptide
POMC	Pro-opiomelanocortin
MSH	Melanocyte stimulating hormone
CART	Cocaine and amphetamine-regulated transcript

164.1 Introduction

The various components of the metabolic syndrome include: dyslipidemia, hypertension, hypergly-cemia, insulin resistance, polycystic ovary syndrome, fatty liver, cholesterol gallstones, asthma, sleep disturbances, and some forms of cancer.

The incidence of metabolic syndrome is increasing and by the year 2010, in the United States alone there may be about 50–75 million people with the disease. An early stage of the metabolic

U.N. Das (✉)
UND Life Sciences 13800 Fairhill Road, #321, Shaker Heights, OH, 44120, USA
Jawaharlal Nehru Technological University, Kakinada- 533 003, Andhra Pradesh, India
e-mail: Undurti@hotmail.com

V.R. Preedy et al. (eds.), *Handbook of Behavior, Food and Nutrition*,
DOI 10.1007/978-0-387-92271-3_164, © Springer Science+Business Media, LLC 2011

Table 164.1 Key features of metabolic syndrome

I. Key clinical features are:
  1. Abdominal obesity
  2. Insulin resistance
  3. Hyperlipidemia
  4. Hypertension
  5. Type 2 diabetes mellitus
  6. Atheroslcerosis
  7. Decreased heart rate variability

II. Key biochemical features are:
  1. Hyperinsulinemia and hyperglycemia
  2. Low plasma endothelial nitric oxide levels
  3. Low plasma adiponectin levels
  4. Hyperleptin emia
  5. Low plasma levels of antioxidants
  6. High plasma levels of lipid peroxides and resistin
  7. Elevated plasma ADMA (asymmetrical dimethyl arginine)
  8. Elevated plasma IL-6, TNF-α, MIF (macrophage migration inhibitory factor), HMGB-1 (high mobility group box-1), hs-CRP (high sensitive –reactive protein), and adhesion molecules
  9. Low plasma BDNF and visfatin
  10. Low plasma GLP-1 (glucagon-like peptide-1) and gastric inhibitory polypeptide (GIP)

syndrome is characterized by insulin resistance restricted to muscle tissue whereas adipose tissue is not resistant to insulin (Grundy et al. 2004). This explains why exercise is beneficial in the prevention and treatment of insulin resistance since it decreases insulin resistance and enhances glucose utilization in the muscles. In addition, exercise is anti-inflammatory in nature (Table 164.1) (Das 2004, 2006a).

164.2 Low-grade Systemic Inflammation Occurs in Metabolic Syndrome

Obesity, insulin resistance, hypertension, hyperlipidemia, and coronary heart disease (CHD) are all associated with low-grade systemic inflammation since plasma levels of C-reactive protein (CRP), tumor necrosis factor-α (TNF-α), and interleukin-6 (IL-6), markers of inflammation, are elevated (reviewed in Das 2008), whereas anti-inflammatory molecules adiponectin, IL-4, IL-10, and eNO (endothelial nitric oxide) are decreased in these conditions (Das 2002a). The exact reason why low-grade systemic inflammation occurs in metabolic syndrome is not clear. But it is interesting to note that glucose is pro-inflammatory whereas insulin is anti-inflammatory in nature.

164.3 Glucose Can Initiate and Perpetuate Inflammation

Hyperglycemia is one of the major components of the metabolic syndrome, and metabolic syndrome is a low-grade systemic inflammatory condition; it is therefore likely that hyperglycemia has proinflammatory actions. Glucose ingestion (75 g in 300 mL water) in healthy human subjects resulted in an increase in intranuclear nuclear factor kappaB (NF-kB) binding, the reduction of inhibitor kappaB alpha (IkBα) protein, and an increase in the activity of inhibitor kappaB kinase (IKK) and the expression of IKKalpha and IKKbeta, the enzymes that phosphorylate IkBα in mononuclear cells.

Glucose intake caused an increase in the expression of TNF-α messenger RNA in mononuclear cells. Membranous p47(phox) subunit, an index of nicotinamide adenine dinucleotide phosphate (NADPH) oxidase expression and activation, also increased after glucose intake (Aljada et al. 2004, 2006). These data are consistent with the prediction that hyperglycemia initiates and perpetuates inflammation.

Rat pancreatic islets or clonal rat BRIN BD11 β cells incubated with 16.7 mmol/L glucose for 1 h produced significantly increased amounts of free radicals that were inhibited by NADPH oxidase inhibitor (Morgan et al. 2007). Pre-exposure of U937 histiocytes to high glucose concentrations markedly increased the lipopolysaccharide-induced secretion of proinflammatory cytokines--> and chemokines and the cellular inducible nitric oxide level compared with pre-exposure to normal glucose (Nareika et al. 2007). Similarly, exposure of human microvascular endothelial cells to various concentrations of glucose from low to physiological levels (0–5 mmol/L), production of G6P (glucose-6-phosphate), lactate, NAD(P)H, and CO_2 increased as expected, while oxygen consumption rate was reduced. These changes were found to be oxidative stress mediated endothelial inflammation induced by excess glucose as a result of G6P accumulation (Sweet et al. 2009). These results clearly suggest that glucose is proinflammatory in nature.

164.4 Hyperglycemia Induces Oxidative Stress in Adipose and β Cells

It is interesting that hyperglycemia induced adipose tissue developed severe insulin resistance and produced a number of acute phase reactants at high levels (Lin et al. 2001) that is mediated by the induction of reactive oxygen species (ROS). Hyperglycemia induced a significant increase in ROS in adipocytes isolated from streptozotocin-treated diabetic mice. Hyperglycemia-induced proinflammatory response in adipose tissue was reduced significantly by agents that lower the mitochondrial membrane potential, or by overexpression of uncoupling protein 1 or superoxide dismutase. On the other hand, hyperpolarization of the mitochondrial membrane, such as overexpression of the mitochondrial dicarboxylate carrier resulted in increased ROS formation and decreased insulin sensitivity, even under normoglycemic conditions (Lin et al. 2005). These results highlight the importance of ROS production in adipocytes and the associated insulin resistance and inflammatory response.

Both hyperglycemia and the proinflammatory cytokine IL-1β induced up-regulation of c-Myc and heme-oxygenase-1 in β cells. Hyperglycemia stimulated islet (β cell) c-Myc and heme-oxygenase-1 expression without affecting NF-kB activity or iNOS and IkBα mRNA levels. Fas mRNA levels only increased after prolonged incubation with 30 mmol/L glucose. Short (such as overnight) exposure to hydrogen peroxide mimicked the effects of hyperglycemia on heme-oxyge-nase-1 and c-Myc mRNA levels without activating NF-kB, while the antioxidant N-acetyl-L-cysteine inhibited the stimulation of heme-oxygenas-1 and c-Myc expression by 30 mmol/L glucose and/or hydrogen peroxide. These results suggest that hyperglycemia and hydrogen peroxide do not activate NF-kB in cultured rat islets, suggesting that the stimulation of islet c-Myc and heme-oxygenase-1 expression by 30 mmol/L glucose results from activation of a distinct, probably oxidative, stress-dependent signaling pathway (Elouil et al. 2005). Thus, hyperglycemia-induced proinflammatory event in different cells may follow different pathways. This proposal is supported by the observation that both TNF-α and glucocorticoid dexamethasone-induced insulin resistance is associated with enhanced levels of ROS, and methods designed to suppress ROS generation improves insulin resistance in obese, insulin-resistant mice and restored glucose homeostasis (Houstis et al. 2006). Since insulin resistance is one of the hallmarks of obesity, type 2 diabetes mellitus, and the metabolic syndrome, it suggests that ROS plays a significant role in these conditions. Hyperglycemia induces oxidative stress not only in pancreatic β cells and adipose tissue but also in endothelial cells. This enhanced oxidative stress in endothelial cells could be responsible for endothelial dysfunction seen in metabolic syndrome.

164.5 Insulin Is Anti-inflammatory in Nature

In contrast, insulin has anti-inflammatory properties (Das 2000, 2001). Insulin suppresses the production of proinflammatory cytokines, ROS, MIF (macrophage migration inhibitory factor), and augments the production of anti-inflammatory cytokines and eNO. In thermally injured rats (30% total body surface area, TBSA), insulin administration significantly decreased dose dependently serum proinflammatory cytokines IL-1β at 1, 5, and 7 days, IL-6 at 1 day, MIF at 5 and 7 days, and TNF at 1 and 2 days after injury when compared with controls. Insulin increased anti-inflammatory cytokines IL-2 and IL-4 at 5 and 7 days after trauma and IL-10 at 2, 5, and 7 days after trauma when compared with controls. Proinflammatory signal transcription factors STAT-5 and C/EBP-beta mRNA were significantly decreased 1 and 2 days post-trauma; insulin increased anti-inflammatory signal transcription factor mRNA expression of SOCS-3 and RANTES 7 days after the injury (Jeschke et al. 2002). These data lend support to the original hypothesis (Das 2000, 2001) that insulin attenuates the inflammatory response and thus restores systemic homeostasis that could be critical for organ function and survival in critically ill patients. Furthermore, insulin significantly improved hepatic protein synthesis by increasing albumin and decreasing c-reactive protein; decreased the hepatic inflammatory response signal cascade by decreasing hepatic proinflammatory cytokines mRNA and proteins IL-1β and TNF levels; and increased hepatic cytokine mRNA and protein expression of IL-2 and IL-10 at a pretranslational level when compared with controls in rats that received thermal injury. Insulin increased hepatocyte proliferation along with Bcl-2 concentration, while decreasing hepatocyte apoptosis along with decreased caspases-3 and -9 concentration and thus improved liver morphology ($P < 0.05$). Thus, insulin attenuates the inflammatory events (Kelin et al. 2004). Similar results have been noted in thermally injured children who received insulin (Jeschke et al. 2004).

High-dose insulin treatment (short-acting insulin 1 IU/kg/h with 30% glucose 1.5 ml/kg/h administered separately) that was targeted to maintain blood glucose levels at 6.0–8.0 mmol/L produced a significant fall in C-reactive protein and free fatty acid levels postoperatively in patients with unstable angina pectoris who underwent urgent coronary artery bypass surgery. Though the proinflammatory cytokine response [interleukin-6 (IL-6), interleukin-8 (IL-8) and TNF-α] levels did not differ between the insulin group and the controls and no beneficial effects on myocardial injury were detected, these results suggested that high-dose insulin treatment has potential anti-inflammatory properties independent of its ability to lower blood glucose levels (Koskenkari et al. 2006). Similar attenuation of the systemic inflammatory response was noted in infants undergoing cardiopulmonary bypass who received intensive insulin therapy (Gu et al. 2008).

In a nonhyperglycemic mouse model of endotoxemia, continuous administration of a low dose of human insulin induced phosphorylation of Akt in muscle and adipose tissues but did not exacerbate lipopolysaccharide (LPS)-induced hypoglycemia. Insulin decreased plasma levels of IL-6, TNF-α, monocyte chemotactic protein 1 (MCP1)/JE, and keratinocyte chemoattractant, and decreased mortality. The PI3K inhibitor wortmannin abolished the insulin-mediated activation of Akt and the reduction of chemokine and interleukin-6 levels suggesting that insulin reduces LPS-induced inflammation in a PI3K/Akt-dependent manner without affecting blood glucose levels (Kidd et al. 2008). In a study designed to evaluate whether insulin attenuates TNF-α induction in acute myocardial ischemia/reperfusion injury both in vitro and in vivo, we observed that insulin inhibited ischemia-reperfusion-induced TNF-α production through the Akt-activated and eNOS-NO-dependent pathway (Li et al. 2008). These results strongly suggest that insulin has cardioprotective and prosurvival effects in the critically ill and, in general, possesses cytoprotective actions. But it should be noted that in some studies the protective effect of intensive insulin therapy in patients after cardiac surgery could not be related to a change in cytokine balance from a proinflammatory to an anti-inflammatory pattern (Hoedemaekers et al. 2005). This discrepancy in the results could be attributed to the differences in the study population, the insulin protocol used, and the underlying clinical conditions.

The fact that glucose and insulin have opposite actions on inflammation and since food intake is regulated by the hypothalamus, a function that is possible only if the hypothalamus is able to sense blood glucose levels and regulate gut function and insulin secretion, it is likely that the glucose-sensing mechanism of the hypothalamus may involve ROS signaling. Vagus seems to facilitate cross-talk among the gut, adipose tissue, pancreas, and hypothalamus, while cytokines modulate hypothalamic neuronal firing rate. In addition, the presence of insulin receptors in the brain and the known interactions between insulin, ROS, cytokines, and glucose homeostasis (as discussed above) suggest that hypothalamus function is regulated by ROS. For a better understanding of the existence of low-grade systemic inflammation in metabolic syndrome and the role played by hypothalamus in glucose homeostasis, it is important to briefly review the role of the hypothalamus in food intake and glucose homeostasis.

164.6 Hypothalamus Regulates Food Intake

Appetite is controlled by an appetite stimulating neuropeptide Y (NPY), an agouti-related peptide (AgRP), and the appetite inhibitory molecules pro-opiomelanocortin (POMC), the precursor for α-melanocyte stimulating hormone (α-MSH), and cocaine and amphetamine-regulated transcript (CART), which are expressed within the hypothalamus and act together to regulate energy balance. NPY is predominantly localized in the hypothalamic arcuate nuclei (ARC) and NPY neurons project to the paraventricular nucleus (PVN), dorsomedial nucleus (DMN), the perifornical region, and the lateral hypothalamic area (LHA) (Grove and Smith 2003). NPY neurons respond to alterations in the concentrations of plasma glucose, insulin, and leptin. Increased food intake increases the circulating concentrations of leptin that are sensed by the leptin receptors expressed on ARC and DMN neurons leading to a fall in hypothalamic NPY mRNA that results in decreased food intake. AgRP that is coexpressed with NPY in the ARC is an endogenous antagonist of anorexigenic melanocortin receptors MC3-R and MC4-R in the PVN and other hypothalamic regions. α-MSH is an endogenous anorexigenic peptide that acts on the melanocortin receptors to suppress food intake. CART, localized within the POMC neurons in the hypothalamus, also suppresses food intake (McMillen et al. 2005).

164.7 Appetite Regulatory Centers Develop During the Perinatal Period

Hypothalamic appetite regulatory centers develop predominantly during the perinatal period. For instance, NPY is present within the fetal ARC from as early as 14.5 days gestation; NPY/AgRP projections between the ARC and DMN develop around 10–11 days after birth whereas NPY containing projections to the PVN develop around 15–16 days (Grove and Smith 2003; McMillen et al. 2005). Hence, factors that influence the growth and development of the brain will have a significant impact on the development of appetite regulatory centers that, in turn, could determine food intake in later life.

For instance, postnatal over nutrition in rats led to an increased early weight gain and fat deposition, hyperphagia, obesity, hyperleptinemia, hyperglycemia, hyperinsulinemia, and insulin resistance. These indices of the metabolic syndrome were accompanied by decreased mean areas of neuronal nuclei and cytoplasm within the PVN, VMN, and ARC and a significant increase in the number of NPY containing neurons within the ARC, and decreased immunostaining for both POMC and α-MSH (McMillen et al. 2005; Davidowa et al. 2003; Fahrenkrog et al. 2004). In contrast, when rats are undernourished during the perinatal period the offspring develop significant hyperphagia and obesity when maintained on a high fat diet and showed an increase in the relative mass of retroperitoneal fat. Thus, the amount and type of food consumed during the suckling period determines food intake and preferences in later life.

The neuropeptides NPY, AgRP, POMC, and CART showed significant changes in their concentrations in the hypothalamic nuclei of fetal sheep in response to intrafetal infusion of glucose between 130 and 140 days of gestation by which time these peptides are highly expressed (Muhlhausler et al. 2005). These results suggest that neuropeptides that regulate appetite centers and their responses to stimuli are "programmed" in the fetal and perinatal stages of development. This ultimately influences the dietary preferences and the development of obesity and the metabolic syndrome in later life. This implies that early life feeding pattern and growth "program" the hypothalamic centers and their neurotransmitters that could have a life-long impact on food intake and thus influence the future development of the metabolic syndrome in a given subject.

164.8 Ventromedial Hypothalamic Lesion Produces Features of Metabolic Syndrome

Hyperphagia and excessive weight gain, fasting hyperglycemia, hyperinsulinemia, hypertriglyceridemia, and impaired glucose tolerance, which are features of the metabolic syndrome are seen when the ventromedial hypothalamus (VMH) is injured in rats (Axen et al. 1994; Keno et al. 1994). Intraventricular administration of antibodies to neuropeptide Y (NPY) abolished the hyperphagia and *ob* mRNA (leptin mRNA) in these animals, suggesting that enhanced NPY is responsible for hyperphagia and obesity seen in VMH lesioned animals, and the *ob* gene is upregulated even in nongenetically obese animals (Dube et al. 1995; Funahashi et al. 1995). Paraventricular, ventromedial (VMH), and lateral hypothalamic areas showed increased NPY concentrations in streptozotocin-induced diabetic rats. These diabetic animals also showed a significant decrease in extracellular concentrations of noradrenaline (NA), serotonin (5-HT), and their metabolites. and a pronounced increase in extracellular GABA, in the VMH. Long-term infusion of norepinephrine plus serotonin into the VMH impairs pancreatic islet function inasmuch as VMH norepinephrine and serotonin levels are elevated in hyperinsulinemic and insulin-resistant animals (reviewed in Das 2008). Streptozotocin-induced diabetes caused an increase in NA concentrations in the PVN with a concurrent increase in serum corticosterone and an increase in the concentrations of NA, dopamine, and serotonin in the ARC. It also increased NA concentrations in the lateral hypothalamus, VMH, and suprachiasmatic nucleus that reverted to normal with insulin treatment, while leptin treatment was ineffective (Das 2008).

The activity of glucokinase (GK), the critical glucose sensor of pancreatic β cells, is high in the arcuate nucleus; moderate or low in the ventromedial nucleus, lateral hypothalamic area, and paraventricular nucleus; and very low in the cortex. GK activity and GK mRNA level in the arcuate nucleus of streptozotocin-treated rats were lower than those of control rats, suggesting that prolonged hyperglycemia induced by diabetes decreased the activity of GK in the arcuate nucleus. This decrease in glucokinase activity in the hypothalamic neurons may interfere with the central regulatory mechanisms of insulin secretion by pancreatic β cells. Thus, hypothalamic neurons and neurotransmitters and GK play a critical role in the regulation of insulin secretion and in the pathobiology of the metabolic syndrome, suggesting that the latter may very well be a disorder of the brain (Das 2008).

164.9 Insulin and Insulin Receptors in the Brain

Brain is rich in insulin receptors especially in the olfactory bulb, the hypothalamus, and the pituitary, and insulin signaling has a role in the regulation of food intake, neuronal growth, and differentiation; it also regulates neurotransmitter release and synaptic plasticity in the CNS (Wan et al. 1997; Bruning et al. 2000; Hill et al. 1986). Insulin infusion into the VMN and PVN increased body temperature and energy expenditure and reduced food intake (Menendez and Atrens 1991; McGowan et al. 1992). Infusion of insulin-specific antibodies or antisense oligonucleotides directed against the insulin receptor in the third ventricle reduced hepatic sensitivity to circulating insulin and increased hepatic glucose production, suggesting that insulin in the brain regulates liver glucose metabolism (McGowan 1992). IRS-2 is abundant in the arcuate nucleus, and insulin administration induced tyrosine phosphorylation of IRS-2 and increased the production of phosphatidylinositol 3,4,5-trisphosphate (PI_3). Mice lacking IRS-2 in the hypothalamus exhibited hyperphagia and enhanced body fat deposition (Lin et al. 2004). ICV insulin infusion blocked the effects of both fasting and streptozotocin-induced diabetes to increase expression of NPY mRNA in the arcuate nucleus, while insulin increased hypothalamic POMC mRNA content. The melanocortin receptor antagonist, blocked the ability of ICV (intracerebroventricular) insulin to suppress food intake (Benoit et al. 2002). Subthreshold doses of insulin and leptin showed additive effects on short-term food intake, while both insulin and leptin suppressed NPY/AgRP neurons in the arcuate nucleus and concomitantly activated POMC/CART neurons. These results suggest that there is a cross talk between insulin and leptin apart from sharing the common ability to suppress anabolic, while activating catabolic, regulatory neurocircuitry.

164.10 Mechanism(s) of Action of Insulin in the Brain

Insulin activates ATP-sensitive K⁺ channels (K_{ATP} channels) of hypothalamic neurons, especially in the mediobasal hypothalamus (Spanswick et al. 2000). Activation of K_{ATP} channels is suppressed by increased intracellular ATP levels in response to oxidation of glucose or other substrates. This raises intracellular concentrations of K⁺, leading to membrane depolarization and increased firing rate. Thus, glucose-excited neurons are those that are activated (i.e., depolarized) by increased local concentrations of glucose. However, some studies showed that these effects are not seen at physiological glucose levels, suggesting that these neurons are downstream of NPY and POMC neurons and potentially play an integrating role for peripheral and central energy homeostasis. Leptin, like insulin, activates K_{ATP} channels in glucose-responsive hypothalamic neurons (Mirshamsi et al. 2004). Glucose-responsive neurons from Zucker fatty (*fa/fa*) rats that develop obesity, which have a leptin receptor mutation, are insensitive to both insulin and leptin. This may explain why ICV insulin inhibits neither food intake nor NPY gene expression in these *fa/fa* rats.

GLUT-4 and GLUT-8, the glucose transporters, and glucokinase, the glucose sensor of the β-cell, are present in several areas of the brain. In the arcuate nucleus, >75% of NPY-positive neurons express glucokinase (Lynch et al. 2000). Intracarotid glucose infusions increased hypothalamic glucokinase expression (Dunn-Meynell et al. 2002), suggesting that glucokinase could function as a glucose-sensor in both glucose-responsive (also referred to as glucose-excited) and glucose-sensitive (also referred to as glucose-inhibited) neurons. Since many glucokinase-expressing neurons coexpress K_{ATP} channels, and coexpression of GLUT-4 with insulin receptor mRNA is reported in glucose-responsive neurons, interactions among glucose-sensors, K_{ATP} channels and various neuropeptides is expected.

Thus, insulin interacts with neuropeptides and regulates food intake that may have relevance to the development of obesity and metabolic syndrome. Disruption of the neuron-specific insulin receptor gene (NIRKO) in mice increased food intake, developed diet-sensitive obesity with increases in body fat and plasma leptin levels, insulin resistance, hyperinsulinemia and hypertriglyceridemia, features that are seen in metabolic syndrome without interfering with the development of brain and neuronal function (Bruning et al. 2000) lending strong support to the concept that a decrease in the number of insulin receptors, deficiencies in the functioning of insulin receptors, and insulin lack or resistance in the brain leads to the development of metabolic syndrome even when the pancreatic β cells are normal (Table 164.2). This is further supported by the observation that intraventricular injection of insulin inhibits food intake (McGowan et al. 1992).

Food-deprivation induced increase in NPY levels in the paraventricular nucleus (PVN) returned to the control range following insulin injections, which did not alter blood glucose levels. Both insulin and insulin-like growth factor-II (IGF-II) decreased the release of NPY in a dose dependent fashion from the PVN *in vitro*, suggesting that the site of insulin action on the hypothalamic NPY network is at the level of NPY nerve terminals and that both insulin and IGF-II decrease NPY release from the PVN (Sahu et al. 1995). Since NPY is a potent orexigenic signal and as insulin and IGF-II decrease hypothalamic NPY, it is suggested that presence of adequate amounts of insulin, insulin receptors, and IGF-II in the brain reduces appetite, and thus controls obesity and hyperglycemia. This interaction among insulin (and insulin receptors), IGF-II, and neuropeptides depends on the health of the neurons in the brain, their receptors, and the presence of adequate synaptic connections among them.

Plasma concentrations of proinflammatory markers are increased in metabolic syndrome. These proinflammatory molecules: TNF-α, IL-6, and CRP, cause endothelial dysfunction. Mice with targeted disruption of eNOS are not only hypertensive and insulin resistant but also showed features of the metabolic syndrome such as hyperlipidemia, hyperleptinemia, hyperuricemia, and hyperfibrinogenemia and glucose intolerance but were not obese (Cook et al. 2003). These features are similar to those seen in the NIRKO mice. Since insulin stimulates the production of eNO and inhibits TNF-α production (Das 2008) and NIRKO mice show several features of the metabolic syndrome, it is postulated that a decrease in the number of insulin receptors, defects in the functioning of insulin receptors, and insulin lack or resistance in the neuronal cells lead to the development of

Table 164.2 Neuron-specific insulin receptor knockout (NIRKO) mice

1. Brain is rich in insulin receptors
2. Insulin and insulin receptors are necessary for normal growth and development of the brain
3. Insulin is also essential for neuronal growth and synapse formation
4. Insulin receptors in the brain are particularly rich in the hypothalamus
5. When these neuron-specific insulin receptors are knocked out by genetic manipulation these animals develop all the features of the metabolic syndrome
6. This suggests that insulin receptors in the brain have the ability to signal pancreatic β cells to secrete adequate amounts of insulin as the situation demands.

metabolic syndrome even when pancreatic β cells are normal. Thus, metabolic syndrome could be a disorder of the brain.

But the major question is: "When and how is metabolic syndrome initiated?" Evidence is available that suggests that the metabolic syndrome may have its origins in the perinatal period.

164.11 Perinatal Programming of the Metabolic Syndrome

Stimuli or insults induced during the perinatal period can have lifetime consequences and is called "programming". Hormonal signals or nutritional factors may serve as programming stimuli. Smallness and thinness at birth, continued slow growth in early childhood, followed by acceleration of growth so that height and weight approach the population means is considered as the most unfavorable growth pattern that results in fetal adaptations that may programme the development of metabolic syndrome in later life (Das 2008). This implies that perinatal nutrition is a crucial determinant of adult diseases. Since the development of brain occurs during the period between second trimester to 5 years of age and again during adolescence, it is likely that nutrition during these periods plays a significant role in this process. Factors that are essential for brain growth and development, regulation of synapse formation, and neurotransmission include: polyunsaturated fatty acids (PUFAs) and their metabolites, various cytokines, insulin and various neuropeptides, and monoaminergic neurotransmitters.

164.12 Essential Fatty Acids

Essential fatty acids (EFAs) are important constituents of all cell membranes. EFAs confer on membranes properties of fluidity and thus determine and influence the behavior of membrane-bound enzymes and receptors. There are two types of naturally occurring EFAs in the body, the ω-6 series derived from *cis*-linoleic acid (LA, 18:2) and the ω-3 series derived from α-linolenic acid (ALA, 18:3). LA and ALA are converted to their respective long-chain metabolites and several eicosanoids that have significant biological actions (see Fig. 164.1 for metabolism). The long-chain metabolites of EFAs (also called as polyunsaturated fatty acids, PUFAs) can give rise to both pro- (such as prostaglandins, thromboxanes, and leukotrienes) and anti-inflammatory (such as lipoxins, resolvins, protectins, and maresins) molecules. Hence, the balance between these mutually antagonistic compounds could determine the final outcome of the disease process.

164.13 PUFAs, Insulin, and Acetylcholine Function as Endogenous Neuroprotectors

Human infants accumulate PUFAs such as arachidonic acid (AA), eicosapentaenoic acid (EPA), and docosahexaenoic acid (DHA) from maternal/placental transfer, consumption of human milk, and synthesis from LA and ALA. AA regulates energy metabolism in the cerebral cortex by stimulating glucose uptake in cerebral cortical astrocytes and enhances acetylcholine (Ach) release in the brain (Das 2002b). DHA also enhances cerebral ACh levels and improves learning ability in rats. ACh modulates long-term potentiation and synaptic plasticity in neuronal circuits and interacts with dopamine

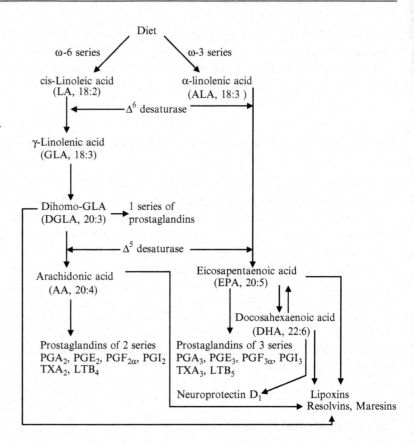

Fig. 164.1 Metabolism of essential fatty acids. Resolvins, protectins, lipoxins, and maresins formed from PUFAs have anti-inflammatory actions and participate in the resolution of inflammation. Neuroprotectin D₁ formed from DHA has anti-inflammatory and cytoprotective actions. EPA can be converted to DHA. DHA can be retroconverted to EPA

receptor in the hippocampus. In obesity, a decrease in the number of dopamine receptors or dopamine concentrations occurs and obesity is common in type 2 diabetes and metabolic syndrome (reviewed in Das 2008).

Insulin augments the activities of desaturases, enzymes involved in the desaturation and elongation of LA and ALA to their respective long-chain metabolites, and this increases the formation of AA, EPA, and DHA. Insulin-like growth factor-1 (IGF-1), insulin and AA, EPA, and DHA antagonize neuronal death induced by TNF-α and thus show neuroprotective and cytoprotective actions (reviewed in Das 2008). Furthermore, PUFAs are potent inhibitors of IL-6 and TNF-α production (Kumar and Das 1994), and they also regulate superoxide anion generation and enhance the production of eNO. NO is anti-inflammatory in nature and quenches superoxide anion. IGF-I and insulin enhance ACh release from rat cortical slices. ACh inhibits the synthesis and release of TNF-α both in vitro and in vivo and thus, has anti-inflammatory actions and is also a potent stimulator of eNO synthesis. These data suggest that insulin enhances the formation of PUFAs that, in turn, enhance ACh levels in the brain and inhibit the production of TNF-α. Thus, insulin, ACh, and PUFAs suppress TNF-α production and augment the synthesis of eNO. ACh and eNO are not only neuroprotective in nature but also interact with other neurotransmitters. Thus, insulin, ACh, and PUFAs protect brain from insults induced by TNF-α and other molecules. In addition, incorporation of significant amounts of PUFAs into the cell membranes increases their fluidity that, in turn, enhances the number of insulin receptors on the membranes and the affinity of insulin to its receptors. Thus PUFAs can attenuate insulin resistance (Das 2008).

Since human brain is rich in AA, EPA, and DHA, one of their important functions in the brain could be to ensure the presence of adequate number of insulin receptors and protect neurons from insults. Hence, it is reasonable to propose that when adequate amounts of PUFAs are not incorporated into the neuronal cell membranes during growth and development it may cause a defect in the expression or function of insulin receptors in the brain that could lead to the development of metabolic syndrome as seen in the NIRKO mice. Furthermore, systemic injections of insulin in rats resulted in an increase in extracellular ACh in the amygdala (Hajnal et al. 1998). ACh modulates dopamine release that, in turn, regulates appetite. As already discussed above, ACh inhibits the production of proinflammatory cytokines (IL-1, IL-2 and TNF-α) in the brain and thus protects the neurons from neurotoxic injury.

AA and DHA activate syntaxin.-->3, a plasma membrane protein that has an important role in the growth of neurites (Darios and Davletov 2006). AA, DHA, and EPA bind to RAR-RXR, LXR, FXR and other nuclear receptor heterodimers and thus modulate development of the brain.

164.14 TNF-α, AA/EPA/DHA, Insulin, and Neuronal Growth and Synapse Formation

Perinatal supply of ω-3 fatty acids influences brain gene expression later in life and is critical to the development and maturation of several brain centers that are specifically involved in the regulation of appetite and satiety. Supplementation of AA and EPA/DHA increased the expression of serotonin receptor in the hypothalamus (Berger et al. 2002). 5-HT$_4$ receptor increases in expression have been shown to augment hippocampal acetylcholine outflow. It was reported that AA and EPA/DHA feeding enhanced the expression of POMC in the hippocampus, suggesting that AA/EPA/DHA influence appetite and satiety and thus control energy metabolism.

TNF-α produced by glial cells enhances synaptic efficacy by increasing surface expression of AMPA receptors. Continued presence of TNF-α is required for preservation of synaptic strength at excitatory synapses (reviewed in Das 2008). TNF-α production is suppressed by EPA/DHA, whereas excess TNF-α induces apoptosis of neurons. Insulin is not only needed for neuronal growth and differentiation and synaptic plasticity in the CNS but also stimulates the formation of AA/EPA/DHA and suppresses TNF-α production. Both insulin and AA/EPA/DHA stimulate eNO formation. This close interaction and feedback regulation among TNF-α, EPA/DHA, insulin, and neuronal growth and synapse formation suggests that growth of neurons and synaptic formation will be optimum only when all these factors are present in physiological concentrations. In contrast, when AA/EPA/DHA concentrations are suboptimal, TNF-α levels tend to be high. High TNF-α concentration are neurotoxic and hence could cause damage to VMH neurons that could lead to the development of the metabolic syndrome.

164.15 Maternal Diet Influences Fetal Leptin Levels

Low birth weight is associated with high prevalence of metabolic syndrome in later life (reviewed in Das 2008). Babies with low birth weights have 10 times greater chance of developing metabolic syndrome compared to those whose birth weight was normal. In addition, postnatal nutrition and growth also play a role in the development of metabolic syndrome in later life. Maternal protein restriction or increased consumption of saturated and/or trans-fatty acids and energy rich diets (maternal overnutrition) during pregnancy decrease the formation of PUFAs. Perinatal protein depletion leads to almost complete absence of activities of the enzymes in fetal liver and placenta that are necessary for the elongation and desaturation of LA and ALA. Thus, both protein deficiency and high-energy diet leads to maternal and fetal deficiency of EPA, DHA, and AA.

A diet rich in PUFAs increases leptin levels in diet-induced obese adult rats, suggesting that variation in the type of diet during pregnancy and lactation might significantly modulate fetal and neonatal growth and development by leptin-associated mechanisms since leptin influences NPY/AgRP and POMC/CART neurons and their connections (reviewed in Das 2008). Plasma leptin levels were found to be low in the lactating dams fed an EFA-deficient diet and their suckling pups compared with controls. The suckling pups showed decreased concentrations of leptin even in their adipose tissue, suggesting that maternal EFA deficiency can produce a decrease in leptin levels in several tissues, possibly even in the hypothalamus. These low leptin levels during the perinatal period alter NPY/AgRP and POMC/CART homeostasis that may lead to the hypothalamic "body weight/appetite/satiety set point" set at a higher level that is long-lasting and potentially irreversible onto adulthood. Thus, maternal malnutrition, low perinatal PUFAs, and consequent low leptin concentrations could lead to the development of metabolic syndrome in adulthood (Das 2008).

164.16 Gastric Bypass-induced Weight Loss Could be due to Changes in the Hypothalamic Neuropeptides and Monoamines

If it is true that metabolic syndrome is a disorder of the brain, then it is necessary to show that diet-induced obesity and weight loss are due to changes in hypothalamic neuropeptides and monoamines. Roux-en-gastric bypass (RYGB) and other bariatric operations are being increasingly adopted to induce weight loss. RYGB produces on an average 49–65% weight loss within 2–5 years and ameliorates diabetes, hyperlipidemia, and other obesity-related metabolic abnormalities. In order to understand the molecular mechanisms involved in weight loss and amelioration of metabolic abnormalities in diet-induced obese animals that shed weight after RYGB operation, we developed a surgical rat model of human RYGB (Meguid et al. 2004; Middleton et al. 2004 and Xu et al. 2004).

Weight loss achieved by RYGB and PF (pair fed rats that received the same amount of diet that RYGB animals consumed) in obese rats was accompanied by a decrease in NPY in ARC, pPVN (parvocellular part of paraventricular nucleus of hypothalamus), and mPVN (magnocellular part of PVN) and an increase in α-MSH in ARC, pPVN, and mPVN compared with obese controls. 5HT-$_{1B}$-receptor in pPVN and mPVN increased in RYGB and PF compared to obese control (Romanova et al. 2004). Thus, weight loss seen after RYGB and diet control in PF groups is due to specific changes in hypothalamic peptides. Serotonin innervation is widely present in the hypothalamus and it innervates NPY neurons both in the ARC and PVN. Serotonin suppresses food intake. Hence, weight loss seen in RYGB and PF groups could be attributed to alterations in the concentrations of specific hypothalamic signaling peptides that regulate appetite, food intake, and satiety.

Even in tumor bearing anorectic rats, which showed significant weight loss due to tumor burden, similar results were seen: an increase of serotonin in PVN and VMN and a concomitant decrease of dopamine in PVN, VMN, and LHA (lateral hypothalamus), and of NPY in LHA, VMN, and PVN; a decrease in NPY in ARC and of POMC (proopiomelanocortin) in ARC and PVN (Romanova et al. 2004; Ramos et al. 2004); these abnormalities reverted to normal after tumor resection. Even the concentrations of IL-6 and TNF-α that were found to be elevated in ARC in tumor-bearing rats reverted to near normal in tumor-bearing rats that were fed fish oil (a rich source of EPA and DHA). In addition, a significant decrease in the concentrations of NPY and POMC in ARC were noted in fish oil fed nontumor-bearing rats, indicating that EPA/DHA regulate the levels of hypothalamic neuropeptides and monoamines.

164.17 Conclusions

Based on the preceding discussion, it is evident that availability of adequate amounts of EPA, DHA, and AA during the perinatal period is crucial to prevent the development of metabolic syndrome in later life. This could be in the form of supplementation of PUFAs to pregnant and lactating women, adequate breast-feeding to the newborn, followed by EPA, DHA, and AA supplementation to infants, children, and adolescents. The negative correlation noted between breast-feeding and insulin resistance and type 2 DM supports this view since human breast milk contains significant amounts of PUFAs. When infants receive inadequate amounts of PUFAs, optimal neural development is unlikely. As a result, the development, expression, and maintenance of NPY/AgRP, POMC/CART neurons, and insulin receptors will be defective; plasma, tissue, and hypothalamic concentrations of leptin will be inadequate, whereas the concentrations of proinflammatory cytokine TNF-α will be high, which may affect neuronal plasticity. A high TNF-α level may result in inadequate development of the critical hypothalamic neurons predisposing to the development of metabolic syndrome as seen in the NIRKO mice, VMH lesioned rats, and Lep^{ob}/Lep^{ob} mice. Thus, a marginal deficiency of PUFAs during the critical phases of fetal and infant growth can have a major effect on subsequent health. This is analogous to the observation that DHA deficiency in the perinatal period results in hypertension in later life, even when animals were subsequently replete with this fatty acid (Weisinger et al. 2001).

PUFAs also regulate food intake by modulating the concentrations of endogenous lipids N-acyl-ethanolamine (NAEs, anandamide) and 2-acylglycerols, and the ligands of cannabinoid (CB) receptors. These polyunsaturated NAEs bind to CB1 and CB2 (cannabinoid) receptors and regulate food intake. Furthermore, defective leptin signaling elevated hypothalamic levels of endocannabinoids in obese db/db and ob/ob mice and Zucker rats. Leptin treatment reduced anandamide and 2-arachidonoyl glycerol concentrations in the hypothalamus. EPA and DHA modulate leptin gene expression and levels both in vitro and in vivo. This suggests that PUFAs, endocannabinoids, and leptins act in concert with neurotransmitters NPY/AgRP and POMC/CART to control food intake, obesity, and metabolic syndrome.

Direct support to the concept that unsaturated fatty acids regulate hypothalamic neurons involved in the control of food intake and energy homeostasis comes from the observation that infusion of oleic acid (18:1 ω-9) in the third ventricle resulted in a marked decline in plasma insulin concentration and a decrease in the plasma glucose concentration compared with control within 1 h from the start of the infusion (Obici et al. 2002), suggesting that intracerebroventricular (ICV) oleic acid enhances insulin sensitivity. These results confirm that unsaturated fatty acids decrease systemic insulin levels and markedly stimulate insulin action on glucose homeostasis. Oleic acid suppressed the rate of glucose production by activating K_{ATP} channels in the hypothalamus similar to leptin and insulin.

Fatty acid synthase inhibitors reduced food intake and hypothalamic NPY mRNA levels (Loftus et al. 2000) by increasing the concentration of malonyl CoA, an inhibitor of the entry of long-chain CoAs into the mitochondria via inhibition of the activity of the enzyme carnitine palmitoyl-transferase-1. This results in elevation of cytoplasmic long-chain fatty acyl CoAs and diacylglycerol that play a role in signaling to the cells about the availability of fuels. Malonyl-CoA mediates nutrient-stimulated insulin secretion in the pancreatic β cell. Since glucose-sensing neurons and β cells have several similarities, such as expression of glucokinase and the ATP-sensitive K^+ channels, it is likely that malonyl-CoA may also signal fuel status in the hypothalamic neurons as it would in the β cells. In addition, both fatty acid synthase inhibitors and ICV injection of oleic acid inhibited hypothalamic expression of NPY, indicating that PUFA content of the hypothalamic neurons regulates the expression of NPY and other neuropeptides and, thus, modulates food intake, glucose homeostasis, and the development of metabolic syndrome.

Regulation of ATP-sensitive K$^+$ channels seems to be a common pathway by which nutrients modulate neuronal sensing of fuels. A primary increase in hypothalamic glucose levels lowers blood glucose through inhibition of glucose production and this effect of glucose requires its conversion to lactate followed by stimulation of pyruvate metabolism, which activates ATP-sensitive K$^+$ channels. Pyruvate has antioxidant and anti-inflammatory actions (pyruvate inhibits NF-κB activation, TNF-α, IL-6, MIF, and HMGB1 production) and is an insulin secretagogue (Das 2006b). This implies that glucose and pyruvate influence neuronal glucose sensing by a free radical dependent process since both modulate free radical generation.

Although ATP production and consequent closure of ATP-sensitive K$^+$ channels and calcium influx is considered as the main metabolic signal for this purpose, glucose-excited signaling in β cells and hypothalamic neurons is not totally dependent on ATP generation. In some hypothalamic arcuate neurons, ATP-sensitive K$^+$ channels function independent of ATP level and glucose-independent depolarization might occur through an ATP-sensitive channel-independent mechanism. Transient increase in glucose metabolism generates NADH and FADH$_2$ from the mitochondria and their use increases superoxide anion production (also called mitochondrial reactive oxygen species, mROS). Hypothalamic slices *ex vivo* exposed to 5–20 mmol/L glucose generated ROS. Glucose-induced increased neuronal activity in arcuate nucleus and insulin release are suppressed by antioxidants, suggesting that the brain glucose-sensing mechanism involves ROS signaling (reviewed in Das 2008). This is supported by the observation that ATP-sensitive K$^+$ channels control transmitter release in dorsal striatum through an H$_2$O$_2$-dependent mechanism and as several ROS-sensitive and nonselective cationic channels are known to exist. It is likely that glucose-sensing mechanisms could be similar, if not identical, in glucose responsive cells: pancreatic β cells and hypothalamic neurons. Thus, hypothalamic pyruvate, a metabolite of glucose metabolism; ROS; and PUFAs not only play a significant role in the regulation of nutrient sensing by hypothalamic neurons and β cells, but may interact among themselves. Ghrelin-induced feeding behavior that is controlled by arcuate neurons that coexpress NPY/AgRP also seem to be mediated by free radicals (Andrews et al. 2008). Thus, free radicals seem to be the common mechanism by which ghrelin, NPY/AgRP, glucose, and insulin (and possibly POMC neurons) act on hypothalamus to bring about their actions on food intake, satiety, appetite, and finally glucose homeostasis (Fig. 164.2).

Peripheral tissues (such as muscle, adipose cells, etc.), pancreatic β cells, and the hypothalamic neurons need to communicate with each other to maintain energy homeostasis. For instance, immediately after food intake gut peptides such as ghrelin, cholecystokinin (CCK), etc., are released that interact with hypothalamic neurons and signal hunger and satiety sensations. CCK reduces food intake by acting at CCK-1 receptors on vagal afferent neurons. Leptin mRNA has been reported in vagal afferent neurons, some of which also express CCK-1 receptor, suggesting that leptin, alone or in cooperation with CCK, might activate vagal afferent neurons and influence food intake via a vagal route. A much higher prevalence of CCK and leptin sensitivity amongst cultured vagal afferent neurons that innervate stomach or duodenum than there was in the overall vagal afferent population was reported. Almost all leptin-responsive gastric and duodenal vagal afferents also were sensitive to CCK. Leptin, infused into the upper GI tract arterial supply, reduced meal size, and enhanced satiation evoked by CCK, indicating that vagal afferent neurons are activated by leptin, and that this activation participates in meal termination by enhancing vagal sensitivity to CCK (reviewed in Das 2008). Injection of adeno-associated viral vectors encoding leptin (rAAV-lep) rAAV-lep injection increased hypothalamic leptin expression in the complete absence of peripheral leptin in *ob/ob* mice; suppressed body weight and adiposity; voluntarily decreased dark-phase food intake; suppressed plasma levels of adiponectin, TNF-α, free fatty acids, and insulin concomitant with normoglycemia and elevated ghrelin levels for an extended period. Leptin administration rapidly decreased plasma gastric ghrelin and adipocyte adiponectin but not TNF-α level, thereby demonstrating a

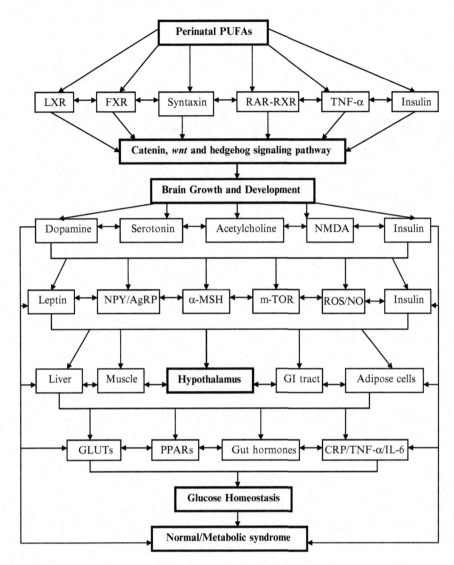

Fig. 164.2 Scheme showing the relationship among PUFAs and various tissues and factors involved in the pathobiology of the metabolic syndrome

peripheral restraining action of leptin on the secretion of hormones of varied origins. Whereas ghrelin administration readily stimulated feeding in controls, it was completely ineffective in rAAV-lep-treated wt mice. Thus, leptin expressed locally in the hypothalamus counteracted the central orexigenic effects of peripheral ghrelin, suggesting that leptin and ghrelin interact with each other and thus regulate energy homeostasis and metabolism. It was reported that incubation of the hypothalamic explants with ghrelin significantly increased NPY and AGRP mRNA expression, suggesting that ghrelin and NPY interact with each other. Ghrelin facilitates both cholinergic and tachykininergic excitatory pathways, consistent with activity within the enteric nervous system and possibly the vagus nerve (reviewed in Das 2008). These evidences suggest that sympathetic and parasympathetic (especially vagus nerve) nerves carry messages from the peripheral tissues and β cells to the hypothalamus and *vice versa* where all the messages are integrated, codified, and relayed to the target tissues to maintain overall energy balance (Fig. 164.3).

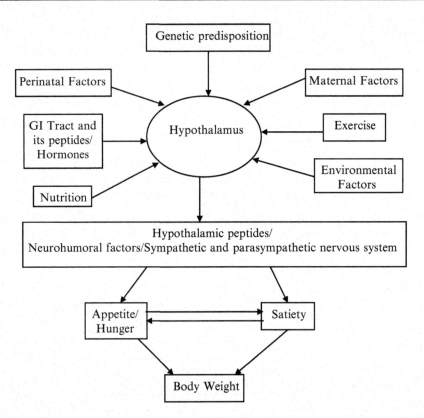

Fig. 164.3 Scheme showing the simplified relationship between genetic factors, maternal factors, diet, GI tract, and hypothalamus to body weight

This is supported by the observation that adenovirus-mediated expression of PPAR-γ2 in the liver induces acute hepatic steatosis while markedly reducing peripheral adiposity, changes that were accompanied by increased energy expenditure and improved systemic insulin sensitivity. Interestingly, hepatic vagotomy and selective afferent blockage of the hepatic vagus reversed these changes, whereas thiazolidinedione, a PPAR-γ agonist, enhanced these changes (reviewed in Das 2008). Thus, a neuronal pathway consisting of the afferent vagus from the liver and efferent sympathetic nerves to adipose tissues is involved in the regulation of energy expenditure, systemic insulin sensitivity, glucose metabolism, and fat distribution between the liver and the periphery. In this context, it should be noted that proinflammatory cytokine production is regulated by the efferent vagus nerve. Acetylcholine (ACh), the principal vagal neurotransmitter, has been shown to inhibit the production of TNF, IL-1, MIF, and HMGB1, and activation of NF-κB expression (reviewed in Das 2008). Since ACh is both a neurotransmitter and regulates serotonin, dopamine, and other neuropeptides, whereas PUFAs influence ACh release and insulin sensitivity (Das 2008), it is clear that a complex network of interaction(s) exists among all these molecules in the regulation of energy homeostasis. Furthermore, brain insulin resistance exists in peripheral insulin resistance, especially in regions subserving appetite and reward; exercise enhanced the sensitivity of hypothalamus to the actions of leptin and insulin and the appetite-suppressive actions of exercise are mediated by the hypothalamus (Das 2008). These evidences emphasize the role of hypothalamus in the pathobiology of metabolic syndrome.

Summary Points

- The incidence of metabolic syndrome is assuming epidemic proportions in almost all countries in the world.
- Low-grade systemic inflammation occurs in metabolic syndrome.
- Glucose has proinflammatory actions while insulin is anti-inflammatory in nature.
- The anti-inflammatory nature of insulin suggests that hyperinsulinemia seen in insulin resistance may be a protective phenomena and this also explains its cardioprotective and cytoprotective actions.
- The hypothalamic centers that regulate appetite, food intake, and satiety are formed during the fetal period; enhanced maternal and early perinatal nutrition programs the hypothalamic centers and this influences food preferences in later life.
- Features of metabolic syndrome are seen when ventromedial hypothalamus is damaged suggesting that it could be a disorder of the brain.
- Insulin receptors are present in the brain and intracerebroventricular injection of insulin reduces food intake and suppresses NPY/AgRP and activates POMC/CART neurons.
- Insulin activates K_{ATP} channels in the neurons and modulates the levels of reactive oxygen species and nitric oxide, and thus regulates glucose homeostasis.
- PUFAs are essential for brain growth and development and modulate the production and actions of acetylcholine, dopamine and other neurotransmitters and monoamines. PUFAs are also neuroprotective in nature.
- Maternal diet influences plasma leptin levels that, in turn, modulates NPY/AgRP and POMC/CART homeostasis
- Gastric bypass and diet restriction induced weight loss could be due to alterations in hypothalamic neuropeptides and monoamines.

Key Points

- Glucose is needed for the energy needs of all tissues of the body.
- Glucose needs to enter the cell for its conversion to ATP (adenosine triphosphate), the main source of energy to all cells of the body.
- Insulin has the property to push glucose into the cells.
- Insulin to produce its actions binds to its receptor, insulin receptor, which leads to the generation of a series of signals that bring about the actions of insulin in the cell.
- Once the glucose enters the cell, though its receptors called GLUT (glucose transporters) receptors plasma glucose levels decrease.
- When glucose fails to enter the cell due to a defect in insulin action and abnormalities in GLUTs, plasma glucose will increase while the cells are starved of glucose.
- Insulin is produced by pancreatic β cells in response to food intake and increase in plasma glucose levels.
- Failure to produce adequate amounts of insulin leads to inadequate utilization of glucose by cells and this results in an increase in plasma glucose. Called hyperglycemia, this is a key feature of type 2 diabetes mellitus and the metabolic syndrome.
- Other features associated with metabolic syndrome are obesity, abnormities in plasma lipid levels, and low-grade inflammation.

- Metabolic syndrome is considered a low grade systemic inflammatory condition.
- Hyperglycemia enhances the production of free radicals, and proinflammatory cytokines.
- Insulin shows anti-inflammatory actions.
- Lesions of the ventromedial hypothalamus (VMH) in experimental animals produce all the features of the metabolic syndrome
- Neuron-specific insulin receptor knockout (NIRKO) mice also show many features of the metabolic syndrome.
- Mice with targeted disruption of endothelial nitric oxides synthase (eNOS) are not only hypertensive and insulin resistant but also show features of the metabolic syndrome.
- The brain is rich in insulin receptors, including the hypothalamus.
- Administration of insulin into the hypothalamus reduces food intake and plasma glucose.
- Hypothalamic centers that regulate food intake, appetite, and satiety are formed during the perinatal period.
- Maternal diet and perinatal nutrition programs the hypothalamic centers, hypothalamic neuropeptides, and monoamines.
- Polyunsaturated fatty acids (PUFAs) are essential for brain growth and development and can modulate the production of leptin and other neuropeptides.
- Intraventricular administration of oleic acid decreases food intake, reduces plasma glucose and leptin levels, and ameliorates diabetes mellitus.
- Cross-talk among gut, liver, pancreas, and hypothalamus occurs through vagal fibers.
- Acetylcholine, the principal vagal neurotransmitter, shows anti-inflammatory actions and regulates various hypothalamic monoamines.
- Insulin, PUFAs, and acetylcholine enhance endothelial nitric oxide generation, and have anti-inflammatory and neuroprotective actions.
- Glucose, insulin, and PUFAs act on K_{ATP} channels in glucose-responsive hypothalamic neurons.
- Brain glucose-sensing mechanism involves reactive oxygen species (ROS) signaling that act on ATP-sensitive K^+ channels.
- The strategy of providing adequate PUFAs during the perinatal period may prevent the development of the metabolic syndrome by suppressing low-grade systemic inflammation, ensuring the presence of adequate number of insulin receptors in the brain, and adequacy of hypothalamic neuropeptides and monoamines.

Acknowledgments Dr U N Das received the Ramalingaswami fellowship of the Department of Biotechnology, India, during the tenure of this study.

References

Aljada A, Ghanim H, Mohanty P, Hofmeyer D, Chaudhuri A, Dandona P. Metabolism. 2006;55:1177–85.
Aljada A, Mohanty P, Ghanim H, Abdo T, Tripathy D, Chaudhuri A, Dandona P. Am J Clin Nutr. 2004;79:682–90.
Andrews ZB, Liu Z-W, Wallingford N, Erion DM, Borok E, Friedman JM, Tschop MH, Shanabrough M, Cline G, Shulman GI, Coppola A, Gao X-B, Horvath TL, Diano S. Nature. 2008;454:846–51.
Axen KV, Li X, Fung K, Sclafani A. Am J Physiol. 1994;266 (3 Pt 2):R921–8.
Benoit SC, Air EL, Coolen LM, Strauss R, Jackman A, Clegg DJ, Seeley RJ, Woods SC. J Neurosci. 2002;22:9048–52.
Berger A, Mutch DM, German JB, Roberts MA. Lipids Health Dis. 2002;1:2.

Bruning JC, Gautam D, Burks DJ, Gillette J, Schubert M, Orban PC, Klein R, Krone W, Muller-Wieland D, Kahn CR. Science. 2000;289:2122–5.

Cook S, Hugli O, Egli M, Vollenweder P, Burcelin R, Nicod P, Thorens B, Scherrer U. Swiss Med Wkly. 2003;133:360–3.

Darios F, Davletov B. Nature. 2006;440:813–7.

Das UN. Diabetologia. 2000;43:1081–2.

Das UN. Nutrition. 2001;17:409–13.

Das UN. Exp Biol Med. 2002a;227:989–97.

Das UN. Lancet. 2002b;360:490.

Das UN. Nutrition. 2004;20:323–6.

Das UN. Eur Heart J. 2006a;27:1385–6.

Das UN. Nutrition. 2006b;22:965–72.

Das UN. Curr Nutr Food Sci. 2008;4:73–108.

Davidowa H, Li Y, Plagemann A. Eur J Neurosci. 2003;18:613–21.

Dube MG, Kalra PS, Crowley WR, Kalra SP. Brain Res. 1995;690:275–8.

Dunn-Meynell AA, Routh VH, Kang L, Gaspers L, Levin BE. Diabetes. 2002;51:2056–65.

Elouil H, Cardozo AK, Eizirik DL, Henquin JC, Jonas JC. Diabetologia. 2005;48:496–505.

Fahrenkrog S, Harder T, Stolaczyk E, Melchior K, Franke K, Dudenhausen JW, Plagemann A. J Nutr. 2004;134:648–54.

Funahashi T, Shimomura I, Hiraoka H, Arai T, Takahashi M, Nakamura T, Nozaki S, Yamashita S, Takemura K, Tokunaga K, et al. Biochem Biophys Res Commun. 1995;211:469–75.

Grove KL, Smith MS. Physiol Behav. 2003;79:47–63.

Grundy SM, Brewer Jr B, Cleema JI, Smith SC, Lenfant C for the conference participants. NHLBI/AHA conference proceedings. Circulation. 2004;109:433–8.

Gu CH, Cui Q, Wang YY, Wang J, Dou YW, Zhao R, Liu Y, Wang J, Pei JM, Yi DH. Cytokine. 2008;44:96–100.

Hajnal A, Pothos EN, Lenard L, Hoebel BG. Effects of feeding and insulin on extracellular acetylcholine in the amygdala of freely moving rats. Brain Res. 1998;785:41–8.

Hill JM, Lesniak MA, Pert CB, Roth J. Neuroscience. 1986;17:1127–38.

Hoedemaekers CW, Pickkers P, Netea MG, van Deuren M, Van der Hoeven JG. Crit Care. 2005;9:R790–7.

Houstis N, Rosen ED, Lander S. Nature. 2006;440:944–8.

Jeschke MG, Einspanier R, Kelin D, Jauch KW. Mol Med. 2002;8:443–50.

Jeschke MG, Klein D, Herndon DN. Ann Surg. 2004;239:553–60.

Keno Y, Tokunaga K, Fujioka S, Kobatake T, Kotani K, Yoshida S, Nishida M, Shimomura I, Matsuo T, Odaka H, et al. Metabolism. 1994;43:32–7.

Kidd LB, Schabbauer GA, Luyendyk JP, Holscher TD, Tilley RE, Tencati M, Mackman N. J Pharmacol Exp Ther. 2008;326:348–53.

Klein D, Shubert T, Horch RE, Jauch KW, Jeschke MG. Ann Surg. 2004;240:340–9.

Koskenkari JK, Kaukoranta PK, Rimpilainen J, Vainionpaa V, Ohtonen PP, Surcel HM, Juvonen T, Ala-Kokko TI. Acta Anaesthesiol Scand. 2006;50:962–9.

Kumar SG, Das UN. Prostaglandins Leukotr Essen Fatty Acids. 1994;50:331–4.

Li J, Zhang H, Wu F, Nan Y, Ma H, Guo W, Wang H, Ren J, Das UN, Gao F. Crit Care Med. 2008;36:1551–8.

Lin X, Taguchi A, Park S, Kushner JA, Li F, Li Y, White MF. J Clin Invest. 2004;114:908–16.

Lin Y, erg AH, Iyengar P, Lam TK, Giacca A, Combs TP, Rajala MW, Du X, Rollman B, Li W, Hawkins M, Barzilai N, Rhodes CJ, Fantus IG, Brownlee M, Scherer PE. J Biol Chem. 2005;280:4617–26.

Lin Y, Rajala MW, Berge JP, Moller DE, Barzilai N, Scherer PE. J Biol Chem. 2001;276:42077–83.

Loftus TM, Jaworsky DE, Frehywot GL, Townsend CA, Ronnett GV, Lane MD, Kuhajda FP. Science. 2000;288:2379–81.

Lynch RM, Tompkins LS, Brooks HL, Dunn-Meynell AA, Levin BE. Diabetes. 2000;49:693–700.

McGowan MK, Andrews KM, Grossman SP. Physiol Behav. 1992;51:753–66.

McMillen IC, Adam CL, Muhlhausler BS. J Physiol. 2005;565:9–17.

Meguid MM, Ramos EJB, Suzuki S, Xu Y, George ZM, Das UN, Hughes K, Quinn R, Chen C, Marx W, Cunningham PRG. J Gastrointestinal Surg. 2004;8:621–30.

Menendez JA, Atrens DM. Brain Res. 1991;555:193–201.

Middleton FA, Ramos EJB, Xu Y, Diab H, Zhao X, Das UN, Meguid MM. Nutrition. 2004;20:14–25.

Mirshamsi S, Laidlaw HA, Ning K, Anderson E, Burgess LA, Gray A, Sutherland C, Ashford ML. BMC Neurosci. 2004;5:54.

Morgan D, Oliveira-Emilio HR, Keane D, Hirata AE, Santos da Rocha M, Bordin S, Curi R, Newsholme P, Carpinelli AR. Diabetologia. 2007;50:359–69.

Muhlhausler BS, Adam CL, Marracco EM, Findlay PA, Roberts CI, McFarlane JR, Kauter KG, McMillen IC. J Physiol. 2005;565:185–95.

Nareika A, Maldonado A, He L, Game BA, Slate EH, Sanders JJ, London SD, Lopes-Virella MF, Huang Y. J Periodontal Res. 2007;42:31–8.

Obici S, Feng Z, Morgan K, Stein D, Karkanias G, Rossetti L. Diabetes. 2002;51:271–5.

Ramos EJB, Suzuki S, Meguid MM, Laviano A, Sato T, Chen C, Das UN. Surgery. 2004;136:270–6.

Romanova I, Ramos EJB, Xu Y, Quinn R, Chan C, George ZM, Inui A, Das UN, Meguid MM. J Am Coll Surg. 2004;199:887–95.

Sahu A, Dube MG, Phelps CP, Sninsky CA, Kalra PS, Kalra SP. Endocrinology. 1995;136:5718–24.

Spanswick D, Smith MA, Mirshamsi S, Routh VH, Ashford ML. Nat Neurosci. 2000;3:757–8.

Sweet IR, Gilbert M, Maloney E, Hockenbery DM, Schwartz MW, Kim F. Diabetologia. 2009;52:921–31.

Wan Q, Xiong ZG, Man HY, Ackerley CA, Braunton J, Lu WY, Becker LE, MacDonald JF, Wang YT. Nature. 1997;388:686–90.

Weisinger HS, Armitage JA, Sinclair AJ, Vingrys AJ, Burns PL, Weisinger RS. Nat Med. 2001;7:258–9.

Xu Y, Ramos EJB, Middleton F, Romanova I, Quinn R, Chen C, Das UN, Inui A, Meguid MM. Surgery. 2004;136:246–52.

Chapter 165
Schizophrenia and the Metabolic Syndrome

Jared Edward Reser

165.1 Introduction

It has been well known for at least 2 decades that schizophrenia is associated with excess mortality, premature death, and increased standard mortality from both natural and unnatural causes (Allebeck 1989). Patients with schizophrenia are at high risk of death from unnatural causes such as suicides and accidents; however, unnatural causes do not account for even half of the excess mortality. It is increasingly recognized that patients with schizophrenia are at increased risk for natural causes of death, primarily life-shortening illnesses (Marder et al. 2004). Epidemiological data have for decades evinced that natural causes afflict patients with schizophrenia much earlier than they do people in the general population. In fact, one meta-analysis concluded that at least 60% of the excess mortality in patients with schizophrenia is attributable to physical illness (Brown 1997). This well-received study also found that only 28% of the excess mortality is attributable to suicide and only 12% to accidents, leaving even more room than initially expected for the contribution of illness. Individuals with schizophrenia have been shown to die younger from a variety of cardiovascular, infectious, gastrointestinal, respiratory, urogenital, and metabolic conditions. It is not clear if there is a common contributing pathological factor that underlies these epidemiological correlations. Probably the best candidate for such a unifying factor is the metabolic syndrome, a cluster of commonly comorbid metabolic derangements that tend to exacerbate one another and tend to afflict individuals with schizophrenia. It is not clear why the metabolic syndrome is relatively prevalent in populations with schizophrenia, but taken together, various points of evidence regarding this association are beginning to elucidate how the two are related and what can be done in regard to prevention.

Most medical professionals do not think of the metabolic syndrome when they hear the word schizophrenia. Schizophrenia is a psychiatric diagnosis that is characterized by abnormalities in the perception or expression of reality. It can present in different ways but commonly manifests as auditory hallucinations, paranoid or bizarre delusions, or disorganized speech and thinking. The impairment in sensory gating, emotional inhibition, and the organization of complex behaviors cause individuals with schizophrenia to have significant impairments in social and occupational abilities. Onset of symptoms typically occurs in young adulthood with between 0.4% and 0.6% of the worldwide population affected (Bhugra 2006). It has become clear that the psychological symptoms are accompanied by a variety of somatic symptoms and health issues. In a study of over 168,000 affected

J.E. Reser (✉)
University of Southern California, Psychology Department, SGM 501, 3620 South McClintock Ave.,
Los Angeles, CA 90089-1061, USA
e-mail: jared@jaredreser.com; reser@usc.edu

V.R. Preedy et al. (eds.), *Handbook of Behavior, Food and Nutrition*,
DOI 10.1007/978-0-387-92271-3_165, © Springer Science+Business Media, LLC 2011

Table 165.1 The key features of schizophrenia

Thought	Hallucinations, delusions, paranoid ideation, bizarre thinking
Behavior	Disorganized speech, emotional outbursts, social and occupational dysfunction, long term unemployment, homelessness, poverty
Causes	Both genetic and environmental, high heritability, stress, prenatal stress, drug abuse, social disadvantage
Brain physiology	Increased dopamine activity in the mesolimbic pathway, hypometabolic states in the prefrontal and temporal cortices and hippocampus
Comorbid conditions	Major depression, anxiety disorders, metabolic disorders, substance abuse

The key features of schizophrenia with selected aspects

patients in Sweden, schizophrenia was associated with an average life expectancy of approximately 80–85% of that of the general population (Hannerz et al. 2001). It is currently thought that a large proportion of this excess mortality can be attributed to metabolic disease.

Before the explicit ties to the metabolic syndrome were made, it was noted by epidemiologists that cardiovascular disease plays a large role in the premature deaths of schizophrenic patients. It was estimated that cardiovascular disease was responsible for as much as 50% of the excess mortality (Osby et al. 2000). Moreover, nearly 20% of deaths in schizophrenia can be attributed to ischemic heart disease, the most common cause of death in both sexes (Newman and Bland 1991). Today it is thought that even though there may be many contributing factors to cardiovascular disease in schizophrenia (such as cardiac arrhythmia and toxic cardiomyopathy), the major contributing factors may be metabolic disturbances – shared, common comorbidities in cardiovascular disease and schizophrenia. Since this realization, it has been well documented that individuals with schizophrenia are markedly susceptible to a specific group of metabolic disturbances that tend to present together in human and animal populations as the metabolic syndrome. It is thought that susceptibility to metabolic disease may be due to many different aspects common to schizophrenia, the most probable include inactive lifestyle, poor dietary choices, severe stress, and the side effects of psychotropic medications (Wirshing and Meyer 2003) (Table 165.1).

165.2 The Metabolic Syndrome in Schizophrenia

The metabolic syndrome has been a significant construct in the field of cardiology and endocrinology for at least 2 decades, but has become of interest to a variety of different fields in the last decade because of the ongoing, worldwide epidemic of obesity and diabetes. The metabolic syndrome is comprised of a group of clinical features that include atherogenic dyslipidemia (low high density lipoprotein (HDL) and elevated fasting triglycerides), hypertension, increased abdominal or visceral adiposity, and impaired fasting glucose or diabetes mellitus (Expert Panel on Detection 2001) (Table 165.2).

In 2005, the Adult Treatment Panel III of the National Cholesterol Education Program defined diagnosis as the presence of three or more of the five states listed in Table 165.3. The International Diabetes Federation, the European Group for the Study of Insulin Resistance, the World Health Organization, and others have each identified unique sets of diagnostic criteria. This disparity in diagnostic definition has created some concern and confusion; however, all three systems are relatively similar. There is broad overlap between the definitions, especially those of the World Health Organization and National Cholesterol Education Program. These similarities led researchers to find that, using data from the third National Health and Nutrition Examination Survey, NCEP and WHO criteria led to identical diagnoses for a group of 8,608 subjects in 86.2% of subjects. Not surprisingly,

Table 165.2 The key features of the metabolic syndrome

Obesity	Increased total body fat, abdominal or central fat distribution, increased visceral fat
Insulin resistance	Hyperinsulinemia
Dyslipidemia	Hypertriglyceridemia, decreased HDL cholesterol, increased LDL cholesterol
Impaired glucose tolerance	Type 2 diabetes mellitus
Hypertension	High or deranged blood pressure

The defining disorders of the metabolic syndrome and their components

Table 165.3 Criteria for the metabolic syndrome

Increased waist circumference	>102 cm in men, >88 cm in women
Elevated triglycerides	>150 mg/dl or 1.7 mmol/l
Decreased HDL cholesterol	<40 mg/dl in men, <50 mg/dl in women
Blood pressure	>130/85 mgHg or active treatment for hypertension
Fasting glucose	>110 mg/dl or active treatment for hyperglycemia

The National Cholesterol Education Program's criteria for diagnosis of the metabolic syndrome and their defining measures. Three of the five risk factors must be present for a diagnosis

differences in susceptibility to individual features caused the prevalence estimates between the two definitions to differ for some subpopulations, including sex and race (Ford and Giles 2003). It is not known if schizophrenia is another subpopulation whose prevalence might be affected arbitrarily by differences in susceptibility to certain features over others, although it is certainly possible.

The metabolic syndrome is highly prevalent in the general population. Based on the estimates derived from the third National Health and Nutrition Examination Survey it is thought that around 47 million people in the US meet the diagnostic criteria (Ford and Giles 2003). The age-adjusted prevalence in the US is 23.7% with the lowest prevalence of 6.7% for individuals between the ages of 20 and 29 and the highest prevalence of 43.5% for individuals aged 60 and higher. Both schizophrenia and a closely related psychiatric illness, schizoaffective disorder, are associated with a drastically increased risk for the metabolic syndrome and together have an age-adjusted prevalence of 42.6% for males and 48.5% for females (Cohn et al. 2004). Ethnicity as a predictor persists even after controlling for age, BMI, and socioeconomic status. For instance, Hispanics have the highest age adjusted prevalence of 31.9%. The age adjusted prevalence for schizophrenia is thought to be above 40%, significantly higher than the highest prevalence by ethnicity (Cohn et al. 2004).

McEvoy et al. (2005) confirmed in a large and well-controlled study that the metabolic syndrome is much more prevalent in patients with schizophrenia than among individuals from the general population, even after controlling for body mass and a variety of demographic variables. The order of the significance of this finding persuaded researchers to state that schizophrenia patients may represent a patient population with one of the highest metabolic syndrome prevalence rates of the major patient groups studied today. This study also showed that female patients with schizophrenia may constitute one of the subpopulations most vulnerable to central obesity and type 2 diabetes mellitus. Despite this and other fine studies in this area, there is no consensus about the prevalence of the metabolic syndrome in schizophrenia, in it subsets, or in associated psychotic disorders. It will be very informative to have the cross-sectional, longitudinal, and component feature data, and this may be available in a more reliable form in the near future.

The etiology of the metabolic syndrome, like that of schizophrenia, is still mysterious and controversial. There are a large number of secondary factors, aside from the key features, that are closely associated with the metabolic syndrome (Ryan and Thakore 2002), see Table 165.4. A review of these by Hansen (1999) identifies a wide assortment including: autonomic neuropathy, altered adipose tissue

Table 165.4 Secondary associations with the metabolic syndrome

Adipose tissue abnormalities: hyperleptinemia, altered lipoprotein lipase activity
Alcohol consumption
Pituitary adrenal abnormalities: hypercoritisolemia, impaired glucocorticoid receptor function
Reduced physical activity
Reduced ability to cope with stress, elevated stress hormone levels
Genetic predisposition, high heritability
Smoking
Increased food intake: hyperphagia, increased dietary fat content
Sex hormone abnormalities

A brief list of some of the secondary abnormalities associated with the diagnosis of the metabolic syndrome

physiology, difficulty coping with stress, excess alcohol consumption, hypercortisolemia, hyperphagia, impaired glucocorticoid receptor function, increased dietary fat content, reduced growth hormone, reduced physical activity, sex hormone abnormalities, and smoking. Factor analyses of the key and secondary features suggest that there is no unifying etiological feature (Zimmet et al. 1999). Many of these features are known to be quite commonplace in schizophrenia (Ryan and Thakore 2002). There has been very little research though, on whether populations of nonschizophrenic individuals with the metabolic syndrome exhibit symptoms particular to schizophrenia.

Individuals with schizophrenia may have increased risk for the metabolic syndrome because of patterns of unhealthy lifestyle choices common to schizophrenia and other psychotic disorders. Heavy alcohol (Mortensen and Juel 1993) and cigarette (Masterson and O'Shea 1984) use, along with poor diet, high fat consumption, lack of exercise and low physical activity (Brown et al. 1999) are all strongly associated with schizophrenia and have been for decades. These lifestyle factors are also powerful risk factors for the metabolic syndrome. It is clear that there is an increased need for lifestyle therapy intervention in this population. Diminishing substance abuse and increasing physical activity have long been treatment goals in schizophrenia therapy designed to ameliorate the psychological symptoms and improve mood. Now it is obvious that these goals will do more for this population than previously appreciated because they will also help to treat the metabolic symptoms.

It is becoming clear that the high prevalence of the metabolic syndrome in schizophrenia is due to more than just the behavioral propensities of patients or the antipsychotic drugs that the majority of patients have been prescribed. Several family history studies, and even decades old historical studies have found weighty, positive associations between schizophrenia and diabetes. Studies have also shown that first episode drug-naïve patients have an increased prevalence of central obesity, impaired fasting glucose, and insulin resistance suggesting that metabolic disturbances may be an inherent genetic component of the schizophrenia phenotype (de Leon and Diaz 2007; Spelman et al. 2007). Some well controlled studies have even shown that diabetes is more common in patients not taking antipsychotics than in those that were receiving them (Mukherjee et al. 1996). This represented powerful evidence suggesting that the association between schizophrenia and the metabolic syndrome is due to more than just the commonly accepted environmental influences. Some recent articles have even stated explicitly that there is evidence indicating that, "patients with schizophrenia might have an inherent predisposition towards the metabolic syndrome in a similar manner seen with certain ethnic groups" (McEvoy et al. 2005). In fact, genes responsible for schizophrenia and the metabolic syndrome seem to transmit together across generations. There is an increased frequency of the metabolic syndrome in the nonschizophrenic relatives of patients with schizophrenia (Mukherjee et al. 1989). Also, many of the individual facets of the metabolic syndrome have been closely tied to first episode or drug naïve schizophrenia as Table 165.5 demonstrates.

Table 165.5 Metabolic disorders and schizophrenia

Cardiovascular disease	Kendrick (1996); Davidson (2002) Ryan and Thakore (2002)
Insulin resistance	Felker et al. (1996); Ryan and Thakore (2002); Ristow (2004)
HPA axis up-regulation	Walker et al. (1996); Walker and Diforio (1997)
Metabolic syndrome	Ryan and Thakore (2002); Heiskanen et al. (2003)
Obesity	Allison et al. (1999); Davidson (2002)

A list of some of the features of the metabolic syndrome that have been associated with drug naïve or first episode schizophrenia

165.3 Schizophrenia and Diabetes

Studies indicate that diabetes mellitus may be twice as prevalent in schizophrenia (14%) as it is in the general population (7%) (Dixon et al. 2000). Additionally, impaired glucose tolerance and insulin resistance are also more common (Jeste et al. 1996). It is still not clear to what extent schizophrenia and diabetes present comorbidly because of shared genetic backgrounds, or if they are associated environmentally through weight gain. Prior to the onset of schizophrenia, there is not strong evidence for preexisting obesity (Weiser et al. 2004), an observation which provides some support for the latter assumption given that susceptibility of children and adults to the metabolic syndrome increases with worsening obesity. This does not necessarily detract from the significance of genetic contribution though, especially since individuals with schizophrenia are more likely to have obese parents. Furthermore, some studies have shown that even though there may not be a predisposition towards obesity prior to onset, it seems there is a prodromal predisposition for visceral adiposity (Zhang et al. 2004). It is possible that this inclination becomes fully expressed as obesity and diabetes after onset due to epigenetic factors, lifestyle, medications or interactions between all three.

The number of published prevalence studies of the metabolic syndrome in schizophrenia patients is not large, but it documents that the association is probably larger than the association between schizophrenia and diabetes mellitus (Heiskanen et al. 2003; Basu et al. 2004). Why this might be is unclear. The association between diabetes mellitus and schizophrenia has come under scrutiny recently because of new data associating atypical antipsychotics (also known as second generation antipsychotics) with new onset diabetes and the dangerous state of diabetic ketoacidosis (American Diabetes Association et al. 2004). Atypical antipsychotics have been known to work well to alleviate the symptoms of schizophrenia, and other forms of psychosis, but have received negative attention in the literature because of the significant weight gain liabilities associated with certain drugs (Meyer 2001).

165.4 Antipsychotic Medications

Atypical antipsychotics have been immensely effective in treating schizophrenia. Ironically though, they have been implicated in greatly accelerating the progression of the metabolic syndrome. More specifically, they have been heavily associated with cardiac irregularities, dyslipidemia, glucose intolerance, and weight gain (Ryan and Thakore 2002). The proportion of patients on antipsychotics with the metabolic syndrome ranges between 20% and 60% and in most cases is double the prevalence in the general population (De Hert et al. 2006; Haupt 2006). The evidence is the strongest for clozapine and olanzapine (Shirzadi and Ghaemi 2006) and suggestive but weaker for other antipsychotics (Newcomer and Haupt 2006).

It has been difficult for researchers to come to conclusions about the adverse effects of antipsychotics without the much needed randomized, controlled trials with prospective designs. Prior antipsychotic treatment and other medications confound the findings of many of the studies. Recent studies done with first episode schizophrenia avoided some of these confounds because all of the participants were drug naïve and had no prior antipsychotic prescription. One such study, using historic data, found that even though there was no difference in prevalence of the metabolic syndrome between first episode schizophrenics from 15–20 years ago compared with first episode moderns, the incidence of the metabolic syndrome was three times higher in the modern group that took atypical antipsychotics compared to the historic group that took first-generation antipsychotics (Hert et al. 2008). A number of findings have reinforced the consensus that first generation antipsychotics were far less likely to lead to metabolic complications. Another first episode study compared individual medications and showed that the test groups receiving olanzapine had the highest prevalence of the metabolic syndrome at 20–25%, followed by risperidone at 9–24% and finally haloperidol at 0–3% (Saddichha et al. 2008). Other studies have identified clozapine as being among the worst of these agents.

There are still many unknowns in this arena but fortunately there are also some thoughtful articles aimed at educating health professionals about what is known. The American Diabetes Association published a consensus paper on antipsychotic drugs and metabolic outcome that provides clear and helpful guidelines for health monitoring and medication selection for patients needing atypical antipsychotic drugs (American Diabetes Association et al. 2004). Despite many strong findings, it is important to point out that the influence of antipsychotic drugs comprises only a piece of this puzzle. As stated earlier, metabolic abnormalities have consistently been associated with schizophrenia even before the era of antipsychotic medications (Raphael 1921; Homel et al. 2002).

165.5 Schizophrenia and Cardiovascular Disease

As stated earlier, cardiovascular disease is one of the primary causes of morbidity and mortality in patients with schizophrenia (Meyer and Nasrallah 2003). Patients are known to commonly exhibit several different markers for cardiovascular risk. Both individuals treated with atypical antipsychotics and those who are drug free have a high propensity for platelet aggregation differences which makes them more likely to produce thrombus. Thrombus production is crucial during wound healing but overproduction can lead to life-threatening pathology including myocardial infarction. Exactly why and how this increased platelet aggregation occurs is unclear. Other unhealthy cardiac features that are associated with schizophrenia include: abnormal heart variation, prolonged phase of cardiac depolarization, decreased variations in cardiac rate, high sinus rhythm resting heart rate, long periodicity of endogenous ultradian rhythm of heart rate, and others. Interestingly, most of these features were abnormal in both individuals treated with antipsychotic drugs and those that were never treated. These findings lead one to conclude that there are multiple sources of evidence for abnormal autonomic control of heart rate, each of them related to cardiovascular risk, and many of them particular to the condition of schizophrenia specifically because they seem to be independent of the effects of antipsychotic medication.

The autonomic basis for these cardiovascular effects may be related to the extreme liability of both the sympathetic and parasympathetic divisions of the autonomic nervous system in untreated schizophrenia. It has been found that treatment with antipsychotic drugs actually has the effect of normalizing these swift autonomic swings. Such major autonomic dysregulation in untreated individuals could be inextricably tied to the development of the metabolic syndrome for several reasons including the following three: insulin is known to stimulate sympathetic activity, habitually elevated

Table 165.6   Therapeutic intervention for the metabolic syndrome

Obesity	Behavior modification, caloric restriction, regular exercise
Atherogenic diet	Reduce trans fats, saturated fats, dietary cholesterol and total fat
Cigarette smoking	Complete smoking cessation
Low HDL	Advise adding fibrate or nicotinic acid to diet
Hypertension	Lifestyle therapy, advise antihypertensive drugs
High LDL	Advise LDL cholesterol lowering drugs
Elevated glucose	Lifestyle therapy, advise hypoglycemic agents
Physical inactivity	Sixty minutes of moderate-intensity exercise daily
Prothrombotic state	Advise low-dose aspirin therapy

A very brief summary of clinical recommendations for individual facets of the metabolic syndrome

levels of sympathetic activity induce insulin resistance in skeletal muscle, increased sympathetic tone is associated with obesity and visceral fat deposition. The autonomic dysregulation may also lead to risk factors for the metabolic syndrome via a separate route. Chronic arousal of the sympathetic branch of the autonomic nervous system causes upregulation in the hypothalamic-pituitary-adrenal axis which in turn increases levels of circulating cortisol. Chronically elevated cortisol levels, a major finding in schizophrenia, influence and accelerate, at multiple etiologic stages, insulin resistance, abdominal obesity and dyslipidemia. An article by Rosmond and Bjorntorp (2000) provides compelling support for the wealth of evidence tying autonomic and hypothalamic-pituitary-adrenal axis dysregulation to risk factors for the metabolic syndrome.

Physician efficacy in moderating lifestyle risk factors for cardiovascular disease such as physical activity, diet and smoking can be very low even in healthy populations. Due to their psychological symptoms such as high levels of emotion and low capacity for inhibition, influencing lifestyle factors is probably more difficult in populations of patients with psychiatric histories, especially ones with schizophrenia. This makes it even more important to treat the other risk factors: hyperlipidemia, obesity, and glucose intolerance. In other words, because patients with schizophrenia can be relatively resistant to lifestyle therapy, the medications and the role of the prescribing physician are of upmost importance. There are a daunting number of antihypertensive, hypoglycemic, and cholesterol lowering drugs to keep track of, each with multiple contraindications and implications for medication evaluation. Table 165.6 summarizes some of the major therapeutic interventions for individual features of the metabolic syndrome, including behavioral goals and medications. These are forms of intervention that any medical professional treating schizophrenia should be aware of.

165.6   Applications to Other Areas of Health and Disease

It is clear that patients with schizophrenia are susceptible to a variety of medical illnesses and that these are responsible for a large proportion of the excess mortality observed. A large proportion of these disturbances map on neatly to the various features of the metabolic syndrome. It is not obvious whether the metabolic disorders are an integral part of schizophrenia or whether both are caused by a third, unidentified mechanism. The close association probably has at least a small genetic foundation and is further exacerbated by unhealthy lifestyle choices and the commonly prescribed antipsychotics. The existence of serious metabolic disease in schizophrenia has major implications for public health. It is very important that mental health professionals are made cognizant of the metabolic issues in patients with schizophrenia and instructed in how to address them proactively. Serious efforts should be made to instruct and educate psychologists and psychiatrists to investigate, recognize, and actively monitor metabolic conditions in their patients with schizophrenia as well as readily refer these patients to primary care physicians. It is also important to increase awareness among psychiatrists of the fact that these conditions can be iatrogenically exacerbated during antipsychotic therapy.

A great deal of evidence suggests that the existence of the metabolic syndrome in schizophrenia, as in other populations, is contingent upon a high fat diet and living in a Westernized culture (Thakore et al. 2002). The metabolic syndrome is reaching pandemic proportions worldwide and this is thought to be closely related to the absence of physical exercise and abundant and cheap supply of calorie dense foods. Another chapter in this book, "Nutrition, Behavior and the Developmental Origins of the Metabolic Syndrome," discusses how immoderate eating habits and reductions in physical activity have the capacity to greatly exacerbate metabolic disturbances in humans from Westernized cultures. Now that we no longer forage throughout the day for lean meats, fruit and vegetables we are susceptible to obesity and metabolic disease, just like laboratory animals that are caged and fed ad libitum. Many of the topics highlighted by that chapter, including the Westernization of diet, the genetic associations between different metabolic abnormalities, the discussion of "thrifty genotypes" and the influences of epigenetic programming may also be relevant to the present discussion.

There are several well refined animal models of schizophrenia. Most of these induce schizophrenic symptoms in rats or mice by using the same cues thought largely responsible for inducing schizophrenia in humans stress and hypercortisolemia. Rats that are stressed, either prenatally or postnatally, exhibit many of the fundamental symptoms of schizophrenia including impulsivity, habituation deficits, sensory gating deficiencies and reduced hippocampal size. There is truly a paucity of research on the metabolic abnormalities in these animals and the present literature on schizophrenia and the metabolic syndrome has all but ignored this model. Researching the metabolic features of the animal models of schizophrenia should be far less expensive and easier to control and manipulate than many of the current studies looking at these features in humans. Of course, further studies with people are urgently needed as well though, and an emphasis should be placed on drug-naïve, longitudinal designs.

Comprehensive reviews in clinical endocrinology have established that, as our population ages, the metabolic syndrome will be an increasingly important concern. The incidence of schizophrenia does not increase with advancing age yet very little is known about the incidence of the metabolic syndrome in aging individuals with a past diagnosis of schizophrenia. As this chapter has illustrated, we know a good deal but there are still many unknowns. The formulation of treatment standards for the metabolic syndrome remains a highly contentious topic even in individuals without schizophrenia. Increasing the efficacy of lifestyle therapy, decreasing the metabolic disturbances associated with antipsychotics and disentangling people from their genetic propensities for schizophrenia and the metabolic syndrome all remain formidable and complicated problems for the future. It is clear; however, that the careful monitoring of metabolic health in patients with schizophrenia, especially those on atypical antipsychotics, could help markedly in early detection and prevention of the metabolic syndrome.

Summary Points

- Schizophrenia is a life-shortening illness with excess mortality attributable to increased frequency of specific natural and unnatural causes.
- Schizophrenia carries increased risk of a variety of metabolic disorders.
- High visceral fat, type 2 diabetes mellitus and cardiovascular disorders occur with increased frequency in schizophrenia.

- Unhealthy lifestyle, poor diet and lack of exercise probably contribute to the metabolic syndrome and metabolic abnormalities in schizophrenia.
- An inherent susceptibility to stress and elevated levels of cortisol probably exacerbate both psychiatric and metabolic disturbances.
- Atypical, or second generation, antipsychotics have been largely implicated in the onset of obesity, diabetes mellitus and the exaggeration of metabolic complications.
- New findings in this literature have important implications for public health and the treatment of schizophrenia.

Definitions

Antipsychotics: Medications used to treat schizophrenia or other psychotic conditions often manipulating dopamine function to decrease hallucinations, delusions, and other symptoms. Also referred to as neuroleptic drugs.

Dyslipidimia: A disruption of the levels of lipids in the blood. In western societies, most dyslipidemias are hyperlipidemias; an elevation of lipids often due to diet, lifestyle or prolonged elevations of insulin.

Glucose tolerance: The ability of the body to adapt to a relatively large dose of glucose. This ability is usually diminished in diabetics and is used to diagnose diabetes mellitus. A fasting subject ingests around 75 g of glucose and blood glucose is measured at intervals. In diabetics the concentration is higher and takes longer to return to baseline value.

Hypercortisolemia: A state marked by elevated levels of circulating cortisol, an essential glucocorticoid steroid hormone, the major hormone secreted by the adrenal glands.

Hyperglycemia: A complex metabolic condition characterized by high levels of blood glucose in the circulation, usually a result of insufficient or ineffective insulin production in either type 1 or type 2 diabetes mellitus.

Hyperphagia: An abnormal appetite or increased consumption of food, often associated with abnormalities in the hypothalamus.

Hypertension: High blood pressure or force of blood on the vessel walls of the arteries.

Hypothalamic-Pituitary-Adrenal axis: This is a neuroendocrine system in the body responsible for regulating stress physiology. Brain areas that sense threat, signal the hypothalamus which communicates hormonally to the pituitary which in turn signals the adrenal glands to secrete adrenaline and cortisol.

Insulin resistance: A condition in which cells, especially those comprising muscle, fat and liver tissue, fail to be properly receptive to the messages of the hormone insulin. Because insulin promotes the extraction of glucose from the blood, allowing cells to meet their metabolic needs, insulin resistance is associated with elevated levels of blood glucose.

Metabolic syndrome: A combination of metabolic disorders that commonly present together and increase the risk of developing diabetes and cardiovascular disease.

Schizophrenia: A group of psychotic disorders characterized by impairments in sensory gating, emotional inhibition and the organization of complex behaviors.

Visceral fat: The accumulation of fat around the internal organs of the torso. It is associated with the "apple shape," belly fat, central obesity and a high waist to hip ratio.

References

Allebeck P. Schizophrenia Bull. 1989;15:81–9.

Allison DB, Fontaine KR, Heo M. J Clin Psychiat. 1999;60:215–20.

American Diabetes Association, American Psychiatric Association, American Association of Clinical Endocrinologists, North American Association for the Study of Obesity. J Clin Psychiat. 2004;65:267–72.

Basu R, Brar JS, Chengappa KNR, John V, Parepally H, Gershon S, Schlicht P, Kupfer D. Bipolar Disord. 2004;6:314–8.

Bhugra D. PLoS Med. 2006;2:372–3.

Brown S. Brit J Psychiatry. 1997;171:502–508

Brown S, Birtwistle J, Roe L, Thompson C. Psychol Med. 1999;29:697–701.

Cohn T, Prud'homme D, Steiner D, Kameh H, Remington G. Can J Psychiat. 2004;49:753–60.

Davidson M. J Clin Psychiat. 2002;63:5–11.

De Hert M, van Eyck D, De Nayer A. Int Clin Psychopharmacol. 2006;21:S11–5.

De Leon J, Diaz FJ. Schizophr Res. 2007;96:185–97.

Dixon L, Weiden P, Delahanty J, Goldberg R, Postrado L, Lucksted A, Lehman A. Schizophrenia Bull. 2000;26:903–12.

Expert Panel on Detection, Evaluation, and Treatment of High Blood Cholesterol in Adults. JAMA. 2001;285:2486–97.

Ford ES, Giles WH. Diabetes Care. 2003;26:575–81.

Felker B, Yazel JJ, Short D. Psychiat Serv. 1996;47:1356–63.

Gothelf D, Falk B, Singer P. Am J Psychiat. 2002;159:1055–7.

Hannerz H, Borgå P, Borritz M. Public Health. 2001;115:32837.

Hansen BC. Ann NY Acad Sci. 1999;829:1–24.

Haupt DW. Eur Neuropsychopharmacol. 2006;16:S149–55.

Heiskanen T, Niskanen L, Lyytikainen R, Saarinen PI, Hintikka J. J Clin Psychiat. 2003;64:575–9.

Hert MD, Schreurs V, Sweers K, Van Eyck D, Hanssens L, Sinko S, Wampers M, Scheen A, Peuskens J, van Winkel R. Schizophrenia Res. 2008;101:295–303.

Homel P, Casey D, Allison DB. Schizophrenia Res. 2002;55:277–84.

Jeste DV, Gladsjo JA, Lindamer LA, Lacro JP. Schizophrenia Bull. 1996;22:412–30.

Kendrick T. Br J Psychiat. 1996;169:733–9.

Marder SR, Essock SM, Miller AL, Buchanan RW, Casey DE et al. Am J Psychiat. 2004;161:1334–49.

Masterson E, O'Shea B. Brit J Psychiat. 1984;43:643–9.

McEvoy JP, Meyer JM, Goff DC, Nasrallah HA, Davis SM, Sullivan L, Meltzer HY, Hsiao J, Stroup TS, Lieberman JA. Schizophrenia Res. 2005;80:19–32.

Meyer JM. J Clin Psychiat. 2001;62:27–34.

Meyer JM, Nasrallah HA. Medical illness and schizophrenia.Washington, DC: American Psychiatric Press; 2003.

Mortensen PB, Juel K. Brit J Psychiat. 1993;163:183–9.

Mukherjee S, Schnur DB, Reddy R. Lancet. 1989;1:495.

Mukherjee S, Decina P, Bocola V, Saraceni F, Scapicchio PL. Compr Psychiat. 1996;37:68–73.

Newcomer JW, Haupt DW. Can J Psychiat. 2006;51:480–91.

Newman SC, Bland RC. Can J Psychait. 1991;36:239–45.

Osby U, Correia N, Brandt L, Ekbom A, Sparen P. Schizophrenia Res. 2000;45:21–8.

Raphael RP. Arch Neurol Psychiat. 1921;5:687–709.

Reser JE. Med Hypotheses. 2007;69:383–94.

Ristow M. J Mol Med. 2004;82:510–29.

Rosmond R, Bjorntorp P. J Intern Med. 2000;247:188–97.

Ryan MC, Thakore JH. Life Sci. 2002;71:239–57.

Saddichha S, Manjunatha N, Ameen S, Akhtar S. Schizophrenia Res. 2008;101:266–72.

Shirzadi AA, Ghaemi SN. Harv Rev Psychiat. 2006;14:152–64.

Spelman LM, Walsh PI, Sharifi N, Collins P, Thakore JH. Diabet Med. 2007;24:481–5.

Thakore JH, Mann JN, Vlahos I, Martin A, Reznek R. J Int Assoc Study Obesity. 2002;26:137–41.

Walker EF, Diforio D. Psychol Rev. 1997;104:667–85.

Walker EF, Neumann C, Baum KM, Davis D, Diforio D, Bergman A. Dev Psychopathol. 1996;8:647–55.

Weiser M, Knobler H, Lubin G, Nahon D, Kravitz E, Caspi A, Noy S, Knobler HY, Davidson M. J Clin Psychiat. 2004;65:1546–9.

Wirshing DA, Meyer JM. In: Meyer JM, Nasrallah H, editors. Medical illness and schizophrenia.Washington, DC: American Psychiatric Press; 2003. pp. 39–58.

Zhang ZJ, Yao ZJ, Liu W, Fang Q, Reynolds GP. Brit J Psychiat. 2004;18:58–62.

Zimmet P, Boyko EJ, Collier GR, De Courten M. Ann NY Acad Sci. 1999;892:25–44.

Chapter 166
Nutrition, Behavior, and the Developmental Origins of the Metabolic Syndrome

Jared Edward Reser

Abbreviations

LDL   Low density lipoprotein
FOAD   Fetal origins of adult disease

166.1 Introduction

A handful of unifying perspectives have guided theory and even research related to the metabolic syndrome and its associated abnormalities. A broad look at the most popular of these adds another dimension to the clinical knowledgebase that we have and also helps us to better characterize findings and unknowns. This chapter will take such an approach and attempt to highlight some of the outstanding perspectives in an attempt to reconcile the metabolic syndrome with the goals and frame of reference of this book. First, of course, it is important to have a handle on what the metabolic syndrome represents nosologically and why it can be such a difficult construct to get a firm grip on.

The metabolic syndrome is a combination of medical disorders that present in a clustered fashion and result in increased risk for cardiovascular disease and diabetes. Also known as syndrome x, and the insulin resistance syndrome, this multifactorial disease was identified over 80 years ago but has shown a striking increase, worldwide, in the last 2 decades. The rise in international prevalence and clinical interest is closely associated with the global epidemic of obesity and diabetes; however, the metabolic syndrome includes other comorbid disorders, including cardiovascular disease. Symptoms and features include: glucose intolerance (type 2 diabetes, impaired glucose tolerance or impaired fasting glycemia); high blood pressure (hypertension); central obesity (visceral adiposity); increased LDL cholesterol; and dyslipidemia (elevated triglycerides) (Table 166.1). These conditions have a tendency to co-occur in individuals more often than they present alone. For this reason, they have been grouped into the encompassing diagnosis of the metabolic syndrome which is known to present in a variety of different ways in different people. Partly because the constellation of metabolic abnormalities can be slightly different for virtually every person, there is still some contention over which features are central etiologically.

J.E. Reser (✉)
University of Southern California, Psychology Department, SGM 501, 3620 South McClintock Ave.
Los Angeles, CA 90089-1061, USA
e-mail: jared@jaredreser.com; reser@usc.edu

V.R. Preedy et al. (eds.), *Handbook of Behavior, Food and Nutrition*,
DOI 10.1007/978-0-387-92271-3_166, © Springer Science+Business Media, LLC 2011

Table 166.1 The key features of the metabolic syndrome

Obesity	Increased total body fat, abdominal or central fat distribution, increased visceral fat
Insulin resistance	Hyperinsulinemia
Dyslipidemia	Hypertriglyceridemia, decreased HDL cholesterol, increased LDL cholesterol
Impaired glucose tolerance	Type 2 diabetes mellitus
Hypertension	High or deranged blood pressure

The defining disorders of the metabolic syndrome and their components

Table 166.2 Diagnosis of the metabolic syndrome

Increased waist circumference	>102 cm in men, >88 cm in women
Elevated triglycerides	>150 mg/dL or 1.7 mmol/L
Decreased HDL cholesterol	<40 mg/dL in men, <50 mg/dL in women
Blood pressure	>130/85 mgHg or active treatment for hypertension
Fasting glucose	>110 mg/dL or active treatment for hyperglycemia

The National Cholesterol Program requires that at least three of the above five criteria be met for a diagnosis of the metabolic syndrome

In 2005 the Adult Treatment Panel III of the National Cholesterol Education Program (2001) defined diagnosis as three or more of five states listed in Table 166.2. The International Diabetes Federation, the European Group for the Study of Insulin Resistance, and the World Health Organization, and others have each identified unique sets of diagnostic criteria. This disparity in diagnostic definition has created some concern and confusion, although all three systems are relatively similar.

Making comparisons of prevalence for different populations is difficult because different published studies utilize different diagnostic criteria, although a standardized, international definition should abet these difficulties. Sex and ethnic origin predict large amounts of variation in prevalence. The prevalence is also highly age-dependent. Prevalence in the USA (in the national health and nutrition examination survey) increased from 7% in participants between the ages of 20 and 29 to 44% in participants between 60 and 69 (Ford et al. 2002). The majority of diagnoses are given to older, obese individuals who have a degree of insulin resistance. Until recently, the metabolic syndrome was regarded as a disease of old age, yet now, with increasing rates of obesity and diabetes in young people, it is commonly diagnosed in children. As in adults, susceptibility of children to the metabolic syndrome increases with worsening obesity.

The etiology and pathophysiology of the metabolic syndrome are extremely complex and have only partially been elucidated. Currently, it is debated whether obesity or insulin resistance is the cause of the metabolic syndrome, or if it can be attributed to a more obscure metabolic derangement (Table 166.3). The disorder, like its features, is highly heritable, and the large genetic component helps health practitioners to identify at-risk individuals if their family medical history is known. The main treatments include calorie restriction and dieting, physical exercise, and occasional drug prescription. The individual diseases that make up the metabolic syndrome are usually treated individually; diuretics and ACE inhibitors for hypertension, cholesterol drugs for elevated LDL cholesterol, and triglyceride levels and various drugs for insulin resistance. More information about treatment and clinical recommendations is given in Table 166.4.

The prevalence of the metabolic syndrome has increased severalfold in the last few decades. In these same decades, fast food and processed foods have become internationally ubiquitous, and physical exercise has been engineered out of our daily routines. It is clear that the metabolic syndrome is a product of the modern environment which has done much to increase sedentary behavior and the overconsumption of unhealthy foods. It is thought that humans were not "designed" to live this type of lifestyle, which is to say that we were not naturally selected to have genes that prepare us for it. Our hunting and gathering ancestors were probably only rarely afflicted by such unhealthy lifestyles or their metabolic consequences.

Table 166.3 Behavior and the metabolic syndrome

Pituitary adrenal abnormalities: hypercortisolemia, stress behavior
Reduced physical activity, sedentariness
Reduced ability to cope with stress, elevated stress hormone levels
Substance abuse: smoking, alcohol, others
Increased food intake: hyperphagia, increased dietary fat content
Sex hormone abnormalities

A brief list of some of the behavioral abnormalities closely associated with the metabolic syndrome

Table 166.4 Therapeutic intervention for the metabolic syndrome

Obesity	Behavior modification, caloric restriction, regular exercise
Atherogenic diet	Reduce trans fats, saturated fats, dietary cholesterol, and total fat
Cigarette smoking	Complete smoking cessation
HDL	Advise adding fibrate or nicotinic acid to diet
Hypertension	Lifestyle therapy, advice antihypertensive drugs
LDL	Advice LDL cholesterol-lowering drugs
Elevated glucose	Lifestyle therapy, advice hypoglycemic agents
Physical inactivity	60 min of moderate-intensity exercise daily
Prothrombotic state	Advice low dose aspirin therapy

A very brief summary of clinical recommendations for the individual disorders of the metabolic syndrome

166.2 The Thrifty Genotype

The same genes that cause humans to be susceptible to diabetes, heart disease, and obesity in modern times may have protected us from starvation and famine during ancestral times. This hypothesis was first put forward in 1962 by James Neel in an article entitled: "Diabetes mellitus: a 'thrifty' genotype rendered detrimental by 'progress.'" Neel coined the phrase "thrifty genotype" referring to the probably very large complement of genes that would have helped our ancestors' metabolisms to be economical and prudent with the foods that they hunted and gathered (Neel 1982). Not only did their meals contain a smaller proportion of sugar and fat, but our ancestors also had to engage in prolonged physical activities to obtain them. Interestingly, adopting a "paleolithic diet" consisting primarily of fruit, vegetables, and meat is an increasingly popular dietary regimen. Neel pointed out that not only are our bodies engineered to expect a different diet, but they are also probably expecting extreme food shortages, something modern people only very rarely encounter. His thesis, refined in subsequent articles, was that adaptations that allowed organisms to minimize metabolism and providently lay down fat reserves would produce a survival advantage during periods of nutritional scarcity (Neel 1999). A good deal of research has indicated that the environment of human adaptedness, and wild environments in general, are marked by periods of "boom and bust" where periods of plenty are interspersed among periods of food shortage or famine. This concept was initially generated to allow an evolutionary explanation for the existence of diabetes, but has since been generalized toward the metabolic syndrome and become widely adopted. The mainstay of this conceptual standpoint is that our inherited propensity for energy conservation probably only translates into obesity and metabolic disease in modern times and may have protected individuals, particularly those with the "thriftiest genotypes" from starvation in ancestral times (Table 166.5).

Thrifty benefits have been attributed to the individual components of the metabolic syndrome. A smaller, weaker, yet less energy-expensive heart may confer the ability to minimize energy expenditure in the heart in order to mitigate the risk of starvation (Barker 1998; Barker et al. 2002). In modern times people that express this once adaptive phenotype no longer enjoy the benefits because the excess of fat and cholesterol consumed by these individuals puts a serious strain on their "thrifty" heart, making

Table 166.5 Diet and behavior, then and now

Prehistoric foraging individual	Modern day individual
Caloric uncertainty	Caloric stability
Moderate to high physical activity	Low physical activity
Dietary balance	Dietary excess
Insulin sensitivity in muscle cells	Insulin resistance in muscle cells
Metabolic efficiency	Metabolic dysregulation
Reproductive advantage	Presumed reproductive disadvantage

A comparison of health and ecological features between a typical forager and modern individual on a Westernized diet with an inactive lifestyle

them susceptible to heart or cardiovascular disease (Ridley 2003). A similar tradeoff is presumed to exist for insulin signaling. The beta cells of the pancreas release insulin in response to carbohydrate intake facilitating the metabolism of carbohydrates. An exaggerated pancreatic response (seen in the metabolic syndrome) results in hyperinsulinemia (high circulating levels of insulin) that leads to increased lipogenic activity and ultimately the storage of fats in adipose tissue. Such metabolic tendencies for increased adiposity may have helped individuals in the past to be frugal with fats and to store more fat, yet today they lead to obesity. Type 2 diabetes mellitus has been characterized as a disorder that is a prototypic example of this kind of evolutionary tradeoff. It has been thought for decades now that, on a cellular and organ system level, the disorder represents a thrifty condition – insulin resistance – that would have only rarely manifested as disease in the ancestral environment, because at that time individuals had no access to refined sugar or processed foods. The current literature holds that insulin resistance, brought about by genes for type 2 diabetes, represents a finely tuned physiological state and that its cellular and molecular pathways have been refined by natural selection over millions of years to help organisms conserve blood sugar. Insulin causes cells to rapidly take up blood sugars and increase the rate of their cellular processes thereby increasing total metabolic output. The defective insulin receptors, seen in cells of people with insulin resistance, might have helped to conserve these blood sugars in the past, but now that our diets feature dramatically higher levels of refined sugar; insulin resistance results in blood sugar levels that are vastly too high. Elevated blood sugar, hyperglycemia, can cause a variety of systemic and organ problems through the glycation and damaging of important biomolecules, seen frequently in diabetes. In all of these examples, biological mechanisms malfunction badly once they are forced to face our unhealthy modern diets (Table 166.6). It is now thought that many individual physiological pathways involved in the metabolic syndrome may represent ancient methods of energy conservancy (Eriksson et al. 2001).

Population genomics has identified some very interesting trends in geographic susceptibility to the metabolic syndrome, which provide corroborating evidence for the thrifty genotype theory. This widely accepted interpretation emphasizes that populations of preagricultural, foraging individuals who live in areas where, until recently, food has been relatively unpredictable have much higher prevalence of thrifty genes (Neel 1982). The traits that these genes code for probably helped these individuals survive during prolonged periods of scarcity or were maintained because historically these individuals were not exposed to high calorie diets (Valencia et al. 1999). Today, the incidence of the metabolic disease remains highest among populations where an economy of foraging existed until recently. Unfortunately, people in these areas such as Native Americans, Aboriginal Australians, and Pacific Islanders have an unusually high prevalence of the metabolic syndrome now that they have been exposed to the modern "diet of affluence." This genetic variation between human populations is akin to other known forms of anthropological adaptation to environment. Unknown tomany, there are several examples of selective pressures acting on humans even in the last 50,000 years. Lactase persistence is one example, where populations in Europe and elsewhere

Table 166.6 Medical risks associated with a westernized diet

Metabolic state	Implications for foragers	Implications for moderns
Adiposity	Healthy fat retention	Excessive fat retention
Insulin resistance	Healthy levels of blood sugar	Excessive levels of blood sugar
Beta cell Responsiveness	Metabolism of carbohydrates	Hyperinsulinemia
Thrifty heart	Healthy, efficient heart	Heart burdened by high body fat
Glucose intolerance	Normoglycemia	Hyperglycemia

A comparison between a typical forager and an obese modern individual with respect to the end result of individual metabolic states

retained the ability to digest lactose into adulthood because of the domestication of cattle and the importance of the ability to derive calories from milk.

The Pima Indians in Arizona and the Nauru people from the Micronesian South Pacific Islands appear to have particularly thrifty genotypes (Dowse et al. 1991). Both populations are thought to have endured repeated episodes of food shortage and starvation. They live and have long lived in relatively isolated, unpredictable, and in the case of the Pima, desolate areas. Fascinatingly, the Nauru people have traveled among remote islands in the Pacific during many, several-week-long canoe voyages. Historical accounts attest that many individuals in these canoes died of starvation during the trips, perhaps creating a Nauru founder population of highly starvation adapted people. When exposed to a Western lifestyle in the twentieth century, obesity and type 2 diabetes increased drastically in the Pima and Nauru. For some time, these two groups had among the highest age and sex-adjusted incidence rates of type 2 diabetes, around 25 per 1,000 people per year for the Pima (Schulz et al. 2006).

A variety of animal studies echo these genographic studies in humans. Diabetes commonly afflicts zoo animals, and an epidemic has been described of captive populations of primates, whose lifestyle approximates the sedentary, high-calorie lifestyle of First World urban humans (Diamond 2003). Ecological support for the thrifty genotype hypothesis comes from studies with leptin-deficient (ob/ob) and leptin receptor-deficient (db/db) mice (Coleman 1979). Heterozygous animals, which have a significant tendency toward obesity and diabetes when fed ad libitum, survived longer during fasting than the wild-type animals, even when matched for body weight. This trend has been observed outside of the laboratory too. Certain animals that are well adapted to frequent food shortages, such as desert mammals, show increased susceptibility to the features of the metabolic syndrome when they are able to feed ad libitum. The Israeli sand rat is a prime example. It is highly predisposed to developing metabolic disease including insulin resistance, obesity, and diabetes when put on the western lab rat diet. The symptoms reverse quickly when its food is restricted or it is placed back in its natural environment (Haines et al. 1965). Fascinatingly, it is known that the facets of the metabolic syndrome in humans, including diabetes, can be reversed by diet, exercise, and weight loss. This decline and even disappearance of diabetes symptoms happened to thousands of Parisians during the 1870–1871 famine associated with the siege of Paris (Zimmet 1997).

Even though the thrifty gene hypothesis has been challenged in its particulars, the aspects discussed here have been well accepted in the medical and ethological literatures. The thrifty genotype model is not meant to account for all instances of metabolic disease, but does seem to offer a high degree of explanatory power for the metabolic pandemic of modern times. Far from being a liability, a tendency to be fine tuned for having a lower metabolism would have been an asset to survival in the Plio-Pleistocene because it would have helped individuals to conserve calories. That individual species, or some individuals within a species, have this tendency has important biomedical ramifications, and further research and experimentation in this area should help to clarify the underpinnings and tradeoffs involved in energy homeostasis. Several successful animal models, like the ones mentioned, are thought to have helped to elucidate some of the key genes and pathways involved in impaired energy balance regulation. Interestingly, the genes that one is born with are not the only predisposing factors, as the next section will illustrate; the environment can play a large role as well.

166.3 The Developmental Origins of the Metabolic Syndrome

It is now widely accepted that the risk for a number of metabolic diseases may be affected by circumstances before birth. Professor David Barker and colleagues have produced a large amount of data, since 1994, showing that low birth weight increases susceptibility to noninsulin-dependent diabetes mellitus, hypertension, and coronary heart disease (Barker 1998) later in life. By analyzing epidemiological data for cohorts whose birth records are available, and following these individuals into adulthood, Barker, Hales and others have shown that birthweight, length, body proportions, and placental weight are highly associated with later metabolic disease incidence (Philips 1998) or risk factors for those diseases (hypertension, glucose intolerance, hyperlipidemia) (Barker, 1994, 1998). In addition to having increased adipose tissue mass in adulthood, low birth weight individuals have a tendency to store adipose tissue centrally and have a lower lean mass. Reduced muscle has been reported to contribute heavily to a lowered basal metabolic rate and is expected to reduce capacity for exercise (Kensara et al. 2005). These associations between birth size and disease are often apparent from childhood, hold in a large number of different populations, and have given rise to the term "fetal origins of adult disease" (FOAD) (Law and Shiell 1996; McKeigue 1997).

The biological changes responsible for metabolic alterations are attributed to epigenetic programming, also called phenotypic plasticity. Epigenetic programming occurs when an environmental cue creates a change in gene expression. Even small changes in gene expression and protein regulation, early on, can cause large phenotypic changes with time. Developmental geneticists closely adhere to the idea that a single genotype can give rise to, or canalize, a variety of different phenotypes depending on the programming effects of the early environment. Intrauterine programming is a well-established biological phenomenon, and there are many well-known examples, affecting organisms from plants to humans. In this case, an environmental stimulus, experienced during gestation, is thought to lead to impaired fetal growth and diminution in size at birth, although "catch-up" growth in childhood is the norm. This stimulus or cue also leads to altered homeostatic mechanisms such as the regulation of blood pressure or insulin sensitivity, which in turn results in susceptibility to the metabolic syndrome later in life. Exactly what this cue or stimulus is, has been open to debate. The majority of models in this literature point to undernutrition (Langley 1997) but some emphasize the contribution of other forces, such as placental dysfunction, or excessive fetal exposure to glucocorticoids.

Evidence for undernutrition as the underlying, environmental stimulus in this association comes from three sources: (1) the aforementioned epidemiological associations; (2) animal models; and (3) historical pseudo-experiments. Birth weight is readily altered in experimental animals by manipulating maternal nutrition during fetal development. A reliable way to decrease a rat's size at birth is by reducing the proportion of protein in the diet of their pregnant mothers. Like humans and other mammals, these rats show catch-up growth in youth, but soon thereafter exhibit tendencies toward obesity, elevated blood pressure (Langley and Jackson 1994), and impairments in glucose tolerance (Desai et al. 1995). Glucose intolerance seen in low-protein exposed offspring is contributed to by a reduction in pancreatic beta cell mass, reduced insulin secretion, and peripheral tissue insulin resistance. These symptoms are worsened by the presence of obesity in an additive manner (Petry et al. 1997) and, as in humans, worsened symptoms lead to reduced longevity in rats and mice (Ozanne and Hales 2004).

Restriction of total calories during pregnancy, without respect to protein composition, has been shown to result in rat offspring that are hyperphagic, hyperinsulinemic, obese, hypertensive, and significantly less physically active (Harding 2001). Again, analogous to what we see in our own species, these symptoms are accentuated by a highly palatable or high-fat diet later in life. High levels of catch-up growth after early deprivation have been shown to be related to skeletal muscle insulin resistance, reduced thermogenesis, and increased insulin sensitivity in adipose tissue (Cettour-Rose et al. 2005). Another parallel in this domain that is directly relevant to human health is the finding that diets of saturated fats lead to detrimental effects on glucose homeostasis in fetally deprived rats whereas diets containing polyunsaturated fatty acids had beneficial effects (Siemelink et al. 2002). Similar studies designed to reduce maternal nutrition during pregnancy have led to comparable results in rats, mice, guinea pigs, and sheep.

Peripheral signals that indicate the size of adipose stores such as circulating factors and the hormone leptin are received and integrated by the central nervous system, primarily at the hypothalamus and brainstem. If adipose stores are sufficient or large, changes in these signaling systems, such as the increase in leptin hormone, induce the nervous system to inhibit feeding and promote energy expenditure. Offspring of undernutrition pregnancies have been shown to demonstrate leptin insensitivity, high body weight, and increased food intake in adult life (Harding 2001). Whether early food restriction acts at the level of the hypothalamus to predispose to this "thrifty behavior" is currently not clear. There is very little doubt though that maternal undernutrition in animals leads to diminished size, altered behavior, and permanent alterations in metabolism, and that this is consistent with disease susceptibility observed in human studies.

The second source of evidence for the efficacy of maternal undernutrition in the programming of the metabolic syndrome comes from historical pseudo-experiments. A popular example, the Dutch Hunger Winter, was a season of extreme food shortage in the Netherlands between 1944 and 1945. Ravelli and colleagues compared data on 300,000 19-year-old males that were born before, during, or after this famine (Ravelli et al. 1976). The study revealed that the nutritional limitations imposed by severe nutritional deprivation lead to offspring with reduced birth size, and increased risk of glucose intolerance, and obesity in adult life. The cohorts that were most affected were the offspring of the mothers whose first two trimesters of pregnancy coincided with the famine. Similar historical pseudo-experiments, with well documented medical data that are consistent with the findings of the Dutch Hunger Winter, have occurred in Asia and elsewhere.

Another body of literature has taken this programming concept a step further and attributed adaptive or evolutionary value to sensitivity to programming (Barker et al. 2002). Evolutionary significance has been attributed to the programming that occurs due to nutritional deprivation, and even to altogether different programming models, such as early life stress. Neonatal rats, when exposed to various stressors, show permanent changes in hypothalamic structure and systemic responses to stress (Barbazanges et al. 1996; Francis et al. 1996) and these responses have been characterized as representing predictive actions to better prepare the animal for predation risk and environmental adversity (Zhang et al. 2004). In a similar manner, the thrifty phenotype hypothesis contends that the permanent changes in metabolic homeostasis represent evolutionarily adaptive programming that decreases susceptibility to starvation.

166.4 The Thrifty Phenotype

It is clear that Hales and Barker, like Neel before them, appreciated the evolutionary implications of their hypotheses. They explicitly proposed that this metabolic response to a nutritionally poor early environment was a predictive, adaptive response that would maximize chances of surviving postnatally in conditions of ongoing deprivation. Also, like Neel, they appreciated the fact that this prediction represents a tradeoff and is subject to being inaccurate. If, unexpectedly, the postnatal environment provides plentiful nutrition these individuals will be at increased risk of metabolic disease.

The phenotypic characteristics of many organisms ranging from plants to insects to mammals are known to show plastic responses to environmental events, many of which are thought to represent adaptive, defensive responses, or reproductive strategies (Via and Lande 1985). This phenotypic plasticity through differential gene expression is often cued by maternal condition and is known to create profound alterations in the phenotypes of developing organisms. The thrifty phenotype hypothesis (Hales and Barker 1992, 2003 2001) has been used widely by researchers from different disciplines to interpret studies showing that maternal malnutrition is a strong risk factor for the metabolic syndrome (Wells). According to this hypothesis, phenotypes that are programmed by prenatal malnutrition to express low metabolic rates enjoy a survival advantage under deprived circumstances; however, if such a thrifty fetus is born into an environment marked by nutritional abundance, it will face increased risk of negative health consequences (Bateson et al. 2004). Conversely, robust phenotypes that express larger size and rapid metabolism are thought to increase reproductive success when resources are more plentiful, but are more susceptible to starvation if exposed to nutritional shortage. Specialists now believe that the association between maternal malnourishment and the offspring's proclivity for a low metabolism is adaptive specifically because the mother's deprived condition during pregnancy is often predictive of the environment into which the fetus will be born. It has been established that many animals share similar metabolic responses to environmental cues and this requires us to concede that our own tendency to react plastically may derive from phylogenetically earlier forms because of a shared evolutionary history (Crespi and Denver 2005).

Epigenetic processes are the biological basis for programming effects. Chemicals such as acetyl or methyl groups attach themselves to promoter regions of genes in specific tissues. Fine and intricate control of gene expression has been taken to suggest that the programming effects have been maintained through evolution because of their adaptive advantage rather than representing maladaptive effects of developmental disruption such as teratogenesis (Hanson and Gluckman 2008). It has been shown that, in animals, these epigenetic effects, for instance DNA methylation, can be passed down to successive generations along with the altered phenotypic expressions. In fact, due to alterations in the epigenome that are maintained during the creation of gametes, the effects of early life undernutrition may be transmitted to subsequent generations without repetition of the immediate insult in the second generation (Drake and Walker 2004). Many researchers believe that there may be an adaptive advantage in long term intergenerational programming, and that information about a grandparent's environment will help a developing animal in its "environmental forecasting."

Many fully grown animals are well known to demonstrate consistent adaptive responses to starvation that help to minimize energy expenditure, even of the order of a few days. Starvation evokes several immediate physiological changes, the most dramatic of which include suppression of metabolic rate, increased adiposity, reduction of thyroid and growth hormone levels, a reduction in fertility (through the suppression of gonadal function), and an increased activation of the hypothalamic–pituitary–adrenal axis (Schwartz et al. 1995; Flier 1998). Unlike animals programmed prenatally for thrift though, these predictive metabolic measures reverse largely after the animal resumes its normal diet. It is also well accepted that seasonal cycles of metabolic alterations occur in hibernating mammals. Many animals that hibernate are insulin insensitive for months before they go into hibernation and exhibit increased adiposity. When they wake up in the spring they are lean and insulin sensitive once again (Scott and Grant 2006). These other examples of phenotypic plasticity are comparable to intrauterine programming in many ways and researchers could potentially learn much from contrasting these models.

The brains of experimental animals that were exposed to early nutritional deprivation seem to be buffered from growth restriction in moderate cases, but can show definite changes in severe ones.

Reductions in the number of cells in certain regions as well as in synapses and white matter evince that programming effects, that may involve thrift, take place in the brain as well. Recent studies using imaging techniques show that gray matter is reduced in humans subjected to intrauterine growth restriction, and that catch up growth may not occur (Tolsa et al. 2004). The present author has offered explanatory hypotheses for these and related observations elsewhere (Reser 2006). It is possible that a large number of different metabolic and organ systems may be affected by epigenetic programming involving predictive adaptive responses. Further, integrative research, incorporating the viewpoints from different levels of biological and medical analysis, should help to provide a clearer picture of what we refer to today as "thrift."

166.5 Applications to Other Areas of Health and Disease

The thrifty genotype hypothesis posits that certain human genes that are associated with increased risk for metabolic disease today were naturally selected in the past because they helped their bearers to be more "thrifty" with energy stores. According to this hypothesis, phenotypes that express low metabolic rates enjoy a survival advantage under deprived circumstances. However, they face increased risk of negative health consequences when sugars and fats are artificially abundant, as they are in many countries today. The thrifty phenotype hypothesis posits that all of us have windows of susceptibility to thrifty programming that enable us to create permanent readjustments in homeostatic systems in an obsolete attempt to aid survival.

Today, the costs of the metabolic syndrome are well documented and well understood, but the prehistoric, defensive manifestations are obscured, at least at first glance, because of discrepancies between the ancestral environment and the modern environment. Many traits that are known to have been defensive in the ancestral environment are now seen as maladaptive in the present (an "environmental mismatch") and the science of evolutionary medicine attempts to identify and characterize these traits. Researchers have identified many such "pathological" conditions such as anxiety, cystic fibrosis, diarrhea, fever, inflammation, pain, sneezing, sickle cell anemia, and vomiting and have helped to show that they actually represent evolved defenses that would have promoted survival and the likelihood of reproductive success (Williams and Nesse 1998).

The merits of the thrifty genotype and phenotype hypotheses include the implications that they generate for understanding past, current, and future trends in disease (Pollard). The historical and evolutionary forces that are apparent are still largely abstract when measured against our biomedical knowledge, and it is clear that during our journey of reconciling the two, they will continue to influence and provide predictions for each other. The notion that the human genome bears witness to past struggles for survival against starvation allows us a new context within which to view the responses of the human body. A person's physiological response to dieting will reflect our ancestors' adaptive responses to seasonal hunger, just as their response to abundant calories and fats will reflect our ancestors' beneficial responses to harvest seasons. Furthermore, the thrifty phenotype hypothesis informs us that early, prenatal effects and even effects that were inherited from grandparents can cause the same anachronistic responses.

The cause of fetal malnutrition in present day populations is different from what it used to be. In the ancestral past the majority of examples of fetal malnutrition and intrauterine growth restriction probably would have come from starvation. Today, especially in affluent countries, it primarily stems from circulatory problems that are secondary to uteroplacental dysfunction, a relatively rare but epidemiologically constant condition. These modern fetuses, restricted by uteroplacental dysfunction, misinterpret their situation and prepare for nutritional scarcity when they will, in fact, encounter the opposite scenario.

Anthony Philipps explains that these findings have important implications for obstetrics and prenatal nutrition. It is imperative that circulatory assessments be made earlier in pregnancy, that more reliable ways to ascertain placental villous blood flow are developed, and that more sophisticated fetal growth measures are devised and used widely.

The identification and mapping of both thrifty genes and epigenetic markers will help to evaluate these hypotheses, but more importantly, will help inform medical research. Many critical aspects remain to be explored: (1) Where are the alleles for thrifty genes? (2) At what points during development do these windows of susceptibility exist? (3) What are the signaling pathways through which an environmental cue is translated into a developmental response? (4) Which developmental responses persist beyond a single generation and how? (5) How long do we have to wait, and how many people have to die prematurely from the metabolic syndrome for natural selection to remove the thrifty genes from our gene pool?

The observations discussed here have been extensively replicated and the theories discussed have been widely espoused but both are – and perhaps for good reason – still discussed, questioned, and debated. Many of these observations are not invariable and the causal pathways are still quite far from being transparent. It is thought that the concepts of the "thrifty genotype" and "thrifty phenotype" can be consistent and reconciled with one another. Sometimes, though, it is clear that they are mutually exclusive explanatory alternatives such as when it is not known if a low birth weight is inherited or acquired. Validity and applicability of these hypotheses is certainly open for dispute. Thrifty genes may not be identified for decades and even given the recent advances in genetic analysis are a rather nebulous concept today. One would assume that thrifty alleles would influence processes such as lipolysis, fuel oxidation, and skeletal muscle glucose metabolism, but it is difficult to say. The 2007 genome-wide association studies on type 2 diabetes mellitus provided promising data, and more refined genetic tools will provide a more complete picture of the genetic and epigenetic complexity of the metabolic syndrome.

Animal models are not always directly comparable to the human situation, but should continue to offer insight into mechanism. Long-term studies in humans are expensive and time-consuming but they will help to clarify the pertinent issues too. It is evident that this line of research has major ramifications for public health policy. Health care funding may be more prudently spent on informing and improving pregnancy care rather than on the contingent metabolic disorders which manifest decades later and cost many times more to treat. If overeating and sedentary behavior are determined during prenatal development to the degree that this literature implies, this may explain why public health initiatives to improve exercise and dieting in adults with metabolic symptoms are largely ineffective.

There is a large literature that addresses these concepts from different angles, and much is known about the similarities in predisposition for metabolic disease between people and animals (Gluckman and Hanson 2004). There is still much that is unknown though, and whether the broad, ultimate, evolutionary hypotheses have to be largely altered or just fine tuned, it is becoming clear that metabolic disease may very simply stem from the fact that our behavior, diet, and nutrition are so different from the way they used to be.

Summary Points for the Developmental Origins of the Metabolic Syndrome

- The metabolic syndrome represents a cluster of metabolic derangements that are risk factors for obesity, type 2 diabetes mellitus, and cardiovascular disease.
- There is currently a worldwide epidemic of obesity and diabetes that is due to unhealthy eating and poor exercise. These are probably issues that our hunting and gathering ancestors would rarely have been exposed to, because they were probably rarely exposed to excess, but commonly exposed to famine.

- The human gene pool probably contains many thrifty genes that would have helped our ancient ancestors to survive food shortages and starvation. For example, a tendency to efficiently take up ingested fats into fat stores would have increased the likelihood of survival.
- The physiological states that cause us to be susceptible to facets of the metabolic syndrome probably all had ecological utility in the past. This is supported by animal models.
- Many mammals and it seems humans too can be programmed for thrift if they are exposed to severe undernutrition early in development. This programming may be a predictive adaptive response to environmental cues signaling that the environment is nutritionally poor.
- The thrifty phenotype that is created from these programming effects is highly susceptible to metabolic disease.
- Future findings in this literature should have serious implications for public health and the treatment of the metabolic syndrome.

Definitions

Dyslipidemia: Refers to a disruption of the levels of lipid in the blood. In western societies, most dyslipidemias are hyperlipidemias; an elevation of lipids, often due to diet, lifestyle, or prolonged elevations of insulin.

Glucose tolerance: The ability of the body to adapt to a relatively large dose of glucose. This ability is usually diminished in diabetics and is used to diagnose diabetes mellitus. A fasting subject ingests around 75 g of glucose, and blood glucose is measured at intervals. In diabetics the concentration is higher and takes longer to return to baseline value.

Genotype: The genetic constitution of a cell or organism. The genotype contains the information, in the form of DNA, which dictates how the cell or organism develops and interacts with its environment.

Hypercortisolemia: High amounts of circulating cortisol, an essential glucocorticoid steroid hormone, and the major hormone secreted by the adrenal glands.

Hyperglycemia: A complex metabolic condition characterized by high levels of blood glucose in the circulation, usually a result of insufficient or ineffective insulin production in either type 1 or type 2 diabetes mellitus.

Hyperphagia: Refers to an abnormal appetite or increased eating of food, often associated with abnormalities in the hypothalamus.

Hypertension: High blood pressure or force of blood on the vessel walls of the arteries.

Hypothalamic–pituitary–adrenal axis: This is a neuroendocrine system in the body responsible for regulating stress physiology. Brain areas that sense threat signal the hypothalamus, which communicates hormonally to the pituitary which hormonally signals the adrenal glands to secrete adrenaline and cortisol.

Insulin resistance: A condition in which cells, especially those comprising muscle, fat, and liver tissue fail to be properly receptive to the messages of the hormone insulin. Because insulin promotes the extraction of glucose from the blood, allowing cells to meet their metabolic needs, insulin resistance is associated with elevated levels of blood glucose.

Metabolic syndrome: A combination of metabolic disorders that commonly present together, and increase the risk of developing diabetes and cardiovascular disease.

Phenotype: An observable characteristic of an organism, such as a trait, property, or behavior. Phenotypes develop from the interaction between an organism's genes and its environment.

Visceral fat: The accumulation of fat around the internal organs of the torso. It is associated with the "apple shape," belly fat, central obesity, and a high waist to hip ratio.

References

Barbazanges A, Piazza PV, Le Moal M, Maccari S. J Neurosci. 1996;16:3943–9.
Barker DJP. Fetal Maternal Med Rev. 1994;6:71–80.
Barker DJP. Mothers, babies and health in later life. London: Churchill Livingstone; 1998.
Barker D, Eriksson J, Forsen T, Osmond C. Int J Epidemiol. 2002;31:1235–9.
Bateson P, Barker D, Clutton-Brock T, Deb D, D'Udine B, Foley R, Gluckman P, Godfrey K, Kirkwood T, Mirazon Lahr M, McNamara J, Metcalfe N, Monaghan P, Spencer H, Sultan S. Nature 2004;430:419–21.
Cettour-Rose P, Samec S, Russell AP, Summermatter S, Mainieri D, Carrillo-Theander C. Diabetes 2005;54:751–6.
Coleman D. Science 1979;203:663–5.
Crespi EJ, Denver RJ. Am J Hum Biol. 2005;17:44–54.
Desai M, Crowther NJ, Ozanne SE, Lucas A, Hales CN. Biochem SocTrans. 1995;23:31–5.
Diamond J. Nature2003;423:599–602.
Dowse GK, Zimmet PZ, King H. Diabetes Care. 1991;14:968–74.
Drake AJ, Walker BR. J Endocrinol. 2004;180:1–16.
Eriksson J, Forsen T, Tuomilehto J, Osmond C, Barker D. Br Med J. 2001;322:949–53.
Expert Panel on Detection, Evaluation, and Treatment of High Blood Cholesterol in Adults. JAMA 2001;285:2486–97.
Flier JS. J Clin Endocrinol Metab. 1998;83:1407–13.
Ford ES, Giles WH, Dietz WH. JAMA 2002;287:356–9.
Francis D, Diorio J, LaPlante P, Weaver S, Seckl JR, Meaney MJ. Ann NY Acad Sci. 1996;794:136–52.
Gluckman P, Hanson M. Trends Endocrinol Metab. 2004;15:183–7.
Haines H, Hackel D, Schmidt-Nielsen K. Am J Physiol. 1965;208:297–300.
Hales CN, Barker DJ. Diabetologia 1992;35:595–601.
Hales CN, Barker DJ. Br Med Bull. 2001;60:5–20.
Hanson MA, Gluckman PD. Basic Clin Pharmacol. 2008;102:90–3.
Harding, JE. Int J Epidemiol. 2001;30:15–23.
Kensara OA, Wootton SA, Phillips DI, Patel M, Jackson AA, Elia M. Am J Clin Nutr. 2005;82:980–7.
Langley-Evans SC. J Hypertens.1997;15:537–44.
Langley SC, Jackson AA. Clin Sci. 1994;86:217–22.
Law CM, Shiell AW. J Hypertens. 1996;14:935–41.
McKeigue P. In: Kuh D, Ben-Shlomo Y, editors. A life course approach to chronic disease epidemiology. Oxford: Oxford University Press; 1997. p. 78–100.
Neel JV. Am J Hum Genet. 1962;14:353–62.
Neel JV. In: Kobberling J, Tattersall R, editors. The genetics of diabetes mellitus. Amsterdam: Academic; 1982. p. 137–47.
Neel JV. Nutr Rev. 1999;57:2–9.
Nesse R, Williams G. Sci Am. 1998;279:58–65.
Ozanne SE, Hales CN. Nature 2004;427:411–2.
Petry CJ, Ozanne SE, Wang CL, Hales CN. Clin Sci Lond. 1997;93:147–52.
Phillips DI. Diabetes Care. 1998;21:150–5.
Pollard TM. Western diseases: an evolutionary perspective. Cambridge UK: Cambridge University Press; 2008. p. 5–9.
Ravelli, GP, Stein ZA, Susser MW. N Engl J Med. 1976;295:349–53.
Reser JE. Med Hypotheses. 2006;67:529–44.
Ridley M. Nature via nurture: genes experience and what makes us human. New York: Harper Collins; 2003.
Scott EM, Grant PJ. Diabetologia 2006;49:1462–6.
Schulz LO, Bennett PH, Ravussin E, Kidd JR, Kidd KK. Diabetes Care. 2006;29:1866–71.
Schwartz MW, Dallman MF, Woods SC. Am J Physiol. 1995;269:949–57.
Siemelink M, Verhoef A, Dormans JA, Span PN, Piersma AH. Diabetologia 2002;45:1397–403.
Tolsa CB, Zimine S, Warfield SK, Freschi M, Rossignol AS, Lazeyras F, Hanquinet S, Pfizenmaier M, Huppi PS. Pediat Res. 2004;56:131–8.
Valencia M, Bennett P, Ravussin E, Esparza J, Fox C, Schulz L. Nutr Rev. 1999;57:55–7.
Via S, Lande R. Evolution 1985;39:505–22.
Vickers MH, Breier BH, McCarthy D, Gluckman PD. Am J Physiol Endocrinol Metab. 2000;279:83–7.
Wells J. J Theor Biol. 2003;7:221:143–61.
Zhang T, Parent C, Weaver I, Meaney M. Ann NY Acad Sci.2004;1032:85–103.
Zimmet P. In: Fischer E, Moller G, editors. The medical challenge: complex traits. Munich: Piper; 1997. p. 55–110.

Part XXVIII
Obesity

Chapter 167
The Relationship Between Television Viewing and Overweight and Obesity in Young Children: A Review of Existing Explanations

Vickii B. Jenvey

Abbreviations

ABS	Australian Bureau of Statistics
BMI	Body Mass Index
kg	Kilogram
kgs	Kilograms
m	Meter
m^2	Meter squared
TV	Television
WHO	World Health Organization
$\geq$	Greater than or equal to
>	Greater than
<	Less than

167.1 Introduction

Data collected worldwide point to an increase in childhood overweight and obesity. Studies in both developed and developing countries [for example, Australia (Bauer 2002) and Peoples' Republic of China (PRC) (Jiang et al. 2006)] show that the proportion of children who can be considered obese has continued to increase over the past three decades. It is often proposed that outcomes of early obesity can predispose children to life-long health problems, including the early onset of Type II diabetes, and early onset of risk factors associated with the later-life development of cardiovascular disease (Teran-Garcia et al. 2008). Additionally, obesity in early childhood has been linked to ostracism and early development of low self-esteem (Schmitz et al. 2002), with the critical factor being peer acceptance (Iobst et al. 2009). Parallel to this rise in overweight and obesity among children of all ages is the apparent increase in sedentary leisure pursuits, such as watching television (TV), surfing the Internet, and playing computer games, because of increased access to all forms of electronic media. Watching TV is a low-level activity and is ubiquitous among young children in both developed and developing countries (see, for example, Larson and Verma 1999). For Australian children's TV consumption see for example, Jenvey (2003) in which

V.B. Jenvey (✉)
School of Psychology, Psychiatry, Monash University, Building 17, Clayton, Victoria 3800, Australia
e-mail: vickii.jenvey@monash.edu.au

V.R. Preedy et al. (eds.), *Handbook of Behavior, Food and Nutrition*,
DOI 10.1007/978-0-387-92271-3_167, © Springer Science+Business Media, LLC 2011

Australian children's usual play and leisure patterns in different social contexts were surveyed, and the Australian Bureau of Statistics (ABS) Survey of Australian children's usual leisure activities (ABS 2004). It is not surprising, therefore, that researchers have attempted to identify an association between TV viewing and increasing levels of obesity among children in those countries. While some studies have investigated relationships between the amount of time children spend accessing all forms of electronic media (computers, computer games, electronic games, TV, and watching DVDs) (for a review, see Marshall et al. 2004), the majority of research has focused on adverse health outcomes associated with frequent TV viewing by children from an early age (Anderson et al. 1998; Landhuis et al. 2008).

167.2 Children Who Are Overweight and Obese

Obesity is assessed by calculating body mass index (BMI). To calculate children's BMI, their weight and height are measured, and BMI is derived from dividing children's weight (in kilograms) by their height (in meters squared). Children whose BMI is more than or equal to 25 kg/m^2 are classified as overweight or obese if BMI is more than or equal to 30 kg/m^2 (Cole et al. 2000). Children's weight and height are compared with established international norms, so that meaningful comparisons of children's growth can be made across different countries (Bar-On 2002). There are separate norms for boys and girls, and each child's weight and height are compared with norms established for children of the same age. While BMI provides a quick and internationally agreed-upon means of determining which children can be classified as overweight or obese, other parameters of children's growth should be considered to determine obesity [World Health Organization (WHO) 1995]. In addition to weight and height, measurement of children's mid-upper arm circumference and skin fold thickness (subscapular and mid-upper arm) should be taken to ascertain, respectively, children's muscle mass and fat stores (WHO 1995). Table 167.1 displays recommended anthropometric measures to most reliably characterize children's growth relative to a normative sample.

Consistency or change in children's and youth's BMI measures throughout development continue to be used as dependent measures to investigate associations between amount of TV viewing and obesity in early childhood. Despite this widespread practice, other researchers point to the inappropriateness of BMI measure to detect individual gains in body mass that result from inherited differences in body composition and bone structure among different ethnic groups. Additionally, even successive BMI measures do not adequately characterize individual differences in children's growth rates, particularly during the early childhood period (Lloyd et al. 2009).

Table 167.1 Anthropometric measures used to characterize overweight and obesity in early childhood

Anthropometric measure	Utility and source
Body Mass Index (BMI)	Efficient, shorthand way to characterize growth/ changes in growth in young children (Weight/Height^2) (Cole et al. 2000)
Mid-upper-arm circumference	Measures muscle mass – better to characterize changes in young children's growth over time (Kanda et al. 1997)
Skin fold thickness (Triceps, Subscapular)	Argued to be most reliable measure of young children's fat stores (WHO Expert Committee 1995)

This table displays the most commonly used and internationally agreed upon measures to characterize changes in children's growth over time, including measures of children's height, weight, muscle mass, and fat stores

167.3 Amount of Time Children Spend Watching Television

In a cross-national investigation of children's leisure pursuits it was found that time spent by children of different ages, including young children 5–8 years, in different countries ranged between 1.5–2.5 h/day (Larson and Verma 1999). Australian parents report similar amounts of TV viewing (average of 15 h/week) among their children, including preschool and early school-age children (Wake et al. 2003). This latter study also included time spent in computer-based activity, which was still less than the time spent watching TV. Additionally, results from a survey of frequency and type of leisure activities of a sample of more than two million 5–15 year-old Australian children (ABS 2004) showed that watching TV and videos was the most popular leisure activity of young Australians, with 98% of children engaged in that activity during their leisure time. In a 2-week period during school term, children spent, on average, 22 h per fortnight watching TV and videos. Time spent watching TV and videos exceeded time spent in other leisure pursuits such as reading or playing electronic games (8 h/fortnight) and more physically active pursuits such as bike riding (6 h/ fortnight) or skateboarding and rollerblading (5 h/fortnight).

When these data are considered in addition to time spent by children accessing other more recent forms of computer-based activities, it is reasonable to assume that young children are spending a sizeable proportion of their leisure time in sedentary, electronic media consumption. In fact, children persist in TV viewing even with the advent of more personalized, interactive media such as Internet and computer games. Thus, time spent accessing these more recent forms of electronic media occurs *in addition to* time spent watching TV (Roberts et al. 1999; ABS 2004). Owing to the fact that TV has been part of children's leisure for several decades, there is a larger body of research investigating the impact of TV viewing on young children's development than exists on more recent forms of computer-based technology taken up by contemporary children. Table 167.2 shows estimated daily or weekly TV viewing among children from different countries.

167.4 Potential Adverse Impact of Watching Television on Young Children's Growth and Development

It is argued that the amount of time young children spend watching TV, displaces time that otherwise might be spent in more physically active leisure pursuits (Dietz and Gortmaker 1985). The second concern is related to the program and advertisement content of TV watched by young children. Television content said to be associated with adverse developmental outcomes for children include programs containing advertisements for food products of poor nutritional quality, which are placed strategically during peak viewing times by children (Kelly et al. 2008; Taras et al. 1989). A third hypothesis proposes an interaction of sedentariness of TV viewing and susceptibility of young children to the persuasive intent

Table 167.2 Estimated hours of television (TV) viewing in early childhood

Estimates of hours of TV viewing	Population and source
22 h/fortnight	Australian children 5–15 years (ABS 2004)
1.5–2.5 h/day	Cross-national comparison (Larson and Verma 1999)
15 h/week	Australian children 3–6 years (Wake et al. 2003)

This table summarizes research estimates (in hours) of amount of time spent by children watching TV across different populations. Estimates are fairly consistent across different populations of children worldwide

Table 167.3 Main explanations and underlying processes associating time spent watching (TV) in early childhood and the development of overweight and obesity

Explanation and source	Proposed underlying processes
Energy displacement (Dietz and Gortmaker 1985)	Time spent watching TV supplants time available for more physically active leisure activities, and energy intake (in the form of food) exceeds energy expenditure (in the form of physical activity) and results in overweight and obesity
Exposure to saturation amounts of TV advertisements for foods of poor nutritional quality (Wilson et al. 1999)	Amount of time spent watching TV ensures high level of exposure to certain food products.
	Young children become familiar with the product brands and pester parents, who, in turn, buy those products, to be eaten by their children
In addition to energy displacement, young children's cognitive immaturity impedes detection of the persuasive intent of the food advertisements (Kelly et al. 2008)	Reduction in physical activity relative to energy requirements coupled with an increase in consumption of food products advertised on TV. Such products consistently high in saturated fats, sugars and excessive amounts of salt.
	Young children, because of their cognitive immaturity are susceptible to the persuasive intent of the advertisements

This table outlines the three main explanations of associations between amount of TV viewed by young children and the development of overweight and obesity in childhood. Specifically three main explanations are (a) energy displacement, (b) cognitive immaturity of young children and their susceptibility to persuasive intent of advertisements for *snack* and *junk* foods, and (c) combination of energy displacement and vulnerability to persuasive messages in *snack* and *junk* food advertisements broadcast during children's TV programs

of advertisements for foods of poor nutritional quality, that are frequently advertised during designated children's TV viewing time (Kelly et al. 2008). Each of these explanations will be discussed more fully in the following sections, and they are presented in Table 167.3.

167.5 Relationship Between Young Children's Television Viewing and Low Physical Activity Levels

A relationship has been found among overweight and obesity, hours of TV viewing, and reduced physical activity among young (3–6 years-old) children (Jago et al. 2005). The more time children spent watching TV, the more overweight or obese they were, and this effect was more pronounced among older children (6–7 years-old) in the cohort. Researchers explained these findings by proposing that TV viewing supplants time spent in physical activity, thereby leading to reduced energy expenditure relative to energy intake, and the development of obesity (Jago et al. 2005). Key features of the energy displacement hypothesis are presented in Table 167.4.

On the other hand, Jackson, Djafarian, Stewart and Speakman (2009) found an association between increased hours of TV viewing and elevated body fatness among preschool children, but this association was not mediated by reduced physical activity. A weak but statistically significant association was found between hours of TV viewing and reduced physical activity among 3–4-year-old children (DuRant et al. 1994), while another study showed no relationship between physical activity and TV viewing among Mexican children living in Mexico City (Hernandez et al. 1999). Thus, there is a lack of consistency in findings from one study to another. In a follow-up study in adolescence of the potential adverse developmental outcomes of TV viewing in early childhood in two cohorts of children in Massachusetts and Kansas, USA, Anderson, Huston, Schmitt, Linebarger and Wright (2001) found no relationship between frequent TV viewing in early childhood and the development of obesity in adolescence. In fact, the single weak but statistically significant relationship was found between

Table 167.4 Key features of energy displacement hypothesis

* Increased time spent in early childhood in sedentary leisure activity of watching TV
* Increased time watching TV occurs at expense of other physical activity
* Children with increased sedentary behavior require lower energy consumption (food), but food intake remains same
* Food intake exceeds daily requirements for decreased physical activity
* Overweight and obesity result from energy intake exceeding energy expenditure

This table outlines one explanation of underlying mechanism by which children develop overweight and obesity in early childhood. Increased hours spent watching TV reduces time available for more physical activities, yet food consumption remains constant, leading to surplus energy intake to energy requirements, in turn resulting in development of overweight and obesity

amount of sedentary behavior (hours spent TV viewing) during adolescence for girls but not boys. The authors interpreted these results as further evidence of findings from multiple studies that females become more sedentary than males during adolescence. Consequently, time that could potentially be taken up with more active leisure pursuits becomes displaced with TV watching for adolescent girls (Anderson et al. 2001).

These equivocal results are not surprising, given the problem that, in large-scale epidemiological studies of factors that contribute to children's and adolescents' growth, it has been difficult to establish a link between physical inactivity and overweight and obesity (see: for example: Krassas et al. 2001, Hernanadez et al. 1999). What is overlooked in these studies is that TV viewing in early childhood does not always displace all forms of physical activity, and young children have been shown to maintain relatively stable levels of physical activity in addition to watching quite a few hours of TV during their usual leisure times (Rey-Lopez et al. 2008). Absence of a clear relationship between time spent watching TV and overweight and obesity among children in these different studies is likely to be linked to methods adopted commonly for data collection of the amount and type of participants' leisure activities. Many of the studies required children or their parents to keep a diary of their daily activities [e.g. Anderson et al. (2001) (early childhood phase of study); Wake and Hesketh 2003], while other samples of children's activity levels are derived from a short-term and an ultimately limited sample of children's regular activity (e.g. ABS 2004). Retrospective diary methods of information gathering have the potential problem of social desirability bias. That is, children and parents report what they should be doing rather than what they are actually doing, and often diaries are completed retrospectively, sometimes several days after a reported activity took place. Further, many studies that investigate links between amount of TV viewing and overweight and obesity in children and youth rely on measurements of TV viewing time that do not report the psychometric properties of the measure used, how the measure was administered, and how data were coded and tabulated. Such methodological problems inevitably compromise the reliability and validity of results that report statistically significant associations between TV viewing and activity levels (Bryant et al. 2007). Perhaps data collection daily at home or school, completed by children themselves, their parents, or their teachers, in the presence of researchers, might overcome problems with diaries completed retrospectively after too much time has elapsed. Such methods are, however, potentially intrusive into family or school life, are very labor-intensive, and dictate large research budgets. Other potential methodological problems include differences in the way children's activity levels are characterized in the different studies. The diverse behaviors of which children's physical activity is comprised has led researchers to recommend that activities be stratified as high activity (e.g. running; jumping, team sports), medium activity (e.g. walking round school playground during recess), and low activity (e.g. occasional movements during play activity) (Goran et al. 1997). Other researchers note that the intensity of the activity may also affect the amount of energy expended during an activity (Strauss et al. 2001).

Contradictory findings should also be considered in light of evidence that the same young children who report that their usual play activity is watching TV when at home alone or in the company of siblings and friends also report that they engage in vigorous outdoor-active play, such as riding bicycles, playing sports, and other physically active games, such as chasey or rough-and-tumble play (Jenvey 2003). It should be noted that children reported less time spent in more vigorous physical activity but also reported that their physical activity was more intense (Jenvey 2003). Moreover, the results of a large-scale survey of Australian children's leisure activities (ABS 2004) support Jenvey's (2003) findings. In the ABS survey, although young children (5–8 year-olds) spent a lot of leisure time in sedentary activities, mainly watching TV, playing computer games, and accessing the Internet, more than 60% of that age group also participated in organized sports and cultural activities, that included learning and practicing folk dancing (ABS 2004).

Larson (2001) notes that even young contemporary children from both developed and developing countries have far more leisure time than children of previous generations, whose time was taken up with household chores and contributing to income-generating activities. Increased technological assistance reduced repetitive manual labor associated with feeding, transportation, and providing a suitable home for children. When many children in developing countries were no longer needed to contribute to such activities, they had more free time available for all forms of leisure activity. Subsequently, children in developing countries also began to spend more of their leisure time watching TV (Larson 2001).

Additional research evidence indicates that certain inherited propensities to develop high leptin levels and fat-mass are implicated in the development of obesity in early childhood (Comuzzie et al. 2003). This latter finding indicates that some children will be more susceptible to early-onset obesity, and low levels of physical activity will have differential developmental outcomes for children according to their inherited predispositions.

Thus, a direct relationship between inactivity resulting from frequent TV viewing in early childhood and the development of obesity is not clearly established. Other factors, such as amount and type of all leisure activities each child engages in, and the level and intensity of the physical activity, together with inherited propensities that differentially predispose some children to the development of obesity in early childhood need also to be taken into account when attempting to ascertain the reasons for increasing levels of obesity among young children worldwide. As well as the amount of time children spend watching TV, it is also important to consider the content of the TV that young children watch.

167.6 Food Advertisements During Designated Children's Television Time and Amount and Type of Food Consumed by Young Children

Before considering the processes by which young children are influenced by advertisements on TV, it is important to consider just how many food advertisements are placed during times when young children are most likely to be watching. As much as 30% of non-program content during children's designated TV time in both Australia (Wilson et al. 1999) and New Zealand (Hill et al. 2006) contains advertisements for food, and the types of products advertised are of poor nutritional quality. That is, food types that are commonly referred to as "snack foods" that can be purchased in attractive packaging at supermarkets and "fast foods" made and sold at fast food outlets are frequently advertised during designated children's TV times. The types of foods advertised to Australian and New Zealand children on TV are similar to products advertised during peak periods of children's viewing in USA (see, for example, Kuribyashi et al. 2001; Harrison and Marske 2005) and for advertisement content on British TV during times of peak viewing by young children (for example, Pine and Nash

Table 167.5 Estimates of proportion of children's television (TV) programs that contain food advertisements

Proportion of food advertisements/children's TV programs[a]	Population and source
Approx. 30% of programs	New Zealand children (Wilson et al. 1999)
Approx. 30% of programs	Australian children (Hill et al. 2006).
Approx. 35% of programs	US children (Kuribyashi et al. 2001)
>25% of programs	British children (Pine and Nash 2003)

This table summarizes research estimates (as percentage of total TV program time), the proportion of designated children's TV programs that contain advertisements for *snack* and *junk* foods and which are broadcast in four different English-speaking populations. Proportional estimates show consistently high proportion of programme content in four different developed countries

[a]In all estimates, majority of food products advertised were most likely to contain levels of salt, saturated fats, and sugars that exceeded recommended daily allowances for children in target age ranges

2003). Table 167.5 summarizes estimates of the level of exposure of children to televised food advertisements across different child populations.

The foods advertised during children's TV programs were more likely to contain levels of salt, saturated fats, and sugars that exceeded recommended daily allowances for children of the ages in the target audiences (Harrison and Marske 2005). They also advertised highly processed foods that were low in dietary fiber (Kuribyashi et al. 2001). The latter compared the contents of food advertisements placed in Saturday morning children's programs with contents of food advertisements placed in Saturday evening adult programs across four free-to-air US TV stations. When the food types advertised during periods of peak viewing by children were compared with types of food products advertised during periods of peak viewing by adults, it was found that there were more food commercials shown during the peak (early morning) children's program hours; they were more repetitious and took up a higher proportion of the overall program time than food advertisements screened in the evenings during prime-time adult programming. Overall, food products advertised during Saturday morning programs, a period of peak viewing by young children, contained significantly higher levels of sugar and saturated fat than products advertised during Saturday evening programs, when the majority of the audience was adult (Kuribyashi et al. 2001).

While it is important to establish the frequency of exposure of young children to certain food types while they watch TV, it is equally important to consider how such advertising might affect children's food preferences, eating patterns, and general nutrition. Evidence from research in different countries indicates that both amount and type of food provided to young children by their parents, grandparents, and even older siblings are the most significant influence on the development of food preferences and eating patterns in early childhood (Cullen et al. 2000). Thus, if parents usually purchase and consume *snack foods* and *junk foods*, then such foods will be readily available to children in their homes. Messages contained in advertising content might reinforce young children's preference to consume foods available already in their home. Even when young children respond to the persuasive intent of the advertisements, it is not clear how young children might then influence their parents to purchase foods advertised on TV, if such foods are not usually provided by their parents or other family members in their homes. Taras, Sallis, Patterson, Nader and Nelson (1989) did show a more direct link between young children's exposure to certain food advertisements on TV and the types of foods they consumed. Mothers of 3–8 year-olds completed a questionnaire on children's TV viewing patterns and the nature of their requests for certain food products commonly advertised on TV (Taras et al. 1989). The more often children saw programs containing advertisements for certain food types, the more frequently they requested that their parents purchase the products. Different relationships were found for exposure to sporting goods advertisements and children's requests for sporting goods. The more time children spent watching TV generally, the less frequently they requested that their parents purchase sporting goods promoted in advertisements they viewed on TV. The design of this study did not control for other potential confounds in the data. For example, children who watch a lot of TV are also exposed to advertisements for all sorts of products, but the type of food advertised (mostly snack, and processed packaged food) is relatively cheap, when compared with toys, sporting goods, and other products also advertised frequently during children's TV programs. Perhaps the more snack food that was requested by children, purchased subsequently by parents, and thus consumed by children occurred because of its cheapness relative to other advertised products (e.g. toys and sporting goods).

Additionally, there was no mention of how frequently parents succumbed to their children's demands to purchase products they saw advertised on TV. This is often referred to as the "pester factor", and is apparently one of the intentions of advertising that targets young children. Nevertheless, while advertisers identify its existence, and it is asserted that children's demands play a role in parents' response to their children's requests for certain products, there is little evidence to support this viewpoint (Jenvey and Jenvey 2003). It is likely that parents who monitor what their young children watch on TV would be far more vigilant about responding to their children's requests for the types of foods advertised (Jenvey and Jenvey 2003). Yet, few studies have surveyed parents of young children about this issue. A second omission from Tallis et al.'s (1999) study was information about the availability of those foods in children's households. Results of other studies show that types of foods available in young children's households, together with their parents' own consumption of food of poor nutritional quality, have a significant role in shaping the food preferences and diet of their young children (Guidetti and Cavazza 2008).

It is proposed that the psychological processes that underlie children being influenced by the media about food, attitudes to food, diet, and exercise involve the dual processes of imitation and modeling (Bandura 1986). At first, children tend to imitate the behaviors of influential adults in their environment. Reinforcement of behaviors of influential others occurs vicariously. Children are rewarded by watching others being rewarded, and are likely to use these people as models upon whom they can base their own behavior, in the expectation that they themselves will be rewarded directly for similar behavior. This process explains why children might show a preference for food advertised on TV, especially if the food is endorsed by popular TV characters, or high profile media, or sporting personalities. This process is understood well by corporate marketers, and is one of the reasons why popular actors, sporting and other media personalities are used for both questionable advertising campaigns (e.g. junk foods advertisements targeted at young children), as well as more prosocial campaigns that contain community service messages (e.g. support programs for child cancer sufferers and road safety campaigns).

Imitation and modeling also explain why parents, and mothers especially, act as important role models in the development of children's food preferences and eating habits. There is evidence to support the influence of parent's modeling both healthy and unhealthy eating habits and food preferences (Guidetta and Cavazzo 2008). Among young 3–8 year-old children, parents or immediate family members are the most significant role models for children's behaviors (Black et al. 2001; Cullen et al. 2000), and this understanding of the importance of parents and even grandparents modeling appropriate nutrition and exercise habits for their offspring has been incorporated into successful intervention programs to improve infant and young children's nutrition and physical activity, as well as to prevent or reverse the early onset of overweight and obesity (Black et al. 2001). Furthermore, in an epidemiological study of factors that contribute to fruit and vegetable consumption by 6–12-year-olds, the most significant predictors of fruit and vegetable consumption by children were, in order, the provision of fruits and vegetables in children's homes, parents' intake of fruit and vegetables, and parents' knowledge of childhood nutrition and dietary recommendations (Blanchette and Brug 2005). In this study, children's TV viewing, including exposure to televised food advertisements and the availability of convenience food at children's schools were less significant predictors of the amount of fruits and vegetables children consumed (Blanchette and Brug 2005).

Thus, these latter factors were far less predictive of poor nutrition than parental factors, and they formed a complex of other factors related to both availability of snack foods in places other than children's homes and, less significantly, to passive TV consumption and exposure to food advertisements, the content of which are not fully described in the study.

Thus, the extent to which young children are influenced by this mode of advertising is still dependent upon: (a) whether parents provide such food for their children, (b) whether parents also model those poor dietary preferences, and (c) how well young children are able to persuade their parents to purchase the snack foods and junk foods frequently advertised on TV which are not usually present in children's households.

A consideration of other cognitive processes of young children may also explain why young, preschool, and early school-aged children may be more susceptible to the persuasive intent of TV advertisements for certain types of food products. It is often the case that advertisements are embedded in thematically related children's TV programs, and that their persuasive intent is not obvious to young children (Kunkel and McIlrath 2003). It has been demonstrated that young children (< 4–5 years) have difficulty distinguishing advertising content from program content on TV, and that they do not understand the persuasive intent of the advertisements (Kunkel and McIlrath 2003). Characteristics of young children's cognition are shown in Table 167.6.

As children mature cognitively, however, they begin to understand the persuasive intent of advertisements (Oates et al. 2002). Nevertheless, these authors noted that, in their study, a sizeable proportion (approximately 25%) of 10-year-olds were unaware of the persuasive intent of advertisements (Oates et al. 2002). What is important to understand is what differentiated the 25% of 4–5 year-olds, who understood the persuasive intent of advertisements from the 75% who did not. Similarly, it is important to find out why 25% of 10-year-olds still did not yet understand the persuasive intent of advertisements, when compared with the majority of their age group, who readily understood the persuasive intent of advertisements. To determine the validity of these findings, it is important to consider whether the minority of 10-year-olds who remain susceptible to the persuasive intent of TV commercials had other cognitive delays, for example, in perspective taking or global cognitive functioning. Additionally, there is no report of whether the group of 10-year-olds watched TV alone or in the company of adults or other children, who might have afforded them opportunities to discuss the content and function of advertisements they watched so that they could develop a more critical response to what they watch on TV.

It is a much-replicated finding that TV advertising, the intent of which is to influence young children to persuade their parents to purchase and consume products such as *snack* or *junk* foods, is placed frequently during programs that attract large numbers of child viewers (Kunkel and McIlrath 2003). There is also evidence that very young children are often unaware that the intent of advertisements is to

Table 167.6 Key features of cognitive immaturity of 3–6-year-olds

- Children's thinking characterized by primitive, pre-logical thinking
- Self-centered perspective that makes them unable to see events from another's viewpoint
- Have literal interpretation of what they see and hear
- What they view on TV is taken at face value
- Respond to content in advertisements and are unable to determine that the persuasive message only represents viewpoint of person or character in advertisement

This table outlines how young children, because of their stage of cognitive development, are unable to detect the intention of food advertisements to influence young children to purchase and consume products advertised

persuade children to themselves purchase and consume their products or to demand that their parents purchase such products. It has yet to be established, however, that there is a direct link between types of products advertised to children during children's TV programs, and parents' purchase and children's consumption of such food products to explain the development of overweight and obesity in many young children. It appears more likely that young children begin to consume nutritionally poor food in certain households where such foods are already available and where parents do not monitor what their young children watch on TV. Additionally, evidence is still needed to show that parents, older siblings, or grandparents are more responsive to young children's requests to buy junk foods, and those foods then are consumed by children instead of more nutritious foods. It is also critical to find out whether young children, who develop poor eating habits and food preferences from being exposed to excessive advertising of *junk* food when they watch TV, are also less likely to engage in physically active leisure pursuits that, in turn, leads to the development of early onset of obesity. Time displaced by watching TV may lead to reduced engagement in physical activity together with increased exposure to junk food advertisements and increases in parents' purchase of such foods *may* result in children eating more nutritionally poor food at the expense of more nutritionally appropriate food. This explanation suggests a multidimensional process rather than a one-dimensional process that leads to early and sustained development of overweight and obesity in early childhood.

Despite the plausibility of the different explanations reviewed, results from research investigating an association between TV and other passive media consumption and early onset of overweight and obesity in young children have been equivocal. Researchers have yet to delineate clearly the underlying mechanisms that link TV viewing with the development of overweight and obesity in early childhood. Methodological shortfalls in existing research include an over-reliance on BMI to characterize children's growth. Other studies lack adequate data on all leisure activities of children, the level and intensity of children's physical activities and reliable and valid documentation of children's TV viewing time. Within the family context there is a lack of information about the amount and type of food parents provided to their young children, including snacks; existing nutritional practices within families; parents' own eating habits and food preferences; and parents' level of physical activity. Table 167.7 summarizes recurrent methodological and conceptual shortfalls in existing research.

How increased TV viewing may be linked to the development of overweight and obesity and thereby the diseases that result from the onset of overweight and obesity in early childhood has yet

Table 167.7 Conceptual and methodological shortfalls of each explanation

Explanation	Conceptual problems	Methodological problems
Energy displacement	Characterizing and measuring typical activity in children	Need measures of all activities and their intensity
	Valid and reliable measure of time spent watching television (TV)	Need reliable and valid method of data collection for amount of time spent watching TV
Exposure to saturation amounts of TV advertisements for foods of poor nutritional quality	Establishing a link between children's awareness of products advertised and their requests to parents to buy same products	Find out whether products already purchased by parents and available in home
		Distinguish between knowledge of product and frequency of purchase
Energy Displacement + Cognitive Immaturity of Young Children	How reduced physical activity co-occurs with susceptibility to persuasive intent of advertisements	Measuring activity levels and children's cognition appropriately

This table lists, some of the recurrent conceptual and methodological shortfalls in existing research on each of the three main explanations that link TV viewing to the development of overweight and obesity in young children

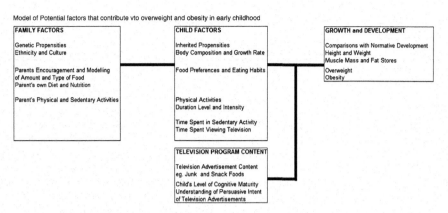

Fig. 167.1 There are several potential biological, behavioral and social factors, in addition to excessive TV watching, that impact on children's growth and development, resulting in overweight and obesity

to be delineated. In Fig. 167.1, a multidimensional model is proposed to explain potential factors that best explain the underlying processes that make some young children more vulnerable to the development of overweight and obesity in early childhood.

Factors identified in Fig. 167.1 should be investigated within one study of a representative sample of young children, and the use of longitudinal research design would also overcome some of the underlying conceptual and methodological shortfalls in research to date. Using a multidimensional model as the basis for future investigations of processes by which young children become overweight and obese would then permit researchers to investigate interactions among variables and identify pathways that lead to the onset of overweight and obesity in early childhood.

Existing research tends to focus on a limited number of variables to investigate relationships between TV watching in early childhood and the development of overweight and obesity. Children do not develop in isolation, and their growth and development is not only affected by inherited propensities and individual behavioral differences but also their family and other social contexts in which growth and development take place.

167.7 Applications to Other Areas of Children's Health and Disease

There is conflicting evidence of an association between time young children spend watching TV and contemporaneous or later-onset development of overweight and obesity. Additionally, existing physiological and cognitive models are not yet able to characterize the processes through which TV viewing contributes to overweight and obesity in early and later stages of development. Thus, any suggested applications of research findings reviewed in this chapter to other areas of young children's health and disease remain tentative. Potential applications of research to other areas of children's health and disease are shown in Table 167.8.

It should be noted, however, that there is almost as much evidence showing no association between TV viewing and overweight and obesity during early childhood. If advertising agencies can produce advertisements that actually do influence young children to buy and consume food products of poor nutritional quality and to develop preferences for such food products, then similar advertising strategies could be implemented to promote more healthy food preferences for young children. For example, advertisements could be developed to persuade children, for example, to eat more healthy foods

Table 167.8 Potential applications to other areas of health and disease in young children

Behaviors associated with television (TV) viewing	Health and well-being	Disease
Increased sedentariness and reduced physical activity	May lead to overweight and obesity	May be related to early symptoms of cardiovascular disease
		Joint and muscular-skeletal problems
		Onset of diabetes
Energy consumption disproportionate to energy requirement	May lead to overweight and obesity	May be related to early symptoms of cardiovascular disease
		Joint and muscular-skeletal problems
		Onset of diabetes
Body image and self-esteem difficulties	May lead to adverse psychological effects related to overweight and obesity	Potential future mental health problems
Over-exposure to TV advertisements for *junk* and *snack* foods	May lead to poor diet, if types of food then consumed by children	Dietary imbalances
		Poor nutrition and later-life health problems
Susceptibility to persuasive intent of advertisement for food of poor nutritional quality	May lead to poor diet, if types of food then consumed by children	Dietary imbalances
		Poor nutrition and later- life health problems
Young children's susceptibility to persuasive intent of advertisements for food of poor nutritional quality	Cognitive strategies used in advertisements to persuade children about nutritionally poor products could be harnessed by health authorities to promote the attractiveness of appropriate foods to young children	Promotion of healthy eating at a young age
		Reduction of overweight and obesity in early childhood
		Potential reduction of future diseases linked to overweight and obesity

This table outlines some of the potential applications to other areas of children's health of research in which an association between amount of TV viewing in early childhood and the onset of overweight and obesity. Caution is recommended, because of the contradictory findings in existing research. Potential applications of findings to the promotion of healthy eating and preventative programs are listed

or to promote knowledge about good nutrition, adequate levels of physical activity, and alternative activities to occupy leisure hours that might otherwise be spent by young children watching TV.

167.8 Conclusion

The ubiquity, frequency, and sedentary nature of TV viewing that occupies a sizeable proportion of young children's leisure time in both developed and developing countries is considered by many researchers to be implicated in the increasing percentage of young children worldwide who are overweight and obese. Three commonly proposed explanations of the underlying processes that link TV viewing to the development of obesity in young children were evaluated. There were inconclusive findings to support the proposal that TV viewing displaces time available for more vigorous activity, reduced energy expenditure relative to energy intake, and the development of early-onset overweight or obesity. Additionally, there was inconclusive evidence to support the proposition that all young children are susceptible to persuasive intent of advertisements for food products of poor nutritional quality that appear frequently during children's TV, and that, arguably, contribute to unhealthy food preferences and eating patterns which predispose young children to the early onset of obesity. An interaction of energy displacement and susceptibility to develop preferences for unhealthy foods advertised when young children are most likely to be watching TV was identified as a more plausible explanation of the proposed link between TV watching and obesity in young children, but more evidence is needed to support an interactive explanation. It was recommended that future research address both conceptual and methodological shortfalls in existing studies and a proposed multidimensional model to investigate all potential factors that contribute to the development of overweight and obesity in early childhood. Potential applications to other areas of children's health and disease were also discussed.

Summary Points

- Apparent increase in obesity at all stages of development. Increasing proportion of young (3–6 year-old) children overweight and obese. Trends in overweight and obesity found in diverse populations of children worldwide. Trend evident in developed and developing countries.
- Ubiquity of TV viewing as leisure activity among younger age group, documented in both developed and developing countries. This finding represents one of the main reasons for investigating any association between amount of time young children spend watching TV and the development of overweight and obesity in early childhood.
- Three main explanations proposed for linking amount of TV viewing with overweight and obesity in early childhood. These are: (1) Energy displacement explanation; (2) Cognitive immaturity of young children explanation; and (3) Combination of energy displacement and cognitive immaturity of young children.
- *Energy displacement* explanation: Time spent watching TV supplants time spent in other more physically active leisure, especially vigorous physical activities that require greater energy expenditure. Energy consumed (by food) exceeds energy required (for less physical activity and increased sedentariness), which in turn leads to early onset of overweight and obesity.
- *Cognitive immaturity* of young children (< 6 years) makes them more susceptible than older children to the persuasive intent of advertisements for *snack* and *junk* foods that are frequently broadcast during TV programs designed for and watched by very young children. Snack and junk foods are highly processed and contain proportions of saturated fats and sugar that far exceed recommended daily allowances in young children's diets. Marketers develop food products and packaging designed to influence children's food preferences and to encourage young children to pester parents to purchase such foods. Buying these products and regularly including them in daily food intake can lead to dietary imbalance, resulting in overweight and obesity when young children consume *snack* and *junk* foods at expense of other food groups. It is argued that younger children are more susceptible to such advertisements because they have difficulty in discriminating between TV content and advertising content, and thus remain unable to detect the persuasive pitch in advertisements because of self-centered cognition.
- *Energy displacement and cognitive immaturity of young children, in concert*, lead to preferences for and consumption of more processed, fat and sugar-laden foods of the types commonly advertised during designated children's TV programs. Increased sedentariness compounds adverse outcomes of poor food choices, leading to more rapid development of overweight and obesity.
- *Persuasive Intent of Advertisements*: Content of the advertisements often contain subtle and covert messages, designed to take advantage of young children's cognitive immaturity, especially in their inability to grasp the intentions or viewpoint of another, including intentions or viewpoints of real or fictitious characters who appear in food products marketed to children during children's TV programs. This leaves young children unable to determine that they are being persuaded, for example, to eat a certain type of food.
- While each of three explanations has some plausibility, evidence in support of all three is equivocal. Some studies report a significant association between TV viewing and development of

overweight and obesity in early childhood. However, several recent studies report no significant association between times spent watching TV or frequency of exposure to advertisements for *snack* and *junk* foods. Contradictory findings can be attributed to both conceptual and methodological shortfalls in many existing studies.

- One of the main methodological problems is the widespread use of BMI, measured at different periods during children's early development to characterize overweight and obesity of children across developmental periods. Besides measuring children's weight relative to their height compared with children of same age and sex, international expert committees recommend measuring children's skin fold thickness (to characterize fat stores) and upper arm and calf circumferences (to assess children's muscle mass). In addition, differences in growth rates on all parameters vary according to children's ethnicity and inherited predispositions, which are often omitted from studies.

- Other methodological shortfalls relate to how the potential range of all children's activities are measured, and whether intensity of physical activity is accounted for. The way in which TV viewing is measured often is not reported, and daily food intakes often are recorded retrospectively via parents' completing a questionnaire.

- There is a dearth of information that directly assesses associations between the actual types of foods advertised on TV and children's requests to parents to purchase those foods. Additionally, there is a lack of information about whether snack and junk foods are readily available in households, whether they are provided usually by parents for children to eat, or whether parents themselves eat such foods in the presence of their young children. There is also a near-absence in studies to investigate parents' and other family members' food preferences and eating habits and how much TV other family members watch.

- A multidimensional model is proposed to investigate more comprehensively the myriad of potential interacting factors that contribute to the development of overweight and obesity in young children. Within such a research model, factors that need to be considered are: (a) the inherited propensities of children that might contribute to increased fat stores; (b) differences in rate and dimensions of growth among different ethnic groups between and within populations; (c) the amount and types of foods provided in children's homes by their parents, together with parents own food preferences, eating habits, and exercise regimens; and (d) the use of valid and reliable measures to quantify children's TV viewing and food consumption.

- Only when methodological and conceptual shortfalls in existing studies are addressed in future research can there be an adequate understanding of the processes that lead to overweight and obesity in early childhood. Once process is delineated, then there will be potential applications of such findings to develop intervention and prevention programs to reduce adverse health outcomes associated with the development of overweight and obesity in young children. Such programs should adopt a multipronged approach to address all potential contributing factors.

- *Intervention and Prevention*: To improve general cardiovascular fitness and to increase bone density; reduce risk of later development of cardiovascular problems; Type II diabetes and kidney disease. To intervene or prevent certain psychological problems associated with overweight and obesity in childhood, including early onset of depression; problems with body image and self-esteem; and to prevent social isolation and withdrawal from activities with peers. In relation to advertising *snack* and *junk* foods during children's TV programs, public health programs could be implemented to reduce advertising hours and scrutinize content for advertisements shown during TV programs aimed at young children. Additionally, if advertisements were shown to be capable of promoting nutritious food preferences and sensible eating habits as well as to educate young children about appropriate nutrition.

Definitions and Explanations of Key Terms

Body mass index: Represents a shorthand way of characterizing children's growth. It is calculated after obtaining height and weight, and height is divided by weight squared to yield a BMI value that can be compared with normative values for child's age and sex. Is argued to be a problematic measure when used to characterize growth changes in children, especially during early childhood, as it does not take into account body types of different ethnic groups

Mid-upper arm circumference (MUAC): Recommended as indicative of children's growth. Measures muscle mass. Measured by finding median point between child's shoulder and elbow. Measured using flexible tape measure. Value is compared with normative data. Comparatively low measures, when compared with normative group can indicate protein malnourishment in young children.

Skin fold thickness: Considered reliable index of children's fat stores. Special calipers are used to measure (in cms/mms) children's fat mass from under their upper arm and just below their scapula. Subscapular skin fold argued to be the best indication of children's fat stores, and when compared with normative data can indicate under- or over-nourishment.

Imitation: Young children learn behaviors, which become stable over time, firstly by imitating models of those behaviors displayed by people deemed to be important in children's lives (role models), and parents are often the most powerful role models whom young children imitate. Additionally, influential or well-known figures also act as behavioral models for children to imitate. This explains why young children are likely to imitate behaviors, even opinions or beliefs expressed in advertisements featuring well-known personalities. If such models, for example, are seen by young children to eat certain food products or express a favorable opinion about a food product, then young children will tend to imitate that behavior (eat the product, if available or adopt the same opinion about a product that is expressed in the food advertisement. Reinforcement to repeat and stabilize such behaviors occurs through vicarious reinforcement (i.e. watching role models being reinforced for their behaviors).

Modeling: A more pervasive behavior than direct imitation. Young children begin to generalize behaviors initially imitated to other wider contexts. For example, preferences for, or opinions about, certain food products that are modeled by influential role models, in TV food advertisements, will be repeated by children, firstly in the context of the food advertisement but later in other contexts.

Cognitive immaturity of 3–6 year-olds: Young children are said to be cognitively immature, because their cognition is perception-dominated and egocentric.

Persuasive intent of advertisements: Content of the advertisements often contain subtle and covert messages designed to take advantage of young children's cognitive immaturity, especially in their inability to grasp the intentions or viewpoint of another, including, intentions or viewpoints of real or fictitious characters, who appear in food products marketed to children during children's TV programs. This leaves young children unable to determine that they are being persuaded, for example, to eat a certain type of food.

Key Points About Associations Between Television Viewing by Young Children and Development of Overweight and Obesity

- There is evidence of worldwide increase in proportion of young children (3–6 year old) who are overweight or obese compared with children of earlier generations.
- Trend exists in both developed and developing countries.

- Much replicated finding that most common free time activity of children worldwide, including younger children, is watching TV. Trend identified in both developed and developing countries. Thus, children's TV viewing patterns frequently targeted in research investigation as contributory factor in the development of overweight and obesity among young children.
- Apparent association between TV viewing and overweight and obesity explained in terms of three probable mechanisms: (1) Increased sedentariness, with attendant energy displacement. (2) Over-exposure to persuasive advertisements for food products of poor nutritional quality that are screened during designated children's TV programs. (3) Young children's cognitive immaturity renders them more susceptible to the persuasive intent contained in advertisements for snack and junk foods frequently broadcast when they watch TV. This exposure said to affect young children's food preferences and eating habits, leading to dietary imbalances associated with development of overweight and obesity.
- Studies yield mixed results when attempting to identify association between TV viewing-overweight and obesity.
- Reasons for conflicting findings attributable to conceptual and methodological problems in research studies to date.
- Conceptual problems include how best to characterize and measure children's growth parameters over time, especially during early childhood.
- BMI, most commonly used measure, has been criticized because it does not account for ethnic differences in growth patterns, and is not fully sensitive to subtle growth changes in early childhood.
- Methods for collecting TV viewing consistently lack adequate reliability and validity, thereby confounding studies' results.
- How best to characterize all activities, in addition to children's TV viewing during early childhood is still to be determined.
- Methods for collecting food consumption often are unreliable because they are collected retrospectively and are subject to social desirability bias.

References

Anderson RE, Crespo CJ, Bartlett SJ, Cheskin KM, Pratt M. JAMA 1998;279:938–42.
Anderson DR, Huston AC, Schmitt KL, Linebarger DL, Wright JC. Monogr Soc Res Child Dev. 2001;66:1–47.
Australian Bureau of Statistics. Children's participation in leisure cultural and activities, Australia. 2004. http://www.abs.gov.au/ausstats/abs@nsf/b06660592430724fca2568b5007b8619/0b14d8. Retrieved 12/02/06.
Bandura A. Social foundations of thought and action: a social cognitive theory. New Jersey: Prentice-Hall; 1986.
Bar-On ME. Arch Dis Child. 2002;83:289–92.
Baur LA. Asia Pac J Clin Nutr. 2002;11:524–8.
Black MM, Siegal E, Abel Y, Bentley ME. Pediatrics 2001;107:e67. http://www.pediatrics.org.cgi/content/full/107/e67. retrieved 10/09/07
Blanchette L, Brug J. J Hum Nutr Diet. 2005;18:431–43.
Bryant MJ, Lucove JC, Evenson, K.R, Marshall S. Obes Rev. 2007;8:197–209.
Cole TJ, Belizzi MC, Flegal KM Dietz WH. Br Med J. 2000;320:1240–3.
Comuzzie AG, Mitchell BD, Cole S, Martin LJ, Hsueh WC, Rainwater DL, Almasy L, Stern MP, Hixson J, MacCluer JW, Blangero J. Hum Biol. 2003;75:635–46.
Cullen KW, Baranowski T, Rittenberry L, Olvera N. Health Educ Res. 2000;15:81–590.
Dietz WH, Gortmaker SL. Pediatrics 1985;75:807–11.
DuRant RH, Baronowski T, Johnson M, Thompson WO. Pediatrics 1994;94:49–455.
Freedman DS, Dietz WH, Srinivasan SR Berenson GS. Pediatrics 1999;103:1175–82.

Goran MI, Hunter G, Nagy, TR, Johnson R. Int J Obes. 1997;21:171–8.

Guidetti M, Cavazzo N. Appetite 2008;50:83–90.

Harrison K, Marske AL. Am J Public Health. 2005;95:1568–74.

Hernandez B, Gortmaker SL, Colditz GA, Petersaon KE, Laird NM, Parra-Cabrera D. Int J Obes. 1999;23:845–54.

Iobst EA, Ritchley PN, Nabors LA, Stutz R, Ghee K, Smith DT. Int J Obes. 2009;52:1–7.

Jackson DM, Djafarian K, Stewart J, Speakman JR. Am J Clin Nutr. 2009;89:1031–6.

Jago R, Baranowski T, Baranowski JC, Thompson D, Greaves KA. Int J Obes. 2005;29:557–64.

Jenvey VB. Australian children's toy and play preferences: 1989–2005. In: Berg LE, Nelson A, Svensson K, editors. Toy research in late twentieth century: toys in educational and sociocultural contexts. Stockholm: SITREC, Swedish Institute of Technology; 2003a. p. 105–21.

Jenvey VB, Jenvey HL. Family, other sociocultural and media influences on preschool children's nutrition: a review and recommendations for intervention. Canberra: Department of Health and Ageing; 2003b.

Jiang J, Rosenqvist U, Wong H, Greiner, T, Ma Y, Toschke A. Int J Pediatr Obes. 2006;1:103–8.

Kanda A, Watanabe, Y, Kawaguchi T. Pub Health. 1997;111:29–32.

Katzmarzyk PT, Malina RM, Song TM, Bouchard C. J Adolesc Health. 1998;23:318–25.

Kelly B, Hattersley L, King L, Flood V. Health Promot Int. 2008;23:337–44.

Krassas GE, Tzotzas T, Tsametis C, Konstantinidis T. J Pediatr Endocrinol Metab. 2001;14:1327–33.

Kunkel D, McIlrath M. In: Palmer EL, Young BM, editors. The faces of televisual media: teaching violence, selling to children. 2nd ed. Mahwah: Lawrence Erlbaum; 2003. p. 287–300.

Kuribayashi A, Roberts MC, Johnson RJ. Child Health Care. 2001;30:309–22.

Landhuis CE, Poulton CE, Welch D, Hancox R. Pediatrics 2007;120:532–7.

Larson RW. Curr Dir Psychol Sci. 2001;10:160–4.

Larson RW, Verma S. Psychol Bull. 1999;125:701–36.

Lloyd LJ, Langley-Evans SC, McMullen S. Int J Obes. 2009. E-published 12/05/09. Retrieved 16/05/09.

Marshall SJ, Biddle SJH, Gorley T, Cameron N, Murdey I. Int J Obes Relat Metab Disord. 2004.

Oates C, Blades M, Gunter B. J Consum Behav. 2002;1:238–45.

Piaget J. Play, dreams and imitation in childhood. New York: W. Norton; 1962.

Pine KJ, Nash A. J Dev Behav Pediatr. 2003;24:219–24.

Rey-Lopez JP, Vincente-Rodriguez G, Biosca M, Moreno LA. Nutr Metab Cardiovasc Dis. 2008;18:242–51.

Roberts D, Foeher U, Rideout V, Brodie M. Kids and media @ the new millennium: a comprehensive analysis of children's media use. Washington, DC: The Henry Kaiser Foundation; 1999.

Ross JG, Pate RR, Casperson CJ, Danberg CL, Svilar M. Int J Phys Educ Recr Dance. 1987;58:85–92.

Schmitz KH, Leslie A, Lytle RD, Phillips GA, Murray DM, Birnbaum A, Kubik MY. Prev Med. 2002;34:266–78.

Strauss RS, Rodzilsky D, Burack G, Colin M. Arch Pediatr Adolesc Med. 2001;155:897–902.

Taras HL, Sallis JF, Patterson TL, Nader PR. J Dev Behav Pediatr. 1989;10:176–80.

Terran-Garcia M, Rankinen T, Bouchard C. J Appl Physiol. 2008;105:988–1001.

Wake M, Hesketh K, Waters E. J Paediatr Child Health. 2003;39:130–4.

World Health Organisation (WHO) Expert Committee on Anthropometry. Geneva: WHO; 1995.

Wilson N, Quigley R, Mansoor O. Aust NZ J Public Health. 1999;23:647–50.

Wilson N, Signal L, Nicholls S, Thomson G. Prev Med. 2006;42:96–101.

Chapter 168
The Dopamine Transporter Gene (DAT1) in Obesity and Binge Eating Disorders

Karen Wight, Caroline Reid-Westoby, and Caroline Davis

Abbreviations

AD(H)D	Attention deficit/(hyperactivity) disorder
BED	Binge eating disorder
BMI	Body mass index
DAT	Dopamine transporter
DAT1	Dopamine transporter gene
DSM-IV-TR	Diagnostic Statistical Manual of Mental Disorders – Fourth Edition
RDS	Reward deficiency syndrome
UTR	Untranslated region
VNTR	Variable number tandem repeat

168.1 Introduction

Experts have often attributed escalating obesity rates to a clash between our genes – adapted to survive seasonal food shortages or possible famines in times past – and the current abundant food environment (Cummings and Schwartz 2003; Peters 2003). According to the *thrifty genotype hypothesis*, obesity can be viewed as a natural response to our modern surroundings with its excess of energy sources (Cummings and Schwartz 2003; Peters 2003). We have a biological drive to eat beyond caloric need when food is available and to store energy as fat, as this would have been beneficial years ago, leading to improved chances of survival when food was scarce. Nowadays, this inherent motivation is problematic, given that the availability, variety, and portion sizes of food have greatly increased (Jeffery and Utter 2003; Nestle 2003) – factors associated with higher caloric intakes and elevated obesity rates (Nestle 2003).

Despite drastic changes to our environment, some individuals are able to maintain a healthy weight. It is critical to determine what differentiates this fraction of the population from the large and escalating proportion who chronically overeat. The various forms of overeating are derived from one of two separate drives according to the *homeostatic–hedonic model* – motives based on needing food and

K. Wight (✉)
Faculty of Health, York University, 223 Bethune College, 4700 Keele Street, Toronto, Canada
and
Centre for Addiction and Mental Health, University of Toronto, Toronto, Canada
e-mail: kapatte@yorku.ca

V.R. Preedy et al. (eds.), *Handbook of Behavior, Food and Nutrition*,
DOI 10.1007/978-0-387-92271-3_168, © Springer Science+Business Media, LLC 2011

motives based on wanting food, respectively (Saper et al. 2002). The involvement of the hypothalamic pathways in the former has long been recognized; whereas, less is known about *hedonic* or *non-homeostatic eating*, which refers to eating for reasons other than caloric need, such as emotional states ("comfort eating") or environmental cues (e.g., seeing others eating, the sight and smell of food stimuli). Experts believe the action of the neurotransmitter *dopamine* on the brain's *common reward pathway* is primarily accountable for hedonic motivations for food intake, with the opioid system playing a more minor role. Individual variations in the tendency to overeat can be attributed – at least in part – to the genetically determined action and availability of dopamine. Among the dopamine-related genes studied, the gene encoding the dopamine transporter (DAT1) has received particular attention in relation to eating behavior. The purpose of this chapter is to review the literature on the role of the DAT1 in obesity and binge eating disorders.

168.2 Binge Eating

Reward-based motivations seem to overpower homeostatic drives in some individuals, given the frequent snacking, binge eating, and higher caloric intakes seen among many obese individuals despite their adequate energy stores. *Binge eating* represents an extreme phenotype of hedonic over-eating and is a significant risk factor for substantial weight gain over time (Fairburn et al. 2000). It is defined as the consumption of an abnormally large amount of food within a limited time span in the absence of physical hunger, and is associated with feelings of loss of control. Individuals typically engage in binge eating when alone because they often feel embarrassed and guilty about their behavior. Binge eating represents a defining behavioral symptom of both *binge eating disorder* (BED) and *bulimia nervosa*.

According to the Diagnostic Statistical Manual of Mental Disorders – Fourth Edition (DSM-IV-TR; see Table 168.1), BED is characterized by regular binge episodes (2–3/week) for a minimum of 6 months, without the use of compensatory behaviors such as purging, excessive exercise, diet pills, laxatives and/or diuretics for the purpose of weight loss, as often associated with bulimia nervosa (American Psychiatric Association 2000). Individuals with the disorder also tend to overeat throughout the day in addition to their binge episodes, and as a result, are usually obese – defined as having a

Table 168.1 Diagnostic criteria for binge eating disorder (Created from DSM-IV-TR criteria APA 2000)

A. Recurrent episodes of binge eating. An episode is characterized by:
- Eating, in a discrete period of time (e.g., 2 h), and amount of food that is definitely larger than most people would eat in a similar period of time under similar circumstances
- Feelings of loss of control over the amount or the type of food being consumed during the episode (e.g., feeling one cannot stop eating)

B. Binge eating episodes associated with at least three of the following:
- Eating alone because of feelings of embarrassment regarding eating
- Eating large quantities of food when not feeling physically hungry
- Eating until feeling uncomfortably full
- Eating much more rapidly than normal
- Feelings of disgust with oneself, depression, and/or guilt after a binge

C. Marked distress regarding binge eating

D. Binge eating occurs, on average, at least 2 days a week for 6 months

E. The binge eating is not associated with regular use of inappropriate compensatory behaviors, such as purging, fasting or excessive exercise, and does not occur exclusively during the course of bulimia nervosa or anorexia nervosa

Body Mass Index (BMI) over 30 kg/m². In a longitudinal study of BED, the proportion of obese individuals rose from 22% to 39% over 5 years – validating binge eating as a significant risk factor for substantial weight gain over time (Fairburn et al. 2000). At a weight loss clinic, as many as 30% of obese attendees met diagnostic criteria for BED (Striegel-Moore and Franko 2003; Yanovski 2003). Current opinion varies on how individuals with BED differ from obese adults who do not binge eat. A recent study found no difference between the groups on many personality variables, leading to the speculation that the distinction exists at the biobehavioral level (Davis et al. 2008).

Much of our understanding of BED stemmed from research on bulimia nervosa, as the former represents a relatively modern phenomenon. Bulimia nervosa is also characterized by recurrent episodes of binge eating; however, unlike BED sufferers, individuals with bulimia nervosa engage in extreme weight-control behaviors, such as self-induced vomiting, strict dieting, and the misuse of laxatives or diuretics (Fairburn et al. 2000). Bulimia nervosa patients are typically of normal body weight as a result of compensatory acts. Many of the underlying mechanisms for binge eating in bulimia nervosa resemble those contributing to BED.

Among both BED and bulimia nervosa sufferers, negative affect (e.g., anxiety, depression) has been acknowledged as a primary risk factor for binge eating (Stice et al. 2000). Largely accounting for the susceptibility to such depressive and anxious states associated with binge eating are genetically determined levels of brain neurotransmitters. Similarly, the brain neurotransmitters play a role in impulsivity and impulse control disorders – such as substance abuse, pathological gambling, conduct disorder, and attention deficit/(hyperactivity) disorder (AD[H]D) – which are often comorbid with binge eating disorders (Blum et al. 2000). A genetic contribution to binge eating is also suggested in twin studies testing for a familial transmission of the behavior (Bulik et al. 2003; Reichborn-Kjennerud et al. 2004). Moreover, candidate genes association studies support the role of certain genes in a predisposition to binge eating disorders. To date, the bulk of this research has focused on the genes contributing to the dopamine reward system.

168.3 Dopamine

The dopamine system is involved in several motor activities and cognitive functions. Dopamine neurons in the *mesolimbic* and *mesocortical* pathways – considered the brain's reward system – originate in the ventral tegmental area and, respectively, project to limbic structures including the nucleus accumbens and amygdala, and to the frontal cortex (Koob 1992; see Fig. 168.1). Along the mesolimbic pathway, dopamine is responsible for regulating our emotional capacity to feel pleasure and our desire and motivation to seek out rewarding experiences (Berridge 2003). The pleasure felt in response to these experiences reinforces certain behaviors and directs attention to relevant environmental cues by associating them with feelings of reward (Blum et al. 1996). Dopamine release in the nucleus accumbens (the "reward centre" of the brain) acts to promote an appetitive/approach response to reward cues that are contingent on carrying out a specific action (Nicola et al. 2005). For example, inactivation of the ventral tegmental area (the major dopaminergic input to the striatum) abolishes neuronal firing in the nucleus accumbens and reward-seeking responses to reinforcing stimuli such as food (Yun et al. 2004). These responses can also be reduced by administration of dopamine receptor antagonists (Nicola et al. 2005). On the other hand, a stimulant injection in the nucleus accumbens potentiates dopamine release and reward-related behavioral responding (Zangen et al. 2006).

Similar to the majority of bodily systems, dopamine response varies considerably across individuals (Davis and Fox 2008). In the case of the mesocorticolimbic pathways, those with inherently higher levels of dopamine availability are likely to have a larger hedonic capacity and a stronger

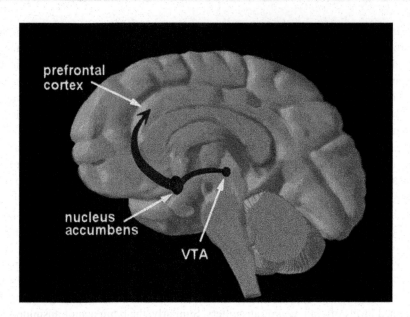

Fig. 168.1 Common reward pathway. All rewarding stimuli (e.g., food, sex) activate the same brain pathway: the mesolimbic pathway from the ventral tegmental area (*VTA*) to the nucleus accumbens, as well as the corticolimbic pathway from the nucleus accumbens up to the prefrontal cortex (Image adapted from National Institution on Drug Addiction (*NIDA*) at www.drugabuse.gov. NIDA cites this image as public domain and copyright permissions not required)

motivation to approach potentially pleasurable outcomes (Davis et al. 2004). In other words, they may experience greater pleasure from rewards, such as food, and therefore engage in more behaviors that will lead to its acquisition and consumption. Alternatively, a sluggish dopamine system is reflected in an anhedonic demeanor and a relative insensitivity to reward (Depue and Collins 1999).

Reduced dopamine availability is believed to place some individuals at increased risk of addictive behaviors according to the *reward deficiency syndrome* (RDS) (Blum et al. 2000). Basically, due to a breakdown in the brain "reward cascade," these individuals are said to require a "dopamine-fix" to feel good, and therefore, they are more likely to seek out stimuli that increase available dopamine such as illicit drugs (e.g., cocaine). The subcortical brain's response to reward does not appear to differentiate among being provoked by illicit drugs, natural reinforcers such as food or sex, or behavioral addictions such as gambling or shopping (Kelley et al. 2005). Nowadays, relative to drugs of abuse, highly caloric food represents an easily accessible, inexpensive, and reliable method to boost a sluggish dopamine system (Wang et al. 2004), and as a result, is one of the most common forms of self-medication (Davis et al. 2004).

The high comorbidity established clinically between substance-related and binge eating disorders supports the hypothesis of a shared biological basis. Moreover, chronic drug abuse and binge eating share many physiological and behavioral similarities, leading some experts to argue that non-homeostatic overeating is also appropriately modeled as an addictive behavior (Davis et al. 2004; Wang et al. 2004). Therefore, based on the RDS theory, researchers speculate dysfunctional dopamine availability due to variations in dopamine genes may predispose individuals to binge eating behaviors.

However, conflicting evidence suggests that an *elevated* dopamine signal also places individuals at risk for binge eating due to a stronger appetitive response to food cues. Consistent with these data, women who have high sensitivity to reward (and likely greater dopamine availability) were found to report stronger food cravings (Franken and Muris 2005) and are more likely to overeat and binge eat (Davis and Fox 2008; Davis et al. 2004) compared with their less hedonic counterparts. Some experts propose that, similar to the response seen in substance abuse addicts, a downregulation may occur among obese individuals as their brain's way of compensating for chronically elevated dopamine levels produced by overeating, and this may account for the conflicting findings of low dopamine levels (Davis et al. 2004). Considering both theories, Davis and Fox (2008) suggest a dual vulnerability for overeating where low or high dopamine availability confers risk – albeit, in different individuals and perhaps with different levels of severity. Indisputably, several routes to obesity and binge eating exist, and are based on various biological vulnerability factors, including variations in the dopamine system.

168.4 Dopamine Transporter

Dopamine availability is highly polygenic, and primarily determined by the affinity and density of the dopamine transporters (DATs) and receptors, and the amount of dopamine synthesized and secreted into the synapse (Need et al. 2006). The DAT is a member of a family of sodium (Na$^+$) and chlorine (Cl$^-$) ion-dependent neurotransmitter transporters that is highly expressed in the human striatum and prefrontal cortex where it regulates the duration of dopamine activity (see Fig. 168.2; Cragg and Rice 2004). Specifically, as a membrane-spanning protein, the DAT functions by binding to dopamine to clear it from the synapse and transport it back into the neuron. Therefore, a greater density of DAT is believed to predict less dopamine reaching the postsynaptic cell (Table 168.2).

The human DAT1 gene (SLC6A3) that encodes for the DAT protein has been mapped to the short arm of chromosome 5 (5p15.3) and carries 15 exons (Giros et al. 1992; Vandenbergh et al. 1992).

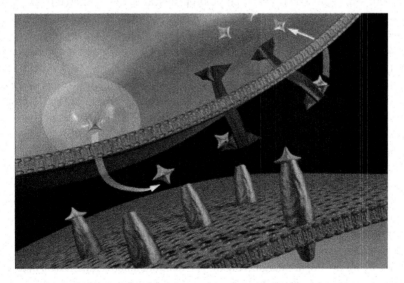

Fig. 168.2 Dopamine transporter at synapse. As synaptic vesicles release dopamine into the synapse, some dopamine binds to the dopamine receptors on the postsynaptic neuron and some of the neurotransmitter is transferred back into the presynaptic neuron by the dopamine transporters (*DATs*). (Image adapted from National Institution on Drug Addiction (*NIDA*) at www.drugabuse.gov NIDA cites this image as public domain and copyright permissions not required)

Table 168.2 Key features of the dopamine transporter (DAT)

	Dopamine transporter (DAT)
Form:	Membrane-spanning protein and member of family of Na⁺ and Cl⁻ ion-dependent neurotransmitter transporters
Location:	Highly expressed in human striatum and prefrontal cortex
Function:	Regulates the duration and strength of the DA signal
Action:	Binds to DA to clear it from synapse and transport it back into the presynaptic neuron
Predicted effect on DA levels:	Greater density of DAT → ↑ DA reuptake → ↓ DA availability

DA dopamine, *Na⁺* sodium, *Cl⁻* chlorine

Table 168.3 Key features of the dopamine transporter gene (DAT1)

	Dopamine transporter gene (DAT1; SLC6A3)
Form:	Carries 15 exons; highly polymorphic
Location:	Short arm of chromosome 5 (5p15.3)
Function:	Encodes DAT protein
Key polymorphism:	Functional 40-base pair VNTR in 3′ UTR in exon 15
Predicted effect on DA levels:	10-repeat → ↑ DAT binding site density → ↓ DA availability (Relative to 9-repeat)

DA dopamine, *DAT* dopamine transporter

Of the polymorphisms identified, a 40-base pair *variable number of tandem repeat* (VNTR) in the 3′ untranslated region (3′ UTR) in exon 15 has been the most extensively studied (Fuke et al. 2001; Heinz et al. 2000; Mill et al. 2002). VNTR polymorphisms are series of altered fragment lengths that are related to each other by sequences of variable number of tandem repeated DNA segments in an interval between two restriction sites. For this VNTR, repeat numbers vary from 3 to 13, with the 9- and 10-repeat alleles occurring with the greatest frequency in the majority of human populations (Giros et al. 1992; Vandenbergh et al. 1992).

Although there have been some inconsistent findings concerning the functional effect of the DAT1 VNTR polymorphism, it is generally agreed upon that the 10-repeat variant is associated with particularly efficient DATs (Mill et al. 2002). According to the best available evidence, the 10-repeat variant yields an approximately 50–90% elevated DAT binding site density in comparison to the 9-repeat allele (VanNess et al. 2005). That is, the 10-repeat variant produces a greater amount of DAT protein, diminishing activity in the dopamine pathways due to heightened transportation of dopamine from the synapse back into the presynaptic neuron. For this reason, the 10-repeat variant has been considered the "high-risk" allele for certain psychiatric syndromes and conditions, and widely investigated due to its central role in the regulation of striatal dopamine availability – a crucial determinant of motivation (Table 168.3) (Yang et al. 2007).

Evidence supports a shared genetic causative mechanism between binge eating and substance dependence involving the dopaminergic system. As mentioned above, the DAT is the main mechanism for dopamine clearance from the synapse in dopaminergic neurons found in the midbrain. Researchers have established a relationship between the DAT1 genetic variants and individual differences in vulnerability to addictive behaviors including smoking (Jorm et al. 2000), alcohol dependence and withdrawal (Sander et al. 1997), and cocaine abuse (Crits-Christoph et al. 2008). The DAT1 has also recently been linked to compulsive overeating and obesity (Epstein et al. 2004).

168.5 DAT1, Obesity, and Binge Eating

Consuming a well-prepared dish is among the most enjoyable experiences in life, and because humans find food so rewarding, we are strongly motivated to acquire it. If feeding were exclusively regulated by homeostatic mechanisms, most people would likely be at their ideal body weight, and would view eating in similar ways to breathing, for example, as an essential but uninteresting part of life. However, many individuals consume more food than is required for survival and compelling evidence suggests that individual differences in food reinforcement play a role in overeating and subsequent obesity. The reinforcing value of food is associated with dopaminergic system activity (Epstein et al. 2007). In fact, consumption of food causes a rise in dopamine levels (Hernandez and Hoebel 1990).

Altering brain dopamine levels has been found to affect eating, where dopamine agonists generally diminish caloric intake (Leddy et al. 2004) and dopamine antagonists increase consumption and body weight (Wellman 2005); although, there is great individual variation in the population in response to these drugs (Davis et al. 2007). In line with this direction of evidence, some genetic studies report that genotypes and alleles associated with *lower* dopamine availability are overexpressed among obese individuals. For instance, in a sample of participants with an African American background, the likelihood of obesity was 5.16 times greater among individuals possessing the homozygous 10-repeat genotype of the DAT1 3′ UTR VNTR compared to that of the 9/9 or 9/10 genotypes; although, no association was found among non-Hispanic white participants (Epstein et al. 2002). Similarly, Epstein et al. (2004) found that participants who demonstrated high levels of food reinforcement (as assessed by a behavioral choice questionnaire) and possessed the 10/10 genotype had significantly greater caloric intakes in a food consumption task compared to subjects in the other groups. However, subjects in these studies were regular smokers and this limits the generalizability of the findings. Long-term tobacco exposure results in an upregulation of DAT activity (Li et al. 2004), which leaves less available dopamine and can increase sensitivity to food reinforcement. Therefore, these findings may not be replicable among participants without a history of smoking. To this effect, a study conducted recently among a larger sample of nonsmokers did not find any significant association between the DAT1 and energy intake, or between the DAT1 and food reinforcement (Epstein et al. 2007).

In contrast, some evidence suggests that obese individuals possess *higher* levels of dopamine availability. For example, using single position emission computational topography (SPECT) to measure striatal DAT availability among 50 healthy volunteers, Chen et al. (2008) found a significant negative association between age and BMI with striatal DAT availability, and BMI was the only significant predictor for DAT density. In other words, higher BMIs predicted lower DAT density, which in turn, is associated with greater dopamine levels. Elevated dopamine availability is believed to lead to greater hedonic capacity and a stronger motivation to approach food. In support of this theory, obese individuals have been reported to find food more rewarding compared to their leaner counterparts (Saelens and Epstein 1996). Specific to binge eating, a case-control study of Japanese women found an excess of short alleles (7- and 9-repeats) of the DAT 3′ UTR VNTR among patients with clinically significant binge eating behaviors (Shinohara et al. 2004). These results suggest that a strong dopamine signal, due to a decrease in the DAT protein, increased the reinforcing value of food, leading to a tendency to binge eat.

In order to test the appetitive response to elevated dopamine levels, many studies have used stimulant medications. The DAT is of specific interest in these studies as it represents the primary site of action of psychomotor stimulants such as cocaine, methylphenidate, and amphetamines, which bind to the transporters, thereby inhibiting the reuptake of dopamine into the cell and increasing its availability in the synapse. In particular, response to methylphenidate – better known by the brand name

Table 168.4 A proposed theory of associations among the dopamine transporter, the dopamine signal, and psychobehavioral response (Adapted from first printing in Davis et al. 2007)

10-repeat allele	↑ DAT Protein → ↓ synaptic DA	Increased risk for AD(H)D and therapeutic response to methylphenidate; increased response to exogenous stimulants
9-repeat allele	↓ DAT Protein → ↑ synaptic DA	Increased risk for binge eating
↓ DA signal	↓ Hedonic tone and ↓ sensitivity to reward	Increased risk for drug addiction
↑ DA signal	↑ Hedonic tone and ↑ sensitivity to reward	Increased risk for overeating

DA dopamine, *DAT* dopamine transporter

Ritalin and the most common treatment for AD(H)D – has often been studied and results generally indicate that ingestion of a small oral dose of the drug increased desire to eat in response to palatable food cues among human participants (Volkow et al. 2002). However, very high stimulation of dopamine pathways produced by chronic drug abuse typically curbs appetite (Cochrane et al. 1998). The same effect is seen in animal studies where drugs causing a substantial rise in dopamine induce anorexia (Bina and Cincotta 2000; Kuo 2002).

To further examine this relationship, Davis and colleagues (Davis et al. 2007) conducted the first study testing the suppression of appetite due to methylphenidate in relation to DAT1 genotype variation. Participants' "favorite snack" was provided as a food cue to judge appetite ratings. The results revealed that individuals with BED possessing at least one copy of the 9-repeat allele had a significant decrease in appetite ratings in response to the methylphenidate, in comparison to control participants with the 9-repeat variants or to BED and controls with the 10/10 genotype – all three of whom had negligible differences in appetite ratings between drug and placebo conditions. Results support the role of genetic factors influencing dopamine availability in regulating appetitive response to methylphenidate. A study by Leddy et al. (2004) also revealed a varied response to methylphenidate in a small sample of obese adults. Following a large dose of the drug, participants were fairly equally divided among showing a large decrease, a small or moderate decrease, or even an increase in caloric intake, and these effects did not correlate with initial body weight.

Some experts interpret the varied DAT relationship with obesity and binge eating to indicate that dopamine activation and subjective response have an inverted-U relationship (Volkow et al. 1999). That is, a moderate boost in dopamine levels is believed to foster appetitive motivation; whereas, the opposite may occur with greater augmentation to very high dopamine levels, causing a suppression effect in the case of eating (Davis et al. 2007). Davis et al. (2007) have proposed that such a nonlinear relationship would assist in understanding some of the apparent contradictions in the literature regarding the relationship between dopamine activation and eating behavior. Evident variations in dopamine availability and responses to dopamine-related medications have important implications for obesity and binge eating treatment. Further examination of the dopamine-eating behavior relationship will assist in allowing better targeting of interventions to individual susceptibility (Table 168.4).

168.6 Implications for Treatment of Binge Eating and Obesity

Behavioral neurogenetic research has begun, and will continue, to enhance our understanding of individual susceptibility to binge eating and obesity in order to develop effective treatment and prevention efforts. This chapter has reported evidence highlighting the heterogeneity of obesity in terms of its diverse risk pathways, despite a long history of researchers and clinicians regarding all obese individuals as one homogeneous group. For this reason, individualized treatment approaches are required and should be determined by factors such as the causes and forms of overeating, biological contributors, and comorbid conditions. Individuals engaging in binge eating represent one subgroup requiring specialized interventions.

Treatment for binge eating in bulimia nervosa typically includes antidepressant medications to target the negative affect and comorbid mood disorders that often underlie and trigger binge behaviors. In terms of general obesity treatments, and of particular relevance, some of the weight loss medications endorsed by the US Food and Drug Administration stimulate norepinephrine and dopamine release in a manner similar to methylphenidate (Rucker et al. 2007). The studies discussed above indicate that the effectiveness and appropriate dosages of these pharmaceutical treatments are largely dependent on patients' baseline dopamine availability and genetic makeup. This chapter focuses on the role of the DAT; however, dopamine availability and drug response depends on variations in several related genes. In the future, with a greater understanding of the polygenic contributors to dopamine availability and treatment response, genetic testing may allow for better targeting of appropriate medications and dosages.

Large-scale clinical trials support the success of some of these drugs in reducing food intake and cravings, and fostering significant long-term weight loss (Rucker et al. 2007). Although, while these medications may be effective among some individuals in controlling eating behavior, the drawback is that they operate on the same systems which moderate mood. This is particularly concerning considering the high prevalence of depression and anxiety disorders found among patients with bulimia nervosa, BED and obesity. For this reason, some of these medications have recently been removed from the market.

In terms of implications for non-pharmacological interventions, other naturally rewarding but healthier activities should be encouraged. For instance, social activities, sex, and exercise are associated with a moderate increase in dopamine. Greater positive reinforcement should be given to individuals for engaging in healthy eating and physical activities. The recently increased attention in controlling food advertising is also promising as commercials often conceptualize high-fat or fast foods as treats or rewards, and therefore, likely enhance the motivation to eat them and the reinforcing value derived from their consumption. Moreover, the food consumed today has progressively moved toward high sugar and processed fare, some of which resembles drugs more closely than the natural whole foods our ancestors consumed. In fact, highly palatable, high-fat foods provoke a larger increase in dopamine relative to the consumption of healthier foods (Berridge 2003). Tackling our obesogenic environment is a necessary but particularly difficult route, and results will not likely be evident for several years. Currently, one of the most promising approaches appears to be first treating the comorbid disorders, such as depression and AD(H)D, which may contribute to, or exacerbate, binge eating.

168.7 Applications to Other Areas of Health and Disease: AD(H)D

The DAT1 has also been implicated in AD(H)D – a lifespan disorder characterized by developmentally age-inappropriate signs of impulsiveness, inattention, and/or hyperactivity (APA 2000). Relatively recently, it has been recognized that AD(H)D and obesity often coexist (Agranat-Meged et al. 2005). The occurrence of AD(H)D is especially high among individuals with Class III or morbid obesity (BMI > 40 kg/m^2), representing almost half of the sample in one study (42.6%) (Altfas 2002). Adding to the problem is the particular difficulty these individuals have adhering to weight loss programs – as evidenced by the greater clinic visits and longer treatment duration found among adults with AD(H)D attending a weight loss program relative to their non-AD(H)D counterparts (Altfas 2002). Among children with AD(H)D, the prevalence of overweight and obesity is also significantly greater than the age-matched population. For instance, in a study of obese school-aged children, over half (57.7%) suffered from co-morbid AD(H)D (Agranat-Meged et al. 2005).

Recent reports indicate that overeating, and binge eating in particular, moderate the relationship between AD(H)D and obesity (Davis et al. 2006). Adults with AD(H)D were found to have a higher prevalence of BED compared to the general population (Mattos et al. 2004), and similarly, a sample of adolescents with AD(H)D was more likely to engage in binge eating than controls (Neumark-Sztainer et al. 1995). AD(H)D symptoms could plausibly predispose individuals specifically to binge eating.

The comorbidities suggest that symptoms or biological factors associated with the disorder increase the risk of weight gain and binge eating. Genetic and neuroimaging research generated the dopamine-dysfunction hypothesis for the etiology of AD(H)D, leading some researchers to propose the AD(H)D-obesity link partially results from sub-optimal dopamine levels (Davis et al. 2006). In support of this theory, several reports indicate that DAT density is approximately 70% greater in AD(H)D cases compared to healthy controls (Yang et al. 2007). In addition, numerous studies and meta-analyses have reported a significant association between the 10-repeat variant of the DAT1 VNTR in the 3′ UTR and the disorder (e.g., Yang et al. 2007), leading to its designation as the "high-risk allele" for AD(H)D; although, there has been some conflicting evidence.

Similar to the varied appetitive response to methylphenidate, the DAT1 appears to regulate treatment response to methylphenidate among AD(H)D patients. Studies indicate the poorest response occurs among individuals homozygous for the 9-repeat allele, whereas the best treatment response is associated with the 10/10 genotype (Bellgrove et al. 2005). As discussed above, the greater effectiveness of treatment in 10-repeat individuals is proposed to occur because it ameliorates a hypodopaminergic state mediated by DAT1. Results have direct implications for treatment approaches for AD(H)D, as well as for the binge eating behaviors found among many of these patients. Awareness of the association and the biological mechanisms will assist in obesity prevention among individuals diagnosed with AD(H)D, and obesity and binge eating treatment among individuals whose previous efforts have been hindered by AD(H)D symptoms.

168.8 Conclusion

The strong links with weight gain and the serious medical and psychiatric morbidities associated with binge eating and related disorders, indicate the behavior demands further exploration. Binge eating emerged in our society relatively recently, in part as a response to environmental factors, such as the altered food composition, decline of family meals, and increased depression rates. There is little doubt that the environment plays an important role in sustaining, if not increasing, current obesity and overeating rates. Nevertheless, not everyone in our obesogenic environment regularly overeats or has difficulty maintaining a healthy weight, suggesting that gene-environment interactions are likely to contribute to individual vulnerability.

The purpose of this chapter was to discuss the role of the DAT1 – encoding the protein responsible for regulating the strength and duration of the dopamine signal, and one of several genes that have been linked to food intake and body weight. Dopamine is an important and necessary neurotransmitter involved in eating behavior. Without it, we would have little motivation to eat because doing so would provide us little pleasure, as witnessed in rat gene knock-out studies. Hedonic motivations often appear to overpower homeostatic mechanisms regulating energy consumption, leading to consumption beyond caloric need. Based on this evidence, interventions aimed at regions within the reward system will likely be required to control eating behavior among individuals engaging in binge eating in order to achieve and maintain a healthy body weight. To date, a comprehensive strategy to address obesity and/or binge eating disorders has yet to be established; although, recent and continuing advances in molecular genetics and neuroscience have greatly improved our understanding of the physiology of energy intake and have brought us closer to developing effective treatments. In the future, using a genetic approach to study eating behavior may enable us to identify susceptible individuals and allow for early intervention to prevent binge eating and weight gain, as well as their many comorbid disorders.

Summary Points

- Binge eating represents an extreme form of hedonic overeating and is defined as the consumption of an abnormally large amount of food in a limited time span in the absence of hunger. Binge eating is a central symptom of both bulimia nervosa and BED.
- Bulimia nervosa is characterized by recurrent episodes of binge eating and extreme weight-control behaviors such as purging, dieting, excessive exercise, and/or diet pill, laxative or diuretic use; whereas, individuals with BED engage in regular binge eating without the use of compensatory behaviors and are typically obese as a result.
- Evidence indicates a genetic contribution to predisposition to binge eating and associated disorders, with the majority of neurogenetic research focusing on the role of the brain neurotransmitter dopamine.
- Dopamine is responsible for regulating our motivation to seek out rewarding experiences and directing attention to relevant environmental cues by associating them with feelings of reward or pleasure.
- The action of dopamine on the brain's "Common Reward Pathway" is primary accountable for hedonic motivations for eating. Dopamine availability along these pathways varies considerably across individuals in the population, and this variation is believed to be partly attributable for individual differences in the tendency to binge eat.
- Two routes are evidenced to lead to bingeing. Based on the RDS model, individuals engage in compulsive overeating as a means to self-medicate low dopamine levels; whereas, a conflicting theory proposes that high dopamine levels are to blame as they cause a greater hedonic capacity and motivation to eat. Dopamine availability is highly polygenic and largely determined by factors including the affinity and density of dopamine transporters and receptors.
- The DAT is expressed in the striatum and prefrontal cortex, where it regulates the strength and duration of the dopamine signal by binding to synaptic dopamine and transporting it back into the neuron.
- The DAT1 gene that encodes the DAT protein contains a functional VNTR polymorphism in the 3′ UTR with the 10- and 9-repeat alleles occurring with the greatest frequency in the general population.
- The 10-repeat variant is associated with an elevated DAT binding site density (i.e., heightened dopamine reuptake and therefore, lower dopamine availability) compared to DATs encoded by the 9-repeat variant.
- In support of the RDS theory, some evidence indicates the 10-repeat allele – associated with lower dopamine availability – is overexpressed among obese individuals; although, more research is required as existing literature is likely confounded by the influence of comorbid smoking behaviors.
- In contrast, women engaging in binge eating behaviors were found to have a higher prevalence of the 9-repeat allele, which has also been associated with higher BMIs.
- An inverted-U relationship is hypothesized between dopamine availability and subjective response, based on studies using stimulant medications to boost dopamine in order to test the appetitive effect. That is, a moderate rise in dopamine levels is believed to increase appetite, whereas, very high dopamine augmentation likely suppresses eating.

Definitions of Key Terms

Binge eating: Binge eating is defined as the consumption of an amount of food that is unquestionably larger than most people would eat under normal circumstances within a discrete period of time (i.e., less than 2 h; APA 2000).

Binge eating disorder (BED): BED is characterized by recurrent episodes of binge eating (2–3 times per week for a minimum of 6 months) without the use of inappropriate compensatory behaviors, such as self-induced vomiting, misuse of laxatives or diet pills, fasting, or excessive exercising (APA 2000).

Bulimia nervosa: Bulimia nervosa is an eating disorder characterized by binge eating and inappropriate compensatory methods to prevent weight gain. In order to meet diagnostic criteria, a person must engage in binge eating and compensatory behaviors on average at least twice a week for the past 3 months (APA 2000).

Dopamine: Dopamine is a neurotransmitter that plays an important role in motivation and pleasure. Dopamine is characterized as a catecholamine (a molecule that acts as a neurotransmitter and/or hormone). It affects brain processes that control movement, emotional response, and ability to experience pleasure and pain.

Common reward pathway: Also referred to as the *mesocorticolimbic* pathway, the Common Reward Pathway is a circuitry in the brain that regulates and activates behaviors necessary for survival, such as feeding, sex, and maternal behavior. This pathway also underlies the development and maintenance of addictions.

Dopamine transporter (DAT): The DAT is a membrane-spanning protein that binds to synaptic dopamine. The DAT clears dopamine from the synapse, reuptaking it back into the presynaptic neuron, which ultimately leads to the termination of the dopamine signal.

DAT1 gene: The human DAT1 gene (SLC6A3) encodes for the DAT protein. It has been mapped to the short arm of chromosome 5 (5p15.3) and carries 15 exons. The gene is highly polymorphic, containing a functional VNTR in the 3′ UTR which is associated with DAT density.

Reward Deficiency Syndrome (RDS): According the RDS theory, deficient levels of dopamine in the reward pathways of the brain leave individuals susceptible to engaging in addictive behaviors as a means of increasing available dopamine.

Hedonic/non-homeostatic eating: As opposed to homeostatic eating, hedonic eating refers to food consumption driven by reasons other than survival, for example, to comfort emotional states (e.g., boredom, depressed mood) or for enjoyment in social situations.

Thrifty Gene hypothesis: The Thrifty Gene hypothesis postulates that genes predisposing individuals to overeating and obesity evolved because they were once beneficial. The ability to store excess energy as fat in times of food abundance was advantageous in order to increase one's chances of survival during times of famine.

Variable Number Tandem Repeat (VNTR): A VNTR is a gene polymorphism where a sequence of nucleotides is repeated a number of times in an interval between two restriction sites, causing different fragment lengths. The number of times the sequence is repeated varies within the population.

References

Agranat-Meged AN, Deitcher C, Goldzweig G, Leibenson L, Stein M, Galili-Weisstub E. Int J Eat Disord. 2005;37:357–9.

Altfas JR. BMC Psychiatry. 2002;2:9.

American Psychiatric Association. Diagnostic and statistical manual. 4th ed. Text revision. Washington, DC: American Psychiatric Association Press; 2000.

Bellgrove MA, Hawi Z, Kirley A, Fitzgerald M, Gill M, Robertson IH. Neuropsychopharmacology. 2005;30:2290–7.

Berridge KC. Brain Cogn. 2003;52:106–28.

Bina KG, Cincotta AH. Neuroendocrinology. 2000;71:68–78.

Blum K, Braverman ER, Holder JM, Lubar JF, Monastra VJ, Miller D, Lubar JO, Chen TJ, Comings DE. J Psychoactive Drugs. 2000;32 (Suppl. i–iv):1–112.

Blum K, Sheridan PJ, Wood RC, Braverman ER, Chen TJ, Cull JG, Comings DE. J R Soc Med. 1996;89:396–400.

Bulik CM, Sullivan PF, Kendler KS. Int J Eat Disord. 2003;33:293–8.

Chen PS, Yang YK, Yeh TL, Lee I-H, Yao WJ, Chiu NT, Lu RB. NeuroImage. 2008;40(1):275–9.

Cochrane C, Malcolm R, Brewerton T. Addict Behav. 1998;23:201–7.

Cragg SJ, Rice ME. Trends Neurosci. 2004;27:270–7.

Crits-Christoph P, Newberg A, Wintering N, Ploessl K, Gibbons MB, Ring-Kurtz S, Gallop R, Present J. Drug Alcohol Depend. 2008;98:70–6.

Cummings DE, Schwartz MW. Annu Rev Med. 2003;54:453–71.

Davis C, Fox J. Appetite. 2008;50:43–9.

Davis C, Levitan RD, Kaplan AS, Carter J, Reid C, Curtis C, Patte K, Hwang R, Kennedy JL. Prog Neuropsychopharmacol Biol Psychiatry. 2008;32:620–8.

Davis C, Levitan RD, Kaplan AS, Carter J, Reid C, Curtis C, Patte K, Kennedy JL. Neuropsychopharmacology 2007;32:2199–206.

Davis C, Levitan RD, Smith M, Tweed S, Curtis C. Eat Behav. 2006;7:266–74.

Davis C, Strachan S, Berkson M. Appetite. 2004;42:131–8.

Depue RA, Collins PF. Behavioral and Brain Sciences. 1999;22:491–569.

Epstein LH, Jaroni JL, Paluch RA, Leddy JJ, Vahue HE, Hawk L, Wileyto EP, Shields PG, Lerman C. Obes Res. 2002;10:1232–40.

Epstein LH, Temple JL, Neaderhiser BJ, Salis RJ, Erbe RW, Leddy JJ. Behav Neurosci. 2007;121:877–86.

Epstein LH, Wright SM, Paluch RA, Leddy JJ, Hawk LW, Jr., Jaroni JL, Saad FG, Crystal-Mansour S, Shields PG, Lerman C. Am J Clin Nutr. 2004;80:82–8.

Fairburn CG, Cooper Z, Doll HA, Norman P, O'Connor M. Arch Gen Psychiatry. 2000;57:659–65.

Franken IH, Muris P. Appetite. 2005;45:198–201.

Fuke S, Suo S, Takahashi N, Koike H, Sasagawa N, Ishiura S. Pharmacogenomics J. 2001;1:152–6.

Giros B, el Mestikawy S, Godinot N, Zheng K, Han H, Yang-Feng T, Caron MG. Mol Pharmacol. 1992;42:383–90.

Heinz A, Goldman D, Jones DW, Palmour R, Hommer D, Gorey JG, Lee KS, Linnoila M, Weinberger DR. Neuropsychopharmacology. 2000;22:133–9.

Hernandez L, Hoebel BG. Brain Res Bull. 1990;25:975–9.

Jeffery RW, Utter J. Obes Res. 2003;11 (Suppl.):12S–22S.

Jorm AF, Henderson AS, Jacomb PA, Christensen H, Korten AE, Rodgers B, Tan X, Easteal S. Am J Med Genet. 2000;96:331–4.

Kelley AE, Schiltz CA, Landry CF. Physiol Behav. 2005;86:11–4.

Koob GF. Trends in Pharmacological Science. 1992;13:177–84.

Kuo DY. J Biomed Sci. 2002;9:126–32.

Leddy JJ, Epstein LH, Jaroni JL, Roemmich JN, Paluch RA, Goldfield GS, Lerman C. Obes Res. 2004;12:224–32.

Li LB, Chen N, Ramamoorthy S, Chi L, Cui XN, Wang LC, et al. J Biol Chem. 2004;279:21012–20.

Mattos P, Saboya E, Ayrao V, Segenreich D, Duchesne M, Coutinho G. Rev Bras Psiquiatr. 2004;26:248–50.

Mill J, Asherson P, Browes C, D'Souza U, Craig I. Am J Med Genet. 2002;114:975–9.

Need AC, Ahmadi KR, Spector TD, Goldstein DB. Ann Hum Genet. 2006;70:293–303.

Nestle M. J Am Diet Assoc. 2003;103:39–40.

Neumark-Sztainer D, Story M, Resnick MD, Garwick A, Blum RW. Arch Pediatr Adolesc Med. 1995;149:1330–5.

Nicola SM, Taha SA, Kim SW, Fields HL. Neuroscience. 2005;135:1025–33.

Peters JC. Obes Res. 2003;11 (Suppl.):7S–11S.

Reichborn-Kjennerud T, Bulik CM, Tambs K, Harris JR. Int J Eat Disord. 2004;36:307–14.

Rucker D, Padwal R, Li SK, Curioni C, Lau DC. BMJ. 2007;335:1194–9.

Saelens BE, Epstein LH. Appetite. 1996;27:41–50.

Sander T, Harms H, Podschus J, Finckh U, Nickel B, Rolfs A, Rommelspacher H, Schmidt LG. Biol Psychiatry. 1997;41:299–304.

Saper CB, Chou TC, Elmquist JK. Neuron. 2002;36:199–211.

Shinohara M, Mizushima H, Hirano M, Shioe K, Nakazawa M, Hiejima Y, Ono Y, Kanba S. J Psychiatry Neurosci. 2004;29:134–7.

Stice E, Akutagawa D, Gaggar A, Agras WS. Int J Eat Disord. 2000;27:218–29.

Striegel-Moore RH, Franko DL. Int J Eat Disord. 2003;34 (Suppl.):S19–29.

Vandenbergh DJ, Persico AM, Hawkins AL, Griffin CA, Li X, Jabs EW, Uhl GR. Genomics. 1992;14:1104–6.

VanNess SH, Owens MJ, Kilts CD. BMC Genet. 2005;6:55.

Volkow ND, Wang G-J, Fowler JS, Logan J, Gatley SJ, Gifford A, Hitzemann R, Ding Y-S, Pappas N. American Journal of Psychiatry. 1999;156:1440–3.

Volkow ND, Wang GJ, Fowler JS, Logan J, Franceschi D, Maynard L, Ding YS, Gatley SJ, Gifford A, Zhu W, Swanson JM. Synapse. 2002;43:181–7.

Wang GJ, Volkow ND, Thanos PK, Fowler JS. J Addict Dis. 2004;23:39–53.

Wellman PJ. Curr Drug Targets. 2005;6:191–9.

Yang B, Chan RC, Jing J, Li T, Sham P, Chen RY. Am J Med Genet B Neuropsychiatr Genet. 2007;144B:541–50.

Yanovski SZ. Int J Eat Disord. 2003;34 (Suppl.):S117–20.

Yun IA, Wakabayashi KT, Fields HL, Nicola SM. J Neurosci. 2004;24:2923–33.

Zangen A, Solinas M, Ikemoto S, Goldberg SR, Wise RA. J Neurosci. 2006;26:4901–7.

Chapter 169
Feeding and Satiety Signals in Prader-Willi Syndrome: Relation to Obesity, Diet, and Behavior

Maithe Tauber, Emmanuelle Mimoun, Patrick Ritz, and Gwenaelle Diene

Abbreviations

AgRP	Agouti-Related Peptide
AP	Area Postrema
ARC	Arcuate Nucleus
BBB	Blood Brain Barrier
BMI	Body Mass Index
CNS	Central Nervous System
DMH	Dorsomedial Hypothalamus
FISH	Fluorescence In Situ Hybridization
fMRI	Functional MRI
FTT	Failure to Thrive
GH	Growth Hormone
GHR	Ghrelin Receptor
GnRH	Gonadotrophin Releasing Hormone
IQ	Intelligence Quotient
mPFC	Medial Prefrontal Cortex
MRI	Magnetic Resonance Imaging
NA	Nucleus Accumbens
NPY	Neuropeptide Y
NTS	Nucleus Tractus Solitarius
OFC	Orbitofrontal Cortex
OXM	Oxyntomodulin
PFC	Pre Frontal Cortex
PP	Pancreatic Polypeptide
PVN	Paraventricular Nucleus
PWS	Prader-Willi Syndrome
PYY	Peptide YY
UPD	UniParental Disomy

M. Tauber (✉)
Centre de référence du syndrome de Prader-Willi, Hôpital des Enfants, 330 av de Grande Bretagne, TSA 70034, 31059 Toulouse Cedex 9, France
e-mail: tauber.mt@chu-toulouse.fr

V.R. Preedy et al. (eds.), *Handbook of Behavior, Food and Nutrition*,
DOI 10.1007/978-0-387-92271-3_169, © Springer Science+Business Media, LLC 2011

VMH   Ventromedial Hypothalamus
VTA   Ventral Tegmental Area
VTA   Ventral Tegmental Area

169.1 Introduction

Prader-Willi syndrome (PWS) is a complex multisystem genetic disorder that arises from the lack of expression of paternally inherited imprinted genes on chromosome 15q11-q13. The syndrome has characteristic phenotypes (Gunay-Aygun et al. 2001), including severe neonatal hypotonia, early onset of hyperphagia, and the development of morbid obesity, short stature, hypogonadism, learning disabilities, behavioral problems, and psychiatric disturbances with severe consequences that pose difficult management issues for patients, families, and caregivers. Recent epidemiological surveys have estimated the lower limit of birth incidence at about 1 in 30,000, and the population prevalence at about 1 in 50,000. Other recent studies have highlighted the high rates and varied causes of morbidity and mortality throughout the natural history of the disease, mainly due to obesity complications (Schrander-Stumpel et al. 2004; Tauber et al. 2008). Early diagnosis and an integrated multidisciplinary approach improve quality of life, prevent complications (particularly childhood obesity), and prolong life expectancy (Bachere et al. 2008).

169.2 Diagnosis of PWS

In the past few years, the diagnosis has been increasingly made during the first months of life. As clinical signs vary with age, the diagnostic criteria from Holm et al. (Holm et al. 1993) have been modified to improve the description of the signs that should lead to genetic testing (see Table 169.1) (Gunay-Aygun et al. 2001).

There are different methods for confirming the diagnosis and identifying the genetic subtype using peripheral blood lymphocytes. DNA methylation analysis is the only technique that can both confirm and reject the diagnosis of PWS and should therefore be the initial investigation of choice. Parental samples are not required for this analysis. If DNA methylation analysis shows only a maternal pattern, then PWS is confirmed. Further methods may then be performed to determine the genetic subtype and to guide genetic counseling, particularly with regard to the risk of recurrence. Fluorescence In Situ

Table 169.1 Indications for DNA testing (Copyright 2008, the Endocrine Society)

Age at assessment	Features sufficient to prompt DNA testing
Birth to 2 years	• Hypotonia with poor suck
2–6 years	• Hypotonia with a history of poor suck
	• Global developmental delay
	• Short stature and/or growth failure associated with accelerated weight gain[a]
6–12 years	• Hypotonia with a history of poor suck (hypotonia often persists)
	• Global developmental delay
	• Excessive eating (hyperphagia, obsession with food) with central obesity if uncontrolled
13 years through adulthood	• Cognitive impairment, usually mild mental retardation
	• Excessive eating (hyperphagia, obsession with food) with central obesity if uncontrolled
	• Hypothalamic hypogonadism and/or typical behavior problems (including temper tantrums and obsessive-compulsive features)

[a]This item was added by the authors (Goldstone et al. 2008)

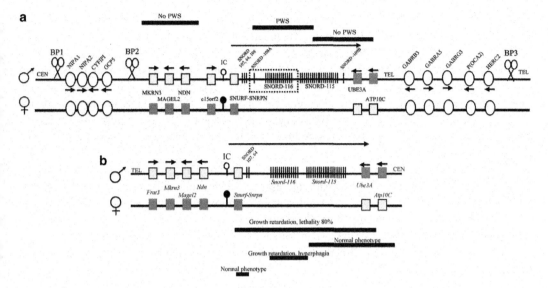

Fig. 169.1 PWS chromosomal region on 15q11-q13 (not to scale) (**a**) and murine orthologous region (**b**). Imprinted genes are white boxes (paternal allele expressed) and grey boxes (maternal allele expressed) and nonimprinted genes are white ovals. Vertical bars indicate snoRNA C/D genes. BP1, BP2, and BP3 indicate common breakpoint (BP) regions for deletions: type I deletions are between BB1 and BP3, and type II deletions are between BP2 and BP3. Arrows indicate transcription direction and horizontal black bars represent some informative deletions. Empty and plain circles indicate, respectively, the hypo- and hypermethylated region overlapping imprinting center (IC). A frame indicates the minimal critical region likely to contain a gene of major interest for PWS (SNORD116 cluster)

Hybridization (FISH) and high-resolution chromosome analysis can detect chromosome 15q11-q13 deletions in PWS.

As a whole, 70% of patients present with a deletion, 25% with maternal uniparental disomy (UPD), 1–3% with imprinting defects, and the remaining few with translocation involving chromosome 15. Most cases are sporadic but a high recurrence risk is associated with imprinting defects.

Figure 169.1 shows the complexity of the chromosomal PWS region in man (A) and mouse (B).

169.3 Description of Nutritional Phases

The two classical phases: PWS has been classically described as having two phases: (1) poor feeding and frequent failure to thrive in infancy (FTT), and (2) onset of hyperphagia leading to obesity (Gunay-Aygun et al. 2001). Phase 1 occurs from birth to early infancy when infants with PWS have severe hypotonia and a poor ability to suck and often require tube feeding. FTT refers to the lack of weight gain despite normal calorie intake. Phase 2 is described as beginning between 1 and 6 years, usually between 2 and 4 years (Gunay-Aygun et al. 2001). Recent examination of the natural history suggests a more complex progression leading to four main nutritional phases with subphases in the first two (McCune H 2005).

169.3.1 Four Nutritional Phases

Not all PWS individuals go through all the phases and subphases, which may be further altered by the use of GH (see Sect. 169.7).

In the first phase, the infant is hypotonic and is not yet obese. Subphase 1a consists of feeding difficulties with or without FTT. In subphase 1b, the infant grows steadily along a growth curve, at a normal rate.

In the second phase, which occurs between 18 and 36 months of age, body weight and BMI start to increase very rapidly. In subphase 2a, the child's weight increases in such a way that it crosses one, two, or more weight percentiles without a significant increase in calorie intake. In subphase 2b, the child increases his or her daily calorie intake, becomes more autonomous and turns overweight or obese, and displays an abnormally increased interest in food. Still, the appetite is not insatiable and unrelenting as it is in phase 3.

Phase 3 starts as early as 3 years of age or as late as 15 years. This is the classical phase that most people typically associate with PWS, with aggressive food-seeking and markedly reduced satiety. Patients in phase 3 have delayed meal termination and require significantly greater calorie intake to experience loss of hunger compared with those without PWS.

In phase 4, an individual may still have an increased appetite, but it is not as aggressive and unrelenting as previously observed and seems to occur only in a subset of adults typically after 30 years of age.

169.4 Eating Behavior and Food Preferences

Children with PWS present a particular meal pattern with a slower initial eating rate but much longer meal duration and nondecelerating eating curves. They are also distinguished by an early return of hunger after the previous meal, with early meal initiation. These findings were demonstrated by Lindgren et al. (Lindgren et al. 2000) using an elegant protocol to study nine subjects with PWS (compared with obese and normal weight subjects). These subjects were served a copious lunch on a hidden scale built into a table and connected to a computer. The authors concluded that the eating behavior of patients with PWS might be due to decreased satiation rather than increased hunger.

Given free access to food, patients with PWS will consume approximately three times more than control subjects, according to Zipf and Bernston (Zipf and Berntson 1987). These authors examined food intake patterns in ten patients with PWS and nine age- and weight-matched obese children by making standard chicken-salad sandwich quarters continuously available for one hour. Moreover, this overeating occurs despite delayed gastric emptying, leading to extremely morbid obesity.

Exploring food preferences, Fieldstone et al. (Fieldstone et al. 1997) elaborated a taste test with three types of foods (high carbohydrate, high protein, and high fat) reduced to spread consistency. PWS subjects preferred high carbohydrate foods over high protein foods and high protein foods over high fat foods. Moreover, the preference for high carbohydrate foods was significantly higher in PWS subjects than in obese controls. In addition, PWS patients are more likely than controls with and without mental retardation to eat nonfood items (pica) and contaminated foods and to make inappropriate food combinations.

Overall, the drive for food remains a life-long source of stress for individuals with PWS and their families. Complications of obesity remain the major cause of deaths in adults with PWS in relation with cardiovascular or respiratory failures. These patients are also at risk of choking due to a swallowing defect combined with their abnormal voracity or gastric perforation after consuming high quantities of food, even in the absence of obesity (Stevenson et al. 2007).

169.5   Evaluation of Hyperphagia and Feeding Disorders in Patients with PWS

Measuring hyperphagia in PWS has long been a research challenge. The abnormal feeding behavior in PWS includes a morbid obsession with food, food stealing, money stealing to buy food, hoarding and foraging, pica behavior, reduced satiety, and early return of hunger after the last meal (Goldstone 2004).

As described above, the first studies on PWS eating behavior provided unlimited access to food to patients and measured the number of sandwich quarters consumed. This methodology was questioned, and specific questionnaires were subsequently developed. In 2003, Russell and Oliver (Russell and Oliver 2003) proposed a 16-item informant-based Food Related Problem Questionnaire with three subscales (preoccupation with food, impairment of satiety, and other food-related 'challenging' behavior) for people with PWS. More recently, Dykens et al. (Dykens et al. 2007) developed a 13-item Hyperphagia Questionnaire to be filled out by parents or caregivers. The development of this questionnaire sets a landmark for future research on the eating behavior of patients with PWS (see article by Dykens in chapter 2.1). It also provides insight into the connections between the various behavioral features of the syndrome, as well as the connections between behavioral and neuronal or biochemical features.

Further research should focus on the role of maladaptive behaviors or emotional problems in the manifestation of hyperphagia in PWS and the mechanisms associated with individual variability, including genetic subtypes, neurobiological factors, emotional functioning, development and aging, and therapeutic interventions.

169.6   Mechanisms Involved in Hyperphagia and Feeding Problems

169.6.1   Feeding and Satiety Signals

PWS has been described as a genetic hypothalamic syndrome, although the phenotype and pathophysiology of the so-called hypothalamic dysfunction have yet to be reported in detail. The necdin gene, which is located in the 4 Mbp PWS chromosomal region, has been clearly implicated in preventing apoptosis of hypothalamic gonadotrophin-releasing hormone (GnRH) neurons. The Magel 2 gene (another candidate gene close to necdin in the PWS region) seems to be involved in hypocretin regulation and sleep control, with an involvement of hypothalamic neurons. Nevertheless, paternal deletion of the three genes – necdin, MKRN-3, and Magel 2 – does not result in the PWS phenotype in humans (Kanber et al. 2009).

Recently, the major components of the distributed neural system controlling food intake and energy balance were extensively reviewed. Over the past 10 years, the limited view of a few mainly hypothalamic centers has gradually been modified by evidence of a much more complex and distributed system including various corticolimbic areas. It is now recognized that cognitive, hedonic, and emotional neural processes play important roles in energy intake and expenditure and in the resulting energy balance, and that hormones modulate many of these processes. This model fits very well with what is known about the integrated dysfunctions in PWS that encompass the hypothalamus and brain regions involved in cognitive, social, and affective processes.

169.6.2 Elevated Ghrelin Levels in PWS

The most striking and specific defect in the satiety signals in PWS is the high circulating level of the orexigenic stomach-derived hormone ghrelin. Ghrelin is a 28-amino acid acylated peptide, first isolated from stomach in 1999, with a strong orexigenic effect, and it is the most potent GH secretagogue through its hypothalamic actions. Ghrelin is now considered a pleiotropic hormone with various secreting organs (duodenum, pancreas, pituitary, hypothalamus, testis, ovary, bone, and cartilage) and a wide range of target tissues depending on its acylation status (hypothalamus, stomach and gut, pancreas, adipose and cardiovascular tissues, testis, ovaries, and muscle), acting through distinct receptors (Hosoda et al. 2006). A specific enzyme, Gastric O acyl transferase (GOAT), was recently reported to be involved in ghrelin acylation and may have an important regulatory role. In addition, the ghrelin antisense strand gene GHRLOS, a recently reported candidate non-coding RNA gene, may have a regulatory and functional role in the ghrelin axis.

There are two reservoirs of ghrelin: the gastrointestinal tract and the central nervous system (CNS). Most circulating ghrelin is released by the stomach into the general circulation and can cross the blood–brain barrier (BBB) in a highly regulated process (Banks et al. 2002). In the CNS, ghrelin is produced in the major site for feeding regulation, the arcuate nucleus (ARC), and by a group of neurons adjacent to the third ventricle between four hypothalamic nuclei: dorsomedial (DMH), ventromedial (VMH), paraventricular (PVN), and ARC. Interestingly, these neurons also express ghrelin receptor GHR1a, which specifically binds acylated ghrelin. Receptors have also been identified in other areas such as the dorsovagal complex which includes nucleus tractus solitary (NTS), area postrema (AP), and dorsal motor nucleus of the vagus. In these areas, the density of GHRs is higher in fasting rats than in fed ones. The vagal nerve obviously plays a crucial but not mandatory role in driving the central actions of ghrelin (Date et al. 2002).

Regarding its role at the level of the ARC, ghrelin demonstrated opposite effects to leptin, another hormone involved in the control of food intake and energy homeostasis that is secreted by adipocytes and acts on the same hypothalamic neurons (Schwartz and Morton 2002). Ghrelin increases NPY and AgRP release. Leptin also plays a role in neuronal plasticity and particularly in the implementation of neuronal pathways in early life; its levels appear to be normal in people with PWS.

Circulating ghrelin levels have been shown to be low in obesity, suggesting that conversely to leptin, there is no ghrelin resistance in obesity. Individuals with PWS, unlike those with other known causes of obesity, have hyperghrelinemia (Cummings et al. 2002; Haqq et al. 2003; Tauber et al. 2004), which could explain at least two major endocrine dysfunctions observed in these patients: obesity and GH deficiency (described in 40–100% of the patients and explaining the short stature). GH deficiency could be explained by ghrelin resistance, whereas obesity could result from a preserved action of ghrelin on appetite centers, possibly due to different receptors or modulators. Nevertheless, ghrelin levels were reported to be negatively correlated with visceral adiposity, fasting insulin, and the homeostasis model assessment insulin resistance index (Goldstone et al. 2005) in adults with PWS. Ghrelin levels decreased with age, in controls, and in patients with PWS (Cummings et al. 2002; Haqq et al. 2003). Most of the studies documented an inverse correlation between ghrelin levels and BMI in the individuals with PWS (Haqq et al. 2003; Tauber et al. 2004). Our group recently described the changes in plasma ghrelin over the course of life in PWS and controls and showed that ghrelin dysregulation in PWS occurs very early in life and precedes the onset of obesity (Feigerlova et al. 2008). Thus, plasma ghrelin levels were high from birth to adulthood in patients with PWS, regardless of age, but the physiological decrease with age was preserved.

Recent data suggest that ghrelin does more than regulate energy homeostasis and that it is involved in the gustatory pathways, locomotor activity, dopamine/serotonin reward networks, and neuronal plasticity.

Ghrelin acts on hippocampal neurons to induce the formation of new synapses in the CA1 region correlated with enhanced spatial learning. Ghrelin-deficient mice exhibited impaired spatial learning that was corrected by ghrelin administration (Diano et al. 2006). These findings are consistent with the idea that ghrelin is involved in the appetitive phase of ingestive behavior, when it is important to find food in the environment. It is plausible that the ghrelin-induced changes in hippocampal function facilitate the recall of stored representations of prior experience with food. This is indicated by human subjects reporting a vivid, plastic image of their preferred meal upon intravenous ghrelin infusion. In addition, ghrelin activates dopamine neurons in the ventral tegmental area (VTA), increases dopamine turnover in the nucleus accumbens, and directly stimulates food intake when locally administered to the VTA. As local ghrelin receptor blockade in the VTA blunted rebound feeding following fasting, these observations suggest that enhancement of reward processing in the mesolimbic dopamine system is an integrated part of endogenous ghrelin orexigenic action (Olszewski et al. 2007).

While the well-known preprandial rise and postprandial fall in plasma ghrelin levels initially supported the hypothesis of a physiological role for ghrelin in meal initiation in humans, these more recent data favor a role of ghrelin in meal anticipation as shown in Fig. 169.2 (Frecka and Mattes 2008).

In humans, ghrelin bursts occur after the peak of hunger, and are related to habitual meal patterns (Frecka and Mattes 2008) and contents. Ghrelin levels may rise in anticipation of eating rather than eliciting feeding. These findings support the implementation of regular schedules for meal times and meal contents to control the eating behavior of patients with PWS. Ghrelin has been shown to be involved in food searching, food storage, foraging, and hoarding in hamsters.

Ghrelin also interacts with other important neuro-hormones possibly involved in PWS: lateral hypothalamic orexin neurons appear to mediate the orexigenic effects of ghrelin, and intra cerebro ventricular ghrelin activates magnocellular ocytocin neurons (Olszewski et al. 2007). Ghrelin may also support feeding driven by energy needs rather than reward (Bomberg et al. 2007).

Although somatostatin acutely suppresses plasma ghrelin concentrations in PWS patients, appetite is not reduced. A recent study found no benefit on weight or appetite in PWS from chronic administration of a long-acting somatostatin analogue (De Waele et al. 2008). This may suggest that early high

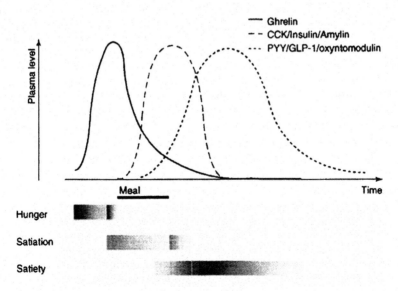

Fig. 169.2 Evolution of ghrelin, CCK, insulin, amylin, PYY, GLP-1, and OXM in humans before, during, and after mealtime

ghrelin levels set up an abnormal tuning for food seeking and anticipation of meals in patients with PWS, which cannot then be turned off. An alternative explanation could be that hyperghrelinemia is secondary to a primary defect that is not corrected by somatostatin. Recent evidence in human subjects suggests that both peptide YY (PYY) and oxyntomodulin (OXM, a product of differential processing of proglucagon in brain and gut) suppress circulating concentrations of ghrelin when given peripherally, whereas pancreatic polypeptide (PP) has no effect (Batterham et al. 2003a) Table 169.4.

169.6.3 Decreased Levels of Pancreatic Polypeptide

Levels of the anorexigenic gut hormone PP are reduced in PWS (Goldstone 2004). PP was discovered in 1975 and isolated from chicken pancreatic extracts. It is a 36-amino-acid peptide and a member of the PP-fold peptide family (also including NPY and PYY). The PP-fold family binds to receptors Y1–Y6, but PP binds with greatest affinity to the Y4 and Y5 receptors. It is produced in the endocrine type F cells, which are located in the peripheries of the pancreatic islets. Pancreatic polypeptide cannot cross the BBB and thus its central effects may be mediated in regions where the BBB is incomplete, such as the hypothalamus, AP, and adjacent brainstem areas (Katsuura et al. 2002). The release of PP appears to require an intact vagal cholinergic reflex. Peptide YY inhibits fluid and electrolyte secretion in the small bowel and delays intestinal meal transport. It may act as an "ileal brake," slowing gastric emptying and intestinal transit, so that nutrients can be absorbed in the small bowel. In humans, intravenous infusion of PP reduced food intake by 21.8% at a free-choice buffet, but did not affect gastric emptying (Batterham et al. 2003b).

Basal PP levels are elevated in anorexia nervosa, and in patients with advanced malignant disease. People with PWS had a blunted PP response to meals and short-term infusions of peripheral PP given to these subjects were shown to reduce subsequent food intake by 12% (Berntson et al. 1993). More recently, further evidence of PP's role in weight regulation came from a prospective study in Pima Indians. PP meal profiles were measured at baseline, and at a 5-year follow-up, and then correlated with change in weight. An increase in postprandial PP levels was associated with decreased weight gain, but surprisingly high fasting PP levels were associated with increased weight gain (Koska et al. 2004). These results suggest that different receptors may be activated. The precise role of PP in appetite regulation is not yet resolved. PP may be involved in the pathophysiology of obesity and dysregulation of body weight via effects on the parasympathetic nervous system.

Interestingly, the two main abnormal signals, one orexigenic (ghrelin) and the second involved in satiety control (PP), may explain the major feeding disturbances described in people with PWS. Part of their action requires an intact vagal nerve reflex and they both regulate gastric emptying. Both hormones are elevated in anorexia nervosa. A decreased parasympathetic tone has long been described in PWS together with a defect in gastric emptying and other gut dysfunctions possibly related to these hormone dysfunctions.

Besides a permanent state of hunger, people with PWS have disturbances in the anticipation of hunger and the representation of meal content, combined with satiety signal abnormalities involving the hypothalamus, corticolimbic networks, and the vagal system.

Table 169.2 summarizes the findings of studies on hypothalamic neuropeptides and their signaling inputs in PWS. It seems likely that in addition to these hormonal abnormalities in PWS, there are overriding brain defects, including hypothalamic, which lead to resistance to peripheral satiety signals (Goldstone 2004). The possibility of therapeutic avenues for reducing hyperphagia in PWS may depend on the existence of relative rather than absolute resistance to peripheral satiety signals.

Table 169.2 Summarized findings of studies on hypothalamic neuropeptides and their signalling inputs in PWS (Adapted from *Trends in Endocrinology and Metabolism*, Vol 15, Prader-Willi syndrome: advances in genetics, pathophysiology and treatment, pages 12–20. Copyright (2004) with permission from Elsevier)

• Normal leptin secretion	• Normal distribution and colocalization of neuropeptide Y (NPY) and agouti-related protein (AgRP) in infundibular nucleus (INF).
• Long isoform leptin receptor mRNA expressed in lymphocytes	
• Increased fasting plasma ghrelin	• Normal increase in NPY, measured by either immunocytochemical (ICC) staining or mRNA expression, or AGRP (ICC staining) in INF during illness.
• Reduced postprandial secretion of pancreatic polypeptide (PP)	
• Reduced fasting and postprandial insulin secretion	
• Normal cholecystokinin (CCK) secretion	• Reduced NPY (ICC or mRNA expression) in INF, compared with control, but not non-PWS obese adults, corrected for the duration of premorbid illness.
• Normal distribution of oxytocin and vasopressin neurons in the paraventricular nucleus (PVN).	
• Reduced number of total (38%) and oxytocin (42%)-containing neurons in the PVN.	• Normal AGRP (ICC staining) in INF, compared to control and non-PWS obese adults, corrected for the duration of premorbid illness.
• Normal number of neurons containing cocaine and amphetamine-regulated transcript (CART) in the INF, PVN, and lateral hypothalamic area (LHA).	• Deficiency of POMC-containing neurons in INF, CART-neurons in INF, PVN, and LHA is not complete.

169.6.4 Dysregulation of Serotonin Receptors

Sno RNAs located in the chromosomal region of PWS (Fig. 169.1) are candidate genes for the disease. It has been hypothesized that the Sno RNA HB-52 negatively regulates editing of the 5HT-2C receptor pre-RNA. Indeed, this post transcriptional regulation of this serotonin receptor involved in cognition and cessation of feeding changes its activity. The lack of editing in PWS through the increasing intrinsic activity of the receptor may explain some of the features of this disease. A recent study performed in a mouse model (PWS IC +/−) seems to confirm this hypothesis, although the link with the lack of Sno RNA HB 52 was not established in the publication (see below the chapter on animal models).

169.6.5 Abnormalities in Hypothalamus Histology

Quantitative neuroanatomical studies of postmortem human hypothalamic tissue from patients with PWS in the Netherlands Brain Bank have yet to find any pathological abnormalities in orexigenic neuropeptide Y or agouti-related protein, anorexigenic POMC neurons or GH-releasing hormone neurons in the infundibular nucleus, or orexin/hypocretin neurons in the lateral hypothalamus. Nevertheless, interpretation may be complicated by small numbers and the effects of premortem illness (Goldstone et al. 2003). However, appropriate changes in neuropeptide Y, agouti-related protein, and GH-releasing hormone were found in PWS subjects in cases of illness, obesity, and exogenous GH therapy. This suggests normal neuronal function in their response to alterations in peripheral signals. Cerebrospinal fluid orexin concentrations have nevertheless been reported to be low in cases of PWS with hypersomnia (Nevsimalova et al. 2005). Reduced immunostaining of processed vasopressin, its processing enzyme, prohormone convertase 2, and its molecular chaperone polypeptide 7B2 has also been found in the PVN and supraoptic nucleus of hypothalami from subjects with PWS, though diabetes insipidus is not a recognized clinical problem (Gabreels et al. 1998).

The total and oxytocin cell number is reduced in the hypothalamic PVN of adults with PWS, which may play a primary causative role in hyperphagia. Oxytocin and the PVN have anorexigenic roles in rodents. A 29% reduction in PVN oxytocin neurons was also seen in necdin knockout mice, though these mice are not obese (Muscatelli et al. 2000). Interestingly, oxytocin is an anorexigenic hormone with other newly described actions, particularly regarding social skills, trust, and pair bonding. Peripheral levels are normal although there was discordant data on oxytocin in CSF levels (Fig. 169.3).

169.6.6 Recent Neuroimaging Data

Several morphological neuroimaging abnormalities have been described in PWS: according to Miller et al. (Miller et al. 2007a), ventriculomegaly (100% of 20 patients with PWS aged 3 months to 39 years), decreased volume of brain tissue in the parietal-occipital lobe (50%), sylvian fissure

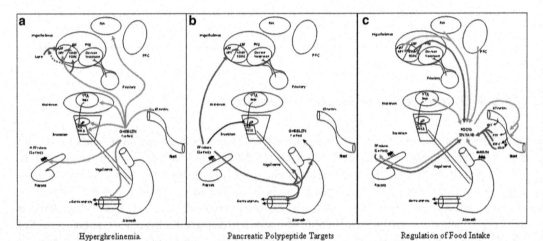

Fig. 169.3 Features of feeding and satiety regulation. *Green arrows* stand for stimulation. *Red arrows* stand for inhibition. Sets of three black arrows stand for secretion. The *nucleus accumbens* (NA) is a collection of neurons within the forebrain that is thought to be involved in the reward circuit, and by which neuronal activity is modulated by dopaminergic input from the ventral tegmental area (VTA). The *prefrontal cortex* (PFC) is the anterior part of the frontal lobes of the brain. (**a**) Hyperghrelinemia. Ghrelin is secreted mainly by the stomach, but also by duodenum, pancreas, hypothalamus, testis, ovary, bone, and cartilage. Patients with PWS have greatly increased circulating levels of ghrelin. The effects of ghrelin on eating behavior are mediated via the arcuate nucleus (ARC) and the solitary tract nucleus (NTS) to merge in the hypothalamus. There, ghrelin opposes the actions of leptin through disinhibition of second line neuropeptides such as neuropeptide Y (NPY) and agouti gene-related peptide (AgRP). Ghrelin activates dopamine neurons in the ventral tegmental area (VTA) and increases dopamine turnover in the nucleus accumbens. Ghrelin also partly exerts its effect through vagal afferent loops. It increases fasting gastro-intestinal motility and the rate of gastric emptying. In PWS, it is hypothesized that a peripheral resistance to ghrelin opposes its stimulating actions (represented by # in the figure), which fits with clinical observations (patients with PWS have decreased GI motility, delayed gastric emptying and decreased PP release). (**b**) Pancreatic Polypeptide Targets. The inhibitory effect of PP on food intake might be indirect and regulated via vagal input to the stomach, pancreas, and other gastrointestinal organs. PP could also enter the brain to bind to AP and influence the adjacent nuclei, such as NTS and Dorso-Medial Nucleus to inhibit gastric emptying, which in turn suppresses food intake. Patients with PWS have reduced PP release both basally and postprandially. PP infusion in subjects with PWS reduced the levels of ghrelin. (**c**) Food Intake Regulation. Peripheral injection of PP inhibits food intake in both humans and mice. In Prader-Willi subjects, intravenous (i.v.) infusion of PP was reported to increase serum PP levels and significantly reduce food intake. GLP-1 is secreted within the circulation by the L-cells of the intestine, together with PYY and OXM; this secretion is stimulated by food intake. CCK is released by the I-cells of the intestine. These peptides all regulate negatively food intake. The ARC appears to be necessary for the stimulatory action of ghrelin on food intake

polymicrogyria (60%), and incomplete insular closure (65%) were found on 3D MRI scans, compared with 21 normal weight sibling controls and 16 individuals with early-onset morbid obesity of unknown etiology. On volumetric MRI, the same author (Miller et al. 2009) found that patients with PWS had smaller cerebellar volumes than a control group of 15 siblings. In several other studies, subjects with PWS had a higher prevalence of pituitary morphological abnormalities than did control subjects, without correlation with hormonal deficiencies (Tauber et al. 2000).

These abnormalities may play a role not only in cognitive, behavioral and neuroendocrine defects in PWS, but in hyperphagia as well. Indeed, recent functional neuroimaging techniques such as positron emission tomography and functional MRI (fMRI) in PWS have revealed abnormal brain activation patterns in corticolimbic structures, such as the amygdala and the prefrontal, orbitofrontal (OFC), and insular cortex, in response to food stimuli after ingestion of oral glucose or a meal (Shapira et al. 2005; Holsen et al. 2006; Miller et al. 2007b). These patterns suggest abnormal reward and motivational responses to food that may underlie the hyperphagia in individuals with PWS.

Hypothalamus dysfunction seems to be central in hyperphagia and underlies other abnormal functioning in PWS (temperature dysregulation, sleep–wake cycle abnormalities, and metabolic and endocrine disorders (Dimitropoulos and Schultz 2008)). Dimitropoulos et al. performed fMRIs on nine individuals with PWS (8–38 years old) IQ- and BMI-matched to ten controls, all in a hunger state, while they performed perceptual discrimination tasks on pictures of pairs of objects and high- or low-calorie foods. The authors showed that patients with PWS displayed a greater activation in the bilateral hypothalamus and right amygdala than controls for high-calorie foods. The OFC was more activated by high-calorie than low-calorie foods in the PWS subjects. The authors thus concluded to a hyper-activation of neural circuitry involving motivation, reward, taste, and food-seeking behaviors (hypothalamus, amygdala, OFC).

The lack of satiety in patients with PWS has also been investigated through fMRI (Shapira et al. 2005) by examining the regions related to satiation (insula, ventromedial prefrontal cortex, and nucleus accumbens). The activation of these regions was delayed after a glucose oral load in PWS patients compared with obese and lean controls. Hyperphagia thus appears to be linked to at least two mechanisms, since patients with PWS (vs. healthy weight controls) who were presented with visual food stimuli after eating a meal showed hyperfunction in limbic and paralimbic regions that drive eating behavior (e.g., the amygdala) and in regions that regulate food intake (e.g., the medial prefrontal cortex (mPFC)) (Holsen et al. 2006) (see article by Ogura in chapter 2.5).

In conclusion, although it has been clearly established that reward and motivation neural pathways and satiety dysfunction are involved in PWS hyperphagia, evidence has gradually emerged that the eating behavior of the patients with PWS arises from a complex mechanism combining insufficient neural development, hormonal dysfunctions, and an overall behavioral disorder involving psychiatric manifestations of the syndrome. In addition to the universal presence of the propensity to overeating and compulsive and ritualistic behaviors, people with PWS show pronounced emotional liability, and a striking inability to control their emotions, which predisposes them to temper outbursts. The frequent anger is often in response to frustration and to the feeling of not being understood, and it may be due to disturbances in understanding others, which in turn could be related to theory of mind and empathy.

169.6.7 Data from Animal Models

Most of the models that reproduce the genetic defects of PWS result in severe growth defect, feeding difficulties, and high lethality within the first days of life. However, surviving mice do not become obese.

Ding et al. (Ding et al. 2008) recently reported a new mouse model with great homologies with the PWS phenotype, but without the occurrence of obesity. This Snord116del mouse model seems to reproduce the abnormal feeding behavior and endocrine disorders described in humans with PWS. The hyperphagia of these mice is associated with prolonged meal times, pointing to a delay in meal termination that is most likely due to an inability to sense satiety. Interestingly, they also have elevated ghrelin, high insulin sensitivity, and low IGF-1, with growth delay that develops soon after birth. They may also have abnormal GH release though this has not been proved.

The authors concluded that the primary mechanism for hyperphagia in PWS is not a defect in energy homeostasis control, but in sensing satiety. They further concluded that the higher cognitive regions of the brain, such as the mPFC, which is involved in interpreting the incentive values of food, and those involved in planning complicated schemes to obtain food, may be changed secondary to the prolonged perception of hunger/lack of satiety. This is in line with the hypothesis developed by Holland (Holland et al. 2003) and with our own hypothesis on the impact of early hypergrhelinemia in the development and implementation of satiety circuits (Feigerlova et al. 2008).

Another interesting finding was reported by Doe et al. (Doe et al. 2009) using the imprinted centre deletion model. The authors studied abnormal editing of the 5HT2C receptor and alterations in its effect. Indeed, mice show impulsive responding, increased locomotor activity, and reactivity to palatable foodstuffs. Use of drugs confirmed the role of this serotonin receptor in these alterations.

The link between the lack of snoRNA genes and abnormal editing has yet to be proven. Although two patients have been described with the PWS phenotype and deletion of snoRNA HB85 (Sahoo et al. 2008; de Smith et al. 2009), an effect of snoRNA HB52 cannot be completely eliminated.

169.7 Management of Hyperphagia and Obesity

Obesity management in people with PWS involves strict and permanent environmental control, with early institution of a low-calorie, well-balanced diet, with regular exercise, rigorous supervision, restriction of access to food and money (after consideration of the legal and ethical obligations), and appropriate psychological and behavioral counseling for the patient and family. Early discussion with parents about the inevitability of hyperphagia, even during infancy, is essential to prepare them for the need to prevent obesity by setting firm limits and strictly controlling the food environment and the daily schedule (hour and contents of the meals). As an example of how important these steps can be, a young institutionalized adult declared that her anxiety and insomnia were improved the day she learned that the kitchen would be locked at night instead of simply being watched by a guardian who could possibly be away from his post for a short time. This aspect of management should thus be reemphasized at every visit, for our opinion is that total autonomy with regards to food is impossible and unrelated to the IQ of the patients.

Anecdotally, pharmacological treatment, including the available anorexigenic agents, has not been of benefit in treating hyperphagia, though there are few published placebo-controlled studies. Studies of the potential benefits of newer agents such as endo-cannabinoid antagonists were awaited in PWS, but recent concerns about psychiatric side effects led to withdrawal of these drugs. Restrictive bariatric surgery, such as gastric banding or bypass, has not been shown to reduce hyperphagia or achieve long-term weight reduction and is associated with unacceptable morbidity and mortality (Scheimann et al. 2008). While some of the studies of biliopancreatic diversion have reported successful weight loss, complications from the resulting intestinal malabsorption were frequent. Intragastric balloons are a risk for these patients and deaths have been reported (Grugni et al. 2008).

Physical activity in PWS is significantly reduced and is related to obesity, hypersomnolence, and persistent reduced lean mass and poor muscle tone. The resting metabolic rate is reduced relative to body size and this is related to the abnormal body composition, which further contributes to a reduction in 24-h energy expenditure (van Mil et al. 2000). Increased physical activity and exercise programs are beneficial in improving body composition in PWS.

169.8   GH Effects on Obesity and Body Composition

Body composition studies have shown both increased body fat and reduced muscle in PWS from infancy to adulthood (Carrel et al. 2004) with a selective relative reduction in visceral adiposity in PWS adults of both sexes (Goldstone et al. 2001). This may explain the relative hypoinsulinemia and normal triglyceride levels, with preservation of insulin sensitivity and protective elevation in adiponectin levels in these patients given their overall obesity.

GH treatment is routinely used for short stature in children with PWS in the USA, and since 2000 for treatment of short stature or abnormal body composition in Europe. As the age at diagnosis has markedly decreased in the past few years and is currently 3 months, the age for starting GH treatment has also decreased. Only a few publications have reported the possible benefits of early treatment on motility scores, cognitive function, and increased head circumference (Festen et al. 2008). The main effects of GH are the improvement in height, velocity, and adult height; the maintenance of lean body mass; and better control of BMI with a decrease in fat mass. It may also delay the occurrence of nutritional phase 3. By modifying the body shape of these children and increasing their motility, GH improves their socialization and, in some of them, lowers depressions scores (Whitman et al. 2002). Part of the GH effects may be related to the decrease in ghrelin under GH treatment (Hauffa and Petersenn 2008). Figure 169.4 shows the effect of GH in a boy who started treatment at 7 years with secondary normalization of BMI and body shape.

The benefits of GH cannot be obtained without integrated multidisciplinary care (Table 169.3).

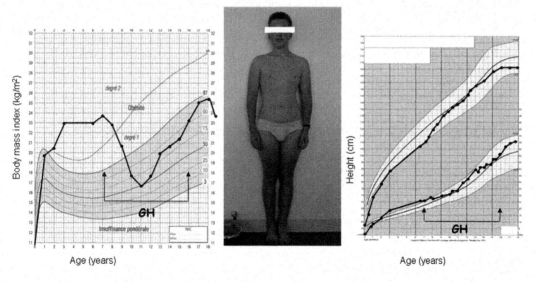

Fig. 169.4 Evolution of BMI chart, growth curve, and body shape in a boy with PWS treated by GH from the age of 7

Table 169.3 Ideal multidisciplinary team for children and adults with PWS (Copyright 2008, the Endocrine Society)

For children	For adults
Neonatologist	
Medical Geneticist[a]	Medical Geneticist[a]
Paediatric Endocrinologist[a]	Endocrinologist/Diabetologist[a]
Neuropediatrician	Gynaecologist/Urologist[a]
Speech and language specialist	Cardiologist
ENT specialist	
Psychiatrist[a]	Psychiatrist[a]
Orthopaedist[a]	Orthopaedist[a]
Surgeon (for orchidopexy)	
Pneumologist	Pneumologist
Sleep disorder specialist	Sleep disorder specialist
Dentist	
Ophthalmologist	
Gastroenterologist	Gastroenterologist
Dietician[a]	Dietician[a]
Speech therapist	
Physical therapist	Physical therapist
Psychologist[a]	Psychologist[a]
Social worker[a]	Social worker[a]

[a]Indicates those particularly involved in transition

Figure 169.5 shows the effects of GH in a boy with PWS with morbid and uncontrolled obesity at 2 years due to poor family compliance with the diet. GH treatment was started in order to try to control the BMI, which nevertheless continued to increase with the aggravation of obstructive sleep apneas. This prompted us to stop the GH treatment and focus on parental guidance. Thanks to the strong collaborative work of all the caregivers, particularly the psychiatrist, family compliance was obtained. The child lost weight, normalized his BMI, and corrected his sleep respiratory disorder, and therefore resumed GH treatment.

Interruption of GH treatment at growth completion is required in most countries, though it may have a deleterious effect on BMI and body composition. Continuing GH in the adult is based on the potential benefits to bone mineralization, body composition, and maintenance of lean mass and muscular function. The effect on quality of life is difficult to prove, however, given the lack of an appropriate evaluation tool.

169.9 Transition from Childhood to Adolescence and Adulthood

The transition phase from childhood to adolescence and adulthood is of great importance in these patients. During the transition appointment, medical issues and psychosocial aspects concerning the patient are discussed. In the case of young adults, the emphasis is put on issues related to the processes of adolescence such as puberty, choice of profession, daily activities, relationships, and sexuality.

The prevalence of obesity in adults with PWS who received GH treatment in childhood is significantly reduced compared with those who did not receive it (personal data).

In conclusion, studies are needed to improve our knowledge of the natural history of hyperphagia and feeding disturbance in patients with PWS. Ongoing research on feeding and satiety signals such as ghrelin, PP, and ocytocin will help to unravel the mechanisms of the feeding behavior in these patients.

Fig. 169.5 Evolution of BMI in a young boy: effects of reinforced multidisciplinary care in a context of compliance difficulties

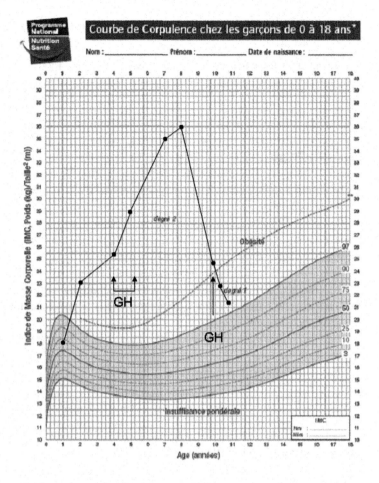

Table 169.4 Key facts of ghrelin

Circulating gut peptide
Orexigenic
Stimulate growth hormone secretion
Acylated in the Serine 3 amino acid
Circulating ghrelin increases before meals and decreases after
Low levels in obese people vs. controls
Elevated levels in PWS and anorexia
Balance between leptin and ghrelin at the level of arcuate nucleus neurons in the hypothalamus

Table 169.5 Key facts of growth hormone

GH is a peptide secreted by the anterior pituitary under hypothalamic control (GHRH, ghrelin, and somatostatin)
Induces somatic growth before cartilage fusion
Acts on different tissues: adipose tissue, muscles, bone
Has metabolic effects (lipid, glucose metabolisms), anabolic effect
GH secretion is decreased in some children having short stature. Treatment increases height and normalizes adult height
GH treatment is based on daily subcutaneous injections

Functional neuroimaging may open new perspectives on pathophysiology and treatment. Last, the effects of early diagnosis, the outcomes of GH treatment, and multidisciplinary care need to be analyzed properly in order to determine the best possible care for patients with PWS (Tables 169.4 and 169.5).

169.10 Applications to Other Areas of Health and Disease

Acquiring knowledge in hormones and signals controlling food and satiety signals in PWS may open new perspectives on pathophysiologics and therapeutical issues for persons with nonsyndromic obesity.

Summary Points

- *Two main features* characterize hyperphagia in PWS: a reduced satiety and an early return of excessive hunger.
- *Two main hormonal dysfunctions* might explain hyperphagia: hyperghrelinemia and decreased pancreatic polypeptide.
- *Oxytocin deficit* may be involved in hyperphagia.
- *Two neuronal networks* may be involved in the eating behavior of PWS: the cortico-limbic structures implied in reward mechanisms and the paralimbic regions that drive food behavior.
- *Better characterization of eating behavior* will help understanding hyperphagia pathophysiology and defining treatment goals.
- *Data on animal models* are insufficient to explain human clinical and biological findings.
- It is likely that the implementation of *early diagnosis, multidisciplinary care, and GH treatment* altogether will optimize patients' quality of life.

Definitions and Explanations of Key Terms

Hyperphagia: Eating disorder in which an individual eats abnormally large amounts of food in little time.

Orexigenic: Hormones that trigger a desire to eat. Ghrelin is the only real orexigenic peptide, since AgRP and NPY release is related to ghrelin activity.

Satiety: Time during which an individual does not feel the desire to eat. Satiety is related to the sensation of fullness without being tantamount to it. PP, CCK, GLP-1 and OXM are peptides which release triggers a satiety feeling.

Hypothalamic syndrome: Although there is no consensus definition of the hypothalamic syndrome, it is usually described as the collection of appetite disorders, hyperphagia and obesity, or anorexia, thirst abnormalities, tiredness, temperature dysregulation, sleep disorders, and behavioral difficulties. In the course of evolution, endocrine abnormalities usually develop, characterized by hyperprolactinemia and pituitary deficits (gonadotrophic, somatotropic, corticotropic, and thyrotropic). Central precocious puberty can also occur. Several causes can be involved: tumors, genetic syndromes such as Prader-Willi, infectious or inflammatory diseases, and idiopathic.

Reward networks: Collection of brain structures which attempts to regulate and control behavior by inducing pleasurable effects. It principally involves the mesolimbic (which goes from the ventral tegmental area via the medial forebrain bundle to nucleus accumbens, where mainly dopamine is released) and the mesocortical pathway (which connects the ventral tegmentum to the cerebral cortex).

References

Bachere N, Diene G, Delagnes V, Molinas C, Moulin P, Tauber M. Horm Res. 2008;69:45–52.

Banks WA, Tschop M, Robinson SM, Heiman ML. J Pharmacol Exp Ther. 2002;302:822–7.

Batterham RL, Cohen MA, Ellis SM, Le Roux CW, Withers DJ, Frost GS, Ghatei MA, Bloom SR. N Engl J Med. 2003a;349: 941–8.

Batterham RL, Le Roux CW, Cohen MA, Park AJ, Ellis SM, Patterson M, Frost GS, Ghatei MA, Bloom SR. J Clin Endocrinol Metab. 2003b;88:3989–92.

Berntson GG, Zipf WB, O'Dorisio TM, Hoffman JA, Chance RE. Peptides. 1993;14:497–503.

Bomberg EM, Grace MK, Wirth MM, Levine AS, Olszewski PK. Neuroreport. 2007;18:591–5.

Carrel AL, Moerchen V, Myers SE, Bekx MT, Whitman BY, Allen DB. J Pediatr. 2004;145:744–9.

Cummings DE, Clement K, Purnell JQ, Vaisse C, Foster KE, Frayo RS, Schwartz MW, Basdevant A, Weigle DS. Nat Med. 2002;8:643–4.

Date Y, Murakami N, Toshinai K, Matsukura S, Niijima A, Matsuo H, Kangawa K, Nakazato M. Gastroenterology. 2002;123:1120–8.

de Smith AJ, Purmann C, Walters RG, Ellis RJ, Holder SE, Van Haelst MM, Brady AF, Fairbrother UL, Dattani M, Keogh JM, Henning E, Yeo GS, O'Rahilly S, Froguel P, Farooqi IS, Blakemore AI. Hum Mol Genet. 2009;18:3257–65.

De Waele K, Ishkanian SL, Bogarin R, Miranda CA, Ghatei MA, Bloom SR, Pacaud D, Chanoine JP. Eur J Endocrinol. 2008;159:381–8.

Diano S, Farr SA, Benoit SC, McNay EC, da Silva I, Horvath B, Gaskin FS, Nonaka N, Jaeger LB, Banks WA, Morley JE, Pinto S, Sherwin RS, Xu L, Yamada KA, Sleeman MW, Tschop MH, Horvath TL. Nat Neurosci. 2006;9:381–8.

Dimitropoulos A, Schultz RT. J Autism Dev Disord. 2008;38:1642–53.

Ding F, Li HH, Zhang S, Solomon NM, Camper SA, Cohen P, Francke U. PLoS ONE. 2008;3:e1709.

Doe CM, Relkovic D, Garfield AS, Dalley JW, Theobald DE, Humby T, Wilkinson LS, Isles AR. Hum Mol Genet. 2009;18:2140–8.

Dykens EM, Maxwell MA, Pantino E, Kossler R, Roof E. Obesity (Silver Spring). 2007;15:1816–26.

Feigerlova E, Diene G, Conte-Auriol F, Molinas C, Gennero I, Salles JP, Arnaud C, Tauber M. J Clin Endocrinol Metab. 2008;93:2800–5.

Festen DA, de Lind van Wijngaarden R, van Eekelen M, Otten BJ, Wit JM, Duivenvoorden HJ, Hokken-Koelega AC. Clin Endocrinol (Oxf). 2008;69:443–51.

Fieldstone A, Zipf WB, Schwartz HC, Berntson GG. Int J Obes Relat Metab Disord. 1997;21:1046–52.

Frecka JM, Mattes RD. Am J Physiol Gastrointest Liver Physiol. 2008;294:G699–707.

Gabreels BA, Swaab DF, de Kleijn DP, Seidah NG, Van de Loo JW, Van de Ven WJ, Martens GJ, van Leeuwen FW. J Clin Endocrinol Metab. 1998;83:591–9.

Goldstone AP. Trends Endocrinol Metab. 2004;15:12–20.

Goldstone AP, Thomas EL, Brynes AE, Bell JD, Frost G, Saeed N, Hajnal JV, Howard JK, Holland A, Bloom SR. J Clin Endocrinol Metab. 2001;86:4330–8.

Goldstone AP, Unmehopa UA, Swaab DF. Clin Endocrinol (Oxf). 2003;58:743–55.

Goldstone AP, Patterson M, Kalingag N, Ghatei MA, Brynes AE, Bloom SR, Grossman AB, Korbonits M. J Clin Endocrinol Metab. 2005;90:2681–90.

Goldstone AP, Holland AJ, Hauffa BP, Hokken-Koelega AC, Tauber M. J Clin Endocrinol Metab. 2008;93:4183–97.

Grugni G, Crino A, Bosio L, Corrias A, Cuttini M, De Toni T, Di Battista E, Franzese A, Gargantini L, Greggio N, Iughetti L, Livieri C, Naselli A, Pagano C, Pozzan G, Ragusa L, Salvatoni A, Trifiro G, Beccaria L, Bellizzi M, Bellone J, Brunani A, Cappa M, Caselli G, Cerioni V, Delvecchio M, Giardino D, Ianni F, Memo L, Pilotta A, Pomara C, Radetti G, Sacco M, Sanzari A, Sartorio A, Tonini G, Vettor R, Zaglia F, Chiumello G. Am J Med Genet A. 2008;146:861–72.

Gunay-Aygun M, Schwartz S, Heeger S, O'Riordan MA, Cassidy SB. Pediatrics. 2001;108:E92.

Haqq AM, Farooqi IS, O'Rahilly S, Stadler DD, Rosenfeld RG, Pratt KL, LaFranchi SH, Purnell JQ. J Clin Endocrinol Metab. 2003;88:174–8.

Hauffa BP, Petersenn S. Clin Endocrinol (Oxf). 2009;71:155–6.

Holland A, Whittington J, Hinton E. Lancet. 2003;362:989–91.

Holm VA, Cassidy SB, Butler MG, Hanchett JM, Greenswag LR, Whitman BY, Greenberg F. Pediatrics. 1993;91:398–402.

Holsen LM, Zarcone JR, Brooks WM, Butler MG, Thompson TI, Ahluwalia JS, Nollen NL, Savage CR. Obesity (Silver Spring). 2006;14:1028–37.

Hosoda H, Kojima M, Kangawa K. J Pharmacol Sci. 2006;100:398–410.

Kanber D, Giltay J, Wieczorek D, Zogel C, Hochstenbach R, Caliebe A, Kuechler A, Horsthemke B, Buiting K. Eur J Hum Genet. 2009;17:582–90.

Katsuura G, Asakawa A, Inui A. Peptides. 2002;23:323–9.

Koska J, DelParigi A, de Courten B, Weyer C, Tataranni PA. Diabetes. 2004;53:3091–6.

Lindgren AC, Barkeling B, Hagg A, Ritzen EM, Marcus C, Rossner S. J Pediatr. 2000;137:50–5.

McCune H, Driscoll DJ, Prader-Willi syndrome. In: Ekvall SW, Ekvall VF, eds. Pediatric nutrition in chronic diseases and developmental disorders, 2nd ed., New York: Oxford University press: 2005, pp. 128–32.

Miller JL, Couch JA, Schmalfuss I, He G, Liu Y, Driscoll DJ. Am J Med Genet A. 2007a;143:476–83.

Miller JL, James GA, Goldstone AP, Couch JA, He G, Driscoll DJ, Liu Y. J Neurol Neurosurg Psychiatry. 2007b;78:615–9.

Miller JL, Couch J, Schwenk K, Long M, Towler S, Theriaque DW, He G, Liu Y, Driscoll DJ, Leonard CM. Dev Neuropsychol. 2009;34:272–83.

Muscatelli F, Abrous DN, Massacrier A, Boccaccio I, Le Moal M, Cau P, Cremer H. Hum Mol Genet. 2000;9:3101–10.

Nevsimalova S, Vankova J, Stepanova I, Seemanova E, Mignot E, Nishino S. Eur J Neurol. 2005;12:70–2.

Olszewski PK, Bomberg EM, Martell A, Grace MK, Levine AS. Neuroreport. 2007;18:499–503.

Russell H, Oliver C. Br J Clin Psychol. 2003;42:379–92.

Sahoo T, del Gaudio D, German JR, Shinawi M, Peters SU, Person RE, Garnica A, Cheung SW, Beaudet AL. Nat Genet. 2008;40:719–21.

Scheimann AO, Butler MG, Gourash L, Cuffari C, Klish W. J Pediatr Gastroenterol Nutr. 2008;46:80–3.

Schrander-Stumpel CT, Curfs LM, Sastrowijoto P, Cassidy SB, Schrander JJ, Fryns JP. Am J Med Genet A. 2004;124A:333–8.

Schwartz MW, Morton GJ. Nature. 2002;418:595–7.

Shapira NA, Lessig MC, He AG, James GA, Driscoll DJ, Liu Y. J Neurol Neurosurg Psychiatry. 2005;76:260–2.

Stevenson DA, Heinemann J, Angulo M, Butler MG, Loker J, Rupe N, Kendell P, Cassidy SB, Scheimann A. J Pediatr Gastroenterol Nutr. 2007;45:272–4.

Tauber M, Barbeau C, Jouret B, Pienkowski C, Malzac P, Moncla A, Rochiccioli P. Horm Res. 2000;53:279–87.

Tauber M, Conte Auriol F, Moulin P, Molinas C, Delagnes V, Salles JP. Horm Res. 2004;62:49–54.

Tauber M, Diene G, Molinas C, Hebert M. Am J Med Genet A. 2008;146:881–7

van Mil EA, Westerterp KR, Gerver WJ, Curfs LM, Schrander-Stumpel CT, Kester AD, Saris WH. Am J Clin Nutr. 2000;71:752–6.

Whitman BY, Myers S, Carrel A, Allen D. Pediatrics. 2002;109:E35.

Zipf WB, Berntson GG. Am J Clin Nutr. 1987;46:277–81.

Part XXIX
Diabetes

Chapter 170
Insulin and Clinical Eating Disorders in Diabetes

Masato Takii

Abbreviations

IDDM	Insulin-dependent diabetes
AN	Anorexia nervosa
DSM-III	Diagnostic and Statistical Manual of Mental Disorders, Third Edition
DSM-III-R	Diagnostic and Statistical Manual of Mental Disorders, Revised Third Edition
BN	Bulimia nervosa
ED-NOS	Eating disorder not otherwise specified
DSM-IV	Diagnostic and Statistical Manual of Mental Disorders, Fourth Edition
ICB	Inappropriate compensatory behavior in order to prevent weight gain
BED	Binge-eating disorder
DKA	Diabetic ketoacidosis
NIDDM	Non-insulin-dependent diabetes

170.1 Introduction

Type 1 diabetes is a disease characterized by a total absence of insulin production because the pancreatic β cells have been destroyed by an autoimmune mechanism. Problems associated with the regulation of blood sugar and the long-term complications are well known. An eating disorder is a disease in which a person has an abnormal eating behavior associated with an excessive fixation on body weight. Because type 1 diabetes patients who develop an eating disorder have great difficulty maintaining a therapeutic dietary regimen and often place priority on weight control over metabolic control, they face severe obstacles to proper diabetes control. As with eating disorders in the general population, an eating disorder concurrent with type 1 diabetes is most commonly seen in young women.

The research on the concurrence of an eating disorder and type 1 diabetes has been done since about 1980, mostly in Europe and North America. Empirical studies in this field have focused on the prevalence of eating disorders, poor metabolic control, the high risk of diabetic long-term complications, and nonadherence to the diabetes treatment regimen through behaviors such as insulin omission.

M. Takii (✉)
Department of Psychosomatic Medicine, Graduate School of Medical Sciences, Kyushu University,
3-1-1 Maidashi, Higashi-ku, Fukuoka, 812-8582, Japan
e-mail: Takii@cephal.med.kyushu-u.ac.jp

V.R. Preedy et al. (eds.), *Handbook of Behavior, Food and Nutrition*,
DOI 10.1007/978-0-387-92271-3_170, © Springer Science+Business Media, LLC 2011

Table 170.1 Key features of type 1 diabetes

1. Type 1 diabetes results from extremely decreased insulin production by the pancreas because the beta cells (insulin secretion cells) are destroyed by an autoimmune mechanism.
2. The main treatment for type 1 diabetes is to supply extrinsic insulin. Persons with type 1 diabetes must take supplementary insulin by injections for the rest of their lives.
3. The onset age of type 1 diabetes is usually young, most often in childhood or the adolescent period, and the onset is fairly rapid.
4. Various self-care efforts are necessary for patients to maintain good glycemic control and to prevent diabetes-related complications.
5. Because the burden of having this severe disease and the requirements of managing it are often too heavy for young patients, they tend to have psychological and behavioral problems.
6. These problems lead to a deterioration of the metabolic control of the diabetes and to early onset of long-term diabetic complications that severely affect the quality of life of the patients.

This table lists the key facts of type 1 diabetes including the etiology by an autoimmune mechanism, the necessity of insulin supplementation for treatment, the young onset age of the disease, the difficulty of controlling it, and the risk for psychological/behavioral and medical problems

This report focuses on current findings and theories related to the epidemiology, clinical condition, mechanism of the onset of the eating disorder, and the treatment approach for patients with clinical eating disorders concurrent with type 1 diabetes. In addition, studies of eating disorders complicated with type 2 diabetes will be introduced.

The Department of Psychosomatic Medicine at Kyushu University specializes in the treatment of both eating disorders and diabetes. Diabetes patients who have psychological problems are referred from all over Japan. Over the past 15 years, we have treated more than 150 type 1 diabetes patients with a concurrent clinical eating disorder. Studies done in our department concerning the clinical condition and treatment of these patients are described in this chapter.

Also discussed are self-destructive behaviors associated with insulin omission and poor insulin manipulation, which are often deeply related to eating disorders and are among the most severe problematic behaviors of diabetes patients (Table 170.1).

170.2 Epidemiology/Clinical Condition

170.2.1 Early Review

Marcus and Wing (1990) did a literature review of the clinical condition of 57 patients with an eating disorder concurrent with insulin-dependent diabetes (IDDM). A summary is as follows:

1. Co-occurrence of these disorders is common.
2. The diagnosis of IDDM occurs before that of an eating disorder in the preponderance (90%) of the cases.
3. Ninety-five percent of the cases of eating disorders among IDDM patients have occurred in women.
4. Sixty-two percent of eating-disordered IDDM patients reported deliberate manipulation of insulin to promote weight loss. Regular elimination of insulin doses would be predicted to have negative consequences for glycemic control.
5. Poor glycemic control was reported in 75% of patients with eating disorders, and major diabetic complications may be prevalent as well.
6. The relationship between diabetes and anorexia nervosa (AN)/bulimia shows a kind of synergism in which one disorder worsens the other and where successful therapeutic interventions may consequently prove exceedingly difficult.

170.2.2 Prevalence of the Eating Disorders of Type 1 Diabetes Patients

A relatively large number of studies investigating the prevalence of the eating disorders of patients with type 1 diabetes have been published since late 1980s (Steel et al. 1987; Rodin et al. 1991; Fairburn et al. 1991; Peveler et al. 1992; Jones et al. 2000). Whether or not eating disorder frequency was higher in female patients of type 1 diabetes than nondiabetic peers was controversial.

Relatively more studies suggested that eating disorder frequency is higher in women with type 1 diabetes than in women in general (Steel et al. 1987; Rodin et al. 1991). For example, Rodin et al. (1991) reported a diagnosis of an eating disorder for 13- to 18-year-old women with type 1 diabetes in 13% of their sample (103 cases), based on DSM-III criteria (AN 1% and bulimia 12%) and in 5% of the sample based on the more severe DSM-III-R criteria (American Psychiatric Association 1987) (all bulimia nervosa (BN)).

Other studies have found that the eating disorder frequency does not differ from that of women in general (Fairburn et al. 1991; Peveler et al. 1992). Fairburn et al. (1991) diagnosed eating disorders in 11% of 54 women with IDDM aged 17–25 years (BN 5.5% and "eating disorder not otherwise specified (ED-NOS)" 5.5%) and in 7.5% of nondiabetic, control women (BN 3% and ED-NOS 4.5%) based on DSM-III-R criteria. No significant difference was found between the groups. ED-NOSs were defined as eating disorders other than AN or BN.

The differences in prevalences may have been because of differences in the method of diagnosis, the eating disorder diagnostic criteria, and/or the sample. The DSM-IV diagnostic criteria (American Psychiatric Association 1994) for the first time accepted insulin omission as an "inappropriate compensatory behavior in order to prevent weight gain" (ICB), which is necessary for a diagnosis of BN. The use of the earlier criteria may have led to underestimation of the prevalence of the eating disorders of type 1 diabetes patients (Affenito and Adams 2001).

Jones et al. (2000) conducted a large, multisite case-controlled study of 356 girls aged 12–19 years with type 1 diabetes and 1,098 case-matched controls. They used a two-stage design with both self-report questionnaires and structured diagnostic interviews of eating disorders and found that eating disorders that met the DSM-IV diagnostic criteria were 2.4 times more common in girls with diabetes (5 BN cases and 31 ED-NOS cases) than in their nondiabetic peers (10% vs 4%).

170.2.3 Classification of the Eating Disorders Associated with Type 1 Diabetes

Research indicates that eating disorders associated with binge eating, such as BN and binge-eating disorder (BED), are the most common types of eating disorders among girls with diabetes and that restricting eating disorders are much less common conditions (Jones et al. 2000; Affenito et al. 1997). BED is classified as an ED-NOS. Although BN and BED have frequent binge eating in common, the primary difference between BN and BED is the regular use of an ICB by BN patients, such as insulin omission, self-induced vomiting, misuse of laxatives, fasting, or excessive exercise (American Psychiatric Association 1994).

In a meta-analysis, Nielsen (2002) reported that although AN was not increased in females with type 1 diabetes compared with their nondiabetic peers, BN (OR = 2.9), ED-NOS (OR = 1.8), and subthreshold eating disorders (OR = 1.9) were increased.

Since 1994, we have treated 158 type 1 diabetes patients with clinical eating disorders: 151 female and 7 male. The classification of the eating disorders of female patients, based on DSM-IV, were

Table 170.2 Demographic and clinical features of female type 1 diabetes patients with bulimia nervosa (BN), with binge-eating disorder (BED), and without an eating disorder (CONTROL) (Adapted from Takii et al. 1999)

	BN (N = 22)	BED (N = 11)	CONTROL (N = 32)	P
Age (years)	23.2 ± 4.4	24.8 ± 7.5	23.9 ± 3.8	NS
Onset of DM (years)	14.5 ± 5.4	20.1 ± 8.2	15.9 ± 5.9	NS
Duration of DM (years)	8.7 ± 5.7	4.7 ± 1.8	7.9 ± 5.5	NS
Onset of BE (years)	18.2 ± 4.2	22.4 ± 7.0	(-)	<0.05
Duration of BE (years)	5.0 ± 3.9	2.5 ± 1.6	(-)	<0.05
BMI (kg/m^2)	21.6 ± 2.5	23.6 ± 2.7	20.7 ± 2.2	<0.05[a]
HbA1c (%)	12.3 ± 2.6	9.7 ± 2.1	6.2 ± 0.8	<0.0001[b]
Retinopathy (%)	40.9	0.0	6.3	<0.001
Neuropathy (%)	45.4	9.0	6.3	<0.005
EDI	93.5 ± 26.9	57.4 ± 25.0	36.2 ± 15.3	<0.0001[b]
SDS	53.3 ± 7.2	42.8 ± 7.2	37.1 ± 6.8	<0.0001[b]
Trait-Anxiety scale in STAI	58.9 ± 7.1	47.9 ± 9.0	42.2 ± 8.3	<0.0001[c]
Any co-occurring mental disorder	18 (81.8%)	5 (45.5%)	ND	<0.05
GAF	45.7 ± 7.7	56.5 ± 8.8	ND	<0.001

Female type 1 diabetes patients with bulimia nervosa (BN) have the most severe medical consequences of diabetes, psychopathology related to eating disorders, and general psychological disturbances; those without eating disorders (CONTROL) have the least; and those with binge-eating disorder (BED) are between BN and CONTROL
DM type 1 diabetes, *BE* binge eating, *EDI* eating disorder inventory, *SDS* self-rating depression scale, *STAI* state-trait anxiety inventory, *GAF* global assessment of functioning, *ND* not determined
Data are means ± SD. NS, *p* > 0.05
Differences were determined by one-way ANOVA followed by Bonferroni's adjusted t-test or by chi-square test
[a]BED > BN and CONTROL
[b]BN > BED > CONTROL
[c]BN > BED and CONTROL

100 cases of BN (66.2%), 35 cases of BED (23.2%), 11 cases of AN (7.3%), and five cases of ED-NOS other than BED (3.3%). Of the 11 cases of AN, only 1 was the restricting type, with the remaining 10 the binge-eating/purging type. For males, one case of BN (14.3%) and six cases of BED (85.7%) were found. Although the high proportion of binge-eating-associated eating disorders was similar to previous studies, the preponderance of BN patients may reflect sample bias because of the urgent necessity to give specialized treatment for the patient's severe medical condition: BN patients with type 1 diabetes have been shown to have the most severe medical problems in comparison with patients with other eating disorders such as BED, as will be presented in the following sections (Takii et al. 1999) (Table 170.2).

170.2.4 Psychopathological Aspects

170.2.4.1 Psychopathology Associated with the Eating Disorder

For young women with type 1 diabetes, some studies have shown that the psychopathology related to the eating disorder is more pronounced than for persons without diabetes (Rosmark et al. 1986; Fairburn et al. 1991).

Our research has shown that type 1 diabetes patients with a clinical eating disorder manifest significantly more severe eating disorder psychopathology than patients with an episode of binge eating but without a clinical eating disorder (abnormal eating habits), and that patients with abnormal eating habits manifest significantly more severe eating disorder psychopathology than patients with normal eating habits (Tsukahara et al. 2009).

We also reported that female type 1 diabetes patients with BN had a significantly more severe eating disorder psychopathology than patients with BED and that patients with BED had a significantly more severe eating disorder psychopathology than patients without eating disorders (Takii et al. 1999) (Table 170.2).

170.2.4.2 General Psychopathology

Mood disorders have been reported to be common in patients with an eating disorder (Kennedy et al. 1994). They are also common in patients with diabetes (Talbot and Nouwen 2000). Vila et al. (1995) found that almost half of the 52 teenaged girls with type 1 diabetes and an eating disorder also reported significant depressive symptoms.

Our research has shown that type 1 diabetes patients with a clinical eating disorder had significantly more severe depression, anxiety, and diabetes-related distrust than patients with abnormal eating habits and that patients with abnormal eating habits had significantly more severe psychopathology than patients with normal eating habits (Tsukahara et al. 2009).

We also reported that female type 1 diabetes patients with BN manifested significantly more severe depression, anxiety, a higher rate of co-occurring mental disorders, and poorer psychosocial functioning than patients with BED and that patients with BED were significantly more depressive than patients without eating disorders (Takii et al. 1999) (Table 170.2).

170.2.5 Behavioral Problems

170.2.5.1 Noncompliance

Rodin et al. (1991) reported that patients with an eating disorder reported significantly more non-compliance with almost all aspects of their diabetes treatment, such as testing of blood and urine, taking insulin on schedule, following a dietary plan, maintaining blood sugar, fitting exercise into the treatment plan, and remembering to do everything specified for controlling IDDM.

170.2.5.2 Insulin Omission

Insulin omission is a problematic behavior in which diabetes patients deliberately omit or reduce their insulin dosage. Many studies have focused on the rates of insulin omission of female diabetes patients, the extreme disturbance of insulin omission to metabolic control, and the relationship between insulin omission and eating disorders (Rodin et al. 1991; Polonsky et al. 1994; Biggs et al. 1994; Affenito et al. 1997; Takii et al. 1999, 2002a, 2008; Goebel-Fabbri et al. 2008).

Polonsky et al. (1994) reported that 31% of women with IDDM reported intentional insulin omission and that approximately half of them reported omitting insulin for weight-management purposes (weight-related omitters). Weight-related omitters evidenced significantly greater psychological distress, poorer regimen adherence (including more frequent omission), poorer glycemic control, and higher rates of long-term diabetic complications than did non-weight-related omitters or nonomitters. Non-weight-related omitters tended to fall between weight-related omitters and nonomitters on most measures of psychological functioning, adherence, and glycemic control.

In a meta-analysis, Nielsen (2002) reported that insulin omission is increased when eating disorders coexist with type 1 diabetes (OR = 12.6).

As mentioned above, the DSM-IV diagnostic criteria (American Psychiatric Association 1994) have for the first time accepted insulin omission as an ICB, which is necessary for the diagnosis of BN. According to the criteria, insulin omission or reduction at least twice a week could be considered an ICB by BN patients. However, we found that, when type 1 diabetic females with BN omit insulin, they nearly always do it more frequently and in a more extreme way: omission of at least one-quarter of the prescribed insulin (Takii et al. 2002a, 2008). We define this degree of insulin omission as "severe insulin omission."

170.2.5.3 ICBs (Purging Behaviors) of Type 1 Diabetes Patients with an Eating Disorder

Rodin et al. (1991) reported the methods of inducing weight loss used by adolescent females with IDDM with and without an eating disorder. Of 13 patients with an eating disorder by DSM-III criteria, 7 (54%) omitted insulin, 9 (69%) dieted, 4 (31%) self-induced vomiting, 3 (23%) did extreme exercise to lose weight, and 1 (8%) abused laxatives. Of the 90 patients without an eating disorder, 5 (6%) omitted insulin, 30 (33%) dieted, 4 (4%) did self-induced vomiting, 17 (19%) did extreme exercise to lose weight, and 1 (1%) abused laxatives.

In a study of 55 female patients with BN, we reported that 44 (80.0%) did severe insulin omission, (omission of at least one-quarter of the prescribed insulin) 27 (49.1%) did self-induced vomiting, and 11 (20.0%) abused laxative (Takii et al. 2002a). In classifying the patients by type of ICB, we found that 22 patients did only severe insulin omission, 22 did both severe insulin omission and another ICB, and 11 did not engage in severe insulin omission but had another ICB. Table 170.3 shows a comparison of the clinical characteristics of these three groups and a group of female BED patients. We found that type 1 diabetic females with BN are not a homogenous group and that they can be classified into three distinctive subgroups by type of ICB. Individuals with severe insulin omission and another ICB (BN-IP) had the most severe medical problems, such as the poorest metabolic control and the highest rate of diabetic complications, and had severe psychological/behavioral pathology. Individuals without severe insulin omission and with another ICB (BN-NI) manifested the highest psychological distress. Individuals with only severe insulin omission (BN-I) had comparatively mild distress despite having the poorest metabolic control. The apparent comparative lack of distress of patients with only severe insulin omission as an ICB may largely result from taking the easy way of reducing their body weight, insulin omission, as an avoidance mechanism.

170.2.6 Medical Problems

170.2.6.1 Poor Glycemic Control

Many studies have shown that HbA1c levels are significantly higher in type 1 diabetes patients with an eating disorder than in patients without (Marcus and Wing 1990; Affenito et al. 1997; Rydall et al. 1997; Takii et al. 1999; Jones et al. 2000; Rodin et al. 2002; Goebel-Fabbri et al. 2002). For example, among 356 adolescent females with type 1 diabetes, Jones et al. (2000) reported that the HbA1c of 36 who had eating disorders (9.4 ± 1.8%) was significantly higher than that of the other patients (8.6 ± 1.6%). We reported that the HbA1c of 22 type 1 diabetic females with BN (12.3 ± 2.6%) was significantly higher than that of 11 female patients with BED (9.7 ± 2.1%), and that the HbA1c of

Table 170.3 Demographic and clinical features of female type 1 diabetes patients categorized by type of bulimia nervosa (BN) and binge-eating disorder (BED) (Adapted from Takii et al. 2002a. Copyright 2002 by the American Diabetes Association, Inc.)

	BED	BN-I	BN-IP	BN-NI	p
N	24	22	22	11	
Age (years)	25.2 ± 5.4	22.3 ± 4.4	23.7 ± 4.7	22.3 ± 3.1	NS
Onset of type 1 diabetes (years)	17.5 ± 8.1	15.9 ± 5.8	13.1 ± 5.4	14.0 ± 4.4	NS
Duration of type 1 diabetes (years)	7.1 ± 5.7	6.4 ± 3.8	10.5 ± 7.0	8.3 ± 5.1	NS
Onset of eating disorder (years)	21.7 ± 5.7	17.9 ± 4.5	17.5 ± 3.6	17.9 ± 2.3	<0.01[a]
Duration of eating disorder (years)	3.5 ± 3.1	4.2 ± 3.5	6.3 ± 4.0	4.4 ± 3.0	NS
BMI (kg/m^2)	24.1 ± 2.6	22.1 ± 2.7	20.4 ± 2.2	22.3 ± 2.7	<0.0001[b]
HbA1c (%)	9.8 ± 1.7	12.4 ± 2.1	13.0 ± 3.1	9.7 ± 2.4	<0.0001[c]
Neuropathy (%)	16.7	28.6	72.7	54.5	<0.001
Retinopathy (%)	8.3	19.0	54.5	45.5	<0.005
Nephropathy (%)	8.3	4.8	27.3	0	<0.05
EDI	63.9 ± 24.6	85.8 ± 35.9	93.7 ± 26.9	103.1 ± 25.2	<0.005[d]
SDS	44.5 ± 7.3	48.5 ± 8.3	53.4 ± 10.0	55.8 ± 8.2	<0.001[e]
STAI-T	50.9 ± 9.8	53.5 ± 9.5	59.5 ± 10.4	62.5 ± 9.3	<0.005 [e]
MPS	99.1±17.7	92.5 ± 23.0	102.3 ± 16.6	122.8 ± 25.0	<0.05[f]

Female type 1 diabetes patients with bulimia nervosa (BN) are not a homogenous group. They can be classified into three distinctive subgroups by type of inappropriate compensatory behavior in order to prevent weight gain
BED Binge-eating disorder, *BN* bulimia nervosa, *BN-I* BN-insulin omission, *BN-IP* BN-insulin omission/other purging, *BN-NI* BN-no insulin omission, *EDI* eating disorder inventory, *SDS* self-rating depression scale, *STAI* state-trait anxiety inventory, *MPS* multiple-dimension perfectionism scale (Frost)
Data are means ± SD. NS, $p > 0.05$
Differences were determined by one-way ANOVA followed by Bonferroni's adjusted t-test or by chi-square test
[a]BED > BN-I, BN-IP, BN-NI
[b]BED > BN-I, BN-IP
[c]BN-I, BN-IP > BED, BN-NI
[d]BN-I, BN-IP, BN-NI > BED
[e]BN-NI > BED, BN-I; BN-IP>BED
[f]BN-NI > BED, BN-I, BN-IP

patients with BED was significantly higher than that of patients without an eating disorder (6.2 ± 0.8%) (Takii et al. 1999) (Table 170.2).

170.2.6.2 Factors Related to the Exacerbation of Glycemic Control

We examined the psychological/behavioral predictors of elevated HbA1c of females with type 1 diabetes and BN or BED by multiple regression analysis (Takii et al. 1999). "Severe insulin omission" was found to be the factor most predictive of a higher HbA1c level, with a large amount eaten (2,000+ calories) in one binge-eating session the next most predictive.

170.2.6.3 Short- and Medium-term Complications

Unstable and poor metabolic control (so-called brittle diabetes), recurrent diabetic ketoacidosis (DKA), and severe hypoglycemic attacks easily occur in diabetes patients with a concurrent eating disorder (Rodin and Daneman 1992) and are likely to be associated with the need for more frequent hospitalization (Glasgow et al. 1991). Because most eating disorders are accompanied by binge eating and insulin omission, it is natural that these patients have extreme hyperglycemia. Female type 1 diabetes patients who have frequently repeated DKA can be strongly suspected of severe insulin omission associated with a severe eating disorder. An irregular diet or the irregular use of insulin injections (based on excessive attachment to body weight) often lead to unstable metabolic control, which can in turn lead to severe hypoglycemic attacks. However, in our experience, severe hypoglycemia attacks are not often seen in type 1 diabetes patients with a clinical eating disorder.

170.2.6.4 Long-term Complications

A considerable number of studies have indicated that a concurrent eating disorder or disordered eating can lead to an increased risk of the long-term complications of diabetes (Steel et al. 1987; Affenito et al. 1997; Rydall et al. 1997; Takii et al. 1999; Goebel-Fabbri et al. 2002).

In a meta-analysis, Nielsen (2000) reported that a coexisting eating disorder with type 1 diabetes increases the overall common odds ratio for retinopathy to 4.8. Of the various problematic behavioral factors related to eating disorders, we found the duration of severe insulin omission (omission of at least one-quarter of the prescribed insulin) to be the factor most closely associated with the retinopathy and nephropathy of type 1 diabetic females with clinical eating disorders (Takii et al. 2008). As mentioned above, severe insulin omission is the factor most predictive of the HbA1c of patients with concurrent type 1 diabetes and an eating disorder (Takii et al. 1999). The duration of severe insulin omission was related to the duration of poorest glycemic control. This finding may help patients who deliberately omit insulin to become aware of the medical risks of insulin omission.

170.2.7 Longitudinal Course of an Eating Disorder in Diabetes

Reports related to the long-term course of eating disorders and disordered eating by patients with type 1 diabetes are rare. Rydall et al. (1997) reported the 4- to 5-year course of type 1 diabetic females who were 12–18 years old at study entry. Intentional omission or underdosing of insulin and dieting for weight loss increased in prevalence from baseline to follow-up. Binge eating, self-induced vomiting, and dieting for weight loss tended to persist at follow-up if they were present at base line. Herpertz et al. (2001) assessed a sample of 36 diabetic patients with an eating disorder (type 1 diabetes: $n = 13$, Type 2 diabetes: $n = 23$) over a period of about 2 years. They reported that the eating disorder tended to persist over time, with a considerable shift within the different types of eating disorders. Nielsen et al. (2002) combined information from earlier studies to estimate mortality and reported a standardized mortality rate of 4.06% for type 1 diabetes, 8.86% for AN, and 14.5% for concurrent cases.

170.2.8 Eating Disorders Complicated with Type 2 Diabetes

In comparison with studies of eating disorders concurrent with type 1 diabetes, such studies of type 2 diabetes patients are rare. Herpertz et al. (1998) reported that although there was no difference in the prevalence of all eating disorders between IDDM (36.3 ± 10.6 years of age) and non-insulin-dependent diabetes (NIDDM) (54.2 ± 8.1 years of age) (point prevalence 5.5% vs 6.5%, lifetime prevalence 10.0% vs 9.9%), the prevalence of BN was higher in IDDM patients (point prevalence 1.5% vs 0.3%, lifetime prevalence 3.2% vs 1.9%) and BED was more frequent in NIDDM patients (point prevalence 1.8% vs 3.7%, lifetime prevalence 2.6% vs 5.9%). They also reported that type 2 diabetes patients with an eating disorder showed a greater psychopathology compared to patients without an eating disorder and that the diagnosis of an eating disorder did not seem to have a special influence on glycemic control (Herpertz et al. 2000). Papelbaum et al. (2005) reported that 20% of patients with type 2 diabetes (52.9 ± 6.8 years of age) displayed an eating disorder, that BED was the predominant eating disorder diagnosis (10%), and that the presence of an eating disorder was associated with a significant increase in the frequency of anxiety disorders.

170.3 The Mechanism of Eating Disorder Onset

170.3.1 Various Etiological Factors Peculiar to Type 1 Diabetes

Eating disorders are generally considered to have multiple etiologies including biological, psychological, familial, cultural, and social factors. Along with these general factors, many hypotheses have been proposed for the relationship between type 1 diabetes and the onset of an eating disorder. For example, "chronic dietary restraint" (Marcus and Wing 1990; Rodin and Daneman 1992; Polonsky 1996; Daneman et al. 1998; Goebel-Fabbri et al. 2002), "weight gain associated with appropriate diabetes self-care" (Marcus and Wing 1990; Rodin and Daneman 1992; Polonsky 1996; Daneman et al. 1998; Goebel-Fabbri et al. 2002), "uniquely effective forms of purging (insulin omission)" (Marcus and Wing 1990; Rodin and Daneman 1992; Polonsky 1996; Daneman et al. 1998; Goebel-Fabbri et al. 2002), "altered family dynamics" (Marcus and Wing 1990; Anderson 1990; Rodin and Daneman 1992; Maharaj et al. 1998), "greater prevalence of depressed and fluctuating moods" (Marcus and Wing 1990; Polonsky 1996; Goebel-Fabbri et al. 2002), "effects of type 1 diabetes on psychological development" (Marcus and Wing 1990), and "feeling out of control" (Schwartz et al. 2002). However, except for a few studies (Maharaj et al. 1998; Schwartz et al. 2002), empirical support is lacking.

The factors Marcus and Wing (1990) reported as the reasons that patients with type 1 diabetes would be vulnerable to eating disorders are as follows.

1. Factors related to the treatment of type 1 diabetes, such as being required to focus on diet and limit weight gain, weight gain by insulin therapy and good glycemic control, and the presence of a purging behavior peculiar to diabetes called insulin omission.
2. Type 1 diabetes may affect the psychological well-being of adolescents. Diabetes can interfere significantly with adolescent development by affecting body image, causing feelings of being different, and/or exacerbating dependence/independence conflict.
3. A family relationship such as a tendency among some parents to be overprotective or overinvolved with their youngster, rigidity, and a lack of conflict resolution.
4. Effects of chronic stress caused by chronic disease, which lead to lower self-esteem, affect body image, feelings of mastery or competence, necessitate changes in diet, and/or affect family environment.

Daneman et al. (1998) developed a model demonstrating how diabetic-related factors, such as weight gain after the initiation of insulin treatment or intensive diabetes management, dietary restriction for the nutritional management of diabetes, and insulin omission, interact to lead to eating disorders. Furthermore, in an empirical study, Maharaj et al. (1998) found that the eating disturbances of adolescent girls with diabetes are associated with significantly more family dysfunction. Diabetic girls with eating disturbances reported less support, poorer communication, and less trust in their relationships with their parents than did diabetic girls without eating disturbances. Schwartz et al. (2002) reported that a lower sense of overall control and a lower sense of bodily control were both directly related to more severe eating-disordered symptoms.

170.3.2 The "Compulsive Self-care → Binge Eating" Hypothesis

We have proposed two etiology hypotheses. Figure 170.1 shows the "Compulsive self-care → binge eating" hypothesis. There is tremendous social pressure on diabetes patients to limit the amount of food they eat and to not become fat, which may lead them to feel cornered and cause them to endure serious distress. Such thoughts can be enhanced by well intentioned, but poorly considered diabetes education. If the patient is overly conscientious and the family is too strict, the patient may feel trapped and that they must engage in overly strict diabetes management. These patients often do compulsive self-care for a period of time after the onset of diabetes. During this time, they are often treated like "honor students" by the medical staff.

However, frustration gradually increases, and the patient becomes unable to tolerate the strict regimen. Binge eating often starts without a special trigger and escalates quickly. Furthermore, weight gain by the binge eating causes a fear of becoming fat, which often leads to inappropriate compensatory behaviors in order to prevent weight gain (ICB), such as insulin omission and self-induced vomiting.

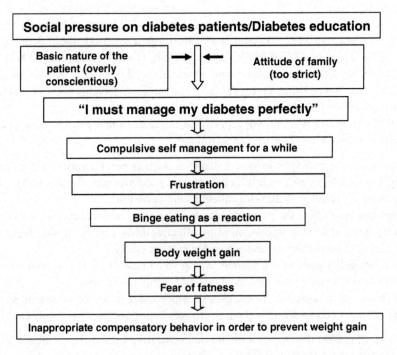

Fig. 170.1 The "Compulsive self-care → binge eating" hypothesis. This figure shows the flow of how female patients with type 1 diabetes who initially engage in compulsive self-care begin to binge and develop an eating disorder

170.3.3 Trauma Hypothesis

We have also developed what we call our Trauma hypothesis. The age at which type 1 diabetes begins most frequently, from infancy to the adolescent years, is a time when the self is not yet well formed. The patients have not developed adult mechanisms to cope with stress in general. At this critical time, the patient is suddenly confronted by a serious disease and the need to face a strict self-care regimen, which often leaves the patient overwhelmed by the diabetes. Unless the patient is able to accept and control it, the diabetes may be experienced with remarkable pain. For these distressed young patients, key people surrounding them sometimes fail to give effective psychological support and, on the contrary, they may take an attitude lacking in understanding; scolding and blaming.

Because of a lack of understanding of type 1 diabetes, diabetes patients are often subject to prejudice, discrimination, and special handling, which can be quite hurtful to the patient. This can lead to feelings of ineffectualness, despair, and a sense of guilt for not being able to deal with the diabetes. Suffering from a sense of alienation and/or feeling of isolation with no outside assistance, diabetes patients may develop severe trauma.

The eating disorder may give the patient relief from this state of despair. It gives the patient a perverted psychological structure in which they no longer care about anything but body weight/shape. Moreover, because the patient thinks about nothing else while they eat binge, they are temporarily freed from stress.

170.4 Self-destructive Behaviors Associated with Insulin Self-administration

By the proper self-administration of insulin, the quality of life and the treatment outcome of patients with type 1 diabetes can be remarkably improved. However, while there are patients who are able to accept this powerful drug and to manage it for the betterment of their life, there are patients who do not use sufficient insulin (insulin omission) or who use insulin extremely inadequately, which can cause serious medical problems (self-destructive behaviors). The most miserable psychosocial problems of type 1 diabetes patients are self-destructive behaviors such as recurrent diabetic ketoacidosis (DKA), frequent severe hypoglycemia, and brittle diabetes (Rubin and Peyrot 1992; Schade et al. 1985). These behaviors are often deeply associated with insulin manipulation. Self-destructive behaviors seem to coincide with severe psychosocial disturbance; either individual psychopathology (Schade et al. 1985), family dysfunction (White et al. 1984), or both (Golden et al. 1985). Self-destructive behaviors and eating disorders probably overlap to a significant degree; both clinical conditions are deeply associated with insulin manipulation (Table 170.4).

170.4.1 Recurrent Diabetic Ketoacidosis

As mentioned above, a comparatively high percentage of female patients with type 1 diabetes omit or reduce insulin to control body weight. Furthermore, some patients with a concurrent clinical eating disorder inject much less insulin than prescribed by the doctor, and they often seem to be on the threshold of DKA. In such cases, DKA will develop from only a slight precipitant, such as an insulin

Table 170.4 Key features of self-destructive behaviors

1. Type 1 diabetes patients sometimes exhibit self-destructive behaviors that result in recurrent diabetic ketoacidosis, frequent severe hypoglycemic attacks, and brittle diabetes.
2. These behaviors are often done with insulin manipulation including insulin omission and overdosing.
3. These behaviors lead to extreme instability of glycemic control, life-threatening episodes, and frequent hospitalizations.
4. These behaviors seem to coincide with severe psychological disturbance of individual psychopathology, family dysfunction, or both.
5. The main reason for these behaviors seems to be an intention to escape from an environment with much stress and to gain the concern of others by creating a serious physical condition that requires hospitalization.
6. Self-destructive behaviors and eating disorders probably overlap to a significant degree; both clinical conditions are deeply associated with insulin manipulation.

This table lists the key factors involved in self-destructive behaviors including the types of these behaviors, the etiological role of insulin manipulation, medical outcomes, psychological disturbance of the patient and family, the patient's psychological intention to engage in these behaviors, and the overlap between eating disorders

resistance increase by a worsened physical situation (sick day), failure to inject the insulin at the proper time because of failure to bring an injection device or by loss of their precarious mental balance because of mental instability. Moreover, patients may repeat DKA in order to escape from severe psychosocial disturbances.

170.4.2 Frequent Severe Hypoglycemic Attacks

Frequent severe hypoglycemic attacks can be caused by the intentional injection of too large a quantity of insulin for the purpose of escaping from the stresses of life. When patients who are psychologically immature and susceptible to stress are continually exposed to a harsh and hopeless environment, it is natural in a sense to escape by taking advantage of their disease. Feeling that they have no place in the family, through hospital admission they can escape form the family and the vicious cycle of family problems. However, even in cases in which the environment is not so terrible, extremely psychologically immature patients often cause repeated, severe hypoglycemia in order to escape from the pressures of diabetes and their life in general by causing themselves to lose consciousness.

170.4.3 Brittle Diabetes

Brittle diabetes overlaps widely with recurrent DKA and frequent severe hypoglycemic attacks. It is defined as "unexplained large changes in blood glucose concentration" (Woodyatt 1934) or "unable to maintain a normal lifestyle because of frequent disruptions secondary to severe hyperglycemic and/or hypoglycemic episodes" (Schade et al. 1985). In their study of brittle diabetes and recurrent DKA, Schade et al. (1985) reported that most type 1 diabetic patients who were thought to have brittle diabetes or insulin resistance were afterward found to have omitted insulin or had poor insulin manipulation. They also reported that, of 30 patients, eight were diagnosed with factitious disease and eight malingering. The most common causes of these self-destructive behaviors seem to be (1) to escape from an environment with much stress and difficulty, (2) severe personality disorder, and (3) insulin omission because of anxiety to weight gain (Fig. 170.2).

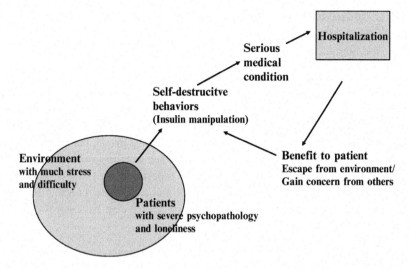

Fig. 170.2 The mechanism of the self-destructive behaviors of diabetes patients. Self-destructive behaviors include recurrent diabetic ketoacidosis, frequent severe hypoglycemia, and brittle diabetes. An intention to escape from an environment with much stress and to gain concern from others by creating a serious physical condition that requires hospitalization seems to be the main reason for the self-destructive behaviors of diabetes patients

170.4.4 Management

Patients tend to hide their problematic behaviors because of an intensive sense of guilt or a fear of being criticized or deserted by people significant to them. Even when the medical staff suspect insulin misapplication, the patient may strongly deny it and the family may show strong resistance to admitting it. As a result, an unexplained inability to control blood glucose can often be attributed to insulin resistance. It is important that the medical staff recognize this psychological problem and recommend psychological treatment by a mental health specialist.

170.5 Treatment Approach for Type 1 Diabetes Patients with Eating Disorders

170.5.1 Treatment for the Clinical Eating Disorders of Patients with Type 1 Diabetes

Previous studies have indicated the difficulties of dealing with type 1 diabetes patients with eating disorders and the urgent necessity for developing effective treatments (Marcus and Wing 1990; Rubin and Peyrot 1992). However, interventions specifically for these patients have rarely been reported, and most have been case studies. Peveler and Fairburn (1992) provided a detailed description of management and outcome, in a report of the treatment of a series of six females with type 1 diabetes and BN in which they used modified cognitive–behavioral therapy for BN, mainly on an outpatient basis. Although the treatment usually resulted in improved eating habits and glycemic control, the success rate was lower than for nondiabetic BN patients. Moreover, the improved glycemic control of their patients seems to have been insufficient to prevent long-term complications.

170.5.2 Psychoeducation Program for Type 1 Diabetes Patients with Disturbed Eating

Several group psychoeducation programs for patients with disturbed eating attitudes, not clinical eating disorders, have also been reported. Olmsted et al. (2002) evaluated the effect of a six-session psychoeducation program for young women with type 1 diabetes and disordered eating attitudes and behaviors that included a "nondeprivational" approach and recommendations that all types of foods be eaten in normal amounts. Compared with a treatment-as-usual group, the psychoeducation group was associated with a reduction in eating disturbance, but not with improvement in the frequency of insulin omission or HbA1c levels. Alloway et al. (2001) reported that a six-session group psychoeducation program, which is based on a program for BN and subclinical bulimia that was modified slightly to adapt to type 1 diabetes, was no more effective than a wait-list control group for treating subclinical disordered eating by women with type 1 diabetes.

170.5.3 Treatment for Type 1 Diabetes Patients with Clinical Eating Disorders in the Department of Psychosomatic Medicine, Kyushu University

We have acquired much experience in the treatment of type 1 diabetes patients with clinical eating disorders, having treated more than 150 of such patients, referred from throughout Japan, from 1994 to 2009. The majority were engaged in recurrent binge eating, either BN or BED. We reported that patients with BN clearly showed more severe psychological and medical pathology than patients with BED (Takii et al. 1999). This finding of pathological difference may be useful for developing a comprehensive treatment system that allows intervention to be tailored to the pathological severity of the individual patient. We have developed two forms of intervention: "outpatient counseling at first visit" (Takii et al. 2002b) and "integrated inpatient therapy" (Takii et al. 2003).

170.5.3.1 Outpatient Counseling at First Visit

Each patient underwent "outpatient counseling at first visit". The main purpose of the counseling is to empathize with the patient's distress from living with diabetes and to reduce the stress associated with their self-care regimen. Table 170.5 presents a summary of the elements of "outpatient counseling at first visit".

After the first visit, the patient returns to the referring physician for follow-up treatment. We reported that a great majority of the 10 BED patients significantly improved their eating pathology and glycemic control with a single session of our "outpatient counseling at first visit" as a turning point (Takii et al. 2002b) (Fig. 170.3). The reasons for this surprisingly good response are that these patients originally had mild psychopathology: Their binge eating was to a considerable extent due to the stress of the strict food regimen for the diabetes and their fixation on body weight/shape was comparatively mild. This counseling is performed for about 3 h by a doctor familiar with this area. The patients, for the first time since having developed type 1 diabetes, feel that they are understood deeply and accepted by significant others. They are given hope that they can live with diabetes through knowing how to more easily control it, in contrast with what they had previously thought. We tell them that type 1 diabetes is a disease in which there is no problem except that no insulin is produced and that they can gain good glycemic control only by proper insulin injection, without having to engage in a

Table 170.5 A summary of the elements of "outpatient counseling at first visit"

1. Bring out feelings about diabetes by listening for a sufficient amount of time that the patient gets a feeling of "validation" (to be deeply understood and accepted by the therapist).
2. Help the patient recover from the injured self-esteem. "It is very natural to be worried about diabetes and to long for eating when one's food is restricted".
3. Contradict too pessimistic an image of diabetes and present a hopeful and acceptable image of it. "Type 1 diabetes is no more than a deficiency of endogenous insulin. It is possible to have excellent glycemic control without special dietary/exercise therapy, if insulin is injected properly".
4. Teach the patient the importance of finding the easiest and most suitable diabetes self-care. "The patient cannot keep up excessive dieting or over exercising".
5. Encourage recovery/improvement of communication between the patient and family members, especially the mother.
6. Not demand that the patient attend our hospital as an outpatient or be hospitalized.

The main purpose of the counseling is to empathize with the patient's distress from living with diabetes and to reduce the stress associated with their self-care regimen

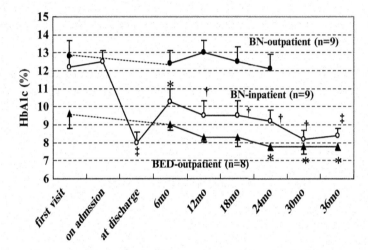

Fig. 170.3 HbA1c course of BN patients who had "Integrated inpatient therapy", BN patients who did not, and BED patients who did not. In BN patients who had the inpatient therapy (BN-inpatient:○), the HbA1c levels at discharge, 6, 12, 18, 24, 30, and 36 months after discharge were significantly lower than at first visit. In BED patients who did not have inpatient therapy (BED-outpatient: ▲), the HbA1c levels at 24, 30, and 36 months after first visit were significantly lower than at first visit. In BN patients who did not have the inpatient therapy (BN-outpatient:●), HbA1c level was not different between the first visit and any follow-up. All patients had "Outpatient counseling at first visit." Data are means ± S.E. $*p < 0.05$, $†p < 0.01$, $‡p < 0,001$ (Adapted from Takii et al. 2002b. Copyright 2002 by Elsevier Science B.V.)

strict dietary regimen. Patients who are able to have such an experience through our counseling can relatively easily change their attitudes toward food/body weight and diabetes.

After a period of observation by the referring physician, patients without sufficient improvement are encouraged to undergo "integrated inpatient therapy" in our hospital. We reported that none of 19 patients with BN showed sufficient improvement at this stage, and nine agreed to undergo "integrated inpatient therapy" (Takii et al. 2003) (Fig. 170.3).

170.5.3.2 Integrated Inpatient Therapy

The main points of this inpatient therapy are (1) to rest the mind and body in a supportive and lenient but regulated ward environment, (2) revision of cognitions and behaviors such as fixed ideas about diet and body weight or poor eating behaviors (3) acceptance of diabetes based on the experience that good glycemic control can be obtained without oppressive effort, and (4) the repair of family relationships based on insights by the patient. Table 170.6 presents a summary of the elements of our "Integrated Inpatient Therapy" (Takii et al. 2003).

On the day of admission, the patient is encouraged to decide the initial caloric intake, with the understanding that she should be able to and will be expected to eat the whole meal. In the conflict between the fear of becoming fat and the desire to eat, the patients waver considerably, but eventually most choose a comparatively small amount of food, such as 1,400 kcal a day. Similarly, the initial insulin injection dose is decided in consultation with the patient. In general, to eat all of the supplied meal is the easiest way for patients with an eating disorder to eat successfully.

However, in spite of the agreement, the majority of patients at first tend to leave part of the meal because of over-concern about body weight. The therapist calls the patient's attention to the fact that strict dieting is what has led to continued binge eating and instructs her not to leave any food uneaten. If the patient continues to resist eating all of her meal, the therapist does not advance to the next step of the treatment schedule: The patient's struggle to eliminate avoidance behaviors is the most important element of the inpatient treatment.

Even with this intervention, some patients regress from time to time when the meal is increased, either by leaving part of the meal or by secretly decreasing the insulin dose. The therapist must be aware of and stop this type of avoidance and again explain the rational behind eating the full portion

Table 170.6 A summary of the elements of "Integrated inpatient therapy" for type 1 diabetes patients with an eating disorder (Adapted from Takii et al. 2003. Copyright 2003 by Elsevier Inc.)

I. Recovery period for the mind and body
   a. Recovery from mental and physical fatigue and depression
   b. Normalization of biorhythms
II. Modification of behaviors and cognition
   a. Improvement of eating behavior
     Therapist control stage
       Decision, by the patient, of the initial calorie intake and insulin dose
       Completely and regularly eating meals
       Not eating snacks or confectioneries
       Incremental increases in the volume of the meal (200 kcal at a time) to a suitable-sized hospital meal (approximately 40 kcal/kg standard body weight each day)
     Patient control stage
       Free ingestion training
       Snack training
       Eating out training
       Staying at home training
   b. Promoting glycemic control competence
     Self-measurement of blood glucose
     Self-injection of insulin
     Practical coaching and training in adjustment of the insulin dose
   c. Modification of cognitive aspects
     Individual counseling
     Group therapy for eating disorders
III. Restoration of family relationships
   a. Spontaneous restoration process
   b. Family counseling
   c. Coaching family members: especially in how to understand and cope with the patient

In therapist control stage, patients are guarded from their eating disorder psychopathology by the therapeutic framework. In patient control stage, by phased removals of hospital staff control, the patient has to face by herself the stimuli that led her to eating disorder-related behaviors and she has to control her mind and behavior

and injecting the full dose of decided insulin. Through the process of making patients stick to their agreements on eating and insulin injection, they come to learn that they can control their body weight and diabetes with a normal food intake, that there is no need of food restriction, or to engage in a purging behavior, and that there will be good changes such as recovering a feeling of timely hunger and fullness, contrary to their expectations.

In therapist control stage, patients are guarded from their eating disorder psychopathology by the therapeutic framework, such as eating all of the food supplied, the prohibition of purging behaviors, not eating snacks, and the relatively restricted life in the hospital. In patient control stage, by phased removals of hospital staff control, the patient has to face by herself the stimuli that led her to eating disorder-related behaviors and she has to control her mind and behavior. These phased removals of control are as follows. (1) Free ingestion training: as the restriction that the patient must completely eat the meal is lifted, she must choose how much and what kind of food she eats; (2) Snack training: training in self-control in eating snack foods; (3) Eating out training: allowing the patient to eat in restaurants; and (4) Staying at home training: rehearsal for living in her own family/community circumstance. Although the patient often suffers setbacks, becoming unstable and/or having failures, including binge eating, these experiences are very good practical learning opportunities that help the patient face and overcome problems. The therapist does not allow the patient to escape from problems, but helps her attain a deep understanding and coaches her as to how to overcome them.

Along with a decreasing fixation on food and body weight, the patient often comes to reflect on herself, the relationship between significant people and herself, and her association with diabetes. The introspective environment of the ward and counseling twice a week facilitate the process. The patient comes to communicate with parents by letters and telephone calls (their place of residence is generally far from the hospital), which leads to a spontaneous restoration process for the family relationship. The therapist follows the process and holds family counseling to facilitate the process. The experience of being able to control diabetes without any special hardships tends to lead the patient to reconcile themselves to their diabetes.

After discharge from our hospital, the patients again return to the referring physician. We reported that the HbA1c levels of nine BN patients who underwent the inpatient therapy were significantly lower at discharge, 6, 12, 18, 24, 30, and 36 months after discharge than at first visit (Takii et al. 2003) (Fig. 170.3). Moreover, the patients had significantly lower psychological test scores related to eating disorder psychopathology, depressiveness, and anxiety; a reduced frequency and amount of binge eating; and fewer patients exhibited purging behaviors at 36 months after discharge than at first visit (Takii et al. 2003). Ten BN patients who did not undergo the inpatient therapy had no significant psychological/behavioral or medical improvement (Takii et al. 2003) (Fig. 170.3).

The effectiveness of the "integrated inpatient therapy" for type 1 diabetes patients with BN can be largely attributed to the therapeutic framework and intervention of the therapist, which block the avoidance behaviors against becoming fat. Because type 1 diabetes patients with BN have such an extreme fixation on body weight/shape, the therapeutic framework and intervention of a therapist, which block the avoidance behaviors, are essential in the treatment of type 1 diabetes patients with BN.

170.5.3.3 Long-term Psychotherapy and Adjustments of the Patient's Circumstances

Although most type 1 diabetes patients with BN respond to the integrated inpatient therapy, some patients who have marked psychopathology tend to regress repeatedly, in spite of multiple episodes of inpatient therapy. The marked psychopathology includes severe personality disorder, trauma, and a marked delay of psychological/emotional development: For some patients, it seems as if their psychological development stopped after they developed type 1 diabetes. It is difficult for such

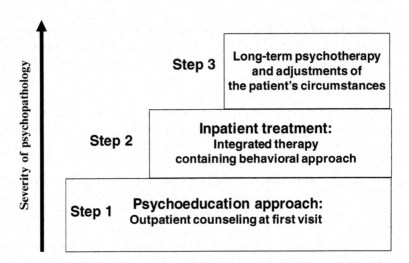

Fig. 170.4 Step-by-step treatment system for type 1 diabetes patients with a clinical eating disorder according to the severity of psychopathology. The number of steps necessary for successful treatment depends on the severity of the patient's psychopathology

patients to improve their eating disorders and control of diabetes without a reduction of their extreme psychopathology. It is important for the therapist to persevere in offering long-term psychotherapy and to strive to adjust the family circumstances to facilitate the patient's psychological growth.

Figure 170.4 shows the step-by-step treatment system of our department for type 1 diabetes patients with a clinical eating disorder, which is done according to the severity of patient's psychopathology.

170.6 Early Awareness and the Prevention of Eating Disorders by Type 1 Diabetes Patients

The treatment of diabetes patients with eating disorders has been reported to be extremely difficult. Moreover, even if the treatment is successful, huge expenditures of time and energy are required before the eating disorder and diabetic control become sufficiently improved. Prevention is much preferable to treatment.

Marcus and Wing (1990) suggested that emotional support and effective information in the context of a sound relationship may prevent problems as well as ameliorate mildly disturbed eating behavior. They emphasized that it is crucial to promote the development of a strong therapeutic relationship in which patients are encouraged to discuss their concerns about body shape and weight. They also indicated that diabetes patients need sound information about weight regulation and that adolescent IDDM patients need special help in learning to eat and drink in social situations, with a view to minimizing feelings of being different.

Rodin et al. (2002) suggested that current diabetes treatment approaches, which emphasize normalizing eating behavior and matching insulin administration to caloric intake, may lessen the experience of deprivation and reduce the risk of eating disturbances. From the suspicion that eating disorders are often not recognized in the diabetes clinic setting, they recommended that health-care professionals who treat young women with type 1 diabetes maintain a high index of suspicion for the presence of an eating disturbance, particularly among those who present with persistently poor metabolic control, repeated episodes of diabetic ketoacidosis, and/or weight and body shape concerns.

Rapaport et al. (1996) listed the following potential markers for the development of an eating disorder by a patient with diabetes: Frequent diabetic ketoacidosis, elevated HbA1c, anxiety about – or avoidance of – being weighed, frequent and severe hypoglycemia, nonadherence, brittle diabetes, delay in puberty or sexual maturation or failure to grow, bingeing with food or alcohol, and severe stress in the family. These markers are of special concern among young women.

We recently reported that the development of type 1 diabetes in preadolescence or adolescence seems to place girls at risk for the subsequent development of AN or BN (Takii et al. in print). Careful attention should be paid to these high-risk patients.

References

Affenito SG, Adams CH. Nutr Rev. 2001;59:179–82.
Affenito SG, Backstrand JR, Welch GW, Lammi-Keefe CJ, Rodriguez NR, Adams CH. Diab Care. 1997;20:182–4.
Alloway SC, Toth EL, Mccargar LJ. Can J Diet Pract Res. 2001;62:188–92.
American Psychiatric Association. Diagnostic and statistical manual of mental disorders. Revised 3rd edn. Washington, DC: American Psychiatric Association; 1987.
American Psychiatric Association. Diagnostic and statistical manual of mental disorders. 4th edn. Washington, DC: American Psychiatric Association; 1994.
Anderson BJ. In: Holmes CS, editor. Neuropsychological and behavioral aspects of diabetes. New York: Springer-Verlag; 1990. p. 85–101.
Biggs MM, Basco MR, Patterson G, Raskin P. Diab Care. 1994;17:1186–9.
Daneman D, Olmsted M, Rydall A, Maharaj S, Rodin G. Horm Res. 1998;50:79–86.
Fairburn CG, Peveler RC, Davies B, Mann JI, Mayou RA. BMJ. 1991;303:17–20.
Glasgow AM, Weissberg-Benchell I, Tynan WD, Epstein SF, Driscoll CD, Turek J, Beliveau E. Pediatrics. 1991;88:98–104.
Goebel-Fabbri AE, Fikkan J, Connell A, Vangsness L, Anderson BJ. Treat Endocrinol. 2002;1:155–62.
Goebel-Fabbri AN, Fikkan J, Franko DL, Pearson K, Anderson BJ, Weinger K. Diab Care. 2008;31:415–9.
Golden MP, Herrold AJ, Orr DP. J Pediatr. 1985;107:195–200.
Herpertz S, Wagener R, Albus C, Kocnar M, Wagner R, Best F, Schleppinghoff BS, Filz H-P, Förster K, Thomas W, Mann K, Köhle K, Senf W. J Psychosom Res. 1998;44:503–15.
Herpertz S, Albus C, Lichtblau K, Kohle K, Mann K, Senf W. Int J Eat Disord. 2000;28:68–77.
Herpertz S, Albus C, Kielmann R, Hagemann-Patt H, Lichtblau K, Köhle K, Mann K, Senf W. J Psychosom Res. 2001;51:673–8.
Jones JM, Lawson ML, Danemann D, Olmsted MP, Rodin G. BMJ. 2000;320:1563–6.
Kennedy SH, Kaplan AS, Garfinkel PE, Rockert W, Toner B. J Psychosom Res. 1994;38:773–82.
Maharaj SI, Rodin GM, Olmsted MP, Daneman D. J Psychosom Res. 1998;44:470–90.
Marcus MD, Wing RR. In: Holmes CS, editor. Neuropsychological and behavioral aspects of diabetes. New York: Springer-Verlag; 1990. p.102–121.
Nielsen S. Eur Eat Disorders Rev. 2002;10:241–54.
Nielsen S, Emborg C, Molbak AG. Diab Care. 2002;25:309–12.
Olmsted MP, Daneman D, Rydall AC, Lawson ML, Rodin G. Int J Eat Disord. 2002;32:230–9.
Papelbaum M, Appolinário JC, Moreira RO, Ellinger VCM, Kupfer R, Coutinho. Res Bras Psiquiatr. 2005;27:135–8.
Peveler RC, Fairburn CG, Boller I, Dunger D. Diab Care. 1992;15:1356–60.
Peveler RC, Fairburn CG. Int J Eat Disord. 1992;11:45–53.
Polonsky WH. In: Powers MA, editor. Handbook of diabetes medical nutrition therapy. 2nd edn. Sudbury: Jones & Bartlett Publishers; 1996. p. 585–601.
Polonsky WH, Anderson BJ, Lohrer PA, Aponte JE, Jacobson AM, Cole CF. Diab Care. 1994;17:1178–85.
Rapaport WS, LaGreca AM, Levin P. In: Anderson BJ, Rubin RR, editors. Practical psychology for diabetes clinicians. Alexandria: American Diabetes Association;1996. p. 133–141.
Rodin G, Craven J, Littlefield C, Murray M, Daneman D. Psychosomatics. 1991;32:171–6.
Rodin GM, Daneman D. Diab Care. 1992;15:1402–12.
Rodin GM, Olmsted MP, Rydall AC, Maharaj SI, Colton PA, Jones JM, Biancucci LA, Daneman D. J psychosom Res. 2002;53:943–9.
Rosmark B, Berne C, Holmgren S, Lago C, Renholm G, Sohlberg S. J Clin Psychiatry. 1986;47:547–50.

Rubin RR, Peyrot M. Diab Care. 1992;15:1640–57.

Rydall AC, Rodin GM, Olmsted MP, Devenyi RG, Daneman D. N Engl J Med. 1997;336:1849–54.

Schade DS, Drumm DA, Duckworth WC, Eaton RP. Diab Care. 1985;8:12–20.

Schwartz SA, Weissberg-Benchell J, Perlmuter LC. Diab Care. 2002;25:1987–91.

Steel JM, Young RJ, Lloyd GG, Clarke BF. Br Med J. 1987;294:859–62.

Takii M, Komaki G, Uchigata Y, Maeda M, Omori Y, Kubo C. J psychosom Res. 1999;47:221–31.

Takii M, Uchigata Y, Nozaki T, Nishikata H, Kawai K, Komaki G, Iwamoto Y, Kubo C. Diab Care. 2002a;25:1571–5.

Takii M, Uchigata Y, Komaki G, Nozaki T, Kawai K, Nishikata H, Kawai H, Morioka K, Iwamoto Y, Kubo C. In: Sivik T, Byrne D, Lipsitt D, Christodoulou G, Dienstfrey H, editors. Psycho-neuro-endocrino-immunology. Amsterdam: Elsevier Science; 2002b. p. 291–296.

Takii M, Uchigata Y, Komaki G, Nozaki T, Kawai H, Iwamoto Y, Kubo C. J Psychosom Res. 2003;55:349–56.

Takii M, Uchigata Y, Tokunaga S, Amemiya N, Kinukawa N, Nozaki T, Iwamoto Y, Kubo C. Int J Eat Disord. 2008;41:259–64.

Takii M, Uchigata Y, Kishimoto J, Morita C, Hata T, Nozaki T, Kawai K, Iwamoto Y, Sudo N, Kubo C. Pediatr Diabetes. In print.

Talbot F, Nouwen A. Diab Care. 2000;23:1556–62.

Tsukahara S, Uchigata Y, Ishido K, Takii M, Iwamoto Y. J Jpn Diab Soc. 2009;52:13–21.

Vila G, Robert JJ, Nollet-Clemencon C, Vera L, Crosnier H, Rault G, Jos J, Mouren-Simeoni MC. Eur Child Adolesc Psychiatry. 1995;4:270–9.

White K, Kolman ML, Wexler P, Polin G, Winter RJ. Pediatrics. 1984;73:749–55.

Woodyatt RT. In: Cecil RL, editor. A textbook of medicine. 3rd edn. Philadelphia: W. B. Saunders Company; 1934. p. 628.

Chapter 171
Comparing Abnormal Eating Behavior in Type 1 and 2 Diabetic Patients

Patrick Ritz, Monelle Bertrand, and Hélène Hanaire

Abbreviation

ED-NOS   Eating disorder not otherwise specified

171.1 Introduction

Diabetes is classically divided into type 1 and type 2. Type 1 diabetes concerns less than 10% of diabetic people, who are typically young, thin, with an intense endocrine pancreatic failure. To closely regulate plasma glucose concentrations within narrow limits, the treatment is an obligatory complex schedule of multiple daily insulin injections and a mandatory monitoring of carbohydrate intake and of capillary blood glucose, to adjust insulin doses. Type 2 diabetes affects the vast majority of diabetic people, and is closely associated to overweight and obesity. The pathophysiology of type 2 diabetes is a combination of endocrine pancreatic failure (making insulin injections necessary during the course of the disease) and insulin-resistance, which is closely associated to fat intake, low physical activity, genetic background, and increased fat mass. The basis of the treatment of type 2 diabetes is the control of body weight through adaptation of the diet, and of physical activity, which remains necessary even when drugs are prescribed.

It is therefore obvious that patients suffering from diabetes have to change their predisease diet. Furthermore, diabetes affects patients who have "learned" to behave with food and eating, and an important question is to ask whether diabetes itself and/or diabetes care affects eating behavior. Indeed, diabetes management does place emphasis on strict dietary adherence, which could reinforce pre-existing "abnormal" eating behavior or indeed promote them in otherwise normal eating behavior patients (Goodwin et al. 2003). This review summarizes the knowledge about "abnormal" eating behavior in type 1 and type 2 diabetic patients. It is obvious from this literature search that the definitions used vary between authors. It sometimes crosses over with other concerns (such as body shape and image in adolescents) so that "insulin omission" is also considered in "eating behavior." It is also noticeable that most of the information come from a limited number of authors, studying mostly young females, with very little known about young males.

P. Ritz (✉)
Unité de Nutrition, CHU Larrey, TSA 30030, F-31059 Toulouse cedex 9, France
e-mail: Ritz.p@chu-toulouse.fr

V.R. Preedy et al. (eds.), *Handbook of Behavior, Food and Nutrition*,
DOI 10.1007/978-0-387-92271-3_171, © Springer Science+Business Media, LLC 2011

171.2 Definitions of "Abnormal" Eating Behavior

171.2.1 DSM Criteria

Strictly speaking, "abnormal" eating behavior can be approached as eating behavior disorders. Those are based on the diagnostic criteria proposed by the DSM panel of the American Psychiatric Association Tables 171.1 and 171.2 (APS 1994). Binge eating is one such disorder. It refers to the episodic consumption of an objectively large quantity of food that is accompanied by a loss of control during the consumption. When no such loss of control is felt, it is termed episodic overeating. It can be distinguished from bulimia nervosa by the absence of frequent inappropriate compensatory

Table 171.1 Diagnostic criteria of bulimia nervosa

- Recurrent episodes of binge eating characterized by both:
  1. Eating, in a discrete period of time (e.g., within any 2-hour period), an amount of food that is definitely larger than most people would eat during a similar period of time and under similar circumstances
  2. A sense of lack of control over eating during the episode, defined by a feeling that one cannot stop eating or control what or how much one is eating
- Recurrent inappropriate compensatory behavior to prevent weight gain
  1. Self-induced vomiting
  2. Misuse of laxatives, diuretics, enemas, or other medications
  3. Fasting
  4. Excessive exercise
- The binge eating and inappropriate compensatory behavior both occur, on average, at least twice a week for 3 months.
- Self evaluation is unduly influenced by body shape and weight.
- The disturbance does not occur exclusively during episodes of anorexia nervosa.

Type
- Purging type: During the current episode of bulimia nervosa, the person has regularly engaged in self-induced vomiting or the misuse of laxatives, diuretics, or enemas.
- Nonpurging type: During the current episode of bulimia nervosa, the person has used inappropriate compensatory behavior but has not regularly engaged in self-induced vomiting or misused laxatives, diuretics, or enemas.

This table describes the clinical traits for the diagnosis pf bulimia nervosa according to DSM IV

Table 171.2 Diagnostic criteria of EDNOS (eating disorders not otherwise specified) (Adapted from APS, 2000)

Eating disorder not otherwise specified includes disorders of eating that do not meet the criteria for any specific eating disorder.
  1. For female patients, all of the criteria for anorexia nervosa are met except that the patient has regular menses.
  2. All of the criteria for anorexia nervosa are met except that, despite significant weight loss, the patient's current weight is in the normal range.
  3. All of the criteria for bulimia nervosa are met except that the binge eating and inappropriate compensatory mechanisms occur less than twice a week or for less than 3 months.
  4. The patient has normal body weight and regularly uses inappropriate compensatory behavior after eating small amounts of food (e.g., self-induced vomiting after consuming two cookies).
  5. Repeatedly chewing and spitting out, but not swallowing, large amounts of food.

Binge-eating disorder is recurrent episodes of binge eating in the absence if regular inappropriate compensatory behavior characteristic of bulimia nervosa. It is often, but not always, associated with obesity symptoms.

Night eating syndrome includes morning anorexia, increased appetite in the evening, and insomnia. Often obese, these patients can have complete or partial amnesia for eating during the night.

This table describes the clinical traits for the diagnosis of eating disorders not otherwise specified according to DSM IV behaviors, whether purging (vomiting, excessive laxative and diuretic use) or nonpurging (excessive exercise, intentional fasting), both of which are characteristic of bulimia (Dingemans et al. 2002).

171.2.2 Other Definitions Arising from the Type 1 Diabetes Literature

Gary Rodin and coauthors (Colton et al. 2004) from the Department of Psychiatry, Toronto (Canada) have extensively studied behaviors in young type 1 females and have extended the definition to include fasting and dieting; self-induced vomiting; the abuse of laxatives, diet pills, diuretics, and other medications; and the use of intense, excessive exercise for weight control. The psychological traits and symptoms include preoccupation with body weight and shape, distortions of body image, and severely disturbed attitudes toward food, calories, and eating.

More specifically, they described eating disorder not otherwise specified (ED-NOS) and subthreshold eating disorders. A specific aspect of the definition of ED-NOS concerns diabetic patients (item 5), probably because weight concerns are very important in type 1 diabetic patients in whom body weight increases dramatically as a consequence of diabetes care (Colton et al. 2004).

ED-NOS is defined in the situations where there are:

1. All the criteria for anorexia nervosa except for amenorrhea; or
2. All the criteria for anorexia nervosa except the subject does not report a fear of weight gain or does not report a disturbance in the way in which their body weight and/or shape is experienced; or
3. All the criteria for bulimia nervosa except that the subject does not report self-evaluation being unduly influenced by shape and/or weight; or
4. All the criteria for bulimia nervosa except that the frequency of binge-eating and purging behavior occurred at least once per week for 3 months, or two times per week over the previous 4 weeks; or
5. An individual regularly engages in inappropriate compensatory behavior in the absence of binge eating (e.g., recurrent self-induced vomiting or insulin omission for shape and weight control at least one time per week for the past 3 months, or twice weekly over the previous 4 weeks); or
6. An individual engages in recurrent episodes of objective binge eating (at least one time per week for the past 3 months, or twice weekly over the previous 4 weeks).

Subthreshold eating disorders are defined in situations where:

1. An individual engages in occasional (three or more times) binge eating, and/or purging over the past 3 months; or
2. An individual whose self-evaluation is unduly influenced by shape or weight, and who regularly engages in extreme dietary restraint (<500 kcal/day); or
3. An individual whose self-evaluation is unduly influenced by shape or weight, and who regularly engages in intense, excessive exercise for the purpose of weight control (at least five times weekly) over the past 3 months.

171.2.3 Definitions from Obesity and Type 2 Literature

In the obesity literature, eating behavior has also been defined with tools assessing dietary restraint, disinhibition, hunger, and emotional and external eating patterns (Mela 1996).

Dietary restraint refers to the intention to restrict and control food intake to attain or maintain a desirable body weight. It can be assessed by questions such as "I often stop eating before being fully satisfied in order to control the amount of food I eat". Disinhibition refers to overeating associated with a loss of control during eating and can be addressed by questions such as "Sometimes what I'm eating is so good I continue on eating even if I'm not hungry". Hunger represents perceived hunger sensations and can be assessed by questions such as "I cannot go on a diet for the simple reason that I get too hungry".

Emotional and external eating refers to the fact that compared with their lean counterparts, obese human subjects are argued to be more reactive to external cues (time, presence of food, situational effects, etc.) and less sensitive to internal hunger and satiety signals than their lean counterparts. According to this view, high external responsiveness would, given an environment of an easily accessible, abundant, and highly palatable food supply, encourage overeating and, hence, the development of obesity.

171.3 Description of "Abnormal" Eating Behavior and Type 1 Diabetes

Gary Rodin and coauthors have produced a large number of studies (Colton et al. 2004; Jones et al. 2000; Rodin et al. 2002; Colton et al. 2007a, b; Rydall et al. 1997; Olmsted et al. 2002) on eating behavior and type 1 diabetes. They mostly studied young type 1 diabetic females. An important concern in these women is that diabetes care leads to weight gain, as reflected by BMI being greater in diabetic women than in controls (22.7 vs. 20.6 kg/m²; Jones et al. 2000). According to Rodin and colleagues this raises preoccupations about body size and shape and leads to an adjustment of eating behaviors in order to deal with these concerns.

In the two largest reports from this group (on more than 350 individuals aged 12–19 years), DSM criteria are present with an odd-ratio of 2.4 as compared to control subjects (Jones et al. 2000; Rodin et al. 2002). There were no people suffering from anorexia nervosa and very few from bulimia (although with an odds ratio of 3 vs. controls). A total of 10% of the subjects (vs. 4% in the controls) are presenting DSM or ED-NOS criteria. The odds ratio of subthreshold eating disorders is 1.9 versus controls. Binge eating occurs in 3% of the patients (vs. 0.3% in controls; Colton et al. 2004), a figure also reported by Peveler et al. (5% in adult type 1 diabetic women, 2005).

In a smaller group of patients (n = 101) with similar BMIs as controls, the prevalence of ED-NOS is 8% and about eight times more frequent that in controls (Colton et al. 2004). If all eating behavior abnormalities are considered, about 20% of these young diabetic people are concerned (Colton et al. 2007a). Dieting in the month preceding the evaluation occurs in 15%, intense exercise in 10% (ten times more than in controls; Colton et al. 2004).

These data are summarized in Table 171.3.

It appears that diabetes care itself promotes "abnormal" eating behaviors since from this 20% figure, there are 10% more new cases after 1 year follow-up (Colton et al. 2007b) and the prevalence is close to 49% after 5 years of follow-up (Colton et al. 2007a). These follow-up data are summarized in Table 171.4.

Another cohort of 90 women (both adults and adolescents) was studied by Peveler et al. in England (Peveler et al. 2005). They found 8 out of 57 subjects presenting with either DSM or ED-NOS or subthreshold eating behavior disorders. It is noticeable that adult women omitted significantly more insulin injections to control weight (37%) than adolescents (15%). This figure was 1% in preteens, 11–14% in adolescents, and about 33% of the young adults studied by Rodin (2002). The 8–12 years follow-up of the British group told that insulin omission was stable in adults but doubled in adolescents (Peveler et al. 2005). Jones et al. showed that insulin omission was closely associated with "abnormal" eating behavior, since the prevalence was 42% in persons with disturbed eating patterns

Table 171.3 Prevalence of eating disorders in type 1 diabetes subjects

Reference	N subjects	Compared to	Full DSM IV (% of group)	AN (N)	BN (N)	BED (N)	EDNOS (N)	IO (N)	SIV (N)	Laxative abuse (N)	Males (N)	Dieting (N)
Peveler et al. (2005)	54 young adults		8%	1	3	3	1	20	6	6	0	
Peveler et al. (2005)	33 young adolescents		8%	0	0	0	0	5	2	0	0	
Herpetz et al. (1998)	341	Controls	5%	1	5	6	6	2			153	
Jones et al. (2000)	361	Controls	10%	0	3	108	32	39	7	2	0	12
Colton et al. (2004)	101	Controls	11%	0	0	3	8	2	0	0	0	11

This table describes the prevalence of eating disorders in the cohorts of patients with type 1 diabetes published in the literature

N is the number of observations in the cohort

AN anorexia nervosa, BN bulimia nervosa, BED binge eating disorder, EDNOS eating disorder not otherwise specified, IO insulin omission, SIV self induced vomiting

Definitions are given in Tables 171.1 and 171.2

Table 171.4 Progression of eating disorders in type 1 diabetes subjects at follow-up

Reference	N subjects at follow up/ initial number	Compared to	Full DSM IV	AN (N)	BN (N)	BED (N)	EDNOS (N)	IO (N)	SIV (N)	Laxative abuse (N)	Males (N)
Peveler et al. (2005)	37/54 young adults	12 years later		1/1	1/3	1/3	0/1	21/20	7/6	8/6	0
Peveler et al. (2005)	26/33 young adolescents	8 years later	10/8	0/01/0	0/0	0/0	1/0	10/5	4/2	2/0	0
Colton et al. (2007a)	126	5 years later	13		3	6	3	3	3		

This table describes the progression of eating disorders in the cohorts of patients with type 1 diabetes published in the literature

N is the number of observations in the cohort

Data are compared to that existing in the initial cohort, the best comparator for Colton et al. is the data from the same author in Table 171.3

AN anorexia nervosa, BN bulimia nervosa, BED binge eating disorder, EDNOS eating disorder not otherwise specified, IO insulin omission, SIV self induced vomiting

Definitions are given in Tables 171.1 and 171.2

(Rodin et al. 2002). Similarly, self-induced vomiting doubled in adolescents (2–4 out of 33 subjects); while it was stable in adults (6 in 57 persons; Peveler et al. 2005).

"Abnormal" eating behaviors are also related to mood disorders that may be secondary to diabetes and/or its complications, which make it difficult to tell which is the chicken from the egg (Rodin et al. 2002). Although there may be a "genetic" component is these behaviors, Rodin et al. (2002) have shown that mothers of these adolescents bring them less support, and that the subjects show less trust in the relationship with their parents than patients without disturbed behaviors.

These "abnormal" behaviors are important to diagnose because they are associated with poorer metabolic control (9.4% glycated hemoglobin, vs. 8.6% in patients without "abnormal" eating behaviors), greater risk of ketoacidosis, and microvascular complications. In particular, diabetic retinopathy is present in 84% of patients with an "abnormal" eating behavior, and 24% of patients without (Rodin et al. 2002; Rydall et al. 1997).

Treatment of "abnormal" eating behavior has been rarely studied. Rodin and colleagues show that a 6-session psychoeducation program improves signs of ED-NOS but not insulin omission or metabolic control (Olmsted et al. 2002).

Data in males are scarce. Ryan et al. (2008) report 43 type 1 diabetic subjects, with 27 males. No patient, male or female, met the full DSM criteria. However, over one-quarter (26%) of males presented with disordered eating behavior, either overeating or binge eating. It is noticeable that patients were older than in other cohorts. Of all patients exhibiting disordered behavior, 22% reported occasionally fasting or exercising excessively to lose weight; however, these episodes were infrequent and considered normal. Herpertz (1998) reported data from 143 German male subjects, with a lower prevalence of disturbed behaviors than in females (that was reported to be 10.8–16.9%; DSM plus ED-NOS criteria).

171.4 Comparison of "Abnormal" Eating Behavior in Type 2 and Type 1 Diabetes

Goodwin et al. (2003) in their assessment of 3,000 primary care patients observed that an eating disorder (based on DSM-IV criteria) was the only psychological condition associated with an increased diabetes risk. Goodwin et al. (2003) also found that diabetes was the only disease of the seven most common diseases evaluated that carried significantly increased odds of developing an eating disorder. Reports of "abnormal" eating behavior in type 2 diabetes suggest that binge eating has ranged between 5% and 21% and that the percentage of patients meeting full DSM criteria has ranged between 1.5% and 26% (Mannucci et al. 2002; Kenardy et al. 1994; Papelbaum et al. 2005; Crow et al. 2001). Observed overeating and binge-eating rates were 27% in French males and 11% in women mildly higher than those observed in other European diabetic populations (Ryan et al. 2008). This was higher than the prevalence in the French nondiabetic population, although caution should be taken with this information since the diabetic sample was rather small (n = 96). Mannucci et al. reported rates of full DSM criteria in 2.5% of type diabetes patients (similar to that in non diabetic or obese Italian patients), and binge eating in 7.5% females and 2.6% males (2002). Herpertz in Germany showed a 6.5–9% prevalence of DSM plus ED-NOS criteria (1998). Such rates may, however, be lower than rates observed in the United States (Kenardy et al. 1994; Papelbaum et al. 2005; Crow et al. 2001) but given the heterogeneity of measurements tools used across these studies it is difficult to compare results meaningfully (Table 171.5).

One-quarter of the Diabetes Prevention Program cohort of patients at risk for type 2 diabetes (n = 274) was studied by Delahanty et al. (2002) and showed a binge-eating rate of 19%.

Type 2 diabetic patients are significantly more dietary restrained than type 1 diabetic patients. Restraint was found to increase in line with BMI (Ryan et al. 2008; Herpetz et al. 1998). Dietary disinhibition score was generally low and similar between diabetic groups as it was for hunger (Ryan et al. 2008). It is noteworthy that both reported disinhibition and hunger were significantly higher in patients with "abnormal" eating behavior than in those without, while dietary restraint was similar. However, dietary restraint increases from the diagnosis to after 6 months in type 1 diabetic patients (Ritz 2008).

Although dietary restraint is not regarded as a DSM or ED-NOS criteria, the restraint theory proposes that increased restraint can facilitate the development of unusual eating habits as a result of stress incurred by the need to control body weight. In diabetic patients, any food intake may be considered to be a result of the "balance between their desire to eat and their wish to diet." A lapse in this self-control (a disinhibition effect) – for whatever reason – can result in overeating. In contrast to "normal" eaters,

Table 171.5 Prevalence of Binge eating in patients at risk or with type 2 diabetes

Reference	% of cohort without Binge eating	% of cohort with episodic over-eating	% of cohort with Binge eating
Delahanty et al. (2002)	59	22	19
Ryan et al. (2008) – Men	73	9	18
Ryan et al. (2008) – Women	74	0	11
Manucci et al. (2002)	94.7		5.3
Herpetz et al. (1998)			2.5–3.4

This table describes the prevalence of binge eating in the published cohorts of type 2 diabetic patients

who are influenced by a sophisticated internal regulatory system that modulates external factors such as smell to initiate or end food intake, restrained eaters try to dominate all external factors. As a result, the food intake of restrained eaters becomes uncontrolled and unrelated to either their appetite or nutritional requirements. This situation, with its eventual subsequent disinhibition, could result in periods of significant overeating. Golay et al. (2001) emphasized the importance of using food diaries to reveal patients' eating habits as well as the need to help them to understand what a meal is and to reestablish a regular eating pattern.

171.5 Conclusion

"Abnormal" eating behaviors are prevalent in both type 1 and type 2 diabetic subjects. In type 1 subjects, classical criteria of DSM and ED-NOS are more prevalent than in the general population, and progress with the disease during adolescence to reach high rates in adults. Other less classical behaviors related to body size and shape concerns develop with the course of the disease, such as insulin omission or self-induced vomiting. Since these behaviors are associated with greater complication rates and poorer metabolic control, they should be searched systematically. Indeed, omitting the diagnosis leads to lack of treatment, although more research is needed about therapeutic approaches. The possibility of a gender effect warrants further exploration in larger patient cohorts. In type 2 patients, binge eating and overeating appear to be frequent and can be subject to specific approaches such as cognitive and behavioral therapy (Golay et al. 2001).

Dietary restraint, disinhibition, and hunger rates are high in both type 1 and type 2 patients. These parameters have been associated in a complex bidirectional relationship with body-weight management. Whether the systematic evaluation of those parameters should be performed remains a matter of debate.

All the studies reported have used somewhat different definitions of "abnormal" eating behaviors, and different tools to address prevalence. Future studies should pay attention to these aspects in order to compare data from different cohorts.

The authors display no conflict of interest between them and with industrial partners related to this work.

Summary Points

- Disordered eating behavior is frequent in type 1 diabetic patients.
- Disordered eating behavior is associated with a higher rate of microvascular complications in type 1 diabetic patients.
- Disordered eating behavior is related to dysregulation of body shape and image in type 1 diabetic patients.

- Disordered eating behavior is characterized by other traits in type 1 diabetic patients, such as intense exercise practice and self-induced vomiting to control body shape and image.
- Disordered eating behavior is probably underdiagnosed in type 1 diabetic patients
- Disordered eating behaviors are different in type 1 and type 2 diabetic patients
- Binge eating disorder is the most frequent disorder in type 2 diabetic patients
- Emotional eating, dietary restraint, and disinhibition are eating behaviors that are often observed in obese patients. Whether they are more frequent in diabetic obese patients remains to be established.

Definitions

Type 1 diabetes: A metabolic disorder characterized by an autoimmune aggression of the pancreatic cells producing insulin. Symptoms are those of hyperglycemia (polyuria, thirst) and those of insulin deficiency (weight loss, muscle mass loss). Patients require exogenous insulin as a treatment.

Microvascular complications: In all types of diabetes chronic hyperglycemia damage small vessels. Organs such as the eyes, the kidney, and nerves are damaged.

Self-induced vomiting: This is a symptom specific of type 1 diabetes. Some patients act so as to vomit in the wish that it will help controlling body weight.

Insulin omission: Voluntary omission of the treatment with insulin

The Diabetes Prevention Program: A trial design to prevent type 2 diabetes by lifestyle modifications (healthy diet, reduction of body weight, increase in physical activity).

References

American Psychiatric Association (APS). Diagnostic and statistical manual of mental disorders. 4th ed. Washington, DC: American Psychiatric Association; 1994.

American Psychiatric Association (APS). Diagnostic and statistical manual of mental disorders. 4th ed, text rev. Washington, DC: American Psychiatric Association; 2000.

Colton P, Olmsted M, Daneman G, Rydall A, Rodin G. 2004;27:1654–9.

Colton P, Olmsted M, Daneman G, Rydall A, Rodin G. Diabetes Care. 2007a;30:2861–2.

Colton P, Olmsted M, Daneman G, Rydall A, Rodin G. Diabet Med. 2007b;24:424–9.

Crow S, Kendall D, Praus B, Thuras P. Int J Eat Disord. 2001;30:222–6.

Delahanty LM, Meigs JB, Hayden D, Williamson DA, Nathan DM, and THE DPP RESEARCH group. Diabetes Care. 2002;25:1992–8.

Dingemans AE, Bruna MJ, van Furth EF. Int J Obes Relat Metab Disord. 2002;26:299–307.

Golay A, Fossati M, Volery M, Rieker A. Diabetes Metabol. 2001;27:71–7.

Goodwin RD, Hoven CW, Spitzer RL. Int J Eat Disord. 2003;33:85–91.

Herpetz S, Albus C, Wagener R, Kocnar M. Comorbidity of diabetes and eating disorders. Diabetes Care. 1998;21:1110–5.

Jones JM, Lawson ML, Daneman D, Olmsted MP, Rodin G. Brit Med J. 2000;320:1563–6.

Kenardy J, Mensch M, Bowen K, Pearson SA. Diabetes Care. 1994;17:1197–9.

Mannucci E, Tesi F, Ricca V, Pierazzuoli E, Barciulli E, Moretti S. Int J Obes Relat Metab Disord. 2002;26:848–53.

Mela DJ. Proc Nutr Soc. 1996;55:803–8.

Olmsted MP, Daneman C, Rydal AC, Lawson ML, Rodin G. Int J Eat Disord. 2002;32:230–9.

Papelbaum M, Appolinario JC, Moreira Rde O, Ellinger VC, Kupfer R, Coutinho WF. Rev Bras Psiquiatr. 2005;27:135–8.

Peveler RC, Bryden KS, Neil HAW, Fairburn CG, Mayou RA, Dunger DB, Turner HM. Diabetes Care. 2005;28:84–8.

Rodin GM, Olmsted MP, Rydall AC, Maharaj SI, Colton PA, Jones JM, Biancucci LA, Daneman D. J Psychosomatic Res. 2002;53:943–9.

Ryan M, Gallanagh J, Livingstone MB, Gaillard C, Ritz P. Diabet Metabol. 2008;34:581–6.

Rydall AC, Rodin GM, Olmsted MP, Devenyi RG, Daneman D. N Engl J Med. 1997;336:1849–54.

Chapter 172
Binge Eating in Overweight and Obese Individuals with Type 2 Diabetes

Amy A. Gorin, Heather M. Niemeier, and Anna Schierberl Scherr

Abbreviations

NIDDM	Non-insulin-dependent diabetes mellitus
BED	Binge eating disorder
HbA_{1c}	Glycosylated hemoglobin
NIH	National Institutes of Health
DSM-IV	Diagnostic and Statistical Manual of Mental Disorders, 4th Edition

172.1 Introduction

Type 2 diabetes, or non-insulin-dependent diabetes mellitus (NIDDM), is a chronic metabolic disorder that results from the body's inability to produce or effectively use insulin. While serious complications such as cardiovascular disease, retinopathy, neuropathy, and nephropathy can occur, successful management is possible through medication, healthy lifestyle choices, and weight loss when indicated. Because of the link between dietary choices and the development and management of diabetes, understanding disordered eating patterns in this patient population is clinically relevant. This chapter focuses on binge eating – one of the most common forms of disordered eating – and its relationship with type 2 diabetes.

172.2 Binge Eating: Definitions and Prevalence

Binge eating disorder (BED) is characterized by recurrent binge eating episodes during which an individual consumes a large amount of food in a relatively short period of time and feels a loss of control over eating (American Psychiatric Assocation (APA) 1994). Accompanying characteristics may include eating rapidly, eating until feeling uncomfortably full, eating large amounts of food when not physically hungry, eating alone because of embarrassment about how much food is being consumed, and feeling disgusted, depressed, or guilty after overeating. To meet diagnostic criteria as

A.A. Gorin (✉)
Department of Psychology, Center for Health, Intervention, and Prevention, University of Connecticut,
2006 Hillside Road, Storrs, CT 06269-1248, USA
e-mail: amy.gorin@uconn.edu

V.R. Preedy et al. (eds.), *Handbook of Behavior, Food and Nutrition*,
DOI 10.1007/978-0-387-92271-3_172, © Springer Science+Business Media, LLC 2011

defined by the American Psychiatric Association's Diagnostic and Statistical Manual of Mental Disorders, 4th Edition (DSM-IV) (APA 1994), binge eating episodes must occur on average two or more times per week for a period of 6 months or more and must occur in the absence of compensatory behaviors such as purging, fasting, or excessive exercise.

BED is present in approximately 1–5% of the general population (Hay 1998; de Zwaan 2001; Striegel-Moore and Franco 2003; Hudson et al. 2007) and is much more common in individuals who are overweight or obese than in normal-weight individuals (Fairburn et al. 1998; Dingemans et al. 2002). While the exact prevalence of BED in obese adults is unknown, a recent study with a community sample found that 16% of obese individuals screened positive for BED (Grucza et al. 2007) and there is some evidence that binge eating is more likely to be present as the degree of obesity increases (Telch et al. 1988; de Zwaan 2001; De Freitas et al. 2008). Some of the highest rates of BED have been found among overweight and obese individuals seeking weight-loss treatment, with rates between 20% and 30% often reported (de Zwaan 2001; Dingemans et al. 2002; Castellini et al. 2008).

Given that the vast majority of individuals with type 2 diabetes are overweight or obese, it is not surprising that binge eating rates in this population are also elevated (Wing et al. 1989; Herpertz et al. 1998; Crow et al. 2001; Kenardy et al. 2001; Mannucci et al. 2002; Meneghini et al. 2006; Allison et al. 2007; Gorin et al. 2008). In a sample of 215 women with type 2 diabetes, 21% reported binge eating at least once per week and 14% met diagnostic criteria for BED (Kenardy et al. 2001). More recent work examining the connection between binge eating and diabetes has come from Look AHEAD, an National Institutes of Health (NIH)-funded multisite, randomized, controlled trial examining the long-term effect of intentional weight loss on cardiovascular disease in overweight and obese individuals with type 2 diabetes. At study entry, 11.7% of the 5145 Look AHEAD participants self-reported having one or more binge eating episodes in the prior 6 months and 2.6% met diagnostic criteria for BED (Gorin et al. 2008). In a subsample of 845 participants who underwent more formal diagnostic interviews, 1.4% were found to meet the full BED criteria (Allison et al. 2007). These numbers illustrate some important points (Table 172.1). First, there is often a discrepancy in BED rates when comparing self-report assessments to standardized diagnostic interviews, with higher BED rates typically found with self-report questionnaires (Streigel-Moore and Franco 2003). Second, many

Table 172.1 Issues to consider in evaluating research on binge eating

Diagnosis via self-report vs. clinical interview	Inconsistencies in the prevalence of BED across studies often are due to differences in assessment methods. Self-report questionnaires, while often briefer and more cost-effective than other methods, may yield higher rates of binge eating than more stringent, structured, interview-based methods (Striegel-Moore and Franco 2003). Brief self-report measures, however, may be more practical in clinical settings and for repeated use when tracking individuals longitudinally.
Binge eating disorder vs. Binge eating behavior	The DSM-IV criteria for BED require an average of 2 binge episodes per week over a 6 month period. Many researchers have suggested that this frequency criterion is arbitrary and that subthreshold cases are equally important to study. Thus, some researchers have expanded their investigations to include as binge eaters any individuals who report binge eating behavior regardless of frequency.
Community vs. treatment-seeking samples	Much of the work on binge eating has been done on overweight and obese individuals presenting for weight-loss treatment, a population with much higher rates of binge eating than found in the general public. Studies on treatment-seeking samples may confound the psychological and physical risk of binge eating with the negative effects of excessive weight. More research on both community and clinical samples is needed to understand the unique impact of binge eating on health.

This table outlines issues that need to be considered when examining research on binge eating. Research findings will be influenced by whether a binge eating diagnosis is made via self-report or clinical interviews, whether the research focuses on binge eating disorder or binge eating behavior more broadly defined, and whether the study includes a community sample or treatment-seeking individuals.

individuals engage in binge eating at subthreshold levels, making binge eating one of the most common forms of disordered eating in overweight and obese individuals with and without type 2 diabetes. Finally, rates of binge eating may vary according to whether the investigation focuses on a clinical or community sample, with the highest rates typically observed in weight loss-seeking samples.

172.3 Demographic, Psychological, and Health Risk Factors Associated with Binge Eating

Overweight and obese individuals who binge eat tend to be younger and are more likely to be college educated than their non-binge eating peers (Wing et al. 1989; Sherwood et al. 1999; Kenardy et al. 2001; Meneghini et al. 2006; Gorin et al. 2008). In treatment-seeking samples, BED is also more likely to be diagnosed in women than in men (Hay 1998; Grucza et al. 2007); however, this gender difference is smaller than that observed in other eating disorders and in community samples in which equivalent rates are often found (Striegel-Moore and Franco 2003; Grucza et al. 2007). Binge eating is present across racial and ethnic groups (Taylor et al. 2007; Nicado et al. 2007), with some evidence that Caucasian and African-American individuals are more prone to binge eating than other ethnicities, a trend that has emerged in both diabetic and nondiabetic samples (Meneghini et al. 2006; Gorin et al. 2008; Allison et al. 2007, Striegel-Moore and Franco 2008).

In addition to demographic differences, the psychological profiles of binge eaters tend to differ from their non-binge eating peers. Binge eating is often accompanied by body image disparagement, interpersonal difficulties, and low levels of self-esteem (Kuehnel and Wadden 1994; Eldredge et al. 1998; Striegel-Moore et al. 1998), perhaps creating a vulnerability for the development of other psychological disorders. Indeed, there is a high degree of comorbidity between binge eating and depressive disorders. Telch and Stice (1999) found that women with BED were twice as likely as weight-matched non-BED women to have a lifetime prevalence of major depressive disorder (49% vs. 28%, respectively) and these findings have been replicated by others (e.g., Kolotkin et al. 1987; Mussell et al. 1995). Connections between binge eating and bipolar disorder, anxiety disorders, and substance abuse have also been reported (Swinbourne and Touyz 2007; Wildes et al. 2008). In addition to elevated risk of many Axis I disorders, individuals who binge eat appear more likely to have a lifetime prevalence of a personality disorder (Telch and Stice 1999).

On indicators of physical health, binge eating is associated with increased adiposity, which may result in a higher risk of developing weight-related health problems such as type 2 diabetes, increased blood pressure, high cholesterol, gallbladder disease, gastrointestinal issues, and so on for those who binge eat (e.g., Telch et al. 1988; Herpertz et al. 1998; Cremonini et al. 2009). While excessive weight is assumed to be the pathway linking binge eating with negative health outcomes, some initial studies suggest that binge eating and body weight exert independent negative effects on health (e.g., Kenardy et al. 2001; Cremonini et al. 2009). Specific to type 2 diabetes, Kenardy and colleagues (2001) found a relationship between binge eating severity and HbA_{1c} levels that remained significant even after controlling for body weight and exercise habits (see Table 172.2). A similar relationship was reported by Meneghini et al. (2006). In a sample of 140 obese diabetics, binge eaters had worse glycemic control and, among individuals who reported binge eating, there was a positive correlation between binge eating severity and HbA_{1c} levels. However, there are some conflicting reports regarding binge eating and its association with glycemic control. Ryan and colleagues (2008), for example, found that binge eating status was not associated with HbA_{1c} among 94 adults with diabetes. Similarly, in Look AHEAD, we found no difference between binge eaters and non-binge eaters in HbA_{1c} levels or on other diabetes-specific measures such as diabetes treatment regimens (Gorin et al. 2008). With

Table 172.2 Key features of HbA$_{1c}$: glycosylated hemoglobin

1. Glycosylated (or glycated) hemoglobin (HbA$_{1c}$) is produced in red blood cells when blood sugar attaches to hemoglobin
2. A HbA$_{1c}$ blood test identifies the average plasma glucose concentration over the prior 2–3 months, serving as a good indicator of diabetes management
3. Higher HbA$_{1c}$ values suggest higher levels of blood glucose. Levels between 4 and 6% are considered normal, however, among individuals with diabetes, levels at or below 7% are often considered ideal
4. Higher HbA$_{1c}$ levels, particularly over an extended period of time, indicate greater risk of developing diabetes complications
5. Individuals with type 2 diabetes should have their HbA$_{1c}$ tested at least two times a year

This table lists the key facts of HbA$_{1c}$ when used as a measure of diabetes control

Table 172.3 Key facts about binge eating in community and clinical samples

Prevalence	• Binge eating disorder is found in 1–5% of community samples
	• Unlike other eating disorders, nearly equal rates of binge eating are found in men and women
	• The highest rates of binge eating are typically found in overweight and obese individuals presenting for weight-loss treatment
	• Overweight and obese individuals who have type 2 diabetes have rates of binge eating that are on par to the general overweight and obese population
Related comorbidities	• Individuals who binge eat tend to have higher rates of depressive disorders, personality disorders, and more issues with self-esteem and body image
	• Binge eating is associated with weight gain over time and consequently with increased risk of weight-related comorbidities
	• In overweight and obese individuals with type 2 diabetes, binge eating is associated with worse reported physical health but is not consistently associated with glycemic control
Treatment options	• If an individual who binge eats is also overweight or obese and wants to lose weight, a lifestyle management program that promotes weight loss through behavioral strategies is likely to both reduce binge eating behaviors and produce modest weight loss
	• In individuals with type 2 diabetes, recent evidence suggests that binge eating is not associated with weight-loss outcomes unless the behavior begins or persists during treatment
	• In individuals with and without type 2 diabetes, binge eating should be monitored throughout weight-loss treatment and additional support should be provided if the behavior continues
	• Additional treatment options for binge eating are cognitive behavioral treatment, interpersonal therapy, dialectical behavior therapy, and some antidepressants

Key features of binge eating, including prevalence rates, commonly associated psychological and physical comorbidities, and treatment options are described in this table

over 5,000 participants, this is the largest and most representative study conducted to date examining the diabetes–binge eating connection. While the link between binge eating and glycemic control is questionable, several studies suggest that overweight and obese diabetes patients who binge eat self-report worse physical health than their non-binge eating counterparts (e.g., Kenardy et al. 2001; Gorin et al. 2008; Table 172.3).

172.4 Treating Overweight and Obese Patients Who Binge Eat

There is debate in the eating disorders and obesity literatures about how best to approach treatment in individuals who present with both binge eating and excessive weight. The primary question is whether binge eating needs to be addressed prior to initiating a weight-loss program (DeAngelis 2002). Those who advocate treating binge eating first often express concerns that the highly structured nature of

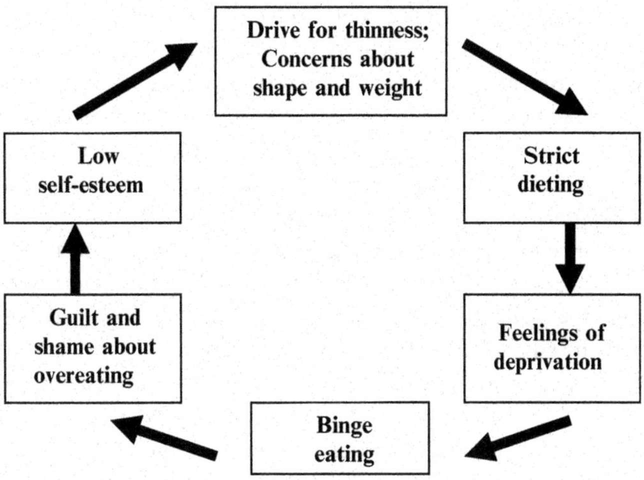

Fig. 172.1 Cognitive behavioral model of binge eating. This figure outlines the cognitive behavioral model of binge eating in which binge eating is believed to result from a cycle of concerns about weight and shape, strict dieting, and deprivation that leads to binge episodes followed by feelings of guilt and decreased self-esteem

behavioral weight-loss treatment will exacerbate binge eating in individuals with a predisposition for the behavior (e.g., Kenardy et al. 2001). This concern is consistent with the cognitive behavioral model of binge eating (Fig. 172.1), which conceptualizes binge eating as a result of a vicious cycle that begins with a thinness-obsessed culture that creates excessive concerns about weight and shape. In individuals predisposed to binge eating, these concerns lead to strict dieting and unrealistic food rules, which are impossible to maintain. Lack of adherence to these self-imposed rules leads to an abstinence violation effect, in which a small lapse in dieting gives way to a loss of control over eating and binge eating. Behavioral weight-loss treatment and its emphasis on caloric restriction, physical activity prescriptions, and increased attention to eating and weight through self-monitoring of food intake, physical activity, and frequent self-weighing may appear contraindicated for those patients engaging in binge eating.

There is some empirical evidence to suggest that binge eaters do not respond as well to weight-loss treatment and have poorer compliance than non-binge eaters. Pagoto and colleagues (2007) recently reported that binge eating was associated with poorer weight-loss outcomes among individuals participating in a hospital-based structured lifestyle program. Clinically significant weight losses were achieved by 37% of non-binge eaters compared to only 16% of individuals who reported binge eating at the start of treatment. Others have found that individuals who binge eat tend to report more extensive weight-loss histories, greater difficulties with weight control, and more unhealthy weight control practices than their non-binge eating peers, findings have emerged in both diabetic and nondiabetic samples (Venditti et al. 1996; Sherwood et al. 1999; Johnsen et al. 2003).

While findings such as these are concerning, most of the available evidence suggests that behavioral weight-loss treatment does not exacerbate or precipitate binge eating (Wadden et al. 2004; Butryn and Wadden 2005), that binge eating status is not associated with weight-loss outcomes (Sherwood et al. 1999; Teixeria et al. 2005; Delinsky et al. 2006), and that binge eating may in fact improve with weight-loss treatment (Wing et al. 1989; National Task Force 2000). For example, to examine whether behavioral weight-loss approaches precipitate binge eating, Wadden et al. (2004) randomly assigned 123 obese women reporting no binge eating at baseline to a 1,000 kcal diet using liquid meal replacement, a 1,200–1,500 kcal diet using conventional foods, or a nondieting program. Following treatment, there were no differences between the groups on binge eating behavior and those in the active weight-loss programs lost more weight and reported less depression than those in the nondieting condition. Furthermore, in a study of participants in a self-help program for weight loss with a relatively high prevalence of self-reported binge eating (41% of participants), Delinsky and colleagues (2006) found no relationship between binge eating and weight-loss outcomes. Indeed there is evidence that participation in behavioral weight loss can improve binge eating behavior (e.g., Agras et al. 1994; Porzelius et al. 1995). Given that weight loss is a cornerstone of effective diabetes management, this is welcome news for binge eaters with type 2 diabetes.

The most recent evidence to suggest that behavioral weight-loss treatment is appropriate for individuals with type 2 diabetes has come out of the Look AHEAD study. In this trial, overweight and obese individuals with type 2 diabetes were randomly assigned to an intensive lifestyle intervention or to a diabetes support and education control condition. The goals of the lifestyle intervention (modeled after the Diabetes Prevention Program) were to produce a mean weight loss of ≥7% of initial weight through caloric restriction and increased physical activity (Wadden et al. 2006). Binge eating behavior was assessed prior to starting the program and 1 year later. We found that about 10% of participants reported binge eating in the 6 months prior to starting the program and that the majority of these individuals (67%) were no longer engaging in binge eating at the 1-year follow-up. We also found that very few individuals, less than 4%, started binge eating during the first year of treatment, suggesting as others have found that behavioral weight-loss treatment does not generally lead to initiation of binge eating behavior (National Task Force on Prevention and Treatment of Obesity 2000; Butryn and Wadden 2005). Finally, we found that binge eating interfered with weight loss only in the small minority of participants for whom binge eating started, or persisted during treatment (see Fig. 172.2). The attenuated weight losses in those who started or continued to binge eat during treatment likely reflect the smaller decreases in caloric intake achieved in these individuals (Fig. 172.3).

Taken together, the findings from Look AHEAD further confirm the current recommendations (National Task Force on Prevention and Treatment of Obesity 2000) that individuals who binge eat

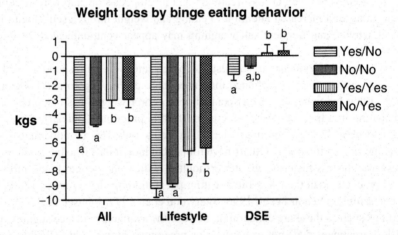

Fig. 172.2 One-year weight loss by binge eating status in overweight and obese individuals with type 2 diabetes participating in the Look AHEAD trial. This figure shows the amount of weight loss (means and standard deviations) overweight and obese individuals with type 2 diabetes achieved in the Look AHEAD trial. Individuals who reported binge eating at baseline but not at year 1 lost just as much weight as individuals who were not binge eating at either time point and lost more weight than those who reported binge eating at only year 1 or who were binge eating at baseline and year 1. Yes/No = reported binge eating at baseline but not 1-year; No/No = did not report binge eating at either time point; Yes/Yes = reported binge eating at both time points; No/Yes = did not report binge eating at baseline but did at 1-year (Originally published in Gorin et al. (2008, 1450). Copyright 2008, American Medical Association. All rights reserved)

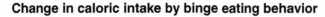

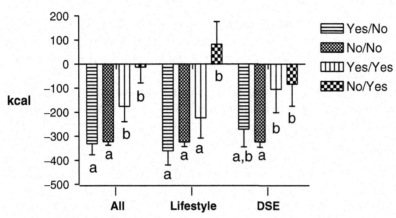

Fig. 172.3 One-year change in reported caloric intake by binge eating status in overweight and obese individuals with type 2 diabetes participating in the Look AHEAD trial. This figure shows changes in caloric intake (means and standard deviations) reported by overweight and obese individuals with type 2 diabetes in the Look AHEAD trial. Individuals who reported binge eating at baseline but not at year 1 decreased their daily intake just as much as individuals who were not binge eating at either time point and decreased their daily intake more than those who reported binge eating at only year 1 or who were binge eating at baseline and year 1. Yes/No = endorsed binge eating at baseline but not 1-year; No/No = did not endorse binge eating at either time point; Yes/Yes = endorsed binge eating at both time points; No/Yes = did not endorse binge eating at baseline but did at 1-year (Originally published in Gorin et al. (2008, 1451). Copyright 2008, American Medical Association. All rights reserved)

should not be discouraged from entering behavioral weight-loss programs. However, it is important to note that individuals who continued to binge eat and those who started to binge eat during treatment did not fare as well. Thus, it would appear useful to assess binge eating throughout treatment, not simply at entry into a program, and provide additional support as needed. Treatments for binge eating with proven effectiveness include several psychotherapies (cognitive behavioral, interpersonal, and dialectical behavior therapy) and antidepressants (Vocks et al. 2009), which may be considered as a supplement or alternative to behavioral weight-loss treatment.

172.5 Applications to Other Areas of Health and Disease

Binge eating is found in a large percentage of overweight and obese individuals with and without type 2 diabetes. If presenting for weight loss, these individuals are best served by a structured lifestyle modification program, with improvements likely to occur in both binge eating and weight status. Moreover, the modest weight losses of 5–10% of initial body weight typically produced by behaviorally based lifestyle modification programs will likely improve overall health parameters. Known benefits of weight losses of this size include a significant reduction in the likelihood of developing type 2 diabetes and hypertension and improvements in diabetes control, urinary incontinence, hyperlipidemia, and overall quality of life (e.g., Diabetes Prevention Program Research Group 2002; Subak et al. 2009). While psychotherapy and pharmacotherapy options have also been shown to be effective in treating binge eating (Vocks et al. 2009), these alternatives do not produce weight loss, which is an important component of successful diabetes management.

Summary Points

- Binge eating is one of the most common forms of eating pathology. Rates range from 1–5% in the general population to 20–30% in individuals entering weight-loss treatment. Binge eating rates in overweight and obese individuals with type 2 diabetes appear similar to the general overweight and obese population.
- Binge eating, by leading to excessive weight gain, may be associated with many obesity-related physical comorbidities such as hypertension and dyslipidemia. In overweight and obese individuals with type 2 diabetes, binge eating is associated with worse self-reported physical health but is not consistently associated with glycemic control.
- There is disagreement about how to treat overweight binge eaters. Some believe that the structured format of behavioral weight-loss treatment is inappropriate for this population. However, research suggests that most individuals who binge eat stop doing so during weight-loss treatment and have outcomes equivalent to non-binge eaters.
- Specific to type 2 diabetes, a recent study found that binge eating was only associated with poorer weight-loss outcomes if an individual started, or continued, to binge eat during a behavioral weight-loss program.

Definition of Key Terms

Binge eating disorder: Disorder recognized as a diagnosis of further study in the American Psychiatric Association's DSM-IV. Characterized by recurrent episodes of binge eating (eating a large amount of food in a discrete period of time while feeling a loss of control) and a lack of compensatory behaviors.

Behavioral weight-loss treatment: A structured lifestyle modification program, typically offered in academic clinics or university-based practices, which provides diet and physical activity prescriptions supported by training in key behavioral techniques such as self-monitoring, stimulus control, problem solving, and goal setting.

Diabetes Prevention Program: A landmark study published in 2002 demonstrating that a behaviorally based weight-loss program that produced modest weight losses (approximately 7% of initial body weight) and increased moderate intensity physical activity was more effective than metformin in reducing the risk of developing type 2 diabetes.

Look AHEAD trial: An ongoing randomized, controlled trial sponsored by NIH that is examining the long-term effects of intentional weight loss on cardiovascular outcomes in individuals with type 2 diabetes. Over 5,000 participants are enrolled in this 12-year, 16-center study (www. lookaheadtrial.org).

References

Agras WS, Telch CF, Arnow BA, Eldredge K, Wilfley DE, Raeburn SD, Henderson J, Marnell M. Behav Ther. 1994;25:209–38.

Allison KC, Crow SJ, Reeves RR, West DS, Foreyt JP, DiLillo VG, Wadden TA, Jeffery RW, Van Dorsten B, Stunkard AJ. Obesity 2007;15:1287–93.

American Psychiatric Association. Diagnostic and statistical manual of mental disorders. 4th ed. Washington, DC: Author; 1994.

Butryn ML, Wadden TA. Int J Eat Disord. 2005;37:285–93.

Castellini G, Lapi F, Ravaldi C, Vannacci A, Rotella CM, Faravelli C, Ricca V. Compr Psychiatry. 2008;49:359–63.

Cremonini F, Camilleri M, Clark MM, Beebe TJ, Locke GR, Zinsmeister AR, Herrick LM, Talley NJ. Int J Obes. 2009;33:342–53.

Crow S, Kendall D, Praus B, Thuras P. Int J Eat Disord. 2001;30:222–6.

DeAngelis T. Monit on Psych. 2002;33.

De Freitas SR, Appolinario JC, Souza ADM, Sichieri R. Int J Eat Disord. 2008;41:471–8.

Delinsky SS, Latner JD, Wilson GT. Obesity 2006;14:1244–9.

de Zwaan M. Int J Obes. 2001;25:S51–5.

Diabetes Prevention Program Research Group. N Engl J Med. 2002;346:393–403.

Dingemans AE, Bruna MJ, van Furth EF. Int J Obes. 2002;26:299–307.

Eldredge KL, Locke KD, Horowitz LM. Int J Eat Disord. 1998;23:383–90.

Fairburn CG, Doll HA, Welch SL, Hay PJ, Davies BA, O'Connor ME. Arch Gen Psychiatry. 1998;55:425–32.

Giovanni C, Lapi F, Ravaldi C, Vannacci A, Rotella CM, Faravelli C, Ricca V. Compr Psychiatry. 2008;24:359–63.

Gorin AA, Niemeier HM, Hogan P, Coday M, Davis C, Dilillo VG, Gluck ME, Wadden TA, West DS, Wlliamson D, Yanovski SZ. Arch Gen Psychiatry. 2008;65:1447–55.

Grucza RA, Przybeck TR, Cloninger CR. Compr Psychiatry. 2007;48:124–31.

Guerdjikova AI, McElroy SL, Kotwal R, Keck PE Jr. Eat Weight Disord. 2007;12:e19–23.

Hay P. Int J Eat Disord. 1998;2:371–82.

Herpertz S, Albus C, Wagener R, Kocnar M, Wagner R, Henning A, Best F, Foerster H, Schulze Schleppinghoff B, Thomas W, Kohle K, Mann K, Senf W. Diabetes Care. 1998;21:1110–6.

Hudson JI, Hiripi E, Pope HG Jr, Kessler RC. Biol Psych. 2007;61:348–58.

Johnsen LA, Gorin A, Stone AA, le Grange D. Eat Behav. 2003;3:295–305.

Kenardy J, Mensch M, Bowen K, Green B, Walton J, Dalton M. Eat Behav. 2001;20:222–6.

Kolotkin RL, Revis ES, Kirkley BG, Janick L. J Consult Clin Psych. 1987;55:872–6.

Kuehnel RH, Wadden TA. Int J Eat Disord. 1994;15:321–9.

Mannucci E, Tesi F, Ricca V, Pierazzuoli E, Barciulli E, Moretti S, Di Bernardo M, Travaglini R, Carrara S, Zucchi T, Placidi GF, Rotella CM. Int J Obes. 2002;26:848–53.

Meneghini LF, Spadola J, Florez H. Diabetes Care. 2006;29:2760.

Mussell MP, Mitchell JE, Weller CL, Raymond NC, Crow SJ, Crosby RD. Int J Eat Disord. 1995;17:395–401.

National Task Force on Prevention and Treatment of Obesity. Arch Intern Med. 2000;160:2581–9.

Nicado EG, Hong S, Takeuchi DT. Int J Eat Disord. 2007;40:S22–6.

Pagoto S, Bodenlos JS, Kantor L, Gitkind M, Curtin C, Ma Y. Obesity 2007;15:2557–9.

Porzelius LK, Houston C, Smith M, Arfkin C, Fisher E. Behav Ther. 1995;26:119–34.

Ryan M, Gallanagh J, Livinstone MB, Gaillard C, Ritz P. Diabetes Metab. 2008;34:581–6.

Sherwood NE, Jeffery RW, Wing RR. Int J Obes Relat Metab Disord. 1999;23:485–93.

Striegel-Moore RH, Franko DL. Int J Eat Disord. 2003;34:S19–29.

Striegel-Moore RH, Franko DL. Ann Rev Clin Psych. 2008;4:305–24.

Striegel-Moore RH, Wilson GT, Wilfley DE, Elder KA, Brownell KD. Int J Eat Disord. 1998;23:27–37.

Subak LL, Wing R, West DS, Franklin F, Vittinghoff E, Creasman JM, Richter HE, Myers D, Burgio KL, Gorin AA, Macer J, Kusek JW, Grady D; PRIDE Investigators. N Engl J Med. 2009;360:481–90.

Swinbourne JM, Touyz SW. Eur Eat Disord Rev. 2007;15:253–74.

Taylor JY, Caldwell CH, Baser RE, Faison N, Jackson JS. Prevalence of eating disorders among blacks in National Survey of American Life. Int J Eat Disord. 2007;40:S10–4.

Teixeria PJ, Going SB, Sardinha LB, Lohman TB. Obes Rev. 2005;6:43–65.

Telch CF, Stice E. J Consult Clin Psych. 1999;66:768–76.

Telch CF, Agras WS, Rossiter EM. Int J Eat Disord. 1988;23:7–15.

Venditti EM, Wing RR, Jakicic JM, Butler BA, Marcus MD. J Consult Clin Psych. 1996;64:400–5.

Vocks S, Tuschen-Caffier B, Pietrowsky R, Rustenbach SJ, Kersting A, Herpertz S. Int J Eat Disord. 2009.

Wadden TA, Foster GD, Sarwer DB, Anderson DA, Gladis M, Sanderson RS, Letchak RV, Berkowitz RI, Phelan S. Am J Clin Nutr. 2004;80:560–8.

Wadden TA, West DS, Delahanty L, Jakicic J, Rejeski J, Williamson D, Berkowitz RI, Kelley DE, Tomchee C, Hill JO, Kumanyika S, Look AHEAD Research Group. Obesity 2006;14:737–52.

Wildes JE, Marcus MD, Fagiolini A. Psychiatry Res. 2008;161:51–8.

Wing RR, Marcus M, Epstein L, Blair E, Burton L. Int J Eat Disord. 1989;8:671–9.

Part XXX
Nutrient Excess and Toxicity

Chapter 173
High Blood Glucose and Damage to Neuronal Tissue

Robert R. Miller Jr.

Abbreviations

AChE	Acetylcholine esterase
BDNF	Brain-derived neurotrophic factor
ChAT	Choline acetyltransferase
DHA	Docosahexaenoic acid
10-FTHF DH	10-formyltetrahydrofolate dehydrogenase
10-FTHF hydrolase	10-formyltetrahydrofolate hydrolase
GDNF	Glial cell line-derived neurotrophic factor
GFAP	Glial fibrillary acidic protein
GLUTS	Glucose transporters
HoCys	Homocysteine
5-Methyl THF	5-methyltetrahydrofolate
NTDs	Neural tube defects
NMDA	N-methyl-D-aspartate
SAH	S-adenosylhomocysteine
SAM	S-adenosylmethionine
STZ	Streptozocin
TBARS	Thiobarbituric acid reactive substances
T1D	Type-1 diabetes
T2D	Type-2 diabetes

173.1 Introduction

Type-1 diabetes (T1D; insulin-dependent), type-2 diabetes (T2D; non-insulin-dependent), and gestational diabetes can damage and impair the nervous system. Type-1 and type-2 diabetics have a 25-fold increase in the risk of retinopathy-associated blindness (Wolff 1993), a 4- to 12-fold increased risk of stroke and ischemia-induced cerebral damage (Scott et al. 1999; Bemur et al. 2007), and

R.R. Miller Jr. (✉)
Biology Department, Hillsdale College, 278 N. West St., Dow Science 213,
Hillsdale, MI 49242-1205, USA
e-mail: bob.miller@hillsdale.edu

V.R. Preedy et al. (eds.), *Handbook of Behavior, Food and Nutrition*,
DOI 10.1007/978-0-387-92271-3_173, © Springer Science+Business Media, LLC 2011

approximately 50% of all type-1 and type-2 diabetics undergo some form of neuropathy (Negi et al. 2008). Among the various risk factors associated with stroke and ischemia, both mild and severe hyperglycemia within 24 h of the onset of cerebral ischemia exacerbates cerebral damage and increases mortality (Lanier 1999).

Hertz (2008) has recently reviewed how glucose is used as virtually the only metabolic fuel in adult neurons, astrocytes, and oligodendrites. Glucose-6-phosphate is anaerobically metabolized to pyruvate via glycolysis. Because neurons and oligodendrites lack pyruvate decarboxylase, astrocytes must convert pyruvate to acetyl coenzyme-A and then aerobically convert acetyl coenzyme-A to α-ketobutyrate. Under aerobic conditions, astrocytes supply neurons with α-ketobutyrate so neurons can complete aerobic respiration via the Kreb's cycle, or the astrocytes can convert α-ketobutyrate to glutamate and then decarboxylate glutamate to glutamine. Astrocytes then release glutamine to nearby neurons and neurons deaminate the incorporated glutamine to glutamate. Neurons can use glutamate as a neural transmitter, which when released, activates nearby N-methyl-D-aspartate (NMDA) receptors and opens Ca^{+2} channels.

During ischemia, astrocytes, oligodendrites, and neurons convert pyruvate to lactate (acidosis). Because of oxygen-debt, neurons are unable to oxidatively deaminate glutamate to α-ketobutyrate and release excessively high glutamate levels and overstimulate nearby neurons via NMDA receptors (Hertz 2008). Coupled with the overstimulation of NMDA receptors and increased cytoplasmic Ca^{+2} levels, changes in the nearby microvascular system are observed associated with local inflammatory responses that include neutrophil recruitment and the formation of reactive oxygen species (oxygen radicals, hydroxyl radicals, and peroxynitrite radicals). Reactive oxygen species can be generated by enhanced neutrophil NADPH oxidase and xanthine oxidase activities and by activation of neuronal nitrous oxide synthase. Any Fe^{+2}-containing enzyme, such as a cytochrome released from mitochondria into the cytoplasm of cells undergoing apoptosis, or any enzyme that produces H_2O_2 can potentially generate hydroxyl radicals (HO^-) at the expense of oxygen radicals (O^-). This is especially true if the newly produced H_2O_2 cannot be converted to H_2O and O_2 by either catalase or glutathione peroxidase. As H_2O_2 levels increase, H_2O_2 can decompose into HO^- via the Harber–Weiss reaction (Miller 2004).

$$H_2O_2 + Fe^{+2} \rightarrow OH^- + HO^- + Fe^{+3} \rightarrow \text{Fenton Reaction}$$

$$+Fe^{+3} + 2O^- \rightarrow Fe^{+2} + O_2 \rightarrow \text{Reduction of ferricion}$$

$$H_2O_2 + 2O^- \rightarrow OH^- + HO^- + Fe^{+3} \rightarrow \text{Harber-Weiss reaction}$$

All of these events initiate oxidative stress, oxidative damage via membrane lipid peroxidation, necrosis, apoptosis, mitochondrial involvement, and have recently been reviewed (Wolff 1993; Gonzalez-Zulueta et al. 1998; Vincent et al. 2005; Negi et al. 2008; Bemur et al. 2007; Norenberg and Rao 2007; Hertz 2008; Friedlander 2009). This article will review articles largely excluded from these reviews.

173.2 Type-1 Diabetes: Cognitive Impairment, Neuropathy, and Astrogliosis

Type-1 diabetic children, who suffer prolonged periods of hyperglycemia and momentary episodes of hypoglycemia, exhibit cognitive deficits (Northam et al. 2001; Hershey et al. 2005) and regional differences in brain anatomy as compared to nondiabetics (Sharma et al. 2003; Perantie et al. 2007).

Hershey et al. (2005) reported deficits in spatial memory as a function of hypoglycemia in type-1 diabetic children as compared to controls, and Malone et al. (2008) reported reduced neuron dendritic branching, reduced spine density within the parietal cortex, and hyperglycemia-induced spatial memory deficits in streptozocin (STZ)-treated rats. Exposure of rats to STZ, an agent that destroys pancreatic β-cells, caused reductions in hippocampus-dependent spatial learning, which was associated with hyperglycemia-induced increased brain sorbitol levels, increased brain inositol levels, and decreased brain taurine levels in male rats as compared to controls (Malone et al. 2008). Type-2 diabetics may also have abnormally low taurine levels in brain due to enhanced excretion of taurine (Sankarasubbaiyan et al. 2001). Beauguis et al. (2008) reported elevated expression of hypothalamic hormones, including oxytocin and vasopressin, and elevated plasma glucocorticosteroid levels, and astrogliosis within the hippocampus of STZ-injected female mice. Astrogliosis was measured by the induction of glial fibrillary acidic protein (GFAP) and is associated with neuropathy (Beauguis et al. 2008).

By the use of magnetic resonance imaging, Sharma et al. (2003) demonstrated reduced brain volume in adults (18–50 years old) who suffered T1D for a period exceeding 10 years as compared to controls. Also by use of magnetic resonance imaging, Perantie et al. (2007) reported smaller gray matter volume in the left temporal region in diabetic children (7–17 years old) who suffered from periods of severe hypoglycemia as compared to hypoglycemia-naive diabetic peers. Reduced gray matter within the left superior temporal and angular gyri has been reported in adults who suffered from T1D (Musen et al. 2006) and this same region of the human brain has been associated with episodic memory (Cabeza et al. 2004). Meanwhile, hyperglycemia in type-1 diabetic children was associated with reduced gray matter in the right cuneus and precuneus, reduced white matter in the right posterior parietal region, and increased gray matter volume in the right prefrontal lobes as compared to nondiabetic siblings (Perantie et al. 2007).

Neurons express GLUT-3 (glucose transporter-3), while astrocytes express GLUT-1 and GLUT-2. Consequently, nerves, retina, and kidneys will undergo an intense hyperglycemia-induced D-glucose influx in type-1 and type-2 diabetics because GLUT-1, GLUT-2, and GLUT-3 are insulin-insensitive as compared to GLUT-4 (Anderson et al. 2001). This D-glucose influx causes sorbitol synthesizes by the polyol pathway during neuropathy because hexokinase, which normally converts glucose to glucose-6-phosphate, becomes saturated and excess glucose is then converted to sorbitol via aldose reductase. The polyol pathway and subsequent formation of glycated proteins (advanced glycation end products; Wolff 1993) is active during diabetic retinopathy (Sun et al. 2006; Negi et al. 2008) and Sun et al. (2006) reported that the use of an aldose reductase inhibitor (ARI-809) ameliorated the severity of diabetic retinopathy.

173.3 Type-1 Diabetes: Peripheral Neuropathy and Glial Cell Line-Derived Neurotrophic Factor (GDNF)

Gastrointestinal dysfunction occurs in many diabetics and gastrointestinal tract motility changes involve losses of peripheral neurons (neuropathy). Increased apoptosis rates have been observed in neurons within dorsal root ganglion in STZ-treated rats (Guo et al. 2004) and the neuropathy has been associated with a reduction in neurotrophic factors (Leinninger et al. 2004). One such neurotrophic factor is GDNF. After being released by glial cells, GDNF binds to Ret tyrosine kinase receptors on neuron membranes and stimulates MAPK (Mitogen-Activated Protein Kinase) and P13K signaling pathways. Activation of the P13K pathway causes phosphorylation of Akt and inhibits the translocation of the forkhead box O3a (FOXO3a) transcription factor, which blocks apoptosis by inhibiting the transcription of the proapoptotic genes *Bim* and *Puma* (Srinivasan et al. 2005;

Anitha et al. 2006). Anitha et al. (2006) reported increased apoptosis rates in myenteric neurons, reduced Akt-phosphorylation in myenteric neurons, and delayed gastric emptying (increased intestinal transit time) in STZ-treated diabetic rats, and these hyperglycemia-related events were reversed with exogenous GDNF.

173.4 Type-1 Diabetes: Acetylcholine

The neural transmitter acetylcholine plays an essential role in learning and memory within the basalis magnocellularis and activates cholinergic innervation to the neocortex (Winkler et al. 1995). Thus, choline uptake, enzymes that modulate acetylcholine levels, and acetylcholine receptors are of interest. Mooradian (1987) reported that choline transport across the blood–brain barrier is reduced in STZ-induced diabetic rats. Type-1 and type-2 diabetic mothers have significantly lower plasma choline phosphoglyceride docosahexaenoic acid (DHA) levels in umbilical cords and in circulating red blood cells of pregnant women as compared to nondiabetic mothers (Min et al. 2005a, b). Improved spatial cognition with dietary DHA supplementation was associated with increased *Fos* expression within the CA1 nucleus within the hippocampus of nondiabetic rats (Tanabe et al. 2004), and a significant correlation coefficient between blood DHA levels and Peabody Picture Vocabulary Test scores (a test of listening comprehension and vocabulary acquisition) (r = 0.46; $p < 0.018$) was observed in healthy 4-year-old children (Ryan and Nelson 2008).

Once choline enters, neurons convert choline to acetylcholine via choline acetyltransferease. However, choline acetyltransferase (ChAT) activities were reduced in the hippocampus of STZ-treated rats as compared to controls (Blokland and Jolies 1993; Terwel et al. 1995). Terwel et al. (1995) observed decreased septum masses as hippocampal ChAT activities decreased in STZ-treated rats, and Blokland and Jolies (1993) reported impaired spatial discrimination performances as hippocampal ChAT activities decreased in STZ-treated rats. While Welsh and Wecker (1991) failed to report significant differences in choline or acetylcholine levels in either the striatum or hippocampus within brain slices obtained from STZ-injected rats, reduced release of acetylcholine in striatal slices of STZ-injected rats was reported.

Not only is the synthesis and release of acetylcholine reduced within the hippocampal region of STZ-treated rats, the degradation of acetylcholine to acetate and choline via acetylcholine esterase (AChE) is inhibited in STZ-treated (Ashokkumar et al. 2006) and alloxan-treated rats (Khandkar et al. 1995; Ghareeb and Hussen 2008). Like STZ, alloxan kills pancreatic β-cells and induces T1D. Ashokkumar et al. (2006) reported that brain AChE activities decreased as brain thiobarbituric acid reactive substances (TBARS) levels increased in STZ-treated rats. TBARS are a measure of oxidative stress and are lipid peroxidation intermediates. Ghareeb and Hussen (2008) reported that brain glutathione-S-transferase activities decreased as brain membrane-bound and soluble-AChE activities decreased in alloxan-treated rats. Oxidative stress is also supported by Ates et al. (2007) who reported increased lipid peroxidation levels, as measured by malondialdehyde, increased nitric oxide levels, and reduced glutathione levels in the hippocampus, cortex, cerebellum, brain stem, and spinal cord of STZ-treated rats as compared to controls. Administering the antioxidant, resveratrol, ameliorated hyperglycemia-induced oxidative stress in STZ-treated rats (Ates et al. 2007). Kamboj et al. (2008) reported that N-acetylcysteine attenuated hyperglycemia-induced decreased glutathione levels, decreased total thiol levels, and decreased AChE activities within the cerebral cortex, cerebellum, and brain stem of STZ-treated rats as compared to controls. N-acetylcysteine is a precursor of cysteine and exerts antioxidant effects by either reacting directly with electrophiles or by facilitating the generation of the antioxidant, glutathione (Song et al. 2004). Kamboj et al. (2008) also reported cognitive deficits and reduced activities of several antioxidant enzymes including superoxide dimutase, catalase, and glutathione reductase within the cerebral cortex, cerebellum, and brain stem in STZ-treated rats as compared to controls. Thus, the loss of the "cholinergic phenotype" in the brains of type-1 diabetics correlates with the generation of reactive oxygen species and oxidative stress.

173.5 Type-2 Diabetes: Acetylcholine

Gautam et al. (2009) recently demonstrated that the failure of acetylcholine to stimulate brain neuronal M3 muscuranic acetylcholine receptors caused pronounced hypoplasia of the anterior pituitary gland. They produced brain-specific M3 muscuranic acetylcholine receptor knockout mice that exhibited a dwarf phenotype, abnormally small anterior pituitary glands, and reduced ability to synthesize and release serum growth hormone, prolactin, and gonadotropic hormone. Treatment of these M3 receptor-deficient knockout mice with CJC-1295, a synthetic gonadotropic hormone-releasing factor, restored normal pituitary size and serum gonadotropic hormone levels. Thus, acetylcholine and M3 muscuranic acetylcholine receptors within the hypothalamus play a role in the development of anterior pituitary.

While anterior pituitary development requires cholinergic neurons and the stimulation of M3 muscuranic acetylcholine receptors, overstimulation of M3 muscuranic acetylcholine receptors within the peripheral nervous system is associated with T2D. Most animals that model T2D, as reflected by obesity and hyperinsulinemia, have increased vagal cholinergic activities and are mediated by G-protein-coupled muscuranic receptor subtypes (M1–M5) within the parasympathetic nervous system (Caulfield and Birdsall 1998). Gautam et al. (2006) mimicked T2D by inducing obesity, glucose intolerance, and insulin resistance in male $M3R^{-/-}$ and $M3R^{-/-}ob^{-/-}$ mice by either feeding mice high-fat diets or by destroying glucose-receptive neurons in the ventromedial nucleus of the hypothalamus with gold thioglucose. The $M3R^{-/-}$ mice lacked G-protein coupled M3 muscuranic receptors and the $M3R^{-/-}ob^{-/-}$ mice lacked M3 muscuranic receptors and were also leptin deficient. In all experimental animals, the lack of M3 muscuranic receptors protected animals against overeating, hyperglycemia, hyperinsulinemia, and all mice lacking M3 muscuranic receptors had increased fatty acid β-oxidation rates. Thus, while fetal and neonatal animals may require M3 muscuranic receptor stimulation for anterior pituitary development, antagonists of peripheral M3 muscuranic receptors may help control T2D.

173.6 Type-2 Diabetes: Cognitive Impairment and Neuropathy

Individuals who suffer from T2D frequently exhibit insulin resistance, leptin resistance, hypertriglyceridemia, and obesity (Van Gaal et al. 1999; Ma et al. 2002; Margetic et al. 2002). Plasma leptin levels were correlated to plasma insulin levels, cholesterol levels, and triglyceride levels in 107 elderly women (67–78 years old) and the correlation coefficients (r) were 0.56 ($p \leq 0.001$), 0.23 ($p \leq 0.05$), 0.25 ($p \leq 0.01$), respectively (Zamboni et al. 2004). Elevated circulating triglyceride levels among individuals suffering from T2D have been associated with poor cognitive performance (Perimuter et al. 1988). Insights into this complex and poorly understood set of relationships have come from studying lean and obese mice. Triolein (a triglyceride) injected directly into the brains of lean CD-1 male mice impaired the NMDA receptor-mediated maintenance of hippocampal long-term synaptic potential as measured by three different measures of cognitive paradigms. The injection of free-palmitate into brains failed to induce cognitive deficits. Meanwhile, lowering blood triglyceride levels, through the administration of gemfibrozil, reversed cognitive impairments and improved measures of oxidative stress in the brains of obese mice. Thus, hypertriglyceridemia somehow inhibits hippocampal long-term potentiation by blocking NMDA receptor activation and NMDA receptor-induced Ca^{+2} influxes into neurons (Farr et al. 2008).

173.7 Type-2 Diabetes: BDGF and VGF

Some individuals have a predisposition in developing T2D and this predisposition may involve brain-derived neurotrophic factor (BDNF). BDNF is a member of the neurotrophin family that includes nerve growth factor, neurotrophin-3, and neurotrophin-4/5 (Skup 1994; Barbacid 1995; Lewin and Barde 1996; Lindsay et al. 1994). BDNF promotes neurite outgrowth, provides tropic support for neurons in both the central and peripheral nervous system, and has been successfully used in the treatment of several neurological disorders (Sendtner et al. 1996; Yuen et al. 1996) and the injection of BDNF into obese mice ameliorated hyperglycemia (Ono et al. 1997; Tonra et al. 1999; Nakagawa et al. 2000). The recent creation of the transgenic mouse strain, $Timo^{-/-}$, has resulted in reduced and disrupted hippocampal *Bdnf* expression and is associated with obesity and hyperglycemia (Sha et al. 2007). Recently, the injection of BDNF into predisposed obese and hyperglycemic mice ($db^{-/-}$), which possess abnormal leptin receptors, blocked the onset of T2D (Yamanaka et al. 2008). Thus, reduced *Bdnf* expression appears associated with the onset of T2D.

VGF (nonacronymic protein) was originally identified as a neutrophin-regulated gene product in PC12 cells (Levi et al. 1985) and is robustly induced by BDNF and neurotrophin-3 and marginally induced by fibroblast growth factors and insulin (Levi et al. 1985, 2004; Salton et al. 2000). In the rat brain, VGF isoforms are distributed throughout the brain, spinal cord, and pancreas with very high abundance in the hypothalamus and hippocampus (Chakraborty et al. 2006). Interest in VGF grew markedly after VGF-deficient mice were created that are lean, hypermetabolic, and resistant to obesity (Hahm et al. 1999). Targeted deletion of the *Vgf* gene, through the creation of several strains of knock-out mice, promoted reduced circulating blood glucose and reduced circulating insulin levels in leptin-deficient $ob^{-/-}$ mice and in $MCR4^{-/-}$ mice, who fail to express hypothalamic melanocortin-4-receptors (Watson et al. 2005). Watson et al. (2005) hypothesized that VGF-ablation induced greater glucose use, greater insulin sensitivity, and obesity-resistance in mice predisposed to T2D.

Vgf gene expression produces *Vgf*-mRNA and a VGF precursor protein that is processed, cleaved, and secreted through a regulated pathway into a number of VGF peptides/isoforms (Chakraborty et al. 2006). Bartolomucci et al. (2006) isolated TLQP-21, which is a VGF-peptide, from rat brains. Surprisingly, chronic injection of TLQP-21 into the brains of rats fed high-fat diets, reduced circulating leptin levels and caused reduced body mass as compared to rats fed only high-fat diets (Bartolomucci et al. 2006). Thus, VGF-derived peptides may up- or downregulate appetite, metabolism, and leptin resistance through complex signaling pathways and are dependent on the presence of VGF isoform.

173.8 Gestational Diabetes

Neural tube defects (NTDs) are the most common abnormality seen within a fetus during gestational diabetes and a major source of neonatal mortality (Becerra et al. 1990; Ramos-Arroyo et al. 1992). Spina bifida, which is a failure of the neural tube to fuse in posterior regions, is the most common form of NTDs and is observed in infants of diabetic mothers (McLeod and Ray 2002). After neural tube fusion, the proliferation of neuroepithelial cells, the outward migration of cells, the differentiation of both neural tube cells and neural crest cells, and cell death via apoptosis of nonfunctional neurons follow.

Gao and Gao (2007) reported that STZ-induced gestational diabetes caused decreased cell proliferation, as measured by bromodeoxyuridine incorporation into proliferating cells, and increased apoptosis rates in neuroepithelial cells within embryonic mouse spinal cords. Apoptosis was measured by terminal deoxynucleotidyl transferase-mediated dUTP nick end-labeled DNA fragments (TUNEL), and by monitoring activated caspase-3 levels via Western blots. Previously, Reece et al. (1985) observed decreased numbers of mitotic cells throughout the neuroepithelium but with a predominance at the site of failed neural tube closure in rat embryos cultured in male rat serum containing high D-glucose (7,500 mg/L) levels as compared to controls cultured with less glucose (1,250 mg/L).

A high incidence of congenital NTDs and reduced levels of *Pax-3* mRNA have been reported in mouse embryos collected from hyperglycemic dames whose diabetes was induced with either STZ or phlorizen treatments (Fine et al. 1999). *Pax-3* codes for a transcription factor necessary for neural tube development and reduced *Pax-3* expression was associated with apoptosis, as measured by TUNEL-labeled DNA fragments, within the neuroepithelium of mouse neural tubes (Fine et al. 1999). Jia et al. (2008) recently isolated and cultured neural progenitor cells from the cerebral cortex of mouse embryos (stage 12.2). When the neural progenitor cells were cultured in medium that contained high D-glucose levels (45 mM), increased reactive oxygen species levels, increased Annexin-V levels, and increased nuclear cAbl and p53 levels were observed as compared to control cells cultured in medium that contained less D-glucose (25 mM). Activated Annexin-V promotes membrane blebbing during apoptosis by carrying phosphatidylserine from the cytoplasmic side of the cell membrane to the external side of the cell membrane. Meanwhile, c-Abl is a Src-related nonreceptor tyrosine kinase that can move from the cytoplasm to the nucleus via actin cytoskeletal filaments. Nuclear c-Abl appears to contribute to p53-dependent apoptosis (Yuan et al. 1996).

173.9 Gestational Diabetes: Arachidonic Acid

Gestational diabetes is associated with abnormally low arachidonic acid levels and DHA levels in maternal red blood cells and umbilical cords (Min et al. 2005b). Because the n-3 isomer of arachidonic acid (20:4, n-3) can be elongated and desaturated to DHA (22:6, n-3) (Reitz 1992) and because the n-6 isomer of arachidonic acid (20:4, n-6) can be metabolized to a wide variety of potent signaling compounds, known as prostaglandins (Anggard and Samuelsson 1965), maternal deficiencies in arachidonic acid (both 20:4, n-3 and 20:4, n-6) may have profound effects on fetal development. In response to this hypothesis, subcutaneous injections of arachidonic acid into pregnant STZ-treated rats failed to alter maternal blood glucose levels, maternal weight gain, or embryonic weights. However, the incidence of NTDs was reduced from 11% to 3.8% ($p < 0.005$), the frequency of cleft palate was reduced from 11% to 4% ($p < 0.005$), and the incidence of micrognatha was reduced from 7% to 0.8% ($p < 0.001$) as compared to controls (Goldman et al. 1985). Unfortunately, it is unclear whether Goldman et al. (1985) injected the n-3 isomer of arachidonic acid, the n-6 isomer of arachidonic acid, or a mixture of both isomers (n-3 and n-6).

173.10 Gestational Diabetes: Increased Fetal Brain Insulin-Binding Sites

Insulin, insulin receptors, and glucose transporters (GLUTs) exist within the brain (Baskin et al. 1987; Schwartz et al. 1992). In order to test the effect of gestational diabetes on the density of insulin receptors, the density GLUTs, and the frequency of GLUTs within various regions of the embryonic rat brain, Leloup et al. (2004) implanted catheters into the jugular veins of pregnant mice and infused the dames with either saline or 30% glucose solutions for a period of 48 h. Just before birth (21.5 days), the infusions were halted and rat fetuses were removed by cesarean sections. The major result was an increased density of insulin receptors in the ventromedial hypothalamus, the arcuate nucleus, the lateral hypothalamus, and in extrahypothalamic areas within the ventromedial hypothalamus in fetal brains obtained from hyperglycemic dames as compared to controls. Among the predominant neural GLUTs identified were GLUT-1 (endothelial and glial cells) and GLUT-3 (neuronal cells). GLUT-2 and GLUT-4 were also identified but at lower levels on astrocytes and neurons within the hypothalamus and spinal cord. The authors concluded that the effect of gestational diabetes was on the density of insulin receptors within the specific fetal brain areas and not on the GLUTs because no relationship could be found between GLUT densities and hyperinsulinism within specific areas of the fetal brain (Leloup et al. 2004).

173.11 Embryonic Diabetes: Apoptosis, Lipid Peroxidation, and Homocysteine

We have also been studying the effects of hyperglycemia in developing chick embryos (Miller et al. 2005; Coes et al. 2008; Miller et al. 2009). For some, this seems like an unlikely choice of animal to model a human condition. However, unlike the mammalian embryo, the avian embryo (cleidoic egg) is a closed system that offers the ability to solely observe embryonic responses to a teratogen as compared to combined maternal responses, fetal responses, and maternal-to-fetal transport systems. It has also been argued that adult birds may naturally reflect a hyperglycemic condition as compared to mammals (Hazelwood 1986). This last argument is partially based on the normally high, at least by mammalian standards, avian serum D-glucose levels (2,000–2,500 mg/L) (Hazelwood 2000).

We have made chick embryos hyperglycemic by injecting D-glucose, L-glucose, or pig anti-insulin antibodies into the air sac of fertile chicken eggs during the first 3 days of avian development. Controls were injected with avian saline (0.72% NaCl, v/v) (Miller et al. 2005; Coles et al. 2008; Miller et al. 2009). After incubation, we collected blood, brains, and livers from embryos at 11 days (theoretical stage 37; Hamburger and Hamilton 1951) and at 18 days of development (theoretical stage 44; Hamburger and Hamilton 1951). Chicks normally hatch in 21 days. Thus, 11 days of chick development is comparable to mid-second trimester and 18 days of development is comparable to mid-third trimester of human development. Our injection period of the first 3 days of chick development (E_{0-2}) is comparable to 0–38 days of human development (≤ 5.4 weeks). Early pregnancy factor can be detected in maternal serum 24–48 h after fertilization, while human chorionic gonadotropin levels within maternal urine cannot be detected until the second week of human pregnancy corresponding with implantation (Nahhas and Barnea 1990). Hence, our injection period in chick embryos corresponds to before and shortly after most women learn of their pregnancies.

The injection of either exogenous D-glucose or L-glucose, concentrations ranging from 9.29 to 18.58 μmol/kg egg, caused embryonic hyperglycemia, reduced embryo masses, and reductions in the % living chick embryos at 18 days of development (Miller et al. 2005). Also noted were increased serum alanine transaminase activities (a marker of liver trauma), increased hepatic caspase-3 activities (a marker of apoptosis), increased hepatic liver lipid hydroperoxides levels, and decreased arachidonic acid (20:4, n-6) levels within hepatic membrane phospholipids of all embryos injected with either exogenous D-glucose or L-glucose as compared to controls. Also noted was decreased DHA (22:6, n-3) levels within hepatic membrane phospholipids when eggs were injected with 18.58 μmol D-glucose/kg egg, 9.29 μmol L-glucose/kg egg, or 18.58 μmol L-glucose/kg egg as compared to controls. The hyperglycemia-induced reductions in long-chain polyunsaturated membrane fatty acids, increased hepatic lipid hydroperoxide levels, and increased hepatic caspase-3 activities all indicate hyperglycemia-induced apoptosis and membrane lipid peroxidation within hepatic membranes.

Within chick brains at 18 days of development, decreased brain masses, increased brain caspase-3 activities (indicating apoptosis), and increased brain lipid hydroperoxides levels were all observed in exogenous D-glucose- or L-glucose-treated embryos as compared to controls. While the authors did not monitor the effects of hyperglycemia on brain membrane fatty acid composition, it appears likely that hyperglycemia-induced increased apoptosis rates and hyperglycemia-induced lipid peroxidation occurred in developing chick brains at 18 days of development (theoretical stage 44; Hamburger and Hamilton 1951) (Miller et al. 2005).

These observations were extended into an earlier developmental stage (11 days of development; theoretical stage 37; Hamburger and Hamilton 1951). L-glucose (9.29 μmol/kg egg) was injected into the air sac of fertile chicken eggs during the first 3 days of embryonic development (E_{0-2}), which promoted embryonic hyperglycemia, reduced embryo viability, increased membrane lipid peroxidation, increased brain homocysteine (HoCys) levels, and decreased S-adenosylmethionine (SAM)/S-adenosylhomocysteine (SAH) ratios at 11 days of development (Coles et al. 2008). Exogenous L-glucose, which inhibits GLUTs from binding endogenous D-glucose, caused a 1.7-fold increase in serum D-glucose levels ($p \leq 0.05$), a 1.4-fold decrease in percentage of living embryos ($p \leq 0.05$), a 1.1-fold decrease in embryo masses ($p \leq 0.05$), and a 1.4-fold decrease in embryonic brain masses ($p \leq 0.05$) as compared to controls. Exogenous L-glucose also caused a 3.8-fold increase in brain lipid hydroperoxide levels, a 1.9-fold ($p \leq 0.05$) decrease in Σ unsaturated/saturated brain membrane fatty acids ratios, and a 1.8-fold ($p \leq 0.05$) decrease in Σ long-chain/short-chain membrane fatty acids ratios as compared to controls. L-glucose-treated embryos had decreased levels of brain membrane arachidonic acid (20:4, n-6) and DHA (22–6, n-3) as compared to controls ($p \leq 0.05$). These observations are consistent with the hypothesis of hyperglycemia-induced brain membrane lipid peroxidation (Coles et al. 2008).

Exogenous L-glucose also caused a 12-fold increase in brain HoCys levels, a 2.5-fold decrease in SAM levels, and a twofold increase in SAH levels as compared to controls ($p \leq 0.05$) at 11 days of chick development. These hyperglycemia-induced alterations in HoCys, SAM, and SAH levels indicate methylation difficulties and were somewhat attenuated by exogenous folic acid (181.2 μmol/kg egg) (Coles et al. 2008). Hyperglycemia-induced hyperhomocysteinemia is also of great interest because HoCys is both an agonist and antagonist to the NMDA receptor (Lipton et al. 1997) and hyperhomocysteinemia has been observed in both type-1 (Khare et al. 2005) and type-2 diabetics (Onat et al. 2008).

Because hyperglycemia-induced membrane lipid peroxidation was observed in embryonic chick livers (Miller et al. 2005) and brains (Coles et al. 2008), it is tempting to test whether an exogenous antioxidant can ameliorate hyperglycemia-induced membrane lipid peroxidation. The antioxidant, resveratrol, ameliorated hyperglycemia-induced oxidative stress in STZ-treated rats (Ates et al. 2007). While other exogenous antioxidants may work, it is unlikely that exogenous resveratrol can ameliorate membrane lipid peroxidation and increased apoptosis rates within developing chick embryos. Hancock and Miller (2006) reported that while moderate (2.95 nmol/kg egg) to high levels of exogenous *trans*-resveratrol (29.50 nmol/kg egg) attenuated ethanol-induced decreased brain membrane arachidonic acid (20:4, n-6) and DHA (22-6, n-3) levels as compared to controls, these same dosages of *trans*-resveratrol failed to attenuate ethanol-induced increased brain lipid hydroperoxide levels and increased brain caspase-3 activities (Hancock and Miller 2006).

While *trans*-reveratrol is an antioxidant, *trans*-resveratrol also inhibits angiogenesis. *Trans*-resveratrol inhibited bovine endothelial cell growth by inhibiting fibroblast growth factor-2 induced phospho-ryation of MAP kinases in a dose-dependent manner (Brakenhielm et al. 2001). In vivo studies using chick embryos, demonstrated that discs containing 1–100 mg per disc of *trans*-resveratrol produced avascular zones within chick chorio-allantoic membranes (Brakenhielm et al. 2001). The dosages of Brakenhielm et al. (2001) (1–100 µg of *trans*-resveratrol/disc) are similar to the dosages used by Hancock and Miller (2006). Interestingly, hyperglycemia-induced increased brain HoCys levels in developing chick brains (Coles et al. 2008) may also be a threat to the developing blood–brain barrier because HoCys is also known to inhibit endothelial cell proliferation and acts as an antiangiogenic molecule (Nagai et al. 2001; Rodriquez-Nieto et al. 2002).

173.12 Embryonic Diabetes: Homocysteine Metabolism and Oxidative Stress

The knowledge of hyperglycemia-induced increased brain and hepatic HoCys levels (Coles et al. 2008) was alarming to us because we have previously demonstrated that exogenous HoCys caused increased apoptosis rates (as measured by increased caspase-3 activities), increased brain membrane lipid peroxida-tion rates (as measured by increased levels of brain lipid hydroperoxides and decreased brain membrane long-chain polyunsaturated fatty acid levels), and decreased chick embryo viability at 11 days of develop-ment (Miller et al. 2003, 2006). We reported that exogenous HoCys-induced reductions in brain SAM/SAH ratios were partially attenuated by exogenous glycine (Miller et al. 2006). Elevated HoCys levels can cause oxidative stress because two HoCys molecules can undergo auto-oxidation and form a dimer (HoCys:oxidized disulfide) by liberating two hydrogen ions and two electrons. In doing so, hydrogen peroxide and hydroxyl radicals can be generated (Hayden and Tyagi 2004) and these reactive oxygen species can promote membrane lipid peroxidation and subsequent necrosis and apoptosis (Miller 2004).

HoCys is metabolized by the transsulfuration pathway and by the remethylation pathway (Fig. 173.1). In the remethylation pathway, methylcobalamine, which receives the methyl group from SAM, 5-methyltetrahydrofolate (5-methyl THF), or betaine (trimethyl glycine), methylates HoCys to methionine. Methionine is subsequently converted to SAM (Selhub 1999). Hence, folate deficiencies inhibit the remethylation of HoCys to methionine and cause hyperhomocysteinemia and have been associated with a variety of pathological problems (Carmel and Jacobson 2001), and folate deficiencies are well associated with increased incidence of NTDs (Boyles et al. 2006). Many methylases within a cell use SAM as the methyl donor. So as methylase activities continue during hyperhomocysteinemia, SAM levels decline while SAH levels increase (Selhub 1999). Consequently, NTDs may be caused by hyperhomocysteinemia and not by folate deficiencies.

Two enzymes in the remethylation pathway are 10-formyltetrahydrofolate dehydrogenase (10-FTHF DH) and 10-formyltetrahydrofolate hydrolase (10-FTHF hydrolase) (Fig. 173.2). Both enzymes cata-lyze the conversion of 10-formyltetrahydrofolate to CO_2 and tetrahydrofolate (THF). The difference between the two enzymes is that 10-FTHF DH requires NADPH while 10-FTHF hydrolase does not require NADPH. In the glycine cleavage system within the remethylation pathway, T-protein requires THF as a coenzyme and synthesizes N^5,N^{10}-methylenetetrahydrofolate, which is converted to the methyl donor, 5-methyl THF (Kikuchi 1973; van der Put et al. 2001). Low 5-methyl THF levels could not only inhibit the remethylation of HoCys to methionine, but also alter SAM/SAH levels because methionine is used to produce SAM, SAM is converted to SAH, and SAH is hydrolyzed to HoCys (Selhub 1999).

HoCys is also removed in the transsulfuration pathway (Fig. 173.1). The first and irreversible reaction is catalyzed by a pyridoxial-5'-phosphate (vitamin B_6) containing enzyme, cystathionine

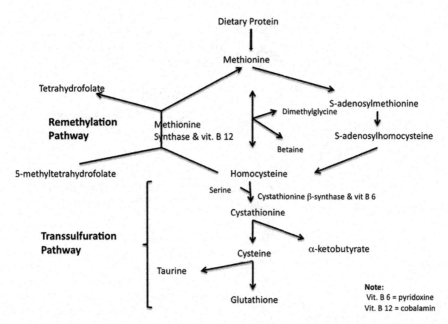

Fig. 173.1 Homocysteine removal via remethylation and transsulfuration pathways. *Vit. B6* pyridoxine, *Vit. B12* cobalamin

β-synthase that condenses serine and HoCys to form crystathionine. Cystathionine is subsequently hydrolyzed by another pyridoxial-5'-phosphate containing enzyme, cystathionine γ-synthase, thus forming α-ketobutyrate and cysteine and excess cysteine is converted to taurine (Selhub 1999). Thus, as cystathionine β-synthase activity decreases and the rest of the transsulfuration pathway slows, increased HoCys levels and decreased taurine levels are observed.

We have recently studied whether embryonic hyperglycemia reduces the enzymatic activities of two enzymes in the remethylation pathway, 10-FTHF DH and 10-formyltethydrofolate hydrolase (10-FTHF hydrolase) (Fig. 173.2) and whether embryonic hyperglycemia slows the transsulfuration pathway, as measured by brain and hepatic taurine levels (Fig. 173.1). We injected white Leghorn chicken eggs with either 9.29 μmol L-glucose/kg egg (avian saline was the solvent) or avian saline (0.72% NaCl, w/v) during the first 3 days of avian development (E $_{0-2}$). At 11 days of development (theoretical stage 37; Hamburger and Hamilton 1951), blood from chorio-allantoic vessels was collected and serum isolated by centrifugation (10,000× g for 1 min). The mass of each chick embryo was measured followed by decapitation. Brains and livers were excised, tissue mass measured, and stored at −80°C for subsequent biochemical analysis. Serum D-glucose levels were measured according to Coles et al. (2008) and brain and hepatic taurine levels were measured by high performance liquid chromatography as described by Barnett et al. (2009). The enzymatic activities of brain and hepatic 10-FTHF DH and 10 FTHF hydrolase activities were also measured according to Barnett et al. (2009).

Exogenous L-glucose injected into early chick embryos (E $_{0-2}$) caused serum D-glucose levels to increase by approximately 2.6 fold ($p < 0.0001$) at 11 days of development (Table 173.1). Presumably, L-glucose inhibited the GLUTs from binding and transporting d-glucose from the developing circulatory system into cells. L-glucose-induced hyperglycemia was also associated with reduced embryo masses ($p \leq 0.0001$) and reduced brain masses ($p = 0.006$) as compared to controls. However, L-glucose-induced hyperglycemia was not associated with reduced hepatic mass or reduced % living embryos as compared to controls (Table 173.1) (Miller et al. 2009).

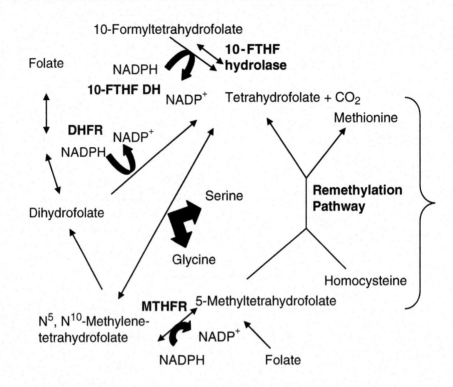

10-FTHF DH: 10-formyltetrahydrofolate dehydrogenase
10-FTHF hydrolase: 10-formyltetrahydrofolate hydrolase
MTHFR: N^5, N^{10}-methylenetetrahydrofolate reductase
DHFR: dihydrofolate reductase

Fig. 173.2 The remethylation pathway and folate metabolism. *10-FTHF DH* 10-formyltetrahydrofolate dehydrogenase, *10-FTHF hydrolase* 10-formyltetrahydrofolate hydrolase, *MTHFR* N^5,N^{10}-methylenetetrahydrofolate reductase, *DHFR* dihydrofolate reductase

Exogenous L-glucose-induced hyperglycemia caused approximately a 2.4-fold reduction in brain 10-FTHF DH activities ($p = 0.0035$) and a 2.5-fold reduction in hepatic 10-FTHF DH activities ($p = 0.0035$) as compared to controls (Table 173.2). Hyperglycemia failed to significantly affect either brain or liver 10-FTHF hydrolase activities. When serum D-glucose levels were correlated to brain 10-FTHF activities, the Pearson product moment (r) was -0.56 [F = (1, 13) 5.89; $p = 0.03$] (Fig. 173.3). When serum D-glucose levels were correlated to hepatic 10-FTHF activities, the Pearson product moment (r) was -0.55 [F = (1, 13) 5.63; $p = 0.04$] (Miller et al. 2009) (Fig. 173.4).

Exogenous L-glucose-induced hyperglycemia also caused approximately a 1.8-fold reduction in brain taurine levels ($p \leq 0.007$) and a 2.0-fold reduction in hepatic taurine ($p < 0.01$) as compared to controls (Table 173.2). When serum D-glucose levels were correlated to brain taurine levels, the Pearson product moment (r) was -0.60 [F = (1, 12) 6.68; $p = 0.02$] (Fig. 173.5). When serum d-glucose levels were correlated to hepatic taurine levels, the Pearson product moment (r) was -0.61 [F = (1, 9) 5.40; $p = 0.045$] (Fig. 173.6). Thus, exogenous l-glucose-induced hyperglycemia is inhibiting both the remethylation and the transsulfuration pathways in embryonic chick brains and livers at 11 days of development (Miller et al. 2009).

Table 173.1 The effect of exogenous L-glucose on chick embryo viability at 11 days of development

	Controls (avian saline)	Exogenous L-glucose (9.29 µmol/kg egg)	Statistical analyses
% living embryos	80.11 ± 6.95% N = 4 different sets of injections where 16–20 eggs were injected during each set	81.89 ± 10.85% N = 4 different sets of injections where 16–20 eggs were injected during each set	t = 0.28 df = 6 p = 0.79
Embryo mass (g)	3.367 ± 0.196 g N = 12	2.873 ± 0.291 g N = 12	t = 4.62 df = 22 p ≤ 0.0001
Liver mass (mg)	54 ± 7 mg N = 12	52 ± 13 mg N = 12	t = 0.33 df = 22 p = 0.74
Brain mass (mg)	607 ± 71 mg N = 12	497 ± 92 mg N = 12	t = 3.09 df = 22 p = 0.006
Serum D-glucose levels	1112.65 ± 256.25 mg/L (6.18 ± 1.52 mM) N = 12	2915.12 ± 735.12 mg/L (16.18 ± 4.08 mM) N = 12	t = 6.49 df = 22 p < 0.0001

Fertile white Leghorn chicken eggs were injected with approximately 25 µL of either avian saline (0.72% NaCl) or 9.29 µmol L-glucose/kg egg in avian saline during the first 3 days of development (E_{0-2}) into the air sac of each egg. After sealing each injection sight with paraffin wax, all embryos were incubated in a forced air incubator at 37.5°C and turned every 4 h with the humidity ranging from 70% to 90%. At 11 days of development (theoretical stage 37, Hamburger and Hamilton 1951), blood was collected from chorio-allantoic blood vessels and serum isolated by centrifugation (10,000× g for 1 min). The mass of each chick embryo was determined followed by decapitation. Brains and livers were excised, tissue mass measured, and stored at –80°C for subsequent biochemical analysis. Serum D-glucose levels were measured according to Coles et al. (2008).
Data presented as mean ± standard deviation

Table 173.2 The effects of exogenous L-glucose on brain and hepatic taurine levels, brain and hepatic 10-formyltetrahydrofolate dehydrogenase (10-FTHF DH), and 10-formyltetrahydrofolate hydrolase (10-FTHF hydrolase) activities at 11 days of development

	Controls (avian saline)	Exogenous L-glucose (9.29 µmol/kg egg)	Statistical analyses
Brain 10-FTHF DH activities (µmol/min/mg brain protein)	6.31 ± 2.50 N = 9	2.57 ± 2.13 N = 9	t = 3.42 df = 16 p = 0.0035
Hepatic-10 FTHF DH activities (µmol/min/mg hepatic protein)	6.32 ± 2.50 N = 9	2.57 ± 2.10 N = 9	t = 3.42 df = 16 p = 0.0035
Brain 10-FTHF hydrolase activities (µmol/min/mg brain protein)	2.37 ± 0.69 N = 10	2.36 ± 0.94 N = 13	t = 0.04 df = 21 p = 0.97
Hepatic-10 FTHF hydrolase activities (µmol/min/mg hepatic protein)	2.23 ± 1.65 N = 10	3.14 ± 2.51 N = 11	t = 0.97 df = 19 p = 0.34
Brain taurine levels (nmol/mg brain)	1.89 ± 0.74 N = 7	1.04 ± 0.22 N = 8	t = 3.20 df = 13 p ≤ 0.007
Hepatic taurine levels (nmol/mg liver)	10.69 ± 3.63 N = 6	5.48 ± 2.29 N = 6	t = 5.21 df = 10 p < 0.01

Brain and hepatic taurine levels were measured by high-performance liquid chromatography as described by Barnett et al. (2009). The enzymatic activities of brain and hepatic 10-FTHF DH and 10-FTHF hydolase were measured according to Barnett et al. (2009)
Data presented as mean ± standard deviation

Fig. 173.3 The relationship between brain 10-formyl tetrahydrofolate dehydrogenase (10-FTHF DH) activities and serum D-glucose levels in embryonic chicks at 11 days of development. $r = -0.56$ [$F = (1, 13)$ 5.89; $p = 0.03$], $y = 6.977 - 0.001 (X)$; $R^2 = 0.312$

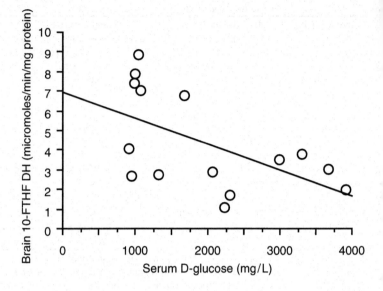

$r = -0.56$ [$F = (1, 13)$ 5.89; $p = 0.03$]

$y = 6.977 - 0.001 (X)$; $R^2 = 0.312$

Fig. 173.4 The relationship between hepatic 10-formyl tetrahydrofolate dehydrogenase (10-FTHF DH) activities and serum D-glucose levels in embryonic chicks at 11 days of development. $r = -0.55$ [$F = (1, 13)$ 5.63; $p = 0.04$], $y = 6.395 - 0.0001 (X)$; $R^2 = 0.302$

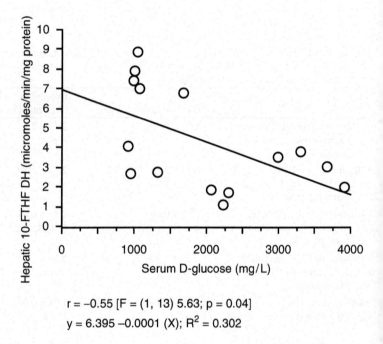

$r = -0.55$ [$F = (1, 13)$ 5.63; $p = 0.04$]

$y = 6.395 - 0.0001 (X)$; $R^2 = 0.302$

Hyperglycemia-induced inhibition of the remethylation and transsulfuration pathways explain increased brain and hepatic HoCys levels within embryonic chicks (Coles et al. 2008). This also raises questions as to whether exogenous 5-methyl THF or taurine ameliorates hyperglycemia-induced hyperhomocysteinemia, oxidative stress, and apoptosis in embryonic brains and livers.

Fig. 173.5 The relationship between brain taurine levels and serum D-glucose levels in embryonic chicks at 11 days of development. $r = -0.60$ [$F = (1, 12)$ 6.68; $p = 0.02$], $y = 2.236 - (3.837 \times 10^{-4})\, X$; $R^2 = 0.358$

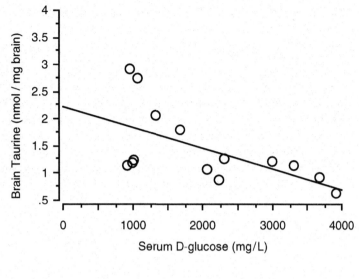

$r = -0.60$ [$F = (1, 12)$ 6.68; $p = 0.02$]

$y = 2.236 - (3.837 \times 10^{-4})\, X$; $R^2 = 0.358$

Fig. 173.6 The relationship between hepatic taurine levels and serum D-glucose levels in embryonic chicks at 11 days of development. $r = -0.61$ [$F = (1, 9)$ 5.40; $p = 0.045$], $y = 12.799 - (0.002)\, X$; $R^2 = 0.375$

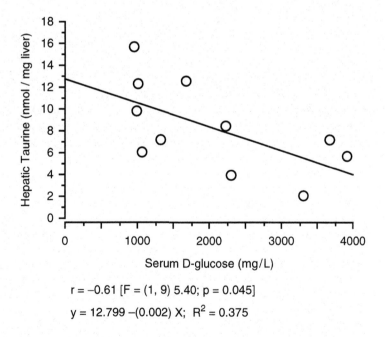

$r = -0.61$ [$F = (1, 9)$ 5.40; $p = 0.045$]

$y = 12.799 - (0.002)\, X$; $R^2 = 0.375$

Chen et al. (1998) reported that taurine is essential for proliferation and neurite extension when culturing human fetal neurons isolated from the cerebral hemispheres in glial-free media and the folate pathway is well associated with the prevention of NTDs (Boyles et al. 2006).

173.13 Applications to Other Areas of Health and Disease

Oxidative stress, enhanced rates of apoptosis, and elevated HoCys levels are also observed in the brains of alcoholics and the brains of fetuses exposed to alcohol. Hyperhomocysteinemia is also seen in a number of serious and debilitating diseases (Carmel and Jacobson 2001) and exogenous HoCys is teratogenic in at least embryonic chicks (Miller et al. 2003, 2006). Consequently, exploring the regulation of folate metabolism; the regulation of the transsulfuration pathway; the use of antioxidants; the use of exogenous folates and possibly taurine; and a better understanding of how neurotrophic factors regulate developing neurons may not only provide us with a better understanding of the physiology and development of the nervous system, but may provide important clinical insights into several serious and debilitating diseases.

Summary Points

- Type-1 and type-2 diabetics have increased risk of ischemia-induced vascular damage. During oxygen-deprivation (ischemia), neurons are unable to convert glutamate to α-ketobutyrate and release excessively high glutamate levels. This causes increased cytoplasmic Ca^{+2} levels, increased reactive oxygen species levels, increased oxidative-stress, increased membrane lipid peroxidation, and apoptosis.
- Type-1 diabetics (insulin-dependent) exhibit spatial and episodic memory deficits and are associated with neuropathy within the hippocampus, hypothalamus, and possess reduced gray matter within the temporal lobes.
- Peripheral neuropathy in STZ-treated rats causes reduced (GDNF) levels, reduced activation of Ret tyrosine kinase receptors, and increased apoptosis rates.
- Type-1 diabetics (insulin-dependent) have reduced choline acetyltransferease activities, reduced AChE activities, and reduced acetylcholine levels and are associated with oxidative stress within the hippocampus and cerebral cortex (Table 173.3).
- During fetal/neonatal development, acetylcholine must stimulate brain neuronal M3 muscuranic acetylcholine receptors in order to prevent an underdevelopment of the anterior pituitary gland. However, the lack of M3 muscuranic acetylcholine receptor activation protects against the onset of type-2 (non-insulin-dependent) diabetes.

Table 173.3 Key features of neuropathy in type-1 diabetics

1. Neuropathy can occur as a result of momentary oxygen deprivation during ischemia-induced vascular damage and type-1 and type-2 diabetics are prone to ischemia-induced vascular damage.
2. During oxygen deprivation, neurons cannot convert glutamate to α-ketobutyrate and overstimulate nearby neurons with excessively high levels of glutamate via the N-methyl-D-aspartate receptor.
3. During neuropathy, reactive oxygen species are produced causing oxidative-stress and are seen during necrosis and apoptosis.
4. Oxidative stress causes membrane lipid peroxidation and is observed during necrosis and apoptosis.
5. Reduced utilization of cholinergenic neurons is seen during oxidative stress and is associated with cognitive deficits.
6. Reduced levels of a tropic factor, such as glial cell line derived-neurotrophic factor, has been observed in peripheral neuropathy in streptozocin (STZ)-treated rats.
7. Elevated levels of circulating homocysteine in type-1 diabetics and decreased brain taurine levels are seen in STZ-treated rats.

This table lists key facts associated with neuronal damage (neuropathy) in type-1 diabetics and animals used to model type-1 diabetes

- Type-2 diabetics (non-insulin-dependent) are frequently obese, insulin-resistant, leptin-resistant, have elevated circulating triglycerides levels, and exhibit poor cognitive performance. Recent injection of triglycerides into the brains of lean mice impaired the NMDA receptor-mediated maintenance of hippocampal long-term synaptic potential (Table 173.4).
- Reduced and disrupted expression of hippocampal *BDNF* is associated with the onset of T2D. While VGF (nonacronymic protein)-deficient mice tend to resist the onset of T2D, exogenous TLQP-21 (a VGF isoform) reduced circulating leptin levels and ameliorated obesity in mice.
- Gestational diabetes stimulates c-Abl- and p53-induced signaling, reduced *Pax-3* expression, and increases apoptosis rates within mouse neural tube neuroepithelial cells.
- Gestational diabetes is frequently associated with abnormally low maternal arachidonic acid (20:4, n-3 and 20:4, n-6) and DHA (22:6, n-3) levels. Meanwhile, exogenous arachidonic acid injected into STZ-treated pregnant rats ameliorated the frequency of gestational diabetes-induced NTDs (Table 173.5).
- Gestational diabetes in pregnant rats caused increased density of insulin receptors within the ventromedial hypothalamus and lateral hypothalamus of fetal rats brains. However, no relationship between the densities of various GLUTs to hyperinsulinemia within various regions of the fetal brain was observed.
- Hyperglycemia in embryonic chicks has been induced and is associated with increased membrane lipid peroxidation rates, increased apoptosis rates, decreased SAM/SAH, and elevated HoCys levels within embryonic brains and livers.

Table 173.4   Key features of neuropathy in type-2 diabetics

1. Neuropathy can occur as a result of momentary oxygen deprivation during ischemia-induced vascular damage and type-1 and type-2 diabetics (T2D)are prone to ischemia-induced vascular damage.
2. During oxygen deprivation, neurons cannot convert glutamate to α-ketobutyrate and overstimulate nearby neurons with excessively high levels of glutamate via the *N*-methyl-D-aspartate receptor.
3. During neuropathy, reactive oxygen species are produced causing oxidative-stress and are seen during necrosis and apoptosis.
4. Oxidative stress causes membrane lipid peroxidation and is observed during necrosis and apoptosis.
5. Overstimulation of M3 muscuranic acetylcholine receptors in the peripheral nervous system has been associated T2D.
6. Reduced levels of a tropic factor, such as brain-derived neurotrophic factor, have been observed in obese, hyperglycemic mice.
7. Elevated levels of circulating homocysteine and the overexcretion of taurine are seen in type-2 diabetics.

This table lists key facts associated with neuronal damage (neuropathy) in type-2 diabetics and animals used to model T2D

Table 173.5   Key features of neuropathy in gestational (embryonic) diabetics

1. Neuropathy can occur before the vascular system fully develops because neuralation begins prior to angiogenesis.
2. While embryonic-derived neurons can undergo in vitro glutamate toxicity, the exact role of glutamate and the *N*-methyl-D-aspartate receptor in gestational/embryonic diabetes is unclear.
3. During neuropathy, reactive oxygen species are produced causing oxidative stress and are seen during necrosis and apoptosis.
4. Oxidative stress causes membrane lipid peroxidation and is observed during necrosis and apoptosis.
5. The role of acetylcholine and acetylcholine receptors during gestational (embryonic) neuropathy is unclear.
6. While reduced levels of tropic factors are possible, exact roles in embryonic neuropathy are unclear.
7. Elevated homocysteine levels and decreased taurine levels are seen in brains and livers of hyperglycemic chick embryos.

This table lists key facts associated with neuronal damage (neuropathy) in animals used to model gestational (embryonic) diabetes

- Elevated embryonic HoCys levels are teratogenic, cause NTDs, stimulate oxidative stress, and stimulate apoptosis in developing chick brains. In chicks, hyperglycemia-induced brain HoCys levels correlate with a hyperglycemia-induced inhibition of the folate-mediated remethylation pathway and inhibited taurine synthesis via the transsulfuration pathway.
- Oxidative stress, enhanced apoptosis rates, and elevated HoCys levels are observed in the brains of alcoholics and in embryonic brains exposed to alcohol. Consequently, exploring the regulation of folate metabolism and the transsulfuration pathway may provide us with a better understanding of hyperglycemia-induced neuropathy and alcohol-induced neuropathy.

Definitions of Key Terms

Apoptosis: Apoptosis and necrosis are two different forms of cell death and can occur at the same time. Necrosis begins with increased membrane fluidity via membrane lipid peroxidation and can be initiated by reactive oxygen species. The ultimate loss of cell membrane integrity spreads to all eukaryotic membranes and results in a total failure of all organelles, inhibition of protein synthesis, and random DNA fragmentation. Apoptosis, sometimes referred as genetically programmed cell death, is dependent on protein synthesis and utilizes a number of proteins including Annexin-V, poly(ADP-ribose)polymerase (PARP), and a number of caspases. PARPs deplete the NAD^+ pool by adding a poly-A tail to DNA fragments and can be detected by deoxynucleotidyl transferease-mediated dUTP nick end-labeled DNA fragments (TUNEL). Apoptosis can be initiated from outside the cell (extrinsic pathway) or inside the cell (intrinsic pathway). While complex, the extrinsic pathway begins with a receptor-ligand interaction at the cell membrane level or a lack of a tropic factor leaving a vacant binding-site on a membrane receptor. This initiates a signal transduction cascade that activates a number of initiator caspases and transcription factors. Ultimately, the activation of Bcl-2 proapoptotic signals, reactive oxygen species, and increased cytoplasmic Ca^{+2} levels activate Bcl-2 family proteins on the outer mitochondrial membrane. Once Bcl-2 family proteins are activated, the intrinsic pathway begins where mitochondria release cytochrome-c and Ca^{+2} into the cytoplasm. This activates the cytoplasmic protein Apaf-1 that binds and activates procaspase-9 and procaspase-3. Procaspase-3 is activated to caspase-3.
Caspase-3: Caspase-3 is a "killer" caspase and a protease. It will bind and cleave any protein that has a DEVD (aspartate-glutamate-valine-aspartate) domain. Whether apoptosis is initiated by the extrinsic pathway, which spreads to the intrinsic pathway, or initiated by direct activation of the intrinsic pathway, caspase-3 is activated and it's enzymatic activity level and/or presence is a convenient measurement of apoptosis rates.
Homocysteine: HoCys is a non-protein-coding amino acid. It is teratogenic in chick embryos and causes both apoptosis and membrane lipid peroxidation. Elevated levels of HoCys are seen in a number of debilitating disorders and can be caused by folate deficiencies and/or inhibition of the transsulfuration pathway.
Ischemia: Type-1 and type-2 diabetics have a 4- to 12-fold increased risk of stroke and ischemia-induced cerebral damage. As the microvascular system becomes occluded, downstream oxygen and glucose levels are momentarily depleted prompting necrosis and energy depletion of downstream cells. Inflammation of the occluded microvascular system is partially due to neutrophil recruitment causing enhanced neutrophil NADPH oxidase and xanthine oxidase activities and the production of reactive oxygen species. Increased oxidative stress is thought to exacerbate ischemia-induced cerebral damage and can promote apoptosis in nearby cells (Bemur et al. 2007).
Lipid peroxidation: Reactive oxygen species can cleave polyunsaturated fatty acids into shorter-chain fatty acids and toxic aldehydes and affect membrane integrity (fluidity).

Oxidative stress: Membrane lipid peroxidation and increased apoptosis rates can ultimately kill cells undergoing oxidative stress. Oxidative stress is exacerbated by decreased levels of antioxidants, such as glutathione, and reduced antioxidant enzyme activity levels. Antioxidant enzymes include superoxide dimutase, catalase, glutathione peroxidase, and glutathione-*S*-transferase.

Reactive oxygen species: Reactive oxygen species include oxygen radicals, hydroxyl radicals, and peroxynitrite radicals. During ischemia, reactive oxygen species can be generated by enhanced neutrophil NADPH oxidase and xanthine oxidase activities and by activation of neuronal nitrous oxide synthase.

Acknowledgments I am very thankful for the superb technical assistance of Ms. Kelly Colesman and Ms. Sarah Yearsley who performed the taurine, 10-FTHF DH, and 10-FTHF hydrolase assays (Tables 173.1 and 173.2; Figs. 173.3, 173.4, 173.5, and 173.6). This article is dedicated to the memories of Grace, Evelyn, and Robert Miller, Sr.

References

Anderson MS, Flowers-Ziegler J, Das UG, Hay WH Jr, Devaskar SU. Am J Regulatory Integrative Comp Physiol. 2001;281:R1545–52.

Anggard E, Samuelsson B. J Biol Chem. 1965;240:3518–21.

Anitha M, Gondha, C, Sutliff R, Parasadanian A, Mwangi S, Sitaraman SV, Srinivasan S. J Clin Invest. 2006;116:344–56.

Ashokkumar N, Pari L, Ramkumar K. Basic Clin Pharm Toxicol. 2006;99:246–50.

Ates O, Cayli SR, Yucel N, Altinoz E, Kocak A, Akif Durak M, Turkoz Y, Yologlu S. J Clin Neuroscience. 2007;14:256–60.

Barbacid M. Curr Opin Cell Biol. 1995;7:148–55.

Barnett RK, Booms, SL, Gura T, Gushrowski M, Miller RR Jr. Comp Biochem Physiol. 2009;150C:107–12.

Bartolomucci A, La Corte G, Possent R, Locatelli V, Rigamonti AE, Torsello A, Bresciani E, Bulgarelli I, Rizzi R, Pavone F, D'Amato FR, Severini, C, Mignogna G, Giorgi A, Schinina ME, Ela G, Brancia C, Ferri G-L, Ciani B, Pascuuci T, Dell'Omo G, Muller EE, Levi A, Moles A. Proc Natl Acad Sci USA. 2006;103:14584–9.

Baskin DG, Figleicz DP, Woods SC, Pore DJ, Dorsa DM. Ann Rev Physiol. 1987;49:335–47.

Beauguis J, Homo-Delarche F, Revsin Y, De Nicola AF, Saravia F. Neuroimmunomodulation 2008;15:61–7.

Becerra JE, Khoury MJ, Cordero, JF, Erickson JD. Pediatrics 85:1–9.

Bemur C, Ste-Marie L, Montogomery J. Neurochem Int. 2007;50:890–904.

Blokland A, Jolies J. Pharmacol Biochem Behav. 1993;44:491–4.

Boyles, AL, Billups, AV, Deak KL, Siegel DG, Mehltretter L, Slifer SH, Bassuk AG, Kessler JA, Reed MC, Nijhout AF, George TM, Enterline DS, Gilbert JR, Speer MC. Env Health Perspect. 2006;114:1547–52.

Brakenhielm E, Cao R, Cao Y. FASEB J. 2001;15:1798–800.

Cabeza R, Prince SE, Daselaar SM, Greenberg DL, Budde M, Dolcos F, Labar KS, Ruben DC. J Cogn Neurosci. 2004;16:1583–94.

Carmel R, Jacobson DW, editors. Homocysteine in health and disease. UK: Cambridge University Press; 2001.

Caulfield MP, Birdsall NJM. Pharmacol Rev. 1998;50:270–90.

Chakraborty TR, Tkalych O, Nanno D, Garcia AL, Devi LA, Salton SRJ. Brain Res. 2006;1089:21–32.

Chen X-C, Pan Z-L, Liu D-S, Han X. Adv Exp Med Biol. 1998;442:397–403.

Coles NW, Weaver KR, Walcher BN, Adams ZF, Miller RR Jr. Comp Biochem Physiol. 2008;150B:338–43.

Farr SA, Yamada, KA, Butterfield DA, Abdul HM, Xu L, Miller NE, Banks WA, Morley JE. Endocrinology 2008;149:2628–36.

Fine EL, Horal M, Chang TI, Fortin G, Locken MR. Diabetes 1999;48:2454–62.

Friedlander RM. New Engl J Med. 2009;348:1365–75.

Gao O, Gao YM. Int J Dev Neurosci. 2007;25:349–357.

Gautam D, Gavrilova O, Jeon J, Pack S, Jou W, Cui Y, Li JH, Wess J. Cell Metab. 2006;4:363–75.

Gautam D, Jeon J, Starost MF, Han S-J, Hamdan FF, Cui Y, Parlow AF, Gavrilova O, Szalayova I, Mezey E, Wess J. Proc Natl Acad Sci USA. 2009;106:6398–403.

Ghareeb DA, Hussen HM. Neurosci Lett. 2008;436:44–7.

Goldman AS, Baker L, Piddington R, Marx B, Herold R, Egler J. Proc Natl Acad Sci USA. 1985;82:8227–31.

Gonzalez-Zulueta M, Ensz, Mukhina G, Lebrovitz RM, Zwacka RM, Engelhardt JF, Oberly LW, Dawson LW, Dawson VL, Dawson TM. J Neurosci. 1998;15:2040–55.

Guo C, Quobatari A, Shangguan Y, Hong S, Wiley JW. Neurogastroenterol Motil. 2004;16:355–45.

Hahm S, Mizuno TM, Wu J, Wisor JP, Priest, CA, Kozak CA, Boozer CN, Peng B, McEvoy RC, Good P, Kelley KA, Takahashi JS, Pintar JE, Roberts, JL, Mobbs CV, Salton SRJ. Neuron 1999;537–48.

Hamburger V, Hamilton HL. J Morphol. 1951;88:49–92.

Hancock ML, Miller RR Jr. Nutr Neurosci. 2006;9:121–9.

Hayden MR, Tyagi SC. J Nutr. 2004;3:4–36.

Hazelwood RL. In: Ouellet H, editor. ACTA XIX Congress Intl. Ornithologia, vol. 2. Ottawa: University of Ottawa Press; 1986. p. 2223–33.

Hazelwood RL. In: Whittow GL, editor. Sturkie's avian physiology. 5th ed. San Diego: Academic; 2000, p. 539–55.

Hershey T, Perantie DC, Warren SL, Zimmerman EC, Sadler M., White NH. Diabetes Care. 2005;28:2372–7.

Hertz L. Neuropharmacology 2008;55:289–309.

Jia DY, Liu HJ, Wang FW, Liu SM, Ling EA, Liu K, Hao AJ. Neurosci Lett. 2008;440:27–31.

Kamboj SS, Chopra K, Sandhir R. Metab Brain Dis. 2008;23:427–43.

Khandkar M, Jee E, Parmar D, Katare. Biochem J. 1995;307:647–9.

Khare A, Shetty S, Ghosh K, Mohanty D, Chatterjee S. Athersoclerosis 2005;180:375–80.

Kikuchi G. Mol Cell Biochem. 1973;1:101–14.

Lanier WL. Can J Anesth. 1999;46:R46–51.

Leinninger GM, Vincent AM, Feldman EL. J Peripher Nerv Sys. 2004;9:26–53.

Leloup C, Magnan C, Alquier T, Mistry S, Offer G, Arnaud E, Kassis N, Ktorza, Penicaud L. Pediatr Res. 2004;56:263–7.

Levi A, Eldridge JD, Paterson BM. Science 1985;229:393–5.

Levi A, Ferri GL, Watson E, Possenti R, Salton SR. Cell Mol Neurobiol. 2004;24:517–33.

Lewin GR, Barde YA. Annu Rev Neurosci. 1996;19:289–317.

Lindsay RM, Wiegand SJ, Altar CA, DiStefano PS. Trends Neurosci. 1994;17:182–90.

Lipton SA, Kim WK, Choi YB, Kumar S, D'Emilia DM, Rayuda PV, Arnelle DR, Stamler JS. Proc Natl Acad Sci USA. 1997;94:5923–8.

Ma XH, Muzumdar R, Yang XM, Gabriely I, Berger R, Barzilai N. J Gerontol Med Sci. 2002;57A:B225–31.

Malone JI, Hanna S, Saporta S, Mervis RF, Park CR, Chong L, Giamond DM. Pediatr Diabetes. 2008;9:531–9.

Margetic S, Cazzola C, Pegg GG, Hill RA. Int J Obes. 2002;26:1407–1433.

McLeod L, Ray JG. Community Genet. 2002;5:33–9.

Mooradian AD. Diabetes 1987;36:1094–7.

Miller RR Jr. In: Preedy VR, Watson RR, editors. Alcohol in disease: nutrient interactions and dietary intake. Boca Raton: CRC; 2004. p. 339–64.

Miller RR Jr, Leanza CM, Phillips EE, Blacquiere KD. Comp Biochem Physiol. 2003;136B:521–32.

Miller RR Jr, Burum AL, Leithart ME, Hart JD. Comp Biochem Physiol. 2005;141B:323–30.

Miller RR Jr, Hay CM, Striegnitz TR, Honsey LE, Coykendall CE, Blacquiere KD. Comp Biochem Physiol. 2006;144C:23–33.

Miller RR Jr, Coleman K, Yearsley S. 2009; Unpublished data.

Min Y, Lowy C, Ghebremeskel K, Thomas B, Offley-Shore B, Crawford M. Am J Clin Nutr. 2005a;82:1162–8.

Min Y, Lowy C, Ghebremeskel K, Thomas B, Crawford M. Diabet Med. 2005b;22:914–20.

Musen G, Lyoo KL, Sparks C, Ryan CM, Jimerson DC, Jacobson AM. Diabetes 2006;55:326–33.

Nagai Y, Tasaki H, Takatsu H, Nihei SI, Yamashita K, Nakashima Y. Biochem Biophys Res Commun. 2001;281:726–31.

Nahhas F, Barnea E. Am J Reprod Immunol. 1990;22:105–8.

Nakagawa T, Tsuchida A, Itakura Y, Nonmura T, Ono M, Hirota F, Inoue T, Nakayama C, Taiji M, Noguchi H. Diabetes 2000;49:436–44.

Negi G, Kumar A, Sharma SS. Current Res Inf Pharm Sci. 2008;9:62–8.

Norenberg MD, Rama Rao KV. Neurochem Int. 2007;50:983–97.

Northam EA, Anderson PJ, Jacobs R, Hughes M, Warne GL, Werther GA. Diabetes Care. 2001;24:1541–6.

Onat A, Hergenc G, Kucukdurmaz Z, Can G, Ayhan E, Bulur S. Clin Nutr. 2008;27:732–9.

Ono M, Ichihara J, Nonomura T, Itakura Y, Taiji M, Nakayama C, Noguchi H. Biochem Biophys Res Acta. 1997;238:633–7.

Perantie DC, Wu J, Koller JM, Lim A, Warren SL, Black KJ, Sadler M, White NH, Hershey T. Diabetes Care. 2007;30:2331–7.

Perimuter LC, Nathan DM, Goldfinger SH, Russo PA, Yates J, Larkin M. J Diabetes Complicat. 1988;2:210–3.

Ramos-Arroyo MA, Rodriquez-Pinella E, Cordero JF. Eur J Epidemiol. 1992;8:503–8.

Reece EA, Pinter E, Leranth CZ, Garcia-Segura M, Sanyal K, Hobbins, JC, Mahoney MJ, Naftolin JC. Teratology 1985;32:363–73.

Reitz RC. In: Watson RR, Watzl B, editors. Nutrition and alcohol. Boca Raton: CRC; 1992. p. 191–204.

Rodriquez-Nieto A, Chavarria T, Martinez-Poveda B, Sanchez-Jime, AR, Medina, MA. Biochem Biophys Res Commun. 2002;293:497–500.

Ryan AS, Nelson EB. Clin Pediatr. 2008;20:1–8.

Salton SR, Ferri GL, Hahm S, Snyder SE, Wilson AJ, Possenti R, Levi A. Front Neuroendocr. 2000;21:199–219.

Sankarasubbaiyan S, Cooper C, Heilig CW. Am J Kidney Dis. 2001;37:1039–43.

Schwartz MW, Figlewicz DP, Baskin DG, Woods SC, Porte DJ. Endocr Rev. 1992;13:387–414.

Scott JF, Robinson GM, French JM, O'Connell JE, Alberti KGMM, Gray CS. Stroke 1999;30:703–99.

Sendtner M, Holtman B, Hughes RA. Neurochem Res. 1996;21:831–41.

Sha H, Xu J, Tang J, Ding J, Gong J, Ge X, Kong D, Gao X. Physiol Genomics. 2007;31:252–63.

Sharma JBR, Lee D, Hachinski V, Chan RKT. Neurology 2003;60(Suppl1):A26C.

Selhub J. Annu Rev Nutr. 1999;19:217–46.

Skup MH. Acta Neurobiol Exp. 1994;54:81–94.

Song M, Kellum JA, Kaldas H, Fink MP. J Pharmacol Exp Ther. 2004;308:307–16.

Srinivasan S, Anitha M, Mwangi S, Heuckeroth RO. Mol Cell Neurosci. 2005;29:118–33.

Sun W, Oates PJ, Coutcher JB, Gerhardinger C, Lorenzi M. Diabetes 2006;55:2757–62.

Tanabe Y, Hashimoto M, Sugioka K, Maruyama M, Fujii Y, Hagiwara R, Hara T, Hossain SM, Shido O. Clin Exp Pharmacol Physiol. 2004;31:700–3.

Terwel D, Prickaerts J, Meng F, Jolies J. Eur J Pharmacol. 1995;287:65–71.

Tonra JR, Ono M, Liu X, Garcia K, Jackson C, Yancopoulos GD, Wiegand SJ, Wong V. Diabetes 1999;48:588–94.

van der Put NMJ, van Straaten HWM, Trijbels FJM, Blom HJ. Exp Biol Med. 2001;226:243–70.

Van Gaal LF, Wauters M, Mertens IL, Considine RV, De Leeuw IH. Int J Obes RelatMetab Disord. 1999;23(Suppl 1):29–36.

Vincent AM, McLean LL, Backus C, Feldman EL. FASEB J. 2005;19:638–640.

Watson E, Hahm S, Mizuno TM, Windsor J, Montgomery C, Scherer PE, Mobbs CV, Salton SRJ. Endocrinology. 2005;146:5151–5163.

Welsh B, Wecker L. Neurochem Res.1991;16:453–60.

Winkler J, Suhr ST, Gage FH, Thal LJ, Fisher LJ. Nature 1995;375:484–7.

Wolff SP. Br Med Bull. 1993;49:642–52.

Yamanaka M, Itakura Y, Tsuchida A, Nakagawa T, Taiji M. Biomedical Res. 2008;29:147–53.

Yuan ZM, Huang Y, Fan MM, Sawyers C, Kharbanda S, Kufee D. J Biol Chem. 1996;271:26457–60.

Yuen EC, Howe CL, Li Y, Holtzman, DM, Mobley WC. Brain Dev. 1996;18:362–8.

Zamboni M, Zoico E, Fantin F, Panagiota Panourgia M, Di Francesco V, Tosoni P, Solerte B, Vettor R, Bosello O. J Gerontol Med Sci. 2004;59A:396–400.

Chapter 174
Neurological Aspects of Dietary Lead

Kim M. Cecil and Diana M. Lindquist

Abbreviations

ADHD	Attention-deficit hyperactivity disorder
ALAD	γ-aminolevulinic acid dehydratase
BE	Belgium
CANTAB	Cambridge Neuropsychological Test Automated Battery
CDC	Centers for Disease Control
CNS	Central nervous system
DE	Germany
DK	Denmark
dL	Deciliter
EPA	Environmental Protection Agency of the United States
EU	European Union
FAO	The Joint Food and Agriculture Organization of the United Nations
FDA	Food and Drug Administration of the United States
FI	Finland
FR	France
GFR	Glomerular filtration rate
HOME	Home Observation for Measurement of the Environment
HE	Greece
IgE	Immunoglobulin E
IQ	Intelligence Quotient
IR	Ireland
IT	Italy
LTP	Long-term potentiation

K.M. Cecil (✉)
Cincinnati Children's Environmental Health Center at the Cincinnati Children's
Hospital Medical Center, Departments of Radiology, Pediatrics, Neuroscience and Environmental Health,
University of Cincinnati College of Medicine, Cincinnati, OH, USA
and
Cincinnati Children's Hospital Medical Center, Department of Radiology/Imaging
Research Center MLC 5033, 3333 Burnet Avenue, Cincinnati, OH 45229, USA
e-mail: kim.cecil@cchmc.org

V.R. Preedy et al. (eds.), *Handbook of Behavior, Food and Nutrition*,
DOI 10.1007/978-0-387-92271-3_174, © Springer Science+Business Media, LLC 2011

μg	Microgram
kg	Kilogram
MRI	Magnetic resonance imaging
MRS	Magnetic resonance spectroscopy
NMDA	N-methyl-D-aspartate
NO	Norway
PKC	Protein Kinase C
ppb	Part per billion
PT	Portugal
PTTI	Provisional Total Tolerable Intake
PTWI	Provisional Tolerable Weekly Intake
SE	Sweden
TEL	Tetraethyl lead
TML	Tetramethyl lead
TSH	Thyroid-stimulating hormone
UK	United Kingdom
US	United States
WHO	World Health Organization

174.1 Introduction

For millennia, lead exposure has harmed human health. While lead is found naturally within the Earth's crust, anthropogenic activities have resulted in widespread contamination of the environment (air, water and soil). Since the late 1970s, public health agencies and associated governmental efforts have dramatically increased the awareness of the toxicity of this element and provided regulation for common sources of lead exposure in a majority of the world's population. The most widely recognized efforts in reduction are associated with elimination of lead additives from the production of paint and petroleum products (gasoline, petrol). However, diet remains a significant source of lead exposure for humans within the modern, industrialized urban centers to the remote Brazilian Amazon. We will review how dietary lead exposures can arise from the ingestion of water, food, vitamins, supplements, pharmaceuticals, and traditional remedies. Lead contamination can occur at any step upon transferring these items from source to the consumer including the contamination of raw materials and implements involved in the preparation, processing, handling, and transport of these items (Table 174.1).

Table 174.1 Dietary sources of lead

- Contaminated drinking water arises from lead contaminated municipal water systems and from leaded pipes and plumbing, often within older homes.
- Food and other ingested items have significant lead levels after grown in lead-contaminated soil or in regions near sources of airborne lead particle emissions such as smelters, incinerators or roads with automobiles using leaded gasoline.
- Contamination of food and other ingested items may occur during the processing, preparation, handling by the producers, and transport to the consumer.
- Contamination of food and beverages may occur after being prepared on leaded cookware, served on lead glazed pottery, ceramics, and crystal and stored in lead-contaminated containers.
- Traditional medicines, pharmaceuticals, supplements, and vitamins are prepared or contaminated with leaded source materials.
- Ingestion of nonfood items related to pica activity provides another source of dietary lead.

This table provides an overview of common sources of lead found in ingested items

Table 174.2 Health effects associated with lead exposure (Adapted from ATSDR 2007)

System	Effect	Vulnerable population
Cardiovascular	Increased risk for hypertension	Adult, General
Developmental	Decrease birth length, stature, head circumference; Delayed sexual maturation	Pediatric, General
Endocrinological	Elevated TSH	Adult, Occupational
Gastrointestinal	Colic	Pediatric, General
Hematological	Decreased ALAD activity	Mixed Age and Source
Immunological	Increased serum IgE	Pediatric, General
Musculoskeletal	Dental caries and bone loss	Mixed Age, General
Neurological	Impaired motor skills, cognition, IQ, attention, executive functioning, social behavioral skills	Pediatric, General
Renal	Decreased GFR	Adult, General
Reproductive	Decreased fertility	Male, Adult Occupational

Lead exposure affects numerous systems within the human body. The effects listed in the table vary in their reversibility. The general population, particularly children, is vulnerable due to multiple sources of lead within the environment.

A number of factors modulate how dietary sources of lead harm the body. Factors such as the form (organic versus inorganic) of lead, age of a person, nutritional status of the individual, and pregnancy influence lead absorption.

Neurological aspects have been examined in cellular and animal models. Complex mechanisms of neurotoxicity are known. For human studies, epidemiologic cohorts have been established and longitudinally monitored to explore cognitive and neurobehavioral aspects of low, moderate, and high lead exposure levels.

While the focus of this work is on the neurological aspects of dietary lead, it is important to recognize that once lead is in the bloodstream, the systemic effects are largely independent of the source whether ingested or inhaled, but rely on the bioavailability pertaining to dose. Lead exposure affects all the major systems within the human body (Table 174.2).

Finally, this review will summarize future directions of research and public policy. Increasing numbers of studies find that low-level lead exposure is associated with adverse cognitive effects. These effects warrant continued action toward identifying sources and reducing lead levels in the environment that potentially threaten human health via ingestion or inhalation.

174.2 Dietary Sources and Intake of Lead

Lead levels within food itself are quite variable due to heterogeneous distribution of lead deposited within the soil and water, the contamination during open shipping of raw items and during processing, the transfer of lead from contaminated storage containers and plastic food wrappers with painted decals, and the transfer from inadequately glazed or heavily worn cookware and ceramic serving dishes. Dietary intake also depends upon cultural practices and individual diet. National regulations regarding lead usage and the practices monitoring compliance can also influence the amount of lead available for dietary consumption. Food lead concentrations have decreased dramatically in most nations primarily due to the reduction of airborne lead emissions and the prohibition of lead solder in storage cans, especially in milk for infant formula. Yet, in 2009 approximately 19 countries continue to use leaded petroleum products. Examining blood lead exposure models at levels above and below the contemporary action level of 10 μg/dL remains relevant toward understanding lead toxicity

Table 174.3 National statistics for dietary intake of lead from food (Adapted from Moschandreas et al. 2002; Marti-Cid et al. 2008; ATSDR 2005; UNEP 2008; EU SCOOP 2004)

Nation State(s)	Average dietary intake in μg/kg of body weight per day	Population
Australia	0.06–0.39	Adult males 25–34 years
	0.02–0.35	Adult females 25–34 years
	0.02–0.43	Boys 12 years
	0.01–0.34	Girls 12 years
	0.03–0.93	Toddlers 2 years
	0.01–1.19	Infant 9 months
Burkina Faso	0.9	52 μg Pb per day for 60 kg average weight
European Union	0.6	42 μg Pb per day for 70 kg average weight
Finland	0.24	17 μg Pb per day for 70 kg average weight
Mexico	3.5	3 μg/kg lead in food
Poland	1.48	Males 103.5 μg Pb per day for 70 kg average weight; 88.5 μg Pb per day for 60 kg average weight
Spain	0.644–0.85	Adult male assuming 70 kg living in Catalonia
USA	0.918	Males over 55 years
	0.895	Males over 20 years
	0.890	Males 13–19 years
	0.946	Females over 55 years
	0.920	Females over 20 years
	0.824	Females 13–19 years
	1.164	Children 7–12 years
	1.952	Children 1–6 years
	3.117	Non-nursing infants
	1.009	US population

This table provides a composite of national statistics reporting contemporary levels of lead intake for individuals in select nations obtained from dietary sources

in all populations. As lead is not degradable and thus, land is the ultimate repository, lead contamination continues to threaten many populations.

The United Nations Environment Program estimated that in 1987 the global average daily intake of lead was about 80 μg/day from food and 40 μg/day from drinking water. More recently, the joint Food and Agriculture Organization of the United Nations (FAO) and World Health Organization Expert Committee on Food Additives established a provisional tolerable weekly intake (PTWI) of 25 μg/kg of body weight, which is the equivalent of 3.5 μg/kg of body weight per day (WHO 2000). Examples of contemporary national estimates of daily intake of lead via food are shown in Table 174.3.

174.2.1 Levels of Lead in Raw Foods

In the European Union, data from national surveys of the adult population find that the major sources of dietary intake include bakery wares, cereals, fruits, vegetables, and beverages (Table 174.4). Levels of dietary lead intake for children were 6–15% above that of adults (not shown).

National surveys tend to focus on adult populations. Children may have lower absolute values of dietary lead intake; however, given their lower body weights, they may have a larger lead burden as they drink more fluids, eat more food, and breathe more air per kg of body weight.

In edible plants, lead contamination may occur from surface deposition of particulate matter or from the soil via the root system using direct foliar uptake and translocation within the plant.

Table 174.4 Daily intake (μg/day) of lead by adults from EU National Surveys (Adapted from EU SCOOP 2004)

Food	UK	DE	NO	BE	DK	FI	FR	HE	IT	IR	PT	SE	Mean
Bakery and cereals	4.0	6.0	2.2		2.35	0.08	9.63	3.2	4.35		0.53	1.43	3.4
Beverage	14	9.7	10.1	18.7	8.61	0.48	13.7		4.2		12.2	1.17	8.9
Cheese, yogurt condensed, powdered milk	0.48	1.3	0.062	0.74	0.19				1.94			0.25	0.71
Confectionary		0.39	0.04		0.74	0.04					0.031		0.30
Crustaceans, bivalves, cephalopods			1.2	0.08			0.79	2.03		0.35	0.51		0.71
Eggs	0.04	0.70	0.42		0.03	0.19	0.12		0.14			0.08	0.21
Fats and oils	0.14	0.74			0.6				0.22		.48		0.44
Fish and fish products	0.28	0.36	0.97		0.16	0.48	0.70	13.8	1.27	0.34	2.22	0.066	1.9
Fruits and vegetables	4.98	14	1.51	17.4	3.98	1.72	25.2	0.29	16.7		117	0.69	18
Meat	1.23	11	3.24		0.99	1.25	1.83	4.21	2.82	0.42		0.74	2.8
Milk, milk products	0.28		0.93	0.95	0.59	2.1	0.32	1.38	0.91			0.3	0.87
Offal	0.09	0.16	0.066	0.01		0.14	0.14	0.23	1.17		0.15		0.24
Ready to eat	0.02		0.008										0.01
Salts and spices		2.2					3.92						3.0
Sweeteners	1.0	0.65	0.047	0.04		0.02	0.47				0.17	0.023	0.30
Sum per Nation	27	47	21	38	18	7	57	25	34	1.1	133	5	**42**

This table provides the amount of lead determined in national surveys of products consumed by adults within the European Union. The data were collected during different periods in the 1990s and 2000s and vary due to study methodology, regional and cultural factors

The bioavailability of lead within the soil depends on pH, amount of organic matter present, amount of additives (i.e. limestone) within the soil, soil moisture levels, cation exchange capacity, and the forms of lead in the soil. For a majority of raw foods, lead is present at low concentration levels. However, contamination during production and processing is responsible for enhanced lead intake via dietary sources. While cocoa beans have the lowest reported values for a raw food, manufactured cocoa and chocolate products have among the highest values reported for all foods (Rankin et al. 2005). Atmospheric emissions of lead particulates contaminate shells, which protect the raw cocoa bean quite well from lead. However, as the beans are harvested, sun dried, and processed, contamination of the cocoa bean can occur upon mixing with the shells. Subsequent transport, distribution, and product formulations also allow for further lead contamination.

In a remote, riverside population within the Brazilian Amazon, with no known documented source of environmental or occupational lead, Barbosa and colleagues found 57% of participants had blood lead levels equal to or higher than 10 µg/dL (Barbosa et al. 2009). The mean blood lead levels were 13.1 ± 8.5 µg/dL (males 15.3 µg/dL vs females 7.9 µg/dL). Upon investigating, the villages with the highest exposures had two sources of lead: the production of farinha and hunting. The artisanal production of farinha (flour) from manioc requires roasting the pulp over fire on metal plates that contain leaded alloy. The young men spend several hours stirring the pulp, inhaling lead vapors, and ultimately consuming the farinha with produced food. Raw manioc had a mean lead concentration of 0.017 µg/g $\pm$ 0.016 (range 0.003–0.04 µg/g) while that for farinha was 0.19 µg/g $\pm$ 0.10 (range 0.09–0.38 µg/g). The lead exposure from hunting arises from contamination of the game from bullets with leaded alloys.

174.2.2 Transfer of Lead to Food from Children's Hands

For Western societies, there is at least a century of human industrialized activity, which produced pervasive contamination of air, soil, and water. Airborne lead particles from industrial sources continue to be deposited in soil and water, and thus, enter the food supply. Household lead contamination occurs in homes previously painted (interior and/or exterior) with leaded paint and/or situated near major highways as the deposition of lead particulates from decades of leaded petroleum product emissions contaminate the soil. In 2000, 1.2 million housing units in the United States with low-income families having children under 6 years of age were reported with deteriorated paint, dust, or bare soil contaminated with lead (Jacobs et al. 2002). Young children, especially toddlers, obtain leaded dust on their hands as they crawl, learn to walk, fall, and move about their residential environment. Freeman demonstrated that children with previously elevated lead levels transferred significant amounts of lead dust to their food (Freeman et al. 2001) by handling food items with their hands. The residential environment, the parents and children's hygiene habits influence the amounts of dietary lead exposure.

174.2.3 Pica Activity

Pica activity, the consumption of nonfood items, particularly in children and pregnant women, greatly increases the risk of lead intake. Pica activity is attributed to cultural and low socioeconomic factors as well as nutritional deficiencies. For children engaging in pica behavior, the soil ingestion rate may be as high as 5 g/day. Blood lead levels ≥ 10 µg/dL in children 6–71 months of age have been associated with yard soil containing lead concentrations exceeding 500 mg/kg (ATSDR 2007).

174.2.4 Lead Contamination of Water

Another dietary source of lead is water used for drinking and in the preparation of beverages, particularly coffee, tea, and infant formulas. Within the United States (US), the Environmental Protection Agency (EPA) monitors municipal water supplies. In 1991, the EPA set an action level for lead in tap water at 0.015 mg/L (15 ppb) with estimates that less than 1% of the public water systems have water entering the distribution system at levels above 5 µg/L (ATSDR 2007). Lead in US drinking water potentially contributes 10–20% of total lead exposure in young children. Lead found in US drinking water is usually derived from corrosion of lead pipes, lead-based solder, and brass, chrome, or bronze plumbing fixtures with older residences. Lead corrosion can occur with soft, acidic water (low pH) and by increasing the dissolved oxygen demand. The temperature and length of time that drinking water resides in a pipe alters the lead concentration within the water. Studies found that 57% of public school buildings in Philadelphia in 2000 and 2001, as well as 22% reported in Seattle during 2004, had lead water levels exceeding recommended levels (Bryant 2004; Sathyanarayana et al. 2006). Lanphear et al. found that children who lived in housing with a water lead concentration greater than 5 ppb had blood lead concentrations that were 20% (1 µg/dL) higher than children living in housing with water lead concentrations below 5 ppb (Lanphear et al. 2002). In Washington DC, increased levels of lead in drinking water were found when the municipal utility changed the disinfectant from free chlorine to chloroamine, which precipitated out lead from leaded plumbing. The incidence of blood lead levels exceeding 10 µg/dL for children less than 30 months increased more than four times (Edwards et al. 2009). Lead in drinking water may be a significant contributor to lead burdens, especially in persons with elevated blood lead levels where no paint or soil source of contamination is found (Levin et al. 2008).

174.2.5 Lead in Traditional Medicines

Traditional medicines, herbal remedies, and other supplements often contain significant amounts of lead either contaminated in processing or directly included in the formulation of the product. Karri et al. found 76 case reports of lead encephalopathy associated with traditional medicine published between 1966 and February 2007 (Karri et al. 2008). For 95% of the reports, the patients involved were infants and young children with outcomes that included death (11%) and residual neurological deficits (21%). Such products are listed in Table 174.5 along with their intended benefit and regional origin. The amounts of lead within the products are variable.

174.2.6 Standards for Lead Intake

The US Food and Drug Administration provisional total tolerable intake levels (PTTI) currently set for young children, for adults, and for pregnant and lactating women are 6, 62.5, and 25 µg/day, respectively. Mindak et al. determined the lead content of 324 multivitamin–mineral products and found that an overall median value for lead exposure was 0.576 µg/day (Mindak et al. 2008). The estimated median and maximum lead exposures varied for young children (less than or equal to 6 years) at 0.123 and 2.88 µg/day, older children (7 years and over) at 0.356 and 1.78 µg/day, adult women at 0.842 and 4.92 µg/day, and for pregnant and lactating women at 0.845 and 8.97 µg/day. In another study, the concentration of lead found in 95 major dietary supplements with an emphasis on botanical-based products, ranged from 20 to 48,600 µg/kg with a median concentration of 403 µg/kg. (Dolan et al. 2003) For 11 products, the lead levels would exceed the tolerable lead intakes for children

Table 174.5 Traditional medicines, herbal remedies and supplements with lead (Adapted from CT 2009 and NY 2009)

Traditional medicines and herbal products	Uses and conditions treated	Region of origin
Albayalde	Vomiting, colic, apathy, lethargy	Mexico, Central America
An Kung Niu Huan Wan (Peaceful Palace Ox Gallstone Pill	Vertigo, delirium, high fevers, measles, restlessness	China
Anzroot	Gastroenteritis	Middle East
Azarcon, also known as Alarcon, Maria Luisa, Coral, Rueda	Gastrointestinal symptoms	Mexico
Ba Bow Sen	Hyperactivity and nightmares in children	China
Bal Chamcha	Problems w/liver, digestion, teething, milk intolerance, irregular stools, colic, regurgitation, bloating, parasites, poor sleep, poor dentition, myalgia	India
Bal Jivan	Baby tonic	India
Bala Goli/Fita	Dissolved in "gripe water"; used for stomach ache	India
Bala Guti	Children's tonic	India
Bala Sogathi	Growth of children, teething, cough, cold, fever, and diarrhea	India
Balguti Kesaria	Tonic tablets for infants with sudha and gold rickets, coryza, cough griping, skin roughness, worms, and dental problems	India
Bao Ning Dan	Traditional remedy for acne, pain, and removing toxins	China
Bezoar Sedative Pills	High grade fever, encephalitis, inflammation, infection, infantile convulsions, and viral meningitis	China
Bint Al Zahab	Diarrhea, colic, constipation, general neonatal use	Middle East, Iran
Bokhoor	Fumes calm infants	Saudia Arabia
Cebagin	Teething powder	Middle East
Chuifong tokuwan	Joint pain, arthritis	Asia
Cordyceps	Hypertension, diabetes, bleeding	China
Deshi Dewa	Fertility	India
Emperor's Tea Pill	Maintain body's natural balance	China
Farouk	Teething powder	Saudi Arabia
Ghasard also known as Ghazard and Qhasard	Aid digestion	India
Greta	Digestive problems	Mexico, Central America
Hai Ge Fen	Gastrointestinal ailments	China
Hepatico Extract	Healthy liver and regularity	China
Jambrulin	Diabetes, sugar control	India
Jeu Wo Dan	Cast dressing	China
Kandu	Intestinal problems	Asian
Kohl also known as Kajal and Surma	Eye cosmetic; Infant eye treatment; skin infections, navel of newborns	Middle East, Africa, South Asia, India
Koo Sar, Koo Soo	Menstrual cramps	Hong Kong
Liga	Digestive and stomach problems	Mexico
Litargirio	Deodorant/antiperspirant	Dominican Republic
Lu Shen Wan	Mumps, fever, infections, sore throat	China
Maha Yograj Guggul	Musculo-skeletal disorders	India
Mahalakshmi Vilas Ras with gold	Cold related symptoms, blood deficiency, wound healing, asthma	India
Mahayogaraj Guggulu	Rheumatic pain	India

(continued)

Table 174.5 (continued)

Traditional medicines and herbal products	Uses and conditions treated	Region of origin
Mahayogaraj Guggulu with silver and Makardhwaj	Rheumatic pain, bile, pigmentation disorders, blood purification, eye problems, weakness	India
Molleja de Pollo Molida	Stomach ache	Mexico
Murrah, al-murrah	Colic, stomach aches, diarrhea	Saudi Arabia
Navratna Rasa	General debility, rickets, calcium deficiency	India
Pay-loo-ah	Rash and high fever	Southeast Asia
Po Ying Tan	Childhood complaints	China
Qing Fen	Cast dressing, pain	China
Rueda	Colic, calm children	China
Santrinj	Teething powder	Saudi Arabia
Sundari Kalp	Menstrual health	India
Saoot	Eye injury, teething, navel of newborns	Middle Eastern
Surma	Teething powder	India
Swarna Mahayograj Guggulu with gold	Rheumatism, gas, cerebrovascular accident, menstrual cycles, menopause, progesterone deficiency, mental disorders, fertility	India
Tibetan Herbal Medicine	Mental retardation	Tibet, India
White Peony Scar Repairing Pills	Scars	Hong Kong
Zhui Feng Tou Gu Wan/ Zhiufeng Tougu Wan	Bone ailments, joint pain, numbness	China

This table provides a reference of traditional medicines, herbal remedies, and supplements known to have significant lead concentrations, their intended usage, and region of origin

and women of child-bearing age. In a survey of lead concentrations in 45 pharmaceutical products by Kauffman, the average mass of lead ingested by the consumer was 0.22 μg/day (Kauffman et al. 2007). The highest lead containing product, a calcium antacid and supplement, was estimated to deliver a maximum daily lead mass of 2.7 μg/day. Lead contamination of calcium supplements has been reported in several studies with older studies tending to find greater lead levels (Bourgoin et al. 1993; Ross et al. 2000; Scelfo and Flegal 2000; Kim et al. 2003). However, overuse of supplements with "safe lead levels" can result in lead intake in excess of current tolerable limits, particularly in vulnerable populations such as children, pregnant, and lactating women.

174.3 Factors Influencing Lead Absorption Within the Body

Lead can be characterized as organic or inorganic depending upon the chemical form. Organic complexes such as tetraethyl lead (TEL) and tetramethyl lead (TML), added to petroleum products for usage as antiknock agents in automobile engines, decompose into trialkyl and dialkyl lead compounds such as lead halides and ammonium lead halides upon atmospheric release and exposure to sunlight. These compounds further react with the air, water, and soil in the environment to produce inorganic forms, which are likely to be ingested as inorganic lead alloys and lead salts. Nearly all forms of lead from anthropogenic sources that are released to soil are inorganic lead compounds. Inorganic lead compounds can be inhaled and swallowed depending on the particle size. In the human body, inorganic lead is metabolized upon forming ligand complexes with amino acids, non-protein thiols, and various proteins (ATSDR 2007). Inorganic lead can be measured in tissues, blood, serum, urine, sweat, saliva, breast milk, cerebrospinal fluid, bone, nails, teeth, and hair.

174.3.1 Nutritional Modifiers

Nutritional factors are often mentioned as important modifiers of the metabolism and toxicity of lead. Essential elements, such as calcium, iron, and zinc, interact with lead as demonstrated in studies of both animal models and humans. These interactions are complex and inter-related. Evidence in the literature (see review (Ros and Mwanri 2003)) supports the nutritional statements listed in Table 174.6; however, some concepts remain controversial.

A recent clinical trial found that for mild-to-moderately lead-poisoned children with sufficient dietary calcium, further supplementation aimed at providing 1,800 mg of calcium per day had no effect on the change in blood lead levels (Markowitz et al. 2004). Another trial evaluated the efficacy of iron and/or zinc supplementation on cognitive performance in school children living in a lead-contaminated city (Rico et al. 2006). For 6 months, children were given 30 mg of iron, 30 mg of zinc, both or placebo daily. At three time points (baseline, end of the trial, and 6 months after the supplementation trial ended) children were evaluated with cognitive tests of memory, attention, visual–spatial abilities, and learning. Among the groups, no consistent or persistent differences in cognitive performance were found. The existing evidence does not support the usage of dietary interventions as a key strategy for a reduction in childhood lead exposure (Ballew and Bowman 2001).

There is a large body of literature supporting the concept that children absorb more lead than adults. Specifically, water-soluble lead absorption appears to be higher in appropriately nourished children than adults, 40–50% versus 3–10%, respectively (ATSDR 2007). However, the fact that blood lead levels rise may be related to bone turnover associated with growth rather than increased absorption within the gastrointestinal tract.

174.3.2 Lead Mobilization from Bone

Without current exposure, women's blood lead levels may rise from the mobilization of lead from bone, which occurs during times of physiological stress such as pregnancy, and lactation in response to calcium demands of the developing fetus and nursing infant (Manton 1985; Gulson et al. 1998). Since lead readily crosses the placenta, fetal lead exposure can be significant and related to adverse postnatal outcomes (reduced birth weight and gestational age, postnatal mental retardation, and impaired neurobehavioral development) as fetal blood lead concentration is highly correlated with

Table 174.6 Nutritional features associated with ingested lead

- Lead ingested during fasting is absorbed at a much higher rate than lead ingested with a regular food intake.
- Retention of lead in children is important due to more rapid gastric emptying times.
- Calcium inhibits the absorption of lead in mammals by binding to and displacing lead from common mucosal carriers in the intestinal tract, though it is short-lived, as calcium must be present with lead.
- Calcium deficiency mobilizes lead from the bone and distributes it via the blood to soft tissues, thereby increasing the concentration of lead in critical organs, particularly the brain.
- For experimental animals, iron deficiency increases lead absorption from the intestinal tract. In humans, the relationship is uncertain.
- Lead and iron compete for critical binding sites; lead further aggravates the features of iron deficiency.
- Iron deficiency and lead toxicity both adversely affect cognitive development. Children with elevated blood lead levels should also be evaluated for iron deficiency, as those at risk for one are likely to be at risk for the other.
- Blood lead levels and activity of zinc-containing heme enzymes, such as ALAD, are inversely related indicating lead can replace zinc in these systems.

The table summarizes how calcium, iron, and zinc influence dietary lead absorption and concentration levels

maternal levels (Goyer 1990). Calcium supplementation at levels of 1200–1,500 mg/day is recommended for pregnant and nursing women. For postmenopausal women and those with osteoporosis, bone mineral resorption can cause lead stored in the bones to be released into the blood.

174.4 Neurological Impact of Lead Exposure

174.4.1 Mechanisms of Action

The neurological impact of lead exposure has been examined in humans, animals, and in vitro systems for several decades (see reviews by Lidsky and Schneider 2003; Toscano and Guilarte 2005; Garza et al. 2006). Significant advancements have been made to our understanding of how lead exerts neurotoxicity to humans and animals. Multiple toxic mechanisms of action for lead are present in the brain, which are often variable in presentation, overlapping in function and opposing in dose–effect relationships. These mechanisms are listed in Table 174.7 (Garza et al. 2006). A common factor among many of these mechanisms is the ability of lead to mimic calcium. In both the developing and adult brain, the ability of lead to substitute for calcium allows selective passage into the brain across the blood–brain barrier. As mentioned previously, intrinsic factors (age, sex, etc.), genetic mechanisms of metal transport, nutritional factors, and dosage factors (form, concentration, duration, and timing) can modulate the lead concentration that reaches the human brain. Lead exposure during distinct periods of neurodevelopment can produce different effects. Chronic "low-level" exposure may also produce different effects from acute "moderate to high-level" exposures. Such modulation of factors can influence human outcomes and contribute to contradictory findings in model systems. While many animal models employ a dietary ingestion method for lead dosing, the majority of human epidemiological studies assume the primary exposure source is inhalation. The neurological aspects of lead exposure are dependent on exposure source as bioavailability modulates dose.

Many contemporary studies have sought to unravel the molecular and biochemical underpinnings associated with the cognitive and behavioral deficits associated with lead exposure. In children, the cognitive and behavioral effects of early, developmental lead exposure are now regarded as irreversible. Animal models, rats, and nonhuman primates with blood lead concentrations on the order of 10–15 µg/dL demonstrate deficits in learning, which are similar to those observed in children associated with lead exposure (Rice 1996; Cory-Slechta 2003).

Table 174.7 Neurotoxic effects and mechanisms of action for lead in the brain

- Apoptosis
- Calcium competition and substitution
- Disruption of calcium homeostasis
- Lipid peroxidation
- Alterations in neurotransmitter synthesis, storage, and release
- Excitotoxicity
- Alterations in the expression and operation of receptors
- Interference with second messenger systems
- Interference with mitochondrial metabolism
- Damage to the oligodendroglia and astroglia
- Zinc substitution in zinc-mediated processes

This table details the mechanisms of action found associated with lead toxicity in model systems

174.4.2 Protein Kinase C

In models of acute exposure, lead directly stimulates Protein Kinase C (PKC) activity at picomolar levels, which are 4–5 orders of magnitude greater than the action of calcium (Markovac and Goldstein 1988). Tomsig and Suszkiw subsequently found that lead, depending on the concentration range, was capable of both activating and inhibiting the enzyme (Tomsig and Suszkiw 1995). PKC influences synaptic transmission via synthesis of neurotransmitters, ligand-receptor interactions, conductance of ion channels, and dendritic branching. Evidence suggests that lead targets the γ-isoform of PKC, a calcium-dependent, neuron-specific isozyme of PKC involved in long-term potentiation, memory function, and spatial learning.

174.4.3 Neurotransmitters: Cholinergic, Dopaminergic, and Glutamatergic

Neurotransmitter systems, particularly cholinergic, dopaminergic, and glutamatergic, have important roles in brain development and cognitive function. Lead exposure decreases neurotransmission. For chronically lead-exposed animals, upregulation of cholinergic, dopaminergic, and glutamatergic receptors are generally consistent with findings of diminished presynaptic function.

Within the central nervous system (CNS), activity within the cholinergic neurons projecting from the basal region of the forebrain to the hippocampus is key for memory and learning activities. Lead blocks the evoked release of acetylcholine and diminishes cholinergic system function. Bielarczyk and colleagues found depression of choline acetyltransferase activity in the cortex and hippocampus of young adult rats exposed to lead only during early development (Bielarczyk et al. 1996). The study also found decreased functional cholinergic innervation in the hippocampus. These reported denervation-like effects in the hippocampus could represent an important factor in long-term learning and cognitive impairments following developmental exposure to low levels of lead (Bielarczyk et al. 1996).

The dopaminergic and glutamatergic systems play a role in many aspects of cognitive functioning including attention, impulsivity, flexibility, learning, and memory. Based on studies of rodents and nonhuman primates, it has been known for some time that the dopamine system is particularly sensitive to lead (Cory-Slechta 1995). Lead may impair regulation of dopamine synthesis and release. The prefrontal cortex has the highest concentration of dopamine of all cortical areas and is the region primarily involved with cognitive and executive functions. For the glutamatergic system, chronic developmental lead exposure increases the threshold of long-term potentiation (LTP) induction with a biphasic dose–effect relationship, and decreased magnitude of LTP. Decreases in stimulated glutamate release are a significant factor contributing to lead-induced changes in LTP. Alterations in the N-methyl-D-aspartate (NMDA) subtype of glutamate receptor can produce deficits in synaptic plasticity that affect learning and memory (Toscano and Guilarte 2005). Developmental lead exposure is able to modify NMDA receptor subunit expression, subunit composition, and synaptic localization resulting in activity changes for calcium-sensitive signaling pathways.

174.4.4 Neurological Symptoms Associated with Lead Encephalopathy

In humans with frank lead encephalopathy, blood lead levels typically exceed 70 μg/dL and manifest with initial symptoms that include headache, loss of memory, hallucinations, muscle tremors, ataxia, dullness, poor attention span, and irritability. At these blood lead levels and above, gastrointestinal distress and other systemic features can also be present. As the condition worsens, seizures, paralysis, coma, and death can occur. In fatal cases, histopathological features include cerebral edema, perivascular glial proliferation, altered capillaries, and neuronal damage consistent with hypoxic–ischemic injury.

Exposures at blood lead levels exceeding 40 μg/dL, typically found in adults with occupational lead exposure, can produce symptoms including headache, malaise, altered mood state, fatigue, lethargy, forgetfulness, irritability, dizziness, and paresthesia. In addition to these features, a significant number of studies have reported neuropsychological effects such as disturbances in manual dexterity, reaction time, visual–motor performance, and cognitive performance.

174.4.5 Pediatric Epidemiological Studies

Human epidemiological studies in children assume that the majority of lead exposure arises from inhalation of automotive emissions and the ingestion of dust from paint residues. However, one study of children demonstrated convincing dose–response deficits in cognitive abilities of lead exposure arising from drinking water (Fulton et al. 1987).

174.4.6 Epidemiological Studies and Intelligence Quotient

Needleman and colleagues investigated pediatric low-level lead exposure in children from Chelsea and Somerville, Massachusetts. This study documented cumulative exposure to lead using a measurement of lead in deciduous teeth, assessed confounding factors, and employed multivariate statistical procedures. Needleman and colleagues reported a covariate-adjusted difference in child IQ of approximately 4.5 points between groups "high" and "low" in tooth lead (Needleman et al. 1979). Teacher ratings of children's behavior in the classroom indicated more behavioral problems and academic difficulties among children with higher concentrations of lead. Many cohort studies were developed to verify these findings and refine study design (i.e. employ blood lead measures). Subsequently, a number of meta-analyses have established that lead is robustly associated with dose-related declines in IQ (Needleman and Gatsonis 1990; Pocock et al. 1994; Schwartz 1994). Lanphear and colleagues conducted a pooled analysis of seven prospective studies that were started prior to 1995 (Lanphear et al. 2005). The analysis involved 1,333 children with complete data on confounding factors used in the multivariable analyses. A significant number ($N = 244$) of children with blood lead concentrations that never exceeded 10 μg/dL were included in the analysis. The participating sites included Boston, MA; Cincinnati, OH; Cleveland, OH; Kosovo, Yugoslavia; Mexico City, Mexico; Port Pirie, Australia; and Rochester, NY. The primary outcome measure was full-scale IQ assessed in school-age children with the Wechsler scales (mean age of testing was 7 years). The median lifetime average blood lead concentration was 12.4 μg/dL (5th–95th percentile 4.1–34.8 μg/dL). The mean IQ of all children was 93.2 (SD 19.2). Multivariable regression analysis resulted in a six-term model including the log of concurrent blood lead, study site, maternal IQ, a measure of caretaking quality (Home Observation for Measurement of the Environment (HOME)), birth weight, and maternal education. Using a log-linear model, the study's authors estimated a decrement of 1.9 points (95% CI 1.2, 2.6) in full-scale IQ for a doubling of concurrent blood lead. However, the IQ point decrements associated with an increase in blood lead from 1 to 10 μg/dL were 6.2 points (95% CI 3.8, 8.6) compared to 1.9 points (95% CI 1.2, 2.6) with an increase in blood lead from 10 to 20 μg/dL. The individual effect estimates indicated steeper slopes in cohorts with lower blood lead levels.

In the Rochester Lead Study analyses using only children with peak blood lead levels less than 10 μg/dL found for each 1 μg/dL increase in concurrent blood lead levels was associated with a statistically significant, covariate-adjusted 1.8 point decline in IQ at 5 years of age (Canfield et al. 2003a). Nonlinear semiparametric smoothing revealed a covariate-adjusted decline of more than 7 IQ points up to 10 μg/dL of childhood average blood lead, whereas a more gradual decline of 2.5 points was associated with an increase in blood lead from 10 to 20 μg/dL.

174.4.7 Neuropsychological Deficits in Pediatric Lead Cohorts

Cognitive abilities, such as attention and executive functions, language, memory and learning, and visuospatial processing have been explored in association with lead exposure. Two of these abilities, attention/executive functions and visual–spatial skills, have demonstrated convincing evidence of diminishment associated with lead exposure (Table 174.8).

174.4.8 Attention Skills

Bellinger and colleagues examined a subset of the Chelsea and Somerville cohorts at 19–20 years of age with a battery of attentional measures (Bellinger et al. 1994). Higher tooth lead concentrations were significantly associated with poorer scores on the Focus-Execute and Shift factors of the battery, supporting the notion that early lead exposure is associated with poorer executive/regulatory functions thought reliant on frontal or prefrontal regions of the brain. Canfield and colleagues evaluated executive functioning and learning in the Rochester Lead Study cohort using the Shape School Task with embedded protocols requiring inhibition and attention switching mental sets (Canfield et al. 2003b). The mean blood lead level at 48 months was 6.5 μg/dL (range 2–21) with 80% of the children below 10 μg/dL. Following covariate adjustment, blood lead concentration at 48 months was negatively associated with children's focused attention, naming efficiency, and inhibition of

Table 174.8 Lead-associated findings reported from pediatric epidemiological cohorts of low-to-moderate lead exposure

- Decreased measures of general intelligence
- Deficits in tests of visual–spatial skills
- Impaired performance on tests of spatial working memory
- Increased errors on test of visual–motor integration
- Impaired performance on tests of spatial memory span
- Increased time required for tests of manual dexterity
- Increased numbers of errors and false alarms on continuous performance test
- Impaired performance on tests of cognitive flexibility
- Deficits with short-term memory
- Impaired performance on test requiring inhibition of automatic responding
- Impaired performance on tests of attention and attention switching
- Decreased academic school performance
- Increased externalizing behaviors, aggressive behaviors, disruptive behaviors
- Increased teacher and parent rankings for hyperactive behavior
- Increased antisocial, delinquent behaviors

This table summarizes the neurobehavioral deficits found from published studies of childhood lead exposure

automatic responding. Children with higher blood lead levels also completed fewer phases of the task and knew fewer color and shape names. At 6 years of age, the Working Memory and Planning protocols from the Cambridge Automated Neuropsychological Test Battery (CANTAB) were administered to assess mnemonic and executive functions (Canfield et al. 2004). Following covariate adjustment, children with higher blood lead concentrations showed impaired performance on tests of spatial working memory, spatial memory span, cognitive flexibility, and planning as indexed by tests of intradimensional and extradimensional shifts and an analogue of the Tower of London task. At 16 years of age, a comprehensive neuropsychological battery was administered to Cincinnati Lead Study participants (Ris et al. 2004). Childhood blood lead levels in the Cincinnati cohort were high with 30% of the cohort having at least one blood lead concentration in excess of 25 µg/dL during the first 5 years of life. After covariate adjustment, the strongest association between lead exposure and cognitive performance was found for attention factor scores derived from a principal components analysis with the findings more prominent among male subjects.

In 1943, Byers and Lord reported problems with attention and aggression in their patients who recovered from acute lead encephalopathy (Byers and Lord 1943). Needleman reported that disturbances in behavior and social conduct are prototypical sequela among victims of lead poisoning (Needleman 2004). Parents frequently report that following recovery from an episode of acute poisoning their child's behavior changed dramatically, and became restless, aggressive, impulsive, and inattentive. In the Yugoslavian prospective study, concurrent blood lead levels were significantly associated with parent ratings on the Destructive Behaviors subscale of the Achenbach CBCL upon covariate adjustment (Wasserman et al. 1998).

Lead levels measured in blood and/or teeth have been associated with teacher ratings of hyperactive behavior, attentional and behavioral problems in many studies (Needleman et al. 1979; Fergusson et al. 1988; Silva et al. 1988; Thomson et al. 1989). Using data from the National Health and Nutrition Examination Survey (1999–2002), Braun and colleagues examined the available blood lead concentrations for 4,704 subjects 4–15 years of age, 4.2% of whom were reported to have ADHD and stimulant medication use (Braun et al. 2006). Following covariate adjustment, higher blood lead concentrations were significantly associated with ADHD. Subjects with blood lead levels > 2 µg/dL were four times more likely to have a diagnosis of ADHD and be on stimulant medication. Braun and colleagues determined that nationally lead exposure accounts for 290,000 excess cases of ADHD in US children.

174.4.9 Visual–Motor Integration Skills

Studies employing specific measures of visual–motor integration skills, such as the Developmental Test of Visual Motor Integration, the Bender Visual-Motor Gestalt Test, demonstrate strong evidence linking deficits with early lead exposure (Winneke et al. 1990; Dietrich et al. 1993; Baghurst et al. 1995; Wasserman et al. 2000). Ris and colleagues observed a significant association between prenatal maternal blood lead levels and deficits in visual–spatial and constructional skills as indexed by Visual-Constructional factor scores for Cincinnati Lead Study participants at 16 years (Ris et al. 2004).

174.4.10 Neuroimaging

Several case reports describe neuroimaging features associated with lead encephalopathy arising from the use of traditional medicines and occupational exposures (Mani et al. 1998; Atre et al. 2006; Karri et al. 2008). In general, blood lead levels within the encephalopathic range can produce focal lesions with abnormal signal, calcified lesions, and edema. The distribution of the lesions is variable, but encompasses every brain lobe, including gray and white matter structures.

For children exposed to lead at low-to-moderate levels, "clinical" neuroimaging modalities (i.e. computerized tomography and magnetic resonance imaging (MRI)) provide very little insight into lead-associated injury responsible for cognitive deficits. Trope and colleagues performed MRI and MRS studies on a sample of 16 subjects with a history of elevated blood lead levels (23–65 µg/dL) prior to 5 years of age (Trope et al. 2001). The average time of evaluation was 8 years. Compared to age-matched controls composed of siblings or cousins without a history of undue lead exposure (i.e., ≤10 µg/dL), lead-exposed subjects exhibited a significant reduction in N-acetyl aspartate:creatine ratios within frontal cortical gray matter. N-acetyl aspartate is a metabolite shown to decrease in processes that involve decreased neuronal and axonal functioning and loss.

Using volumetric MRI, Cecil and colleagues also examined a subset of the Cincinnati Lead Study cohort (Cecil et al. 2008). In studies of 157 subjects between the ages of 19 and 24 years, analyses of whole-brain MRI revealed significant decreases in brain volume associated with childhood blood lead concentrations. Following adjustment for other significant covariates including age at time of imaging and birth weight, the most affected regions were within the frontal gray matter, specifically the anterior cingulate cortex and ventrolateral prefrontal cortex, which are areas associated with executive functions, including mood regulation, decision-making, and interpretation of sensory inputs. Areas of lead-associated gray matter volume loss were larger for males.

Using functional MRI, the influence of childhood lead exposure on language function was examined in a subset of 42 young adults from the Cincinnati Lead Study (Yuan et al. 2006). Subjects performed an integrated verb generation/finger-tapping paradigm. Higher childhood average blood lead levels were significantly associated with reduced activation in Broca's area, a recognized region of speech production in the frontal lobe of the left hemisphere. Higher blood lead levels were also associated with increased activation in the right temporal lobe, the homologue of Wernicke's area, which is associated with speech perception. These associations were statistically significant following adjustment for covariate including birth weight, and marijuana usage as assessed by a positive urine screen. Lead exposure during childhood reorganizes the brain circuitry responsible for language function in a striking, dose-dependent fashion.

174.5 Future Directions of Research and Policy

174.5.1 Research

The complex mechanisms of lead toxicity require further elucidation. Questions remain such as: (a) is there any "safe" level or threshold of exposure? (b) at what ages are humans, specifically children, most vulnerable to lead? (c) can dietary modifications and pharmaceutical interventions help to minimize the neurotoxic effects of lead? As we uncover more about the "normal" functioning of brain systems with emerging imaging technologies, we will also have the opportunity to study how lead perturbs cellular networks, as lead affects numerous neural systems.

Controlled trials of environmental interventions aimed at reducing an existing lead exposure source are necessary to offer options to exposed populations. Continued research understanding the low-level effects of lead exposure needs to be coupled with studies of concurrent exposures to other prevalent neurotoxicants. Examination of the current action level, 10 µg/dL, to possibly lower levels for children is important based upon emerging evidence of low-level lead exposure effects.

Table 174.9 Steps for reducing the harmful effects of lead exposure

- Remediate lead-contaminated soil, especially where children play and where food items are grown.
- Removal or abatement of leaded paint in homes.
- Removal of leaded dust from homes with frequent cleaning.
- Removal of cookware and storage containers containing lead.
- Replace water system lines to homes, plumbing, and pipes within homes.
- Provide nutritious diets with appropriate amounts of iron, zinc, and calcium.
- Provide appropriate monitoring of lead hazards in homes, schools, and other places where children play.
- Eliminate leaded additives in petroleum products, paint, jewelry, cosmetics, and other consumer items in all nations.
- Eliminate usage of traditional medicines, and supplements, which purposely include lead within the formulation.
- Minimize production of industrial materials containing lead.

This table summarizes actions that can be employed to minimize lead exposure

174.5.2 Policy Implications

Lead continues to threaten significant numbers of the world's population, as it remains present in several sources. The goal must be the prevention of lead exposure in all populations (Table 174.9). Elimination of lead additives to petroleum products and paint needs to be enacted in all nations. Primary prevention strategies to eliminate lead hazards in homes and workplaces must be implemented. Lead paint residues, particularly within dust and soil, are often found in the homes located in older, urbanized centers. Screening of high-risk, older housing units in urbanized centers for leaded paint and plumbing is needed to prevent exposure. Lead abatement, while costly, could provide greater savings in special education, medical, and crime-related costs. Lead added to paint continues to be found in toys and other consumer products. Support for regulations and resources for enforcements of existing standards must be strengthened.

Severe restrictions on industrial and all nonessential uses of lead will greatly minimize occupational exposures in addition to the general population. Uniform lead limits are also needed to insure the lowest achievable exposure to lead from pharmaceutical and dietary supplement products (Kauffman et al. 2007).

174.6 Applications to Environmental Neurotoxicants and Human Health

The decades of research in the field of lead neurotoxicity have demonstrated that exposure to lead is associated with neurological and neurobehavioral disorders in adults and children. Exposure to lead during infancy and childhood produces essentially irreversible deficits in cognition, attention, executive functions, intelligence, learning, memory, and increases in externalizing behavioral problems. The success in reducing environmental lead sources was difficult to achieve. Novel approaches with genetics, imaging, and epidemiological statistical modeling developed for investigating lead exposures offer tremendous potential to other toxicants. Confirmed and suspected ubiquitous toxicants such as mercury, traffic-related exhaust particles, tobacco smoke, polychlorinated biphenyls, pesticides, and some plastics may be responsible for human morbidities and disease in children and adults. Applying the lessons learned from lead to existing and emerging toxicants could improve the lives of significant numbers within the world's population.

174.7 Key Facts of Lead Toxicity

- Lead exposures have decreased dramatically due to the elimination of lead additives in petroleum products, paint, and lead solder in food cans.
- Lead remains a health threat as it remains present in our environment, in dust, land and water. Food grown in contaminated soil, handled by children living in home environments with lead dust from leaded paint residues and water obtained from leaded plumbing continue to serve as a source for potential lead exposure in children.
- Traditional medicines, herbal remedies, and supplements can contain significant amounts of lead.
- Factors such as age, sex, fasting status, nutritional deficiencies such as zinc and iron deficiency and pregnancy status for women modulate the amount of lead that enters the blood stream and ultimately, the brain.
- Human epidemiological studies find significant cognitive, neuropsychological, and motor deficits related to blood lead levels, even at levels below the currently set action level of 10 μg/dL.

Summary Points

- Despite efforts to reduce human exposure, lead contamination, particularly via dietary sources, remains a significant global health problem.
- Dietary lead exposures can arise from the ingestion of contaminated water, food, vitamins, supplements, pharmaceuticals, and traditional remedies.
- Lead contamination can occur at any step upon transferring these items from source to the consumer including the contamination of raw materials and implements involved in preparation, processing, handling, and transport of consumed items.
- Factors such as the form (organic versus inorganic) of lead, age of a person, nutritional status of the individual, and pregnancy influence lead absorption.
- Complex mechanisms of lead neurotoxicity are implicated from in vitro, animal, and human epidemiological studies.
- Meta-analyses of pediatric epidemiological cohorts have established that lead is robustly associated with dose-related declines in IQ.
- Recent advanced neuroimaging studies suggest gray matter neuronal volume loss and reorganization of function associated with low-to-moderate childhood lead exposure.

Definition and Explanations of Key Terms

Anthropogenic: Processes or materials are those derived from human activities
Cognitive: Process of thinking, comprehension, reasoning, learning, or understanding
Covariate: It is a variable that is possibly predictive of outcome under study
Epidemiological: Study of factors affecting the health of populations
Executive functions: Processes for planning, cognitive flexibility, abstract thinking, rule acquisition, initiating appropriate actions and inhibiting inappropriate actions, and selecting relevant sensory information
Hippocampus: A structure within the limbic system of the brain thought responsible for long-term memory and spatial navigation

Long-term potentiation: Major cellular mechanism responsible for memory and learning as neurons simultaneously communicate.

Neuropsychological: Refers to brain processes and behaviors relating to mental and behavioral functions

Neurotoxic: An agent which adversely acts on nerve cells

Toxicant: A chemical compound introduced into the environment by human activity that has an affect on organisms

Acknowledgments The authors were supported by grants from the National Institutes of Health, NIEHS R01 ES015559, NCI R01 CA112182, NIMH R03 MH074645, R01 MH078043 and P50 MH077138.

References

Agency for Toxic Substances and Disease Registry (ATSDR). Toxicological Profile for Lead, Atlanta: US Department of Health and Human Services; 2005.

Agency for Toxic Substances and Disease Registry (ATSDR). Toxicological Profile for Lead, Atlanta: US Department of Health and Human Services; 2007.

Atre AL, Shinde PR, Shinde SN, Wadia RS, Nanivadekar AA, Vaid SJ, Shinde RS. Am J Neuroradiol. 2006;27:902–3.

Baghurst PA, McMichael AJ, Tong S, Wigg NR, Vimpani GV, Robertson EF. Epidemiology. 1995;6:104–9.

Ballew C, Bowman B. Nutr Rev. 2001;59:71–9.

Barbosa F, Jr., Fillion M, Lemire M, Passos CJ, Rodrigues JL, Philibert A, Guimaraes JR, Mergler D. Environ Res. 2009;109:594–9.

Bellinger D, Hu H, Titlebaum L, Needleman HL. Arch Environ Health. 1994;49:98–105.

Bielarczyk H, Tian X, Suszkiw JB. Brain Res. 1996;708:108–15.

Bourgoin BP, Evans DR, Cornett JR, Lingard SM, Quattrone AJ. Am J Public Health. 1993;83:1155–60.

Braun JM, Kahn RS, Froehlich T, Auinger P, Lanphear BP. Environ Health Persp. 2006;114:1904–9.

Bryant SD. J Toxicol Clin Toxicol. 2004;42:287–94.

Byers RK, Lord EE. AMA Am J Dis Child. 1943;66:471–94.

Canfield RL, Gendle MH, Cory-Slechta DA. Dev Neuropsychol. 2004;26:513–40.

Canfield RL, Henderson CR, Jr., Cory-Slechta DA, Cox C, Jusko TA, Lanphear BP. New Engl J Med. 2003a;348:1517–26.

Canfield RL, Kreher DA, Cornwell C, Henderson CR, Jr. Child Neuropsychol. 2003b;9:35–53.

Cecil KM, Brubaker CJ, Adler CM, Dietrich KN, Altaye M, Egelhoff JC, Wessel S, Elangovan I, Hornung R, Jarvis K, Lanphear BP. PLoS Med. 2008;5:e112.

Cory-Slechta DA. Annu Rev Pharmacol Toxicol. 1995;35:391–415.

Cory-Slechta DA. Child Neuropsychol. 2003;9:54–75.

CT. Ethnic and Ayurvedics Products Containing Lead. Connecticut: Department of Public Health; 2009. Available at http://www.ct.gov/dph/lib/dph/environmental_health/lead/pdf/Ethinc-Ayurvedics_Products.pdf.

Dietrich KN, Berger OG, Succop PA. Pediatrics. 1993;91:301–7.

Dolan SP, Nortrup DA, Bolger PM, Capar SG. J Agric Food Chem. 2003;51:1307–12.

Edwards M, Triantafyllidou S, Best D. Environ Sci Technol. 2009;43:1618–23.

EU SCOOP. Assessment of the Dietary Exposure to Arsenic, Cadmium, Lead and Mercury of the Population of the EU Member States. Reports on Task for Scientific Cooperation. Report of Experts Participating in Task 3.2.11. Directorate-General Health and Consumer Protection. European Commission, Brussels. 2004. Available at http://ec.europa.eu/food/food/chemicalsafety/contaminants/scoop_3-2-11_heavy_metals_report_en.pdf.

Fergusson DM, Fergusson JE, Horwood LJ, Kinzett NG. J Child Psychol Psycchiatry. 1988;29:811–24.

Freeman NC, Sheldon L, Jimenez M, Melnyk L, Pellizzari E, Berry M. J Expo Anal Environ Epidemiol. 2001;11:407–13.

Fulton M, Raab G, Thomson G, Laxen D, Hunter R, Hepburn W. Lancet. 1987;1:1221–6.

Garza A, Vega R, Soto E. Med Sci Monit. 2006;12:RA57–65.

Goyer RA. Environ Health Persp. 1990;89:101–5.

Gulson BL, Mahaffey KR, Jameson CW, Mizon KJ, Korsch MJ, Cameron MA, Eisman JA. J Lab Clin Med. 1998;131:324–9.

Jacobs DE, Clickner RP, Zhou JY, Viet SM, Marker DA, Rogers JW, Zeldin DC, Broene P, Friedman W. Environ Health Persp. 2002;110:A599–606.

Karri SK, Saper RB, Kales SN. Curr Drug Saf. 2008;3:54–9.

Kauffman JF, Westenberger BJ, Robertson JD, Guthrie J, Jacobs A, Cummins SK. Regul Toxicol Pharmacol. 2007;48:128–34.

Kim M, Kim C, Song I. Food Addit Contam. 2003;20:149–53.

Lanphear BP, Hornung R, Ho M, Howard CR, Eberly S, Knauf K. J Pediatr. 2002;140:40–7.

Lanphear BP, Hornung R, Khoury J, Yolton K, Baghurst P, Bellinger DC, Canfield RL, Dietrich KN, Bornschein R, Greene T, Rothenberg SJ, Needleman HL, Schnaas L, Wasserman G, Graziano J, Roberts R. Environ Health Persp. 2005;113:894–9.

Levin R, Brown MJ, Kashtock ME, Jacobs DE, Whelan EA, Rodman J, Schock MR, Padilla A, Sinks T. Environ Health Persp. 2008;116:1285–93.

Lidsky TI, Schneider JS. Brain. 2003;126:5–19.

Mani J, Chaudhary N, Kanjalkar M, Shah PU. J Neurol Neurosurg PS. 1998;65:797.

Manton WI. Br J Ind Med. 1985;42:168–72.

Markovac J, Goldstein GW. Nature. 1988;334:71–3.

Markowitz ME, Sinnett M, Rosen JF. Pediatrics. 2004;113:e34–9.

Marti-Cid R, Llobet JM, Castell V, Domingo JL. Biol Trace Elem Res. 2008;125:120–32.

Mindak WR, Cheng J, Canas BJ, Bolger PM. J Agric Food Chem. 2008;56:6892–6.

Moschandreas DJ, Karuchit S, Berry MR, O'Rourke MK, Lo D, Lebowitz MD, Robertson G. J Expo Anal Environ Epidemiol. 2002;12:233–43.

Needleman H. Annu Rev Med. 2004;55:209–22.

Needleman HL, Gatsonis CA. JAMA. 1990;263:673–8.

Needleman HL, Gunnoe C, Leviton A, Reed R, Peresie H, Maher C, Barrett P. N Engl J Med. 1979;300:689–95.

NY. Imported herbal medicine products known to contain lead, mercury or arsenic. Department of Health and Mental Hygiene. The City of New York, 2009. Available at http://www.nyc.gov/html/doh/downloads/pdf/lead/lead-herb-almed.pdf.

Pocock SJ, Smith M, Baghurst P. BMJ. 1994;309:1189–97.

Rankin CW, Nriagu JO, Aggarwal JK, Arowolo TA, Adebayo K, Flegal AR. Environ Health Persp. 2005;113:1344–8.

Rice DC. Environ Health Persp. 1996;104 (Suppl 2):337–51.

Rico JA, Kordas K, Lopez P, Rosado JL, Vargas GG, Ronquillo D, Stoltzfus RJ. Pediatrics. 2006;117:e518–27.

Ris MD, Dietrich KN, Succop PA, Berger OG, Bornschein RL. J Int Neuropsychol Soc. 2004;10:261–70.

Ros C, Mwanri L. Asia Pac J Clin Nutr. 2003;12:388–95.

Ross EA, Szabo NJ, Tebbett IR. JAMA. 2000;284:1425–9.

Sathyanarayana S, Beaudet N, Omri K, Karr C. Ambul Pediatr. 2006;6:288–92.

Scelfo GM, Flegal AR. Environ Health Persp. 2000;108:309–13.

Schwartz J. Environ Res. 1994;65:42–55.

Silva PA, Hughes P, Williams S, Faed JM. J Child Psychol Psychiatry. 1988;29:43–52.

Thomson GO, Raab GM, Hepburn WS, Hunter R, Fulton M, Laxen DP. J Child Psychol Psychiatry. 1989;30: 515–28.

Tomsig JL, Suszkiw JB. J Neurochem. 1995;64:2667–73.

Toscano CD, Guilarte TR. Brain Res Brain Res Rev. 2005;49:529–54.

Trope I, Lopez-Villegas D, Cecil KM, Lenkinski RE. Pediatrics. 2001;107:1437–42.

UNEP. Draft final review of scientific information on lead. Geneva, Switzerland: United Nations Environment Programme, Chemicals Branch; 2008.

Wasserman GA, Musabegovic A, Liu X, Kline J, Factor-Litvak P, Graziano JH. J Pediatr. 2000;137:555–61.

Wasserman GA, Staghezza-Jaramillo B, Shrout P, Popovac D, Graziano J. Am J Public Health. 1998;88:481–6.

WHO. Evaluation of certain food additives and contaminants, Vol. 896. Geneva: WHO; 2000.

Winneke G, Brockhaus A, Ewers U, Kramer U, Neuf M. Neurotoxicol Teratol. 1990;12:553–9.

Yuan W, Holland SK, Cecil KM, Dietrich KN, Wessel SD, Altaye M, Hornung RW, Ris MD, Egelhoff JC, Lanphear BP. Pediatrics. 2006;118:971–7.

Chapter 175
Diet- and Mercury-induced Visual Loss

Cian E. Collins

Abbreviations

EPA   The Environmental Protection Agency
MR   Magnetic resonance
SCDS   The Seychelles Child Development Study
VEP   Visual evoked potential

175.1 Introduction

Mercury is a heavy metal emitted into the atmosphere from both natural (such as volcanoes) and human sources (power plants, mining, waste incineration etc.) (http://www.epa.gov/mercury).

Atmospheric mercury in rainwater enters lakes and oceans, where microbial activity converts inorganic mercury into organic methylmercury. Methylmercury is readily absorbed and actively transported into tissues. Thus, methylmercury bioaccumulates in aquatic food chains and concentrations are magnified through the food chain. Larger, longer-living predators (e.g. swordfish, shark) have higher tissue concentrations, while smaller or shorter-lived species (e.g. shellfish, salmon) have very low concentrations. (http://www.epa.gov/mercury/report.htm)

Our knowledge of the effects of methylmercury poisoning on a population is based on two well-known industrial accidents. Industrial pollution of Minamata Bay, Japan in the 1950s poisoned local fish stocks and when local people consumed these contaminated fish, they suffered extensive neurological damage including paraplegia, ataxia, paresthesias, confusion, and in some cases, death (Tsubaki and Takahashi 1986). Visual symptoms reported include sudden bilateral blindness, constricted visual fields, and poor night vision. Seed grain contaminated by mercury mistakenly made its way into the food chain in Iraq in the 1970s and caused similar acute and chronic effects (more than 6000 people hospitalized, 459 deaths, and extensive neurological defects). (Bakir et al. 1973)

C.E. Collins (✉)
Princess Alexandra Eye Pavilion, Chalmers Street, Edinburgh EH3 9HA
e-mail: collinscian@btinternet.com

V.R. Preedy et al. (eds.), *Handbook of Behavior, Food and Nutrition*,
DOI 10.1007/978-0-387-92271-3_175, © Springer Science+Business Media, LLC 2011

175.2 Neurological Findings

In adult monkeys and humans, methylmercury exposure has been linked to constriction of the visual field and abnormal color vision (Korogi et al. 1994). Korogi et al performed MR imaging of the brains of patients with known Minamata disease. The visual cortex, the cerebellar vermis and hemispheres, and the postcentral cortex were significantly atrophic. MR also demonstrated lesions in the calcarine area, cerebellum, and postcentral gyri. Korogi et al later looked at the striate cortex in patients with known Minamata disease and visual field constriction. They found a correlation between the visual field defect and the extent of dilatation of the calcarine fissure. (Korogi et al. 1997).

Ventura et al (Ventura et al. 2004) have reported on electrophysiological findings in patients with a history of mercury intoxication. Full-field ERGs showed that scotopic, photopic, peripheral, and midperipheral retinal functions were affected, and the multifocal ERGs indicated that central retinal function was also significantly depressed.

Electrophysiological testing of workers exposed to mercury vapors found a significant reduction of Visual Evoked Potential (VEP) latency, especially for the N75. (Urban et al. 2003) Further work completed in 2003 identified greater color confusion, greater errors on color, testing and an increased frequency of type III dyschromatopsias (blue–yellow confusion axis) in comparison with the control group. Cavalleri et al (Cavalleri and Gobba 1998) studied a group of workers with high levels of urinary mercury and found a dose-related impairment of color discrimination. Following changes to their work practices, mercury levels 12 months later had fallen to one-tenth of the previous levels and their color vision had returned almost to normal.

Neurological recovery after removal of the source of mercury is variable. Color vision impairment as a result of occupational mercury exposure was noted to be irreversible in one large study (Feitosa-Santana et al. 2008). Mercury-exposed patients had significantly worse color discrimination ($p < 0.02$) than controls, as evaluated by the size of MacAdam's color discrimination ellipses and color discrimination thresholds along protan, deutan, and tritan confusion axes. These changes persisted and were unchanged three years later. Other symptoms such as peripheral neuropathies have been noted to persist with little improvement, even up to 30 years later, after prolonged occupational exposure to inorganic mercury(Letz et al. 2000)

175.3 Children and Mercury Exposure

Children with raised blood mercury concentrations have been studied for changes in visual function testing. Saint-amour et al (Saint-Amour et al. 2006), examining preschool Inuit children living in Nunavik Northern Quebec, reported similar reduced VEP latency to those found in mercury-exposed workers. Many seaside communities depend on fish as a major food source. A large study by Davidson et al. (1998) followed 711 mother and child pairs in the Seychelles over a 5-year period from pregnancy through childhood. Using 6 age-appropriate test of neurodevelopment, no adverse effect was found to be associated with a raised hair mercury level of 6.5 ppm (US average is quoted as 0.47–3.8 ppm).

175.4 Pregnancy and Mercury Exposure

Methylmercury crosses the placenta, and fetal exposure correlates with maternal exposure. Following the Minamata and Iranian disasters, marked neurodevelopmental abnormalities were found in children exposed in-utero to very high levels of mercury. (Gochfeld 2003) Very high doses of methylmercury have been associated with mental retardation, poor motor function, ataxia, and seizures (Harada 1995).

In the mid-1980s, 2 large cohort studies were initiated: one in the Republic of Seychelles called the Seychelles Child Development Study (SCDS) (Van Wijngaarden et al. 2006) and the other in the Faeroe Islands. (Myers and Davidson 1998) In the Seychelles study, of a total of 46 primary end points, only one end point showed a possible adverse association with prenatal methylmercury exposure. The Faeroes study reported adverse associations between prenatal methylmercury exposure and tests of memory, attention, language, and visual–spatial perception measured at 7 years of age.

Seafood species are also rich dietary sources of selenium. Selenium may reduce tissue accumulation of mercury in fish and humans. (Seppanen et al. 2000) The protective effect of selenium may partly account for conflicting results of studies of mercury exposure and neurodevelopmental indexes in children. (Raymond and Ralston 2004)

175.5 Chronic Diet-related Exposure

We recently published an unusual case of diet-related mercury poisoning resulting in visual loss in a 36-year-old man of Caribbean origin living in the UK. (Saldana et al. 2006) His unexplained neurological symptoms (peripheral neuropathies, reduced visual acuity, central scotomas) were eventually linked to his raised blood mercury levels at 13.9 µg/l. The Environmental Protection Agency (EPA) quotes the US average blood mercury to be 1.3 µg/l (http://www.epa.gov/waterscience/fishadvice/advice.html). He underwent electrophysiological testing and multifocal visual evoked potential showed almost abolition of the central responses in both eyes. Multifocal ERG also showed mild reduced amplitudes and delayed responses.

His liking for imported Caribbean fish known to be high in mercury levels (3 or 4 red snapper fish, every day) was identified as the likely source and his change in diet has to date produced little improvement.

A previously published case-report highlights a 53 year-old woman with similar dietary exposure. She had been eating fresh fish between 6 and 12 times per week for more than 10 years and ate swordfish at least twice a week. Her hair mercury levels measured 67.8 ppm (US average is quoted as 0.47–3.8 ppm). She initially presented to her doctor with skin erythema, and later developed stomatitis, headaches, and tinnitus. (Risher John 2004) No further details were provided as to her progress after reducing exposure to mercury.

175.6 Applications to Other Areas of Health and Disease

The EPA states the reference dose, (ie the allowable upper limit of daily intake) for methylmercury of 0.1 ug/kg per day, which is 50 µg/wk for a 70-kg woman. This was calculated from the lower 95% confidence limit at which gestational exposure to mercury may produce abnormal neurological test scores, multiplied by a 10-fold uncertainty factor. The EPA also has published a focused advisory for women of childbearing age, nursing mothers, and young children. (http://www.epa.gov/waterscience/fishadvice/advice.html)

The advisory specifically advises such individuals to avoid shark, swordfish, golden bass, and king mackerel (each containing >50 µg methylmercury per serving); to eat up to 12 oz/wk (two average meals) of a variety of fish and shellfish lower in mercury; and to consult local advisories for locally caught freshwater fish. However, a recent Lancet article showed mothers who consumed more than the US recommendations (340 g or three portions per week) had children who scored better on tests of fine motor, communication, and social skills. (Myers and Davidson 2007)

A large review published in JAMA highlighted the benefits of regular fish consumption (1–2 servings per week of oily fish) in adults (Mozaffarian and Rimm 2006). It identified the reduction in risk of coronary death by 36% and total mortality by 17%.

Summary

- Many studies have tried to identify whether the known benefits of a diet rich in seafood are outweighed by the dangers posed by methyl mercury.
- Large studies on childhood neurodevelopment in communities with a high rate of fish consumption show conflicting results depending on the type of neurological tests used.
- Overall, it is felt that any adverse effects of methylmercury are likely to be minimal alongside the known nutritional advantages of fish oils and omega-3 in a child's neurodevelopment.
- Fish consumption in adults has been shown to confer significant cardiovascular health benefits. Studies suggest people may be avoiding fish consumption due to the risks of methylmercury toxicity and may miss out on the known health benefits of fish consumption.
- Visual changes associated with mercury exposure depend on the duration and degree of exposure.
- Toxic effects on the brain and optic pathways are unfortunately likely to be irreversible.
- Diet-related visual loss is extremely rare and is not a risk to people who keep within the common-sense guidelines

---

Definitions

Inorganic mercury: A heavy metal found in the environment, which is nontoxic and cannot be absorbed in this form

Methylmercury: When mercury is converted into this organic form it can be absorbed and accumulated in tissues resulting in toxicity

Minamata disease: Called after the Minamata area in Japan where it was first described, it is a broad spectrum of neurological disorders caused by exposure to high doses of methylmercury.

Neurodevelopmental testing: A complex series of tests that compare many neurological functions (such as memory, language, motor function and spatial awareness) in subjects with expected age-matched levels in a control population.

Electrophysiological testing: Visual stimuli are introduced to the patient and the electrophysiological responses produced by the photoreceptors are measured by contact skin probes around the eyes. These findings are compared to expected average responses in a control population.

Key facts on mercury exposure and vision

1. Most significant cases of visual loss are as a result of industrial accidents, where there was exposure to very high levels of methylmercury.
2. Most people will only be exposed to methylmercury in any significant quantities if they consume seafood.
3. Certain fish (e.g. those higher up the food chain) will have considerably higher levels of methyl mercury than those short-lived species
4. Recommended guidelines suggest 1–2 servings of oily fish will provide most people with the beneficial effects without being at risk of methylmercury toxicity.

References

Bakir F, et al. Methylmercury poisoning in Iraq. Science. 1973;181:230–41.

Cavalleri A, Gobba F. Color vision impairment in workers exposed to neurotoxic chemicals fabriziomaria Gobbal, Alessandro Cavalleri. Neurotoxicology. 1998;24(2003):693–702.

Davidson G, et al. Effects of prenatal and postnatal methylmercury exposure from fish consumption on neurodevelopment: outcomes at 66 months of age in the Seychelles Child Development Study. JAMA. Feb 17 1998;280(8):701–7.

Feitosa-Santana C, et al. Irreversible color vision losses in patients with chronic mercury vapor intoxication. Vis Neurosci. May-Jun 2008;25(3):487–91.

Gochfeld M. Cases of mercury exposure, bioavailability and absorption. Ecotoxicol Environ Saf. 2003;56:174–9.

Harada M. Minamata disease: methylmercury poisoning in Japan caused by environmental pollution. Crit Rev Toxicol. 1995;25(1):1–24, Review.

Korogi Y, Takahashi M, Shinzato J, Okajima T. Am J Neuroradiol. Sep 1994;15(8):1575–8.

Korogi Y, Takahashi M, Hirai T, Ikushima I, Kitajima M, Sugahara T, Shigematsu Y, Okajima T, Mukuno K. Representation of the visual field in the striate cortex: comparison of MR findings with visual field deficits in organic mercury poisoning (Minamata disease). Am J Neuroradiol. Jun-Jul 1997;18(6):1127–30.

Letz R, Gerr F, Cragle D, et al. Residual neurologic deficits 30 years after occupational exposure to elemental mercury. Neurotoxicology. 2000;21:459–74.

Mozaffarian D, Rimm EB. Fish intake, contaminants, and human health: evaluating the risks and the benefits. JAMA. Oct 18 2006;296(15):1885–99.

Myers GJ, Davidson PW. Prenatal methylmercury exposure and children: neurologic, developmental, and behavioral research. Environ Health Perspect. 1998 Jun;106(Suppl 3):841–7, Review.

Myers GJ, Davidson PW. Maternal fish consumption benefits children's development. Lancet. Feb 17 2007;369(9561):537–8.

Raymond LJ, Ralston NV. Mercury: selenium interactions and health implications. Seychelles Med Dent J. 2004;7:72–7.

Risher JF. Too much of a good thing (fish): methylmercury case study. J Environ Health. Jul/Aug 2004;67(1):9–14.

Saint-Amour D, et al. Alterations of visual evoked potentials in preschool Inuit children exposed to methylmercury and polychlorinated biphenyls from a marine diet. Neurotoxicology. 2006;27:567–78.

Saldana M, Collins C, Gale R, Backhouse O. Diet-related mercury poisoning resulting in visual loss. Br J Ophthalmol. 2006;90: 1432–4.

Seppanen K, Kantola M, Laatikainen R, et al. Effect of supplementation with organic selenium on mercury status as measured by mercury in pubic hair. J Trace Elem Med Biol. 2000;14:84–87.

Tsubaki T, Takahashi H. (editors) Recent advances in minimata disease studies: methylmercury poisoning in Minimata and Nigiita, Japan. Tokyo, Japan; 1986.

Urban P, Gobba F, Nerudova J, Lukas E, Cabelkova Z, Cikrt M. Color discrimination impairment in workers exposed to mercury vapor. Neurotoxicology. 2003 Aug;24(4–5):711–6.

US Environmental Protection Agency. Controlling power plant emissions: emissions progress. Washington: US Environmental Protection Agency; 2009a. http://www.epa.gov/mercury.

US Environmental Protection Agency. Mercury Study report to Congress. Washington: US Environmental Protection Agency; 2009b. http://www.epa.gov/mercury/report.htm.

US Environmental Protection Agency. What you need to know about mercury in fish and shellfish. Washington: US Environmental Protection Agency; 2009c. http://www.epa.gov/waterscience/fishadvice/advice.html.

Van Wijngaarden E, Beck C, Shamlaye CF, Cernichiari E, Davidson PW, Myers GJ, Clarkson TW. Benchmark concentrations for methyl mercury obtained from the 9-year follow-up of the Seychelles Child Development Study. Neurotoxicology. 2006 Sep;27(5):702–9.

Ventura DF, Costa MT, Costa MF, et al. Multifocal and full field electroretinogram changes associated with colour-vision loss in mercury vapour exposure. Visual Neurosci. 2004;21:421–9.

Part XXXI
Aging and Dementia

Chapter 176
Soy, Tofu and Brain Function in the Elderly

Amina Yesufu-Udechuku, Tri Budi W. Rahardjo, and Eef Hogervorst

Abbreviations

AD	Alzheimer's disease
Aβ	Amyloid beta
CASI	Cognitive abilities screening instrument
CI	Cognitive impairment
CVFT	Category verbal fluency test
DHEAS	Dehydroepiandrosterone sulphate
E	Estrogen
E2	17 β-Estradiol
ER	Estrogen receptor
ERα	Estrogen receptor alpha
ERβ	Estrogen receptor beta
FDA	Food and Drug Administration
FFQ	Food Frequency Questionnaire
HAAS	Honolulu Asia Aging Study
LDH	Lactate De-Hydrogenase
MMSE	Mini Mental Status Examination
MRI	Magnetic Resonance Imaging
P	Progesterone
RCT	Randomized Controlled Trials
ROS	Reactive Oxygen Species
SOPHIA	Soy and Postmenopausal Health In Aging Study
SWAN	Study of Women's Health Across the Nation
UK	United Kingdom
USA	United States of America
VaD	Vascular dementia

E. Hogervorst (✉)
School of Sport, Exercise and Health Sciences, Loughborough University,
Ashby Road, Loughborough, Leicestershire, United Kingdom
e-mail: E.Hogervorst@lboro.ac.uk

V.R. Preedy et al. (eds.), *Handbook of Behavior, Food and Nutrition*,
DOI 10.1007/978-0-387-92271-3_176, © Springer Science+Business Media, LLC 2011

176.1 Introduction

Dementia is characterized by severe cognitive decline, which impacts on daily living (American Psychiatric Association 1994). Its most common form is Alzheimer's disease (AD). Dementia is on the increase with an increasing aging population, particularly in developing countries. The human and economic costs of dementia are high and it is therefore important that cheap and easily adaptable preventive measures are identified. Given its biological plausibility (see Sect. 176.8), eating soy could be a potential preventive measure against cognitive impairment. This chapter describes the effect that phytoestrogens have on the brain and cognitive function in the elderly. The incidence of AD is lower in East Asian countries than in Western populations (see Sect. 176.9). Furthermore, East Asian populations consume significantly more soy in their daily diets. It has thus been hypothesized that these observed differences in AD prevalence can be attributed, in part, to the isoflavone-rich diets in Japan and China compared to the USA and Europe and the potential positive effects that isoflavones can have on the brain. However, other healthy lifestyle choices (e.g., consumption of fruit and vegetables, less alcohol consumption, more exercise and a lower body mass index, etc.) could also attribute to lower AD risk in these countries. In this chapter, we review the biochemistry of phytoestrogen, the food it occurs in and its effect on the brain using data derived from animal and cell culture studies, as well as data from observational and treatment studies in humans.

176.2 Soy, Tofu and Phytoestrogens

The soybean is an important part of the diet in East Asian countries, with increasing popularity in Western countries (see Table 176.1). Soy is used in the production of a number of food products, with the most well known being tofu (see Table 176.2). Soy foods contain varying quantities of phytoestrogens.

Phytoestrogens are naturally occurring polyphenolic molecules found in plants. Phytoestrogens are found in abundance in the soybean (and soybean-based products such as tofu) as well as other fruits, vegetables, grains, legumes and clover (Kurzer and Xu 1997). Phytoestrogens, or plant hormones, are very similar to estrogens (E) in their physiochemical and physiological properties (Murkies et al. 1998; Setchell 1998; Kurzer and Xu 1997). The Food Standards Agency (FSA) defined phytoestrogens as 'any plant substance or metabolite that induces biological responses in

Table 176.1 Key facts of soy

1. The soybean is an oilseed that is an important source of protein and vegetable oil and contains omega-3 fatty acids, alpha-Linolenic acid, and is the richest source of isoflavones.
2. Oil (20%) and protein (40%) account for approximately 60% of the weight of the soybean, with the remainder consisting of carbohydrate (35%) and approximately 5% ash (Mohamed and Xu 2003).
3. The majority of the compounds in the soybean are heat-stable, which makes the soybean suitable for high-temperature cooking to produce tofu, soymilk and textured vegetable protein (Mohamed and Xu 2003).
4. Soy-based foods have been eaten in Asian societies for over 1,000 years and are an important part of everyday diet (Murkies et al. 1998).
5. Soy is used to make foods such as tofu, tempe miso, natto as well as other products such as soy milk and soy sauce (Murkies et al. 1998).
6. Soy consumption is substantially higher in Asian societies than in Western countries with populations in Japan, Taiwan and Korea consuming approximately 20–150 mg/day from a variety of soy-based foods, compared to a much lower (approximately 1–3 mg/day) intake in Western populations (Murkies et al. 1998)

This table shows the key facts about soy which includes its composition, origins and uses in diet

Table 176.2 Key facts of Tofu

1. Tofu is of Chinese origin, although the exact origins and discovery have not been confirmed.
2. Tofu is made by coagulating soy milk from the soy-bean curd and using salt or acid coagulants. This is then formed into blocks and processed in a variety of ways to form different types and textures.
3. Tofu is relatively bland in taste and therefore picks up flavours easily. Because of this, it is used in Asian cooking in a wide variety of ways including soups, stews, stir-fries, eaten raw or stuffed with other fillings.
4. Although it originated from China, the spread of Buddhism (which places high importance on proteins and has a strict vegetarian diet) meant that tofu was then introduced into the diet in Korea, Japan, and other parts of East Asia, such as Indonesia, in the late eighth century.
5. In Western countries, tofu was not well known until the middle of the twentieth century with increasing popularity and adoption of vegetarian diets. It is not eaten widely but is popular amongst vegetarians, and promoted as a 'healthy superfood'.
6. Tofu contains isoflavones (a type of phytoestrogen) primarily in the aglycone form which previous research has shown has effects on the human brain similar to that of estrogen (a natural sex hormone).
7. The effects of consuming tofu on brain function are not fully known with studies reporting both positive and negative effects.
8. The effects of tofu consumption on the brain have been attributed to the high quantities of isoflavones (a type of phytoestrogen which mimics the effects of natural estrogen) as well as possibly other chemicals (e.g., formaldehyde) added in the processing of tofu which may be toxic to the brain.
9. It is possible that age, gender, quantity consumed and habitual intake may influence if tofu consumption has a protective or negative effect on cognitive function.

This table lists the key facts about tofu explaining its origins, the differences between populations in its consumption and its effects on cognitive function

vertebrates and can mimic or modulate the actions of endogenous, usually by binding to estrogen receptors' (FSA 2002). Es are naturally occurring hormones that promote secondary female sex characteristics and fertility. However, their role in also maintaining cognition in older women and men is now disputed, despite basic sciences data supporting their potential protective effects on the brain (see book edited by Hogervorst et al., 2009). The role of phytoestrogens in protecting the brain is less well investigated and this chapter aims to review the existing evidence available.

176.3 Phytoestrogen Classification

Phytoestrogens can be classified into three main categories; lignans, coumestans, and isoflavones. The most potent estrogenic aglycone isoflavones, and those mostly discussed in the current chapter, are daidzein and genistein (Fig, 176.1).

Isoflavones resemble estrogens in their heterocyclic phenol structure. The location of the hydroxyl groups allows binding to the estrogen receptor (ER) protein, and the A and C rings of isoflavones are similar to the A and B rings of 17β-estradiol (E2), the most potent E (Ganora 2008).

176.4 Application to Other Areas of Health and Disease

Before we discuss the possible effects of isoflavones on the brain and cognition, it may be important to highlight other more researched benefits (or potential increased risks) of phytoestrogen consumption. East Asians (who show high consumption of soy products) and Western populations show different prevalence rates for certain health conditions (Adlercreutz 1990), which could indirectly impact on cognitive health and risk of secondary dementias (APA 1994). Table 176.3 briefly describes some of these areas of research findings.

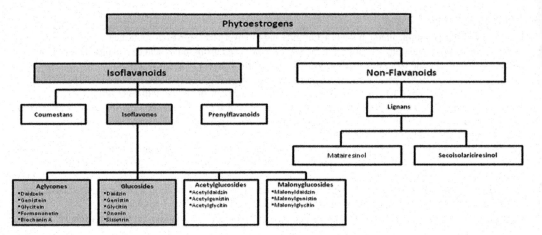

Fig. 176.1 Classification of phytoestrogens. This figure shows the classification of phytoestrogens. This chapter focuses on the isoflavones aglycones and glucosides

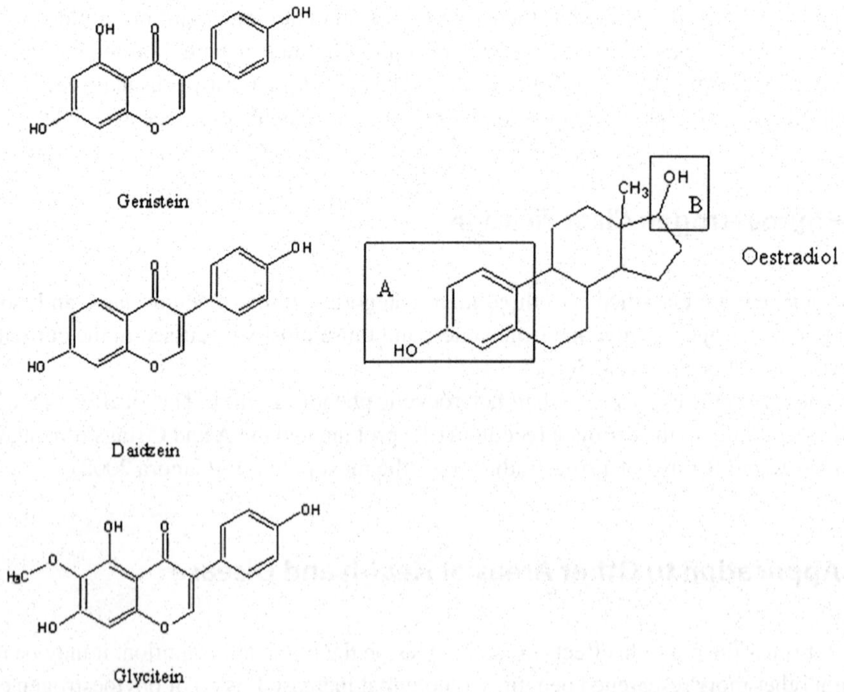

Fig. 176.2 Chemical similarities of aglycone isoflavones and oestradiol. Figure shows the structure of 17β-oestradiol, as well as the aglycone isoflavones genistein, daidzein, and glycitein. Aglycone isoflavone structures possess the phenolic (A) and hydroxyl (B) moieties also seen in estradiol, with a similar distance between the two groups (FSA 2002)

Table 176.3 Application to other areas of health and disease

- Asian population having a lower prevalence and incidence of some cancers, e.g., breast cancer (Wu et al. 2008) and prostate cancer (Dhom 1991).
- High soy intake has been associated with lower incidence of breast cancer (Wu et al. 2008) and prostate cancer (Coward et al. 1993).
- Concern has recently arisen from the reports of in vitro and animal studies finding an *increased* risk of breast cancer with soy isoflavones (Ju et al. 2006).
- Geographic differences in cardiovascular health have also been positively linked to soy intake (Azadbakht et al. 2007), as has a low prevalence of osteoporosis (Chiechi et al. 2002), and some menopausal symptoms (Maskarinec 2003).
- However, most research into the health effects of phytoestrogens has been on the basis of animal models and in vitro cell culture studies with only limited clinical assessments (see Knight and Eden 1996).

This table lists some other areas of health and disease which have shown cross-cultural variation and been linked to soy intake

176.5 Biological Mechanisms Explaining Neuroprotective Effects of Phytoestrogens

A number of studies have shown neuroprotective effects of isoflavones on various biological mechanisms. For full reviews see Murkies et al. (1998); Setchell (1998); and Adlercreutz and Mazur (1997). Isoflavones (and coumestans) thus have the ability to bind to the ERs in the mammalian body, but with less affinity than E2. They have shown greater binding to the ER-beta (ERβ) than the ER-alpha (ERα) receptor sites and can moderately interfere with the endogenous E-responsive signalling (Fitzpatrick 2003). On the other hand, genistein initiates greater gene transcription of ERα compared to ERβ, and also has the ability to bind to the progesterone (P) and androgen receptors (Fitzpatrick 2003) In postmenopausal women, who have very low levels of endogenous estrogens, phytoestrogens have greater potential to bind to ER than in premenopausal women, whose endogenous estrogens levels are much higher which renders greater competition for ER sites (Kuiper et al. 1998). Phytoestrogens can thus behave as estrogenic antagonists in environments with high levels of estrogens (e.g., during the ovulatory phase in premenopausal women), but can act as estrogenic agonists in low estrogenic environments (e.g., in postmenopausal women) (see Boettger-Tong et al. 1998; Murkies et al. 1998).

Although a great deal of attention has been paid to effects of phytoestrogens on peripheral systems, research is limited concerning the influence of phytoestrogens on the nervous system and cognitive function (Linford and Dorsa 2002; Halbreich and Kahn 2000) Phytoestrogens can directly protect the brain and act upon mechanisms thought to be implicated in Alzheimer's disease (AD, the most common form of dementia), such as the formation of tangles by tau protein phosphorylation and accumulation of the toxic amyloid-beta (Aβ) in plaques (Kim 2000). Phytoestrogens have been found to demonstrate a neuroprotective effect by attenuating tau protein phosphorylations (Kim et al. 2000), and by protecting cells against Aβ-induced apoptosis (self-programmed cell death) (Bang et al. 2004). The hippocampus is thought to be implicated in early AD (Reitz et al. 2009). Phytoestrogens have been found to regulate choline acetyltransferase, nerve growth factor, and brain-derived neurotrophic factor in the hippocampus, and also in the frontal cortex of female rats (Pan et al. 1999), which also is thought to play an important role in cognitive aging (see, e.g., Isingrini and Taconnat 2008).

Genistein and daidzein have also been found to protect hippocampal and cortical neurons against several forms of induced neurotoxicity (Occhiuto et al. 2008; Sonee et al. 2004). In an in vivo rat model study (Zeng et al. 2004), genistein reversed Abeta25–35-induced apoptosis and related cell pathology. Abeta25–35-induced apoptosis is associated with an increase in intracellular levels of free Ca^{2+}, the accumulation of reactive oxygen species (ROS), and the activation of caspase-3 and is further characterized by loss of cell viability and neuronal DNA fragmentation. Trieu et al. (1999) reported that cerebral lesions in mice caused by singlet-oxygen-induced cerebral strokes were reduced by 44% with genistein treatment compared to controls, supporting the potential antioxidant effects of soy isoflavones. Genistein was also found to increase the activity of anti-oxidant enzymes (Lee et al. 2005) and has earlier also been shown to have antioxidant effects on neurons exposed to free radical damage (Lee et al. 2005).

We must note that although these studies distinctly show neuroprotective qualities of genistein, other studies have reported that genistein can also induce apoptosis and damage in neurons. The association between phytoestrogens and brain function may therefore not be linear (e.g., more is always better). For example, Choi and Lee (2004) reported that rats consuming a very large dose of genistein (20 mg/day) showed an increase in lactate dehydrogenase (LDH), a marker of neuronal damage, in brain tissue, which was not the case for rats on low genistein regimes (2 mg/day). DNA fragmentation was seen in both treatment groups. It must be noted that these amounts of genistein given to rats in these studies would far exceed the normal amount of isoflavones that are given to human participants in treatment trials or eaten in a normal daily diet. For example, assuming a rat weighed approximately 300 mg and the average human weighs approximately 60 kg, a rat being given a dose of 2 mg/day is then the equivalent of giving a human 1,200 g/day of genistein. As we have previously discussed, even in populations where isoflavone consumption is very high (e.g. 100 mg/day = 0.1 g/day), this toxic dosage would equate to over 12,000 times the quantity of normal daily consumption.

176.6 Different Soy Foods and their Composition

Many databases have been developed to list the isoflavone content of soy foods (Beecher et al. 2000; Horn-Ross et al. 2000). A summary is given in Table 176.4. Soy is the richest source of genistein, is abundant in daidzein, and is the only source of glycitein (Zhao and Brinton 2007). The estrogenic effect of soy has been attributed to genistein and daidzein, as well as the daidzein metabolite, equol. Equol has high estrogenic activity. However, there are individual (genetic) and cross-cultural differences in the ability (or lack of it) to produce equol in the intestines (see discussion). The soy-bean is cultivated and processed in different ways to make products from its different components, and this can have a significant effect on the pharmacokinetics and pharmacodynamics of isoflavones. For example, consumption of tempe (which contains approximately 50% aglycone) was found to result in higher serum peak levels of genistein than 15% aglycone textured vegetable protein. However, soymilk (which also contains ≈ 15% aglycone) was absorbed quicker and reached peak plasma levels faster than both tempe and textured vegetable protein (Cassidy et al. 2006). Alcohol extraction and acid precipitation reduces the isoflavone content of soy protein and the soybean can be altered in its levels of fibre, fat, phytic acid and saponin content by the processing methods used to make the end-product (Oakenfull 2001; Potter 1995)

176.7 Safety and Availability of Dietary Phytoestrogens

Currently, dietary phytoestrogens are a billion-dollar business at least partly accounted for by the fact that four out of five middle-aged women use herbal remedies and dietary supplements, with or without prescription drugs, on a regular basis in order to treat health problems associated with aging. Isoflavones are readily available, either over the counter, or as ingredients in (fortified) foods (Bloedon et al. 2002; Setchell et al. 2001).

Table 176.4 Soy food isoflavone content

Product	Aglycone (microgram per gram)			
	Daidzein	Genistein	Glycitein	Total
Traditional soy foods				
Roasted soybeans ♦	563	869	193	1625
Tofu ♦	146	162	29	337
Tempe ♦	273	320	32	625
Miso (soy bean paste) ♦	272	245	77	593
Natto (fermented soybeans)) ◊				
Soy milk (liquid from boiled pureed soybeans) ◊	50	63	ns	ns
Soy Sauce◊	2	6	ns	ns
Second-generation soy foods				
Soy hotdog ♦	34	82	34	150
Soy bacon ♦	28	69	24	122
Tempe burger ♦	64	196	30	289
Flat noodle ♦	9	37	39	85
Soy parmesan ♦	15	8	41	65
Foods containing soy flour or protein and other foods				
White bread ◊	7	8	ns	ns
Wholegrain bread ◊	2	1	ns	ns
Canned tuna ◊	4	7	ns	ns
Doughnuts ◊	20	32	ns	ns
Pancakes ◊	13	14	ns	ns
Soy/"veggie" Burgers ◊	30	20	ns	ns
Coffee ◊	0.5	tr	ns	ns
"Power"-type bars ◊	18	33	ns	ns
Pizza ◊	2	2	ns	ns

This table shows the quantities of the aglycones genistein, daidzein and glycitein, in the most common soy-based foods. Please note: ns = not stated; tr = trace defined as ≤25 μg/100g (the authors minimum level of reliable detection); ♦ = data sourced from Wang and Murphy (1994); ◊ = data sourced from Horn-Ross et al. (2000)

The US Food and Drug Administration (FDA) recently allowed the food industry to state that soy protein can protect and promote a healthy heart, focusing on its isoflavone and protein content (US Food and Drug Administration 1999). This has resulted in a flooding of the food markets with soy products and supplements, as well as an expected further increase in the sale and use of these compounds. This is worrying as the full implications of soy manufacturing processes or efficacy are not fully understood. In fact, the scarce and conflicting information regarding the metabolism and bioavailability of phytoestrogens in itself should be enough to cause concern over its promotion as a 'health food'. Furthermore, a trend towards manufactured isoflavone supplements, as opposed to isoflavone in a more natural form through isoflavone-rich foods, may have further implications for health.

176.8 East Versus West: Cultural Differences in Soy Consumption and Phytoestrogen Levels

Soy-based foods have been eaten in Asian societies for over 1,000 years and are an important part of everyday diet, thus their consumption is much higher than in Western countries. Populations in Japan, China, Taiwan and Korea are estimated to consume approximately 20–150 mg/day of isoflavones,

Table 176.5 Eastern versus Western intake of isoflavones

Country	Study	Mean intake (mg/day)		
		Isoflavones	Daidzein	Genistein
Japan	Kimira et al. (1998)	39.46	4.62	52.12
Japan	Arai et al. (2000)	NR	16.4	30.1
Finland	Valsta et al. (2003)	0.79	NR	NR
USA	Horn-Ross et al. (2000)	NR	1.28	1.48
Holland	Boker et al. (2002)	NR	0.15	0.16
USA	de Kleijn et al. (2001)	1.54	0.39	0.7

NR not reported
Table gives an example of average isoflavone intake in some Eastern and Western countries as published by a selection of studies

usually from a variety of soy food sources (Murkies et al. 1998), compared to the average American who consumes only 1–3 mg/day (Barnes et al. 1995). Table 176.5 displays findings from various studies which assessed Eastern and Western soy consumption.

In Japan, soy foods and supplements are heavily promoted as "natural" sources of Es with beneficial effects for women and as having a positive influence on healthy aging, therefore soy intake in that part of the world is especially high. The most common types of soy foods eaten in Japan are tofu, miso, natto (Arai et al. 2000), and fried tofu (Wakai et al. 1999). Among the Chinese, Chen et al. (1999) found that the majority (96.7%) of women of a Shanghai sample (*n* = 60) ate soy foods at least once a week (median intake of soy foods = 100.6 g/day). Although many of these samples were small in size (less than 100 participants), the same finding was reported across studies, associating high phytoestrogen intake with East Asian communities. For instance, in our Indonesian study (*n* = 719) virtually everyone ate tofu and tempe (65% of the sample ate tofu at least once a day and 67% ate tempe at least once a day), (Hogervorst 2008).

In the West, most of the phytoestrogens consumed are lignans (de Kleijn et al. 2001; Horn-Ross et al. 2000), whereas isoflavone intake in Western countries is low compared to that in East Asian countries. Isoflavones are derived mainly from second-generation soy foods such as tofu, doughnuts, soy milk, white bread, pancakes or waffles, canned tuna and coffee (Horn-Ross et al. 2000).

176.9 Cross-cultural Dementia Prevalence

If consumption of phytoestrogens is different and if soy can affect the brain, one would expect differences in dementia prevalence in East Asian countries (such as Japan and China) and Western populations (such as the USA or Europe) in the prevalence of cognitive disorders and dementia. This is indeed found to be the case. This difference is not found for all-cause dementia, which seems to be similar across Japan, China and the West (Zhao and Brinton 2007), but specifically for the most common subtypes of dementia, AD and Vascular Dementia (VaD) (Zhao and Brinton 2007). AD rates are lower in Japan and China, and its prevalence is ~2.5 times higher in Western populations. Whereas AD is more prevalent in Western societies than VaD (~2.2 fold), AD and VaD rates in Japan and China are more similar (for an excellent review on this topic see Zhao and Brinton 2007).

The difference between East and West in AD prevalence has thus been hypothesized to be attributed to the isoflavone-rich diets in Japan and China compared to the USA and Europe and the potential positive effects that isoflavones can have on the brain. However, other healthy lifestyles (e.g., consumption of fruit and vegetables, less alcohol consumption, more exercise and a lower body mass index, etc.) could also attribute to lower AD risks in these countries. Studies investigating the association between soy and cognition in the elderly in more detail are described below.

176.10   Observational Studies of Soy Consumption and Cognitive Function

Observational studies assessing the relationship between isoflavone and cognitive function have been few and far between, and have also reported conflicting results. These studies have investigated the relationship between phytoestrogen consumption and various aspects of cognitive function in Western countries with postmenopausal women of non-East Asian descent, older men and postmenopausal women of East Asian descent (Rice et al. 2000; White et al. 2000) as well as multi-ethnic populations younger than 50 years of age (Ostatníková et al. 2007; Huang et al. 2006; Celec et al. 2005).

176.10.1   Observational Studies in Non-Asian Western Populations

Kreijkamp-Kaspers et al. (2007) assessed the effects of habitual intake of low quantities of phytoestrogens through diet on cognition. The sample consisted of 301 Dutch postmenopausal women aged between 60 and 75 years. These were volunteers from an ongoing cohort study assessing nutrition and cancer, as well as a breast screening program, who had a wide range of phytoestrogen intake. A Food Frequency Questionnaire (FFQ) was utilized to compile information on consumption of food containing phytoestrogens. Furthermore, to evaluate approximate levels of phytoestrogens consumed, the researchers assigned a value to the various phytoestrogens (in mg per 100 g of food or drink). The foods were then divided into seven groups based on this phytoestrogen 'score' (see de Kleijn et al. 2001 for methods used), and a median phytoestrogen content was assigned to each group to avoid over- or underestimation of phytoestrogen consumption. In this sample, median intake per day of lignans ranged from 0.65 to 2.29 mg/day, whereas for isoflavones this was 0.18–14.64 mg/day, although the middle two quartiles were significantly lower than the highest (0.34 and 2.99 mg/day). The researchers reported no significant differences between the effects of various levels of isoflavone intake on cognitive tests of memory, processing speed, or executive functions. However, a significant association was found between high lignan intake and processing capacity and speed, as well as executive function.

In the same Dutch sample, Franco et al. (2005) investigated the effects of isoflavones and lignans of the levels found in a typical Western diet on cognitive performance using only the Mini Mental Status Examination (MMSE). However, in these analyses, the investigators were interested in differences between women who had experienced a longer (20–30 years) versus a shorter (8–12 years) period since menopause (postmenopausal time span). They also included natural menopause as a factor that might have affected the relationship between phytoestrogen intake and cognitive function. No significant association was found between isoflavone intake and cognitive function as measured by the MMSE. However, and more pronounced in women with longer postmenopausal time span, a significant association was found between higher lignan intake and better cognitive performance. The authors speculated that this stronger association in women with longer postmenopausal time span could be due to the older age, or other age-related mechanisms, which could have mediated the relationship. However, it must be noted that mean isoflavone intake was very low (0.14 mg/day) in this sample and was substantially lower than those observed in Japanese and Chinese samples showing significant (negative) associations which are discussed below in 176.10.2.

176.10.2 Observational Studies in East-Asian Western Populations

Two large-scale epidemiological studies have assessed the relationship between phytoestrogen consumption, specifically tofu, and cognitive function, in Asian-Americans living in Western communities. These are the Honolulu Asia Ageing Study (HAAS) (White et al. 2000) and the Kame Project (Rice et al. 2000) although the latter has only been published as a peer-reviewed abstract, to our knowledge.

176.10.2.1 The Honolulu Asia Ageing Study

The largest study of the effect of phytoestrogen on cognitive function in both men and women has been the Honolulu Asia Ageing Study (HAAS), consisting of 3,734 Japanese-American participants, aged 70–90 years and living in Hawaii, USA (White et al. 2000). The investigators reported that (contrary to expectations based on its biological plausibility) high midlife soy consumption had a negative association with late life cognitive function. The study found that men aged 71 and above, as well as their wives, who had consumed tofu more than twice a week in midlife and in old age, had a higher risk of dementia and lower cognitive function, but also lower brain weight and more ventricular enlargement than those who consumed less tofu. For example, for men with the lowest tofu intake, the percentage of participants with cognitive impairment (CI) was identified as 4%, as compared to men with the highest tofu intake where 19% had CI. Also, in the low tofu intake group, low brain weight was seen in 12% of cases, compared to 40% of men in the highest tofu intake category. Data suggested that there may be a dose-dependent effect of tofu consumption, i.e., that increased tofu consumption was associated with poorer cognitive function.

The strength of the HAAS study lies in its' coverage of a wide time-span of dietary assessment (data were collected in two assessments, up to nine years apart). Also, some data were collected in midlife, approximately 20 years before cognitive evaluation and magnetic resonance imaging (MRI) scans. However, and as with studies using this methodology, it is unclear if tofu consumption itself was responsible for dementia risk, or whether high tofu intake was an indication of some other unfavourable exposure. For example, the men with high tofu intake, and hence a more traditional diet, were more likely to come from impoverished backgrounds and may have experienced more childhood deprivation which could be related to brain development and later life cognitive function (see also Whalley et al. 2000). In addition, a high-tofu diet could be an indication of a specific dietary pattern that may be harmful to the brain, but separating the individual elements of this diet in order to isolate the contributing factors may prove very difficult. Although these results are of great interest, they were limited, as relatively few subjects consumed very high levels of tofu and confidence intervals around the estimates of effect presented were wide, indicating little precision of results (Grodstein et al. 2000).

176.10.2.2 The Kame Project

The Kame Project (Rice et al. 2000) consisted of Japanese-American men ($n = 634$) and women ($n = 767$) living in Washington State, USA, who were aged 65 years and above. Cross-sectional results showed an association between having a lower cognitive score, as measured by the Cognitive Abilities Screening Instrument (CASI, the same test was also used in the HAAS to identify CI), and high tofu consumption (>3 times a week) as opposed to moderate (1–2 times a week) or low consumption (<1 time a week). In stratified analyses, this negative association remained significant only for women who were hormone replacement users (but not for those who were not hormone users, elderly men or those who consumed moderate to low amounts of tofu). The investigators also found longitudinally (although no overall association was found between tofu consumption and 2 year change of CASI score), that those with modest tofu consumption showed the greatest improvements in CASI scores. These data suggest that there may be optimal levels of phytoestrogens, perhaps interacting with age, gender and E levels. It must be noted that in this and the HAAS study, the investigators did not assess total isoflavone exposure, but only estimated tofu intake. This may be problematic as the authors pointed out that tofu accounted for only approximately half of soy-based isoflavones consumed by this particular population.

176.10.3 Observational Studies in Premenopausal Women

Other observational studies have assessed the relationship between phytoestrogen consumption and cognitive function in premenopausal women. In the Study of Women's Health Across the Nation (SWAN) (Huang et al. 2006), a sub-group of 195 Japanese and 185 Chinese women who were living in the USA and were between 42 to 52 years of age were assessed for this relationship. Various tests of episodic memory, working memory and processing speed were used to assess cognitive function. The investigators found no association between genistein intake (as calculated from the FFQ) and cognitive function. The authors surmised that the effects might only be present in women who are in low-estrogenic states (i.e., postmenopausal women). Comparisons with the other studies mentioned above are difficult, as optimal genistein and daidzein levels were investigated using tertiles, rather than reported in weekly intake of tofu, as in the previous studies mentioned (Rice 2000; White 2000). Furthermore, although the participants were of Japanese and Chinese origin, with higher isoflavone intake than other Western non-Asian populations, mean genistein and daidzein intakes were still only 6.79 and 4.68 µg for Japanese women, and 3.53 and 1.74 µg for Chinese women. An intake of approximately 45,000 µg of isoflavones is needed to significantly affect follicular phase and menstrual cycle length in premenopausal women (Cassidy et al. 1995). Therefore, it is possible that the finding of no association in this study could in part be due to the levels of isoflavone not being sufficiently high enough to have an impact on cognitive function. This could also explain a lack of significant findings in the Kreijkamp-Kaspers study described above. For instance, a 100 g size serving of tofu, which is typical of an Asian diet (see Chen et al. 1999), is equivalent to 33,700 µg, which, when eaten daily, might affect human fertility, physiology and hence possibly the brain, although the exact dosage at which this occurs (if it does) is not entirely clear. This is further complicated as different sources and forms of phytoestrogens were used in the various studies.

176.10.4 Discussion of Findings from Observational Studies

It is hypothesized that the lack of any significant findings in studies assessing Western populations could thus be due to the very low levels of isoflavones consumed in these populations. The participants in Kreijkamp-Kaspers (2007) observational study had at a maximum dietary intake of 15mg/day of soy isoflavones. This is only a quarter or half of that consumed by Japanese women living in Japan, but it was higher than that reported in other Caucasian women living in Western countries (e.g., Franco et al. 2005). This suggests there may be a dose effect and/or an effect of habitual intake, and that the lack of significance in the studies not finding an association may be due to the lower habitual intake of isoflavones consumed.

In line with previous suggestions and theory, the findings from observational studies (whether the association is a positive one, a negative one or no association has been found) thus suggest that an optimal level of phytoestrogens may be needed in order to maintain cognitive function in the middle-aged, but not in the elderly (>65 years of age) in whom high tofu consumption could be negatively associated with cognitive function. However, these studies relied on self-report FFQ, which may not be the most reliable single indicator of soy intake (especially in samples with a very low phytoestrogen intake). There is also a potential problem when comparing studies due to the differences in the type of food questionnaires used. For example, some used dietary self-report methods (recall vs. active food diary), which may cause a problem in distinguishing between cause and effect (i.e., those with cognitive impairment not remembering their intake), as well as introducing biases, such as the 'healthy-user' bias (e.g., eating soy as part of a healthy diet and/or lifestyle). In addition, in these studies, no actual endogenous phytoestrogen levels were measured.

176.11 Soy Consumption and Cognitive Function in an Elderly Indonesian Sample: Findings from our Indonesian Pilot Study

We assessed the relationship between soy intake and cognitive function in an elderly Indonesian sample. The results of the study revealed that tofu and tempe were the most common forms of soy consumed in this sample. We also measured isoflavone levels using saliva samples from the participants. See Table 176.6 for mean soy intake and salivary isoflavone levels.

In our Indonesian sample, similar to findings by White (2000) and Rice (2000), we also reported a negative association between high daily or more tofu intake and memory in participants over the age of 68 years (see Fig. 176.3) (Hogervorst et al. 2008). On the other hand, we found that participants between 52 and 68 years of age appeared to have optimal genistein levels relating to optimal memory function, whereas participants older than 68 years of age with high genistein levels exhibited lower cognitive performance and an increased risk of dementia (Hogervorst et al. 2009) (see Fig. 176.4). This suggests that the role of phytoestrogens on cognitive function may be modified by age and gender.

Another novel finding was that high tempe intake, in the same analyses, was positively associated with cognitive function. We suggested that a possible reason for this could be due to different processing methods used to make these two types of soy foods. Formaldehyde is reported to be added to tofu in Indonesia and can create oxidative damage to frontal cortex and hippocampal tissue (Gurel et al. 2005). Tempe could potentially protect against formaldehyde-induced damage through its antioxidant effects (Rilantono et al. 2000).

However, a pilot study carried out by the University of Indonesia in Jakarta, Depok recently found no trace of formaldehyde in various tofu samples bought in Jakarta (data unpublished). An alternative hypothesis is that the fermentation process used to make tempe can produce folate (Ginting and Arcot 2004) which is known to have protective effects in the brain (Smith 2002) This may be similar to findings of an interaction between estrogens and folate found before, where women who had high

Table 176.6 Frequency and quantity of soy foods eaten and salivary isoflavone levels in our Indonesian sample

Type of food eaten daily or more	Number of Participants (%)
Soy of any type	511 (71)
Tofu (daily or more)	479 (67)
Tempe (daily or more)	491 (68)
Mean Weekly Intake	Mean ± SD
Tofu	9.3 (6.9)
Tempe	9.5 (6.8)
Salivary Phytoestrogen Levels (ppm)	Mean ± SD
Genistein	0.021 (0.009)
Daidzein	0.043 (0.016)
Glycitein	0.041 (0.027)

Table shows the intake of soy foods as well as the mean salivary isoflavone levels for the whole sample. The figures show the number and percentage [N(%)] of participants whom eat these foods at least once a day. The table also shows the mean (and standard deviation or SD) number of times the food are eaten a week. The mean (and SD) salivary isoflavone levels are also displayed

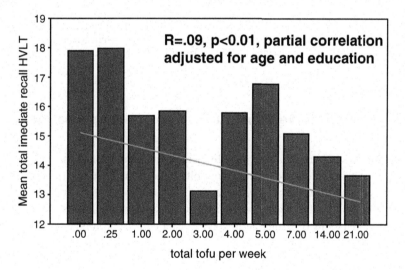

Fig. 176.3 Weekly Tofu intake and memory Score on the Hopkins Verbal Learning Test (HVLT) in an Elderly Indonesian Population. Figure shows the quantity of tofu eaten on a weekly basis in our elderly Indonesian sample plotted against scores on the HVLT verbal memory test. As can be seen a weekly tofu intake increase was associated with lower memory scores

levels of estrogens, but also high levels of folate did not score below the cut-offs scores on the MMSE for dementia (Hogervorst and Smith 2002). These associations need to be investigated in more detail in future studies.

Clearly, observational studies can introduce systematic bias and ultimately treatment studies carry more weight in disentangling cause and effect of (dietary) phytoestrogens versus cognitive outcomes. These studies are thus discussed in more detail in the next section.

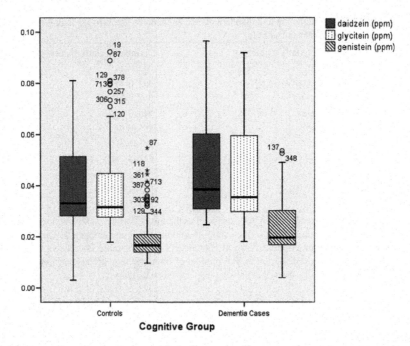

Fig. 176.4 Salivary phytoestrogen levels for the possible dementia cases and control cases in an elderly Indonesian population. Figure shows levels of the phytoestrogens daidzein, genistein and glycitein stratified by possible dementia cases and control cases. Genistein and glycitein levels were significantly higher in cases than in controls ($p < 0.05$)

176.12 Treatment/Intervention Studies in Postmenopausal Women

See Table 176.7 for a summary of all human phytoestrogen treatment studies.

There have been ten randomized placebo-controlled intervention studies (randomized controlled trials or RCTs) assessing the effects of soy isoflavone supplementation on various aspects of cognitive function (see Table 176.7). Of these, eight have assessed postmenopausal women only, of which seven were in Western populations (Fournier et al. 2007; Casini et al. 2006; File et al. 2005; Howes et al. 2004; Kreijkamp-Kaspers et al. 2004; Duffy et al. 2003), and one in a Hong Kong sample (Ho et al. 2007). Another study has assessed older men and postmenopausal women (Gleason et al. 2009) and the tenth study has been with premenopausal women and young men in a UK sample (File et al. 2001). Furthermore, two very short-term (1 week) prospective intervention studies, also with premenopausal women and young men have also been conducted (Ostatníková et al. 2007; Celec et al. 2005).

176.12.1 RCTs Reporting Positive Effects of Isoflavone Consumption on Cognitive Function

Four of the studies assessing postmenopausal women reported beneficial effects of isoflavone treatment on cognitive function (Casini et al. 2006; Duffy et al. 2003; Kritz-Silverstein et al. 2003; File 2005). Two were from the same group of investigators and separately assessed the effects of 60 mg total isoflavones per day on cognitive function, using the same cognitive test battery with postmeno-

Table 176.7 Human intervention studies of soy isoflavones and cognitive function

Study	Location	Design	Duration	Participant Variables	Intervention	Cognitive Measures	Outcomes
Gleason et al. (2009)		RDBP, P	6 months	$n = 30$ healthy PMW and men	1. Soy supplement – 100 mg total isoflavones/day	Verbal and visuospatial memory – Buschke Selective Reminding test, Paragraph Recall, Rey Complex Figure test, Visual Spatial Learning test)	Plama Dadizein and Genistein ↑ with isoflavone consumption
						Language – Boston Naming test Language Fluency – FAS, animal fluency	Isoflavone ↑ visual spatial memory, construction, verbal fluency, speed dexterity; Placebo ↑ executive function; → verbal memory
						Visual-motor function – Rey Complex Figure test copy, Grooved Pegboard	
				Mean age = 74.3 years (Placebo) and 73.0 (Isoflavone)	2. Placebo	Executive function – Stroop Color Word test, Mazes and Trail Making Test B	
Ho et al. (2007)	Hong Kong, China	RDBP, P	6 months	$n = 176$ (168 completed) healthy PMW	1. Soy supplement – 80 mg total isoflavones/day	Learning & Memory Tests: Hong Kong Learning List Test, Rey-Osterrieth Complex Figure Test, WMS-R	0/15 measures were significantly improved
						Executive function: Trail-Making Test, Verbal Fluency Test	
						Verbal fluency: Boston Naming Task	
						Attention and Concentration: Digit Span test	
				Mean age = 63.5 years (55–76 years)	2. Placebo	Motor Control: Finger Tapping test Language: Boston Naming test Visual Perception: Rey-Osterrieth Copy Trial	
				Exclusion criteria: HT in previous 6 months		Global Cognition and Dementia: MMSE	

(continued)

Table 176.7 (continued)

Study	Location	Design	Duration	Participant Variables	Intervention	Cognitive Measures	Outcomes
Fournier et al. (2007)	Pullman, USA	RDBP, P	16 weeks	$n = 79$ healthy PMW	1. Soy milk – 72 mg total isoflavone/ day (37 mg genistein, 31 mg daidzein, 4 mg glycitein)	Working memory: Digit Ordering, Color Matching	0/16 measures were significantly improved
				Mean age = 56.1 years (48–65 years), 1–35 years beyond menopause (mean 7.7 years)	2. Soy supplement – 70 mg total isoflavone/day (33mg genistein, 30 mg daidzein, 7 mg glycitein)	Memory Recall & Recognition: Benton Visual Retention Test, Visual Pattern Recognition	
				Exclusion criteria: HT in previous 6 months	3. Placebo	Memory span (working memory): Forward Digit Span, Corsi Block-Tapping Selective attention: Stroop Test	
Casini et al. (2006)	Milan and Rome, Italy	RDBP, CO	6 months	$n = 76$ PMW	1. Soy supplement – 60 mg total isoflavone/day (40–45% genistein, 40–45% daidzein, 10–20% glycitein)	Psychomotor performance: Digit Symbol test	↑ 6/8 measures of all three cognitive aspects
					2. Placebo	Immediate auditory attention and mental flexibility: Digit Span test Distractibility and visual inattentiveness: Visual Scanning Test	↑ Self-rated mood
				Mean age = 49.5 years; >1 year of menopause (mean 5.7 years) Exclusion criteria: HT use in previous 8 weeks, presence or history endocrinological disorders, use of psychoactive medication		Other non-cognitive measures: Mood, Participant Condition Preference	↑ Preference to isoflavone treatment ($n = 49$)

| File et al. (2005) | London, UK | RDBP, P | 6 weeks | n = 50 healthy PMW

Mean age 58 years (51–66 years); >1 year beyond menopause (mean = 9.1 years, 66% >5 years)

Exclusion criteria: HT in previous 12 months | 1. Soy supplement – 60 mg total isoflavone/day
2. Placebo | Short-term non-verbal memory: CANTAB
Short and long-term verbal memory: Logical memory & Recall Wechsler (revised)
Long-term episodic memory: Picture Recall
Verbal Fluency & Semantic Memory: Category Fluency
Sustained Attention: PASAT
Mental flexibility (simple and complex rule reversal): IDED-CANTAB
Planning Ability: SoC CANTAB | ↑ Short-term nonverbal memory, mental flexibility, planning ability
→ Short & long term verbal memory, long-term episodic memory, verbal fluency & semantic memory, sustained attention |
| Kreijkamp-Kaspers et al. (2004) | Utrecht, Netherlands | RDBP, P | 12 months | n = 175 PMW

Mean age 66.6 years (60–75 years); >1 year of menopause (mean 18 years)

Exclusion criteria: HT in previous 6 months, estrogen related health conditions | 1. Soy protein Supplement – 99 mg total isoflavone/day (52 mg genistein, 41 mg daidzein, 6 mg glycitein)
2. Placebo | Verbal episodic memory: Rey Auditory Verbal Learning test
Visual memory: The Doors test
Short-term/working memory: Digit Span test
Verbal Fluency: Boston Naming Task
Global cognition & dementia: MMSE
Complex attention: Trail Making Test, Digit Symbol Substitution test
Other non-cognitive measures: Depression (Geriatric Depression Scale), Verbal Intelligence (Dutch Adult Reading Test), Bone Mineral Density, Plasma Lipids | → On 16 cognitive measures |

(continued)

Table 176.7 (continued)

Study	Location	Design	Duration	Participant Variables	Intervention	Cognitive Measures	Outcomes
Howes et al. (2004) ♥	New South Wales, Australia	RP, P	6 months	n = 30 PMW	1. Aglycone Isoflavone extract from red clover (25 mg formone-netin 2.5 mg biochanin, < 1 mg daidzein & genistein)	Visuo-spatial intelligence: Block Design	→ On all cognitive measures
				Age > 60 years	2. Placebo	Verbal Memory Digit Recall	
Duffy et al. (2003)	London, UK	RDBP, P	12 weeks	n = 33 healthy PMW	1. Soy supplement – 60 mg total isoflavone/day	Short term verbal episodic memory: Logical Memory & Recall WMS-R	→ Short-Term Verbal & Non-Verbal Memory; Verbal Fluency & Semantic Memory
				Mean age = 57.8 years (50–65 years); >1 year of menopause (mean 8.1 years)	2. Placebo	Short term non-verbal episodic memory: DMTS-CANTAB	
				Exclusion criteria: HT in previous 12 months, use of antibiotics in previous 3 months, use of psychoactive medication, smoking		Long term episodic memory: Picture Recall	↑ Long-Term Episodic Memory; Sustained Attention; Mental Flexibility; Planning Ability
						Verbal Fluency & Semantic Memory – Category Generation	
						Frontal Lobe Functioning (mental flexibility & simple rule reversal) – IDED – CANTAB	
						Frontal Lobe Functioning (planning ability) – SoC-CANTAB	
						Sustained Attention – PASAT	
						Other Non-Cognitive Measures: Mood (Bond & Lader Mood Questionnaire)	

Study	Location	Design	Duration	Sample	Treatment	Cognitive measures	Outcomes
Kritz-Silverstein et al. (2003) ❤	San Diego, USA	RDBP, P	6 months	n = 53 healthy PMW; Mean age = 60.7 years (55–74 years); >2 years of menopause (mean 10.9 years); Exclusion criteria: current HT users	1. Soy supplement – 110 mg total isoflavones/day; 2. Placebo	Short and long-term memory: Logical memory & recall Wechsler; Verbal fluency & semantic memory: Category Fluency; Visuomotor tracking & attention: Halstead-Reitan Trails A & B	→ Short & Long Term Memory; Trail A; ↑ Verbal Fluency & Semantic Memory; Trail B
Ostatnikova (2007)	Bratislava, Slovak Republic	STPI	1 week	n = 86 PRMW and young men (54 females & 32 males) Age range 18–25 years; Exclusion criteria: use of hormonal contraceptives	1. 2 g/kg per day soybeans	Mental rotation: Sub-section of Amthauer Intelligence test (non-verbal); Spatial visualization: Sub-section of Smith & Whetton intelligence scale (non-verbal); Other Non-Cognitive Measures: Salivary Testosterone, Plasma Estradiol	↑ Mental Rotation & Spatial Visualization
Celec et al. (2005)	Bratislava, Slovak Republic	STPI	1 week	n = 16 PRMW; Mean age = 23.4 years	900 g soybean to be eaten with one week (1,080.0–3,780.0 mg isoflavones)	Mental rotation: Sub-section of Amthauer Intelligence test (non-verbal); Spatial visualization: Sub-section of Smith & Whetton intelligence scale (non-verbal); Other Non-Cognitive Measures: Salivary and Plasma Testosterone & Estradiol	↑ Mental Rotation & Spatial Visualization

(continued)

Table 176.7 (continued)

Study	Location	Design	Duration	Participant Variables	Intervention	Cognitive Measures	Outcomes
File et al. (2001)	London, UK	RP	10 weeks	$n = 27$ PRMW and young men (15 males and 12 females)	1. High soy diet (100 mg total isoflavones/day)	Attention: DSS, DC test, PASAT	↑ Short-Term Non-Verbal Memory; Short-Term Verbal Memory; Long-Term Episodic Memory; Mental Flexibility Females only
				Mean age = 25 years	2. Low soy diet (0.5 mg total isoflavones/day)	Immediate episodic memory: Short story (WMS-R)	↑ Frontal Function; Planning Ability
						Short-term non-verbal memory: DMTS-CANTAB	→ Verbal Fluency & Semantic Memory; Sustained Attention
						Long-term episodic memory: Picture Recall	
						Semantic memory: Category Generation Task	
						Mental flexibility (simple and complex rule reversal): IDED-CANTAB	
						Planning ability: SoC CANTAB	
						Frontal function: Letter Fluency	
						Intelligence: NART-R	
						Other non-cognitive measures: Depression (HAD)	
						Mood (Bond & Lader Mood Questionnaire)	

Table shows the study details of human intervention trials assessing the effects of isoflavone consumption on cognitive function. NB: ♥ = Full Paper could not be accessed, only abstract; ↑ = Improvement in performance; → = No change in performance; *CANTAB* Cambridge Neuropsychological Test; Automated Battery, *CBLC* Community Based Longitudinal Cohort Study, *CO* Crossover Design, *CS* Cross-Sectional, *DC* Digit Cancellation Test, *DMTS* Delayed Matching to Sample Test (part of CANTAB), *DSS* Digit-Symbol Substitution, *HAD* Hospital Anxiety & Depression Scale, *HT* Hormone Therapy, *IDED* Attentional Set Shifting, *MMSE* Mini Mental Status Examination, *NART-R* National Adult Reading Test revised version, *P* Parallel Design, *PASAT* Paced Auditory Serial Addition Test, *PMW* Postmenopausal Women, *PRMW* Premenopausal Women, *RDBP* Randomized, double-blind placebo-controlled, *RP* Randomized, placebo-controlled, *SoC* Stockings of Cambridge, *STPI* Short Term Prospective Intervention Study, *WMS-R* Wechsler Memory Scale – Revised

pausal women aged 50–66 years in the UK for a duration of 6 weeks (File et al. 2005) and 12 weeks (Duffy et al. 2003). The investigators found that 60 mg/day isoflavone equivalent was beneficial for cognitive function as assessed by memory tests, as well as on tests of frontal lobe function, such as those assessing mental flexibility and planning ability.

Around the same time as the UK studies were published, the Soy and Postmenopausal Health in Aging Study (SOPHIA) (Kritz-Silverstein et al. 2003) data from the USA were disseminated. This study had also included postmenopausal women aged 55–74 years. However, a higher dose (110 mg/day) of isoflavones was used and for a much longer duration of 6 months. A learning effect was observed over time in both the placebo and isoflavone treatment group, showing improvements in all five cognitive tests used. This improvement was larger in the isoflavone groups for four tests, and significantly greater (23% as opposed to 3%) for the Category Fluency test, even after controlling for age and education. Furthermore, in analysis stratified by age, those in the younger age group (50–59 years) taking the isoflavone supplement showed a greater improvement than those on placebo on a test of visuospatial tracking and attention (Trails B). This effect was not observed in the older group (60–74 years), again suggesting that not only could isoflavones have a beneficial effect on verbal memory in postmenopausal women, but also that the effect of isoflavones may be greater for perimenopausal women than for those who are older and had already experienced menopause. This would be in line with our observational data and those of E studies (Hogervorst et al. 2009). Similarly, another RCT (Casini et al. 2006) reported that postmenopausal women (with a mean age of 49.5 years and an average 5.7 years since menopause), who were given 60 mg/day equivalent of isoflavones as aglycones for a duration of 6 months showed an improvement in cognitive ability, as measured by three cognitive tests, as well as improved mood. When asked, the participants also generally showed a preference for phytoestrogen over placebo (64%). This study has particular value because it provides support for the possible role of phytoestrogens in alleviating or reversing psychological ailments associated with menopause, such as mood and quality of life. Gleason et al. (2009) investigated the effects of 100 mg/day soy isoflavone for a duration of 6 months on cognitive function for both men and women aged 62–89 years. Cognitive function was tested at month 1, 3 and 6 and the investigators reported that the isoflavones group showed greater improvements in visual-spatial memory, construction, verbal memory and speed dexterity. However, the placebo group were faster on two tests of executive function. There was no significant effect on verbal memory for either group. Interestingly, although plasma genistein and daidzein levels showed a rise with increasing isoflavone supplementation, equol levels did not and none of the samples were equol producers. This is important as some investigators have suggested that equol, a highly estrogenic metabolite derived from daidzein in some, but not all, humans, is the most potent derivative for maintaining brain function through its strong estrogenic effects. This study would suggest that this is not necessarily the case. However, the small sample size in this study ($n = 30$) must be taken into consideration.

176.12.2 RCTs Reporting No Effects of Isoflavone Consumption on Cognitive Function

Four studies failed to show any significant effect of isoflavone supplementation on various aspects of cognitive function with postmenopausal women (Fournier et al. 2007; Ho et al. 2007; Howes et al. 2004; Kreijkamp-Kaspers et al. 2004). Using aglycone isoflavone extracts from red clover, (Howes et al. 2004) investigated the effects of 25 mg/day of predominantly biochanin A (which contains less than 2 mg daidzein and genistein) for a duration of 6 months and found no significant effects on tests of visuospatial intelligence and verbal memory in postmenopausal women. The dose used may have thus been too low and, in addition, the women included in this study were all older than 60 years of age. In a study of the longest duration of all RCTs carried out in this area, Kreijkamp-Kaspers et al. (2004) investigated the effects of 12 months of soy protein containing 99 mg equivalent of total isoflavone per day (52 mg genistein, 41 mg daidzein, and 6 mg glycitein) on cognitive function (and other health indicators) in postmenopausal women aged 60–75 years in the Netherlands. No effect of isoflavones supplementation was found on a large number of cognitive tests (see Table 176.2 for full list). However, it must be noted that compared to the earlier reported positive studies, these participants were much older on average (66 years of age), had been menopausal for longer (mean of 18 years), and 19% were also using cholesterol-lowering and antihypertensive medication. Similarly, Ho et al. (2007) did not find any effects of 6 months supplementation with 80 mg/day soy isoflavones on quality of life, as well as various cognitive functions. They had also included postmenopausal women with an average age of 63.5 years, who were also 13.8 years since menopause, on average. Interestingly, this latter study was the only study of a population who habitually ate soy as part of their daily diet (Hong Kong Chinese) and who had a mean dietary intake of 20 mg/day isoflavones. It is thus also possible that no effect was found in this study due to the higher habitual intake of soy in the sample, which could have potentially reduced group differences (Ho et al. 2007).

These data taken together would suggest that age of women, duration of treatment, habitual intake and years since menopause could explain differences found between studies. This reasoning is very similar to that for E treatment (Hogervorst et al. 2009). However, in a US-based study of postmenopausal women with a mean age of 56.1 years, and with an average of 8 years since menopause (Fournier et al. 2007), researchers also found no significant effects of either 72 mg/day total isoflavones (from soy milk) or 70 mg/day total isoflavone (via a soy isoflavone supplement) on various cognitive abilities, including selective attention, working or visuospatial short- or long-term memory when compared to placebo. On the other hand, the large variability in age since menopause (Zhao and Brinton 2007) in this group may have been responsible for a lack of significant findings.

176.13 Dose Effect of Phytoestrogens in a Pilot RCT

In a pilot RCT study (Yesufu 2009) we assessed the 24-h dose effect of phytoestrogens on verbal episodic (word lists) and semantic memory (Category Fluency) in postmenopausal women between 45 to 65 years of age. See Table 176.8 for inclusion and exclusion criteria and Fig. 176.5 for procedure. Participants had been instructed to take one of the allocated pills (half the dose) 24 hours before the morning of testing immediately upon waking, and the other half of the dose immediately before going to bed on the night before testing (10 hours before testing) to obtain maximal phytoestrogen levels. This was done to investigate the potential 24-hour dendritic sprouting effects of E (Woolley and McEwen 1993). Timing of ingestion of the dosages was based on findings by Setchell et al. (2003), who reported the terminal half-life (the interval required for the quantity to decay to half its initial value) of daidzein and genistein to be approximately 8–10 hours. In this pilot study, fifteen participants successfully completed the study. Due to subject drop out (unrelated to side effects), cells were unbalanced and there was an uneven number of participants in each treatment group (placebo $n = 6$; 30 mg, $n = 5$; 100 mg $n = 4$).

Table 176.9 below describes the sample demographics. The mean age of the participants was 55.47 ± 5.74 (range 49–65 years). Most participants had achieved secondary or university level education ($n = 6$ and $n = 8$, respectively), and only one participant had a primary level education. The majority of participants were Caucasian ($n = 12$). Nearly half the sample was currently using medication ($n = 7$), but the majority of participants did not smoke ($n = 14$) and exercised on a regular basis ($n = 14$), indicating a healthy lifestyle. No significant difference was observed between treatment

Table 176.8 Inclusion and exclusion criteria for pilot randomized controlled trial

Inclusion criteria	Exclusion criteria
Aged 45–65 years old	Use of supplementary hormones (including hormonal contraception within the last 3 months)
Good health as assessed by self-report questionnaire	
Postmenopausal (women): last menses longer than 6 months ago	Use of antibiotics in previous 6 months
Surgical or natural Menopause	Previous history of thrombosis
	Benign or malignant growths
	History of breast, ovarian or endometrial cancer
	Psychiatric disorder (e.g., clinical depression)
	Pregnancy
	Dementia (e.g., Alzheimer's disease)
	Epilepsy
	Vision/ear/hearing problems
	Dyslexia
	Premenopausal women
	Regular soy food consumers

This table shows the study inclusion and exclusion criteria for participants in the pilot Randomised Controlled Trial (RCT)

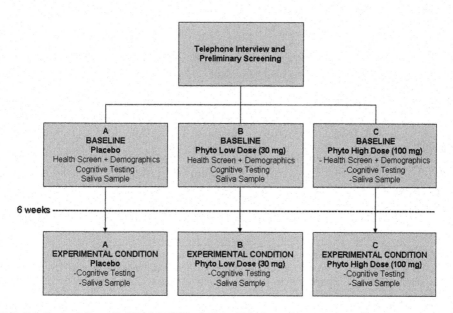

Fig. 176.5 Randomized Controlled Trial (RCT) procedure. This figure shows the recruitment and test procedure for the RCT. After initial telephone screening, participants were allocated to one of the three treatment groups. Baseline data was collected. After a time period of 6 weeks, the participants consumed their treatment or placebo pills and completed the same test battery again

groups in educational attainment, ethnicity, medication use, smoking and exercise. Unfortunately, due to randomization, participants in the 30 mg group were significantly older (61 ± 4.30 years of age) than the participants in the 100 mg (50 ± 1.16 years of age) and placebo (54.50 ± 4.60 years of age) groups [F(14) = 9.10, df = 2, $p = 0.004$].

We found a positive effect of 100 mg total equivalent of isoflavones, as opposed to the 30 mg or placebo treatment on verbal Category Fluency (number of animals in 90 s) (see Fig. 176.6) controlling for

Table 176.9 Pilot randomized controlled trial sample demographic variables

Demographic variables	Whole group	Placebo	30 mg	100 mg	Critical value	df	p value
N	15	6	5	4			
Age, mean ± SD	55.47 (5.74)	54.60 (4.59)	61.00 (4.30)	50.0 (1.15)	9.1	2	0.004*
Education, N (%)					2.82	4	ns
Primary	1 (6.7)	1 (16.7)	0 (0)	0 (0)			
Secondary	6 40.0)	2 (33.3)	3 (60.0)	1 (25.0)			
University or higher	8 (53.3)	3 (50.0)	2 (40.0)	3 (75.0)			
Profession							
Higher manager, admin, professional	1 (6.7)	0 (0)	0 (0)	1 (25.0)	6.83	8	ns
Intermediate – Manager, admin, professional	5 (33.3)	2 (33.3)	1 (20.0)	2 (50.0)			
Supervisory or clerical, junior manager, admin or professional	5 (33.3)	2 (33.3)	2 (40.0)	1 (25.0)			
Student	1 6.7)	1 (16.7)	0 (0)	0 (0)			
State Pensioner, no other earner, casual or lowest grade worker	3 (20.0)	1 (16.7)	2 (40.0)	0 (0)			
Ethnicity							
Caucasian	12 (80.0)	4 (66.7)	1 (16.7)	1 (16.7)	2.58	4	ns
Asian	2 (13.3)	4 (80.0)	1 (20.0)	0 (0)			
Black	1 (6.7)	4 (100)	0 (0)	0 (0)			
On medication at present							
Yes	7 (46.7)	2 (33.3)	4 (66.7)	1 (25.0)	3.42	2	ns
No	8 (53.3)	4 (80.0)	1 (20.0)	3 (75.0)			
Do you smoke?							
Yes	1 (6.7)	0 (0)	0 (0)	1 (25.0)	2.95	2	ns
No	14 (93.3)	6 (100.0)	5 (100.0)	3 (75.0)			
Do you exercise on a regular basis?							
Yes	14 (93.3)	6 (100.0)	4 (80.0)	4 (100.0)	2.14	2	ns
No	1 (6.7)	0 (0)	1 (20.0)	0 (0)			

This table displays the differences between treatment groups in demographic variables. Univariate ANOVA analyses were used to assess the differences between groups in age and chi-square analyses for all other categorical variables. NB: Critical value refers to F = ANOVA, χ^2 = chi-square; p Value = significance; df = degrees of freedom; * Correlation is significant at the 0.01 level (2-tailed); ns = correlation is not significant

age and BMI [F (14) = 4.057, df = 2, p = 0.05]. Analyses exhibited no baseline differences between groups (which had been done six weeks earlier at enrolment). The 100-mg treatment group showed more improvement than the 30-mg group, who also showed greater improvement than the placebo group ($p = 0.05$).

Women in our RCT isoflavone study (participant recruitment is ongoing) were on average younger (mean age 55 years) than those in previous studies reporting no effect or detrimental effects of phytoestrogen consumption. Due to similarities between the sex hormone E and naturally occurring phytoestrogens, this positive effect on cognitive function was expected, as this finding is in line with the 'window of opportunity' theory for estrogens (Gibbs 2006; Henderson et al. 2005; Pinkerton and Henderson 2005). This theory suggests beneficial effects of E on cognition in recently menopausal

Fig. 176.6 Change in
baseline score for the
Category Verbal Fluency Test
(CVFT). This figure shows
the 'change in baseline score'
using box plots (with
medians) between test
session 1 and test session 2
on the CVFT for each
treatment group

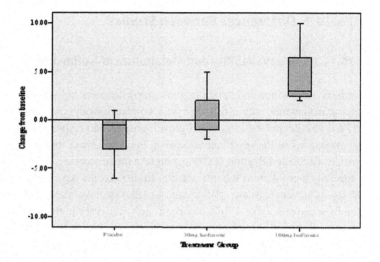

women only and is substantiated by basic science and human observational data. While our results reported are preliminary, they are also similar to other reports finding positive effects of phytoestrogen intake on the Category Fluency test (Kritz-Silverstein et al. 2003). Also reflective of our study was that Kritz-Silverstein et al. (2003) did not find any significant effects on other types of verbal memory either (e.g., story and verbal list recall were also assessed in our study). This may indicate that, similar to estrogenic findings, phytoestrogens may also have test-specific effects. Interestingly, the two longitudinal studies investigating menopausal change on cognition also show the largest differences on the same verbal Fluency task, which may thus be very sensitive to fluctuations in estrogenic metabolite levels (Fuh et al. 2006; Thilers et al. 2006).

176.14 Discussion

It is thought that diet and nutrition could play an important part in age-related health issues, such as cancer, cardiovascular disease, and to maintain cognitive function and prevent AD (American Institute for Cancer Research 1997). In this modern day and age we have turned to dietary supplements as a quick and easy way to obtain the nutrition we believe maintains and promotes good health. Therefore, the dietary supplement industry is now a multi-billion-dollar business based on studies such as those described in this review. However, a worrying increase in hormone-dependent health issues has been observed. Consequently, soy isoflavones have been suggested as a natural alternative to manufactured hormones, such as E, and have already been endorsed as being protective for cardiovascular health (US Food and Drug Administration 1999). The labelling of a product as 'natural' does not necessarily confirm its safety (Ernst 2002) and relatively little is known about the biological behaviours of soy isoflavones in the human body. Furthermore, the effects of a plant hormone in its natural state is not necessarily the same as that of when it is capsulated or has been extracted and processed to create a tablet form (Fitzpatrick 2003). Human phytoestrogen trials have evaluated many health issues (e.g., menopausal symptoms, cardiovascular markers, cancer, bone density and cognitive function), but clinical data remain limited and a discrepancy can be seen between studies in vitro and in vivo, across various in vivo clinical trials as well as observational studies. There are a few possible explanations for discrepancies between studies and reasons why comparing them may be complicated.

176.14.1 Differences Between Studies

176.14.1.1 Bioavailability and Metabolism of Isoflavones

Various composition and structural make-up differences between different types, products and sources of soy isoflavones may affect their in vivo pharmacodynamics in the human body (see Kano et al. 2006). This begins with the initial growth process and response to external stimuli (which may cause the molecules of the soy plant to develop in certain ways that result in more complex phytoestrogen profiles (Zhao and Brinton 2007) and ends in the processing, storage and preparation of foods. This is especially a problem as the intervention studies to date have used various different sources and types of soy isoflavones. Some studies used isolated isoflavones, while others used intact soy protein. As can be seen from Table 176.2, phytoestrogen trials vary in the make-up of their administered phytoestrogens. Variability in composition of the soy used leads to the issue of differences in bioavailability of compounds between studies and hence the possible differences in their overall effect on health. This degree of variation needs to be taken into consideration when comparing and contrasting studies, as well as when forming conclusions based on the findings of these studies.

Knowledge about the bioavailability of ingested isoflavones is of paramount importance as it enables an understanding of the way in which the chemical forms of isoflavones have a positive biological effect on the human body, i.e., their efficacy (Zubik and Meydani 2003) and allows for an evaluation of their safety. However, this knowledge, particularly in reference to the bioavailability of genistein and daidzein as a result of the form consumed (aglycone or glucoside), is in the main part incomplete, contradictory and inconclusive, particularly in human studies, making it difficult to establish firm recommendations with regards to the optimal dosage to maintain health and optimal function.

176.14.1.2 The Effects of Dose and Habitual Intake

As discussed, soy isoflavones may have different estrogenic effects, which could also be dose-dependent, but the effective dose to maintain cognitive function has not been found. Linford and Dorsa (2002) reported that very high concentrations of genistein are toxic to neurons, suggesting optimal and non linear levels. Zeng et al. (2004) reported that the neuroprotective effects of genistein are mediated by two mechanisms dependent on dose. The first one is at a nonmolar level, in which genistein protects neurons via an ER-mediated pathway. The second involves a micromolar level in which genistein behaves as an antioxidant. For instance, treatment with 50 μmol/L did not attenuate neuronal apoptosis induced by the endoplasmic reticulum calcium-ATPase inhibitor thapsigargin and actually enhanced apoptosis of cells, whilst low concentrations of genistein ameliorated apoptosis of neurons. In contrast, another study found that the same dose of genistein did protect HCN1-A and HCN2 cells from death (Sonee et al. 2004). The dose administered could thus greatly influence the efficacy and safety, by either being too low to have a noticeable effect on cognitive function, (e.g., in the SWAN study, Huang et al. 2006), or by being too high over a long exposure period and resulting in possible safety issues, which have not yet been investigated in sufficient detail. Dose, but also tissue-specific issues (see Sect. 176.3) thus need to be considered when assessing different types of health benefits of the isoflavones.

The RCTs to date all tended to use large quantities of daily administered isoflavones, which exceed the amount of daily isoflavone consumed in food in a typical Asian diet. No guidelines exist to assist in this decision and the reasons for this are not at all clear, as they are not based on any known pharmacokinetics of isoflavones. Although a possible influence of dose was found in our RCT, confusion still exists as to whether there is a linear relationship between bioavailability and increasing dose (Setchell et al. 2003; Setchell et al. 2003; Bloedon et al. 2002). Setchell et al. (2003) and Setchell (2000) reported a positive correlation between isoflavone intake and peak concentrations of daidzein and genistein, although this was nonlinear. The same relationship has been seen between bioavailability and intake, with urine analyses showing that, over a 4-day period, a doubling of the dose of isoflavones did not double the total recovery (Setchell et al. 2003). This indicates that consuming a greater quantity of isoflavones does not necessarily result in higher quantities of isoflavones being metabolized, which may reflect a possible saturation or storage effect. Further studies assessing the optimal dosage of isoflavones in tandem with both bioavailability and cognitive function are required in order to have a clearer understanding about the relationship between these factors. The observational studies have not shed any light on this either as amount consumed was not weighted or analyzed. They did, however, suggest that intake of tofu more than 2/3 times a week could already have detrimental associations with cognitive function in the elderly.

The implication of habitual intake of isoflavones is an issue all on its own and may impact on many factors relating to bioavailability (Slavin et al. 1998; Adlercreutz et al. 1982). The regularity of isoflavone consumption could also be of some importance. Significant effects, protective or detrimental, have been reported in populations who regularly consume large amounts of isoflavones (e.g., the HAAS and Kame project), whereas no associations have been found in other sample populations treated with phytoestrogens and/or those who consumed very low and infrequent quantities of isoflavones through their diets. Setchell et al. (2003) suggests that eating soy foods regularly through the day may be more effective for maintaining high serum phytoestrogen levels, and hence may be more beneficial (or detrimental to the elderly as reflected in our Indonesian sample) than eating soy once a day or once a week. However, in a soy treatment study assessing bioavailability as a result of chronic exposure to soy isoflavones over a 10-week period, no difference was found between midpoint and endpoint concentrations of isoflavones in plasma, urine and faeces, which suggests that there were no significant effects of habitual intake (Wiseman et al. 2004). On the other hand, this study may have been too short to appropriately assess 'habitual' intake effects.

176.14.1.3 Characteristics of the Study Population: Age and Menopausal Status

Variations in some characteristics of the study participants (e.g., habitual consumption) may thus influence the effect of isoflavones on cognitive function. Similar to the findings with E, data suggest that it is also possible that age, menopausal status and endogenous hormonal profile may have an impact on the effect of soy isoflavone on cognitive function (Zhao and Brinton 2007). Interestingly, most RCTs finding no, or a negative (e.g., seen in two tests in Gleason et al. 2009), effect of isoflavone treatment on cognitive function had included participants older than 60 years of age (Ho et al. 2007; Howes et al. 2004; Kreijkamp-Kaspers et al. 2004), similar to the observational studies finding negative associations in those over 65 years of age (Rice et al. 2000; White et al. 2000; Hogervorst 2008). Beneficial effects of soy isoflavones were mainly seen for women who were within 10 years of the onset of menopause (bar Gleason et al. 2009) and/or those who had been treated for less than a year with a high dosage, which is also similar to effects seen in E treatment studies (Hogervorst 2006).

Another possible difference between the pre- and postmenopausal studies is the duration of supplementation, as the premenopausal studies tended to use much shorter treatment regimes than the postmenopausal treatment trials (Lu and Anderson 1998; Slavin et al. 1998; Lu et al. 1995). Similar to the effects of E treatment, positive effects of treatment on cognition may be limited up to 2–6 months (Hogervorst et al. 2009).

176.14.1.4 Characteristics of the Study Population: Genetics Determining Phytoestrogen Metabolism

Genetic factors could further influence the metabolism of isoflavones, i.e., due to differences in intestinal microfloral populations (Rowland et al. 1999). It is possible that the colonic microfloral environments of American participants (Zubik and Meydani 2003) may have a higher capacity to hydrolyze glucosides than those of Japanese samples (Izumi et al. 2000), and thus metabolize glucosides better, resulting in these being less bioavailable in the American participants (Zubik and Meydani 2003). Furthermore, the presence of other foods in the digestive system and the composition of those foods may also be factors to consider (Zubik and Meydani 2003). For instance, food-deprived animals were found to absorb isoflavones faster than fed animals (Piskula 2000). In the Izumi et al. (2000) and Zubik and Meydani (2003) studies, participants were fed foods with a different composition matrix before isoflavone consumption, affecting the quantities of aglycones and glucosides, which may have accounted for some of the discrepancies between the studies on cognition which were reviewed earlier.

Another factor causing variation between individuals that has relatively recently been recognized is equol. As previously stated, equol is a metabolite of the isoflavone daidzein produced by gut microflora. Equol's binding ability is of similar strength to genistein, and it has been found to be three times as estrogenic as its parent daidzein in an endometrial tumour line (Markiewicz et al. 1993). Variations exist between animals and humans, as well as between various human populations in the proportion of people who have the ability to produce equol. Due to the variability in gut microflora, only 20–35% of a Western population can produce equol (Wiseman et al. 2004; Morton et al. 1994). It is possible that the effects of isoflavones on various endogenous systems are mediated by the variable of being an equol producer or not (Zhao and Brinton 2007) and, possibly, by age affecting equol production (Frankenfeld et al. 2004). Therefore, equol may be a major player in the effect of soy consumption in the human body, and the failure of human intervention studies to account for this could result in marked differences in individuals' responses to soy consumption. On the other hand, positive effects of soy were also found in a population of non-equol producers (Gleason et al. 2009). This would suggest that other aglycones could mediate the positive effect on cognition (e.g., genistein, and daidzein itself).

176.14.1.5 Other Differences Between Studies

Another factor that needs to be considered when comparing studies and drawing conclusions from the results of RCTs is the types of cognitive tests used. The Fluency test seemed to be particularly sensitive to estrogenic effects (menopausal transition, RCTs with E and phytoestrogens), as well as possibly some specific executive function tests. However, not all studies used the same tests, which makes comparisons complicated. Again, these issues are very similar to those found in studies of the effects of E on the brain (Hogervorst 2009).

176.15 Concluding Remarks

To summarize our research, to our knowledge, we were the first to assess the intake of different types of soy products, as well as endogenous isoflavone levels, in relation to cognitive function in our Indonesian observational study (Hogervorst et al. 2008). In addition, we (Yesufu 2009) were the first to find a beneficial effect of a 24-hour high dose isoflavone supplement (100 mg equivalent of total intake of isoflavones), as opposed to low 30 mg total intake or placebo on Verbal Fluency. Woolley and McEwen (1993) reported that the increase in dendritic sprouting as a result of high levels of Es peaked at two and three days and then decreased over the preceding 7 days. Taking these findings into consideration, with data suggesting optimal levels in the young and middle aged and negative effects of consuming tofu more than two/three times weekly in the elderly, it could be suggested that intermittent intake may be the most favourable regime to render positive effects on the brain in women who are younger than 65 years of age.

To date, most studies assessing the health effects of soy isoflavones have run into conflict and disagreement. Undeniably, there is a huge gap in our knowledge about the effects of phytoestrogens, partly due to the lack of well-controlled large clinical studies. The optimal dose at which a positive effect will be observed is unknown, as well as the toxicity of high doses of isoflavones in humans. The duration of consumption needed to detect if any effect exists, and at what point long-term intake becomes detrimental in whom, is also unclear. Other factors such as genetic/ethnic and environmental variables, isoflavone metabolism and equol production, gender, age and menopausal status, all need to be taken into consideration. Therefore, future studies should aim at addressing these issues and at arriving at a consensus about methodological standards (e.g., type of cognitive test used, isoflavones measurements, etc.) which should be used in order to make the studies more directly comparable. Taking all these points into consideration, the evidence to date is not sufficient to make any recommendations about the use of dietary intake of soy isoflavones to address any human health issues at present. Further focused research needs to be conducted in order to arrive at more definitive conclusions.

Summary Points

- Phytoestrogens are found in abundance in a variety of foods, such as fruits, vegetables and grains. However, very high concentrations can be found in soy. When consumed, they can mimic the effect of estrogens in the body.
- Phytoestrogen consumption has been promoted as beneficial on various health aspects. However, the isoflavone content can vary between different soy foods as a result of their growth process, production and the form they are consumed in. This can affect their metabolism, as well as their effect on the human body.
- It has been suggested that a diet rich in isoflavones (genistein and daidzein) could be implicated in the lower prevalence of Alzheimer's disease in East Asian countries compared to Western countries. East Asian countries consume greater quantities of isoflavones than Western countries from more traditional soy foods, such as tofu and tempe.
- Previous research assessing the relationship between isoflavones and cognition is limited and the effects are not well understood, partly due to conflicting reports from previous studies. Basic cell research has reported both neuroprotective and neurotoxic (but only in very high dosages) effects of genistein and daidzein on biological mechanisms implicated in dementia.
- Observational studies assessing the relationship between isoflavone consumption through diet and cognitive function have either found no relationship in Western populations consuming low levels of isoflavones, or a detrimental effect of high tofu consumption (>2–3/week) in older East Asian populations. This suggests that an optimal level may be required to maintain cognitive function.
- In our observational study in Indonesia, we also reported a negative relationship between high (daily) tofu intake and cognitive function. A positive relationship was observed between high tempe intake and cognitive function in the same analyses. We suggest that processing differences (formaldehyde added to tofu and folate as a by-product of tempe production) may be implicated in these findings.

- However, our results only pertained to women over 68 years of age. This suggests that the effects of phytoestrogens on cognitive function may be modified by age and gender. Participants between 52–68 years appeared to have optimal genistein levels, which was associated with better memory function. However, those over 68 years of age with high genistein levels had lower cognitive scores and a higher risk of dementia.
- Ten RCTs have also assessed this relationship in postmenopausal men and women. Some of these studies have reported beneficial effects on various cognitive functions in women and men. However, others did not find any effect. The data suggests that the duration of treatment (6 months or less), age of women (<65 years), years since menopause and possibly habitual intake could potentially explain differences found between studies.
- Preliminary results of our pilot RCT assessed the 24-hour effects of isoflavone consumption on verbal episodic and semantic memory in postmenopausal women with a mean age of 55 years. We found a positive effect of 100 mg isoflavones (compared to 30 mg or placebo) on verbal Category Fluency. This reflects previous studies reporting a protective effect of high intake in postmenopausal women.
- We propose that possible reasons for discrepancies seen between studies could be due to differences in types and sources of isoflavones (affecting bioavailability and metabolism), dose and the effect of habitual intake, duration of treatment, types of cognitive test used (not all are sensitive), as well as characteristics of the study population (age, internal hormonal status, and genetic factors affecting metabolism).
- To our knowledge, we were the first to assess soy intake and endogenous isoflavone levels in the same sample. We are also the first, to our knowledge, to find beneficial effects of isoflavones on verbal semantic memory after 24 hours. Future research is needed to identify a possible optimal dose at which a positive effect of isoflavones can be observed on cognitive function.

Definition and Explanations of Key Terms or Words

Phytoestrogen: A plant hormone which is physiologically and physiochemically similar to estrogen

Cognition: Mental capacity (Literally 'knowing'), the ability to process information; this includes perception, learning and memory, language and higher executive functions, including complex (but not simple) psychomotor reaction times

Isoflavone: A type of phytoestrogen in the form of glucosides (a sugar group attached to the main part of the molecule which makes it water soluble). When consumed isoflavones can be found in the form of aglycones (no sugar group attached)

Equol: A metabolite of the isoflavone daidzein produced by gut microflora

Estradiol: Most potent estrogen

Estrogenic: A substance which has a biological effect which is similar to that of estrogen

Anti-estrogenic: A substance which competes with estrogens to bind to receptor sites and hence blocks the activity of estrogen

Bioavailability: The part of a substance that remains after it has been digested, absorbed and metabolized by the human body

Agonist: A substance that binds to a receptor and hence affects it's functioning

Antagonist: A chemical that blocks the binding of another chemical to its receptor in an organism without binding to the receptor itself

Pharmacokinetic: The process by which a substance is absorbed, distributed, metabolized and eliminated by the body

Pharmacodynamic: The actions or effects of a substance on a living organism

Acknowledgements We would like to acknowledge the funders, Loughborough University, Universitas Indonesia (Center for Health) and the Alzheimer's Research Trust UK as well as all participants and staff involved in SEMAR.

References

Adlercreutz H. Scan J Clin Lab Inv. 1990;201:3–23.

Adlercreutz H, Fotsis T, Heikkinen R, Dwyer JT, Woods M, Goldin BR, Gorbach SL. Lancet. 1982;2:1295–9.

Adlercreutz H, Mazur W. Ann Med. 1997;29:95–120.

American Institute for Cancer Research. Food nutrition and the prevention of cancer. Washington: World Cancer Research Fund. 1997

American Psychiatric Association. Diagnostic and statistical manual of mental disorders, 4th ed. (DSM-IV) Washington, DC: American Psychiatric Association; 1994.

Arai Y, Uehara M, Sato Y, Kimira M, Eboshida A, Adlercreutz H, Watanabe S. J Epidemiol. 2000; 10 (2):127–35.

Azadbakht L, Kimiagar M, Mehrabi Y, Esmaillzadeh A, Padyab M, Hu FB, Hu FB, Willett WC. Am J Clin Nutr. 2007;85:735–41.

Bang OY, Hong HS, Kim DH, Kim H, Boo JH, Huh K, Mook-Jung I. Neurobiol Dis. 2004;16:21–8.

Barnes S, Peterson TG, Coward L. J Cell Biochem Suppl. 1995; 22:181–7.

Beecher GR, Bhagwat S, Haytowitz D, Holden JM, Murphy PA. J Nutr. 2000;130:666S.

Bloedon LT, Jeffcoat AR, Lopaczynski W, Schell MJ, Black TM, Dix KJ, Thomas BF, Albright C, Busby MG, Crowell JA, Zeisel SH. Am J Clin Nutr. 2002;76:1126–37.

Boettger-Tong H, Murthy L, Chiappetta C, Kirkland JL, Goodwin B, Adlercreutz H, Stancel GM, Mäkelä S. Environ Health Perspect. 1998;106:369–73.

Boker LK, Van der Schouw YT, De Kleijn MJ, Jacques PF, Grobbee DE, Peeters PH. J Nutr. 2002;132:1319–28.

Casini ML, Marelli G, Papaleo E, Ferrari A, D'Ambrosio F, Unfer V. Fertil Steril. 2006;85:972–8.

Cassidy A, Bingham S, Setchell K. Br J Nutr. 1995;74:587–601.

Cassidy A, Brown JE, Hawdon A, Faughnan MS, King LJ, Millward J, Zimmer-Nechemias L, Wolfe B, Setchell KD. J Nutr. 2006;136:45–51.

Celec P, Ostatnikova D, Caganova M, Zuchova S, Hodosy J, Putz Z, Bernadic M, Kúdela M. Gynecol Obstet Invest. 2005;59:62–6.

Chen Z, Zheng W, Custer LJ, Dai Q, Shu XO, Jin F, Franke AA. Nutr Cancer. 1999;33:82–7.

Chiechi LM, Secreto G, D'Amore M, Fanelli M, Venturelli E, Cantatore F, Valerio T, Laselva G, Loizzi P. Maturitas. 2002;42:295–300.

Choi EJ, Lee BH. Life Sci. 2004;75:499–509.

Coward LN, Barnes C, Setchell KD, Barnes S. J Agric Food Chem. 1993;41:1961–7.

de Kleijn MJ, van der Schouw YT, Wilson PW, Adlercreutz H, Mazur W, Grobbee DE, Jacques PF. J Nutr. 2001;131:1826–32.

Dhom G. In: Voight KD, Knabbe C, editors. Endocrine dependent tumors. New York: Raven Press; 1991. pp. 1–42.

Duffy R, Wiseman H, File SE. Pharmacol Biochem Be. 2003;75:721–9.

Ernst E. Ann Intern Med. 2002;136:42–53.

File SE, Hartley DE, Elsabagh S, Duffy R, Wiseman H. Menopause. 2005;12:193–201.

File SE, Jarrett N, Fluck E, Duffy R, Casey K, Wiseman H. Psychopharmacology. 2001;157:430–6.

Fitzpatrick LA. Maturitas. 2003;44:S21–9.

Fournier LR, Ryan Borchers TA, Robison LM, Wiediger M, Park JS, Chew BP, McGuire MK, Sclar DA, Skaer TL, Beerman KA. J Nutr Health Ageing. 2007;11:155–64.

Franco OH, Burger H, Lebrun CE, Peeters PH, Lamberts SW, Grobbee DE, Van Der Schouw. J Nutr. 2005;135:1190–5.

Frankenfeld CL, Atkinson C, Thomas WK, Goode EL, Gonzalez A, Jokela T, Wähälä K, Schwartz SM, Li SS, Lampe JW. Exp Biol Med (Maywood). 2004;229:902–13.

FSA. COT WOrking group on phytoestrogens draft report. Retrieved August 18, 2008, from http://www.food.gov.uk/multimedia/webpage/phytoreportworddocs; 2002***

Fuh JL, Wang SJ, Lee SJ, Lu SR, Juang KD (2006). Maturitas. 53: 447–453

Ganora L. (2008) Phyoestrogens. Retrieved August 16, 2008, from http://www.herbalchem.net/Introductory.htm***

Gibbs RB. In: Rasgun NL, editor. The effects of estrogen on brain function. Baltimore: John Hopkins Press; 2006. pp. 9–45.

Ginting E, Arcot J. J Agric Food Chem. 2004;52:7752–8.

Gleason CE, Carlsson CM, Barnet JH, Meade SA, Setchell KD, Atwood CS, Johnson SC, Ries ML, Asthana S. Age Aging. 2009;38:86–93.

Grodstein F, Mayeux R, Stampfer MJ. J Am CollNutr. 2000;19:207–9.

Gurel A, Coskun O, Armutcu F, Kanter M, Ozen OA. J Chem Neuroanat. 2005;29:173–8.

Halbreich U, Kahn LS. Expert Opin Pharmacother. 2000;1:1385–98.

Henderson VW, Benke KS, Green RC, Cupples LA, Farrer LA, MIRAGE Study Group. J Neurol Neurosurg Psychiatry. 2005;76:103–5.

Ho SC, Chan AS, Ho YP, So EK, Sham A, Zee B, Woo JL (2007) Menopause. 14: 489–499

Hogervorst E. In: Rasgun NL, editor. Effects of estrogen on brain function. Baltimore: John Hopkins University Press; 2006. pp. 46–78.

Hogervorst E, Yesufu A, Sadjimim T, Kreager P, Rahardjo TB. In: Hogervorst E, Henderson AS, Brinton-Diaz R, Gibbs R (eds.) Hormones, cognition and dementia. New York: Cambridge University Press; 2009.

Hogervorst E, Henderson V, Brinton-Diaz R, Gibbs R. Hormones cognition and dementia. Edinburgh: Cambridge University Press; (2009 in press) (Chapter 13) 121–122.

Hogervorst E, Sadjimim T, Yesufu A, Kreager P, Rahardjo TB. Dement Geriatr Cogn. 2008;26:50–7.

Hogervorst E, Smith AD. Neuro Endocrinol Lett. 2002;23:155–60.

Horn-Ross PL, Barnes S, Lee M, Coward L, Mandel JE, Koo J, John EM, Smith M. Cancer Causes Control. 2000;11:289–98.

Horn-Ross PL, Lee M, John EM, Koo J. Cancer Causes Control. 2000;11:299–302.

Howes JB, Bray K, Lorenz L, Smerdel P, Howes LG. Climacteric. 2004;7:70–7.

Huang MH, Luetters C, Buckwalter GJ, Seeman TE, Gold EB, Sternfeld B, Greendale GA. Menopause. 2006;13:621–30.

Isingrini M, Taconnat L. Rev Neurol (Paris). 2008;164:S91–5.

Izumi T, Piskula MK, Osawa S, Obata A, Tobe K, Saito M. The Journal of Nutrition. 2000;130(7):1695–1699.

Ju YH, Allred KF, Allred CD, Helferich WG. Carcinogenesis. 2006;27:1292–9.

Kim H, Xia H, Li L, Gewin J. BioFactors. 2000;12:243–50.

Kimira M, Arai Y, Shimoi K, Watanabe S. J Epidemiol. 1998;8:168–75.

Knight DC, Eden JA. Obstet Gynecol. 1996;87:897–904.

Kreijkamp-Kaspers S, Kok L, Grobbee DE, de Haan EH, Aleman A, Lampe JW van der Schouw YT. JAMA. 2004;292:65–74.

Kreijkamp-Kaspers S, Kok L, Grobbee DE, de Haan EH, Aleman A, van der Schouw YT. J Gerontol A-Biol. 2007;62:556–62.

Kritz-Silverstein D, Von Muhlen D, Barrett-Connor E, Bressel MA. Menopause. 2003;10:196–202.

Kuiper GG, Lemmen JG, Carlsson B, Corton JC, Safe SH, van der Saag PT, van der Burg B, Gustofsson JA. Endocrinology. 1998;139:4252–63.

Kurzer MS, Xu X. Annu Rev Nutr. 1997;17:353–81.

Lee YB, Lee HJ, Sohn HS. J Nutr Biochem. 2005;16:641–9.

Linford NJ, Dorsa DM. Steroids. 2002;67:1029–40.

Lu LJ, Anderson KE. Am J Clin Nutr. 1998;68:1500S–4S.

Lu LJ, Grady JJ, Marshall MV, Ramanujam VM, Anderson KE. Nutr Cancer. 1995;24:311–23.

Markiewicz L, Garey J, Adlercreutz H, Gurpide E. J Steroid Biochem Mol Biol. 1993;45:399–405.

Maskarinec G, Singh S, Meng L, Franke AA. Cancer Epidem Biomark. 1998;7:613–9.

Maskarinec S. Nutrition Bytes. 2003;9:5.

Mohamed A, Xu J. Food Chem. 2003;83:227–36.

Morton MS, Wilcox G, Wahlqvist ML, Griffiths K. J Endocrinol. 1994;142:251–9.

Murkies AL, Wilcox G, Davis SR. J Clin Endocrinol Metab. 1998;83:297–303.

Oakenfull D. J Nutr. 2001;131:2971–2.

Occhiuto F, Zangla G, Samperi S, Palumbo DR, Pino A, De Pasquale R, Circosta C. Phytomedicine. 2008;15:676–82.

Ostatníková D, Celec P, Hodosy J, Hampl R, Putz Z, Kúdela M. Fertil Steril. 2007;88:1632–6.

Pan Y, Anthony M, Clarkson TB. Proc Soc Exp Biol Med. 1999;221:118–25.

Pinkerton JV, Henderson VW. Semin Reprod Med. 2005;23:172–9.

Piskula MK. J Nutr. 2000;130:1766–71.

Potter SM. J Nutr. 1995;125:606S–11S.

Reitz C, Honig L, Vonsattel JP, Tang MX, Mayeux R. J Neurol Neurosurg Psychiatry. 2009;80:715–21.

Rice MM, Graves AB, McCurry SM, Gibbons L, Bowen J, McCormick W, Larson EB (2000) Third international symposium on the role of soy in preventing and treating chronic disease, Washington, DC, Oct 31–Nov 3, 1999, Vol. 130, p. 676S.

Rilantono LI, Yuwono HS, Nugrahadi T. Clin Hemorheol Microcirc. 2000;23:113–7.

Rowland I, Wiseman H, Sanders T, Adlercreutz H, Bowey E. Biochem Soc Trans. 1999;27:304–8.

Setchell KD. Am J Clin Nutr. 1998;68:1333S–46S.

Setchell KD. (2000) Absorption and metabolism of soy isoflavones-from food to dietary supplements and adults to infants J Nutr. 2000;130:654S–5S.

Setchell KD, Brown NM, Desai P, Zimmer-Nechemias L, Wolfe BE, Brashear WT, Kirschner AS, Cassidy A, Heubi JE. J Nutr. 2001;131:1362S–75S.

Setchell KD, Brown NM, Desai PB, Zimmer-Nechimias L, Wolfe B, Jakate AS, Creutzinger V, Heubi JE. J Nutr. 2003;133:1027–35.

Slavin JL, Karr SC, Hutchins AM, Lampe JW. The American Journal of Clinical Nutrition, 68(6 Suppl), 1998;1492S–1495S.

Smith AD (2002) Am. J. Clin. Nutr. 75: 85–786

Sonee M, Sum T, Wang C, Mukherjee SK. Neurotoxicology. 2004;25:885–91.

Thilers PP, Macdonald SW, Herlitz A. Psychoneuroendocrinology. 2006;31:565–76.

Trieu VN, Dong Y, Zheng Y, Uckun FM. Radiat Res. 1999;152:508–16.

US Food and Drug Administration. Federal Register. 1999;64:57699–733.

Valsta LM, Kilkkinen A, Mazur W, Nurmi T, Lampi AM, Ovaskainen ML, Korhonen T, Adlercreutz H, Pietinen P. Br J Nutr. 2003;89:S31–8.

Wang HJ, Murphy P. J Agr Food Chem. 1994;42:1666–73.

Wakai K, Egami I, Kato K, Kawamura T, Tamakoshi A, Lin Y, Nakayama T, Wada M, Ohno Y. Nutr Cancer. 1999;33:139–45.

Whalley LJ, Starr JM, Athawes R, Hunter D, Pattie A, Deary IJ. Neurology. 2000;55:1455–9.

White LR, Petrovitch H, Ross GW, Masaki K, Hardman J, Nelson J, Davis D, Markesbery W. J Am Coll Nutr. 2000;19:242–55.

Wiseman H, Casey K, Bowey EA, Duffy R, Davies M, Rowland IR, Lloyd AS, Murray A, Thompson R, Clarke DB. Am J Clin Nutr. 2004;80:692–9.

Woolley CS, McEwen BS. J Comp Neurol. 1993;336:293–306.

Wu AH, Yu MC, Tseng CC, Pike MC. Br J Cancer. 2008;98:9–14.

Yesufu A. Demographic and modifiable risk factors for age related cognitive impairment and possible dementia. Loughborough University Library; 2009.

Zeng H, Chen Q, Zhao B. Free Radic Biol Med. 2004;36:180–8.

Zhao L, Brinton RD. Expert Rev Neurother. 2007;7:1549–64.

Zubik L, Meydani M. Am J Clin Nutr. 2003;77:1459–65.

Chapter 177
Nutritional Risk in the Elderly with Cognitive Impairment: A Far Eastern Perspective

Kang Soo Lee and Chang Hyung Hong

Abbreviations

AD   Alzheimer's disease
ADL   Activities of daily living
IADL   Instrumental activities of daily living
K-MMSE   Korean version of mini mental state examination
MCI   Mild cognitive impairment
NCF   Normal cognitive function
NSI   Nutrition screening initiative

177.1 Introduction

The 2005 data from the Korea National Statistical Office indicates that by 2018, Korea would become an aged society in which the elderly population, i.e., persons aged more than 65 years, would comprise 14% of the total population. As a result, problems pertaining to the welfare and health of the elderly have become a national concern. With the increase in the elderly population, the incidence of chronic geriatric diseases is also on the rise. Nutrition and diet have gradually become important from the perspective of prevention of geriatric diseases and promotion of the health of the elderly. If malnutrition refers to dietary intake in reference to dietary needs, intakes of several nutrients have been shown to be inadequate among those living in the community. However, diet is only one indicator of nutritional status of elderly people and probably not the best given the methodological assessment issues. Therefore, other indicators such as anthropometric, hematological, biochemical and immunological indices, health conditions and diseases need to be considered in addition in the evaluation of nutritional health. Many efforts have been directed to discovering factors influencing the nutritional status of elderly people to identify people with poor nutritional status or those who are at high risk of nutritional problems. Based on these factors, some simple and easy to apply nutritional assessment tools such as nutrition screening initiative checklist have been developed.

Malnutrition is one of the most prevalent problems in the elderly that is easily overlooked. The nutritional state of the elderly is threatened by several factors including the followings: tooth loss or

C.H. Hong (✉)
Department of Psychiatry and Ajou Institute of Aging, Ajou University School of Medicine,
San 5, Wonchun-dong, Youngtong-gu, Suwon-si, 443-749, Korea
e-mail: antiaging@ajou.ac.kr

V.R. Preedy et al. (eds.), *Handbook of Behavior, Food and Nutrition*,
DOI 10.1007/978-0-387-92271-3_177, © Springer Science+Business Media, LLC 2011

masticatory difficulty; deterioration of physiological functions, including the weakening of digestion and absorption; loss of gustation; effect of medications used for treating various ailments; smoking; habitual drinking; decreased activity; living alone; depression due to death of a spouse; psychological factors such as feelings of neglect; financial difficulties due to reduction in income; and environmental factors (Brownie 2006). Consequently, there is insufficient intake of food by the elderly and the utilization rate in the body also becomes lower; thus, there is a high predisposition to a nutritional risk state. Through various studies, it has been shown that the nutritional state of elderly Koreans is generally not good (Kim et al. 1997; Cho et al. 1997). In particular, the level of malnutrition is higher in the elderly residing in social welfare institutions and the low-income elderly residing at home, and it is known that the nutritional intake state is poor in the elderly who evaluate their own health as being poor or as having more clinical symptoms of diseases (Son et al. 1996; Song et al. 1995).

There is growing attention in the relationships between aging, nutritional status, and cognitive function. Research in this filed has tended to focus on advanced old age, although many of the causal pathway implicated may operate over a much longer period from early life. Nutrition has been found to be associated with cognitive impairment and dementia in older populations. The nutritional risk level of the elderly is associated with cognitive function (Pearson et al. 2001). Impairment of cognitive functions related to the basic activities of daily living (ADL) has been reported to be more rapid over a 1-year follow-up period in malnourished subjects (Vellas et al. 2005). An increased interest in this field has led to the formulation of varied hypotheses regarding the correlation between nutritional factors and cognitive impairment (Donini et al. 2007).

177.2 Nutrition and Alzheimer's Dementia

Nutrition Screening Initiative (NSI) checklist has been developed as part of the US Nutrition Screening Initiative, a collaborative effort between the American Dietetic Association, the American Academy of Family Physicians and the National Council on the Aging, Inc. The NSI checklist is the first step in a two-tiered approach to screening and assessment. The checklist is designed to enhance the older person's understanding of the determinants of nutritional well-being and promote the consideration of nutritional problems by health professionals. This self-administered awareness tool is intended for the public and may need a follow-up by professionals for further nutritional and health assessments. The checklist includes 10 Yes/No items that are given different weights associated with the nutritional well-being of older people. The checklist is not meant to be a clinical diagnostic tool but should predict overall perceived health status and identify persons whose estimated nutrient intakes fall below the recommended dietary allowances (Table 177.2).

Table 177.1 Key features of K-MMSE: Korean Mini Mental State Examination

1. The MMSE developed by Folstein et al. (1975) is the most widely used instrument for measuring global cognitive performance and for identifying individuals with cognitive dysfunction
2. The MMSE, variously modified and translated into several languages, has been used successfully in several independent cross-national studies of dementia epidemiology
3. The original MMSE was somewhat modified in the development of the K-MMSE in order to adapt it to the cultural background in Korea
4. The total K-MMSE score was calculated by summing the correct responses to all the K-MMSE sub items
5. The test scores ranged from 0 to 30
6. A Korean study in the community defined the cutoff point of K-MMSE score during the screening of dementia as 17/18 points

Table 177.2 Key features of nutrition screening Initiative checklist

1. The Nutrition Screening Initiative checklist comprises 10 questions that were designed such that their answer would be "yes" or "no."

2. Based on the evaluation standard for the nutritional risk level, 0–2 points were assigned to a good nutritional state; 3–5 points, moderate nutritional risk state; and more than 6 points, high nutritional risk state.

3. In case of good nutritional state, recheck your nutritional score in 6 months

4. If you are at moderate nutritional risk, see what can be done to improve your eating habits and life style. Recheck your nutritional score in 3 months

5. If you are at high nutritional risk, bring this checklist the next time you see your doctor or other qualified health and social service professional. Ask for help to improve your nutritional health.

6. The NSI checklist is influenced by the type of family members living together, diseases, financial condition, age, physical health condition, and its effects on cognitive function

7. Question 1 (yes = 2 point): I have an illness or condition that made me change the kind and/or amount of food I eat.
Question 2 (yes = 3 point): I eat fewer than 2 meals per day.
Question 3 (yes = 2 point): I eat few fruits or vegetables or milk products
Question 4 (yes = 2 point): I have 3 or more drinks of beer, liquor or wine almost every day.
Question 5 (yes = 2 point): I have tooth or mouth problems that make it hard for me to eat.
Question 6 (yes = 4 point): I don't always have enough money to buy the food I need.
Question 7 (yes = 1 point): I eat alone most of the time.
Question 8 (yes = 1 point): I take 3 or more different prescribed or over-the-counter drugs a day.
Question 9 (yes = 2 point): Without wanting to, I have lost or gained 10 lb in the last 6 months.
Question 10 (yes = 2 point): I am not always physically able to shop, cook, and/or feedmyself.

Nutritional status is potentially important in the etiology of cognitive impairment and dementia. Dementia is associated with weight loss, which precedes the onset of the clinical syndrome and accelerates around the time of diagnosis. Specific nutritional deficits such as vitamin B12 and folate deficiency are recognized to be important potential risk factors, and other dietary factors such as caloric intake and fish consumption have also been implicated as modifying risk. Epidemiological (Masaki et al. 2000; Engelhart et al. 2002) and laboratory studies (Cotman et al. 2002; Kruman et al. 2002) have demonstrated that antioxidants, which are found in abundance in fresh fruits and vegetables, are associated with cognitive function. In addition, it has been reported that nutritional substances or food stuffs such as fish, vitamin, and a moderate amount of alcohol decrease the risk for dementia and Alzheimer's disease (AD) (Kalmijn et al. 1997, 2004; Luchsinger and Mayeux 2004). Several studies have clearly demonstrated that nutritional factors are linked with AD, both as risk or protective factors in the onset of the disease and as elements that are capable of modifying the disease course (Donini et al. 2007). Although dietary intervention is capable of minimizing or preventing weight loss (Franzoni et al. 1996), patients at particular risk of malnutrition are not detected quickly enough; therefore, nutritional screening tools should be included in the multidimensional geriatric evaluation that must be performed in every elderly patient.

177.3 Nutrition and Mild Cognitive Impairment

In 1999, Petersen et al. proposed clinical MCI criteria including essentially preserved activities of daily living. In 2003, Petersen et al. revised original criteria as one including clinical judgment for assessing people of low education and for ADL performance. In terms of the criterion of preserved activities of daily living, the CSHA study found intact ADL to be unnecessary for case definition but the validity of the ADL criterion were also challenged in the other study. These reflect that MCI represents a condition with multiple sources of heterogeneity. Key methodological factors differing across studies of MCI include (1) the fact of MCI diagnoses being assigned on a case-by-case basis in a consensus conference of expert clinicians or assigned purely objectively using neuropsychological, functional, and medical data; (2) the extent to which non-demented older subjects with memory deficits are distinguished from those with cognitive deficits in non-memory domains; (3) the extent to which those with isolated deficits in one cognitive domain are distinguished from those with impairment in multiple cognitive domains; (4) the test score "cutoff" used to define cognitive impairment; (5) the use of norms that adjust for age and other background factors such as years of school, sex, and race/ethnicity; (6) the extent to which subjective memory complaints are considered as a requirement for the diagnosis of MCI; and finally, (7) follow-up diagnosis being made with the knowledge of prior diagnostic status.

Difficulties remain in defining the boundaries between normal ageing and MCI, and between MCI and mild dementia. An international working group on MCI formulated specific recommendations for certain criteria, including: (1) the individual is neither normal nor demented; (2) there is evidence of cognitive deterioration, shown by either objectively measured decline over time or subjective report of decline by self or informant in conjunction with objective cognitive deficits; and (3) activities of daily life are preserved and complex instrumental functions are either intact or minimally impaired. Considering the special situation that low educational level and simple life style are frequent in the Korean rural community, there are many subjects who are neither normal nor demented and whose complex instrumental functions are impaired. Findings of epidemiological studies have shown that subtle difficulties in the performance of everyday activities are common in individuals with MCI. If limitations on complex ADL were present in patients with MCI, the assessment of impairments in everyday life might provide useful complementary information to establish the diagnosis of the syndrome. The use of combined tests has shown to be a promising procedure in order to increase the accuracy of mild dementia diagnoses, as for instance the combination of a cognitive test with a functional evaluation test. An approach that combines both domains of information is often part of a comprehensive clinical assessment and appears, from the present data, to be valuable in prediction of clinical course as well. However, until now no specific instruments for evaluating complex ADL in MCI have been proposed. So, there is a need for a consensus regarding the degree of functional decline that can be considered acceptable in the frame of MCI definition.

Mild cognitive impairment (MCI) defines a transitional stage between normal aging and dementia (Petersen et al. 2001) and reflects a clinical situation where a person has complaints about memory loss and shows objective evidence of cognitive impairment but exhibits no evidence of dementia (Burns and Zaudig 2002). Not many studies have prospectively addressed the role of putative risk factors for MCI. Three short-term longitudinal studies, carried out in subjects with MCI, identified older age, low education, being African American, presence of ApoE 4, cortical atrophy at neuroimaging, signs or symptoms of vascular diseases and depression as risk factors. In a recent 3-year prospective study, the authors found that a previous diagnosis of psychosis, hip fracture and polypharmacy increased the risk of cognitive impairment in non-demented subjects, independent of subsequent development of dementia. Furthermore, three long-term prospective studies described midlife alcohol drinking, elevated serum cholesterol, high diastolic blood pressure, ApoE4, and white matter hyperintensities as risk factors for MCI in late life. In the absence of sensitive and specific biomarkers, risk profiles are of great importance in identifying individuals with the highest probability of incipient disease. To the extent that MCI represents preclinical AD, risk factors for AD should also be risk factors for MCI development or progression. That this degree of correspondence has not been found again reflects the heterogeneity of MCI. These might well represent reversible comorbid conditions, other than neurodegeneration, that caused or contributed to the cognitive impairment, for example, depression, heart failure, anticholinergic drug use (Ganguli 2006).

Over the last decade few studies have examined nutritional risk and low weight in the community-living older adult population. Multifactorial issues that contribute to nutritional risk and malnutrition make it difficult to study. It is apparent that weight loss and nutritional risk are common in this population and can be associated with adverse outcomes. The results of many studies carried out in recent years ascertained that nutritional factors are linked with dementia, especially with AD, both as risk or protective factors in the onset of the disease and elements able to modify the course of the disease (Donini et al. 2007). But in the case of MCI, antioxidant trials are underway, aiming to prove that vitamin E, selegiline, and Ginkgo Biloba slow or stop MCI to AD conversion (Brenner 2003; Mecocci et al. 2004); however, another trial (Petersen et al. 2005) failed to demonstrate a benefit from vitamin E. This approach is in line with previous studies on preceding concepts on MCI with cognitive stimulants and nootropics (Levy 1994; Lockhart and Lestage 2003). The results have been consistently disappointing and in contrast with neurobiological data, which have always been in favor of the role of free radicals and reactive oxygen species in cell death and dementia onset (Qin et al. 2006).

177.4 Nutrition and Functional Status in the Elderly

At the beginning of the disease course, there may be an alteration of nutritional status. This alteration may be explained by a change in dietary intake due to the inability to carry out complex tasks in daily life (e.g., difficulty in shopping, preparing meals, or selecting food). A change in the instrumental activities of daily living (IADL), which assesses independence in performing complex tasks in daily life, is sometimes one of the first signs of the disease. The original criteria for MCI provided for intact ADL, but the current recommendations indicate that the basic ADL should be mainly preserved, and that a "minimal impairment" in IADL may be accepted (Winblad et al. 2004). Recent data suggest that the inclusion of IADL restriction in MCI criteria improves the prediction of subsequent dementia as well as the stability of the MCI condition over time (Peres et al. 2006). Although no consensus has been reached about what composes an ADL restriction in MCI, functional impairments in MCI are focused on the area of instrumental ADL (IADL) tasks – such as managing finances or using a telephone. As IADL tasks are definitely more cognitively demanding tasks than basic ADL tasks, they are more likely to be vulnerable to early cognitive decline due to MCI. Loss in the ability to complete IADL tasks can be among the earliest signs of MCI, even though global functional impairment would still be unnoticeable. Moreover, recent studies suggest that MCI patients with IADL impairment are at higher risk of progression to dementia in the future. MCI patients have significantly worse IADL ratings compared with cognitively unimpaired controls, and those with IADL impairment experience more rapid functional decline and are more likely to convert to dementia compared with those MCI patients without IADL problems. Therefore, an assessment of the completion of IADL tasks in MCI is potentially of great interest, and could serve as a major criterion for differentiating MCI and cognitively normal elderly. Impaired IADL is a strong prognosticator of progression to dementia, with the risk increasing as a function of the number of impaired IADL tasks, particularly specific IADL tasks (e.g., telephone, transport, medication, and finances) in MCI patients, the conversion rate being almost four times higher.

Because functional and nutritional statuses are interrelated, functional impairment can also increase the risk of poor nutrition in MCI. Many of the identified nutritional risk factors of malnutrition are based on functional competencies such as mobility, depression, cognition, food shopping, and food preparation. Considering MCI has little known risk factors and minimal impairment in IADL, nutritional risk assessment will be helpful.

177.5 Nutritional Risk and Cognition: A Far Eastern Perspective

177.5.1 Nutritional Risk and Cognitive Impairment

Elderly Korean people have a low level of education because the sociopolitical circumstances during their childhood and adolescence hindered their access to formal schooling, and the availability of public education was generally lower during the time period between the Second World War and the Korean War. Although the K-MMSE equals the scoring of the MMSE reported by Folstein, considering the special situation that low educational level are frequent in the Korean rural community, the low K-MMSE scores in the MCI subjects could not suggest that these patients may meet criteria for dementia. Another normative study of the K-MMSE in the elderly showed that education level had a greater effect on the K-MMSE than age and sex (Table 177.1).

The MMSE developed by Folstein is the most widely used instrument for measuring global cognitive performance and for identifying individuals with cognitive dysfunction. The elderly exhibit a high prevalence of cognitive dysfunction that may influence their test performance, and therefore their normative data may differ from those in younger subjects. The MMSE, variously modified and translated into several languages, has been used successfully in several independent cross-national studies of dementia epidemiology. The MMSE was modified and translated into Korean by Kang, and the resulting K-MMSE has been widely used in clinical evaluations and research involving patients with dementia in Korea. The original MMSE was somewhat modified in the development of the K-MMSE in order to adapt it to the cultural background in Korea; however, the K-MMSE still shares all of the limitations of the original MMSE. Temporal orientation was assessed according to the two methods used to calculate year and time in Korea: the solar and lunar years. The words "airplane," "pencil," and "pine tree" were used in the memory assessment, with their associated sounds. Serial sevens (sequential subtraction of 7 from 100) were performed to assess the attention of each patient. The repetition phrase item, "no ifs, ands, or buts," was modified to "seeing is believing" with vowel sounds. The three-stage command was modified to "turn the paper over, fold it in half, and give it to me." The total K-MMSE score was calculated by summing the correct responses to all the KMMSE sub items. The test scores ranged from 0 to 30.

The original K-MMSE score was lower in the moderate or high nutritional risk state group of elderly subjects living in the community when compared with the good nutritional state group of elderly subjects. A Korean study in the community defined the cutoff point of K-MMSE score during the screening of dementia as 17/18 points; the sensitivity and specificity of the findings were 91% and 86%, respectively (Kim et al. 2003). Based on these results, we defined cognitive impairment as the group that had a K-MMSE score lower than 17 points, and cognitive non-impairment was defined as the group that had a K-MMSE score higher than 18 points. In the good nutritional state group, the percentage of subjects demonstrating cognitive function impairment was only 13.9%, whereas it was 27.0% in the moderate nutritional risk state group or the high nutritional risk state group. This suggests that malnutrition state is associated with an impairment of cognitive function (Tables 177.3 and Fig 177.1).

This is in agreement with the findings reported in a study of 627 elderly individuals (Pearson et al. 2001). Although the interrelationship between cognitive impairment and nutritional risk are complex and reciprocal; cognitive impairment recedes malnutrition or vice versa. Recent research demonstrates that altered nutritional status appear to predict the severity and progression of cognitive impairment (Vellas et al. 2005). These findings underscore the importance of systematic nutritional assessment at the time of diagnosis and during the follow-up of cognitive impairment cases, especially in those with dementia, in order to implement nutritional intervention as soon as it is deemed necessary (Gillette-Guyonnet et al. 2007). To examine whether cognitive function differs depending

Table 177.3 The relationship between nutritional risk and Mini Mental State Examination in the Far Eastern community elderly subjects (Reprinted from Lee et al.2009. With permission)

K-MMSE score	Good nutritional state (NSI[a] score ≤ 2), n (%)	Moderate or high nutritional risk (NSI[a] score > 2), n (%)	p^b
>17	1485 (86.1)	615 (73.0)	<0.0001
≤17	239 (13.9)	228 (27.0)	

[a]Nutritional Screening Initiative
[b]Chi-square test

Chi-square analysis was performed to assess the risk for cognitive impairment based on the presence or absence of nutritional risk. Table 177.2 shows that the relative frequency of cases with cognitive impairment was higher in the moderate or high nutritional risk level group when compared with that observed in the good nutritional state group ($x^2 = 66.1$, d.f. = 1, $p < 0.0001$)

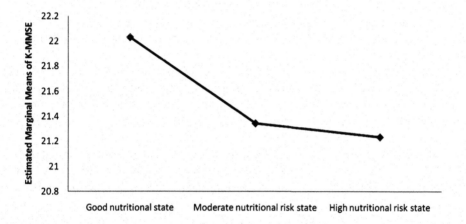

Fig. 177. 1 Estimated marginal means of Mini Mental State Examination according to the nutritional risk in the Far Eastern community elderly subjects. Multiple logistic regression analysis was performed to assess the risk for cognitive impairment based on the presence or absence of nutritional risk after adjustment for age, sex, and educational level. General Linear Model (GLM) univariate analysis was performed, and GLM profile plots were plotted as shown in this figure (Reprinted from Lee et al. 2009. With permission)

on the responses to the ten questions in the NSI checklist, we compared the response rate of NSI checklist items in the low and high K-MMSE groups. It was observed that the low K-MMSE group responded more frequently to the following two items after adjustment of age, sex, education: (1) "I have tooth or mouth problems that make it difficult for me to eat," (2) "I am not always physically able to shop, cook, and feed myself." Tooth problems are not simply limited to oral problems. Additionally, they are not limited by their association with the socio-economic and education levels, lifestyle, and smoking history; they are also related to diverse physical conditions such as the presence of cardiopulmonary diseases. It has been reported that there is an association between most oral problems and lower cognitive function (Avlund et al. 2004). However, the results cannot confirm whether the presence of tooth and other oral problems resulted in malnutrition and consequently impairment in cognitive function, whether cognitive impairment was caused by other factors that led to tooth and oral problems, or whether cognitive impairment resulted in changes in the lifestyle that induced tooth and oral problems. The same problem was also applied to other questions.

177.5.2 Nutritional Risk and Mild Cognitive Impairment

The frequency of MCI was higher in the moderate or high nutritional risk state group of elderly subjects living in a community when compared with the group of elderly subjects in a good nutritional state. In the good nutritional state group, the percentage of MCI subjects was only 47.0%, whereas it was 61.1% in the moderate or high nutritional risk state group. One study showed that the K-MMSE score was lower in the moderate or high nutritional risk state group of elderly subjects living in the community when compared with the good nutritional state group of elderly subjects. In line with this concept, the nutritional risk state is associated with an MCI (Table 177.4).

However, the interrelationships between MCI and nutritional risk are complex and reciprocal; MCI precedes malnutrition or vice versa. On the one hand, nutritional risk influences risk factors or outcomes of MCI. Recent research demonstrates that an altered nutritional status appear to predict the severity and progression of cognitive impairment (Vellas et al. 2005). These findings underline the systematic nutritional assessment in MCI. On the other hand, mild changes in discrete IADLs in MCI increase nutritional risk. By analyzing the functional characteristics of subjects with MCI collected in the ReGAl study, it was found that subjects with MCI had more severe IADL disability than cognitively healthy elderly controls, particularly with regard to shopping, self-administration of drugs, and handling finances. These IADL disabilities were significantly associated with the degree of cognitive impairment, but not with somatic comorbidity. Similarly, in another study (Perneczky et al. 2006), it was found that MCI patients are limited in everyday tasks that involve either memory (i.e., finding things at home, keeping appointments, and remembering information from a conversation or from television) or complex reasoning (i.e., checking bank account, shopping). When compared the response rate of the NSI checklist items in the MCI and NCF elderly groups to examine whether MCI results in different responses to the ten questions in the NSI checklist. The MCI group responded more frequently to the following two items after the adjustment of age, sex, and education: (1) "I do not always have enough money to buy the food I need" and (2) "I am not always physically able to shop, cook, and feed myself (Table 177.5)." Items (1) and (2) generally reflect financial abilities and physical abilities. Because the "yes" response rate to item (1) was too low, the interpretation of the result has limitations. But financial abilities cognitively demand IADLs that are vital to independent functioning in a community (Marson et al. 2000), and they are very sensitive to mild AD (Earnst et al. 2001; Wadley et al. 2003). Financial skills are multidimensional, and they encompass an array of judgmental, conceptual, and pragmatic skills. They have been shown to be affected in the early stages of dementia. The nutritional state is also not limited by the association with the socio-economic and education levels, lifestyle, and

Table 177.4 Multiple logistic regression analysis for mild cognitive impairment with nutritional risk in the Far Eastern community elderly subjects (Reprinted from Lee et al. 2009. With permission)

	β (SE)	p	OR (95% CI)
Intercept	−0.28 (1.44)	0.846	–
Nutritional risk (NSI score ≥ 3)	0.12 (0.06)	0.032	1.13 (1.01–1.26)
Age (year)	0.004 (0.02)	0.849	1.14 (1.10–1.17)
Sex: male	0.24 (0.24)	0.319	1.28 (0.79–2.06)
Education (year)	−0.23 (0.08)	0.007	0.798 (0.679–0.939)
K-SGDS score	0.03 (0.03)	0.317	1.028 (0.974–1.086)

K-SGDS Korean short form Geriatric Depression Scale, *SE* standard erro, *OR* odds ratio, *CI* confidence interval

The nutritional risk increased the risk of mild cognitive impairment (OR = 1.13, 95% CI = 1.01–1.26) after the adjustment for age, sex, educational level, and geriatric depression score

Table 177.5 Relationship between mild cognitive impairment and nutrition screening initiative checklist (ten items) in the Far Eastern community elderly subjects (Reprinted from Lee et al. 2009. With permission)

Items (weighted score)		NCF elderly n (%)	MCI n (%)	p	Odds ratio (OR)
F1. I have an illness or condition that made me change the kind and/or amount of food I eat. (2)	Yes	23 (9.7)	37 (14.6)	0.10	Unadjusted OR = 0.627 (0.361–1.092)
	No	214 (90.3)	216 (85.4)		Adjusted OR = 1.563 (0.890-2.744)
F2. I eat fewer than two meals per day. (3)	Yes	2 (0.8)	3 (1.2)	0.71	Unadjusted OR = 0.709 (0.117–4.282)
	No	235 (99.2)	250 (98.8)		Adjusted OR = 1.532 (0.243–9.658)
F3. I eat few fruits or vegetables or milk products. (2)	Yes	1 (0.4)	4 (1.6)	0.20	Unadjusted OR = 3.791 (0.421–34.165)
	No	236 (99.6)	249 (98.4)		Adjusted OR = 4.717 (0.496–44.832)
F4. I have three or more drinks of beer, liquor, or wine almost every day. (2)	Yes	6 (2.5)	10 (4.0)	0.38	Unadjusted OR = 1.584 (0.567–4.429)
	No	231 (97.5)	243 (96.0)		Adjusted OR = 1.503 (0.513–4.404)
F5. I have tooth or mouth problems that make it hard for me to eat. (2)	Yes	118 (49.8)	135 (53.4)	0.43	Unadjusted OR = 1.154 (0.809–1.645)
	No	119 (50.2)	118 (46.6)		Adjusted OR = 0.963 (0.662–1.400)
F6. I don't always have enough money to buy the food I need. (4)	Yes	2 (0.8)	12 (4.7)	0.01	Unadjusted OR = 5.851(1.295–26.423)
	No	235 (99.2)	241 (95.3)		Adjusted OR = 6.006 (1.316–27.398)
F7. I eat alone most of the time. (1)	Yes	33 (13.9)	40 (15.8)	0.56	Unadjusted OR = 1.161 (0.705–1.913)
	No	204 (86.1)	213 (84.2)		Adjusted OR = 1.064 (0.635–1.782)
F8. I take 3 or more different prescribed or over-the-counter drugs a day. (1)	Yes	20 (8.4)	21 (8.3)	0.96	Unadjusted OR = 0.982 (0.518–1.862)
	No	217 (91.6)	232 (91.7)		Adjusted OR = 1.169 (0.608–2.247)
F9. Without wanting to, I have lost or gained 10 lb in the last 6 months. (2)	Yes	3 (1.3)	3 (1.2)	0.94	Unadjusted OR = 0.936 (0.187–4.684)
	No	234 (98.7)	250 (98.8)		Adjusted OR = 1.325 (0.258–6.807)
F10. I am not always physically able to shop, cook and/or feed myself. (2)	Yes	38 (16.0)	65 (25.7)	0.01	Unadjusted OR = 1.811 (1.158–2.831)
	No	199 (84.0)	188 (74.3)		Adjusted OR = 1.647 (1.025–2.648)

NCF normal cognitive function, *MCI* mild cognitive impairment
The mild cognitive impairment group responded more significantly than the normal cognitive function elderly groups in the following two items: (1) "I do not always have enough money to buy the food I need" and (2) "I am not always physically able to shop, cook, and feed myself" ($p = 0.01$; $p = 0.001$, respectively). Those participants with economic problem or physical disability were significantly more likely than those are not to develop mild cognitive impairment (with economic problem adjusted OR = 6.006, 95 % CI = 1.316–27.398; with physical disability adjusted OR = 1.647, 95 % CI = 1.025–2.648) after adjustment for age, sex, and education

smoking history; it is also related to diverse physical conditions such as the presence of cardiopulmonary diseases. This finding is consistent with the results of previous study that the low cognitive function group (less than the score of K-MMSE 17) responded more frequently to item (1).

177.6 Applications to Other Areas of Health and Disease

Although dietary intervention is capable of minimizing or preventing weight loss, patients at particular risk of malnutrition are not detected quickly enough; therefore, nutritional screening tools should be included in the multidimensional geriatric evaluation that must be performed in every elderly patient.

Because functional and nutritional statuses are interrelated, functional impairment can also increase the risk of poor nutrition in mild cognitive impairment (MCI). Many of the identified nutritional risk factors of malnutrition are based on functional competencies such as mobility, depression, cognition, food shopping, and food preparation. Considering MCI has little known risk factors and minimal impairment in IADL, nutritional risk assessment will be helpful.

Summary Points

- Mini Mental State Examination score was lower in the moderate or high nutritional risk state group of elderly subjects living in the community when compared with the good nutritional state group of elderly subjects.
- The frequency of Mild Cognitive Impairment was higher in the moderate or high nutritional risk state group of elderly subjects living in a community when compared with the group of elderly subjects in a good nutritional state.
- Nutritional factors are linked with Alzheimer's disease, both as risk or protective factors in the onset of the disease and as elements that are capable of modifying the disease course.
- Considering Mild Cognitive Impairment has little known risk factors and minimal impairment in Instrumental Activities of Daily Living, nutritional risk assessment will be helpful.
- Nutrition screening tools should be included in the multidimensional geriatric evaluation that must be performed in every elderly patient.

Key Terms

Mild cognitive impairment: This is a transitional stage between normal aging and dementia and reflects a clinical situation where a person has complaints about memory loss and shows objective evidence of cognitive impairment but exhibits no evidence of dementia.

Nutrition screening initiative: The checklist comprises ten questions that were designed such that their answer would be "yes" or "no." 0–2 points were assigned to a good nutritional state; 3–5 points, moderate nutritional risk state; and more than 6 points, high nutritional risk state.

Acknowledgement This study was supported by a grant of the Korea Healthcare technology R & D Project, Ministry for Health, Welfare & Family Affairs, Republic of Korea (A050079).

References

Avlund K, Holm-Pedersen P, Morse DE, Viitanen M, Winblad B. Gerodonotology. 2004;21:17–26.
Brenner SR. Arch Neurol. 2003;60:292–303.
Brownie S. Int J Nurs Pract. 2006;12:110–8.
Burns A, Zaudig M. Lancet. 2002;360:1963–5.
Cotman CW, Head E, Muggenburg BA, Zicker S, Milgram NW. Neurobiol Aging. 2002;23:809–18.
Cho HS, Oh BH, Kim KS, Kim KW, Park JY, Lee HR, Yoo GJ. J Kor Geriatr. 1997;1(2):120–139.
Donini LM, De Felice MR, Cannella C. Arch Gerontol Geriatr. 2007;44:143–53.
Earnst KS, Wadley VG, Aldridge TM, Steenwyk AB, Hammond AE, Harrell LE, Marson DC. Aging Neuropsychol Cogn. 2001;8:109–19.
Engelhart MJ, Geerlings MI, Ruitenberg A, Van Swieten JC, Hofman A, Witteman JC, Breteler MM. Neurology. 2002;12:1915–21.

Franzoni S, Frisoni GB, Boffelli S, Rozzini R, Trabucchi M. J Am Geriatr Soc. 1996;44:1366–70.

Ganguli M. Alzheimer Dis Assoc Disord. 2006;20:52–7.

Gillette-Guyonnet S, Abellan Van Kan G, Alix E, Andrieu S, Belmin J, Berrut G, Bonnefoy M, Brocker P, Constans T, Ferry M, Ghisolfi-Marque A, Girard L, Gonthier R, Guerin O, Hervy MP, Jouanny P, Laurain MC, Lechowski L, Nourhashemi F, Raynaud-Simon A, Ritz P, Roche J, Rolland Y, Salva T, Vellas B, International Academy on Nutrition and Aging Expert Group. J Nutr Health Aging. 2007;11:38–48.

Kalmijn S, Launer LJ, Ott A, Witteman JC, Hofman A, Breteler MM. Ann Neurol. 1997;42:776–82.

Kalmijn S, Van Boxtel MP, Ocke M, Verschuren WM, Kromhout D, Launer LJ. Neurology. 2004;62:275–80.

Kim MY. J Kor Commu Health Nur Academic Soc. 1997;11(2):94–105.

Kim JM, Shin IS, Yoon JS, Lee HY. J Kor Neuropsychiatr Assoc. 2003;42:124–30.

Kruman II, Kumaravel TS, Lohani A, Pedersen WA, Cutler RG, Kruman Y, Haughey N, Lee J, Evans M, Mattson MP. J Neurosci. 2002;22:1752–62.

Lee KS, Cheong HK, Kim EA, Kim KR, Oh BH, Hong CH. Arch Gerontol Geriatr. 2009;48:95–9.

Levy R. Int Psychogeriatry. 1994;6:63–8.

Lockhart BP, Lestage PJ. Exp Gerontol. 2003;38:119–28.

Luchsinger JA, Mayeux R. Lancet Neurol. 2004;10:579–87.

Marson DC, Sawrie SM, Snyder S, McInturff B, Stalvey T, Boothe A, Aldridge T, Chatterjee A, Harrell LE. Arch Neurol. 2000;27:877–84.

Masaki KH, Losonczy KG, Izmirlian G, Foley DJ, Ross GW, Petrovitch H, Havlik R, White LR. Neurology. 2000;54:1265–72.

Mecocci P, Mariani E, Cornacchiola V, Polidori MC. Neurol Res. 2004;26:598–602.

Pearson JM, Schlettwein-Gsell D, Brzozowska A, Van Staveren WA, Bjornsbo K. J Nutr Health Aging. 2001;5:278–83.

Peres K, Chrysostome V, Fabrigoule C, Orgogozo JM, Dartigues JF, Barberger-Gateau P. Neurology. 2006;67:461–6.

Perneczky R, Pohl C, Sorg C, Hartmann J, Tosic N, Grimmer T, Heitele S, Kurz A. Int J Geriatr Psychiatry. 2006;21:158–62.

Petersen RC, Thomas RG, Grundman M, Bennett D, Doody R, Ferris S, Galasko D, Jin S, Kaye J, Levey A, Pfeiffer E, Sano M, Van Dyck CH, Thal LJ. N Engl J Med. 2005;352:2379–88.

Petersen RC, Doody R, Kurz A, Mohs RC, Morris JC, Rabins PV, Ritchie K, Rossor M, Thal L, Winblad B. Arch Neurol. 2001;58:1985–92.

Qin B, Cartier L, Dubois-Dauphin M, Li B, Serrander L, Krause KH. Neurobiol Aging. 2006;27:1577–87.

Son SM, Park YJ, Koo JO, Mo SM, Yoon HY, Sung CJ. Kor J Commu Nutr. 1996;1:79–88.

Song YS, Chung HK, Cho MS. Kor J Nutr. 1995;28:1100–1166.

Vellas B, Lauque S, GilletteGuyonnet S, Andrieu S, Cortes F, Nourhashemi F, Cantet C, Ousset PJ, Grandjean H, REAL.FR Group. J Nutr Health Aging. 2005;9:75–80.

Wadley VG, Harrell LE, Marson DC. J Am Geriatr Soc. 2003;51:1621–6.

Winblad B, Palmer K, Kivipelto M, Jelic V, Fratiglioni L, Wahlund LO, Nordberg A, Backman L, Albert M, Almkvist O, Arai H, Basun H, Blennow K, De Leon M, DeCarli C, Erkinjuntti T, Giacobini E, Graff C, Hardy J, Jack C, Jorm A, Ritchie K, Van Duijn C, Visser P, Petersen RC. J Intern Med. 2004;256:240–6.

Chapter 178
Aluminium in the Diet, Cognitive Decline and Dementia

Vincenza Frisardi, Vincenzo Solfrizzi, Patrick G. Kehoe, Bruno P. Imbimbo, Gianluigi Vendemiale, Antonio Capurso, and Francesco Panza

Abbreviations

AD	Alzheimer's Disease
VaD	Vascular dementia
MCI	Mild Cognitive Impairment
NFT	Neurofibrillary tangles
SP	Senile plaque
AβPP	Amyloid-β protein precursor
CAA	Cerebral amyloid angiopathy
CNS	Central nervous system
BBB	Blood-brain barrier
Al	Aluminium
SOD	Superoxide dismutase
RR	Relative risk
OR	Odds ratio
MTP	Mitochondrial transition pore
HEDTA	Hydroxyethylethylenediaminetriacetic acid
ER	Endoplasmic reticulum
ROS	Reactive oxygen species
Zn	Zinc
TCA	Tricarboxylic acid
Ca	Calcium
Mg	Magnesium
ALS	Amyotrophic lateral sclerosis
TPN	Total parenteral nutrition
FDA	Food and Drug Administration

V. Frisardi (✉)
Department of Geriatrics, Center for Aging Brain, Memory Unit, University of Bari, Bristol, UK
e-mail: vfrisardi@yahoo.com

V.R. Preedy et al. (eds.), *Handbook of Behavior, Food and Nutrition*,
DOI 10.1007/978-0-387-92271-3_178, © Springer Science+Business Media, LLC 2011

178.1 Introduction

178.1.1 Dementia and Predementia Syndromes

In westernised countries, Alzheimer's disease (AD) and vascular dementia (VaD) are the most common forms of dementia, with estimated incidences of 70% and 15% of all dementia, respectively (Table 178.1). In elderly people, AD is the primary neurodegenerative disorder defined by a loss of memory associated with a progressive deterioration of other cognitive functions that must also contribute to significant decline in a person's level of everyday functioning, eventually to disability and finally contributing to death in a period of time that can range from 2 to 20 years (Table 178.1). After the age of 60 years, the prevalence of AD doubles every 5 years, increasing from a prevalence of 1% among those 60–64 years old to about 40% among those aged 85 years and above (Vickers et al. 1999). Thus, with recent improvements in life expectancy and as a result of increased aging population, AD has become a major public health consideration because of its consequence in terms of social and emotional costs. AD is characterised by two major anatomo-pathological features, intraneuronal protein clusters composed of paired helical filaments consisting of hyperphosphorylated forms of tau protein [neurofibrillary tangles (NFTs)], and extracellular protein aggregates [senile plaques (SPs)]. The SPs contain a diverse array of constituents but the main one being a toxic amyloid β (Aβ) peptide that accumulates most likely as a result of misprocessing of the Aβ protein precursor (AβPP) by β- and γ-secretases as well as reduced levels of clearance of Aβ through the blood-brain barrier (BBB) from the brain (Bell and Zlokovic 2009) and its degradation by a variety of Aβ degrading enzymes within the brain (Miners et al. 2008; Banks et al. 1997). In turn, Aβ aggregates into a variety of molecular configurations (Irvine et al. 2008) which contribute to a pathogenic cascade ultimately leading to neuronal loss. Amongst the various molecular configurations that Aβ can

Table 178.1 Key features of dementia syndromes

1. Dementia is a syndrome definite by impairments in memory and other cognitive functions that are severe enough to cause significant decline from a previous level of social and occupational functioning
2. AD is the most common dementia and primary neurodegenerative disorder in the elderly, gradually leading to a complete psychological and physical dependency and finally to death within one to two decades
3. The diagnosis of AD is essentially a clinical one, and it is based on a typical clinical picture and findings, with a set of clinical criteria often used in research
4. Cognitive function declines over time, and the diagnosis of AD can be considered when the patient has impairments in memory and at least in one other cognitive function (executive dysfunction, agnosia, aphasia, apraxia), severe enough to cause impairment in social or occupational functioning
5. In advanced AD, common symptoms include also confusion, behavioural and gait disturbances, and the patients are increasingly dependent on others in activities of daily living
6. Another common form of dementia is VaD, its clinical presentation varies greatly depending on the causes and location of cerebral damage
7. Large-vessel disease leads commonly to multiple cortical infarcts and a multifocal cortical dementia syndrome
8. Small-vessel disease, usually resulting from hypertension and diabetes, causes periventricular white matter ischemia and lacunar strokes characterised clinically by subcortical dementia with frontal lobe deficits, executive dysfunction, slow information processing, impaired memory, inattention, depressive mood changes, slowing of motor function, Parkinsonian features, small-step gait, urinary disturbances and pseudobulbar palsy
9. The characteristic neuropsychological profile of VaD is believed to include frequently early impairment of attention and executive control function, with slowing of motor performance and information processing, while episodic memory is relatively spared compared to that in AD

This table lists the key facts of dementia syndromes including clinical pictures and criteria of Alzheimer's disease (AD) and vascular dementia (VaD), the most common dementia syndromes

form, including soluble monomers, dimers and oligomers, increasingly complex aggregations are suggested to be more toxic than monomeric forms (Permanne et al. 2002).

Although the 'amyloid cascade hypothesis' is one of the more commonly upheld and cited hypotheses, AD is also recognised to involve a combination of genetic and environmental factors. Moreover, a significant comorbidity of AD and cerebrovascular disease has been demonstrated, suggesting that cerebrovascular disruption may be an important contributor to, and feature of, AD and supporting views of possible pathological and clinical overlap between AD and VaD (Gold 2003; Jellinger 2003). In fact, it has been shown that the major forms of Aβ peptides (Aβ 1–40 and Aβ 1–42) may cause vascular lesions. Cerebral amyloid angiopathy (CAA), which involves the deposition of Aβ 1–40 in the cerebrovascular system and is a major risk factor for stroke, is one such example. CAA is normally present in the majority of AD cases but is only present (in less severe forms) in approximately 30% of non-demented elderly (Love et al. 2009). Other examples include the occurrence of Aβ associated lesions in the arterioles of some animal models (Rhodin et al. 2003), similar to those observed in the brain of AD patients and which may represent the initial phase of a vascular inflammatory response associated with CAA (Banks et al. 2006).

Recently, the term 'predementia syndrome' was proposed to describe all conditions associated with age-related deficits in cognitive function that are reported in the literature. This included a mild stage of cognitive impairment based on a model of normality and pathological characteristics that were considered to be predictive of early stages of dementia (Panza et al. 2006) (Table 178.2). Mild cognitive impairment (MCI) is, at present, the most widely used term to identify non-demented aged persons with a mild memory or cognitive impairment that is not considered to be explained by any recognised medical or psychiatric disorder and which is not severe enough to cause impairment as might be more typically attributed to dementia (Table 178.2). Moreover, 12% of MCI patients develop dementia within 1 year (Panza et al 2005) a prevalence that increases to 20% over 3 years (Petersen et al. 2001). Recently, in the Italian Longitudinal Study on Aging (ILSA), a population-based study involving a sample of 5,632 individuals aged 65–84 years, a progression rate to dementia of MCI of 3.8/100 person-years was found (Solfrizzi et al. 2004). Nevertheless, at present, it still questionable whether these entities are a manifestation of normal aging, are clinically distinguishable from dementing syndromes, or, are part of a continuum with dementia.

Table 178.2 Key features of predementia syndromes

1. The term 'predementia syndromes' identifies all conditions with age-related deficits in cognitive function reported in the literature, including a mild stage of cognitive impairment based on a normality model and pathological conditions considered predictive or early stages of dementia

2. Among predementia syndromes, MCI is, at present, the most widely used term to indicate non-demented aged persons with a mild memory or cognitive impairment that cannot be accounted for any recognised medical or psychiatric condition

3. The general criteria for MCI include: (a) memory complaint, (b) objective memory disorder, (c) absence of other cognitive disorders or repercussions on daily life, (d) normal general cognitive function, (e) absence of dementia

4. MCI definitions can be broadly classified as amnestic (aMCI) and nonamnestic (naMCI)

5. There is now ample evidence that MCI is often a pathology-based condition with a high rate of progression to AD, and aMCI, with a central role for memory disorder and with relative preservation of other cognitive domains, was identified as the predementia syndrome for AD

6. aMCI can be subdivided into a single domain subtype with a pronounced memory deficit or a multiple domain subtype that includes memory impairment along with some impairment in other cognitive domains such as language, executive function, and visuospatial skills

7. The other major MCI subtype is naMCI, which similarly can be subdivided into single and multiple domain subtypes

This table lists the key facts of predementia syndromes including diagnostic criteria and clinical classification of mild cognitive impairment (MCI), the most common predementia syndrome

Table 178.3 Key features of aluminium

1. Aluminium is a nonessential metal present in 8% of the Earth's crust
2. Aluminium has no known function in living cells and produces some toxic effects in elevated concentrations
3. The toxicity of aluminium can be traced to deposition in bone and the central nervous system, which is particularly noticeable in patients with reduced renal function
4. In very high doses, aluminium can cause neurotoxicity, and is associated with altered function of the blood-brain barrier
5. Present studies have not convincingly demonstrated a causal relationship between aluminium and AD. Nevertheless, some studies suggested aluminium exposure as a risk factor for AD, as some brain senile plaques have been found to contain increased levels of the metal

AD Alzheimer's disease
This table lists the key features of aluminium including definition, general health effects, and current research findings on the aluminium and AD

178.1.2 Neurotoxicity of Aluminium and Other Metals

Although knowledge of the pathophysiology of AD has greatly increased during recent decades, and new therapeutic approaches have been proposed, AD is still a chronic and incurable disease, and its causal mechanisms remain unclear. In recent years, interest in the potential role of metals such as iron, copper and zinc, among other trace redox-active transition metals, in the pathogenesis of AD, has grown considerably (Todorich and Connor 2004). The hypothesis that aluminium (Al) exposure is related to AD has prompted several studies and, at present, the relationship is still unresolved and under investigation (Table 178.3). The potential role of Al as a mediator of neurotoxicity was suggested more than 100 years ago after Dollken reported his work with Al in experimental studies on animals (Dollken 1897). Al neurotoxicity was first reported in humans at the beginning of the 1970s when neurodegeneration in patients undergoing chronic hemodialysis was observed (Wills and Savory 1983). The hypothesis that Al could be involved in the pathogenesis of AD arose when Al was detected in SPs and NFTs in brain tissue from AD patients (Crapper et al. 1973). Subsequently, several studies have reported that higher intake of Al increases the production of Aβ in transgenic APP mice (Praticò et al. 2002; El-Rahman 2003). Although further research supported these findings, the role of Al remains controversial, because several other investigations did not find any relationship between Al exposure and risk of AD. In this chapter, we examine the possible role of dietary exposure to Al from drinking water or foods in modulating the risk of age-related changes in cognitive function, predementia and dementia syndromes, as well as the possible molecular epidemiological mechanisms behind the observed associations.

178.2 Environmental Exposure to Aluminium, Including Drinking Water, in Cognitive Decline and Dementia

Al is a non-essential metal present in 8% of the Earth's crust. It is a lightweight, silvery white, soft, malleable metal derived from the refining and smelting of cryolite and bauxite ore (Miessler 2003). Al is omnipresent in everyday life, and may enter the human body in many ways such as the environment, diet or drugs. Several pathological conditions that involve neurobehavioral changes have been reported among the workers involved in the Al industry such as shipbuilding, petroleum processing, and rubber industry. In particular, the potential relationship between Al body burden and CNS function was studied in Al welders where a threshold level for adverse effects was suggested (Riihimäki et al. 2000). In this context, low-exposure and high-exposure groups were defined according to Al concentrations measured in serum (S-Al) and urine (U-Al) and were examined with a neuropsychological test battery. This neuropsychological testing revealed a circumscribed negative dose-dependent effect associated with increased Al body burden, mainly in tasks demanding complex attention, the processing of information using working memory and the analysis and recall of abstract visual patterns. This study indicated that the body burden threshold for adverse effect approximates to a U-Al value of 4–6 micromol/l and an S-Al value of 0.25–0.35 micromol/l among Al welders (Riihimäki et al. 2000). Further evidence in support of the potential of Al-mediated toxicity in humans comes from observations made of the widespread practise of glue sniffing among teenagers (Akay et al. 2008). Here the investigators compared the S-Al of glue sniffing groups and healthy control adolescents and they computed Al levels of different commercial glue preparations (i.e., metal and plastic containers). The S-Al was found to be 63.29 ± 13.20 in glue sniffers compared with 36.7 ± 8.60 ng/ml in control subjects ($P < 0.001$) (Akay et al. 2008).

Unlike occupational exposures, environmental exposure to Al is inevitable or less easy to avoid. The principal route of metal exposure is through diet (food/drinking water) and inhalation of Al as fine particles. It has been estimated that the dietary intake of Al can range from 3 to 30 mg/day, and varies with the composition of the food eaten, country of residence, age and sex (World Health Organization 1997). In the USA, the total dietary Al intake estimates for adult men and women are 8–9 and 7 mg/day, respectively (Pennington and Schoen 1995). The metal can be taken from food (both naturally occurring Al and its additives), from cookware, utensils and food wrappings, containers (including Al drink cans), and from water, aerosols and dusts. However, dietary absorption of Al consumed from food is small (less than 1% of ingested Al is absorbed) if compared with the amounts consumed through the use of Al containing antacids that may provide doses of 50–1,000 mg/day (Reinke et al. 2003). Similarly, the bioavailability of Al from water is higher than from food (0.3% vs 0.1%, respectively); yet, due to differences in daily Al intake, drinking water contributes considerably less to the total Al body burden (Yokel and Florence 2006).

Since Al is used extensively as a coagulant in water treatment, to reduce the number of small particles or as a flocculation agent to remove organic substances and improve the colour of the water, the issue of safe levels of Al in drinking water is of considerable interest to public health officials and regulatory agencies (Flaten 2001). However, other elements present in drinking water, such as fluoride, copper, zinc, iron could also have an effect on cognitive impairment or influence the Al neurotoxicity. Some epidemiological studies, but not all, suggest that silica could be protective against Al damage, because it reduces the oral absorption of Al and/or enhances Al excretion (Gillette-Guyonnet et al. 2005).

The World Health Organization (1997) has recommended that Al concentrations in drinking water should not exceed 0.2 mg/l. The US Environmental Protection Agency set 0.05 mg/l as a limit in 1985, but the European Union has more recently recommended 0.05 mg/l as a guideline with a maximum permissible level of 0.2 mg/l (Shcherbatykh and Carpenter 2007). Numerous epidemiological studies reported their investigations of the relationship between exposure to Al from drinking water and risk of AD (Flaten 2001). The first attempts to relate the actual levels of Al in drinking water to AD were made in 1986, when two parallel Norwegian studies reported higher mortality from dementia (from all causes) in areas with high Al concentration in drinking water (Vogt 1986). A cross-sectional investigation conducted a few years later in England and Wales found that among all other causes of dementia the risk of AD was 1.5 times higher in districts where the mean Al concentration in drinking water exceeded 0.11 mg/l, compared to the districts where Al concentrations were less than 0.01 mg/l (Martyn et al. 1989) (Table 178.4). In the same period, another ecological study conducted in Canada reported an excess of dementia mortality from the north shore of Bonavista Bay; a phenomenon that could be explained only by high Al concentration in the drinking water (165 mg/l) and low pH (5.2) in that area, because no other differences in sex, age or other parameters could be found (Frecker 1991) (Table 178.4).

Table 178.4 Principal cross-sectional studies on the relationships between dietary aluminium (Al) from drinking water and dementia (i.e., Alzheimer's disease, AD)

References	Setting and study design	Subjects	Aluminium assessment	Cognitive functions assessment	Results and conclusions
Longitudinal studies					
Martyn et al. (1989) United Kingdom	Cross-sectional study	1,203 patients with dementia aged under 70 years; 445 (37%) of these subjects had probable AD by 88 country districts data	Al concentrations in water were obtained from water authorities and water companies	Indirect measures by computed tomography scan records	Among all other causes of dementia, the risk of AD was 1.5 times higher in districts where the mean Al concentration in drinking water exceeded 0.11 mg/l, compared to the districts where Al concentrations were less than 0.01 mg/l
Frecker (1991) Canada	Ecological study; 1985 and 1986 survey data from the province of Newfoundland	399 persons dead between 1985 and 1986	Detailed analysis of untreated drinking water samples collected in June and October 1986 from six communities in Bonavista Bay	Indirect measures by death certificates based census population, the prevalence of dementia at death for 1985 and 1986	The highest Al concentration is recorded in the area with the highest dementia mortality
Neri and Hewitt (1991) Canada	Case-control study	2,232 patients aged 55 years or over	Water quality data from the Water Quality Surveillance Programme of the Ontario Ministry of the Environment	Hospital discharge data with a diagnosis of dementia or presenile dementia	The relative risks associated with the consumption of drinking water containing Al concentrations of <0.01, 0.01–0.1, 0.1–0.199 and >0.200 mg/l were estimated to be 1.00, 1.13, 1.26 and 1.46, respectively
McLachlan et al. (1996) Canada	Case-control study; 830 brains of healthy controls and those with neurodegenerative diseases were donated by next of kin to the CBTB between 1981 and 1991, who, at the time of death, were Ontario residents.	680 brains analyzed which 385 with pathological or clinical diagnosis of AD and 295 controls	Al of public drinking water at last residence before death at the first moment; in the second moment Al of 10-year weighted residential exposure prior to death	Histopathologically verified AD	Elevated risk for AD associated with higher levels of Al (>0.1 mg/l) (OR = 1.7, 95% CI 1.2–2.5). For an Al concentration in drinking water of 0.125 mg/l, the OR for risk of AD was 3.6 (95% CI 1.4–9.9); at 150 mg/l the OR was 4.4 (95% CI 0.98–20), and at 0.175 mg/l it was 7.6 (95% CI 0.98–61)

CBTB Canadian Brain Tissue Bank

This table lists the principal findings of cross-sectional clinical, ecological and epidemiological studies on the relationships between dietary Al from drinking water and dementia (i.e., AD), including setting, study design, and Al and cognitive assessment used. OR = Odds Ratio; 95% CI = 95% confidence internal

A case-control study conducted in Ontario, Canada, described dose–response relationships between the Al content of drinking water and risk of AD, using hospital discharge data with a diagnosis of dementia or presenile dementia (Neri and Hewitt 1991) (Table 178.4). The relative risks (RR) associated with the consumption of drinking water containing Al concentrations of < 0.01, 0.01–0.1, 0.1–0.199 and > 0.200 mg/l were estimated to be 1.00, 1.13, 1.26 and 1.46, respectively. Subsequent re-analysis of the data adjusted for age and sex confirmed a stronger dose–response relationship for those over 75 years of age (Smith 1995). Another Canadian investigation studied the relationship between Al, fluoride and other constituents in drinking water and cognitive function (Forbes et al. 1995). The research project was based on the Ontario Longitudinal Study of Aging, where 2,000 men have been followed for about 30 years. Analysis of the data showed that men living in areas with high Al and low fluoride concentrations in drinking water were about three times more likely to have some form of cognitive impairment than those individuals living in the areas with low Al and high fluoride levels (Forbes et al. 1995). The same authors in a previous analysis confirmed that both neutral pH, relatively low Al concentrations, and relatively high fluoride concentrations in drinking water decreased the odds of cognitive impairment by a factor of five (Forbes et al. 1994). Al concentration in drinking water at last residence before death was used as the measure of exposure in a case-control study conducted on autopsy-verified material comparing the patients with AD and controls without brain pathology (McLachlan et al. 1996) (Table 178.4). The results reported elevated risks for histopathologically verified AD associated with higher levels of Al [odds ratios (OR) = 1.7, 95% CI 1.2–2.5, for a level of Al > 0.1 mg/l]. For an Al concentration in drinking water of 0.125 mg/l, the OR for risk of AD was 3.6 (95% CI 1.4–9.9); for 0.150 mg/l, the OR was 4.4 (95% CI 0.98–20); and for 0.175 mg/l, it was 7.6 (95% CI 0.98–61). Despite the fact that results were seemingly biased by selection criteria, the study had several methodological strengths, including the diagnostic quality of the data (McLachlan et al. 1996) (Table 178.4).

In France, a geographic association between Al and silica and cognitive decline or dementia was reported, utilizing the data from the Personnes Agèes QUID (PAQUID) cohort study. In this study, 3,777 subjects aged 65 years and above who were living at home in either a rural or an urban area in southwestern France were followed for up to 8 years, recording all new cases of dementia and AD (Rondeau et al. 2000). In each residential area, the range and mean exposure to Al (0.001–0.459 mg/l, median 0.009 mg/l) and silica (4.2–22.4 mg/l) from drinking water were recognised. The analysis of data adjusted for age, gender, educational level, place of residence, and wine consumption revealed that the risk of dementia was higher for individuals who lived in areas with high levels of Al in water (mean concentration >0.1 mg/l) compared with people residing in areas with Al levels less than 0.1 mg/l (RR: 1.99; 95% CI: 1.20–3.28, $P = 0.007$). Higher silica concentrations (11.25 mg/l), adjusted for age and gender, were associated with a reduced risk of dementia (RR: 0.71; 95% CI: 0.56–0.91, $P = 0.007$) (Rondeau et al. 2000) (Table 178.5). The adjusted RR of AD for individuals exposed to drinking water with Al concentration > 0.10 mg/l was 2.14 (95% CI: 1.21– 3.80, $P = 0.007$). The risk of AD was reduced in the presence of high concentrations of silica (RR: 0.73; 95% CI: 0.55–0.99, $P = 0.04$), and the authors concluded that a concentration of Al in drinking water above 0.1 mg/l may be a risk factor for dementia and AD although no dose-response effect was found (Rondeau et al. 2000) (Table 178.5). Recently, the same group revisited this topic with more precise data on daily Al and silica intake in a larger cohort followed for 15 years adding 400 subjects from the Aluminum-Maladie d'Alzheimer (ALMA+) cohort to the 3,777 elderly subjects from the PAQUID study (Rondeau et al. 2009) (Table 178.5). In this recent study, two measures of exposure to Al and silica were taken into account: geographic and individual exposure from daily consumption of tap water (including water used in making tea, coffee, soup or alcoholic drinks) and bottled water (spring or mineral). Of the whole sample, only 1,925 subjects were considered because they were free of cognitive impairment at baseline and had reliable water consumption data. Whereas geographic exposure

Table 178.5 Principal longitudinal studies on the relationships between dietary aluminium (Al) and dementia (i.e., Alzheimer's disease, AD and vascular dementia, VaD), or predementia syndromes (i.e., age-related cognitive decline, ARCD) in older people

References Longitudinal studies	Setting and study design	Subjects	Aluminium assessment	Cognitive functions assessment	Results and conclusions
Rondeau et al. (2000) France	Longitudinal study (8 years of follow-up); subjects from PAQUID study	3,777 subjects aged 65 years and older	In each residential area the range and mean exposure to Al ($0.001-0.459$ mg/l, median 0.009 mg/l) and silica ($4.2-22.4$ mg/l) from drinking water were recorded	MMSE and other cognitive tests; standardised questionnaire for dementia's diagnosis (DSM III revised criteria); NINCDS/ADRDA criteria for AD; Hachinski score for VaD	The risk of dementia was higher for individuals who lived in areas with high levels of Al in water (>0.1 mg/l) compared with people residing in areas with Al levels less than 0.1 mg/l ($RR = 1.99$, 95% $CI = 1.20-3.28$). Higher silica concentrations (>11.25 mg/l), were associated with a reduced risk of dementia ($RR = 0.71$, 95% CI $0.56-0.91$). The adjusted RR of AD for individuals exposed to Al concentration >0.10 mg/l was 2.14 (95% CI $1.21-3.80$); the risk of AD was reduced in the presence of high concentrations of silica ($RR = 0.73$, 95% CI $0.55-0.99$). No dose-response effect was found
Gillette-Guyonnet et al. (2005) France	Cross-sectional and longitudinal study (7 years of follow-up); multicentre study (EPIDOS)	7,598 women aged >75 years	Questionnaire relative to the daily consumption of tap water and mineral water and the brand of mineral water most frequently consumed	SPMSQ considering women cognitively normal with a score >8; MMSE and Grober and Buschke test; dementia was diagnosed by DSM IV and AD diagnosed by NINCDS/ADRDA criteria.	An inverse association between silica intake from drinking water and AD was found. Women with AD were 2.7 times as likely to have a low daily silica intake (<4 mg/ day). However, this study does not show any evidence for aluminium as a risk factor for AD

Reference	Study design	Subjects	Exposure measure	Cognitive assessment	Findings
Rondeau et al. (2009) France	Longitudinal study (15 years of follow-up); subjects living in 91 drinking-water districts in southern France (PAQUID Cohort), and subjects living at home in one of the 14 drinking-water areas in southwestern France (ALMA+ Cohort)	1,677 subjects aged 65 years or over (PAQUID cohort), and 248 subjects aged 75 years or over (ALMA+ cohort)	Two kinds of drinking water indicators for Al and silica: (1) geographic exposure measure; (2) individual measure by the questionnaire on daily consumption of tap water and bottled water	MMSE and other cognitive tests; standardised questionnaire for diagnosis of dementia (DSM III revised criteria); NINCDS/ADRDA criteria for AD; Hachinski score for VaD; cognitive decline was analyzed in both the PAQUID and the ALMA+ cohorts; dementia and AD were investigated only in the PAQUID cohort	The risk of dementia was higher for subjects with a high daily Al intake (for >0.1 mg/day; RR = 2.26; $P = 0.049$). Conversely, an increase of 10 mg/day in silica intake reduced the risk of dementia (adjusted RR = 0.89; $P = 0.036$). Using the geographic measure of tap-water exposure, Al or silica concentrations were no more associated with the risk of AD, although the tendencies were similar

This table lists the principal findings of longitudinal clinical and epidemiological studies on the relationships between dietary Al (from drinking water or foods) and dementia (i.e., AD and VaD) or predementia syndromes (i.e., ARCD) in older people, including setting, study design, and Al and cognitive assessment used

PAQUID Personnes agées Quid, *MMSE* Mini Mental State Examination, *DSM III* Diagnostic and Statistical Manual of Mental Disorders, Third Edition, *DSM III* Diagnostic and Statistical Manual of Mental Disorders, Third Edition, *NINCDS/ADRDA* National Institute of Neurological and Communicative Disorders and Stroke/Alzheimer's Disease and Related Disorders Association, *DSM IV* Diagnostic and Statistical Manual of Mental Disorders, Fourth Edition, *RR* relative risk, *EPIDOS Study* Epidemiology of Osteoporosis Study, *SPMSQ* Short Portable Mental Status Questionnaire, *ALMA+* Aluminium-Maladie Alzheimer

to Al or silica from tap water was not associated strongly with dementia, given that other territorial factors could influence cognitive decline, the conclusions of the study were that cognitive decline became greater over time in subjects with a higher daily intake of Al from drinking water (>0.1 mg/ day; adjusted RR =2.26; P = 0.005). Moreover, about silica intake, an increase of 10 mg/day was associated with a reduced risk of AD (adjusted RR = 0.89, P = 0,036) (Rondeau et al. 2009) (Table 178.5).

Recently, new evidence has come to the fore in support of the Al-AD hypothesis. First, a case of a 58-year-old woman with a rapidly progressive, fatal neurological illness, who, at autopsy, showed dramatic Aβ deposition of cerebral cortical and leptomeningeal blood vessels, modest numbers of NFTs and Lewy bodies, and evidence of very high Al content in affected brain regions. This neurological injury is potentially linked to Al exposure from drinking water. In fact, this woman was exposed, along with other 20,000 people, to high concentrations of Al in their water supplies, in excess of 500–3,000 times the limit of 0.2 mg/l. (Exley and Esiri 2006). Second, a very recent report that compared baseline and follow-up composition of drinking water and the level of cognitive function and possible risk of AD in women taking part in the Epidemiology of Osteoporosis Study (EPIDOS) found that a low silica concentration was associated with low cognitive performance at baseline. Further multivariate analysis including potential confounding factors showed that women with AD appeared to have been exposed to lower amounts of silica at baseline, suggesting a protective role against AD of silica in drinking water (Gillette-Guyonnet et al. 2005) (Table 178.5).

On balance, all epidemiological studies of Al in drinking water are more or less open to critique, particularly considering the difficulty in producing high-quality data for exposure and especially for the disease (Lovell et al. 1996). A fundamental difficulty in the interpretation of the epidemiological studies indicating increased risk for AD with increased Al concentrations in drinking water is that even at high concentrations (0.1–0.4 mg/l), drinking water accounts for less than 5% of total daily Al intake. Moreover, in contrast with the findings of these epidemiological studies and evidence against the Al-AD hypothesis is the fact that many studies examining antacid exposure that involves 1000-fold higher exposure to Al compared to drinking water or diet and AD, have been largely negative (Lione 1985). Similarly, other studies did not support any association between Al in drinking water and AD. Wettstein and colleagues (1991) compared the cognitive functions of two groups of elderly, long-term residents of Zurich, who lived in two different areas: one, with high Al concentration in drinking water (> 0.10 mg/l), and the other with relatively low Al levels (<0.01 mg/l). The authors found no substantial differences in cognitive impairment between these two groups (Wettstein et al. 1991). However, a limitation of this study was that the methodology relied on only two sources of drinking water, and thus the bioavailability of Al was likely different in the two water sources. Another study that compared 106 men with AD, 99 men with other dementias, 226 men with brain cancer, and 441 men with other diseases of the nervous system reported no association between the prevalence of AD and higher Al concentrations in drinking water (Martyn et al. 1997). In this context, all subjects aged up to 75 years old and the analysis performed employed three different measurements of exposure. No association between AD and either higher Al or lower silica concentrations in drinking water was found and this study represents perhaps some of the strongest evidence against the idea of causal relationship between Al exposure and AD.

178.3 Aluminium in Food and Cognitive Decline

Unlike a lot of studies about drinking water and AD, little investigations have attempted to measure the possible association between Al in food and cognitive decline, most likely due to significant variability in Al content in food and the difficulty to accurately measure levels of exposure and in turn absorption from food. Yet, dietary intake of Al remains the largest route of exposure, since Al consumption from foods is typically ten-fold greater than that from drinking water (Saiyed and Yokel 2005). Al in the food supply comes from natural sources including the natural composition of the food itself, water used in food preparation, and food additives. Some foods, known as Al accumulators (e.g., herbs, tea leaves) may naturally contain more than 5 mg/g of this metal. Intake of dietary Al is higher in the USA than in other countries due to widespread use of Al-containing food additives (Flaten 2001; Saiyed and Yokel 2005). One pilot study that interviewed close relatives about dietary intake of patients in a geriatric centre, with special attention to foods high in Al (such as American cheese, chocolate pudding, doughnuts, pancakes or muffins), showed the crude OR of 2.0 (P value = 0.19) for daily intake of any such high-Al foodstuffs and OR of 8.6 adjusted for total caloric intake, body mass index, education and intake of vitamins A, C and E (Rogers and Simon 1999). Some subcategories of food containing Al additives were also examined; however, due to the smaller samples in these subgroups, the resulting ORs were not statistically significant, except for one food category containing waffles, pancakes, biscuits, muffins and cornbread or corn tortillas. Although interesting, these results require reproducing in other studies with larger samples sizes and more rigorous design.

Several studies have explored the link between tea consumption and risk of AD since it has been known that Al is naturally present in tea leaves. The reported concentration of Al is 0.3% in older leaves and about 0.01% in younger ones (Rao 1994). Typical tea infusions contain 50 times as much as Al as do infusions from coffee. Levels of Al in tea infusions are commonly in the range of 2–6 mg/l (Rao 1994), and thus may contribute up to 50% of the total daily Al intake in the countries with high consumption and small intake of Al from other sources (Pennington1987; Saiyed and Yokel 2005). In a case-control study (Forster et al. 1995), comparing cases of clinically diagnosed presenile dementia of the Alzheimer's type and controls matched for age and sex, exposure to Al from tea was not a significant risk factor for dementia (the OR for dementia among people consuming more than four cups of tea a day was 1.4; 95% CI: 0.8–2.6). Similarly, no relationship was found between exposure to Al from drinking water, or medicinal sources. A case-control study completed in Canada produced a similar OR for the risk of AD (1.4; 95% CI: 0.86–2.28); however, the serving amount of tea was not specified (Canadian Study of Health and Aging 1994). An Australian case-control study (Broe et al. 1990), also reported an OR of 1.42 (95% CI: 0.93–2.17) while another study found no significant relationship between tea consumption and AD (adjusted OR: 0.7, P-value = 0.69). In the latter there was a suggestion that the absence of association may be due to loss of Al during the tea processing and binding of Al to organic compounds, possibly lemon juice (Rogers and Simon 1999). In summary, it would seem that despite relatively high Al content and high dietary consumption, the role of tea as a dietary source of Al in development of AD or similar pathologies remains controversial.

178.4 Possible Mechanisms of Aluminium Neurotoxicity

Although there is compelling evidence in support of a central role of Aβ (including from genetic studies) and tau protein in the pathogenesis of AD, there have been some residual questions whether these abnormalities are causative of the disease or secondary to another etiologic factor (Neve and Robakis 1998). Many lines of evidence have focused on the role of oxidative stress mechanisms and free radical damage in AD pathogenesis (Grant et al. 2002) (Fig. 178.1). Whether oxidative damage increases Aβ peptide production or vice versa is still unresolved. There is ambiguous evidence on the hypothetical molecular mechanisms that might explain Al involvement in the aetiology and pathogenesis of AD. Several experimental models have strongly supported the involvement of Al as a secondary modifying factor or risk factor in the pathogenesis of AD (Bharathi et al. 2008) (Fig. 178.2). There is

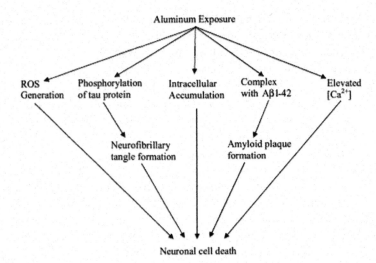

Fig. 178.1 Possible mechanisms whereby aluminium exposure causes neuronal cell death and lead to Alzheimer's disease. This figure shows major hypothesised pathways whereby aluminium exposure leads to neuronal cell death and Alzheimer's disease including aluminium-induced oxidative stress, accumulation of amyloid β (Aβ), phosphorylation of tau protein, elevation of [Ca^{2+}], complex with Ab1–42 peptide, and intracellular accumulation of aluminium (From Shcherbatykh and Carpenter 2007. With permission)

also evidence that Al may alter the normal processing of AβPP and as such the dynamics of Aβ production (Garruto and Brown 1994), via reduced solubility of aluminium-Aβ 1–42 complexes, as well as increased precipitation of β-sheets (Exley 2006) and facilitated Aβ transport across the BBB (Yokel 2006). Several studies suggest that Aβ and oxidative stress are causally linked and Al enhances Aβ production leading to Aβ aggregation into oligomeric forms (Bondy and Kirstein 1996) which might influence the early-onset of AD or its progression (Fig. 178.1).

An appealing feature of the oxidative stress hypothesis for neurodegenerative diseases is that cumulative oxidative damage over time could account for the late-life onset and the slowly progressive nature of such disorders (Shcherbatykh and Carpenter 2007). With the development of transgenic techniques in neuroscience, new research approaches have emerged. It has been demonstrated that chronic dietary administration of Al can increase Aβ levels and accelerate SP deposition in an animal model of AD-like amyloidosis with an exacerbation of brain lipid peroxidation (Praticò et al. 2002). This phenomenon could be limited by addition of the antioxidant addition (vitamin E). Other investigators have shown that exposure to Al affects different neuronal areas, and that melatonin protects against the Al-induced cellular damage (Esparza et al. 2003).

Various mechanisms have been suggested to explain the Al toxicity, taking into account that many biological reactions, if altered, can have profound cellular consequences, eventually contributing to neuronal cell death. The major sites of localisation of these important reactions are mitochondria, lysosomes and the nucleus in the cell; therefore Al toxicity can be mediated across a number of cellular compartments (Dobson et al. 1998). Al could play a role in neurodegeneration by increasing oxidative stress because as a non-redox active metal it may increase the redox active iron concentration in brain, mainly through a Fenton reaction. Al is simultaneously an activator of superoxide dismutase (SOD) and an inhibitor of catalase, and this leads to an increase in the production of hydroxyl radicals (Good et al. 1996). Apoptosis or programmed cell death, which plays a role in normal development and maintenance of tissue homeostasis, is also believed to be the general mechanism by which Al toxicity is mediated in cells. Mitochondrial changes

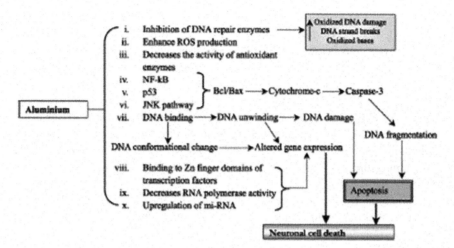

Fig. 178.2 Synopsis of principal mechanisms of neurotoxicity linked to aluminium exposure. This figure shows aluminium (Al) to be one of the principal causes of neurotoxicity, including modulation of inhibition of DNA repair enzymes, enhancement of ROS production, decrease of the activity of antioxidant enzymes, alteration of NF-kB, p53, JNK pathway, DNA binding. Al also binds to Zn finger domains of transcription factors, thereby decreasing RNA polymerase activity and upregulating mi-RNA. All these events lead to genomic instability and cell death (From Bharathi et al. 2008. With permission)

following cytotoxic stimuli represent a primary event in apoptotic cell death. Al has also been demonstrated to accumulate in neurons, where it inhibits the sodium $(Na)^+$/calcium $(Ca)^{2+}$ exchange mechanisms and thereby mediates the accumulation of mitochondrial Ca^{2+} (Bharathi et al. 2008) (Fig. 178.1). This increase in intra-mitochondrial Ca^{2+} levels in turn leads to an opening of the mitochondrial transition pore (MTP), with cytochrome c (an important apoptotic factor) release and subsequent apoptosis resulting from the activation of the caspase family of proteases (Dewitt et al. 2006) (Fig. 178.2).

Although mitochondrial alterations may represent an important step in the apoptotic process, other evidence supported the endoplasmic reticulum (ER) role in regulating this cell death and ER homeostasis changes due to Al. The ER is the major reservoir for calcium and is the main site of the apoptotic mediators including members of the Bcl-2 family of proteins, Bcl-2 and Bcl-XL. Al induces a redistribution of the apoptosis-regulatory proteins within the ER, resulting in Bax being elevated in the ER compared with the cytosol and mediating the reduction of Bcl-2 (D'mello et al. 1994) (Fig. 178.2). Therefore, Al mediates a specific type of apoptosis which is independent from other mitochondrial-targeted apoptotic signals. Moreover, since Al is a Lewis base, it might bind to oxygen donors generated in the cell and binds to vital biomolecules such as nucleic acids, phosphate groups of ATP and/or phosphorylated proteins and carboxylic groups of the molecules (Lankoff et al. 2006). Thus, Al could facilitate genotoxicity, through modification of DNA repair processes and conformational changes that cause DNA to unwind all of which increase the likelihood of DNA damage and changes to gene expression that might lead to neuronal cell death in AD. Further evidence in support of this are reports of Al-mediated decrease of the levels of mRNA from genes of endogenous antioxidant enzymes (Gonzalez-Muñoz et al. 2008). This may be the result of interference with the binding of transcription factors, such as factor IIIA to its corresponding zinc finger domains and in turn inhibition of gene expression (Hanas and Gunn 1996)

The biogenesis of NFTs remains an important question in understanding Alzheimer's neuropathology. Al promotes phosphorylation of the tau protein, the microtubular-associated protein that accumulates into NFTs making it less soluble and increasing the likelihood that the protein will aggregate (Li et al. 1998) (Fig. 178.1). Thus, Al could act to promote the development of NFTs. However, an important consideration is that NFTs are associated with a number of diseases such as dementia pugilistica and other diseases where the causes remain unclear (Bharathi et al. 2008). Furthermore, studies have reported that Al kills isolated neurons secondary to its intracellular accumulation, and that the cell death is neither secondary to generation of reactive oxygen species (ROS) nor accumulation of intracellular calcium. This is despite the capability of Al to cause an elevation in both (Tuneva et al. 2006), suggesting that Al could be directly toxic to some intracellular processes. Considering numerous studies about Al neurotoxicity, Kawahara proposed a comprehensive hypothesis regarding the implications of Al and other trace metals in the pathogenesis of AD (Kawahara 2005) (Fig. 178.3).

Recently, a study investigated the effects of Al on behaviour, neurological function and morphology, using Al-maltolate administered to rabbits via the intracisternal route (Bharathi et al. 2008). The authors concluded that Al caused neurotoxicity in a multifaceted way by modulating the inhibition of DNA repair enzymes, the enhancement of ROS production, the decrease in the activity of antioxidant enzymes, and the alteration in apoptotic pathways as NF-kB, p53 and JNK (Fig. 178.2). Al was also found to bind to Zn finger domains of transcription factors, thereby decreasing RNA polymerase activity and gene expression and also upregulating micro-RNA. All these events lead to genomic instability and cell death. Common mechanisms such as failure in protein folding mechanisms have not yet been fully explored but offer possible models for further testing, particularly where circulating or intracellular forms of these proteins, complexed to Al may be toxic, and work in addition to other primary causes of the neuronal cell death (Bharathi et al. 2008).

178.5 Possible Alzheimer's Disease Treatment Linked to the Aluminium Hypothesis

Metal ligand-based therapeutic approaches for the treatment of AD have been suggested, given the growing number of epidemiological investigations that have identified Al and other metals (especially zinc and copper) as possible risk factors for this disease (Fig. 178.4). Therefore, if metals play a potential role as a cofactor in the pathogenesis of AD, removal of these from the brain might hypothetically modulate neuronal damage and progression of the AD process (Domingo 2006). Among these drugs, the use of fluoride and chelating agents were strong candidates. It was well known that fluoride ions bind with high affinity to Al, while desferrioxamine, an iron chelator, was also shown to be an effective chelating agent for Al.

Desferrioxamine (deferoxamine, DFOA) usually used for the treatment of iron overload, was first employed to enhance Al removal in 1980, and it has been the most effective and safest Al chelator for long-term use and has produced a striking improvement in a patient with severe dialysis encephalopathy (Ackrill et al. 1980). However, the authors noted that both fluoride and chelating agents could have systemic side effects. Due to the high affinity of DFOA for Al ($K = 1,022$), this chelating agent has also been successfully applied to the therapy of Al overload, including the treatment of dialysis encephalopathy (Swartz 1985; Milne et al. 1983), however, important side effects have been reported, including increased susceptibility to infectious diseases, ocular and auditory toxicity, audiovisual neurotoxicity and developmental toxicity if used for prolonged periods at excessive doses (Domingo 1996). The hypothesis that DFOA might slow the clinical progression of the dementia associated with AD was tested in a small study, which

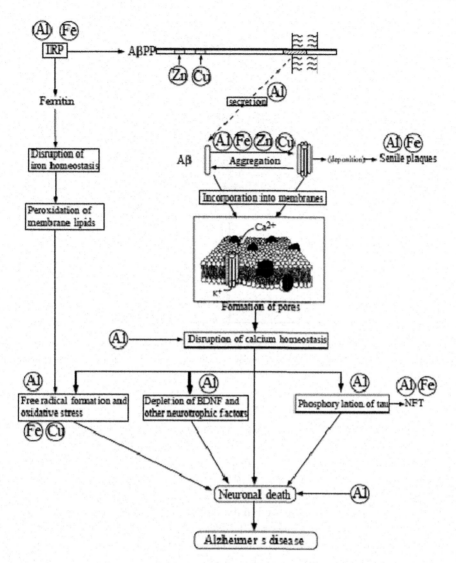

Fig. 178.3 Hypothesis regarding the implications of aluminium (Al) and other trace metals in the pathogenesis of Alzheimer's disease (AD). Al binds to iron regulatory protein (IRP) and influences the expression of amyloid β protein precursor (AβPP) as well as ferritin. Abnormal expression of AβPP will lead to the increased amount of amyloid β (Aβ). Normally secreted Aβ is degraded by various proteases. However, Aβ which is aggregated in the presence of trace metals, including Al, zinc (Zn), iron (Fe), and copper (Cu), could be resistant to proteases and accumulates in the brain. The aggregated Aβ could be easily incorporated into membranes resulting in the formation of ion channels. The abnormal calcium influx through amyloid channels cause the phosphorylation of tau, the depletion of neurotrophic factors such as brain-derived neurotrophic factor (BDNF), and the formation of free radicals, and finally induces neuronal death. Al implicates these neurodegenerative pathways by inhibition of BDNF-induced increase in intracellular calcium levels, by accelerating the phosphorylation of tau, and by stimulating iron-induced lipid peroxidation. Meanwhile, abnormal expression of ferritin caused an altered concentration of free iron ions, and thus, will cause oxidative damage and membrane lipid peroxidation. These events also finally lead to neuronal death. Various genetic and environmental factors may contribute to these pathways. It is possible that Al and other metals are implicated in various stages of these degenerative processes and finally link to the pathogenesis of AD (From Kawahara 2005. With permission)

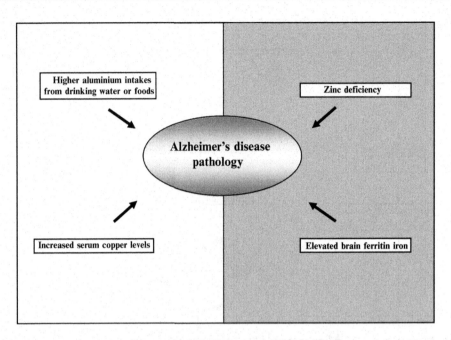

Fig. 178.4 Synopsis of the evidence on the possible effects of metals on Alzheimer's disease pathology. This figure shows the suggested impact of various metals on Alzheimer's disease pathology including aluminium, zinc, copper and iron

investigated 48 patients with probable AD, who were randomly assigned to receive DFOA (125 mg intramuscularly twice daily, 5 days per week, for 24 months), oral placebo (lecithin), or nontreatment (i.e., normal care) (McLachlan et al. 1991). No significant differences in baseline measures of intelligence, memory or speech ability existed between the groups. Activities of daily living were also assessed and video recorded at 6, 12, 18 and 24 month intervals. DFOA administration was associated with a significant reduction in the rate of decline of daily living skills as assessed by both group means and variances, while differences in the rate deterioration of patients receiving either placebo or nontreatment were noted. The mean rate of decline was twice as rapid for the nontreatment group while appetite and weight loss, which was found to be reversible by temporary suspension of DFOA, were the only reported side effects (Kruck et al. 1990). These findings (McLachlan et al. 1991) proved controversial, particularly in relation to the statistical analyses of the results as well as the use of lecithin as placebo, which was administered orally while DFOA was injected intramuscularly (Domingo 2006). Experimental studies on rabbits showed that although a partial reversal of Al-induced neurodegeneration by DFOA was observed, pretreatment of the animals with this chelator was not protective against Al-induced NFT-associated pathology. One possible explanation could also be that the therapeutic effects of DFOA were partly due to mechanisms other than chelation, such as inhibition of free radical formation or inflammation (McLachlan et al. 1991).

   To date, ten natural and synthetic Al(III) ligands and chelators (fluoride, maltol, citrate, EDTA, hydroxyurea, dihydroxyacetone, salicylate, ascorbate, DFOA and Feralex-G), have been investigated alone or in combination (Kruck et al. 2004) for their ability to remove Al(III) from intact human brain cell nuclei, following preincubations with the respective compounds. Although nuclear-bound Al(III) was found to be resistant to removal, the combination of ascorbate plus Feralex-G was found to be particularly effective in removing Al(III) from the nuclear matrix. The mechanism proposed by authors (Kruck et al. 2004), called molecular shuttle chelation, might provide a useful pharmacotherapy in the potential treatment of Al(III) overload. Nonetheless, DFOA has been the only Al chelator successfully tested in the palliative treatment of AD and while it is the main stay of iron and Al chelation therapy, the high cost of this drug, the need for parenteral administration, and various side effects observed have been considered reasonable justification to pursue an orally effective, cheaper and less toxic chelating agent than DFOA where BBB permeability of the compound would be particularly useful in AD.

There are, however, many other effective chelators of trivalent ions available that might already be exerting protective effects through the chelation of Al (House et al. 2004). Among a number of these chelating agents tested in animal models, the most promising were the 1-alkyl-3-hydroxy-2-methylpyrid- 4-ones, and particularly the compound 1,2-dimethyl-3- hydroxypyrid-4-one (deferiprone, L1) (Domingo 1996). Until recent years, aminoacridines have been the group of drugs most frequently used to improve cognitive functions in AD patients. It was even hypothesised that, in addition to the enhancement in cholinergic transmission, their metabolite might chelate Al, thereby offering an additional benefit by diminishing the Al body burden, but these claims have not been substantiated (Domingo 1996).

The possible effects of combined treatments using chelating agents to remove Al from the body have also been investigated based on the rationale that they might be more efficient than monotherapy. In a study of rats, the therapeutic efficacy of combined administration of citric acid and N-2 hydroxyethylethylenediaminetriacetic acid (HEDTA) was measured on the extent to which blood and brain Al concentrations and parameters indicative of haematological disorders as well as brain oxidative stress were altered (Flora et al. 2003). In contrast to DFOA, which is unable to enter the brain, HEDTA which is BBB-permeable resulted in a moderate decrease in rat brain Al concentration. The authors concluded that HEDTA could be a potential antidote for Al overload. However, in order to achieve an optimum effect of chelation therapy, administration of citric acid and HEDTA would be recommended (Flora et al. 2003). In previous studies, injection of citrate following parenteral Al administration depleted tissue Al concentrations (Domingo 2006); however, citrate may be able to increase or decrease Al accumulation, depending on the relative concentrations of Al and citrate within different compartments in the organism (Yokel et al. 1996). Research into this topic continues but it remains to be seen whether this possible therapeutic route might be of any practical importance.

178.6 Applications to Other Areas of Health and Disease

Al, as a known environmental toxicant, has been linked to a variety of pathological conditions such as dialysis encephalopathy, osteomalacia as well as AD. However, its precise role in the pathogenesis of these disorders is not fully understood. Studies using hepatocytes as a model system have examined the impact of Al on aerobic energy production and found that Al-exposed hepatocytes were characterised by lipid and protein oxidation and a dysfunctional tricarboxylic acid (TCA) cycle. Thus Al toxicity was suggested to promote a dysfunctional TCA cycle and impede ATP production, events that may contribute to various Al-induced abnormalities (Mailloux et al. 2006). Al has also been associated with other neurodegenerative diseases and, along with decreased levels of Ca and magnesium (Mg), is suspected to contribute to the pathogenesis of amyotrophic lateral sclerosis (ALS) and Parkinson's disease–related dementia (Shiraki and Yase 1991). The existence of Al in NFTs of patients with ALS/Parkinsonism dementia was also reported at the beginning of the 1960s, when epidemiological surveys in both Kozagawa and Hobara foci revealed the characteristics of Kii ALS as follows: younger age at onset, especially men, familial clustering and presence of Alzheimer's NFTs (Kawahara 2005). Other environmental studies showed that extremely low levels of Ca and Mg in rivers adjacent to the birthplaces of ALS patients inversely and significantly correlated with high mortality rates, Al content, and densities of hippocampal NFTs (Kawahara 2005). Similarly, in experimental animals, low Ca and Mg, but high Al content in diet led to a neuronal loss with axonal swellings and chromatolysis (Kawahara 2005). Recently, a significant loss of dopaminergic neurons was identified exclusively in the substantia nigra of 1-year-old rats derived from colonies fed a low Mg diet over two generations (Kawahara 2005). Overall, some of these interactions may point to a predisposition to develop ALS/Parkinsonism dementia but which are precipitated by their environmental exposures and supporting suggestions that the aetiologies of these conditions are the result of gene-environment interactions (Kawahara 2005).

Dialysis encephalopathy was found to be caused by Al in dialysis solution or Al-containing pharmacological compounds in hemodialysis patients (Alfrey et al. 1976). A more recent case report has demonstrated that Al-containing cement used in bone reconstruction surgery caused fatal encephalopathy (Reusche et al. 2001). There have also been cases of encephalopathy that have developed in dialysis patients after they took Al-containing antacids. The Japanese Ministry of Health, Labour and Welfare recommended that patients on dialysis or with kidney failure should not use Al-containing antacids.

The lipophilic nature of the organic Al salt is a critical determinant of toxicity (Campbell et al. 2001). Human cell lines of neural origin were utilised to study the effect of lipophilic Al acetylacetonate and non-lipophilic Al sulfate on cell proliferation and viability. Although analysis of Al species in the cell culture media demonstrated that there are positively charged Al species present in solutions prepared with both Al salts, only the Al acetylacetonate salt caused changes in cell proliferation and viability. Neuroblastoma (SK-N-SH) cells were also more susceptible to decreased cell proliferation although the lipophilic Al salt was more toxic to the glioblastoma (T98G) cells. While the toxicity of Al acetylacetonate was inhibited in the T98G cells by the addition of phosphate, the same treatment did not reverse cell death in the SK-N-SH cells. Thus, the mechanism of Al toxicity appears to be different in the two cell lines and it is possible that the most susceptible cell type for Al is glial but when these cells are compromised, then there may be a secondary impact upon the neuronal population that eventually leads to neurodegeneration (Campbell et al. 2001).

The Al contamination of total parenteral nutrition (TPN) solutions is a matter of great concern. Bishop et al. reported that the neurological development of premature infants who had received a TPN solution containing a high level of Al was impaired compared with infants who had received an Al-depleted TPN solution (Bishop et al. 1997). Considering that Al in TPN solutions is highly bioavailable and that the renal function of infants is impaired, the Al contamination of TPN solutions could cause serious brain damage. The US Food and Drug Administration (FDA), the North American Society for Pediatric Gastroenterology and Nutrition (Klein et al. 1998), and other societies have recommended the reduction of the contamination of Al in parenteral solutions.

178.7 Conclusions

AD is widely accepted as a multifactorial disease, and genetic as well as environmental factors play significant roles in its pathogenesis. The involvement of Al in the pathogenesis of AD cannot be discarded, especially when there are many reports suggesting links between Al and the Aβ hypothesis

Table 178.6 Key points of clinical and epidemiological studies on the relationships between dietary aluminium (Al) and dementia or predementia syndromes

A. In recent years, an increasing body of epidemiological evidence suggested potential role of metals in the pathogenesis of Alzheimer's Disease (AD). In particular, the aluminium (Al) neurotoxicity has been established, beginning from its presence discovered in the senile plaques and neurofibrillary tangles, the principal histopathological hallmarks of AD
B. Al may enter the human body from several sources, especially from drinking water and food consumption. The epidemiological evidence supporting this association is somewhat stronger for exposure to Al from drinking water, as compared to food. However, other elements present in drinking water, such as fluoride, copper, zinc or iron could also have an effect on cognitive impairment or influence the Al neurotoxicity
C. Metal ligand-based therapeutic approaches for treatment of AD have been suggested, given the growing number of epidemiological investigations that have identified Al and other metals (especially zinc and copper) as possible risk factors for this disease, opening a new route to disease-modifying treatment of AD

This table lists the principal features of clinical and epidemiological studies on the relationships between dietary Al and dementia (i.e., AD), or predementia syndromes (i.e., age-related cognitive decline)

in AD. Overall, the results of molecular epidemiological investigations have suggested an association between chronic exposure to Al and risk of AD. This possible association is biologically plausible and likely to be of moderate significance and may be modified by other inorganic substances, like silica (Rondeau et al. 2000). The evidence supporting this association is stronger for exposure to Al from drinking water, compared to food (Table 178.6). However, this association does not yet satisfy all of Hill's criteria for causation (Hill 1965). Therefore, future studies require stronger methodological designs in order to fully test the validity of previous positive findings and to demonstrate dose–response relationships between Al and AD risk. This might provide new routes to the treatment of AD, with a disease-modifying effect, as opposed to the predominantly symptomatic approaches currently in use.

Summary Points

- An increasing body of molecular epidemiological evidence suggests the potential role of metals in the pathogenesis of Alzheimer's Disease (AD).
- Aluminium (Al) neurotoxicity, in particular, has been identified due to its presence in the senile plaques and neurofibrillary tangles that are the principal neuropathological hallmarks of AD.
- Epidemiological evidence supporting association between Al and AD is stronger for exposure to Al from drinking water, compared to exposure from food, although other elements present in drinking water, such as fluoride, copper, zinc or iron could also have an effect on cognitive impairment or influence any Al-mediated neurotoxicity.
- Metal ligand–based therapeutic approaches that might offer treatment for AD have been suggested, following the epidemiological evidence supporting the involvement of Al and other metals (especially zinc and copper) as possible risk factors for this disease
- The therapeutic efficacy of combined administration of citric acid and N-2 hydroxyethyl-ethylenediaminetriacetic acid (HEDTA) in decreasing blood and brain Al concentrations, other adverse haematological parameters, and brain oxidative stress has been investigated but further research is required to identify whether it can truly offer practical or clinical application.

Definitions

Aluminium: is a nonessential metal present in 8% of the Earth's crust. Despite its natural abundance, aluminium has no known function in living cells and produces some toxic effects in elevated concentrations. Its toxicity can be traced to deposition in bone and the central nervous system, which is particularly noticeable in patients with reduced renal function. In very high doses, aluminium can cause neurotoxicity, and is associated with altered function of the blood-brain barrier

Dementia: is a syndrome defined by impairments in memory and other cognitive functions that are severe enough to cause significant impairment and decline from a previous level of social and occupational functioning

Alzheimer's disease neuropathology: Alzheimer's disease is characterised by a number of pathological hallmarks, the most common being intraneuronal protein clusters composed of paired helical filaments including hyperphosphorylated tau protein (neurofibrillary tangles), and extracellular protein aggregates (senile plaques). The senile plaques are the result of either increased processing of the amyloid-β (Aβ) protein precursor by β- and γ-secretases or reduced degradation of clearance of the resultant toxic Aβ peptide that forms and in turn aggregates and initiates a pathogenic cascade that leads to neuronal loss

Predementia syndrome: this term identifies all conditions with age-related deficits in cognitive function, including a mild stage of cognitive impairment based on a model of normality or also due to pathological conditions considered predictive or early stages of dementia

Mild cognitive impairment (MCI): is a clinical label that includes non-demented aged persons with memory impairment that is more pronounced than what would be expected normal for that age but not severe enough as to cause significant disability

---

Acknowledgement This work was supported by the Italian Longitudinal Study on Aging (ILSA) (Italian National Research Council - CNR-Targeted Project on Ageing - Grants 9400419PF40 and 95973PF40).

References

Ackrill P, Ralston AJ, Day JP, Hodge KC. Lancet. 1980;2:692–3.

Alfrey AC, LeGendre GR, Kaehny WD. New Engl J Med. 1976;294:184–8.

Akay C, Kalman S, Dündaröz R, Sayal A, Aydýn A, Ozkan Y, Gül H. Basic Clin Pharmacol Toxicol. 2008;102:433–6.

Banks WA, Kastin AJ, Maness LM, Banks MF, Shayo M, McLay RN. Ann N Y Acad Sci. 1997;826:190–9.

Banks WA, Niehoff ML, Drago D, Zatta P. Brain Res. 2006;1116:215–21.

Bell RD, Zlokovic BV. Acta Neuropathol. 2009;118:103–13.

Bharathi, Vasudevaraju P, Govindaraju M, Palanisamy AP, Sambamurti K, Rao KSJ. Indian J Med Res. 2008;128:545–56.

Bishop NJ, Morley R, Day JP, Lucas A. New Engl J Med. 1997;336:1557–61.

Bondy SC, Kirstein S. Mol Chem Neuropathol. 1996;27:185–94.

Broe GA, Henderson AS, Creasey H, McCusker E, Korten AE, Jorm AF, Longley W, Anthony JC. Neurology. 1990;40:1698–707.

Campbell A, Hamai D, Bondy SC. Neurotoxicology. 2001;22:63–71.

Canadian Study of Health and Aging. Neurology. 1994;44:2073–80.

Crapper DR, Krishnan SS, Dalton AJ. Science. 1973;180:511–3.

Dewitt DA, Hurd JA, Fox N, Townsend BE, Griffioen KJ, Ghribi O, Savory J. J Alzheimers Dis. 2006;9:195–205.

D'mello SR, Anelli R, Calissano P. Exp Cell Res. 1994;211:232–8.

Dobson CB, Day JP, King SJ, Itzhaki RF. Toxicol Appl Pharmacol. 1998;152:145–52.
Döllken V. Arch Exp Pathol Pharmacol. 1897;98–120.
Domingo JL. Adverse Drug React Toxicol Rev. 1996;15:145–65.
Domingo JL. J Alzheimers Dis. 2006;102 (3):331–41.
El-Rahman SS. Pharmacol Res. 2003;47:189–94.
Esparza JL, Gomez M, Romeu M, Mulero M, Sanchez DJ, Mallol J, Domingo JL. J Pineal Res. 2003;35:32–9.
Exley C. J Alzheimer Dis. 2006;10:173–7.
Exley C, Esiri MM. J Neurol Neurosurg Psychiatry. 2006;77:877–9.
Flaten TP. Brain Res Bull. 2001;55:187–96.
Flora SJ, Mehta A, Satsangi K, Kannan GM, Gupta M. Comp Biochem Physiol C Toxicol Pharmacol. 2003;134:319–28.
Forbes WF, McAiney CA, Hayward LM, Agwani N. Can J Aging. 1994;13:249–67.
Forbes WF, Lessard S, Gentleman JF. Can J Aging. 1995;14:642–56.
Forster DP, Newens AJ, Kay DWK, Edwardson JA. J Epidemiol Community Health. 1995;49:253–8.
Frecker MF. J Epidemiol Community Health. 1991;45:307–11.
Garruto RM, Brown P. Lancet. 1994;343:989–99.
Gillette-Guyonnet S, Andrieu S, Nourhashemi F, de la Guéronnière V, Grandjean H, Vellas B. Am J Clin Nutr. 2005;81:897–902.
Grant WB, Campbell A, Itzhaki RF, Savory J. J Alzheimers Dis. 2002;4:179–89.
Gold G. Int Psychogeriatr. 2003;15 Suppl 1:111–4.
Gonzalez-Muñoz MJ, Meseguer I, Sanchez-Reus MI, Schultz A, Olivero R, Benedí J, Sánchez Muniz FJ. Food Chem Toxicol. 2008;46:1111–8.
Good PF, Werner P, Hsu A, Olanow CW, Perl DP. Am J Pathol. 1996;149:21–8.
Hanas JS, Gunn CG. Nucleic Acids Res. 1996;24:924–30.
Hill AB. Proc R Soc Med. 1965;58:295–300.
House E, Collingwood J, Khan A, Korchazkina O, Berthon G, Exley C. J Alzheimers Dis. 2004;6:291–301.
Irvine GB, El-Agnaf OM, Shankar GM, Walsh DM. Mol Med. 2008;14:451–64.
Jellinger KA. J Alzheimers Dis. 2003;5:247–50.
Kawahara M. J Alzheimer Dis. 2005;8:171–82.
Klein GL, Leichtner AM, Heyman MB. J Pediatr Gastroenterol Nutr. 1998;27:457–60.
Kruck TP, Fisher EA, McLachlan DR. Clin Pharmacol Ther. 1990;48:439–46.
Kruck TP, Cui JG, Percy ME, Lukiw WJ. Cell Mol Neurobiol. 2004;24:443–59.
Lankoff A, Banasik A, Duma A, Ochniak E, Lisowska H, Kuszewski T, Gó d S, Wojcik A. Toxicol Lett. 2006;16:27–36.
Li W, Kenneth KY, Sun W, Paudel HK. Neurochem Res. 1998;23:1467–76.
Lione A. Pharmacol Ther. 1985;29:255–85.
Love S, Miners S, Palmer J, Chalmers K, Kehoe P. Front Biosci. 2009;14:4778–92.
Lovell MA, Ehmann WD, Markesbery WR, Melethil S, Swyt CR, Zatta PF. J Toxicol Environ Health. 1996;48:637–48.
Martyn CN, Osmond C, Edwardson JA, Barker DJP, Harris EC, Lacey RF. Lancet. 1989;333:61–2.
Martyn CN, Coggon DN, Inskip H, Lacey RF, Young WF. Epidemiology. 1997;8:281–6.
Mailloux RJ, Hamel R, Appanna VD. J Biochem Mol Toxicol. 2006;20:198–208.
McLachlan DRC, Bergeron C, Smith JE, Boomer D, Rifat SL. Neurology. 1996;46:401–5.
McLachlan DR, Dalton AJ, Kruck TP, Bell MY, Smith WL, Kalow W, Andrews DF. Lancet. 1991;337:1304–8.
Miessler G, Tarr D. Inorganic chemistry. Prentice Hall. 2003;720.
Milne FJ, Sharf B, Bell P, Meyers AM. Clin Nephrol. 1983;20:202–7.
Miners JS, Baig S, Palmer J, Palmer LE, Kehoe PG, Love S. Brain Pathol. 2008;18:240–252.
Neri LC, Hewitt D. Lancet. 1991;338:390.
Neve RL, Robakis NK. Trends Neurosci. 1998;21:15–9.
Panza F, D'Introno A, Colacicco AM, Capurso C, Del Parigi A, Caselli RJ, Pilotto A, Argentieri G, Scapicchio PL, Scafato E, Capurso A, Solfrizzi V. Am J Geriatr Psychiatry. 2005;13:633–44.
Panza F, D'Introno A, Colacicco AM, Capurso C, Parigi AD, Capurso SA, Caselli RJ, Pilotto A, Scafato E, Capurso A, Solfrizzi V. Neurobiol Aging. 2006;27:933–40.
Pennington JA. Food Addit Contam. 1987;5:161–232.
Pennington JA, Schoen SA. Food Addit Contam. 1995;12:119–28.
Permanne B, Adessi C, Fraga S, Frossard MJ, Saborio GP, Soto C. J Neural Transm Suppl. 2002;62:293–301.
Petersen RC, Doody R, Kurz A, Mohs RC, Morris JC, Rabins PV, Ritchie K, Rossor M, Thal L, Winblad B. Arch Neurol. 2001;58:1985–92.
Praticó'D, Uryu K, Sung S, Tang S, Trojanowski JQ, Lee VM. FASEB J. 2002;16:1138–40.
Rao KSJ. Nahrung. 1994;5:533–7.

Reinke CM, Breitkreutz J, Leuenberger H. Drug Saf. 2003;26:1011–25.

Reusche E, Pilz P, Oberascher G, Lindner B, Egensperger R, Gloeckner K, Trinka E, Iglseder B. Hum Pathol. 2001;32:1136–40.

Riihimäki V, Hänninen H, Akila R, Kovala T, Kuosma E, Paakkulainen H, Valkonen S, Engström B. Scand J Work Environ Health. 2000;26:118–30.

Rhodin JA, Thomas TN, Clark L, Garces A, Bryant M. J Alzheimers Dis. 2003;5:275–86.

Rogers MAM, Simon DG. Age Ageing. 1999;28:205–9.

Rondeau V, Commenges D, Jacqmin-Gadda H, Dartigues JF. Am J Epidemiol. 2000;152:59–66.

Rondeau V, Jacqmin-Gadda H, Commenges D, Helmer C, Dartigues JF. Am J Epidemiol. 2009;169:489–96.

Saiyed SM, Yokel RA. Food Addit Contam. 2005;22:234–44.

Shcherbatykh I, Carpenter DO. J Alzheimer Dis. 2007;11:191–205.

Shiraki H, Yase Y. In: Pierre J Vinken, HL Klawans, GW Bruyn, JM De Jong, editors. Diseases of the motor system. Handbook of clinical neurology 15. Amsterdam: Elsevier Health Sciences; 1991. p. 273–300.

Smith LF. Environmetrics. 1995;6:277–86.

Solfrizzi V, Panza F, Colacicco AM, D'Introno A, Capurso C, Torres F, Grigoletto F, Maggi S, Del Parigi A, Reiman EM, Caselli RJ, Scafato E, Farchi G, Capurso A. Neurology. 2004;63:1882–91.

Swartz RD. Am J Kidney Dis. 1985;6:358–64.

Todorich BM, Connor JR. Ann NY Acad Sci. 2004;1012:171–8.

Tuneva J, Chittur S, Boldyrev AA, Birman I, Carpenter DO. Neurotox Res. 2006;9:1–8.

Vickers JC, Dickson TC, Adlard PA, Saunders HL, King CE, McCormack G. Prog Neurobiol. 1999;60:139–65.

Vogt T (1986) Water quality and health. Study of a possible relation between aluminum in drinking water and dementia (published in Norwegian with English summary). Sociale Og Okonomiske Studier 61, Statistisk Sentralbyra Oslo-Kongsvinger, pp. 60–63.

Wettstein A, Aeppli J, Gautschi K, Peters M. Int Arch Occup Environ Health. 1991;63:97–103.

World Health Organization (WHO)/IPCS. Environ Health Criteria. 1997;194:1–152.

Wills RR, Savory J. Lancet. 1983;2:29–34.

Yokel RA, Ackrill P, Burgess E, Day JP, Domingo JL, Flaten TP, Savory J. J Toxicol Environ Health. 1996;48:667–83.

Yokel RA, Florence RL. Toxicology 2006;227:86–93.

Yokel RA. J Alzheimers Dis. 2006;10:223–53.

Chapter 179
Dietary Fatty Acids, Cognitive Decline, and Dementia

Vincenzo Solfrizzi, Vincenza Frisardi, Cristiano Capurso, Alessia D'Introno,
Anna M. Colacicco, Gianluigi Vendemiale, Antonio Capurso, and Francesco Panza

Abbreviations

AD	Alzheimer's disease
VaD	Vascular dementia
MCI	Mild cognitive impairment
ARCD	Age-related cognitive decline
AACD	Aging-associated cognitive decline
UFA	Unsaturated fatty acids
MUFA	Monounsaturated fatty acids
PUFA	Polyunsaturated fatty acids
LA	Linoleic acid
ALA	α-linolenic acid
DHA	Docosahexaenoic acid
EPA	Eicosapentaenoic acid
APOE	Apolipoprotein E
ARA	Arachidonic acid

179.1 Introduction

179.1.1 Dementia and Predementia Syndromes

Dementia is estimated to affect approximately 6% of the population aged 65 and older, the prevalence increasing exponentially with age, to 40–70% at the age of 95 years and over. In Western countries, the most common forms of dementia are Alzheimer's disease (AD) (Table 179.1) and vascular dementia (VaD) (Table 179.2), with respective frequencies of 70% and 15% of all dementias (Qiu et al. 2007). AD is an age-related progressive neurodegenerative disorder with an enormous unmet medical need, characterized by relatively slow chronic but progressive impairment in cognition, behavior, and functionality. The number of people suffering from AD is rising quickly because there are no effective

V. Solfrizzi (✉)
Department of Geriatrics, Center for Aging Brain, Memory Unit,
University of Bari, Policlinico, Piazza Giulio Cesare, 11, 70124 Bari, Italy
e-mail: v.solfrizzi@geriatria.uniba.it

V.R. Preedy et al. (eds.), *Handbook of Behavior, Food and Nutrition*,
DOI 10.1007/978-0-387-92271-3_179, © Springer Science+Business Media, LLC 2011

Table 179.1 Key features of Alzheimer's disease (AD)

1. AD is the most common dementia and primary neurodegenerative disorder in the elderly
2. AD gradually leads to a complete psychological and physical dependency and finally to death within one to two decades
3. The neuropathology of AD involves aberrant protein processing and is characterized by the presence of both intraneuronal protein clusters composed of paired helical filaments of hyperphosphorilated tau protein (NFTs), and extracellular protein aggregates (SPs)
4. The diagnosis of AD is essentially a clinical one, and it is based on a typical clinical picture and findings, with a set of clinical criteria often used in research
5. From a clinical point of view, AD is a slow, progressive disease that most often starts with episodic memory impairment. However, the patients with preclinical AD show deficits in several cognitive areas, including executive function, verbal and visuospatial abilities, attention, and perceptive speed
6. Cognitive function declines over time, and the diagnosis of AD can be considered when the patient has impairments in memory and at least in one other cognitive function (executive dysfunction, agnosia, aphasia, apraxia), severe enough to cause impairment in social or occupational functioning
7. In advanced AD, common symptoms include also confusion, behavioral and gait disturbances, and the patients are increasingly dependent on others in activities of daily living

NFTs neurofibrillary tangles, *SPs* senile plaques
This table lists the key facts of AD including neuropathological hallmarks, clinical criteria for diagnosis, and the natural history of the disease

Table 179.2 Key features of vascular dementia (VaD)

1. The clinical presentation of VaD varies greatly depending on the causes and location of cerebral damage
2. Large-vessel disease leads commonly to multiple cortical infarcts and a multifocal cortical dementia syndrome
3. Small-vessel disease, usually resulting from hypertension and diabetes, causes periventricular white matter ischemia and lacunar strokes characterized clinically by subcortical dementia with frontal lobe deficits, executive dysfunction, slow information processing, impaired memory, inattention, depressive mood changes, slowing of motor function, Parkinsonian features, small-step gait, urinary disturbances and pseudobulbar palsy
4. The term Vascular Cognitive Disorder (VCD) has been recently proposed and it would become the global diagnostic category for cognitive impairment of vascular origin
5. VCD would include the group of syndromes and diseases characterized by cognitive impairment resulting from a cerebrovascular etiology
6. The main categories of VCD are Vascular Cognitive Impairment (VCI) (i.e., vascular CIND and vascular MCI), VaD, and mixed AD plus CVD. previously termed "mixed dementia"
7. Dementia is defined as executive control deficit producing loss of function for instrumental activities of daily living, while mixed AD plus CVD is defined as preexisting AD worsened by stroke (equivalent to prestroke dementia)
8. VCI is a term referred to all forms of mild to severe cognitive impairment associated with CVD, including vascular CIND and vascular MCI, e.g., predementia syndromes with a presumed primary vascular basis
9. The characteristic neuropsychological profile of VCI is believed to include frequently early impairment of attention and executive control function, with slowing of motor performance and information processing, while episodic memory is relatively spared compared to that in AD

CIND cognitive impairment no dementia, *MCI* mild cognitive impairment, *AD* Alzheimer's disease, *CVD* cerebrovascular disease
This table lists the key features of VaD including clinical and neuropathological classification, and the clinical picture of the disease

treatments for the disorder available. Clinical and epidemiological research has also focused on the identification of risk factors that may be modified in predementia syndromes, at a preclinical or early clinical stage of dementing disorders. The umbrella term "predementia syndromes" includes the transitional phase between mild nondisabling cognitive decline and disabling dementia, an ambiguous diagnostic period during which it is unclear whether mild cognitive deficits predict incipient dementia or not. In fact, the clinical label identifies all conditions with age-related deficits in cognitive function reported in the literature, including a mild stage of cognitive impairment based on a normality model and pathological conditions considered predictive of early stages of dementia (Panza et al. 2005). Such predementia syndromes have been defined for AD and partly for VaD, but have not yet been operationalized for other specific forms of dementia. Therefore, the term "predementia syndromes" includes different conditions and, among them, MCI is at present the most widely used term to indicate non-demented aged persons with no significant disability and a mild memory or cognitive impairment, which cannot be explained by any recognized medical or psychiatric condition (Panza et al. 2005). At present, the term mild cognitive impairment and its abbreviation MCI have frequently been used in studies on the preclinical phases of dementia, although with differing and inconsistent definitions (Petersen et al. 1999, 2001; Winblad et al. 2004) (Table 179.3). There is now ample evidence that MCI is often a pathology-based condition with a high rate of progression to AD (Panza et al. 2005). Therefore, MCI has also been identified as the predementia syndrome for AD. The more recently proposed multiple subtypes of MCI were intended to reflect the heterogeneity of different types of dementia. Actually, the recent subclassifications of MCI according to its cognitive features [dysexecutive MCI and amnestic-MCI (aMCI), or aMCI and non-amnestic MCI (naMCI): single-domain aMCI and multiple-domain aMCI or single-domain naMCI and multiple-domain naMCI] (Winblad et al. 2004), clinical presentation [MCI with parkinsonism, cerebrovascular disease (CVD), depressive symptoms, behavioral and psychological symptoms], or probable etiology (MCI-AD, vascular MCI, or MCI-Lewy body dementia) (Gauthier et al. 2006) all represent an attempt to control this heterogeneity. A critical review has recently made in Stockholm and then in Montreal, in order to define a new consensus on MCI (Winblad et al. 2004). Furthermore, different diagnostic criteria have been proposed for other predementia syndromes, and the terms age-related cognitive decline (ARCD) (American Psychiatric Association 1994) (Table 179.4) and aging-associated cognitive decline (AACD) (Levy 1994) (Table 179.5) have been recently proposed to distinguish individuals with mild cognitive disorders associated with aging, also non-pathological, from noncognitively unimpaired individuals.

Table 179.3   Key features of mild cognitive impairment (MCI)

1. MCI is, at present, the most widely used term to indicate non-demented aged persons with a mild memory or cognitive impairment that cannot be accounted for any recognized medical or psychiatric condition
2. The general criteria for MCI include: a) memory complaint, b) objective memory disorder, c) absence of other cognitive disorders or repercussions on daily life, d) normal general cognitive function, e) absence of dementia
3. MCI definitions can be broadly classified as amnestic (aMCI) and nonamnestic (naMCI)
4. There is now ample evidence that MCI is often a pathology-based condition with a high rate of progression to AD, and aMCI, with a central role for memory disorder and with relative preservation of other cognitive domains, was identified as the predementia syndrome for AD
5. aMCI can be subdivided into a single domain subtype with a pronounced memory deficit or a multiple domain subtype that includes memory impairment along with some impairment in other cognitive domains such as language, executive function, and visuospatial skills
6. The other major MCI subtype is naMCI, which similarly can be subdivided into single and multiple domain subtypes

AD Alzheimer's disease
This table lists the key features of MCI including diagnostic criteria, and clinical classification

Table 179.4   Key features of age-related cognitive impairment (ARCD)

1. ARCD is defined by the DSM-IV as "an objectively identified decline in cognitive functioning consequent to the aging process that is within normal limits given the person's age
2. At present, there are no defined diagnostic criteria for ARCD or other operational definition
3. Few epidemiological studies using this definition have been conducted

DSM IV Diagnostic and Statistical Manual of Mental Disorders, fourth edition
This table lists the key features of MCI including definition, and current research issues on this clinical entity.

Table 179.5 Key features of aging-associated cognitive decline (AACD)

1. In 1994 a task force of the International Psychogeriatric Association (IPA) in collaboration with the World Health Organization (WHO) proposed diagnostic criteria for AACD
2. In these clinical diagnostic criteria, patients score at least one SD below age and education-based standards (e.g., by reference to norms for elderly people) on neuropsychological tests assessing multiple cognitive abilities (memory and learning, attention and concentration, thinking, language, and visuospatial functioning)
3. In the AACD criteria there is no age restriction: though the cognitive decline is more prevalent in old age, its onset may occur earlier in life

SD standard deviation
This table lists the key features of AACD focusing on clinical diagnostic criteria

179.1.2 Possible Prevention of Dementia and Predementia Syndromes

The causes of predementia syndromes and dementia are at present unknown. However, some studies have suggested that these conditions may be prevented (Solfrizzi et al. 2006a, 2008). The role of the diet in cognitive decline has not been extensively investigated, with a few data available on the role of macronutrient intake in the pathogenesis of predementia and dementia syndromes (Solfrizzi et al. 2006a, 2008). Since several dietary factors affect the risk of cardiovascular disease, it can be assumed that they also influence the risk of dementia. Some recent studies have suggested that dietary fatty acids may play a role in the development of cognitive decline associated with aging or dementia (Solfrizzi et al. 2005). This concept is further supported by recent evidence that certain diets have been associated with a lower incidence of AD. In fact, antioxidants, dietary fatty acids, and micronutrients appear to have a role, and evidence is at least suggestive that diets rich in fruits and vegetables and other dietary approaches may permit a beneficial effect on the risk of dementia (Solfrizzi et al. 2006a, 2008).

Fatty acids can be categorized briefly into saturated fatty acids (SFA) and unsaturated fatty acids (UFA). SFA, such as stearic acid, is present in products such as meat, dairy products, cookies, and pastries. Monounsaturated fatty acids (MUFA) are most frequently consumed in olive oil. The principal series of polyunsaturated fatty acids (PUFA) are *n*-6 [i.e., linoleic acid (LA)] and *n*-3 [i.e., α-linolenic acid (ALA), docosahexaenoic acid (DHA), and eicosapentaenoic acid (EPA)]. In our Mediterranean dietary pattern, the main sources of *n*-6 PUFA are vegetable oils, while the principal sources of *n*-3 PUFA are fatty fish (salmon, tuna, and mackerel). In fact, olive oil contains 70–80% MUFA (oleic acid) and 8–10% PUFA (6–7% linoleic acid and 1–2% a-linolenic acid) (Solfrizzi et al. 2005). In this chapter, we examine the possible role of dietary fatty acids in modulating the risk of age-related changes in cognitive function, predementia, and dementia syndromes, as well as the possible mechanisms behind the observed associations. Furthermore, we review current evidence on dietary fatty acid supplementation in predementia and dementia syndromes.

179.2 Dietary Fatty Acids in Predementia Syndromes

179.2.1 Cross-sectional Studies

Recently, an increasing number of epidemiological and clinical studies have addressed the link between UFA intake and cognitive function, most being cross-sectional (Solfrizzi et al. 2005). In the last years, the study approach was to associate single micro- or macronutrients to ARCD, MCI, AD, or VaD. In this picture, several hallmarks of the Mediterranean diet were linked to increased risk or to a protective effect against cognitive impairment (Panza et al. 2004). The typical dietary pattern of a Mediterranean diet is characterized by high intakes of vegetables, fruits and nuts, legumes, cereals, fish, and MUFA, relatively low intakes of meat and dairy products, and moderate consumption of alcohol. In fact, higher levels of consumption of olive oil are considered the hallmark of the traditional Mediterranean diet. In a cross-sectional French study, a positive relationship was found in elderly women between lipid intake and the Mini Mental State Examination (MMSE) score, which evaluates global cognitive functions. A positive relationship was also found between PUFA intake and mobility in elderly men, and between functional variables and alcohol intake in the whole sample. The response rate of this study was very low (around 50%) and these findings, contradictory to the results of the subsequent studies, were explained by the authors with the fact that high intakes of these dietary factors can be considered as an indicator of a better health status (Pradignac et al. 1995) (Table 179.6). Another cross-sectional study from Spain showed that the older subjects with a lower intake of MUFA, SFA, and cholesterol, and higher intakes of total calories, fresh fruit, carbohydrate, thiamine, foliate, vitamin C, and minerals (iron and zinc) had the best performance in global cognitive tests, with a statistical significance after adjustment for age and sex (Ortega et al. 1997) (Table 179.6).

As seen above, MUFA, consequent to the high consumption of extra-virgin olive oil, represent the most important fats in the Mediterranean diet. Cumulative evidence suggests that extra-virgin olive oil may have a role in the protection against cognitive decline, besides coronary disease and several types of cancer, because of its high levels of MUFA and polyphenolic compounds. In the older subjects of the Italian Longitudinal Study on Aging (ILSA), which followed a Mediterranean dietary pattern, total fat is 29% of energy, with a high consumption of olive oil (46 g/d), an MUFA energy intake of 17.6% of total energy, 85% of which is derived from olive oil, and an SFA intake of only 6% (Solfrizzi et al. 1999) (Fig. 179.1). The cross-sectional association between dietary macronutrients and cognitive impairment was examined in elderly subjects aged 65–84 years from the ILSA. After adjustment for educational level, the odds ratios (ORs) of cognitive decline (MMSE score < 24) decreased exponentially with the increase of MUFA energy intakes. Furthermore, selective attention performances were independently associated with MUFA intake (Solfrizzi et al. 1999) (Table 179.6). Recently, in another Northern Italian cross-sectional study on older subjects, the Progetto Veneto Anziani (Pro.V.A. study), in a multiple regression analysis, age and educational level accounted for 29.6% of the MMSE variance, while the contribution of the other variables considered [low-density lipoproteins (LDL) cholesterol, diastolic blood pressure, MUFA, and PUFA] was almost negligible. The authors acknowledged that these results were limited by the fact that total energy intake, which is known to be reduced in patients with cognitive impairment, was not considered, and by the fact that the study was a cross-sectional survey (Manzato et al. 2003). Recently, in the Doetinchem Cohort Study, after adjusting for age, gender, education, alcohol consumption, smoking, and energy intake, higher dietary cholesterol was associated with an increased risk of impaired memory function and cognitive flexibility cognitive function, whereas higher SFA intake was associated, although not significantly, with a 15% to 19% increased risk of impairment in memory function, psychomotor speed, and cognitive flexibility. Fatty fish and marine n-3 PUFA consumption were significantly associated with a 19% to 28% decreased risk of global cognitive function impairment and psychomotor speed. These associations appeared to be independent of differences in cardiovascular risk factors (Kalmijn et al 2004) (Table 179.6).

179.2.2 Longitudinal Studies

To our knowledge, there is an increasing number of longitudinal epidemiological studies on the association between fatty acids and cognitive functioning (Kalmijn et al. 1997a; Hende et al. 2003; Morris et al. 2004, 2005a; Solfrizzi et al. 2005, 2006a, b; Psaltopoulou et al. 2008; Eskelinen et al. 2008;

Table 179.6 Principal cross-sectional studies on the relationships between dietary fatty acids and predementia syndromes in older people

Reference	Setting and study design	Subjects	Dietary assessment	Cognitive outcomes	Results and conclusions
Cross-sectional studies					
Pradignac et al. (1995)	Cross-sectional, population based	441 subjects aged >65 years	Evaluation of dietary intake	MMSE, Geronte scale for the assessment of daily living activities	In men, alcohol intake was associated with improved functional and cognitive parameters, while PUFA intake only with functional status. In women, lipid intakes were related to better cognitive performance. Overweight in both sexes was associated with an improvement in functional status
Ortega et al. (1997)	Cross-sectional	260 subjects aged 65–90 years	Evaluation of dietary intake with a weighed-food record for 7 consecutive days, and biochemical assays	MMSE, PMSQ	A diet poor in fatty acids, saturated fatty acids, and cholesterol, but rich in carbohydrates, fibers, vitamins (folates, vitamins C and E, and β-carotene, and minerals (zinc and iron) seems to improve cognitive skills
Solfrizzi et al. (1999)	Cross-sectional, population based	278 subjects, 65–84 years old	Evaluation of dietary intake with a 77-item FFQ	MMSE, DCT, and BSRT	Inverse relationship between MUFA intake and cognitive decline. Significant inverse association between MUFA intakes and selective attention. No association was found between nutritional variables and episodic memory
Manzato et al. (2003)	Cross-sectional, population based	191 subjects aged ☐ 65 years	Evaluation of plasma phospholipid fatty acid composition	MMSE: subjects with a score between 10 and 17 versus subjects with a score between 28 and 30	Cognitive functioning are affected mainly by age and education, not by dietary fatty acids
Kalmijn et al. (2004)	Cross-sectional, population based	1,613 subjects, 45–70 years old	Evaluation of fatty fish, total fat, cholesterol, SFA MUFA, PUFA (n-6 and n-3) dietary intakes with a 178-item FFQ	Concurrent to the dietary assessment, the VVLT, the CST, an abbreviated SCWT, the LDST, a CFT were administrated	Fatty fish and marine n-3 PUFA consumption was associated with a reduced risk and intake of cholesterol and saturated fatty acids with an increased risk of impaired cognitive function in this middle-aged population

Nurk et al. (2007)	Cross-sectional, population based	2,031 subjects, 70–74 years old	Evaluation of dietary intakes with a 169-item FFQ	Six cognitive tests were administered: m-MMSE, m-DST, m-BD; KOLT; TMT-A, and the S-task of the COWAT	Consumers of fish and fish products had better cognitive function than did non-consumers. The associations between fish and fish product intake and cognition were dose-dependent. The effect of fish on cognition differed according to the type of fish and fish product consumed
Dangour et al. (2009)	Randomized clinical trial (24 months)	867 subjects, 70–79 years old from 20 general practices in England and Wales.	Evaluation of fish consumption variable that took into account both frequency and type of fish consumption	A standardized battery of cognitive tests: CVLT; subjective memory assessment; 3 tests of prospective memory; story recall (immediate and delayed); verbal fluency; letter cancellation; location memory (immediate and delayed); symbol-letter substitution; digit span forwards and backwards; simple and choice reaction time	High levels of fish consumption are associated with better cognitive function in later life. Furthermore, there was an apparent linear trend for increased cognitive function across the five-item fish consumption variable, with highest cognitive function levels found in those individuals who report eating the largest amount of fatty, as opposed to white fish

This table lists the principal findings of cross-sectional clinical and epidemiological studies on the relationships between dietary fatty acids and predementia syndromes (i.e., age-related cognitive decline, ARCD, and mild cognitive impairment, MCI) in older people, including the setting and study design, and the dietary and cognitive assessment used. *FFQ* food frequency questionnaire, *MMSE* Mini-Mental State Examination (global cognitive functioning), *PUFA* = polyunsaturated fatty acids, *PMSQ* Pfeiffer's Mental State Questionnaire (global cognitive functioning), *DCT* Digit Cancellation Test (selective attention), *BSRT* Babcock Recall Story Test (episodic memory); *MUFA* = monounsaturated fatty acids; *SFA* = saturated fatty acids; *VVLT* = Visual Verbal Learning Test (verbal memory), *CST* Concept Shifting Task (mental processing speed), *SCWT* Stroop Color Word Test (selective attention), *LDST* Letter Digit Substitution Test (perceptual-motor speed), *CFT* Category Fluency Test (semantic memory), *m-MMSE* modified Mini-Mental State Examination (global cognitive functioning), *m-DST* modified Digit Symbol Test (perceptual speed), *m-BD* modified Block Design (visuo-spatial and motor skills), *KOLT* Kendrick Object Learning Test (episodic memory), *TMT-A* Trail Making Test, part A (executive function), S-task of the *COWAT* the abridged version of the Controlled Oral Word Association Test (access to semantic memory), *CVLT* Californian Verbal Learning Test (verbal memory)

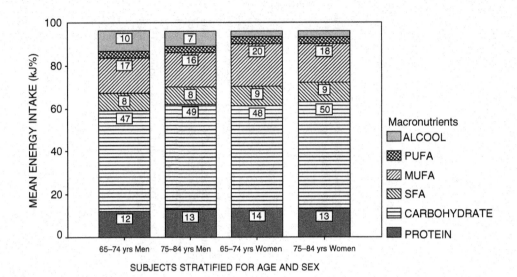

Fig. 179.1 Mean energy intakes from the Italian Longitudinal Study on Aging (*ILSA*). This figure shows the distribution of mean energy intakes (%), stratified for age and gender of the ILSA (Casamassima, Bari, Italy), first prevalence Survey, 1992–1993

Vercambre et al. 2009) (Table 179.7), indicating a crucial need for prospective studies that could confirm initial observations. In particular, one of these prospective studies, the Zutphen Study of 476 men aged 69–89 years, found that high linoleic acid intake was positively associated with cognitive impairment in elderly subjects only in one cross-sectional study after an adjustment for age, education, cigarette smoking, alcohol consumption, and energy intake. High fish consumption, tended to be inversely associated with cognitive impairment and cognitive decline at 3-year follow-up, but not significantly (Kalmijn et al. 1997a) (Table 179.7). Furthermore, in the cohort of the Etude du Viellissement Arteriel (EVA) Study, moderate cognitive decline (a > 2-point of MMSE decrease) and erythrocyte membrane fatty acid composition were evaluated in 264 elderly subjects aged 63–74 years, during a 4-year follow-up. In this study, a lower content of *n*-3 PUFA was significantly associated with a higher risk of cognitive decline. After adjusting for age, gender, educational level and initial MMSE score, stearic acid and total *n*-6 PUFA were consistently associated with an increased risk of cognitive decline. Moreover, a lower content of *n*-3 PUFA was significantly associated with cognitive decline, but after adjustment, this association remained significant only for DHA, and not for EPA (Hende et al. 2003) (Table 179.7). Findings from the CHAP on 2,560 persons aged 65 years and older, showed that in a large population-based sample, a high intake of saturated and trans-unsaturated fat was associated with a greater cognitive decline over a 6-year follow-up. Intake of MUFA was inversely associated with cognitive change among persons with good cognitive function at baseline and among those with stable long-term consumption of margarine, a major food source. Slower decline in cognitive function was associated with higher intake of PUFA, but the association appeared to be due largely to its high content of vitamin E, which shares vegetable oil as a primary food source and which is inversely related to cognitive decline. Finally, cognitive change was not associated with intakes of total fat, animal fat, vegetable fat, or cholesterol (Morris et al. 2004) (Table 179.7). In the same CHAP sample on 3,718 persons aged 65 years and older, high copper intake was associated with a significantly faster rate of cognitive decline but only among persons who also consumed a diet that was high in saturated and trans fats in a 6-year follow-up (Morris et al. 2005a) (Table 179.7). Moreover, in a total of 732 men and women aged 60 years or older, participating

Table 179.7 Principal longitudinal studies on the relationships between dietary fatty acids and predementia syndromes in older people

Reference	Setting and study design	Subjects	Dietary assessment	Cognitive outcomes	Results and conclusions
Longitudinal studies					
Kalmijn et al. (1997a)	Longitudinal, population based (3 years)	476 subjects, aged 69–89 years	Evaluation of dietary intake with the cross-check dietary history method	Cognitive impairment defined as a MMSE score <25 points and cognitive decline as a drop of >2 points of MMSE over a 3-year period	High linoleic acid intake (PUFA) was positively associated with cognitive impairment. High fish consumption was inversely associated with cognitive impairment
Hende et al. (2003)	Longitudinal, population based (4 years)	246 subjects aged 63–74 years	Evaluation of fatty acid composition in erythrocyte membranes	MMSE score with a >2-point of decrease in a 4-year follow-up	Inverse association between cognitive decline and the ratio of n-3 to n-6 PUFA in erythrocyte membranes
Morris et al. (2004)	Longitudinal, population based (6 years)	2,560 subjects, aged 65 years and older	Evaluation of dietary intake with a 139-items FFQ	Cognitive change at 3-year and 6-year follow-ups measured with the EBT of Immediate and Delayed Recall, the MMSE, and the SDMT	A diet high in saturated and trans-unsaturated fat or low in non-hydrogenated unsaturated fats may be associated with cognitive decline among older people
Morris et al. (2005a)	Longitudinal, population based (6 years)	3,718 subjects, aged 65 years and older	Evaluation of dietary intake with a 139-items FFQ	Cognitive change at 3-year and 6-year follow-ups measured with the EBT of Immediate and Delayed Recall, the MMSE, and the SDMT	High copper intake was associated with a significantly faster rate of cognitive decline, but only among persons who also consumed a diet that was high in saturated and trans fats
Morris et al. (2005b)	Longitudinal, population based (6 years)	3,718 subjects, aged 65 years and older	Evaluation of dietary intake with a 139-items FFQ	Cognitive change at 3-year and 6-year follow-ups measured with the EBT of Immediate and Delayed Recall, the MMSE, and the SDMT	Dietary intake of fish was inversely associated with cognitive decline over 6 years. There were no consistent associations with the n-3 fatty acids, although the effect estimates were in the direction of slower decline

(continued)

Table 179.7 (continued)

Reference	Setting and study design	Subjects	Dietary assessment	Cognitive outcomes	Results and conclusions
Solfrizzi et al. (2006a)	Longitudinal, population based (8.5 years)	278 subjects, 65–84 years old from a cohort of 5,632 subjects	Evaluation of MUFA and PUFA dietary intakes with a 77-item FFQ	MMSE	High MUFA, PUFA, and total energy intake were significantly associated with a better cognitive performance in time. The association between high MUFA, PUFA intakes and cognitive performance remained robust even after adjustment for potential confounding variables such as age, sex, educational level, CCI, BMI, and total energy intakes
Solfrizzi et al. (2006b)	Longitudinal, population based (2.6 years)	278 subjects, 65–84 years old from a cohort of 5,632 subjects	Evaluation of MUFA and PUFA dietary intakes with a 77-item FFQ	Incident MCI. Diagnostic criteria for MCI: 1.5 SDs below mean age and education adjusted on the MMSE and 10th percentile below age and education adjusted on memory test, without SMC and intact ADL/IADL	Dietary fatty acids intakes were not associated with incident MCI. However, high PUFA intake appeared to have borderline nonsignificant trend for a protective effect against the development of MCI that may be important.
van Gelder et al. (2007)	Longitudinal, population based (5 years)	210 subjects, 70–89 years old	Information about habitual food consumption was collected using the cross-check dietary history method	MMSE	Fish consumption was associated with less subsequent 5-y cognitive decline than was no fish consumption. Furthermore, a dose-response relation was noted between the combined intake of EPA and DHA and cognitive decline, which suggests that a higher intake of EPA plus DHA was associated with less cognitive decline
Psaltopoulou et al. (2008)	Longitudinal, population based (median 8 years)	732 subjects, 60 years or older	Evaluation of dietary intakes with a 150-item FFQ. A dietary composite score (MeDi score) evaluated adherence to Mediterranean diet	MMSE	No significant association between MeDi score and MMSE scores, whereas a statistically significant inverse association was found between MMSE performance and some individual dietary components, such as seed oil or PUFA intakes

| Vercambre et al. (2008) | Longitudinal, population based (13 years) | 4,809 elderly women, 76–82 years old | Evaluation of dietary intakes with a 208-item FFQ | DECO and IADL | Elderly women that were reported by informants to have undergone recent cognitive decline had, 13 years previously, lower intakes of poultry, fish, and animal fats, as well as higher intakes of dairy desserts and ice-cream. They had lower habitual intakes of dietary fiber and n-3 PUFA, but a higher intake of retinol. Elderly women that were reported by informants to be functionally impaired had, in the past, lower intakes of vegetables and vitamins B2, B6 and B12 |
| Eskilinen et al. (2008) | Longitudinal, population based (21 years) | 1,449 subjects aged 65–80 years | Evaluation of dietary intakes with a 208-item FFQ | The Mayo Clinic AD Research Center criteria were applied for diagnosing MCI; MMSE, CFT, PPBt, LDST, episodic memory with immediate word recall tests; executive function with the Stroop test, and prospective memory with a task by Einstein | Elevated SFA intake at midlife was associated with poorer global cognitive function and prospective memory and with an increased risk of MCI. High intake of PUFA was associated with better semantic memory. Frequent fish consumption was associated with better global cognitive function and semantic memory. Higher PUFA/SFA ratio was associated with better psychomotor speed and executive function |

This table lists the principal findings of longitudinal clinical and epidemiological studies on the relationships between dietary fatty acids and predementia syndromes (i.e., age-related cognitive decline, ARCD, and mild cognitive impairment, MCI) in older people, including the setting and study design, and the dietary and cognitive assessment used

MMSE Mini-Mental State Examination (global cognitive functioning), *PUFA* polyunsaturated fatty acids, *FFQ* food frequency questionnaire, *EBT* East Boston Memory test (immediate and delayed episodic memory), *SDMT* Symbol Digit Modalities Test (perceptual-motor speed), *MUFA* monounsaturated fatty acids, *CCI* Charlson comorbidity index, *BMI* body mass index, *SMC* subjective memory complaint, *ADL* activities of daily living, *IADL* instrumental activities of daily living, *DHA* docosahexaenoic acid, *DECO* DEtérioration COgnitive Observeé scale (observed cognitive deterioration), *CFT* Category Fluency Test (semantic memory), *PPBt* Purdue Peg Board task (psychomotor speed), *LDST* Letter Digit Substitution Test (perceptual-motor speed) in the European Prospective Investigation into Cancer and Nutrition (EPIC), Greece cohort, and residing in the Attica region, 6–13 years follow up showed that seed-oil consumption may adversely affect cognition, whereas adherence to the Mediterranean diet, as well as intake of olive oil, MUFA, and SFA exhibited weakly positive but not significant associations (Psaltopoulou et al. 2008) (Table 179.7). Finally, 4.809 elderly women (born between 1925 and 1930) were studied in a French longitudinal cohort, the Etude Epidémiologique de Femmes de la Mutuelle Générale de l'Education Nationale (E3N) study. Elderly women participating in the E3N cohort who were reported by informants to have undergone recent cognitive decline had, 13 years previously, lower intakes of poultry, fish, and animal fats, as well as higher intakes of dairy desserts and ice-cream. They had lower habitual intakes of dietary fiber and n-3 PUFA, but a higher intake of retinol. Furthermore, elderly women who were reported by informants to be functionally impaired had, in the past, lower intakes of vegetables and vitamins B2, B6, and B12 (Vercambre et al. 2009) (Table 179.7). More recently, in the Cardiovascular Risk Factors, Aging and Dementia (CAIDE) Study from eastern Finland, abundant SFA intake from milk products and spreads at midlife was associated with poorer global cognitive function and prospective memory and with an increased risk of MCI in average follow-up period of 21 years after adjusting for demographic and vascular factors, other fats, and apolipoprotein E (APOE). On the contrary, high PUFA intake was associated with better semantic memory. Also frequent fish consumption was associated with better global cognitive function and semantic memory. Further, higher PUFA/SFA ratio was associated with better psychomotor speed and executive function (Eskelinen et al. 2008) (Table 179.7).

Therefore, on the basis of the previous significant suggestions (Solfrizzi et al. 2005), we tested further the hypothesis that high MUFA and PUFA intakes may protect against the development of cognitive impairment over time in a median follow-up of 8.5 years of the ILSA. The major finding of this study was that high MUFA, PUFA, and total energy intake were significantly associated with a better cognitive performance in time (Figs. 179.2 and 179.3). Total energy intake should be considered

Fig. 179.2 Cognitive profile across time for total energy intake from the Italian Longitudinal Study on Aging (*ILSA*). This figure shows the mean observed Mini-Mental State Examination (*MMSE*) score profile across time for total energy intake (<11,330 kJ/day and ≥11,330 kJ/day at the beginning of the study), ILSA, 1992–2001. The *squared symbols* and *solid line* represent the mean observed MMSE scores for total energy intake, respectively, computed using all observations (*n* = 278 subjects), while the squared symbols and short dashed line represent the mean MMSE scores for total energy intake, computed data from 95 subjects with complete observations

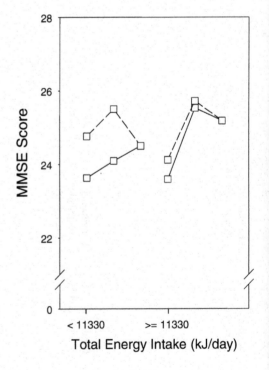

Fig. 179.3 Cognitive profile across time for monounsaturated fatty acids (*MUFA*) intake from the Italian Longitudinal Study on Aging (*ILSA*). This table Mean observed MMSE score profile across time for daily MUFA intake (<53.1 g/day and ≥53.1 g/day at the beginning of the study), ILSA, 1992–2001. The *circle symbols* and *solid* represent the mean observed MMSE scores for MUFA intake, respectively, computed using all observations (*n* = 278 subjects), while the circle symbols and short dashed line represent the mean MMSE scores for MUFA intake, computed data from 95 subjects with complete observations

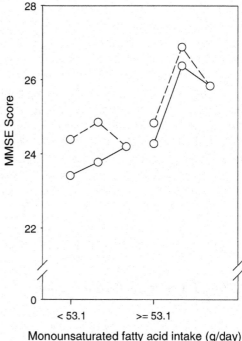

an important confounder of diet-ARCD relationships and, as we proposed in our methodological approach, suggesting that association between macronutrient intake and cognitive decline should be adjusted by total energy intake. No other individual dietary component of our study population was significantly associated with cognitive impairment in time (Solfrizzi et al. 2006a) (Table 179.7). The association between high MUFA, PUFA intakes, and cognitive performance remained robust even after adjustment for potential confounding variables such as age, sex, educational level, Charlson comorbidity index, body mass index, and total energy intakes (Solfrizzi et al. 2006a). Finally, recent findings from the ILSA demonstrated that while dietary fatty acids intakes were not associated with incident MCI, high PUFA intake appeared to have a borderline nonsignificant trend for a protective effect against the development of MCI (Solfrizzi et al. 2006b) (Table 179.7).

179.2.3 Fish Consumption and Cognitive Decline

Epidemiological observational studies reporting associations of fish consumption with cognitive function have shown mixed results; some cross-sectional and longitudinal studies have reported a positive association with higher fish consumption (Morris et al. 2005b; van Gelder et al. 2007; Nurk et al. 2007; Dangour et al. 2009), while others have found no association (Kalmijn et al. 1997a) (Tables 179.6 and 179.7). Fish, particularly fatty fish (e.g., herring, mackerel, salmon, or trout), is the principal source of *n*-3 PUFA in the Mediterranean diet. Very recently, the baseline data from the Older People And *n*-3 Long-chain polyunsaturated fatty acid (OPAL) study, a double-blind randomized placebo-controlled trial examining the effect of daily supplementation with 700 mg *n*-3 PUFA on cognitive performance in healthy older persons aged 70–79, suggested that higher fish consumption is associated with better cognitive function in later life (Dangour et al. 2009) (Table 179.6).

In the Chicago Health and Aging Project (CHAP), dietary intake of fish was inversely associated with cognitive decline over 6 years of follow-up. In this cohort, there was little evidence that the *n*-3 PUFA were associated with cognitive change (Morris et al. 2005b) (Table 179.7). Furthermore, in the Zutphen Elderly Study, fish consumers had significantly less 5-year subsequent cognitive decline than did non-consumers. A linear trend was observed for the relation between the intake of EPA + DHA and cognitive decline, and an average difference of 380 mg/day in EPA plus DHA intake was associated with a 1.1-point difference in cognitive decline (van Gelder et al. 2007) (Table 179.7). Finally, findings from the Hordaland Health Study suggested that subjects whose mean daily intake of fish and fish products was >10 g/day had significantly better mean test scores and a lower prevalence of poor cognitive performance than did those whose intake was <10 g/day. The associations between total intake of seafood and cognition were strongly dose dependent; and the effect was more pronounced for non-processed lean fish and fatty fish (Nurk et al. 2007) (Table 179.6).

179.3 Dietary Fatty Acids and Dementia

179.3.1 Cross-sectional Studies

In 1997, for the first time, a strong dietary link to AD was suggested (Grant 1997) (Table 179.8). The primary finding of this cross-sectional ecological study was that fat and total caloric supply have the highest correlations with AD prevalence rates. In addition, a combination of fat and fish consumption is found to reduce the prevalence of AD in the European and North American countries, i.e., one calorie of fish was found to counter the effects of approximately 4.3 calories of fat. As with most studies of this type, there are a number of potential caveats. In particular, the results of analyses of food supply data with prevalence data that are applied to specific populations should be viewed with caution. However, these ecological evidences were in agreement with various recent epidemiologic studies (Grant 1999).

One of the most interesting findings of a recent study on VaD risk factors conducted on the cohort of the Honolulu-Asia Aging Study (HAAS), in 3,385 older Japanese subjects, was the protective effect of a Western diet against the development of VaD (Ross et al. 1999) (Table 179.8). Oriental populations from Asian countries are known to be more prone to stroke and VaD. A traditional Western diet is high in animal fat and protein and low in complex carbohydrates, compared to the traditional Japanese diet, which is high in complex carbohydrates and low in animal fat and protein. This is an interesting approach in which dietary patterns, not only single micro- or macronutrients, are considered in explaining the possible role of diet in cognitive decline. The mechanism by which an oriental diet leads to VaD remains speculative. The higher risk of stroke could probably be referred to the lower intake of animal fat and protein. As these findings do not allow analysis of separate nutrients, a hypothesis could be that more fat intake may stabilize the integrity of smaller intracranial arterioles, while the quantity and quality of dietary protein may affect small vessel pathology. Furthermore, the increased risk of VaD and stroke in Japan may well be due to the high sodium intake, in the form of soy sauce, pickled fish, etc.

179.3.2 Longitudinal Studies

The possible relationship between dietary fatty acids intake and risk of dementia and AD has been evaluated in a series of longitudinal studies. In fact, the finding that total dietary fat is a possible risk factor for the development of AD has been reported in the Rotterdam Study, although not at a

Table 179.8 Principal cross-sectional studies on the relationships between dietary fatty acids and dementia, or vascular dementia (VaD), or Alzheimer's disease (AD)

Reference	Setting and study design	Subjects	Dietary assessment	Dementia diagnosis	Results and conclusions
Cross-sectional studies					
Grant (1997)	Ecological cross-sectional	18 community-wide studies conducted after 1979 ($\geq$65 years old)	Evaluation of the components of the national diets	Prevalence of AD diagnosed with various clinical criteria	The primary finding is that fat and total caloric supply have the highest correlations with AD prevalence rates. In addition, fish consumption is found to reduce the prevalence of AD in the European and North American countries
Ross et al. (1999)	Cross-sectional, population based	3,734 Japanese American men aged 71 to 93	Evaluation of vascular risk factors, dietary habits, and questionnaire on supplementary vitamin E and C use and alcohol intake	Diagnosis of dementia, VaD (ADDTC criteria), and stroke without dementia	The antioxidant vitamin E and unknown factors related to a Western diet, high in animal fat and protein and low in complex carbohydrates, as opposed to an Oriental diet may be protective against developing VaD

This table lists the principal findings of cross-sectional ecological and epidemiological studies on the relationships between dietary fatty acids and dementia, or VaD, or AD, including the setting and study design, and the dietary and cognitive assessment used

ADDTC California Alzheimer's Disease Diagnostic and Treatment Centers

statistically significant level. In the same study, fish consumption was confirmed to reduce AD risk and LA was inversely correlated with AD. This study suggested that an elevated intake of lipids and saturated fat increased the risk for dementia with a cerebrovascular component (Kalmijn et al. 1997b) (Table 179.9). The cohort of the Rotterdam Study was reexamined in a 6-year follow-up, and a high intake of total fat, saturated fat, trans fat, and cholesterol and low intake of MUFA, PUFA, n-6 PUFA, and n-3 PUFA were not associated with an increased risk of dementia or its subtypes (Engelhart et al. 2002) (Table 179.9). The discrepancy in comparison with the results of the first study was explained by the authors by the shorter follow-up (2.1 years) and a consequent smaller number of incident cases of dementia. Moreover, other limitations of the Rotterdam study included the potential for confounding by intake of other types of fat (e.g., intake of trans fat is associated with both intakes of MUFA and SFA), and the potential for nonlinear associations, with associations of the extremes of intake.

Finally, the findings of the reexamined cohort of the Rotterdam Study are at odds with several recent studies (Luchsinger et al. 2002; Barberger-Gateau et al. 2002; Morris et al. 2003a, b; Laitinen et al. 2006; Barberger-Gateau et al. 2007) (Table 179.9). In fact, a 4-year cohort study in New York, the Washington Heights-Inwood Columbia Aging Project, found that dietary fat was an important risk factor for AD for those with the APOE ε4 allele, but not for those without that allele (Luchsinger et al 2002). Luchsinger and colleagues did not find associations with individual types of fat, but like the Rotterdam study, failed to control for other types of fat, which may have confounded the observed findings. They also confirmed previous ecological findings on the possible role of cereals as a risk reduction factor (Grant 1997).

Furthermore, findings coming from the Personnes Agees QUID (PAQUID) study, a population-based study conducted in France on 1,674 subjects aged 68 years and over, with no apparent dementia at baseline, showed that participants who ate fish or seafood at least once a week had a significantly lower risk of dementia (age and sex adjusted hazard ratio of 0.66, 95% CI: 0.47–0.93) in the 7 subsequent years. After adjusting for education, the hazard ratio was almost unchanged (0.73), but the 95% CI (0.52–1.03), slightly overlapping 1.00, indicated that higher education regarding regular consumption explains in part the protective effect of weekly fish or seafood consumption against dementia. Moreover, in this study no significant association between meat consumption and the risk of dementia was found for weekly consumers, with only a borderline significance for developing AD (hazard ratio: 0.68, 95% CI: 0.47–1.01) (Barberger-Gateau et al. 2002) (Table 179.9).

More recently, two studies from the cohort of the CHAP, increased the evidence of a strict linkage between dementia and fatty acid intake (Morris et al. 2003a, b) (Table 179.9). In fact, in this cohort of 815 subjects, aged 65 years and older, after a mean follow-up of 3.9 years, 131 persons developed AD. A high intake of saturated fat and trans-unsaturated fat may be associated with a higher risk of AD; while a high intake of n-6 PUFA and MUFA may be protective against AD (Morris et al. 2003a). Furthermore, in the same cohort, a higher intake of n-3 PUFA and weekly fish consumption may reduce the risk of incident AD. In fact, in this study, people who ate fish once or more times in a week had a relative risk for AD of 0.4: the absolute risk reduction was about 9.5% (Morris et al. 2003b). More recently, in the CAIDE Study, after an average follow-up of 21 years, moderate intake of PUFA at midlife decreased the risk of dementia, whereas SFA intake was associated with an increased risk, only among the APOE ε4 carriers (Laitinen et al. 2006) (Table 179.9) (Fig. 179.4). Finally, data from the Three-City Study demonstrated that a diet rich in fish, n-3 rich oils, fruits, and vegetables could contribute to decreasing the risk of dementia and AD in older persons whereas consumption of n-6 rich oils could exert detrimental effects when not counterbalanced by sufficient n-3 intake. These effects seem more pronounced among APOE ε4 non-carriers (Barberger-Gateau et al. 2007) (Table 179.9).

Table 179.9 Principal longitudinal studies on the relationships between dietary fatty acids and dementia, or vascular dementia (VaD), or Alzheimer's disease (AD)

Reference	Setting and study design	Subjects	Dietary assessment	Dementia diagnosis	Results and conclusions
Longitudinal studies					
Kalmijn et al. (1997b)	Longitudinal, population based (2.1 years)	5,386 subjects aged 55 and older	Evaluation of dietary intakes with a 170-item FFQ	Diagnosis of AD (NINCDS-ADRDA criteria), VaD (NINDS-AIREN criteria), or dementia with a vascular component	High intakes of total fat, saturated fat, and cholesterol were associated with an increased risk of dementia. Dementia with a vascular component was most strongly related to total fat and saturated fat. Fish consumption was inversely related to incident dementia, and in particular to AD
Engelhart et al. (2002)	Longitudinal, population based (6 years)	5,395 subjects aged 55 and older	Evaluation of dietary intakes with a 100-item FFQ	Diagnosis of dementia (DSM-III-R criteria), AD (NINCDS-ADRDA criteria), and VaD (NINCDS-AIREN criteria)	High intakes of total fat, saturated fat, *trans* fat, and cholesterol and low intake of MUFA, PUFA, *n*-6 PUFA, and *n*-3 PUFA were not associated with an increased risk of dementia, AD, or VaD
Luchsinger et al. (2002)	Longitudinal, population based (4 years)	980 subjects, mean age: 75.3±5.8 years	Evaluation of dietary intake with a 61-item FFQ	Diagnosis of prevalent dementia (DSM-IV criteria) and incident AD (NINCDS-ADRDA criteria)	Higher intake of calories and fats may be associated with higher risk of AD in subjects carrying the apolipoprotein E □4 allele
Barberger-Gateau et al. (2002)	Longitudinal, population based (7 years)	1,674 subjects aged 68 years and over	Evaluation of frequency of consumption of meat and fish and seafood: from daily to never	Diagnosis of incident dementia, including AD (DSM-III-R criteria)	Elderly people who consumed fish [rich in PUFA] or seafood at least once a week are at lower risk of dementia, including AD
Morris et al. (2003a)	Longitudinal, population based (3.9 years)	815 subjects, aged 65 years and older	Evaluation of dietary intake with a 154-item FFQ	Incident diagnosis of AD (NINCDS-ADRDA criteria)	High intake of saturated and *trans*-unsaturated fats may be associated with higher risk of AD; while high intake of *n*-6 PUFA and MUFA may be protective against AD
Morris et al (2003b)	Longitudinal, population based (3.9 years)	815 subjects, aged 65 years and older	Evaluation of dietary intake with a 154-item FFQ	Incident diagnosis of AD (NINCDS-ADRDA criteria)	Higher intake of *n*-3 PUFA and weekly fish consumption may reduce the risk of incident AD

(continued)

Table 179.9 (continued)

Reference	Setting and study design	Subjects	Dietary assessment	Dementia diagnosis	Results and conclusions
Huang et al. (2005)	Longitudinal, population based (5.4 years)	5,201 participants, aged 65 years and older	Evaluation of dietary intake with a 99-item FFQ	Incident diagnosis of dementia (DSM-IV criteria) and AD (NINCDS-ADRDA criteria)	Fatty fish, such as tuna or "other fish" was associated with a lower risk of developing dementia and AD with a dose-response relationship, whereas lean, fried fish was not. Those without an APOE ε4 allele had a 35–45% lower risk with consumption of fatty fish, whereas there was little or no difference for APOE ε4 allele carriers
Schaefer et al. (2006)	Longitudinal, population based (9.1 years)	488 participants from a sample of 899 individuals, median age: 76.0 years	Evaluation of dietary intake with a 125-item FFQ and plasma phosphatidylcholine DHA content	Incident diagnosis of dementia (DSM-IV criteria) and AD (NINCDS-ADRDA criteria)	Higher dietary intakes of DHA and fish did not result protective against all cause dementia and AD. A protective effect of higher plasma DHA was observed against the risk of all cause dementia but not for AD
Laitinen et al. (2006)	Longitudinal, population based (21 years)	1,449 subjects aged 65–80 years	Evaluation of dietary intake with a 154-item FFQ	Incident diagnosis of AD (NINCDS-ADRDA criteria)	Moderate intake of PUFA at midlife was protective, whereas a moderate intake of SFA may increase the risk of dementia and AD, especially among APOE ε4 carriers.
Barberger-Gateau et al. (2007)	Longitudinal, population based (4 years)	9,294 subjects, aged 65 years and older	Evaluation of dietary intakes with a FFQ	Incident diagnosis of dementia (DSM-IV criteria) and AD (NINCDS-ADRDA criteria)	Frequent consumption of fruits and vegetables, fish, and n-3 rich oils may decrease the risk of dementia and AD, especially among APOE ε4 non-carriers

This table lists the principal findings of longitudinal clinical and epidemiological studies on the relationships between dietary fatty acids and dementia, or VaD, or AD, including the setting and study design, and the dietary and cognitive assessment used.

FFQ food frequency questionnaire, *NINCDS-ADRDA* National Institute of Neurological and Communicative Disorders and Stroke and the Alzheimer's Disease and Related Disorders Association, *NINCDS-AIREN* National Institute of Neurological and Communicative Disorders and Stroke and the Association Internationale pour la Recherche at l'Enseignement en Neurosciences, *DSM-III-R* Diagnostic and Statistical Manual of Mental Disorders, third edition revised, *PUFA* polyunsaturated fatty acids, *MUFA* monounsaturated fatty acids, *DSM-IV* Diagnostic and Statistical Manual of Mental Disorders, fourth edition, *APOE* apolipoprotein E, *DHA* docosahexaenoic acid

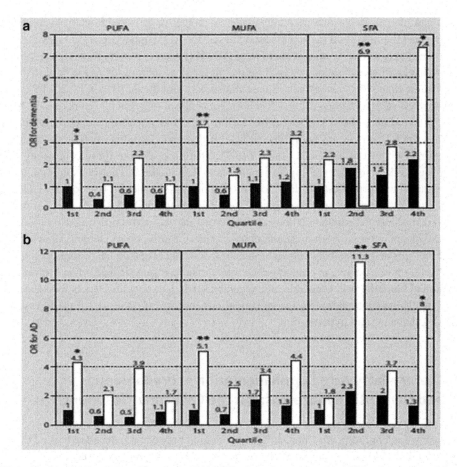

Fig. 179.4 Combined effects of apolipoprotein E (*APOE*) ε4 carrier status and midlife polyunsaturated fatty acids (*PUFA*), monounsaturated fatty acids (*MUFA*), and saturated fatty acids (*SFA*) consumptions in spreads and the risk of dementia (**a**) and Alzheimer's disease (*AD*) (**b**). This figure lists analyses adjusted for age, sex, education, follow-up time, other subtypes of fat from spreads and milk, APOE ε4 and midlife systolic blood pressure (*SBP*), body mass index (*BMI*), cholesterol, smoking, and late-life history of myocardial infarction, stroke and diabetes; *$p < 0.05$, **$p < 0.01$ when compared to the reference group (first fat quartile and APOE ε4 non-carrier); = APOE ε4 non-carriers; = APOE ε4carriers (Reprinted from Laitinen et al. 2006. With permission)

179.3.3 Fish Consumption and Dementia

A lower risk of incident dementia in subjects consuming more fish has nevertheless been reported in several other independent prospective cohort studies (Barberger-Gateau et al. 2002; Morris et al. 2003b; Huang et al. 2005; Barberger-Gateau et al. 2007) (Table 179.9). In particular, data from the Cardiovascular Health Cognition Study (CHCS) showed that consumption of fatty fish more than twice per week was associated with a reduction in risk of dementia by 28%, and AD by 41% in comparison to those who ate fish less than once per month. Stratification by APOE ε4 showed this effect to be selective to those without the ε4 allele (Huang et al. 2005) (Table 179.9). Only one prospective study has not shown a significant benefit of higher fish intake and risk of AD (Schaefer et al. 2006) (Table 179.9). This study was based on a subsample of 488 participants representing about 25% of the main cohort of the Framingham Heart Study in which both dietary DHA intakes were calculated and plasma DHA measurements made. A protective effect of higher plasma DHA was observed against the risk of all cause dementia but not for AD. Higher dietary intakes of DHA and fish did not result protective against dementia and AD. This negative finding for AD per se may have been due to a lack of statistical power because the 50% risk reduction for AD in subjects who consumed fish more than twice a week was almost statistically significant (95% CI 0.20–1.27; P=0.14). Furthermore, several studies suggest that APOE polymorphism may inhibit or prevent the beneficial effect of fish in reducing the risk of cognitive decline in the elderly. Two recent prospective studies indicate that ApoE4 carriers are not protected against dementia by higher fish intake (Huang et al. 2005; Barberger-Gateau et al. 2007) (Table 179.9). Therefore, despite these contrasting findings, there is now considerable evidence suggesting that fatty acid intake and fish consumption may influence dementia and AD risk, but the direction (protection or risk) and the level of this effect remain unclear. In fact, based on the current evidences from human and animal studies, it is not possible to make definitive dietary recommendations in relation to the AD risk on fish consumption and the lower intake of saturated fat from meat and dairy products. Furthermore, individuals who consume a diet high in fruits and vegetables as well as nuts or fish would probably have other lifestyle characteristics that might be effective in reducing AD or VaD risk (e.g., physical activity). However, a high consumption of fats from fish, vegetable oils, vegetables, and nuts should be encouraged because this dietary advice is in accordance with recommendations for lowering the risk of cardiovascular disease, obesity, diabetes, and hypertension.

179.4 Dietary Fatty Acid Supplementation in Predementia and Dementia Syndromes: Is It the Case for a Treatment?

The increasing epidemiological evidence of an association between a reduced risk of AD and a diet high in n-3 PUFA and fish consumption (Panza et al. 2004), is further supported by recent findings that certain diets have been associated with a lower incidence of predementia syndromes (Solfrizzi et al. 2006a, b). Two randomized clinical trials (RCT), using an n-3/n-6 fatty acid compound on 100 AD patients and a supplementation with DHA on 20 nursing home residents with VaD found improvements in mood, cooperation, appetite, sleep, ability to navigate in the home, and short-term memory in the AD-treated group (Yehuda et al. 1996) and improved cognitive scores in the VaD-treated group (Terano et al. 1999) (Table 179.10).

Recently, Freund-Levi and colleagues found that, in 204 patients with moderate AD, the supplementation with DHA and EPA (for a total dose of 1,720 mg DHA/600 mg EPA) for 6 months (OmegAD Study) did not delay the rate of cognitive decline but, in the group of 32 patients with the most mild AD (MMSE >27, Clinical Dementia Rating Score 0.5–1), n-3 PUFA supplementation slowed the decline in MMSE scores (Freund-Levi et al. 2006) (Table 179.10). After the treatment period, all the subjects received open label n-3 PUFA for another 6 months. The subjects in the placebo group of these very mild AD patients also showed a statistically significant slowing of decline when they were switched to treatment between 6 and 12 months, suggesting that n-3 PUFA might be of benefit to slow the progression of the disease in MCI or very mild AD (Freund-Levi et al. 2006). Furthermore, this supplementation did not result in marked effects on neuropsychiatric symptoms in mild to moderate AD patients except for possible positive effects on depressive symptoms and agitation symptoms in subgroups. In fact, there were positive effects on depressive symptoms in non-APOE ε4 carriers and in non-APOE ε4 carriers on agitation symptoms (Freund-Levi et al. 2008) (Table 179.10).

At present, the effect of arachidonic acid (ARA) and DHA (240 mg/day), after a 90-day supplementation, on MCI, organic brain lesions, or AD showed a significant improvement of the immediate

Table 179.10 Principal clinical trials on polyunsaturated fatty acid (PUFA) supplementation in patients with mild cognitive impairment (MCI), vascular dementia (VaD), Alzheimer's disease (AD), and age-related cognitive decline (ARCD)

Reference	Participants	Intervention and duration of exposure	Outcome measures	Effects of interventions
Terano et al. (1999)	20 elderly nursing home residents with VaD	A single dose of 4.3 g of DHA was administered; dose effect was not assessed. The duration of exposure was 12 months	Cognitive functioning was evaluated using HDS-R and MMSE scores at baseline, and after 3, 6, and 12 months	Baseline HDS-R and MMSE scores were 15 to 22, consistent with mild to moderate dementia. HDS-R and MMSE scores improved in the DHA-treated group but not among patients who were not treated with DHA. Comparisons between groups were significant at 3 and 6 months for the HDS-R and at 6 months for the MMSE
Freund-Levi et al. (2006)	204 patients with mild to moderate AD and with acetylcholine esterase inhibitor treatment and a MMSE >15 points	A single dose of 1.7 g of DHA plus 0.6 g of EPA was administered. The duration of exposure was 6 months placebo-controlled and 6 months open for both groups	Primary outcome measures: MMSE and ADAS-cog. Secondary outcome measures: was global function as assessed with the CDR	Administration of n-3 PUFA in patients with mild to moderate AD did not delay the rate of cognitive decline according to the MMSE or ADAS-cog. However, positive effects were observed in a small group of patients with very mild AD (MMSE >27 points)
Kotani et al. (2006)	21 patients with mild cognitive dysfunction (12 MCI patients with supplementation and 9 MCI patients with placebo), 10 patients with organic brain lesions, and 8 patients with AD	A single dose of 240 mg/day of ARA and DHA, or 240 mg/day of olive oil (placebo). The duration of exposure was 3 months	The cognitive functions were evaluated using Japanese version of RBANS at two time points: before and 90 days after the supplementation	The MCI group with supplementation showed a significant improvement of the immediate memory and attention score. Organic group showed a significant improvement of immediate and delayed memory. However, there were no significant improvements of each score in AD and MCI placebo groups
Freund-Levi et al. (2008)	204 patients with mild to moderate AD and with acetylcholine esterase inhibitor treatment and a MMSE >15 points	A single dose of 1.7 g of DHA plus 0.6 g of EPA was administered. The duration of exposure was 6 months placebo-controlled and 6 months open for both groups	Neuropsychiatric symptoms were measured with NPI and MADRS. Care givers' burden and activities of daily living (DAD) were also assessed.	No significant overall treatment effects on neuropsychiatric symptoms, on activities of daily living or on caregiver's burden were found. However, significant positive treatment effects on the scores in the NPI agitation domain in APOE ε4 carriers and in MADRS scores in non-APOE ε4 carriers were found.

(continued)

Table 179.10 (continued)

Reference	Participants	Intervention and duration of exposure	Outcome measures	Effects of interventions
Chiu et al. (2008)	23 patients with mild to moderate AD and 23 patients with MCI	n-3 PUFA 1.8 g/day in monotherapy or placebo (olive oil). The duration of exposure was 24 weeks	Global clinical function measured with CIBIC-plus, cognitive function with ADAS-cog and MMSE, depressive symptoms with HDRS	This supplementation may improve global clinical function (CIBIC-plus) in MCI patients relative to placebo. No associations were found between randomization group and ADAS-cog, MMSE or HDRS scores
Van de Rest et al. (2008a)	Independently living individuals ($n = 302$) aged ≥ 65 years CES-D score < 16 MMSE score > 21	A single dose of 1,800 mg/day EPA+DHA ($n = 96$), 400 mg/day EPA+DHA ($n = 100$), or placebo capsules ($n = 106$); the duration of exposure was 26 weeks	Changes in mental well-being were assessed as the primary outcome with the CES-D, MADRS, GDS-15, and HADS-A	Treatment with neither 1800 mg nor 400 mg EPA+DHA differentially affected any of the measures of mental well-being after 13 or 26 weeks of intervention compared with placebo
Van de Rest et al. (2008b)	Independently living individuals ($n = 302$) aged ≥ 65 years CES-D score < 16 MMSE score > 21	A single dose of 1,800 mg/day EPA+DHA ($n = 96$), 400 mg/ day EPA+DHA ($n = 100$), or placebo capsules ($n = 106$); the duration of exposure was 26 weeks	Cognitive performance was assessed using an extensive neuropsychological test battery that included the cognitive domains of attention (SC-WT; fWDST), sensorimotor speed (TMT-A), memory (WLT; bWDST), and executive function (TMT-B; VFT)	There were no significant differential changes in any of the cognitive domains for either low-dose or high-dose fish oil supplementation compared with placebo; an effect of EPA–DHA supplementation in subjects who carried the APOE ε4 allele was also found, but only on the cognitive domain of attention

This table lists the principal findings of clinical trials on PUFA supplementation in patients with MCI, VaD, AD, and ARCD, including the intervention and duration of exposure, and the outcome measures used

DHA docosahexaenoic acid, *HDS-R* Hasegawa's Dementia rating scale, *MMSE* Mini-mental State Examination, *EPA* eicosapentaenoic acid, *ADAS-cog* cognitive portion of the Alzheimer Disease Assessment Scale, *CDR* Clinical Dementia Rating Scale, *ARA* arachidonic acid, *RBANS* Repeatable Battery for Assessment of Neuropsychological Status, *NPI* Neuropsychiatric Inventory, *MADRS* Montgomery Asberg Depression Scale, *DAD* Disability Assessment for Dementia, *APOE* apolipoprotein E, *CIBIC-plus* Clinician's Interview-Based Impression of Change Scale, *HDRS* Hamilton Depression rating Scale, *DRS-2* Dementia Rating Scale 2, *CDT* Clock Drawing Tests, *ADCS-ADL* Alzheimer's Disease Cooperative Study–Activities of Daily Living, *CES-D* Center for Epidemiologic Studies Depression Scale, *GDS-15* 15-item Geriatric Depression Scale, *HADS-A* Hospital Anxiety and Depression Scale, *SC-WT* Stroop Color–Word Test, *fWDST* forward test of the Wechsler Digit Span Task, *TMT-A* Trail Making Test version A, *WLT* Word Learning Test, *bWDST* backward test of the Wechsler Digit Span Task, *TMT-B* Trail Making Test version B, *VFT* Verbal Fluency Test

memory and attention score for MCI patients, and a significant improvement of immediate and delayed memories for patients with organic brain damages (Kotani et al. 2006) (Table 179.10). Finally, the preliminary results from a 24-week, randomized, double-blind placebo-controlled study on 23 participants with mild or moderate AD and 23 with MCI randomized to receive n-3 PUFA 1.8 g/day or placebo (olive oil), suggested that his supplementation may improve global clinical function, as measured by Clinician's Interview-Based Impression of Change scale which included caregiver-supplied information (CIBIC-plus), relative to placebo. No associations were found between the randomization group and ADAS-cog, MMSE, or Hamilton Depression rating Scale scores. Levels of EPA on erythrocyte membrane, were associated with cognitive function, measured by ADAS-cog, in these patients (Chiu et al. 2008) (Table 179.10). However, in a secondary analysis, participants with MCI showed more improvement of ADAS-cog than those with AD associated with n-3 PUFA administration (Chiu et al. 2008), which support recent reports showing that PUFA supplementation could be more beneficial on cognition in people with very mild AD (Freund-Levi et al. 2006) or MCI Kotani et al. 2006) than in AD patients (Table 179.10).

A few years ago, a Cochrane review concluded that there was a growing body of evidence from biological, observational, and epidemiological studies that suggested a protective effect of n-3 PUFA against dementia. However, the Cochrane review team was unable to locate a single published randomized controlled trial on which to base recommendations for the use of dietary or supplemental n-3 PUFA for the prevention of cognitive impairment or dementia (Lim et al. 2006). However, very recently, a randomized, double-blind, placebo-controlled trial on 302 cognitively healthy (MMSE score > 21) individuals aged 65 years or older investigated the possible impact of n-3 PUFA on the mental well-being and cognitive performance of nondepressed (CES-D score < 16), older individuals (van de Rest et al. 2008a, b) (Table 179.10). In this RCT, participants were randomly assigned to 1.800 mg/d EPA–DHA, 400 mg/d EPA–DHA, or placebo capsules for 26 weeks. In older Dutch subjects, no effect of daily supplementation with low or high doses of EPA-DHA on mental well-being as assessed by depression and anxiety questionnaires was found (van de Rest et al. 2008a). Furthermore, there were no significant differential changes in any of the cognitive domains (attention, sensorimotor speed, memory, and executive function) for either low-dose or high-dose fish oil supplementation compared with placebo (van de Rest et al. 2008b). However, an effect of EPA–DHA supplementation in subjects who carried the APOE-ε4 allele was found, but only on the cognitive domain of attention (van de Rest et al. 2008b). Fish oil may be beneficial in these subjects who are most sensitive to developing dementia. These two substantially negative studies on ARCD may be explained by the samples investigated (nondepressed and noncognitively impaired older subjects). Further trials in depressed patients or ε4-carriers with MCI are needed. Finally, there is another ongoing RCT with cognitive endpoints of n-3 PUFA supplementation in healthy cognitively intact older persons. The OPAL study is a double-blind randomized placebo-controlled trial examining the effect of daily supplementation with 700 mg n-3 PUFA (500 mg DHA and 200 mg EPA) for 24 months on cognitive performance in healthy older persons aged 70–79 with good cognitive function (MMSE equals or greater than 24 out of 30 points at baseline), who are recruited from 20 primary care practices (Dangour et al. 2006). The OPAL study was completed at the end of 2007 and its findings will be published shortly. Thus, epidemiological evidence has suggested a possible association between PUFA (particularly, n-3 PUFA) and reduced risk of cognitive decline and dementia. However, due to the small number of studies that inform this topic, further research is necessary before a strong conclusion can be drawn. Some recent RCTs assessed the cognitive or functional effect of n-3 PUFA supplementation on patients with VaD, AD, MCI, or ARCD in cognitively unimpaired older subjects. These RCTs suggested a positive effect of this intervention only in very mild AD or MCI patients, or in subgroups (e.g., APOE-e4 carriers) for cognitive performance in nondemented subjects or for neuropsychiatric symptoms in mild to moderate AD patients. On the basis of these evidences, we strongly suggest also for predementia syndromes, a high-risk condition for progression to dementia of vascular and degenerative origin, intervention trials using measures of dietary supplementation similar to the OmegAD Study to determine if such supplements will slow cognitive decline.

179.5 Dietary Unsaturated Fatty Acids and Cognitive Decline: Possible Mechanisms

179.5.1 Monounsaturated Fatty Acids and Cognitive Decline

Different pathways could contribute to the neuroprotective as well as the neurotrophic properties of UFA. As seen above, in the older subjects of the ILSA, there was a high consumption of olive oil, with an MUFA energy intake of 17.6%, 85% of which was derived from olive oil (Solfrizzi et al. 1999) (Fig. 179.1). In our population, the prolonged protection of MUFA intake against age-related changes in cognitive functions may be linked to the relevant quota of antioxidant compounds in olive oil, including low-molecular-weight phenols (Solfrizzi et al. 2005). In fact, animal studies suggested that diets high in antioxidant-rich foods, such as spinach, strawberries, and blueberries, rich in anthocyanins and other flavonoids may be beneficial in slowing age-related cognitive decline (Solfrizzi et al. 2005). The possible role of antioxidant compounds from olive oil do not diminish or otherwise alter the argument concerning the fatty acids, because this is only a possible explanation of the role of MUFA on age-related cognitive changes in our population, in which MUFA intake derived for a large part from olive oil.

The neuroprotective effects of dietary UFA could rely on their impact on membrane architecture. In fact, UFA have an important role in maintaining the structural integrity of neuronal membranes, determining the fluidity of synaptosomal membranes and thereby regulating neuronal transmission. Furthermore, essential fatty acids can modify the activity of certain membrane-bound enzymes (phospholipase A2, protein kinase C, and acetyltranferase), and the function of the neurotransmitters' receptors. Finally, free fatty acids, lipid metabolites, and phospholipids modify the function of membrane proteins including ion channels (Solfrizzi et al. 2005). Moreover, fatty acid composition of neuronal membranes in advancing age demonstrated an increase in MUFA content and a decrease in PUFA content (Solfrizzi et al. 2005). n-3 PUFA increase membrane fluidity by replacing n-6 PUFA and cholesterol from the membrane (Solfrizzi et al. 2005) maintaining an optimal membrane fluidity as obligatory for neurotransmitter binding and signaling within the cell (Solfrizzi et al. 2005). There is also evidence associating a dietary deficiency of n-3 PUFA with changes in cortical dopoaminergic function (Solfrizzi et al. 2005) (Fig. 179.5).

179.5.2 Polyunsaturated Fatty Acids and Cognitive Decline

In adult rats, learning and cognitive behavior are related to brain DHA status, which, in turn, is related to the levels of the dietary n-3 PUFA (Moriguchi et al. 2000). In fact, administration of DHA seems to improve learning ability in β-amyloid (Aβ)-infused rats (Hashimoto et al. 2005) and inhibit decline in avoidance learning ability in the AD model rats, associated with an increase in the cortico-hippocampal n-3/n-6 ratio, and a decrease in neuronal apoptotic products (Hashimoto et al. 2002).

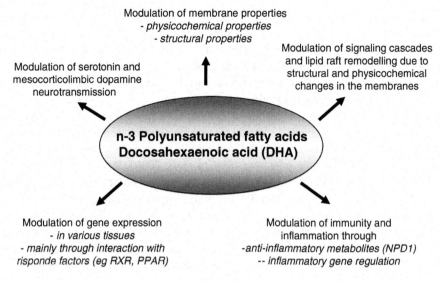

Fig. 179.5 Synopsis of the neuroprotective properties of *n*-3 polyunsaturated fatty acids (*PUFA*) and docosahexaenoic acid (*DHA*). This figure lists various possible molecular mechanisms of *n*-3 PUFA and DHA linked to their neuroprotective properties including modulation of membrane properties, serotonin, and dopamine neurotransmission, signaling cascades and lipid raft remodeling, gene expression, and immunity and inflammation (Modified from Florent-Béchard et al. 2007. With permission)

Similarly, recent studies showed that dietary DHA in an aged AD mouse model could be protective against Aβ production, deposition in plaques and cerebral amyloid angiopathy (Lim et al. 2005; Hooijmans et al. 2007), and increases cerebral blood volume (Hooijmans et al. 2007). In other transgenic AD mouse models, DHA also protects against dendritic pathology (Calon et al. 2004) and prevents neuronal apoptosis induced by soluble Aβ peptides (Florent et al. 2006), increases synaptic protein and phospholipid densities (Cole et al. 2005; Wurtman et al. 2006), and inhibits degradative endopeptidase activities (Park et al. 2003). Some experimental evidence has suggested that essential *n*-3 PUFA effectively lower Aβ production in transgenic mice, as reported in studies from several laboratories (Lim et al. 2005; Cole et al. 2005; Oksman et al. 2006). Yet, plaque burden was reduced in only one study using aged transgenic mice, following 3 months DHA enriched diet (Lim et al. 2005), but not in several other studies that started dietary intervention at a much younger age (Oksman et al. 2006; Hooijmans et al. 2007).

Furthermore, DHA, given its unique structural properties, could allow of the modification of the architectural properties of the membrane, especially the distribution and the abundance of lipid raft microdomains (Florent-Béchard et al. 2007). Lipid rafts are liquid ordered sphingomyelin-rich cholesterol-rich PUFA-poor microdomains. DHA and PUFA enrichment is known to be accompanied by lateral phase separation and local lipid redistribution, subtle membrane remodeling and selective displacement of proteins (Florent-Béchard et al. 2007) (Fig. 179.5). By changing the organization and/or composition of the lipid rafts, DHA could directly modify many signaling pathways such as those initiated at the plasma membrane (Florent-Béchard et al. 2007) (Fig. 179.5).

It is well known that PUFA of both *n*-3 and *n*-6 families control gene expression in a variety of tissues including liver and adipose tissue. However, the underlying mechanisms of the direct effects of dietary PUFA-induced differential gene expression pattern in the brain have been addressed by few studies (Florent-Béchard et al. 2007). Gene regulation by PUFA can occur through interactions with specific or nonspecific ligands such as transcription factors like peroxysome proliferator-activated receptors (PPAR) or retinoid X receptor (RXR) that directly modulate the expression of target genes (Florent-Béchard et al. 2007) (Fig. 179.5). The direct effects of PUFA on gene regulation might be one of the clues to understand the beneficial effects of the n-3 PUFA on the nervous system.

Several clinical and epidemiological studies have identified beneficial effects of PUFA for a variety of inflammatory diseases, yet without mechanistic explanations for these beneficial effects. Resolvins and protectins are recently identified molecules that are generated from n-3 PUFA precursors and can orchestrate the timely resolution of inflammation in model systems. In fact, DHA also serves as a precursor for the biosynthesis of additional bioactive counter-regulatory lipid mediators. For (neuro)protectin D1 (N)PD1 formation, DHA is rapidly released for conversion to 17S-hydroxy-DHA that serves as a biosynthetic precursor (Serhan et al. 2006). In AD, NPD1 biosynthesis is activated by soluble APP-α (Lukiw et al. 2005). In this disorder, levels of DHA, NPD1, and 15-lipoxygenase (15-LOX) are selectively decreased in the hippocampus, providing a plausible mechanism for decreased neuroprotection in AD: less inhibition of apoptosis and subsequently, increased neuronal cell death (Lukiw et al. 2005) (Fig. 179.5). In a placebo-controlled randomized trial, the OmegAD study, AD patients treated with DHA-rich dietary supplements had reduced release of interleukin (IL)-1b, IL-6 and granulocyte colony-stimulating factor from peripheral blood mononuclear cells (Vedin et al. 2008).

The n-3 PUFA from fish may be inversely associated with dementia because it lowers the risk of thrombosis, stroke, cardiovascular disease, and cardiac arrhythmia, reducing the risk of thromboembolism in the brain and consequently of lacunar and large infarcts that can lead to VaD and AD (Solfrizzi et al. 2005). Furthermore, the n-3 PUFA may be important as lipids in the brain, particularly for the possible influence of DHA on the physical properties of the brain that are essential for its function (Solfrizzi et al. 2005). Furthermore, fish oil was a better source than α-linolenic acid for the incorporation of n-3 PUFA into rat brain phospholipid subclasses (Solfrizzi et al. 2005). On the contrary, high linoleic acid intake (n-6 PUFA) may increase the susceptibility of LDL cholesterol to oxidation, which makes it more atherogenic, even if the association between linoleic acid and atherosclerosis is controversial (Solfrizzi et al. 2005). Therefore the ratio of dietary n-3/n-6 PUFA intake may influence the potential role of PUFA on cognitive decline and dementia, the optimal ratio of n-6/n-3 should be <5:1 (de Lorgeril et al. 1998). Finally, a high dietary intake of SFA and cholesterol increases the risk for cardiovascular disease, and therefore for cognitive decline, VaD, and AD (Solfrizzi et al. 2008). On the contrary, treatment for 4 weeks with a Mediterranean-inspired diet rich in n-3 PUFA decreased blood lipids in healthy individuals with a low-risk profile for cardiovascular disease, with a beneficial effect also on vascular function and oxidative stress (Ambring et al. 2004).

179.6 Applications to Other Areas of Health and Disease

About 50–60% of the dry weight portion of the human brain consists of lipids. PUFA constitute approximately 35 percent of that lipid content (Lauritzen et al. 2001). n-3 PUFA, particularly EPA and DHA, play important roles in the development and maintenance of normal central nervous system structure and function. Along with the n-6 PUFA, ARA, DHA is a major constituent of neuronal membranes, making up about 20% of the brain's dry weight (Yehuda et al. 1999). Synapses contain a high concentration of DHA, which appears to play a role in synaptic signal transduction (Jones et al. 1997). The metabolic pathways of the essential fatty acids that play an important role in neuronal signal transduction and release of these fatty acids is involved in the phospholipase A2 cycle following activation of various neurotransmitter receptors. DHA is also important for normal cognitive development. In addition, the anti-inflammatory compounds for which DHA is a precursor may function in the brain to protect against ischemic damage. PUFA in general play important roles in structural and functional maintenance of neuronal membranes, neurotransmission, and eicosanoid biosynthesis (Lauritzen et al. 2001; Tapiero et al. 2002), as well as in the maintenance of membrane fluidity and flexibility and in the modulation of ion channels, receptors, and ATPases. The importance of PUFA in the maintenance of adequate membrane rigidity is evidenced by the loss of fluidity that follows decrease in PUFA (Bourre et al. 1991), leading to changes in the orientation and function of receptors and ion channels, such as calcium and sodium channels.

Several lines of research have suggested that the high ratio of n-6 PUFA to low levels of n-3 PUFA currently consumed in occidental countries promotes a number of chronic diseases. Whether or not the relatively high intake of n-6 PUFA independently contributes to this problem is currently uncertain (Richardson 2003). Because of the slow rate of elongation and further desaturation of the essential fatty acids, the importance of PUFA to many physiological processes, and the overwhelming ratio of n-6 PUFA to n-3 PUFA in the average occidental diet, nutrition experts are increasingly recognizing the need for humans to augment the body's synthesis of n-3 PUFA by consuming foods that are rich in these compounds. According to data from two population-based surveys, the major dietary sources of n-3 PUFA in the US population are fish, fish oil, vegetable oils (principally canola and soybean), walnuts, wheat germ, and some dietary supplements, and the primary dietary sources of n-6 PUFA are meats and dairy products. These surveys, the Continuing Food Survey of Intakes by Individuals 1994–98 (CSFII) and the third National Health and Nutrition Examination (NHANES III) 1988–94 surveys, are the main sources of dietary intake data for the US population.

Other studies specifically addressed the association of n-3 PUFA consumption with risk or incidence of particular neurological diseases other than dementia, e.g., the incidence of multiple sclerosis (MS) (Ghadirian et al. 1998; Zhang et al. 2000), the risk of Parkinson's disease (PD) (Chen et al. 2003), and the risk of cerebral palsy (Petridou et al. 1998). The relationship between dietary intake of n-3 PUFA and incidence of MS was assessed in two reports; one pooled data from two large cohorts of women from the Nurses' Health Study (NHS) and the Nurses' Health Study II (NHS II) (Zhang et al. 2000), and the other used a case-control design (Ghadirian et al. 1998). The prospective cohort study assessed the effect of n-3 PUFA in terms of fish consumption, fish n-3 PUFA, ALA, EPA, and DHA. ALA was associated with a reduced risk of MS in both cohorts that did not reach statistical significance. Intakes of n-3 PUFA, EPA, or DHA were not associated with MS incidence. The case-control study evaluated 197 incident MS cases and 202 age-, sex- and neighborhood-matched controls and found no significant association between fish consumption and risk of MS overall. However, fish consumption was significantly associated with a lower risk of MS in females only (Ghadirian et al. 1998).

The relationship between dietary intake of n-3 PUFA and incidence of PD was assessed in one report that pooled data from two large prospective cohorts, the Health Professionals Follow-up Study and the NHS (Chen et al. 2003). This study assessed the effect of n-3 PUFA in terms of n-3 fats from fish, ALA, EPA, and DHA over a 6- to 8-year period. There was no significant association between fish n-3 PUFA, ALA, EPA, or DHA intake and risk of PD. In a pooled analysis of men and women across two cohorts, ALA was associated with a reduced risk of developing PD (RR = 0.65, 95% CI 0.46, 0.91 for comparison of highest to lowest quintiles of risk). Among women, there was a significant trend but no significant risk reduction for any individual quintile of consumption. This finding is particularly noteworthy given the statistical power of the Health Professionals Follow-up Study and the NHS and the longitudinal analysis of dietary intake in these studies.

One study evaluated the effects of maternal dietary intake on the risk of cerebral palsy in offspring in a case-control study of 91 cases of cerebral palsy identified from statistics of hospitals and rehabilitation centers in Greece and 246 neighborhood controls (Petridou et al. 1998). Mothers of cases and controls were interviewed about their dietary habits during pregnancy using a food-frequency questionnaire. Consumption of fish once a week throughout pregnancy was associated with a lower risk of cerebral palsy compared with no fish intake.

In the Mediterranean countries, the principal source of MUFA is olive oil, probably the most representative food in the traditional Mediterranean diet. The hypocholesterolemic effect of the isoenergetic substitution of dietary MUFA for SFA first generated interest in MUFA-rich fats, which include olive, canola, and high-oleic sunflower oils. However, olive oil has additional biological effects, related in part to MUFA but also to minor components, particularly antioxidant phenolics. Virgin olive oil, a pure olive juice, is particularly rich in phenolics. Increasing epidemiologic and clinical evidences suggest that MUFA as a nutrient, olive oil as a food, and the Mediterranean diet as a food pattern have beneficial effects on obesity, the metabolic syndrome, and diabetes (Perez-Jimenez et al. 2005). A Mediterranean diet rich in virgin olive oil and virgin olive oil per se have been shown to improve classical and novel cardiovascular risk factors, such as lipid profiles, blood pressure, postprandial lipemia, endothelial dysfunction, oxidative stress, inflammation, and thrombosis (Perez-Jimenez et al. 2005). Limited epidemiologic evidences from Mediterranean countries suggest that dietary MUFA and/or olive oil intake might protect against breast, colorectal and prostate cancer. Experimental cellular studies have provided new evidences on the potential protective effect of virgin olive oil on cancer (Perez-Jimenez et al. 2005).

179.7 Conclusions

Recently, several studies have suggested that an increase of SFA could have negative effects on cognitive functions. Furthermore, a clear reduction of risk for cognitive decline has been found in population samples with elevated fish consumption, high intake of MUFA and PUFA, particularly *n*-3 PUFA (Fig. 179.6). Recent findings have demonstrated that while dietary fatty acid intakes were not associated with incident MCI, high PUFA intake appeared to have a borderline nonsignificant trend

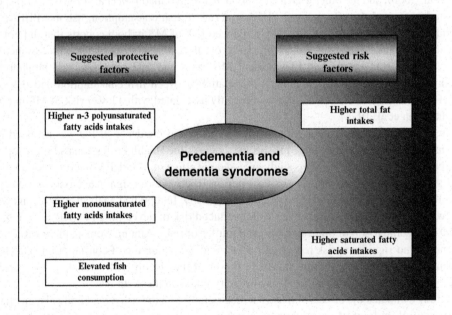

Fig. 179.6 Synopsis of the evidence on the possible effects of dietary fatty acids on predementia and dementia syndromes. This table lists the key possible effects of dietary fatty acids on predementia and dementia syndromes including *n*-3 polyunsaturated fatty acids, monounsaturated fatty acids, saturated fatty acids (*SFA*), and fish consumption

Table 179.11 Key points of studies on the relationships between dietary fatty acids and predementia and dementia syndromes

A. An increasing body of epidemiological evidence suggests that elevated saturated fatty acids (SFA) could have negative effects on age-related cognitive decline (ARCD). On the contrary, a reduction of risk for dementia and mild cognitive impairment (MCI) has been found in population samples with elevated fish consumption, high intake of monounsaturated fatty acids (MUFA) and polyunsaturated fatty acids (PUFA), particularly n-3 PUFA

B. Recent findings from clinical trials with n-3 PUFA supplementation have shown efficacy on depressive symptoms in non-apolipoprotein E (APOE) ε4 carriers, and on cognitive symptoms only in very mild Alzheimer's disease (AD) subgroups, MCI patients, and cognitively unimpaired subjects non-APOE ε4 carriers

C. The evidence coming from clinical trials together with epidemiological findings support the idea that n-3 PUFA may play a role in maintaining adequate cognitive functioning in predementia syndromes, but not when the AD process has already taken over. Therefore, at present, no definitive dietary recommendations on fish and unsaturated fatty acids consumption or lower intake of saturated fat in relation to the risk for predementia and dementia syndromes are possible

This table lists the principal features of clinical and epidemiological studies on the relationships between dietary fatty acids and predementia (MCI and ARCD) and dementia syndromes (AD and vascular dementia), including findings of clinical trials on PUFA supplementation in these patients

for a protective effect against the development of MCI. Nonetheless, at present, no definitive dietary recommendations on fish and UFA consumption or lower intake of saturated fat in relation to the risk for dementia and cognitive decline are possible (Table 179.11). In fact, in a recent randomized controlled trial, n-3 PUFA supplementation did not influence cognitive functioning during a follow-up of 6 months except in a small group of patients with very mild AD and for possible positive effects on depressive symptoms in non-APOE ε4 carriers. These data together with epidemiological evidence support the idea that n-3 PUFA may have a role in the primary and maybe secondary prevention of the disease but not when the disease process has already taken over. However, high levels of consumption of fats from fish, vegetable oils, and vegetables should be encouraged because this dietary advice is in accordance with recommendations for lowering the risk of cardiovascular disease, obesity, diabetes, and hypertension. Therefore, epidemiological studies on the association between diet and cognitive decline suggested a possible role of fatty acids intake in maintaining adequate cognitive functioning and possibly in preventing or delaying the onset of dementia, both of degenerative or vascular origin. Appropriate dietary measures or supplementation with specific macronutrients might open new ways for the prevention and management of cognitive decline and dementia (Solfrizzi et al. 2008).

On the other hand, Scarmeas and colleagues, using an inclusive dietary score (MeDi score) but studying a population with a substantial difference in dietary habits in comparison with Greek (EPIC) (Psaltopoulou et al. 2008) and Italian (ILSA) (Solfrizzi et al. 2006a, b) cohorts, found that higher adherence to the Mediterranean diet is associated with a trend for reduced risk of incident MCI and with reduced risk of MCI progression to AD (Scarmeas et al. 2009). The use of diet-scoring systems such as the MeDi score has undeniable advantages in understanding the role of diet in chronic disease (Solfrizzi et al. 2006c). They may account for the complex biological interactions between different components of a composite dietary pattern, such as a Mediterranean diet, that may be difficult to detect in analyses focusing only on individual components (Trichopoulou et al. 2006). These contrasting findings about the impact of MeDi score or individual macronutrients on ARCD or MCI may suggest an approach not confined only to cognitive skills but extended to functional status and comorbidity. However, we should not renounce a priori the work for a correct estimate of the validity of the MeDi score for cognitive impairment as a criterion. In fact, the evidence about the role of the whole Mediterranean diet on cognitive decline are still scarce (Psaltopoulou et al. 2008; Scarmeas et al. 2009). Therefore, in future studies, it would be indicated, along with measuring this effect by a dietary composite score, also to report the estimates and the impact of the individual components of the diet. In a very recent re-analysis from the ILSA cohort, we showed that high PUFA were associated with reduced risk of incident MCI among who consumed a low MUFA/SFA ratio intake (Solfrizzi et al. 2009). Therefore, it should be advisable to include PUFA in the MeDi score as individual macronutrient (such as MUFA/SFA ratio), among the components presumed to be beneficial, in evaluating the relationship between adherence to Mediterranean diet and ARCD or MCI. In fact, while an increasing body of evidence suggested that elevated fish consumption and high intake of n-3 PUFA may be protective against ARCD and MCI, the traditional Cretan diet, although strongly dependent on high olive oil intake, was never centered on fish consumption. In this context, n-6 PUFA could potentially exert some health benefits. In fact, in a Mediterranean diet, some foods are rich in n-6 PUFA (e.g., walnuts, almonds, hazelnuts), while other foods, although poor in n-6 PUFA, are highly consumed such as cereals, legumes, and, in less amount, some types of meat (pork), and poultry. Furthermore, olive oil contains n–6 and n–3 PUFA in a ratio of 10:1. Therefore, it should be advisable to include PUFA in the MeDi score as individual macronutrient (such as MUFA/SFA ratio), among the components presumed to be beneficial, in evaluating the relationship between adherence to Mediterranean diet and ARCD or MCI (Solfrizzi et al. 2009).

Summary Points

- Dietary and vascular factors are associated with increasing risk of predementia and dementia syndromes.
- Among different dietary patterns, adherence to a traditional Mediterranean diet was associated with a significant reduction in risk for Alzheimer's disease (AD).
- Among dietary factors, a clear reduction of risk of cognitive decline has been found in a population sample with a high intake of polyunsaturated fatty acids (PUFA) and monounsaturated fatty acids (MUFA).
- Cumulative evidence has suggested that elevated saturated fatty acids (SFA) could have negative effects on age-related cognitive decline (ARCD).
- Recent findings have demonstrated that while dietary fatty acids intakes were not associated with incident mild cognitive impairment (MCI), high PUFA intake appeared to have a borderline non-significant trend for a protective effect against the development of MCI.
- Recent findings from clinical trials with n-3 PUFA supplementation, showing efficacy on cognitive and depressive symptoms only in very mild AD subgroups or MCI, suggest a possible role of fatty acid intake in maintaining adequate cognitive functioning and possibly for the prevention and management of cognitive decline and dementia.

Definitions

Unsaturated and saturated fatty acids: Unsaturated fat is fat or fatty acid in which there are one or more double bonds in the fatty acid chain. A fat molecule is monounsaturated if it contains one double bond, and polyunsaturated if it contains more than one double bond. Whendouble bonds are formed, hydrogen atoms are eliminated. Thus,saturated fat is "saturated" with hydrogen atoms.

Dementia: This is a syndrome defined by impairments in memory and other cognitive functions that are severe enough to cause significant decline from a previous level of social and occupational functioning.

Predementia syndrome: This term identifies all conditions with age-related deficits in cognitive function, including a mild stage of cognitive impairment based on a normality model and pathological conditions considered predictive of early stages of dementia

Mild cognitive impairment (MCI): This is a clinical label that includes non-demented aged persons with memory impairment and no significant disability.

Age-related cognitive decline (ARCD): This is defined as an objectively identified decline in cognitive functioning consequent to the aging process that is within normal limits given the person's age, but there are no defined diagnostic criteria, and few epidemiological studies using this definition have been conducted.

Acknowledgments This work was supported by the Italian Longitudinal Study on Aging (ILSA) (Italian National Research Council-CNR-Targeted Project on Ageing-Grants 9400419PF40 and 95973PF40).

References

Ambring A, Friberg P, Axelsen M, Laffrenzen M, Taskinen MR, Basu S, Johansson M Clin Sci. 2004;106:519–25.

American Psychiatric Association Committee on Nomenclature and Statistics. Diagnostic and statistical manual of mental disorders. Washington, DC: American Psychiatric Association; 1994.

Barberger-Gateau P, Letenneur L, Deschamps V, Peres K, Dartigues JF, Renaud S. BMJ. 2002;325:932–3.

Barberger-Gateau P, Raffaitin C, Letenneur L, Berr C, Tzourio C, Dartigues JF, Alperovitch A. Neurology. 2007;69:1921–30.

Bourre JM, Dumont O, Piciotti M, Clement M, Chaudiere J, Bonneil M, Nalbone G, Lafont H, Pascal G, Durand G. In: Simopoulos AP, Kifer RR, Martin RE, Barlow SM, editors. Health effects of omega-3 polyunsaturated fatty acids in seafoods. Vol. 66. Karger/Basel/Switzerland: World Rev. Nutr. Diet.; 1991. p. 103–117.

Calon F, Lim GP, Yang F, Morihara T, Teter B., Ubeda O, Rostaing P, Triller A, Salem N, Ashe KH, Frautschy SA, Cole GM. Neuron. 2004;43:633–45.

Chen H, Zhang SM, Hernan MA, Willett WC, Ascherio A. Am J Epidem. 2003;157:1007–14.

Chiu CC, Su KP, Cheng TC, Liu HC, Chang CJ, Dewey ME, Stewart R, Huang SY. Prog Neuropsychopharmacol Biol Psychiatry. 2008;32:1538–44.

Cole GM, Lim GP, Yang F, Teter B, Begum A, Ma Q, Harris-White ME, Frautschy SA. Neurobiol Aging. 2005;26 (Suppl 1):133–6.

Dangour AD, Clemens F, Elbourne D, Fasey N, Fletcher AE, Hardy P, Holder GE, Huppert FA, Knight R, Letley L, Richards M, Truesdale A, Vickers M, Uauy R. Nutr J. 2006;5:20.

Dangour AD, Allen E, Elbourne D, Fletcher A, Richards M, Uauy R. J Nutr Health Aging 2009;13:198–202.

de Lorgeril M, Salen P, Martin JL, Monjaud I, Boucher P, Mamelle N. Arch Intern Med. 1998;158:1181–7.

Engelhart MJ, Geerlings MI, Ruitenberg A, Van Swieten JC, Hofman A, Witteman JC, Breteler MM. Neurology. 2002;59:1915–21.

Eskelinen MH, Ngandu T, Helkala EL, Tuomilehto J, Nissinen A, Soininen H, Kivipelto M. Int J Geriatr Psychiatry. 2008;23:741–7.

Florent S, Malaplate-Armand C, Youssef I, Kriem B, Koziel V, Escanye M-C, Fifre A, Sponne I, Leininger-Muller B, Olivier J-L, Pillot T, Oster T. J Neurochem. 2006;96:385–95.

Florent-Béchard S, Malaplate-Armand C, Koziel V, Kriem B, Olivier JL, Pillot T, Oster T. J Neurol Sci. 2007;262:27–36.

Freund-Levi Y, Eriksdotter-Jönhagen M, Cederholm T, Basun H, Faxén-Irving G, Garlind A, Vedin I, Vessby B, Wahlund LO, Palmblad J. Arch Neurol. 2006;63:1402–8.

Freund-Levi Y, Basun H, Cederholm T, Faxén-Irving G, Garlind A, Grut M, Vedin I, Palmblad J, Wahlund LO, Eriksdotter-Jönhagen M. Int J Geriatr Psychiatry. 2008;23:161–9.

Gauthier S, Reisberg B, Zaudig M. Lancet. 2006;367:1262–70.

Ghadirian P, Meera J, Ducic S, Shatenstein B, Morisset R, Jain M. Int J Epidem. 1998;27:845–52.

Grant WB. Alzheimers Dis Rev. 1997;2:42–55.

Grant WB. J Alzheimers Dis. 1999;1:197–201.

Hashimoto M, Hossain S, Shimada T, Sugioka K, Yamasaki H, Fujii Y, Ishibashi Y, Oka J, Shido O. J Neurochem. 2002;81:1084–91.

Hashimoto M, Tanabe Y, Fujii Y, Kikuta T, Shibata H, Shido O. J Nutr. 2005;135:549–55.

Hende B, Ducimitiere P, Berr C. Am J Clin Nutr. 2003;77:803–8.

Hooijmans CR, Rutters F, Dederen PJ, Gambarota G, Veltien A, van Groen, T, Broersen LM, Lütjohann D, Heerschap A, Tanila H, Kiliaan AJ. Neurobiol Dis. 2007;28:16–29.

Huang TL, Zandi PP, Tucker KL, Fitzpatrick AL, Kuller LH, Fried LP, Burke GL, Carlson MC. Neurology. 2005;65:1409–14.

Jones C, Arai T, Rapoport S. Neurochem Res. 1997;22:663–70.

Kalmijn S, Feskens EJ, Launer LJ, Kromhout D. Am J Epidemiol. 1997a;145:33–41.

Kalmijn S, Launer LJ, Ott A, Witteman JC, Hofman A, Breteler MM. Ann Neurol. 1997b;42:776–82.

Kalmijn S, van Boxtel MP, Ocke M, Verschuren WM, Kromhout D, Launer LJ. Neurology. 2004;62:275–80.

Kotani S, Sakaguchi E, Warashina S, Matsukawa N, Ishikura Y, Kiso Y, Sakakibara M, Yoshimoto T, Guo J, Yamashima T. Neurosci Res. 2006;56:159–64.

Laitinen MH, Ngandu T, Rovio S, Helkala E-L, Uusitalo U, Viitanen M, Nissinen A, Tuomilehto J, Soininen H, Kivipelto M. Dement Geriatr Cogn Disord. 2006;22:99–107.

Lauritzen L, Hansen HS, Jorgensen MH, Michaelsen KF. Prog Lipid Res. 2001;40:1–94.

Levy R. Int Psychogeriatrics. 1994;6:63–8.

Lim GP, Calon F, Morihara T, Yang F, Teter B, Ubeda O, Salem Jr N, Frautschy SA, Cole GM. J Neurosci. 2005; 25:3032–40.

Lim WS, Gammack JK, Van Niekerk JK, Dangour A (2006) Cochrane Database Syst. Rev: CD005379.

Luchsinger JA, Tang MX, Shea S, Mayeux R. Arch Neurol. 2002;59:1256–63.

Lukiw WJ, Cui JG, Marcheselli VL, Bodker M, Botkjaer A, Gotlinger K, Serhan CN, Bazan NG. J Clin Invest. 2005;115:2774–83.

Manzato E, Roselli della Rovere G, Zambon S, Romanato G, Corti MC, Sartori L, Baggio G, Crepaldi G. Aging Clin Exp Res. 2003;15:83–6.

Moriguchi T, Greiner RS, Salem N. J Neurochem. 2000;75:2563–73.

Morris MC, Evans DA, Bienias JL, Tangney CC, Bennett DA, Aggarwal N, Schneider J, Wilson RS. Arch Neurol. 2003a;60:194–200.

Morris MC, Evans DA, Bienias JL, Tangney CC, Bennett DA, Wilson RS, Aggarwal N, Schneider J. Arch Neurol. 2003b;60:940–6.

Morris MC, Evans DA, Bienias JL, Tangney CC, Bennett DA, Wilson RS. Neurology. 2004;62:1573–9.

Morris MC, Evans DA, Tangney CC, Bienias JL, Schneider JA, Wilson RS, Scherr PA. Arch Neurol. 2005a;63:1085–8.

Morris MC, Evans DA, Tangney CC, Bienias JL, Wilson RS. Arch Neurol. 2005b;62:1849–53.

Nurk E, Drevon CA, Refsum H, Solvoll K, Vollset SE, Nygård O, Nygaard HA, Engedal K, Tell GS, Smith DA. Am J Clin Nutr. 2007;86:1470–8.

Oksman M, Iivonen H, Hogyes E, Amtul Z, Penke B, Leenders I, Broersen L, Lutjohann D, Hartmann T, Tanila H. Neurobiol Dis. 2006;23:563–72.

Ortega RM, Requejo AM, Andres P, Lopez-Sobaler AM, Quintas ME, Redondo MR, Navia B, Rivas T. Am J Clin Nutr. 1997;66:803–9.

Petersen RC, Smith GE, Waring SC, Ivnik RJ, Tangalos EG, Kokmen E. Arch Neurol. 1999;56:303–8.

Petersen RC, Doody R, Kurz A, Mohs RC, Morris JC, Rabins PV, Ritchie K, Rossor M, Thal L, Winblad B. Arch Neurol. 2001;58:1985–92.

Petridou E, Koussouri M, Toupadaki N, Youroukos S, Papavassiliou A, Pantelakis S, Olsen J, Trichopoulos D. Br J Nutr. 1998;79:407–12.

Panza F, Solfrizzi V, Colacicco AM., D'Introno A, Capurso C, Torres F, Del Parigi A, Capurso S, Capurso A. Public Health Nutr. 2004;7:959–63.

Panza F, D'Introno A, Colacicco AM, Capurso C, Del Parigi A, Caselli RJ, Pilotto A, Argentieri G, Scapicchio PL, Scafato E, Capurso A, Solfrizzi V. Am J Geriatr Psychiatry. 2005;13:633–44.

Perez-Jimenez F, Alvarez de Cienfuegos G, Badimon L, Barja G, Battino M, Blanco A, Bonanome A, Colomer R, Corella-Piquer D, Covas I, Chamorro-Quiros J, Escrich E, Gaforio JJ, Garcia Luna PP, Hidalgo L, Kafatos A, Kris-Etherton PM, Lairon D, Lamuela-Raventos R, Lopez-Miranda J, Lopez-Segura F, Martinez-Gonzalez MA, Mata P, Mataix J, Ordovas J, Osada J, Pacheco-Reyes R, Perucho M, Pineda-Priego M, Quiles JL, Ramirez-Tortosa MC, Ruiz-Gutierrez V, Sanchez-Rovira P, Solfrizzi V, Soriguer-Escofet F, de la Torre-Fornell R, Trichopoulos A, Villalba-Montoro JM, Villar-Ortiz JR, Visioli F. Eur J Clin Invest. 2005;35:421–4.

Park IH, Hwang EM, Hong HS, Boo JH, Oh SS, Lee J, Jung MW, Bang OY, Kim SU, Mook-Jung I. Neurobiol Aging. 2003;24:637–43.

Pradignac A, Schlienger JL, Velten M, Mejean L. Aging Clin Exp Res. 1995;7:67–74.

Psaltopoulou T, Kyrozis A, Stathopoulos P, Trichopoulos D, Vassilopoulos D, Trichopoulou A. Public Health Nutr. 2008;11:1–9.

Qiu C, De Ronchi D, Fratiglioni L. Curr Opin Psychiatry. 2007;20:380–5.

Richardson AJ. Scand J Nutr/Naringsforskning. 2003;47:92–8.

Ross GW, Petrovitch H, White LR, Masaki KH, Li CY, Curb JD, Yano K, Rodriguez BL, Foley DJ, Blanchette PL, Havlik R. Neurology. 1999;53:337–43.

Schaefer EJ, Bongard V, Beiser AS, Lamon-Fava S, Robins SJ, Au R, Tucker KL, Kyle DJ, Wilson PW, Wolf PA. Arch Neurol. 2006;63:1545–50.

Serhan CN, Gotlinger K, Hong S, Lu Y, Siegelman J, Baer T, Yang R, Colgan SP, Petasis NA. J Immunol. 2006;176:1848–59.

Solfrizzi V, Panza F, Torres F, Mastroianni F, Del Parigi A, Venezia A, Capurso A. Neurology. 1999;52:1563–69.

Solfrizzi V, D'Introno A, Colacicco AM, Capurso C, Del Parigi A, Capurso S, Gadaleta A, Capurso A, Panza F. Exp Gerontol. 2005;40:257–70.

Solfrizzi V, Colacicco AM, D'Introno A, Capurso C, Torres F, Rizzo C, Capurso A, Panza F. Neurobiol Aging. 2006a; 27:1694–704.

Solfrizzi V, Colacicco AM, D'Introno A, Capurso C, Del Parigi A, Capurso SA, Argentieri G, Capurso A, Panza F. Exp Gerontol. 2006b;41:619–27.

Solfrizzi V, Capurso C, D'Introno A, Colacicco AM, Capurso A, Panza F. J Am Geriatr Soc. 2006c;54:1800–2.

Solfrizzi V, Capurso C, D'Introno A, Colacicco AM, Frisardi V, Santamato A, Ranieri M, Fiore P, Vendemiale G, Seripa D, Pilotto A, Capurso A, Panza F. J Nutr Health Aging. 2008;12:382–6.

Solfrizzi V, Frisardi V, Capurso C, D'Introno A, Colacicco AM, Chiloiro R, Dellegrazie F, Di Palo A, Capurso A, Panza F. J Am Geriatr Soc. 2009;57:1944–6.

Scarmeas N, Stern Y, Mayeux R, Manly JJ, Schupf N, Luchsinger JA. Arch Neurol. 2009;66:216–25.

Tapiero H, Nguyen Ba G, Couvreur P, Tew KD. Biomed Pharmacother. 2002;56:215–22.

Terano T, Fujishiro S, Ban T, Yamamoto K, Tanaka T, Noguchi Y, Tamura Y, Yazawa K, Hirayama T. Lipids. 1999;34(suppl):S345–6.

Trichopoulou A, Orfanos P, Norat T, Bueno-de-Mesquita B, Ocké MC, Peeters PH, van der Schouw YT, Boeing H, Hoffmann K, Boffetta P, Nagel G, Masala G, Krogh V, Panico S, Tumino R, Vineis P, Bamia C, Naska A, Benetou V, Ferrari P, Slimani N, Pera G, Martinez-Garcia C, Navarro C, Rodriguez-Barranco M, Dorronsoro M, Spencer EA, Key TJ, Bingham S, Khaw KT, Kesse E, Clavel-Chapelon F, Boutron-Ruault MC, Berglund G, Wirfalt E, Hallmans G, Johansson I, Tjonneland A, Olsen A, Overvad K, Hundborg HH, Riboli E, Trichopoulos D. BMJ. 2006;330:1329–30.

van Gelder BM, Tijhuis M, Kalmijn S, Kromhout D. Am J Clin Nutr. 2007;85:1142–7.

van de Rest O, Geleijnse JM, Kok FJ, van Staveren WA, Hoefnagels WH, Beekman AT, de Groot LC. Am J Clin Nutr. 2008;88:706–13.

van de Rest O, Geleijnse JM, Kok FJ, van Staveren WA, Dullemeijer C, Olderikkert MG, Beekman AT, de Groot CP. Neurology. 2008;71:430–8.

Vedin I, Cederholm T, Freund Levi Y, Basun H, Garlind A, Faxén Irving G, Jönhagen ME, Vessby, B, Wahlund LO, Palmblad J. Am J Clin Nutr. 2008;87:1616–22.

Vercambre MN, Boutron-Ruault MC, Ritchie K, Clavel-Chapelon F, Berr C. Br J Nutr. 2009;102:419–27.

Winblad B, Palmer K, Kivipelto M, Jelic V, Fratiglioni L, Wahlund LO, Nordberg A, Backman L, Albert M, Almkvist O, Arai H, Basun H, Blennow K, de Leon M, DeCarli C, Erkinjuntti T, Giacobini E, Graff C, Hardy J, Jack C, Jorm A, Ritchie K, van Duijn C, Visser P, Petersen RC. J Intern Med. 2004;256:240–46.

Wurtman RJ, Ulus IH, Cansev M, Watkins CJ, Wang L, Marzloff G. Brain Res. 2006;1088:83–92.

Yehuda S, Rabinovtz S, Carasso RL, Mostofsky DI. Int J Neurosci. 1996;87:141–9.

Yehuda S, Rabinovitz S, Mostofsky DI. J Neurosci Res. 1999;56:565–70.

Zhang SM, Willett WC, Hernan MA, Olek MJ, Ascherio A. Am J Epidem. 2000;152:1056–64.

Chapter 180
Nutritional Issues for Older People and Older People with Dementia in Institutional Environments

Angela B. Kydd

Abbreviations

BAPEN   British Association for Parenteral and Enteral Nutrition
ENHA   European Nutrition for Health Alliance

180.1 Introduction

Nutrition has always been a factor in the care of ill people and chapters on nutrition were common-place, and still are, in nursing textbooks. In the field of gerontology, authors such as Potter and Perry (1993:1094) suggest that when treatments or therapies were lacking, care relied heavily on the *preparation and administration* of food to maintain the body's strength and fight disease. Later nursing texts, for example, Ebersole et al. (2008), devote a chapter to nutrition and again emphasize the importance of ensuring that patients take adequate fluids and diet. The authors stress the problems associated with poor nutrition and provide strategies to ensure that all patients have the opportunity to eat well by giving them assistance and by providing them with an atmosphere conducive to eating. It appears to be simple; people need adequate food and fluids to maintain and to restore health. However, on further exploration of factors affecting the nutritional needs of older people, providing an environment conductive to eating and making mealtimes special are an essential part of nutritional care.

This chapter highlights the problems of poor nutrition for an ever increasing ageing population who are in institutions (hospital or care home). It goes on to examine·why, when there are so many directives for, and standards on, good nutritional care, frail older people and people with dementia are failing to have their nutritional needs met. The conclusion centres on the fact that directives and standards are aimed at managers and qualified staff, yet the direct care of serving food and assisting with meals is carried out by care assistants who have no knowledge of best practices (Table 180.1).

A.B. Kydd (✉)
School of Health Nursing and Midwifery, University of the West of Scotland, Hamilton Campus, Almada Street,
Hamilton, Lanarkshire, ML3 0JB, UK
e-mail: angela.kydd@uws.ac.uk

V.R. Preedy et al. (eds.), *Handbook of Behavior, Food and Nutrition,*
DOI 10.1007/978-0-387-92271-3_180, © Springer Science+Business Media, LLC 2011

Table 180.1 Key facts of ageing

- Ageing is a complex, natural process potentially involving every molecule, cell and organ in the body.
- In its broadest sense, ageing merely refers to changes that occur during the lifespan and is marked by time.
- Chronological ageing is not a disease, but biological ageing involves internal and external factors that negatively impact on an individual's system
- As individuals grow older, they do lose functional reserve, which means that their bodies do lose the ability to compensate when threatened by disease or hardship
- The term Frailty is common, but there is no consensus on its definition, apart from that it is caused by many factors including anorexia and weight loss and is a state of vulnerability
- Poor nutrition is recognised as one of the physical factors leading to frailty

This table illustrates the difference between chronological age, marked by years, and biological age, marked by factors that negatively impact on an individual's bodily functions. It highlights the important of maintaining an older person's nutritional status as poor nutrition can compromise an individual's ability to combat disease

Table 180.2 Three calls to action from the European Nutrition for Health Alliance (2005)

Action	Recommendation
1	Malnutrition is 'alive and killing'. It must be recognised as a disease in its own right
2	The high prevalence of malnutrition can no longer be tolerated. It is a serious social and economic issue with significant repercussions for individuals and society as a whole
3	Every stakeholder needs to take ownership and action to address the problem. Malnutrition occurs across all settings. Targeted actions are needed to address the root causes of malnutrition and empower individuals to foster 'well nutrition' for themselves

The calls to action were drawn from discussions and recommendations from the ENHA 2005 conference. In identifying malnutrition as a disease, the onus is on stakeholders to see this as a condition that needs treating as much as any other disease or disorder

180.2 The Extent of the Problem of Poor Nutrition in Older People

There is high incidence of malnutrition in the older age groups. This is a cause for major concern and more worryingly, not a new concern. Addressing poor nutrition has been on the health and social care agenda for many years. The statistics make depressing reading.

In 2005, the European Nutrition for Health Alliance (ENHA) published an inaugural conference report which stated that 46% of all hospitalized patients in Europe are malnourished on admission to hospital. The figure rises to 50% for those over the age of 60. The report stated that as one third of all Europeans will be over 60 in 2050, malnutrition is a serious problem and a critical issue for Europe. The recommendations from the conference are presented in Table 180.2.

Statistics from Age Concern England (2006) show a higher incidence, with estimates that 60% of people over 60 are at risk of becoming malnourished.

Prevalence of malnutrition does increase with age (ENHA 2005) but malnutrition is not a normal part of ageing. For those who are not in ill health, a healthy diet can result in many years of active life into old age (Department of Health 2001). Indeed, many people over the age of 65 are healthy and living full lives, with only 7% being classed as "frail" (Fried et al. 2004).

180.3 The Increase in the Numbers of Frail Older People in the UK

The prevalence of frailty increases up to 40% in persons aged 85 and over, and given the dramatic increase of the oldest-old population (those 85 and over), frailty is becoming increasingly common (Table 180.3).

Table 180.3 The ageing population

Year	Population over 65 (%)	Those aged 65–74 (%)	Those aged 75–84 (%)	85 years or older (%)
2006	16.4	8.9	5.5	2
2021	19.2	10.4	6.3	2.5
2051	24.4	10.7	8.8	4.9

Figures from the Office of Health Economics (2009) to illustrate the projected percentage increase in the numbers of frail older people in the United Kingdom (UK)

The incidence of dementia also increases with age. Approximately 2% of persons aged over 65 have some form of dementia, but prevalence rises to 20% in those over 80. In terms of numbers, this means there are currently 670,000 people with dementia in the UK, and this figure is expected to rise to nearly 1,000,000 by 2021 (Barratt 2004). If the above projections are realized, this figure is set to double in 2050.

These statistics have serious implications when coupled with the statistics on the number of older people thought to be malnourished.

180.4 Malnutrition in Institutions

In the early 1990s attention was paid to the fact that older people in institutional care were not having their nutritional needs met. A wealth of publications resulted. In 1991, the Committee on Medical Aspects of Food Policy [COMA] found that nearly 50% of people in care had nutrient deficiencies. In 1992 COMA reported that further research needed to be carried out on the nutritional needs of frail older people. The King's Fund Centre report (Lennard-Jones 1992) suggested the benefit of treating poor nutritional states would only be realised when nutritional assessment on every patient was routine.

In 1995, the Caroline Walker Trust recommended that all older people entering residential care accommodation should have their nutritional needs assessed in the first week after admission, and should be monitored regularly thereafter. This recommendation was reiterated in 1996 by BAPEN. In 1997 the publication *Hungry in Hospital* by the Association of Community Health Councils in England and Wales (ACHEW) identified the need for nurses to assess nutritional status and ensure that frail older people received adequate nutrition. Yet a National study by Finch et al. (1998) reported that of 412 people over the age of 65 living in institutions, 16% of men and 15% of women were underweight.

Currently, there are many recommendations of how to address the problem of poor nutrition of older people in institutions. In 2003, BAPEN developed a valid and reliable nutritional screening tool to identify people who were underweight and those at risk of under-nutrition; the Malnutrition Universal Screening Tool (MUST). Standards to address the nutritional needs of older people in institutions were published by the Nutrition Advisory Group for Elderly People (NAGE) (2005), the Food Standards Agency (2006) and the Commission for Social Care Inspection (2006) in England and NHS Quality Improvement Scotland (2003) and the Care Commission in Scotland (2009).

Best practices and standards for good nutritional care, *all* include the need for qualified and unqualified staff to recognize both the physical and psychosocial aspects of mealtimes and the importance of food and fluids. These have been outlined in Table 180.4 and expanded below.

However, life in institutions frequently centre on the routine tasks to be performed, and rather than be seen as an enjoyable way to break up an otherwise long day, mealtimes are treated as a task to be accomplished at certain times.

Table 180.4 Intrinsic and extrinsic risk factors for malnutrition in care

Domain	Examples of intrinsic risk factors	Examples of extrinsic risk factors
Physical	Arthritic	Fasted prior to surgery
	In pain	Inability to use utensils
	Xerostomia (dry mouth)	Medicines given prior to mealtimes
	Oral thrush or mouth ulcers	Food not hot/cold enough
	Poorly fitting dentures	
	Sensory loss	
	Constipated	
	Nauseated	
	Side effects of medication	
	Difficulties with chewing/swallowing	
Psycho-social	Depression	Dislikes people sharing the table
	Confusion	Poor relationship with staff
	Delirium	Noisy environment
	Dementia	Untrained staff
	Feeling rushed/anxious, frightened/ withdrawn/stressed/agitated	Dislikes food
		Food not suitable for the individual
	Not able to recognize food	Meal served in unsuitable surroundings
	Unable to move food from plate to mouth	such as a clinical area with urinals/vomit bowls in sight
	Unable to accept current situation	
	Dining area not conducive to eating	No sense of occasion

Physical and psychosocial considerations as risk factors for malnutrition

180.5 Meals in Institutions

The recommendations and standards of good nutritional care stress the importance of the intrinsic and extrinsic factors associated with mealtimes and food, yet meals served in institutions are still reported to be an unpleasant experience. Sadly, early literature of life in institutions such as Goffman (1961) on *block treatment* and Miller and Gwynne (1971) on *warehousing* is found in more current literature such as institutional disrespect (Kitwood 1997) and lack of personalised care (Kydd 2006; Kerr et al. 2008).

180.5.1 The Social Environment

The social aspect of meals should not be underestimated, yet mealtimes in some institutions can be anti-social. Staff can appear like wardens, overseeing patients eating, and the environment can be noisy and alarming. Studies (e.g., Mathey et al. 2001; Desai et al. 2007) have shown that when institutionalised mealtimes were changed to more homely environments, the results showed improved food consumption and therefore improved nutritional status in older people. Providing a homely environment includes providing a set dining area, matching crockery, a nicely set table, with glasses for water and a water jug.

180.5.2 Institutional Food

Whilst the social environment of mealtimes is important, so are the food and fluids. Some foods served in institutions can be difficult to eat and fluids are not always offered or available. Some food might be unpalatable or culturally inappropriate for the individual (Kayser-Jones 2000), the

Table 180.5 Personalised strategies to promoting eating

Strategies to increase appetite	Reason
Provide balanced meals	To avoid constipation
Offer a favourite alcoholic drink before the meal (if medications permit)	To stimulate appetite
Do not give medications directly before a meal	The taste can put individuals off their food
Allow the person to eat when hungry	Food is more enjoyable
Encourage physical activity where possible	To work up an appetite
Find out what the individual's favourite foods are	To enhance enjoyment
Encourage the individual to eat one type of food before moving on to the next	To avoid confusion when tastes and textures change
To ascertain which meal should be the largest	To fit in with the individuals pattern of eating
Allow enough time to help individuals to the table or to sit alone if that is their preference	To avoid individuals feeling rushed
Ensure that individuals have their dentures and their mouth is clean	
Ensure that each individual has assistance at hand should they require it	To avoid people becoming frustrated with the effort of trying to manage their food
Provide seasonal food and temperature appropriate foods	Soups are more appetising in the winter and ice-cream in the summer

The above strategies are basic requisites to provide a person-centred approach to care

packaging may be difficult to open (Healthcare Commission 2007), or the portions too big (Vivanti et al. 2008). Antecedents to meals such as medications given just before meals can negatively affect food consumption (de Graaf 1994; Stratton et al. 2003) and strategies to enhance appetite, such as an aperitif before main meals are a rare occurrence. Examples of such strategies are given in Table 180.5.

180.5.3 *Institutional Living*

Routines within institutions can pose threats to promoting each individual's nutritional status. For example, staff shortages at mealtimes can mean that the individuals who need assistance may not get the help they require (Crogan and Scultz 2000). Timing of meals is also important. Food is usually prepared in one main kitchen and meals are given at set times. Unless such foods are prescribed, it is not easy for staff to provide fortified foods or snacks outside of the normal routine mealtimes. Individuals have different times of day to have their main meals and may not be able to eat a large meal at the times served in the institution. Many older people will have lived alone before being admitted into an institution and will have developed eating habits to suit themselves. Focussing on an individual's past routines and personalising care needs should be at the heart of good care and this has to include nutritional care, which must be person centred and have the explicit aim of helping individuals to maintain their own nutritional needs (European Nutrition for Health Alliance 2005). This can be a problem especially at night time when food is not usually available (Kerr et al. 2008).

Table 180.6 outlines some of the considerations necessary to ensure that individuals get the maximum benefit from meals within an institutional setting.

Table 180.6 Considerations at mealtimes

Area	Action	Examples of evidence
Personal care	Well fitting dentures, mouth care, choice of menu, choice of person to sit with (if appropriate)	Barratt (2004)
The social environment of mealtimes	The environment should be homely, the table set nicely and the environment should be calm and non confrontational	Mathey et al. (2001); Desai et al. (2007)
Communal eating	Consideration given to those people who wish to eat alone and those who prefer company	Barratt (2004)
Crockery and cutlery	Disabilities should be minimized. Cutlery and crockery designed to help people eat their food	Marshall (1996); Bartlett (2000)
The food	The food should be identifiable and culturally appropriate for the individual. It should be easy for the individual to eat. Small and nutrient rich	Kayser-Jones (2000); Healthcare Commission (2007); Vivanti et al. (2008)
Time of meal	Personal preferences for meals or snacks	Barratt (2004)
Time of and type of medications	Medications should not be given immediately before meals if possible. Knowledge of drugs/side effects that may affect appetite needs to be included in nutritional assessment and reviewed regularly	de Graaf et al. (1994); Stratton et al. (2003)
The Assistance required	Help should be available to give time to all patients who require assistance	Crogan and Scultz (2000)
Staff training	Staff need to be trained in how to ensure patients receive adequate nutrition	Castellanos et al. (2000); Chang and Lin (2005)

The areas of concern are not exhaustive but serve to illustrate the multifactorial nature of the antecedents to meals and mealtimes

180.5.4 Staff Attitudes

Institutionalised ageism, explained by Bender (2003: 121) as a way of treating everyone in the same manner, serves to devalue the individual. Bender (2003) states that any expressions of preference or individuality are seen as complaints and patients' requests are frequently ignored. People who are physically dependent are more vulnerable to being treated this way and yet these are the people in most need of help. A study by Sormunen et al. (2007) found that the greater the dependence of the resident in a care home, the greater the number of inappropriate treatments they received, and of the inappropriate treatments, a quarter of these occurred during mealtimes, with staff talking over patients and performing tasks for people that the individuals could still do for themselves if given time.

180.6 The Extent of the Problem of Poor Nutrition in People with Dementia

All of the issues of poor nutrition as described above are all relevant to people with dementia living in institutions, but this client group are at greater risk from dehydration and malnutrition (Castellanos et al. 2003). One of the symptoms of dementia is weight loss and is associated with the disease process, poor quality of life and morbidity and mortality (Smith and Greenwood 2008). However, weight loss is also associated with age-related physical problems and psychosocial behaviours of people with dementia in care, and the behaviours and attitudes of staff.

180.7 The Need to Train Frontline Staff

In order to identify people who need extra calories, staff need to be trained and frontline staff who give direct help with meals are usually care assistants, who have little training in the nutritional care of frail older people and older people with dementia (Watson 1997). Training care staff has been shown to have positive effects on the nutritional status of older people with dementia, as staff need to be aware of the multiple factors involved in presenting, serving and assisting people to eat the food offered (Chang and Lin 2005). The challenges in providing adequate nutrition to people with dementia can lie in knowledge of how dementia affects a person's neuromuscular ability to take food to their mouths, chew and swallow (Ikeda et al. 2002), their perceptual difficulties of recognizing food and/or utensils (apraxia), or their ability to identify objects by name (aphasia). They may also lack the cognitive ability to initiate and/or maintain an effective way of eating (Chang and Roberts 2008). This can make following instructions impossible for them, and may lead to confrontations between staff and the individual at mealtimes. Such individuals can have difficulty communicating their likes, dislikes and their lack of comprehension verbally, which can cause them to feel frustrated and incapable, resulting in them communicating their dislikes with aggressive behaviours. In turn, staff who have no training in caring for people with dementia will not view the distress, but will view the individual as a 'problem'. This lack of understanding of what the person with dementia is experiencing can lead to negative attitudes and negative or diminished social interaction with the individual. This treatment depersonalises the individual, leading to what Kitwood (1998) termed 'malignant social psychology'.

Person-centred care, espoused by Kitwood (1997), centres on seeing the person and not the dementia. Promoting independence in eating is preferable and various strategies can be used to promote food intake. Marshall (1996), in writing on mealtimes in institution, speaks of disabling environments and suggests that people could be given greater assistance with eating independently if they had utensils and crockery that compensated for their disabilities.

Table 180.7 illustrates activities and actions to promote an individual's nutritional status.

180.8 Applications to Other Areas of Health and Disease

People who are ill have a compromised nutritional status. Poor nutrition can be the cause of health problems, ranging from relatively minor ailments such as constipation to more serious problems such as anaemia, osteoporosis, coronary heart disease and declining mental health (The Caroline Walker Trust 2004). Malnutrition can exacerbate illness (British Association for Parenteral and Enteral Nutrition [BAPEN] 2006) and prevent recovery from illnesses. The human cost of malnutrition is high, resulting in lengthy hospital stays, poor quality of life and malnutrition can have serious consequences for frail older people (Crogan and Pasvogal 2003). The public cost on disease-related malnutrition is also high; with a projected spend of over £7 billion per annum in 2007 in the UK (BAPEN 2009).

Table 180.7 Activities and actions to ensure adequate nutrition

Activity	Action
Valid nutritional assessment	Medical and nursing staff to ascertain any causes for poor appetite that can be treated, such as pain, illness, side effects from medications, depression
Educating staff, especially those involved in direct care	To provide staff training on food and nutrition for older people and older people with dementia
Providing easy to eat foods at regular times that individual patients like	The social aspects of mealtimes help people orientate to time of day and mix with other residents
Provide high calorie snacks at regular intervals between meals	Foods such as muffins, cakes scones, malt loaf, cheese and biscuits
Provide finger foods	Foods and for people who have compromised manual dexterity and that can be eaten independently. These foods are also suitable for people who find it difficult to sit still while eating.
Offer fortified foods or food supplements when adequate food cannot be taken	Food should always be offered first, food can be fortified and supplements given but not instead of meals.

Assessment is essential in order to follow through on the actions. Meals should be treated as an enjoyable experience. Food should be acceptable, fortified if necessary and supplements given to augment calorific intake

180.9 Conclusion

This chapter highlights that the importance of providing good nutritional care for older people has been well documented in the many recommendations and standards written by experts in Europe and the UK. However, if these standards are to be implemented, they have to be taught to those involved in the direct care of mealtimes. Frontline staff who deal with meals have to not only be aware of the importance of maintaining an individual's nutritional status, but they need to be taught that ensuring good nutrition is more than a physical requirement, it involves knowing that the psychosocial aspects of meals play a major part in helping older people and older people with dementia to maintain dignity, independence and a sense of enjoyment at mealtimes.

Summary Points

- Malnutrition in older people and older people with dementia is a critical issue.
- Recommendations and standards are not being carried out in many institutions.
- Training is essential for staff who provide meals to people in institutional care.
- Frontline staff are usually untrained people who have little knowledge of the strategies that can be used to ensure adequate nutrition.
- Mealtimes involve physical and psychosocial interventions.

Definitions of Key words

Malnutrition: The cellular imbalance between the supply of nutrients and energy and the body's demand for them to ensure growth, maintenance and specific functions. This can result in weight gain or weight loss

Nutrients: Foods that contain the elements necessary for bodily functions. The six categories of nutrients are water, carbohydrates, proteins, lipids, vitamins and minerals.

Undernutrition: When nutrient intake falls below that necessary to sustain health and well-being and results in weight loss.

Fortified drinks: Fluids that have extra nutrients in them.

Finger foods: Foods that can be eaten without the need for crockery or cutlery.

Nutritional screening tool: An assessment carried out to assess people at risk of undernutrition and/or malnutrition.

References

Age Concern. Hungry to be heard: The scandal of malnourished older people in hospital. England, London: Age Concern; 2006.

Association of Community Health Councils in England and Wales [ACHEW]. Hungry in hospital. London: ACHEW; 1997.

Barratt J. Rev Clin Geront. 2004;14:247–51.

Bartlett R. J Dem Care. Sept/Oct2006 ;33–36.

Bender M. Explorations in dementia. London: Jessica Kingsley Publications; 2003

British Association for Parenteral and Enteral Nutrition [BAPEN] (1996) BAPEN, Maidenhead

British Association for Parenteral and Enteral Nutrition [BAPEN]. The MUST Report: Nutritional Screening of Adults: A multi-disciplinary responsibility. Redditch: BAPEN; 2003

British Association for Parenteral and Enteral Nutrition [BAPEN]. Malnutrition among older people in the Community: Policy Recommendations for Change. A UK Policy Report by the European Nutrition for Health Alliance, BAPEN and the International Longevity Centre – UK. BAPEN, Redditch; 2006.

British Association for Parenteral and Enteral Nutrition [BAPEN]. Nutrition Screening Survey in the UK in 2008. Hospitals, care homes and mental health units. A Report by BAPEN, Redditch; 2009.

Care Commission. Eating well in care homes for older people. Dundee: Scottish Commission for the Regulation of Care; 2009

Castellanos V, Silver H, Gallagher-Allred C, Smith T. Nutrition issues in the home, community and long term care setting. Nut Clin Pract. 2003;18:21–36.

Chang C, Lin L. Effects of a feeding skills training programme on nursing assistants and dementia patients. J Clin Nurs. 2005;14:1185–92.

Chang C, Roberts B. Feeding difficulty in older adults with dementia. J Clin Nurs. 2008;17:2266–74.

Commission for Social Care Inspection. Highlight of the day? – improving meals for older people in care homes. 2006. Available at http://www.csi.org.uk/PDF/highlight_of_day.pdf

Committee on Medical Aspects of Food Policy [COMA]. Dietary Reference Values for Food Energy and Nutrients for the United Kingdom (Report on Health and Social Subjects No 41). The Stationery Office, London; 1991.

Committee on Medical Aspects of Food Policy [COMA]. The Nutrition of Elderly People. (Report on Health and Social Subjects No 43) The Stationery Office, London; 1992.

Crogan N, Pasvogal A. J Gerontol A Biol Sci Med Sci. 2003;58:159–64.

Crogan N, Schultz J. J Nurses Staff Dev. 2000;16:216–21.

de Graaf C, Polet P, van Staverton W. J Gerontol. 1994;49 (3):93–9.

Department of Health. National standards framework for older people, London: Department of Health; 2001.

Department of Health. Standards for better health. London: Department of Health; 2004.

Desai J, Winter A, Young K, Greenwood C. J Am Diet Assoc. 2007;107:808–14.

Ebersole P, Hess P, Touhy T, Jett K, Luggen A. Toward healthy aging: human needs and nursing response. 7th ed. Missouri: Mosby Elsevier; 2008. Chap. 9, pp. 194–265.

European Nutrition for Health Alliance. Malnutrition within an ageing population: a call for action. Report on the Inaugural Conference of the European Nutrition for Health Alliance, 14 Sept 2005. Available at http://www.european-nutrition.org/files/pdf_pdf_34.pdf

Finch S, Doyle W, Lowe C, Bates C, Prentice A, Smithers G. National diet and nutrition survey. People aged 65 years and over, 1994–1995. Volume 1: Report of the diet and nutritional survey. The Stationery Office, London; 1998.

Fried L, Furrucci L, Darer J, Williamson J, Anderson G. J Gerontol A Biol Sci Med Sci. 2004;59:255–63.

Food Standards Agency. Food served to older people in residential care. 2006. Available at http://www.food.gov.uk/healthiereating/nutritioncommunity/care

Goffman E. Asylums: essays in the social situation of mental patients and other inmates. New York: Hawthorne; 1961.

Healthcare Commission. Caring for dignity: a national report for dignity in care of older people while in hospital. London: Commission for Healthcare Audit and Inspection; 2007.

Ikeda M, Brown J, Holland A, Fukuhara R, Hodges J. J Neurosurg Psych. 2002;73:371–6.

Kayser-Jones J. Nursing homes: long term care management. 2000;49:56–59, 113–114.

Kerr D, Wilkinson H, Cunningham C. Supporting older people in care homes at night. Edinburgh: Joseph Rowntree Foundation; 2008.

Kitwood T. Dementia reconsidered: the person comes first. Philadelphia: Open University Press; 1997.

Kitwood T. J Clin Ethic. 1998;9:23–34.

Kydd A. Life in limbo: delayed discharge from a policy and patient perspective. PhD thesis, Aberdeen: University of Aberdeen; 2006.

Lennard-Jones J. A positive approach to nutrition as treatment. London: Kings Fund Centre; 1992.

Marshall M. 'I Can't Place This Place at All': working with people with dementia and their carers. Birmingham: Venture; 1996.

Mathey M, Vanneste V, de Graaf c, de Groot L, van Stavaren W. Prev Med. 2001;32:416–23.

NHS Quality Improvement Scotland. Food, fluid and nutritional care in hospitals. Edinburgh: NHS QIS; 2003.

Office of Health Economics. OHE compendium. 20th ed. 2009. Available from http://www.ohe.org/page/knowledge/schools/appendix/aging_population.cfm

Potter P, Perry A. Fundamentals of nursing. 3rd ed. London: Mosby-Year Book; 1993.

Smith K, Greenwood C. Nestle Nutr Works Se. 2008;27:381–403.

Sormunen S, Topo P, Elonieme-Sulkava U. Aging Ment Health. 2007;11:246–55.

Stratton R, Green C, Elia M. Disease-related malnutrition: an evidenced based approach to treatment. Oxford: CABI publishing; 2003.

The Caroline Walker Trust. Eating well for older people. London: The Caroline Walker Trust; 1995.

The Caroline Walker Trust. Eating well for older people. 2nd edn. London: The Caroline Walker Trust; 2004.

Vivanti A, Banks M, Aliakbari J, Suter M, Hannah-Jones M, McBride E. Nutr Diet. 2008;65:36–40.

Watson R. Undernutrition, weight loss and feeding difficulty in elderly patients with dementia: a nursing perspective. Rev Clin Geront. 1997;7:317–26.

Watson R, Manthorpe J, Stimpson A. Learning from carer's experiences: helping older people with dementia to eat and drink. Nursing Older People. 2003;14:23–27.

Printed by Printforce, United Kingdom